Swanson's
FAMILY PRACTICE REVIEW

A Problem-Oriented Approach

Visit our website at **www.mosby.com**

Swanson's
FAMILY
PRACTICE
REVIEW
A Problem-Oriented Approach

ALFRED F. TALLIA, M.D., M.P.H, F.A.A.F.P.
Editor-in-Chief
Associate Professor and Vice Chairman
Department of Family Medicine
University of Medicine and Dentistry of New Jersey—
Robert Wood Johnson Medical School, New Brunswick, New Jersey
Newport Beach, California

DENNIS A. CARDONE, D.O., D.A.B.F.P., C.A.Q.S.M.
Co-Editor
Assistant Professor and Director of Sports Medicine
Department of Family Medicine
University of Medicine and Dentistry of New Jersey—
Robert Wood Johnson Medical School, New Brunswick, New Jersey
Newport Beach, California

DAVID F. HOWARTH, M.D., M.P.H., D.A.B.F.P.
Associate Editor
Associate Professor and Director of Fellowship Programs
Department of Family Medicine
University of Medicine and Dentistry of New Jersey—
Robert Wood Johnson Medical School, New Brunswick, New Jersey
Newport Beach, California

KENNETH H. IBSEN, Ph.D.
Senior Corresponding Editor
Director, Academic Development/CME, Kaplan Medical
Newport Beach, California
Professor Emeritus, Biochemistry
University of California, College of Medicine
Irvine, California

FOURTH EDITION

Kaplan Medical

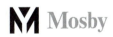 Mosby

A Harcourt Health Sciences Company

St. Louis   London   Philadelphia   Sydney   Toronto

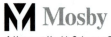
Mosby
A Harcourt Health Sciences Company

Editor: Elizabeth M. Fathman
Developmental Editor: Ellen Baker Geisel
Project Manager: Patricia Tannian
Project Specialist: Suzanne C. Fannin
Book Design Manager: Gail Morey Hudson
Cover Design: Teresa Breckwoldt

FOURTH EDITION
Copyright © 2001 by Mosby, Inc.

Previous editions copyrighted 1991, 1996

NOTICE
Pharmacology is an ever-changing field. Standard safety precautions must be followed, but as new research and clinical experience broaden our knowledge, changes in treatment and drug therapy may become necessary or appropriate. Readers are advised to check the most current product information provided by the manufacturer of each drug to be administered to verify the recommended dose, the method and duration of administration, and contraindications. It is the responsibility of the treating physician, relying on experience and knowledge of the patient, to determine dosages and the best treatment for each individual patient. Neither the publisher nor the editor assumes any liability for any injury and/or damage to persons or property arising from this publication.

Mosby, Inc.
A Harcourt Health Sciences Company
11830 Westline Industrial Drive
St. Louis, Missouri 63146

Printed in the United States of America

Library of Congress Cataloging in Publication Data

Swanson's family practice review : a problem-oriented approach.—4th ed. / Alfred F. Tallia, editor-in-chief . . . [et al.]
      p. ; cm.
    Includes bibliographical references and index.
    ISBN 0-323-00914-X (alk. paper)
      1. Family medicine—Examinations, questions, etc.   I. Title: Family practice review.   II. Tallia, Alfred F.   III. Swanson, Richard W. Family practice review.
    [DNLM: 1. Family Practice—Examination Questions. WB 18.2 S972 2001]
RC58.S93 2001
616'.0076—dc21   00-033875

00 01 02 03 04 CL/KPT 9 8 7 6 5 4 3 2 1

To the memory of

Dr. Richard Swanson

An awesome educator and a beautiful person.

Contributing Authors

DENNIS A. CARDONE, D.O., D.A.B.F.P., C.A.Q.S.M.
Co-Editor
Assistant Professor and Director of Sports Medicine
Department of Family Medicine
University of Medicine and Dentistry of New Jersey—
Robert Wood Johnson Medical School
New Brunswick, New Jersey

FLOYD CULLER, III, M.D., F.A.A.P
Associate Professor and Vice Chairman
Chief of Pediatric Endocrinology, Department of Pediatrics
University of California, Irvine
Irvine, California

MARK NOLAN HILL, M.D., F.A.C.S.
Clinical Associate Professor
Finch University of Health Sciences
Chicago Medical School
North Chicago, Illinois

PAUL HOLTOM, M.D., F.A.C.P.
Associate Professor of Clinical Medicine and Orthopedics
University of Southern California School of Medicine
Los Angeles, California

DAVID HOWARTH, M.D., M.P.H., D.A.B.F.P.
Associate Editor
Associate Professor and Director of Fellowship Programs
Department of Family Medicine
University of Medicine and Dentistry of New Jersey—
Robert Wood Johnson Medical School
New Brunswick, New Jersey

KENNETH H. IBSEN, Ph.D.
Senior Corresponding Editor
Professor Emeritus Biochemistry
University of California College of Medicine
Irvine, California
Director Academic Development/CME
Kaplan Medical/National Medical School Review
Newport Beach, California

DAVID S. KOUNTZ, M.D., F.A.C.P.
Associate Professor of Internal Medicine
Chief, Division of Primary Care, Department of Medicine
Robert Wood Johnson Medical School
New Brunswick, New Jersey

ELMAR P. SAKALA, M.D., M.A., M.P.H., F.A.C.O.G.
Professor of Obstetrics and Gynecology
Director of Medical Education
Department of Obstetrics and Gynecology
Loma Linda University School of Medicine
Loma Linda, California

RODERICK SHANER, M.D., F.A.A.C.A.P.
Clinical Professor of Psychiatry
University of Southern California School of Medicine
Medical Director
Los Angeles County Department of Mental Health
Los Angeles, California

ALFRED F. TALLIA, M.D., M.P.H., F.A.A.F.P.
Editor-in-Chief, Associate Professor and Vice Chairman
Department of Family Medicine
University of Medicine and Dentistry of New Jersey—
Robert Wood Johnson Medical School
New Brunswick, New Jersey

Preface

The third edition of Dr. Swanson's *Family Practice Review* was a marvelous educational tool; the product of a great deal of sweat, sparked by genius. User feedback has shown it to be an effective tool not only for family practice physicians preparing for certification or recertification, but also for physicians preparing for the SPEX and others desiring to hone their familiarity with the basic concepts pertinent to primary care health delivery.

Dr. Swanson's first sentence in the preface to the third edition starts out with the phrase, "The world is constantly changing . . . ." Nothing could be more true for medicine's world. The 5 years since production of the third edition have seen revolutionary changes in medicine, with profound implications for the practitioner. New diagnostic and therapeutic modalities have been introduced, and even the modes of practice have been transfigured. These changes have created a need to update Dr. Swanson's *Family Practice Review.*

In 1996 Dr. Swanson transformed the book into a lecture CME format. Unfortunately, Dr. Swanson passed away in November, 1996. In the spring of 1997, Dr. Alfred F. Tallia, Associate Professor and Vice Chairman of Family Medicine at the University of Medicine and Dentistry of New Jersey—Robert Wood Johnson Medical School, assumed the directorship of the annual live-conference Family Practice CMEs, sponsored by Kaplan/National Medical School Review. Initially the third edition was used as a textbook for this course as well as for the USMLE Step 3 review. Unfortunately, as the years passed, the initial tiny crack between what was written in the book and modern medical practice began to widen until it became significant. Therefore it was decided to have Dr. Tallia and the other faculty of the Family Practice CME activity work together to revise the third edition. Thus the fourth edition was conceived. It is a testimony to the late Dr. Swanson's genius that it takes a team to update and perhaps embellish his effort.

The primary goals of the fourth edition are to update the content while retaining the special essence that has made the third edition such a valued and popular educational instrument. Although the basic format of the third edition is retained, it is now arranged in a more hierarchical fashion designed to make it easier for the readers to find their way through the content. The book is divided into nine chapters, each representing a clinical subdiscipline tested for by the American Board of Family Physicians (ABFP). These chapters comprise a series of problems. Each problem is presented as at least one clinical case, many by several cases. Each case covers an aspect of a differential diagnosis. This way the problems simulate real clinical situations, providing the learner with a sense of reality and enhancing retention. Each case is followed by questions concerning its diagnosis and management. This question section ends with a Short Answer Management Problem that asks the reader to summarize the most pertinent therapeutic factors relevant to the problem.

The question section is followed by an answer section, which provides a detailed discussion relevant to the cases. Finally, each problem has a short summation and a few selected Suggested Readings. The overall process is designed to increase retention and to expand and refine the readers' knowledge of the diagnostic methods, medications, and patient management techniques presented in each case while providing a more holistic concept of the potential significance of the set of symptoms that defined the problem.

The problems and most of the cases were initially chosen by Dr. Swanson and subsequently reaffirmed and updated by the contributors on the basis of thorough needs analyses, including opinions of readers, participants, and faculty in the live CME conferences, expert opinion, and Dr. Swanson's original morbidity and chart studies. Selections were made under the direction of the team of family physicians from Robert Wood Johnson Medical School with input from the contributing specialists. Therefore, while still directed toward the family physician preparing for certification or recertification, these problems represent the core of knowledge that the primary care physician should have, supported by the expertise of the specialists.

Alfred F. Tallia
Kenneth H. Ibsen

Acknowledgments

As Editor-in-Chief, I am indebted to many individuals for their support and assistance in the preparation of the fourth edition of Swanson's *Family Practice Review.* To Dr. Victor Gruber and Mr. Jon Gruber of Kaplan Medical, my thanks for the inspiration and opportunity to edit and write for this edition.

To David E. Swee, M.D., Professor and Chair of Family Medicine at the University of Medicine and Dentistry of New Jersey—Robert Wood Johnson Medical School, my thanks for allowing me and my co-authors and editors the time for this important undertaking.

To my wife, Elizabeth; Dr. Cardone's wife, Silvana; and Dr. Howarth's wife, Allison; and to our families and those of the other authors, our profound thanks for their sacrifice of time and their understanding.

To Sara Schlesinger at my and Dr. Cardone's office, Louis Ignosia at Dr. Howarth's office, and the staff at Kaplan Medical and Mosby, my thanks for their hard work and assistance.

Finally, to Dr. Kenneth Ibsen, Director of Academic Development/Continuing Medical Education at Kaplan Medical, a true scholar and gentleman, without whose tireless efforts of reading and formatting this manuscript, making excellent suggestions, and, in general, keeping us all coordinated and organized this book would not have been completed, my deepest thanks and appreciation.

Alfred F. Tallia, M.D., M.P.H.

Editor-in-Chief

Tips on Passing the Board Examinations

This section briefly discusses the philosophy and techniques of passing board examinations or any other type of medical examination.

First, realize that you are "playing a game." It is, of course, a very important game, but it is nevertheless a game. When answering each question you must ask yourself the following: "What is it that the examiner wants from this question?" Let us turn our attention to the most common type of question, the multiple-choice question (MCQ).

There are many pros and many cons to MCQs, and a brief review of those ideas is in order.

The pros of MCQs are as follows:

1. An MCQ item requires the student to choose among a fixed set of alternatives. In other words, the student simply has to recognize the choices, a far cry from having to memorize them.
2. An MCQ test can sample a broad range of facts and a variety of facts using specific questions requiring a choice among responses.
3. An MCQ test that is well written is more valid and more reliable than any other form of examination; this conclusion is drawn strictly from the number of questions asked.
4. An MCQ test correlates highly with short answer tests; this should turn out to be an advantage for the student.
5. An MCQ test increases the reliability or precision of the score distribution. The score distribution is not dependent on who is marking the examination.

The cons of multiple-choice questions are as follows:

1. An MCQ test lends itself to esoterica. In other words, many examiners go out of their way to ask questions that are at best questionable and at worst completely irrelevant to anything the student will ever encounter in practice.
2. An MCQ test does not allow the student to qualify or explain his or her answer.
3. In an MCQ test the correct answer is provided for recognition, a situation not equivalent to real practice.
4. The answer to a particular question on an MCQ test is dependent not only on the facts tested but also on the manner in which the question is written.

What this book provides the student is a way to "outfox the fox." There is a story about an individual who passed five different specialty board examinations while knowing nothing about the content. This individual, was, however, an expert in taking MCQ tests.

So, how do you outfox the fox? Following these rules will maximize the chances.

Rule 1: Allocate your time appropriately. At the beginning of the examination divide the number of questions by the time allotted. A fair examination will allow approximately 1 minute per question. Pace yourself accordingly and check your progress every half hour.

Rule 2: Do not wait until the end to transfer your answers from the question paper to the answer sheet. You may find that you have run out of time and your answer sheet is blank.

Rule 3: Answer every question in order. Do not leave an answer space blank. If you do, you run the risk of unsequencing your answers and having all answers out of order.

Rule 4: Do not spend more than your allotted time on any one question. If you don't know the answer and no marks are subtracted for wrong answers, simply guess.

Rule 5: Even if marks are subtracted for wrong answers and you can eliminate even one choice, answer the question anyway. The laws of mathematics indicate that you will still come out ahead.

Rule 6: If there is a question in which one choice is significantly longer than the others and you do not know the answer, select the long choice.

Rule 7: If you are faced with an "all of the above" choice, realize that these are right far more often than they are wrong. Choose "all of the above."

Rule 8: Become suspicious if you have more than three choices of the same letter in a row. Two of one choice in a row is common, three is less common, and four is almost unheard of. Something is probably wrong.

Rule 9: Answer choices tend to be very evenly distributed. In other words, the number of correct

(a) choices is close to the number of correct (b) choices, and so on. However, there may be somewhat more choice (e)s than any other, especially if there are a fair number of "all of the above" choices. If you have time, do a quick check to provide yourself with some reassurance.

Rule 10: Never, never change an answer once you have recorded it on the answer sheet unless you have an extraordinary reason for doing so. Many people taking MCQ examinations, especially if they have time on their hands after completing the examination, start second-guessing themselves and thinking of all kinds of unusual exceptions. Resist this temptation.

Rule 11: If you have absolutely no idea regarding the correct answer and marks are not subtracted for guessing, choose (c). It tends to have a slightly higher frequency of being correct.

Rule 12: Before you write anything on the answer sheet, always, always read each and every choice. Do not get caught by seeing what you believe is the correct answer jump out at you. Read all of the choices.

Rule 13: Read each question carefully. Be especially careful to read words such as *not, except,* and so on. Some people find it helpful to carefully underline certain parts of the question containing such words.

Success cannot be guaranteed with these or any other rules. I do, however, believe that these rules will help you achieve better results on your board examinations.

Contents

1 ADULT MEDICINE, 1

Problem 1 **Acute Myocardial Infarction, 1**

"Yes, My Chest Hurts, But I'm Sure the Pain Will Go Away Soon."

Case 1: A 72-Year-Old Male with Acute Chest Pain

Problem 2 **Angina, 7**

"My Chest Pain Is Getting Worse—Am I Dying?"

Case 1: A 55-Year-Old Male with Chest Pain

Case 2: A 76-Year-Old Male with a History of Angina Pectoris

Case 3: A 50-Year-Old Female with Sharp Retrosternal Chest Pain

Case 4: A 65-Year-Old Male with Angina and Hypertension

Problem 3 **Dyslipidemia, 13**

"Where Can I Get Some of That Good Cholesterol?"

Case 1: A 51-Year-Old Male with a High Blood Cholesterol Level

Problem 4 **Congestive Heart Failure, 18**

"I Get So Scared. Sometimes in the Middle of the Night I Can't Catch My Breath."

Case 1: A 78-Year-Old Male with Shortness of Breath

Problem 5 **Hypertension, 21**

"I Feel Fine, But Those Pills Were Distressing Me, So I Stopped Taking Them."

Case 1: An Obese 47-Year-Old Male with Hypertension

Problem 6 **Dysrhythmia, 27**

"Sometimes My Heart Forgets a Beat or Two."

Case 1: A 37-Year-Old Male with "Skipping Heart Beats"

Case 2: A 51-Year-Old Male with Acute Chest Pain

Case 3: A 44-Year-Old White Male with Palpitations

Problem 7 **Obesity, 30**

"My Doctor Has Me on a Diet. So Please Leave the Nuts and Cherry Off of My Banana Split."

Case 1: A 45-Year-Old, 320-Pound Male Complaining of Fatigue

Problem 8 **Pulmonary Embolism, 33**

"A Broken Leg Killed My Wife?"

Case 1: A 65-Year-Old Female with Cyanosis, Shortness of Breath, and Substernal Chest Pain

Problem 9 **Chronic Obstructive Pulmonary Disease, 37**

"I Quit Smoking, So Why Am I Still Coughing?"

Case 1: A 55-Year-Old Male with a Chronic Cough

Case 2: Second-Hand Smoke Is Less Than Beneficial

Case 3: A 23-Year-Old Male with a 10-Day Cough

Problem 10 **Asthma, 44**

Some Wheeze, Some Don't, But It's Still Serious.

Case 1: A 22-Year-Old Male with a Chronic Cough

Case 2: A 24-Year-Old Woman Develops Wheezing and Shortness of Breath

Problem 11 **Pneumonia, 50**

"You Gave Mrs. Jones a Shot. Why Can't I Have One, Too?"

Case 1: A 24-Year-Old University Student with Pneumonia

Case 2: A 55-Year-Old Female Who Takes a Turn for the Worse

Case 3: A 35-Year-Old Renal Transplant Patient with Fever, Dyspnea, and 2 Days of Diarrhea

Case 4: A 75-Year-Old Alcoholic with Fever, Shortness of Breath, Chest Pain, and Cough Productive of Purulent Sputum and Blood

Case 5: A 55-Year-Old Male Smoker with Chronic Obstructive Pulmonary Disease (COPD), High Fever, Chills, Cough, and Shortness of Breath

Problem 12 **Esophageal Motility Disorder, 54**

"It Is My Heart, Isn't It?"

Case 1: A 53-Year-Old Male with Burning Substernal and Retrosternal Pain

Problem 13 **Inflammatory Bowel Disease, 57**

"I Must Have Picked Up a Bug; It's Tearing My Gut Out!"

Case 1: A 32-Year-Old Female with Fever, Weight Loss, and Chronic Diarrhea

Case 2: A 25-Year-Old Male with an 18-Month History of Chronic Abdominal Pain

Case 3: A 31-Year-Old Female with a 6-Month History of Gastrointestinal Complaints

Case 4: A 15-Year-Old Female with a 1-Month History of Abdominal Cramping, Abdominal Bloating, and Increased Flatulence

Problem 14 **Peptic Ulcer Disease,** *62*

"You Mean I Have Bacteria Eating Holes in My Intestines?"

Case 1: A 51-Year-Old Male with Epigastric Pain

Problem 15 **Mononucleosis,** *66*

"Oh, Doctor, You Mean I Have the Kissing Disease? What Will People Think?"

Case 1: A 20-Year-Old College Student with a Fever and a Sore Throat

Problem 16 **Hepatitis and Cirrhosis,** *69*

"My Husband's Beer Belly Is Ballooning."

Case 1: A 50-Year-Old Male with Ascites

Case 2: A 25-Year-Old Male with Abdominal Pain for the Past 3 Weeks

Case 3: A 25-Year-Old Schoolteacher with Icteric Sclera and Right Upper Quadrant Pain

Problem 17 **Irritable Bowel Disease,** *75*

"I Strain So Hard and I Find Mucus on the Toilet Paper."

Case 1: A 38-Year-Old Female with Lower Abdominal Pain and Constipation

Problem 18 **Cancer Pain Management,** *78*

When Not to Say No to Drugs

Case 1: A 75-Year-Old Male with Metastatic Bone Pain Secondary to Advanced Prostate Cancer

Case 2: A 52-Year-Old Male with Metastatic Renal Cell Carcinoma

Case 3: A 66-Year-Old Female with Metastatic Renal Cell Carcinoma

Problem 19 **Management in Palliative Care,** *86*

"Oh Doctor, That Shot Gave Me a New Lease on Life."

Case 1: A 51-Year-Old Female with Severe Nausea, Vomiting, and Anorexia with Advanced Ovarian Cancer

Case 2: A 53-Year-Old Male with Sudden-Onset Left-Sided Weakness

Case 3: A 42-Year-Old Female with Disseminated Breast Cancer

Case 4: A 51-Year-Old Patient with Terminal Colon Cancer

Problem 20 **Diabetes Mellitus,** *92*

"I Must'a Gotten Up 10 Times Last Night To Go Potty."

Case 1: A 17-Year-Old Female with Weight Loss, Polyuria, and Polydipsia

Case 2: A 27-Year-Old Type I Diabetic with Protein in Her Urine

Case 3: A 65-Year-Old Female with a Fasting Sugar of 240 mg/dl

Problem 21 **Miscellaneous Endocrine Disease,** *99*

Too Much or Too Little Messenger or, Perhaps, Poor Reception.

Case 1: A 45-Year-Old Male with "Visual Problems," Headaches, Weight Gain, Sweating, and "Hands and Feet That Are Changing"

Case 2: A 24-year-Old Male with Weakness and Hyperpigmentation

Case 3: A 25-Year-Old Female with Increased Thirst and Urination

Case 4: A 37-Year-Old Overly Tired Hypertensive Female

Case 5: A 22-Year-Old Female with Breast Secretions, Amenorrhea, and Decreased Libido

Case 6: A 42-Year-Old Female with Increased Body Hair and Purple Streaks on Her Abdomen

Problem 22 **Thyroid Disease,** *105*

"What Is It, Doc? Tee 4, Tee 3, or Tea to Stay Awake?"

Case 1: A 38-Year-Old Female with Sweating, Palpitations, Nervousness, Irritability, and Tremor

Case 2: A 25-Year-Old Female with a Higher-Than-Normal T_4 Level

Case 3: A 28-Year-Old Female Who Is Wonderfully Healthy

Case 4: A 65-Year-Old Lethargic Male

Problem 23 **Multiple Sclerosis,** *109*

"I'm So Clumsy and I Can Hardly See Out of My Left Eye. What Could Be Happening?"

Case 1: A 27-Year-Old Female with Weakness, Visual Loss, Ataxia, and Sensory Loss

Problem 24 **Diagnosis and Treatment of Headaches,** *113*

"Acetaminophen Is Just Not Strong Enough!"

Case 1: A 45-Year-Old Male with a Headache

Case 2: A 32-Year-Old Female with a 2-Year History of Recurrent Headaches

Case 3: A 38-Year-Old Female with a 6-Year History of Recurrent Headaches

Case 4: A 24-Year-Old Female with Chronic Headaches Preceded by Nausea and Vomiting

Case 5: A 35-Year-Old Male with a 6-Month History of Recurrent, Steady, Aching, "Viselike" Headaches

Case 6: A 75-Year-Old Female with a Severe Left-Sided Temporal Headache

Case 7: A 35-Year-Old Female with Almost-Constant Migraine Headaches

Case 8: A 62-Year-Old Male with Headaches That Have Been Getting Progressively Worse

Case 9: A 17-Year-Old Male with a Headache from Hell

Problem 25 **Seizure Disorders**, *121*

Seize the Moment.

Case 1: A 65-Year-Old Male with a New-Onset Seizure

Case 2: A 22-Year-Old Male Who Suddenly Lost Consciousness, Became Rigid, and Fell

Case 3: A 12-Year-Old Female Who Stares into Space

Problem 26 **Stroke and Stroke-Related Illness**, *126*

"You Say My Husband Has an Overripe Berry in His Brain?"

Case 1: A 67-Year-Old Male with a Sudden-Onset, Left-Sided Hemiplegia, Dysphagia, and a "Visual Problem"

Case 2: A 42-Year-Old Patient with Mental Status Impairment, Foot Drop, and Left-Sided Hemiplegia and Numbness

Case 3: A 77-Year-Old Female with Nystagmus, Homonymous Hemianopia, Facial Numbness, and Weakness

Case 4: A 42-Year-Old White Male with a Curtain Coming Down Over His Eyes

Problem 27 **Anemia**, *132*

"I Hardly Have Enough Energy to Get Out of Bed."

Case 1: A 35-Year-Old Female with Fatigue

Case 2: A Patient with Anemia and Severely Dysfunctional Uterine Bleeding with Unstable Vital Signs

Case 3: A Pregnant Woman at 22 Weeks' Gestation Who Has a 10.8-g/dl Hemoglobin Level

Case 4: A 55-Year-Old Male Who's been Feeling Fatigued for the Last 3 Months

Case 5: A 78-Year-Old Female Complaining of a "Lack of Energy"

Case 6: A 75-Year-Old Female with Fatigue, Paresthesias, Weakness, and an Unsteady Gait

Problem 28 **Lymphomas and Multiple Myelomas**, *138*

"Isn't Red Sternberg the Man Who Puts Out Oil Well Fires?"

Case 1: A 16-Year-Old Male with a Mass in the Left Supraclavicular Area and Chest Pains

Case 2: A 52-Year-Old Male with Swelling in His Neck and Elbows

Case 3: A 75-Year-Old Male with "Bone Pain" in His "Breast Bone" and Head

Problem 29 **Rheumatoid Arthritis**, *144*

"I Hurt a Bit and Am Kind of Stiff When I Wake Up, but It's Not Serious, Is It?"

Case 1: A 35-Year-Old Female with Malaise, Weight Loss, Vasomotor Disturbance, and Vague Periarticular Pain and Stiffness

Problem 30 **Osteoarthritis**, *148*

"Oh, How I Ache in the Evening."

Case 1: An 80-Year-Old Female with Painful Finger Joints

Problem 31 **Fibromyalgia**, *151*

"It's Awful; I Ache All Over."

Case 1: A 35-Year-Old Female with Total Body Muscle Pain

Problem 32 **Chronic Fatigue Syndrome**, *154*

"Oh, How I Hate to Get Up in the Morning!"

Case 1: A 25-Year-Old Female with Chronic Fatigue

Problem 33 **Gout**, *158*

"Ouch, My Big Toe!"

Case 1: A 45-Year-Old Male with Excruciating Pain in His Left Foot

Case 2: A 55-Year-Old Male with Joint Pain

Problem 34 **Glomerulonephritis**, *162*

"The Blood in My Urine Came from My Sore Throat?"

Case 1: A 29-Year-Old Female with Fatigue, Anorexia, and Bloody Urine

Problem 35 **Urinary Tract Infections and Pyelonephritis**, *168*

"Let's Avoid Dialysis If We Can."

Case 1: A 27-Year-Old Female with Spina Bifida and Bilateral Costovertebral Angle Pain

Case 2: A 34-Year-Old Female with Hematuria, Dysuria, Increased Urinary Frequency, and Nocturia

Problem 36 **Acne**, *172*

"Hit That Zit!"

Case 1: A 15-Year-Old Distressed Adolescent with "The Zits"

Problem 37 **Infertility**, *176*

"Doctor, I'll Just Die If I Don't Have a Baby Now!"

Case 1: A Couple That Has Been Unsuccessful in Conceiving after 18 Months of Trying

Problem 38 **Sleep Disorders**, *181*

"Sweet Sleep, Where Are You?"

Case 1: A 48-Year-Old Male with a 6-Month History of Snoring, Nocturnal Breath Cessation, and Excessive Daytime Sleepiness

Case 2: A 35-Year-Old Male with Weak Muscles after Laughing

Problem 39 **Pain Management**, *186*

"The Only Thing That Helps Is Demerol. How About Another Prescription?"

Case 1: A 21-Year-Old Male with Chronic Back Pain

Problem 40 **Ethics**, *190*

"Beware! There May Be a Surreptitious Price to Pay!"

Case 1: A Pharmaceutical Company That Is Paying for a "Weekend Getaway" for All of the Family Practice Residents

2 OBSTETRICS, 194

Problem 41 **Family-Centered Maternity Care,** *194*

"Doctor, Will You Help Me Make This a Family Affair?"

Case 1: A 26-Year-Old Primigravida Who Wishes to Discuss a Birth Plan

Problem 42 **Pregnancy Can Be Uncomfortable,** *198*

"Read My Lips, Doctor. I'm Never Going to Let This Happen Again."

Case 1: A 23-Year-Old Primigravida with Many Physical Complaints

Case 2: A 29-Year-Old Multigravida with an Unrelenting Backache

Case 3: A Pregnant 37-Year-Old Professional Woman with Varicose Veins

Case 4: A 25-Year-Old Primigravida with Severe Rectal Pain

Case 5: A 28-Year-Old Multigravida with Gastroesophageal Reflux Disease

Case 6: A Pregnant Woman with Swollen Legs

Case 7: A 29-Year-Old Primigravida with Copious Vaginal Discharge

Case 8: A Constipated 29-Year-Old Multigravida

Problem 43 **Routine Prenatal Care,** *203*

"Shouldn't You See Me More Often, Doctor?"

Case 1: A 24-Year-Old Primigravida at 8 Weeks' Gestation

Problem 44 **Management of the First and Second Stages of Labor,** *209*

There Is a Time to Sow, a Time to Reap, and a Time to Deliver.

Case 1: A 28-Year-Old Primigravida in Labor

Problem 45 **Hypertension in Pregnancy,** *212*

"Will the Lid Blow Off?"

Case 1: A 35-Year-Old Primigravida with Hypertension

Case 2: A Hypertensive 25-Year-Old Primigravida Who Is Taking a Thiazide Diuretic

Problem 46 **Diagnosis and Management of Intrauterine Growth Restriction,** *216*

Is It Too Small or Too Immature?

Case 1: A 36-Year-Old Multigravida with a Uterus Too Small for Dates

Problem 47 **Postterm Pregnancy,** *222*

"Is It Late, Doctor?"

Case 1: A 24-Year-Old New Patient Who Allegedly Has Gone Past Her Due Date

Problem 48 **Spontaneous Abortion,** *226*

"Will We Make It to Term?"

Case 1: A 25-Year-Old with Vaginal Bleeding at 11 Weeks' Gestation

Problem 49 **Postpartum Blues, Depression, and Psychoses,** *228*

"A Bundle of Joy: So Why Is Mom So Sad?"

Case 1: A 26-Year-Old Primigravida Who Is Tearful and Depressed 4 Days Postpartum

Case 2: A 28-Year-Old Primigravida Who Is Guilt Driven, Tearful, and Depressed

Case 3: A 29-Year-Old Primigravida Who Is in Orbit

3 WOMEN'S HEALTH, 233

Problem 50 **Osteoporosis,** *233*

"Am I Shrinking?"

Case 1: A 61-Year-Old Female with Severe Back Pain

Problem 51 **Vulvovaginitis,** *238*

"I'm On Fire Below!"

Case 1: A 21-Year-Old Female with a Curdy-White Vaginal Discharge

Case 2: A 25-Year-Old Female with a Gray-Green Malodorous Vaginal Discharge

Case 3: A 29-Year-Old Female with a Gray Malodorous Vaginal Discharge

Problem 52 **Evaluation and Management of Cervical Abnormalities,** *241*

"Papa Smear: Who Is That?"

Case 1: A 26-Year-Old Female with an Abnormal Pap Smear

Case 2: A 28-Year-Old Female with a *Trichomonas vaginalis* Infection

Problem 53 **Premenstrual Syndrome,** *246*

Flowing Along with the Moon

Case 1: A 35-Year-Old Female with Premenstrual Syndrome

Problem 54 **Postmenopausal Symptoms and Their Sequelae,** *249*

"Turn on the Air Conditioner."

Case 1: A 48-Year-Old Female with Hot Flashes

Problem 55 **Dysmenorrhea,** *252*

"Why Do I Get This Terrible Stomachache Every Month?"

Case 1: A 14-Year-Old Female with Lower Midabdominal, Colicky Pain with Her Menstrual Cycle

Case 2: A 24-Year-Old Female with Lower Midabdominal, Colicky Pain with Her Menstrual Cycle

Problem 56 **Dysfunctional Uterine Bleeding,** *256*

"Doctor, I'm Using a Gross of Sanitary Napkins Each Month."

Case 1: A 35-Year-Old Female with Heavy Menstrual Periods

Case 2: A 24-Year-Old Female with Heavy Uterine Bleeding

Problem 57 **Ectopic Pregnancy,** *259*

"I Missed My Period, but I Have Pain and I Am Still Spotting."

Case 1: A 28-Year-Old Female with Pelvic Pain and Vaginal Bleeding

Problem 58 **Management of Contraception,** *263*

"Doctor, I'll Just Die if I Have a Baby Now!"

Case 1: A 23-Year-Old Hypertensive Female Requesting a Prescription for Oral Contraceptive Pills

Case 2: A 21-Year-Old Female with Multiple Sexual Partners

Case 3: A 16-Year-Old Female Who Fears Pregnancy 4 Hours after Sexual Intercourse

Case 4: A 17-Year-Old Female Who Is Being Pressured by Her Boyfriend to Have Sexual Intercourse

Case 5: A 22-Year-Old Para 2, Gravida 2 Female Who Does Not Want to Get Pregnant Again

Problem 59 **Sexually Transmitted Disease,** *270*

"We Had a Great Time, Honey, but That's Your Problem Now."

Case 1: A 24-Year-Old Female with Abdominal Pain, Pelvic Pain, and Adnexal Tenderness

Case 2: A 24-Year-Old Male with a Mucoid Urethral Discharge

Case 3: A 24-Year-Old Male with a Mucoid Urethral Discharge and a History of Greater Urgency and Frequency

Case 4: A 24-year-Old Female with Dysuria and Painful Genital Lesions

Case 5: A 25-Year-Old Female with Vulvar "Growths"

Case 6: A 17-Year-Old Male with a Mucoid Urethral Discharge

4 PSYCHIATRY, BEHAVIORAL SCIENCE, AND COMMUNICATION, 278

Problem 60 **Depressive Disorders,** *278*

When the Blues Become Black

Case 1: A 34-Year-Old Female Who Is Tearful and Sad

Case 2: A 41-Year-Old Male Who Is Chronically Depressed

Case 3: A 35-Year-Old Female Who Is Distressed at Work

Case 4: A Hard-Driving 45-Year-Old Male Who Is "Burned Out"

Case 5: A 61-Year-Old Retired Male Who Is Depressed

Problem 61 **Bipolar Disorder,** *285*

"I Can Do Anything You Can Do, Better."

Case 1: A 42-Year-Old Computer Science Professor Who Has Just Been Anointed by God as the New Head of the Computer Age

Problem 62 **Schizophrenia,** *289*

"You Had Better Do What I Say; I Get My Orders from Lucifer, Himself."

Case 1: A 22-Year-Old Male Brought to the Emergency Room by the Paramedics

Case 2: A 19-Year-Old Hallucinating Male Brought to the Emergency Department by His Parents

Case 3: A Patient with Acute Psychiatric Symptoms but with More Prominent Depression Symptoms

Problem 63 **Alcohol Dependence and Alcohol Abuse,** *294*

"Doc, I'll Never Be an Alcoholic; I Have a Hollow Leg."

Case 1: A 45-Year-Old Male with an Enlarged Liver

Case 2: A Patient with Short-Term Memory Deficits

Problem 64 **Drug Abuse,** *299*

One Minute, Euphoric; the Next, Down in the Dumps

Case 1: A 32-Year-Old Administrator with "Rapidly Swinging Moods"

Problem 65 **Eating Disorders,** *303*

"I Watch My Diet and Run 5 Miles Every Day, but I'm Still So Fat That I Can't Stand Looking in the Mirror."

Case 1: A 19-Year-Old Female with Rapid Weight Loss and an Intense Fear of Gaining Weight

Case 2: A 26-Year-Old Binge-Eating Female Who Vomits to Prevent Weight Gain

Problem 66 **Generalized Anxiety Disorder,** *307*

"My Mom Won't Let Me Play Outside. She Is Afraid I Will Get Run Over by a Truck."

Case 1: A 36-Year-Old Female with Shortness of Breath and Palpitations

Problem 67 **Factitious Disorder,** *310*

"I Most Certainly Need Another Operation. You Must Be Incompetent!"

Case 1: A 26-Year-Old Female with an "Abdomen Full of Scars"

Problem 68 **Somatoform Disorders,** *314*

"Dr. X Told Me It Is Just My Imagination, but I Really Do Hurt Bad."

Case 1: A 27-Year-Old Female with 22 Different Symptoms

Case 2: A 23-Year-Old Female Complaining of Having a "Peculiarly Prominent Jaw"

Case 3: A Mother of Five with a Constant Headache

Case 4: A 27-Year-Old Woman Complaining of Suddenly Becoming Blind

Case 5: A 41-Year-Old Male Requesting a Cancer Checkup

Problem 69 **Panic Disorder,** *320*

"I Just Can't Do It! I Think I Will Die If I Try."

Case 1: A 29-Year-Old Female with a Pounding Heart, Shortness of Breath, Chest Pain, Dizziness, and Feelings That She Is Losing Her Mind

Case 2: A 29-Year-Old Musician with an Intense Fear before Performing

Problem 70 **Social Phobia, Posttraumatic Stress Disorder, and Obsessive-Compulsive Disorder,** *324*

"Sometimes I Just Can't Do What I Should, Other Times I Must Do What I Shouldn't."

Case 1: A 22-Year-Old Law Student Who Is Unable to Answer Questions in Class

Case 2: A 27-Year-Old Woman Who Is Terrified of Flying

Case 3: A 73-Year-Old Male Who Is Anxious and Withdrawn

Case 4: A Compulsive 26-Year-Old Male Who Is Newly Married

Problem 71 **Sexual Dysfunction Disorders,** *330*

"Sex Is Not Wonderful Anymore."

Case 1: A 65-Year-Old Hypertensive Male with Impotence

Case 2: A 24-Year-Old Female Who Is Unable to Have Sexual Intercourse

Problem 72 **Psychotherapy in Family Medicine,** *335*

"Stop the World, I Want to Get Off!"

Case 1: A 29-Year-Old Working Mother with Three Children Who Is Unable to Cope

Case 2: A 39-Year-Old Female with a 4-Month History of Depression

Problem 73 **Patient Use of Alternative Complementary Care,** *340*

"Doctor, I Know It Is a Long Shot, but It Seems to Be My Only Chance."

Case 1: A 35-Year-Old Female with Metastatic Cancer of the Cervix

Problem 74 **Spousal Abuse,** *343*

"A Useless Nothing Like Me Is Lucky to Have Any Man."

Case 1: A 25-Year-Old Female with Pelvic Discomfort, Low Back Pain, Insomnia, and Fatigue

Problem 75 **Ethics and Responsibilities Associated with Referrals and Consultations,** *348*

"I Think I Should Get a Second Opinion!"

Case 1: A 35-Year-Old Female with a 4-Year History of Chronic Abdominal Pain

Case 2: A 28-Year-Old Female Seeking Referral to a Neurologist

Case 3: A 35-Year-Old Female Who Is Admitted to a Hospital by a Surgeon

Problem 76 **How to Break Bad News,** *353*

"Well, Doc, How Did the Tests Come Out?"

Case 1: A 34-Year-Old Female Just Diagnosed with Metastatic Malignant Melanoma

5 CHILDREN AND ADOLESCENTS, 359

Problem 77 **Attention-Deficit Hyperactivity Disorder, Conduct Disorder, and Oppositional Defiant Disorder,** *359*

The Riddle of Ritalin

Case 1: A 6-Year-Old Child Who Is "Always on the Go," "Into Everything," and "Easily Distractible"

Problem 78 **Child Abuse,** *364*

"My Baby Cries Constantly; All I Want to Do Is to Shut Him Up!"

Case 1: A 6-Month-Old Infant Who Fell Off a Sofa and Fractured His Humerus

Case 2: A Scared 1-Year-Old Male Whose Weight Is Below the 5th Percentile for His Age

Case 3: A Blistered 8-Month-Old Baby

Problem 79 **Neonatal Jaundice,** *368*

"Oh My! My Baby Is Yellow."

Case 1: A Full-Term Neonate with Jaundice

Case 2: A Full-Term Infant Who Develops Jaundice on the Fourth Day of His Life

Case 3: An Infant Born at Term Who Develops Jaundice at 18 Hours of Life

Problem 80 **Infantile Colic,** *374*

"My Baby Cries Constantly. Can't You Do Something to Help Her?"

Case 1: An 8-Week-Old Infant with Inconsolable Crying for Many Hours and Days

Problem 81 **Guideline for Newborn, Infant, and Childhood Immunizations,** *377*

"That Shot Made My Baby Ill."

Case 1: A 2-Month-Old Infant with High Fever 8 Hours after Receiving Her First Set of Immunizations

Problem 82 **Infant Feeding,** *379*

"I Just Know My Milk Is Inadequate."

Case 1: An Anxious Mother with a 3-Week-Old Infant and Many Questions Concerning Feeding

Case 2: A 28-Year-Old Primigravida with Mastitis

Case 3: A Mother with a Baby Who Spits Up Her Formula

Case 4: A Mother Trying to Breast Feed

Problem 83 **Failure to Thrive and Short Stature,** *386*

"How Come He Seems So Skinny and Small?"

Case 1: An 8-Month-Old Infant Who Appears Malnourished
Case 2: A 13-Year-Old Female with a Short, Webbed Neck

Problem 84 **Diagnosis and Treatment of Serious Respiratory Syndromes in Infants and Children,** *389*

"Do Something! My Baby Can't Breathe."

Case 1: An 18-Month-Old Infant with an Upper Respiratory Tract Infection
Case 2: A 19-Month-Old Male with a Cough, Wheezing, Dyspnea, and Irritability
Case 3: A 5-Year-Old Child Who Has Been Talking Strangely and Is Anorexic
Case 4: A 6-Year-Old Male in Severe Respiratory Distress
Case 5: A 12-Year-Old Male with Exercise-Induced Asthma

Problem 85 **Otitis Media,** *394*

"My Child Won't Become Deaf, Will He?"

Case 1: A 24-Month-Old Child Who Is Constantly Crying and Who Complains of a Right-Sided Earache
Case 2: An 8-Month-Old Male with an Upper Respiratory Tract Infection but No External Signs of Acute Ear Infection
Case 3: A 7-Month-Old Child with an Upper Respiratory Infection and Erythema of the Tympanic Membrane
Case 4: A 9-Month-Old Child with a Discharge from His Ear

Problem 86 **The Common Cold,** *398*

"Since My Youngest Started Nursery School, All I Do Is Wipe His Runny Nose."

Case 1: A 4-Year-Old Child with a Runny Nose, a Sore Throat, and a Nonproductive Cough

Problem 87 **Streptococcal Infections in Children,** *400*

"You Mean My Little Boy's Sore Throat Can Cause Heart Problems?"

Case 1: A 4-Year-Old Male with an Extremely Sore Throat

Problem 88 **The "Big Five" Viral Exanthems in Children,** *405*

Don't Judge a Rash Too Rashly.

Case 1: A 1-Year-Old Male with a Rash and a Fever
Case 2: A 5-Year-Old Male with a Bright Red Rash on Both Cheeks
Case 3: A 4-Year-Old Female with Pain behind Her Ears and a Maculopapular Rash
Case 4: A Pregnant Woman Exposed to Rubella
Case 5: A 4-Year-Old Male with a Dry Hacking Cough, Coryza, Conjunctivitis, a Temperature of 40° C, and a Fine Maculopapular Rash
Case 6: An 8-Year-Old Male with a Fever of 39° C, Chills, Vomiting, and a Headache

Problem 89 **Childhood Pneumonia,** *410*

"My Baby Has Water in His Lungs?"

Case 1: A 2-Day-Old Infant with Pneumonia
Case 2: A 3-Year-Old Female with Fever, Chills, Nasal Flaring, Subcostal Indrawing, and a Harsh Cough

Problem 90 **Fever Without Focus,** *413*

"My Child Is Fine Except for His Fever."

Case 1: A 9-Month-Old Infant with Fever and No Localized Signs
Case 2: A 2-Year-Old Infant with a Temperature of 39° C, a Sore Ear, and a Convulsion

Problem 91 **Pediatric Gastroenteritis,** *417*

"I'm Sure Glad I Use Disposable Diapers."

Case 1: An 18-Month-Old Infant with Diarrhea
Case 2: A 23-Month-Old Infant with Sunken Eyeballs and Doughy Skin
Case 3: A 3-Year-Old Male with Diarrhea Who Had Been Camping

Problem 92 **Recurrent Abdominal Pain in Childhood,** *421*

"I Just Can't Go to School, My Tummy Aches Again."

Case 1: A 12-Year-Old Female with Recurrent Abdominal Pain

Problem 93 **The Limping Child,** *423*

"Mom! Can You Rub My Legs? They Hurt So."

Case 1: A 9-Year-Old Male with Leg Pain
Case 2: A 13-Year-Old Female with Pain and a Grating Sensation in Her Knee

Problem 94 **Foot and Leg Deformities in Infants and Children,** *428*

"I Would Just Die If I Had a Son with Crooked Legs."

Case 1: An Anxious Mother with a 3-Month-Old Infant with Crooked Feet
Case 2: A 4-Week-Old Pigeon-Toed Infant
Case 3: A 15-Month-Old Bowlegged Infant
Case 4: An 18-Month-Old Infant with Twisted Legs
Case 5: A 6-Month-Old Infant with Crooked Feet
Case 6: A 21-Month-Old Infant with Flat Feet

Problem 95 **Adolescent Development,** *432*

"I'm Good. Just a Few Pimples."

Case 1: A 16-Year-Old Male with Acne

Problem 96 **Enuresis in Children,** *436*

"My 6-Year-Old Son Still Needs Diapers at Night."

Case 1: A 6-Year-Old Male Who Still Wets the Bed

Problem 97 **Allergic Rhinitis,** *439*

"I Don't Want to Play; You're a Stupid Snot Nose!"

Case 1: A 6-Year-Old Male with a Constantly Running Nose

Problem 98 **Diaper Dermatitis,** *443*

"Doctor, His Cheeks Are Too Red."

Case 1: A 2-Month-Old Infant with a Rash on His Cheeks

Case 2: A 1-Month-Old Infant with a 2-Week-Old Diaper Rash

Case 3: An 8-Month-Old Infant with a Long-Term Persistent Diaper Rash

Case 4: A 4-Month-Old Infant with a Diaper Rash Caused by Dirty Diapers

Problem 99 **Cardiac Murmurs in Children,** *446*

"My Baby Has Heart Problems?"

Case 1: A 3-Year-Old Child with a Cardiac Murmur

Case 2: A 6-Month-Old Infant with a Harsh Grade III/VI Pansystolic Heart Murmur

Problem 100 **Use and Abuse of Over-the-Counter Drugs for Infants and Young Children,** *449*

"You Mean That Medicine from the Drug Store Can Be Bad for My Baby?"

Case 1: A 6-Month-Old Infant with an Upper Respiratory Tract Infection

Case 2: A 6-Month-Old Infant with a Persistent Cough

Case 3: A 13-Month-Old Infant with Nausea and Vomiting

Case 4: An 8-Month-Old Infant with Fever, Diarrhea, and Red Cheeks

Problem 101 **Sickle-Cell Disease,** *453*

"Mom, Why Should I Have This Disease? I'm Never Going to See a Malaria Mosquito."

Case 1: An 8-Year-Old Female with Acute Skeletal Pain

6 GENERAL SURGERY AND SURGICAL SPECIALTIES, 458

Problem 102 **Acute Appendicitis,** *458*

The Great Imitator

Case 1: A 29-Year-Old Female with Nausea, Vomiting, and Central Abdominal Pain

Problem 103 **Biliary Tract Disease,** *461*

Stones and Groans but Not Bones

Case 1: A 43-Year-Old Female with Recurrent Right Upper Quadrant Pain

Problem 104 **Common Procedures in Office Surgery,** *465*

"Are You Sure You Can Cut It Out, Right Here in Your Office?"

Case 1: A 37-Year-Old Female with a Skin Lesion on Her Back

Case 2: A 5-Year-Old Child with a Second-Degree Burn on Her Right Hand

Case 3: A 4-Year-Old Male Who Banged His Thumb

Case 4: A 25-Year-Old Female with a Sore Big Toe

Case 5: A 45-Year-Old Male with Rectal Pain

Case 6: A 28-Year-Old Male with Rectal Bleeding

Problem 105 **Pancreatitis,** *470*

"Another Drink Will Settle My Stomach."

Case 1: A 44-Year-Old Male with a History of Very Heavy Alcohol Intake

Problem 106 **Colonic Disorders,** *473*

"Doctor, I Think the Idea of Having a Tube Stuck Up My Rear Is Disgusting."

Case 1: A 48-year-Old Male with Weakness, Fatigue, and Lower Right-Sided Abdominal Fullness

Case 2: A 78-Year-Old Male with Acute and Severe Abdominal Pain

Case 3: A 35-Year-Old Male with Rectal Bleeding and Mucoid Discharge from the Rectum

Problem 107 **Breast Disease,** *479*

"A Lump! Does That Mean Mastectomy?"

Case 1: A 41-Year-Old Female with a Painless Breast Lump

Case 2: A 49-Year-Old Female with a Suspicious Lesion Discovered with Mammography

Case 3: A 42-Year-Old Female with Painful Bilateral Breast Masses That Wax and Wane with Her Period

Case 4: A 23-Year-Old Female with a Firm but Mobile Mass

Case 5: A 33-Year-Old Female with a Small Lump and a Bloody Nipple Discharge

Problem 108 **Pancreatic Carcinoma,** *484*

A Little Organ; Big Problems

Case 1: A 62-Year-Old Male with Abdominal Pain

Problem 109 **Diagnosis and Treatment of Ophthalmologic Problems,** *488*

"Doc, I Can Hardly See."

Case 1: A 32-Year-Old Female with Bilateral Red Eyes, a Sore Throat, and a Cough

Case 2: A 17-Year-Old Female with a 1-Day History of Red Eye

Case 3: A 29-Year-Old Male with Bilateral Red Eyes

Case 4: A 29-Year-Old Female with a Tender, Painful, and Sore Red Eye

Case 5: A 35-Year-Old Female with an Acutely Inflamed and Painful Eye

Case 6: A 36-Year-Old Male with Ankylosing Spondylitis and a Painful Red Eye

Case 7: A 61-Year-Old Male with an Extremely Painful Eye

Case 8: A 23-Year-Old Female with a Painful Eye and Blurred Vision

Problem 110 **Low Back Pain and Whiplash Injuries,** *492*

"Do You Think I'm Hurt Bad Enough for Me to Sue?"

Case 1: A 28-Year-Old Male with Chronic Low Back Pain

Problem 111 **Renal Stones,** *499*

Stones and Groans and, on Occasion, Bones

Case 1: A 30-Year-Old Male with Flank Pain

Problem 112 **Disorders of the Prostate,** *501*

"Doc, I Can Hardly Pee."

Case 1: A 75-Year-Old Male with Nocturia, Hesitancy, and a Slow Flow of Urine

Case 2: A 58-Year-Old Male with Hesitancy of the Urinary Stream and Bone Pain

Case 3: A 24-Year-Old Male with Fever, Suprapubic Discomfort, and Inhibited Urinary Voiding

Problem 113 **Common Ear, Nose, and Throat Problems,** *506*

"Doc, I Can Hardly Hear and My Head Is Spinning."

Case 1: A 38-Year-Old Female with a Feeling of Dizziness and Imbalance

Case 2: A 23-Year-Old Female Who Is Dizzy

Case 3: A 30-Year-Old Male Who Becomes Dizzy When He Rolls Over

Case 4: A 29-Year-Old Female with Unrelenting Dizziness Associated with Nausea and Vomiting

Case 5: A 26-Year-Old Female with Severe Dizziness, Ataxia, and Hearing Loss

Case 6: A 37-Year-Old Female with Intermittent Hearing Loss

Case 7: A 43-Year-Old Male with Hearing Loss Lateralized to the Left Ear

7 GERIATRIC MEDICINE, 513

Problem 114 **Elderly Abuse,** *513*

"I'm a Very Patient Person, but That Old Bitch Simply Will Not Do What She Should."

Case 1: A 72-Year-Old Female with a Sore Right Shoulder and Multiple Bruises

Problem 115 **Ethical Dilemmas,** *516*

"Don't Let Her Know, Doctor. It Will Just Kill Her."

Case 1: An 87-Year-Old Female with a Terminal Malignancy Who Has Not Been Informed of Her Condition by Her Doctors

Case 2: A Terminal 45-Year-Old Female Who Experiences a Cardiopulmonary Arrest

Case 3: A 44-Year-Old Female with Multiple Liver Metastases

Case 4: A 27-Year-Old Female Came Back with a Diagnosis of Malignant Melanoma

Case 5: An Unmarried Pregnant 18-Year-Old Woman

Case 6: A "Brain Dead" Newborn Male

Problem 116 **Senile Dementia and Delirium,** *522*

"Officer, I've Lived in the Same House for the Past 45 Years, but I Can't Seem to Locate It Today. Can You Help Me?"

Case 1: A 78-Year-Old Female with Increasing Confusion, Memory Impairment, and Inability to Look after Herself

Problem 117 **Polymyalgia, Rheumatica, and Temporal Arteritis,** *529*

"Well, Doctor, I Guess Old Age Arthritis Has Finally Caught Up with Me."

Case 1: An 82-Year-Old Female with Aching and Stiffness in the Shoulder and Hip Girdles

Problem 118 **Hypertension Management in the Elderly,** *532*

"Doc, Your Pills Don't Do No Good. That Top Number Still Is Always Much More Than 140."

Case 1: An 80-Year-Old Male with Hypertension

Case 2: A 75-Year-Old African-American Male with Angina Pectoris

Case 3: A Hypertensive 72-year-Old White Female with a Previous Myocardial Infarction and Mild Congestive Heart Failure

Case 4: A Hypertensive 72-Year-Old White Male with Diabetes

Problem 119 **Parkinson's Disease,** *536*

"Doctor, My Hand Just Sits There and Quivers on Its Own."

Case 1: A 75-Year-Old Male with a Slow, Shuffling Gait, Tremors, and Depression

Problem 120 **Constipation in the Elderly,** *540*

"Doctor, I Am Terribly Constipated. I Only Go Two or Three Times a Week."

Case 1: A 78-Year-Old Female with Constipation

Case 2: An 86-Year-Old Male with Stage IV Carcinoma of the Prostate

Problem 121 **Pneumonia Management,** *545*

"I Feel That Nursing Home Is Responsible for My Father's Death from Pneumonia."

Case 1: An 81-Year-Old Male Who Lives by Himself and Has Increasing Confusion and Shortness of Breath

Case 2: An 84-Year-Old Female Who Is Currently Residing in a Long-Term Care Facility and Has Increasing Confusion and Shortness of Breath

Case 3: An 81-Year-Old Female with Dysuria, Frequency, Urgency, and Incontinence

Case 4: A 75-Year-Old Female with Fever, Chills, Confusion, Dysuria, and Diarrhea

Problem 122 **Urinary Incontinence in the Elderly,** *550*

"I'm So Embarrassed. I Haven't Done That Since I Was
5 Years Old."

Case 1: An 88-Year-Old Institutionalized Female with Urinary
Incontinence

Problem 123 **Depression in the Elderly,** *555*

"I'm Dead. They Just Haven't Buried Me Yet!"

Case 1: An 85-Year-Old Female Nursing Home Resident Who
Simply "Stares into Space" and Cries Almost All of the
Time

Problem 124 **Pressure Ulcers,** *559*

"Doctor, the Care in This Place Must Be Terrible. Look, My
Mother Has a Big Sore on Her Back."

Case 1: An 80-Year-Old Female Nursing Home Resident with a
Pressure Ulcer

Case 2: A 78-Year-Old Immobilized Male with a 1-cm Area of
Erythema and Bruising on His Heel

Problem 125 **Polypharmacy and Drug Reactions
in the Elderly,** *566*

"Gee, Mom, Do You Know What All These Different Kinds of
Pills Are For?"

Case 1: A 75-Year-Old Female with a Bagful of Pills

Case 2: An 85-Year-Old Female with a Dangerously High Blood
Pressure of 150/95 mm Hg

Problem 126 **The Propensity and Consequences of Falls
Among the Elderly,** *571*

It's No Longer Just Oopsy Daisy.

Case 1: An 81-Year-Old Female Who Is Repeatedly Falling

8 EPIDEMIOLOGY AND PUBLIC HEALTH, 575

Problem 127 **Recommendations of the U.S. Preventive
Services Task Force on the Periodic Health
Examination,** *575*

What to Test for and When

Case 1: A 45-Year-Old Male with No Specific Complaints or
Concerns

Case 2: A 66-Year-Old Male for Whom You Wish to Reduce the
Chance of Death from Colorectal Cancer

Case 3: A 26-Year-Old Asymptomatic Sexually Active Female

Case 4: A 53-Year-Old Male with a 20-Year History of Smoking
Two Packs of Cigarettes Per Day

Case 5: A 32-Year-Old Male Who Presents for a Health
Maintenance Examination

Case 6: A 45-Year-Old South-Vietnamese Woman with Hot
Flashes

Case 7: A 28-Year-Old Pregnant Woman Seeking Prenatal
Counseling

Case 8: A 20-Year-Old Male with Hay Fever

Case 9: A 65-Year-Old Bisexual Male with Gonorrhea

Problem 128 **The Routine Complete Physical
Examination vs. the Focused Periodic Health
Maintenance Examination,** *584*

"Doctor, Why Do Your Physical Exams Seem Less Thorough? Is
It Because You Became Part of an HMO?"

Case 1: A 51-Year-Old Male Who Presents for a Complete
Physical Examination

Case 2: A 35-Year-Old Female Who Presents for a Health
Maintenance Examination

Problem 129 **Epidemiology,** *587*

"Is It Sensitivity, Specificity, or What?"

Case 1: A 26-Year-Old Medical Student Who Is Having Panic
Attacks Regarding His Upcoming Epidemiology
Examination

Problem 130 **Physician Intervention in Smoking
Cessation,** *594*

"My Father Lived to Be 90 Years Old and He Smoked Like a
Chimney. Why Should I Quit?"

Case 1: A 40-Year-Old Executive Who Smokes Three Packs of
Cigarettes a Day

Problem 131 **Trends in Cancer Epidemiology,** *599*

"Hell, Doctor, It Seems Like Everything Causes Cancer! So Why
Worry?"

Case 1: A 74-Year-Old Farmer with Abdominal Pain

Problem 132 **Cardiovascular Epidemiology,** *602*

"Doctor, I'm African-American, Male, I Smoke, I'm Too Fat, and I
Have High Cholesterol and Uncontrollable Hypertension. I Guess
I Better Write My Will Now."

Case 1: A 52-Year-Old Male with Coronary Artery Disease Who
Has Had Both Coronary Artery Bypass Grafting and
Percutaneous Transluminal Angioplasty Procedures
Done

Problem 133 **Use and Abuse of Laboratory Medicine
for Routine Screening,** *605*

Having Too Much Laboratory Data May Be Perilous.

Case 1: A 45-Year-Old Male Who Requests a Complete
Laboratory Workup

Case 2: A 53-Year-Old Male with a Slightly Elevated Serum
Bilirubin Value

Problem 134 **Human Immunodeficiency Virus and Acquired Immunodeficiency Syndrome, 611**

"Now with the Discovery of These New Drugs I Can Have Sex with No Worries, Right?"

Case 1: A 24-Year-Old Male with a Nonproductive Cough
Case 2: A 32-Year-Old African-American Female with Fever, Lymphadenopathy, a Rash, and Pharyngitis
Case 3: A 31-Year-Old Patient with Full-Blown AIDS
Case 4: A 28-Year-Old Male Who Recently Tested HIV Positive

Problem 135 **Advice for Travelers, 616**

"Oh! I Didn't Drink the Water, but I Never Thought About the Ice."

Case 1: A 51-Year-Old Male Who Is Planning on Traveling to Africa
Case 2: A 73-Year-Old Farmer Who Punctured His Foot on a Rusty Nail

Problem 136 **Diagnosis and Treatment of Influenza, 618**

"Doctor, I Heard That the Flu Shot Caused Guillain-Barré Syndrome, a Very Bad Disease. Why Risk That to Prevent Ordinary, Everyday, Old-Fashioned Flu?"

Case 1: A 73-Year-Old Male with Fever, Headache, and Myalgias

9 EMERGENCY AND SPORTS MEDICINE, 623

Problem 137 **Cardiopulmonary Resuscitation and Emergency Cardiac Care, 623**

"You Are Looking at a Man Who Died Twice."

Case 1: A 55-Year-Old Male Found Collapsed in the Street
Case 2: A 70-kg Man Who Collapsed in the Street
Case 3: A 53-Year-Old Male with a Rapid Heartbeat, Nausea, and Dizziness

Problem 138 **Diagnosis and Management of Trauma, 628**

"I Wish I Had Fastened the Safety Belt!"

Case 1: A 27-Year-Old Female Injured in a Motor Vehicle Accident
Case 2: A 31-Year-Old Male Who Was Involved in a Car-Motorcycle Accident

Problem 139 **Diabetic Ketoacidosis, 631**

"You Mean My Belly Aches because I Haven't Been Taking My Insulin Shots?"

Case 1: A 17-Year-Old Male with Abdominal Pain

Problem 140 **Emergency Treatment of Abdominal Pain in the Elderly, 634**

"In All My Born Days I've Never Had Such a Stomach Ache."

Case 1: An 84-Year-Old Male with Abdominal Pain

Problem 141 **Poison Management, 637**

"It Really Was an Accident. I Just Forgot How Many I Took."

Case 1: A 24-Year-Old Female Brought into the Emergency Department with a Suspected Drug Overdose

Problem 142 **Urticaria and Angioneurotic Edema, 641**

"If There Are Shrimp in That Soup, It Will Kill Me. Keep It Away!"

Case 1: A 24-Year-Old Male Who Developed a Skin Rash while Playing Football
Case 2: A 51-Year-Old Farmer with a Nonhealing Ulcer on the Tip of His Nose
Case 3: A 65-Year-Old Male with a Nonhealing Skin Lesion on His Lower Lip
Case 4: A 45-Year-Old Female with Scaly Patches
Case 5: A 25-Year-Old Female with Pruritic, Polygonal, Flat-Topped Violaceous Papules
Case 6: A 67-Year-Old Farmer with Skin Lesions on His Ears
Case 7: A 57-Year-Old Farmer with Greasy, Warty, Heaped-Up Skin Lesions
Case 8: A 29-Year-Old Farmer with a Brown Skin Lesion

Problem 143 **Fracture Management, 646**

"You Don't Really Expect Me to Wear That Thing for 6 Weeks, Do You?"

Case 1: A 75-Year-Old Female Who Slipped and Fell on Her Outstretched Hand
Case 2: An 18-Year-Old Basketball Player Who Fell on His Outstretched Hand
Case 3: A 25-Year-Old Male with Severe Ankle Pain

Problem 144 **Sprains and Strains, 649**

"Are You Sure It's Not Broken, Doc?"

Case 1: A 28-Year-Old Female with a Swollen Ankle
Case 2: A 26-Year-Old Professional Football Player Whose Knee Buckled
Case 3: A 22-Year-Old Football Player Who Felt a Sharp Pain at the Anteromedial Aspect of His Knee after Being Hit
Case 4: A 23-Year-Old Runner with Anterior Thigh Pain
Case 5: A 14-Year-Old Female Who Sustained a Knee Injury while Pivoting

Problem 145 **Heat- and Cold-Related Injuries, 653**

"He Could Have Won the Race If He Didn't Give Up on the Last Lap."

Case 1: A 51-Year-Old Alcoholic Male Brought into the Emergency Department
Case 2: A 45-Year-Old Male with Blanched Feet
Case 3: A 4-Year-Old Male Who Fell through the Ice
Case 4: A 34-Year-Old Male Who Worked in Temperatures Exceeding 100° F
Case 5: An Exhausted 23-Year-Old Female Marathon Runner
Case 6: A 34-Year-Old Male Who Collapsed while Running the Marathon

CHAPTER 1

Adult Medicine

ACUTE MYOCARDIAL INFARCTION

"Yes, My Chest Hurts, But I'm Sure the Pain Will Go Away Soon."

Case 1 ■ A 72-Year-Old Male with Acute Chest Pain

A 72-year-old farmer is brought to the Emergency Department of his local rural hospital by his wife. Apparently he developed a "twinge of chest pain" while shoveling grain 3 hours ago. He insisted on staying home until "he collapsed on the floor." Even then, he wanted to stay home and rest, but his wife insisted he receive medical care, and she brought him to the Emergency Department. He states that the pain is "almost gone." He is obese, smokes two packs of cigarettes daily, drinks a "goodly amount of beer," and has been told that his serum cholesterol level is "way out of sight." He seems confused on the cholesterol issue, believing that the higher the cholesterol, the better.

He describes dull, aching, viselike pain around his chest, with radiation to the left shoulder. His wife says that she has never seen him in so much pain. He admits that when the pain was at its worst he experienced nausea and vomiting.

On physical examination, he is sweating and diaphoretic. He has vomited twice since coming to the Emergency Department. His blood pressure is 160/100 mm Hg, and his pulse is 120 bpm and irregular. His abdomen is obese, and you believe you can detect an enlarged aorta by deep palpation.

His electrocardiogram (ECG) reveals significant Q waves in V1 to V4 with significant ST segment elevation in the same leads. There are reciprocal ST changes (ST segment depression) in the inferior leads (II, III, and aVF).

SELECT THE BEST ANSWER
TO THE FOLLOWING QUESTIONS

Q1. The most likely diagnosis in this patient is:
   a. acute inferior wall myocardial infarction (MI)
   b. acute anterior wall MI
   c. acute myocardial ischemia
   d. acute pericarditis
   e. musculoskeletal chest wall pain

Q2. Given the history, physical examination, and ECG, your first priority is to:
   a. call the ambulance for immediate transport to another hospital that "knows how to treat this thing"
   b. admit the patient for observation
   c. administer intravenous (IV) streptokinase or t-PA
   d. administer IV heparin
   e. none of the above

Q3. Given your attention to your first priority, you would now:
   a. call the ambulance for immediate transport to another hospital that "knows how to look after this thing"
   b. admit the patient to the Coronary Care Unit (CCU) for observation
   c. administer IV streptokinase or t-PA immediately
   d. administer IV heparin immediately
   e. none of the above

Q4. Which of the following criteria should be met before a patient is given thrombolytic therapy after the history, physical examination, and ECG previously described?
   a. typical chest pain suggestive of MI
   b. ECG changes confirming MI
   c. the absence of other diseases that would explain the symptoms
   d. all of the above
   e. none of the above

Q5. The most correct statement regarding thrombolytic therapy in acute MI is:
   a. patients under age 65 years benefit more than elderly MI victims
   b. no benefits have been realized when therapy has been instituted more than 6 hours after onset of chest pain

c. thrombolytic therapy has improved the prognosis of patients with prior coronary artery bypass graft (CABG)

d. patients with non-Q-wave MI have benefited from thrombolytic therapy as well as patients who sustain Q-wave MIs

e. a 50% reduction in mortality has been realized when therapy is administered within 3 hours of onset of chest pain

Q6. Which of the following statements regarding the use of heparin in patients with acute MI is (are) true?

a. heparin therapy is now used almost routinely with thrombolytic therapy during the acute phase of MI treatment, providing certain criteria are met

b. heparin is recommended whenever there is echocardiographic evidence of left ventricular thrombi

c. heparin should be administered (unless contraindicated) to all patients with acute anterior wall MI

d. heparin is contraindicated in patients with uncontrolled hypertension

e. all of the above

Q7. Which of the following is a (are) contraindication(s) to the use of thrombolytic therapy in patients with acute MI?

a. active gastrointestinal bleeding

b. recent surgery (2 weeks postoperatively)

c. history of cerebrovascular accident

d. atrial fibrillation or mitral stenosis

e. all of the above

Q8. Which of the following statements regarding patients admitted to the CCU after presumed MI is (are) true?

a. patients with suspected MIs should have the left ventricular ejection fraction measured before leaving the unit

b. patients without additional complications (except as discussed in Case 1) should have a submaximal exercise tolerance test with thallium-201 imaging on the fourth or fifth hospital day

c. patients with negative submaximal stress tests should have a maximal exercise stress test performed after 4 to 6 weeks

d. all of the above

e. a and c

Q9. Which of the following is a (are) significant feature(s) of the pathophysiology of MI?

a. endothelial cell wall damage

b. coronary atherosclerosis

c. thromboxane A_2 production

d. all of the above

e. a and b

Q10. Which of the following is (are) true concerning aspirin in the treatment of acute MI?

a. aspirin may serve as a substitute for streptokinase or t-PA

b. aspirin may serve as a substitute for heparin

c. aspirin may serve as a substitute for β-blockers

d. all of the above

e. none of the above

Q11. Which of the following statements regarding thrombolytic therapy is (are) false?

a. thrombolytic therapy limits myocardial necrosis

b. thrombolytic therapy preserves left ventricular function

c. thrombolytic therapy reduces mortality

d. all of the above statements are false

e. none of the above statements is false

Q12. In the United States today, what percentage of patients with acute MI who would potentially qualify for thrombolytic therapy receive it?

a. 95%

b. 80%

c. 60%

d. 30%

e. 5%

Q13. Which of the following statements concerning dysrhythmias and dysrhythmic drugs in patients who have sustained an MI is (are) true?

a. premature ventricular contractions (PVCs) are common and should be treated with lidocaine

b. sustained runs of ventricular tachycardia frequently progress to ventricular fibrillation

c. prophylactic lidocaine is recommended to prevent dysrhythmias in all patients who have sustained an MI

d. none of the above

e. all of the above

Q14. One of the major patient concerns after an MI is the risk of a second or subsequent attack. In which of the following circumstances is the risk of reinfarction and/or mortality following MI significantly increased?

a. left ventricular ejection fraction of 40%

b. exercise-induced ischemia

c. non-Q-wave infarction (subendocardial infarction)

d. a and b
e. all of the above

Q15. Which of the following medications has (have) been shown to be of benefit in some post-MI patients?
a. β-blockers
b. calcium channel blockers
c. aspirin
d. a and c
e. all of the above

Q16. Which of the following statements concerning rehabilitation of the patient after an MI is (are) true?
a. sexual intercourse should not resume for at least 3 months
b. patients who have sustained an MI should stay off work for at least 4 months
c. patients who have sustained an MI may gradually increase activity over 6 to 8 weeks
d. no significant psychologic distress regarding the MI has been shown to occur in the patient's spouse or significant other
e. all of the above

Q17. The major pathophysiologic difference between (a) unstable angina and non-Q-wave or non-transmural infarction and (b) transmural infarction is:
a. the presenting signs and symptoms of the attack
b. the duration and completeness of the occlusion
c. the risk factor profile
d. the male-female ratio
e. the degree of injury pattern surrounding the true ischemic area(s)

Q18. The best single confirmatory investigation for acute MI is:
a. the ECG
b. the height of ST segment elevation in the affected area (in millimeters) and the depth of ST segment depression in the reciprocally affected leads (in millimeters)
c. the creatine kinase isoenzyme MB fraction
d. the presence of dysfunctional heart muscle as demonstrated by echocardiography
e. measurement of radiolabeled antimyosin antibody fragments

Q19. Sudden death as a result of MI is almost always caused by:
a. third-degree heart block resulting from infarction of the atrioventricular (AV) node
b. ventricular tachycardia
c. ventricular fibrillation
d. ventricular standstill
e. none of the above

Q20. Which of the following statements regarding shock and its treatment in acute MI is (are) true?
a. the acute MI patient may develop shock secondary to hypovolemic hypotension
b. the acute MI patient may develop shock secondary to persistent hypotension and a poor cardiac index
c. both forms of shock respond well to treatment with IV fluids (Ringer's lactate or normal saline solution)
d. a and b only
e. all of the above

Q21. Coronary reperfusion with thrombolytic agents has been shown to be of benefit when the onset of the pain occurs up to how many hours (maximum) before the initial assessment?
a. 4
b. 6
c. 12
d. 24
e. 48

Q22. In Case 1 there is a key finding on physical examination of the patient's abdomen that should be further assessed by:
a. an abdominal ultrasound
b. an intravenous pyelogram
c. a digital subtraction angiogram
d. a computed tomography (CT) scan
e. a magnetic resonance imaging (MRI) scan

SHORT ANSWER MANAGEMENT PROBLEM
List the adjunctive agents commonly used in the treatment of acute MI.

ANSWERS

A1. **b.** This patient has most likely suffered an anterior wall MI. The history suggests that he is at high risk for an infarct, and the Q waves in V1 to V4 and ST segment elevation in the anterior chest leads and reciprocal changes in the inferior wall confirm the diagnosis.

An acute inferior wall MI would present with ST segment elevation and possibly Q waves in the inferior leads.

Acute pericarditis would present with ST segment elevation in all leads.

Musculoskeletal chest wall pain does not produce the abnormalities in the ECG that we see in this patient.

A2. **e.** The history, physical examination, and ECG point clearly to acute anterior wall MI. First, ascertain that the patient's airway is patent (without obstruction, vomit, or any blockage) and administer 100% oxygen.

A3. **c.** Administer streptokinase or t-PA. The recommended dose of streptokinase in acute MI is 1.5 million units IV over 30 to 60 minutes.

The two recommended regimens for administration of t-PA are the standard regimen and the front-loaded regimen. The front-loaded regimen, used in the GUSTO trial, may produce a higher early patency rate than the standard regimen.

The standard regimen for the administration of t-PA is 10 mg IV bolus, then 50 mg IV over the first hour, followed by 40 mg IV over the next 2 hours. The front-loaded regimen used in the GUSTO trial is 15 mg IV bolus, then 50 mg IV over 30 minutes, followed by 35 mg over 1 hour for a 100-mg total dose.

A third choice is APSAC (Eminase), delivered as a dose of 30 units (IV bolus) infused over 5 minutes. Reteplase, a recombinant DNA product like t-PA, is also approved for acute MI. A dose of 20 units is infused over 15 minutes. The advantages of the recombinant DNA sources, reteplase and t-PA, are high clot selectivity and the absence of reported allergic reactions.

A4. **d.** Thrombolytic therapy should be administered only when the following criteria are met: (a) typical chest pain suggestive of an MI, (b) ECG changes confirming MI, and (c) the "absence" of other diseases that would explain the symptoms.

An age greater than 70 years was formerly a criterion for exclusion of patients for thrombolytic therapy; this is no longer the case. Contraindications to thrombolytic therapy include (a) active internal bleeding, (b) suspected aortic dissection, (c) prolonged or traumatic cardiopulmonary resuscitation, (d) recent head trauma or known intracranial neoplasm, (e) hemorrhagic retinopathy, (f) pregnancy, (g) systolic blood pressure over 190 mm Hg and/or a diastolic blood pressure over 110 mm Hg, (h) history of cerebrovascular disease, and (i) trauma or surgery within the last 2 weeks.

A5. **e.** Although the benefits of thrombolytic therapy are greatest within the first 1 to 3 hours, a 10% mortality benefit can be achieved up to 12 hours after the onset of pain. Older patients, who have a higher complication rate, actually benefit more from thrombolytic therapy because of a higher hospital mortality. Treatment should be considered for patients up to age 80 years—or even older if the benefit-to-risk ratio seems favorable.

Patients with non-Q-wave infarcts have not consistently benefited from thrombolytic therapy, nor have patients with prior CABG.

A6. **e.** The role of concomitant heparin in the initial treatment of acute MI has become increasingly clear over time. The HART study has shown that early, effective anticoagulation with heparin maintains t-PA-induced coronary artery patency more effectively than aspirin alone. Subgroup analyses have shown that patients receiving therapeutic heparin, as measured by the activated partial thromboplastin time (APTT), have an extremely high patency, approaching 95%, after t-PA administration. Although there is some evidence to the contrary, it may be reasonable to believe that what applies to t-PA and heparin also applies to streptokinase and heparin.

In the GUSTO trial (t-PA vs streptokinase), patients received a 5000-unit heparin bolus followed by 1000 units/hr constant infusion, titrated every 6 hours, to maintain an APTT of 60 to 85 seconds for at least 48 hours.

The two most important indications for concomitant use of heparin are acute anterior wall MI and echocardiographic evidence of left ventricular thrombi.

A7. **e.** The major contraindications to adjunctive heparin therapy in MI are history of major surgery with time from discharge under 14 days, history of cerebrovascular accidents, chronic atrial fibrillation or chronic mitral stenosis, and acute gastrointestinal hemorrhage.

A8. **d.** Once placed in the CCU, the patient should have his left ventricular ejection fraction measured. If no other cardiac conditions are discovered, the patient should have a submaximal stress test before discharge. If this result is negative, a maximal exercise stress tolerance test should be performed after 4 to 6 weeks.

A9. **d.** The pathophysiology of acute MI centers around the formation and rupture of a vulnerable atherosclerotic plaque. The progression of atherosclerosis is as follows:
   a. Superficial atherosclerotic fatty streaks form in the coronary arteries of children
   b. The fatty streaks progress to elevated fibrous plaques by the third and fourth decades of life
   c. These fibrous plaques progress to complex, eccentric, ulcerated, and hemorrhagic plaques by

the fifth and sixth decades, culminating in plaque rupture or intraplaque hemorrhage and coronary artery occlusion

The endothelial injury eventually provides the basis for atherogenesis. The fragile endothelium is damaged by hypertension, elevated low-density lipoprotein (LDL) cholesterol, diabetes, smoking, and other factors.

Simple denudation exposes the vascular collagen, which triggers circulating platelet adhesion and aggregation and a cascade of growth factor release, including thromboxane A_2, prostacyclin, and platelet-derived growth factor. Smooth muscle cell and monocyte proliferation, along with lipid accumulation under the influence of growth factors, leads to severe atherosclerosis. For reasons that are still not entirely clear, some atherosclerotic lesions, particularly those near vessel branch points and possibly triggered by viral infection or other causes of inflammation, become vulnerable and rupture, leading to the acute MI syndrome.

A10. **e.** Aspirin is the only adjunctive agent that has unequivocally been shown to reduce mortality alone or in conjunction with thrombolytic agents in patients with acute MI. The ISIS-II study showed that acetylsalicylic acid (ASA) reduced mortality by 25%. However, when ASA was added to streptokinase, the effect was synergistic, and mortality from MI was reduced by 42%.

Thus aspirin has been shown to reduce rethrombosis and recurrent MI. It is not, however, a substitute for anything; it should be used along with other acute agents in the treatment of MI.

A11. **e.** The cornerstone of treatment of acute MI is thrombolytic therapy. It is an established, effective therapy that limits myocardial necrosis, preserves left ventricular function, and reduces mortality. Presently the following statement can be made: "The use of thrombolytic therapy in acute myocardial infarction has been established to the point where not to use such therapy is considered to be substandard care."*

A12. **d.** Thrombolytic therapy currently is underutilized in the treatment of acute MI in the United States. Despite excellent data supporting thrombolytic therapy, only approximately 30% of patients with acute MI receive it. Of the remaining 70%, only 20% have true contraindications or equivocal ECG changes that would preclude thrombolytic therapy.

---

*From Rakel R, ed: *Conn's current therapy*, Philadelphia, 1994, WB Saunders.

A13. **d.** PVCs occur frequently after acute MI and do not require treatment. Couplets, triplets, multifocal PVCs, and short runs of nonsustained ventricular tachycardia are effectively treated with IV lidocaine. Despite the fact, however, that they are treated with IV lidocaine, no survival advantage has been shown with lidocaine in this setting.

Most clinicians do not treat these nonmalignant ventricular dysrhythmias because they rarely progress to life-threatening situations, and, if they do, they can be treated effectively with cardioversion or defibrillation.

Lidocaine is not recommended in the routine prophylaxis of acute MI. In addition, long-term prophylaxis with oral antiarrhythmics such as flecainide and encainide after acute MI has been shown to increase mortality drastically.

A14. **e.** The risk of subsequent infarction and/or mortality after discharge from the hospital following an MI is increased in patients with (a) postinfarction angina pectoris; (b) non-Q-wave infarction; (c) congestive cardiac failure; (d) left ventricular ejection fraction less than 40%; (e) exercise-induced ischemia diagnosed by ECG or by scintigraphy; and (f) ventricular ectopy (frequency >10 PVCs/min).

A15. **e.** β-Blockers, aspirin, and calcium channel blockers have improved the prognosis in some patients after an MI. β-Blockers appear to reduce the risk of sudden death in patients who are at increased risk. Antiplatelet agents, particularly aspirin, have been shown to be of benefit in patients who have had an MI. Aspirin reduces both rethrombosis and recurrent MI.

Calcium channel blockers (diltiazem and verapamil) have been shown to decrease the risk of reinfarction after a non-Q-wave infarction.

Anticoagulants have not been shown to improve prognosis, although they do reduce peripheral embolization in the early discharge phase.

Antiarrhythmics other than β-blockers have not been shown to be effective as prophylactic agents.

A16. **c.** Patients who have suffered an MI should gradually increase activity levels over a period of 6 to 8 weeks. Patients can return to work by approximately 8 weeks. Patients who have suffered an uncomplicated MI may be safely started in an activity program by 3 to 4 weeks after infarction.

Sexual intercourse can resume within 4 to 6 weeks of the infarction. There does not seem to be any logical reason for the patient to wait 3 months to resume intercourse. A good rule to follow in this case is, "If the patient can climb the stairs to the bedroom, the rest is probably okay too!"

In many patients the psychologic impact of an MI outweighs the physical impact. Also, in a significant percentage of families, the spouse is affected as much as, if not more than, the patient. One of the most common errors in cardiac rehabilitation is not involving the spouse or significant other at every stage of the program.

A17. **b.** The pathophysiologic difference between (a) unstable angina and non-Q-wave or nontransmural infarction on the one hand and (b) transmural infarction on the other is the duration and completeness of the occlusion.

There is no difference between (a) the presenting and symptoms of the attack, (b) the risk factor profile, (c) the male-female ratio, or (d) the "area of injury" surrounding the actual "area of infarction."

A18. **c.** The single best confirmatory test of the choices offered for the diagnosis of acute MI is creatine kinase isoenzyme MB (CK-MB) fraction. Elevation of the ST segment can result from either injury or infarction. It is neither sensitive nor specific enough for the diagnosis of infarction in the absence of Q waves.

For the diagnosis of acute MI, the ECG is sensitive (70% to 90% with more than 1 mm of elevation in two contiguous leads); unfortunately it is less specific.

The presence of dysfunctional heart muscle on echocardiography means that there is likely to be a lowering of both the ejection fraction and the cardiac index; it says nothing about whether an MI has occurred or anything regarding the age of same. Radiolabeled antimyosin antibody fragments are sensitive and specific imaging agents, but scintigraphy must be performed 24 to 48 hours after injection, so this test has very limited clinical utility. In the near future it is likely that determinations of troponin T and I, which are also surrogates for cardiac necrosis and are more specific than CK-MB, will be the standard measure of acute MI.

A19. **c.** Sudden death as a result of acute MI is almost always the result of ventricular fibrillation induced by the electrical instability of the ischemic/infarction zone. Ventricular fibrillation is most common either at the immediate onset of coronary occlusion or at the time of coronary reperfusion (reperfusion arrhythmia).

A20. **d.** Shock in the presence of an acute MI can be of two pathophysiologic varieties. Either there is hypovolemia and associated hypotension (hypovolemic shock), or there is persistent hypotension and a poor cardiac index in the presence of adequate left ventricular filling pressures.

Hypovolemic shock is best treated with volume replacement using either Ringer's lactate or normal saline solution. Care must be taken to avoid "volume overloading," which may produce pulmonary edema and congestive cardiac failure.

Cardiogenic shock is generally associated with severe left ventricular dysfunction and occurs with large infarcts that damage more than 40% of the left ventricle. Treatment is urgent, and mortality is high. The treatments of choice include (a) intraaortic balloon pump placement to increase coronary flow and decrease afterload; (b) coronary reperfusion with percutaneous transluminal coronary angioplasty (PTCA) (the mainstay of treatment); and (c) pharmacologic agents, including morphine, dopamine, and dobutamine.

A21. **c.** One clinical trial has shown unequivocally that there is a significant survival advantage to patients with acute MI, even when thrombolytic agents are given up to 12 hours after the onset of the chest pain.

A22. **a.** The finding on physical examination of the abdomen of "an enlarged aorta" should be further assessed by an abdominal ultrasound study. The patient probably has an aortic aneurysm. Although this finding could also be assessed by CT or MRI, an abdominal ultrasound is considerably less expensive and just as sensitive.

SOLUTION TO THE SHORT ANSWER MANAGEMENT PROBLEM

The commonly used adjunctive agents in acute MI are as follows:
1. Aspirin: 160 mg at the time of infarct and 160 mg every day following. Aspirin reduces rethrombosis and recurrent MI.
2. β-Blockers (e.g., metoprolol): 5 mg IV bolus q5min for three doses, then 50 mg PO q6h for 48 hours, then 100 mg PO bid. β-Blockade is contraindicated with hypotension or bradycardia, severe left ventricular dysfunction, or AV block. It is especially effective for reflex tachycardia or hypertension.
3. Heparin: 5000-unit IV bolus followed by 1000 units/hr. Heparin is begun concomitantly with thrombolytic therapy and continued for 24 to 48 hours.
4. Magnesium sulfate: 8 mmol IV over 5 minutes, then 65 mmol over 24 hours. Benign therapy has been shown to reduce mortality. Side effects include flushing and bradycardia.
5. Morphine sulfate: 2 to 5 mg IV every 5 to 30 minutes and as needed. Morphine sulfate is an excellent analgesic/anxiolytic. It decreases both preload and afterload and myocardial oxygen demand. However, morphine sulfate may cause hypotension.

6. Nitroglycerin: 0.4 mg sublingual followed by 5 to 10 mg/min by IV infusion. The infusion rate can be increased by 10-mg increments to 100 mg/min to control symptoms or to decrease mean blood pressure by 10%.

7. Oxygen: 2 to 4 L/min by nasal cannula is administered to all patients during the initial hours of treatment. Higher flow rates may be necessary in patients with congestive heart failure or frank hypoxia.

8. Warfarin: 10 mg/day for 3 days, then 2.5 to 5 mg/day is indicated for severe left ventricular dysfunction to prevent mural thrombus.

SUMMARY OF THE DIAGNOSIS AND TREATMENT OF ACUTE MYOCARDIAL INFARCTION

1. Signs and symptoms: The pain of MI, unlike angina pectoris, usually occurs at rest. The pain is similar to angina in location and radiation but is more severe and builds up rapidly. Usually it is described as a retrosternal tightness or squeezing sensation or sometimes a dull ache. Radiation to the left shoulder is common. Other symptoms include sweating, weakness, dizziness, nausea, vomiting, and abdominal discomfort. Abdominal discomfort is especially common in inferior wall MIs.

2. ECG changes: The classic evolution of changes is from peaked (hyperacute) T waves, to ST segment elevation, to Q-wave development, to T-wave inversion. This sequence may occur over a few hours or may take several days. (NOTE: If ECG changes are not present, do not assume an MI has not occurred. If signs and symptoms suggest MI, it is an MI until proved otherwise.)

3. Confirmatory evidence: Evidence of infarction is confirmed by elevation of the CK-MB fraction for 3 days.

4. Other diagnostic procedures: Scintigraphic studies, including technetium-99 and thallium-201 imaging and radionuclide angiography, as well as echocardiography, may help document the extent of the damage.

5. Treatment:
   a. Supplementary oxygen
   b. Morphine sulfate for pain relief as well as for its preload- and afterload-reducing properties
   c. Thrombolytic therapy: streptokinase, APSAC, reteplase, or t-PA
   d. Heparin therapy: initiate concomitantly with thrombolytic agent

   e. β-Blockade: limits extent of infarction
   f. Nitroglycerin: ideal for pain control as well as its preload-reducing properties
   g. Warfarin: consider if severe left ventricular dysfunction to prevent mural thrombosis
   h. Consider magnesium sulfate as analgesic/anxiolytic
   i. Aspirin: one stat; 160 mg/day
   (NOTE: Lidocaine prophylaxis is not indicated for the prevention of dysrhythmias.)

6. Post-MI:
   a. Submaximal stress ECG test before discharge
   b. Discharge medications: aspirin; β-blocker, possibly acetylcholinesterase inhibitor if there was a large infarct or thrombolytic therapy was administered
   c. Exercise program within 3 to 4 weeks
   d. Return to work within 8 weeks
   e. Sexual intercourse in 4 weeks
   f. Involvement of the spouse or significant other is critical

SUGGESTED READINGS

Thompson MA, Ross AM: Acute myocardial infarction. In Rakel R, ed: *Conn's current therapy,* Philadelphia, 1994, WB Saunders.

Tierney LM, McPhee SJ, Papadakis MA, eds: *Current medical diagnosis and treatment, 2000,* ed 39, Stamford, Conn, 1999, Appleton & Lange.

PROBLEM · 2

ANGINA

"My Chest Pain Is Getting Worse—Am I Dying?"

Case 1 ■ A 55-Year-Old Male with Chest Pain

A 55-year-old male comes to your office for assessment of left-sided shoulder pain. The pain begins after any strenuous activity, including walking. The pain is described as follows: (1) *quality:* dull, aching; (2) *quantity:* 8/10 when doing any activity—otherwise 0/10; (3) *chronology:* began about 8 months ago and has been getting worse ever since; (4) *continuous/intermittent:* intermittent; (5) *aggravating factors:* exercise of any kind; (6) *relieving factors:* rest; (7) *associated manifestations:* occasional nausea; (8) *pain history:* no pain before 8 months ago; no other significant history of pain syndromes; (9) *radiation:* appears to be radiating to the left shoulder area; (10) *location:* mainly retrosternal; (11) *quality of life:* definitely affecting quality of life by limiting activity.

The patient tells you that the pain seems somehow

worse today. For the first time, it did not go away after he stopped walking.

The patient's blood pressure is 120/80 mm Hg; his pulse is 72 bpm and regular. His heart sounds are normal. There are no extra sounds and no murmurs.

SELECT THE BEST ANSWER TO THE FOLLOWING QUESTIONS

Q1. Which of the following statements regarding this patient's chest pain is false?
  a. the patient may have suffered a myocardial infarction (MI)
  b. the patient's chest pain may be caused by angina pectoris
  c. the patient's chest pain may be caused by esophageal motor disorder
  d. the administration of sublingual nitroglycerin is a very sensitive test to distinguish angina pectoris from esophageal causes
  e. the patient should be admitted to the Coronary Care Unit (CCU) until the origin of the pain is firmly established

Q2. The patient is admitted for observation to the CCU. His pain subsides with intravenous (IV) nitroglycerin. His creatine kinase isoenzyme MB (CK-MB) fraction is normal. Which of the following investigations is not indicated at this time?
  a. an exercise tolerance test
  b. coronary angiography
  c. an upper gastrointestinal series
  d. a plasma lipid profile
  e. a fasting blood sugar level

Q3. The patient subsequently has an exercise tolerance test. This test reveals a 2.5-mm ST segment depression at 5 METS of activity as the patient achieved 50% of his age-predicted maximum heart rate. Which of the following statements regarding this test result is (are) true?
  a. it probably indicates angina pectoris
  b. coronary angiography is indicated
  c. a hypotensive response with stress testing suggests severe ischemia and severe (probably multivessel) coronary artery disease
  d. a and b
  e. all of the above statements are true

Q4. Which of the following medications would not be indicated as a first-line therapy for the treatment of this patient?
  a. diltiazem
  b. propranolol
  c. isosorbide dinitrate
  d. prazosin
  e. labetalol

Case 2 ■ A 76-Year-Old Male with a History of Angina Pectoris

A 76-year-old male with a history of angina pectoris is brought to the Emergency Department by his wife. For the past 3 days he has been having increasing chest pain. The chest pain has been occurring at rest and while in bed at night as well as while walking (he is able to walk only very slowly). The pain has been getting progressively worse over the last 8 hours.

On physical examination, his blood pressure is 120/70 mm Hg. His pulse is 96 bpm and regular.

His electrocardiogram (ECG) shows ST segment depression of 1.5 mm. Flattening of the T waves is seen across the precordial leads.

Q5. Which of the following statements regarding this patient is (are) true?
  a. this patient has unstable angina
  b. IV nitroglycerin is the treatment of first choice
  c. the patient probably has complex coronary artery stenosis
  d. this patient should be given one aspirin daily
  e. all of the above are true

Case 3 ■ A 50-Year-Old Female with Sharp Retrosternal Chest Pain

A 50-year-old female comes to the Emergency Department with a sharp retrosternal chest pain that awoke her. This is the fourth episode in as many nights, but she is sure that she is not having a heart attack because she saw her physician only 3 weeks ago. At that time, he gave her a "clean bill of health." She was told that her ECG, blood pressure, and cholesterol levels were completely normal. She is a nonsmoker and has no family history of coronary artery disease.

On physical examination, her blood pressure is 100/70 mm Hg. Her pulse is 96 bpm and regular, and the remainder of the cardiovascular and respiratory examinations is normal.

Her ECG reveals a significant ST segment elevation in the anterior limb leads. Within 1 hour, the ST segment has returned to normal. CK-MB fraction levels done over the next 3 days are normal.

Q6. Which of the following statements regarding this patient is (are) true?
  a. this patient probably has Prinzmetal's angina
  b. calcium channel blockers are the treatment of choice for this type of angina

c. β-blockers are contraindicated in this type of angina

d. all of the above

e. none of the above

Q7. Which of the following statements regarding percutaneous coronary angioplasty and mortality from coronary artery disease is true?

a. percutaneous coronary angioplasty increases longevity

b. percutaneous coronary angioplasty improves both morbidity and mortality from coronary artery disease

c. percutaneous coronary angioplasty is of no proven benefit

d. the use of glycoprotein IIb/IIIa inhibitors has markedly reduced the rates of acute vessel closure

e. optimal lesions for angioplasty are proximal in location, noneccentric, and located at branch (bifurcation) points in the vessel

Q8. In which of the following patients would percutaneous coronary angioplasty most likely be used?

a. a patient with left main stem disease

b. a patient with triple-vessel disease

c. a patient with a ventricular aneurysm

d. a patient with one-vessel disease

e. any of the above are good indications for percutaneous coronary angioplasty

Q9. Which of the following is least likely to be used as a combination therapy in patients with angina pectoris?

a. nitroglycerin-atenolol-nifedipine

b. nitroglycerin-enalapril-nifedipine

c. nitroglycerin-propranolol-verapamil

d. nitroglycerin-metoprolol-diltiazem

e. nitroglycerin-propranolol-nifedipine

Q10. Which of the following drugs is considered the most potent vasodilator?

a. nifedipine

b. verapamil

c. metoprolol

d. atenolol

e. propranolol

Q11. Coronary artery bypass graft (CABG) surgery may be indicated as the treatment of choice for angina pectoris with which of the following angina patients?

a. a patient with triple-vessel disease

b. a patient with one-vessel disease

c. a patient with two-vessel disease

d. CABG may be first-line therapy in any of the above

e. b or c

Case 4 ■ A 65-Year-Old Male with Angina and Hypertension

A 65-year-old male comes to your office with a history strongly suggestive of angina pectoris. He also has a long history of hypertension. On physical examination, his blood pressure is 170/100 mm Hg. Exercise tolerance testing reveals a 2.5-mm ST segment depression. A 2D/M mode echocardiogram reveals apical akinesis and an estimated ejection fraction of 45%.

Q12. Which of the following medications would you consider as the agent(s) of first choice in the treatment of this patient?

a. hydrochlorothiazide

b. verapamil

c. clonidine

d. atenolol

e. b and/or d

f. a and/or b

g. c and/or d

Q13. Which of the following investigations should be performed on a patient with possible angina pectoris?

a. complete blood count (CBC)

b. chest x-ray

c. fasting lipid profile

d. thyroid function testing

e. all of the above

Q14. The pathophysiology of angina pectoris is best explained by which of the following?

a. significantly increased peripheral vascular resistance

b. a balance between oxygen supply and oxygen demand

c. an imbalance of oxygen supply and oxygen demand plus or minus coronary artery spasm

d. significant peripheral venous and arterial vasoconstriction

e. none of the above

Q15. Which of the following criteria indicate(s) a diagnosis of unstable angina pectoris?

a. new onset angina (2 months) that is either severe or frequent (three episodes daily) or both

b. patients with accelerating angina

c. patients with angina at rest

d. b and c

e. all of the above

SHORT ANSWER MANAGEMENT PROBLEM
Briefly describe the phenomenon of asymptomatic coronary artery ischemia.

ANSWERS

A1. **d.** Acute chest pain is a very common and often difficult diagnostic problem. MI must be assumed until proven otherwise in patients with any significant risk factors. Pain from esophageal motor disorder is often confused with pain from myocardial ischemia. This differential diagnosis is often exceedingly difficult; many times (a) quality of pain, (b) quantity of pain, (c) radiation of pain, and (d) some aggravating factors are the same in both conditions. Although many physicians believe that relief with nitroglycerin is specific for myocardial ischemia and MI, this is not the case. Sublingual nitroglycerin will relieve pain from esophageal motor disorder as well as it will relieve pain from myocardial ischemia and myocardial injury.

A2. **b.** We are not yet far enough down the diagnostic pathway leading to angina pectoris to justify the invasive procedure of coronary angiography. A normal CK-MB fraction essentially rules out MI. However, the origin of this patient's chest pain is still unclear and must be pursued in a systematic manner. At this time the following are the major diagnostic considerations:
   a. Myocardial ischemia
   b. Esophageal motor disorder
   c. Musculoskeletal chest wall pain

Because this patient has other significant risk factors, he should be assumed to have a cardiovascular cause for his pain until proven otherwise. Thus all possible testable risk factors should be checked. Because this patient has a relatively high pretest probability of having coronary artery disease (Bayes' theorem), a treadmill exercise stress test should be performed. On the other hand, an upper gastrointestinal series may determine any contribution from reflux esophagitis. It is most reasonable to do these tests in sequence.

A3. **e.** The 2.5-mm ST segment depression quite likely represents severe coronary ischemia. Although we are not told the results of blood pressure monitoring during this patient's exercise tolerance test, it is certainly true that a "hypotensive response" indicates severe ischemia. The other information provided—pain at less than 6 METS and at less than 70% of his predicted maximal heart rate—is sensitive to cardiac ischemia. With this information, coronary angiography should now be performed.

A4. **d.** Medications indicated for treating angina pectoris include three classes of drugs:
   a. β-Blockers
   b. Nitrates
   c. Calcium channel blockers

The drugs listed include one calcium channel blocker (diltiazem), two nitrates (isosorbide dinitrate and nitroglycerin), and one β-blocker (propranolol). The list also includes one peripheral β-adrenergic agonist (prazosin), which is not a drug of choice for the treatment of angina pectoris. There are ongoing trials to evaluate the efficacy of aggressive lipid-lowering with statins as another modality to reduce cardiac ischemia, presumably by improving endothelial function. The first of these studies should be available in the next several years.

A5. **e.** The history given by this patient is one of unstable angina pectoris. *Unstable angina pectoris* is the term used to describe accelerating or "crescendo" angina in a patient who has previously had stable angina. Unstable angina can be diagnosed when the angina occurs with less exertion or at rest, lasts longer, and is less responsive to medication. IV nitroglycerin is the first treatment that should be given. If more pain relief is needed, IV or subcutaneous morphine may be used. One baby aspirin should also be given at this time.

Unstable angina is often associated with complex coronary artery stenosis consisting of plaque ulceration, hemorrhage, and/or thrombosis. The unstable situation may rapidly progress to complete occlusion and infarction or may heal, with reendothelialization and a return to a stable angina, albeit most likely with a more severe pattern of ischemia.

Nitrates are first-line therapy for the initial presentation of unstable angina. Nonparenteral therapy with sublingual or oral nitrates or nitroglycerin ointment may be sufficient. As a general rule, however, if there is any doubt as to the most appropriate route, use the IV preparation. IV β-blockers are an alternative.

Once the acute episode is controlled, therapy can be initiated or changed using a combination of nitrates, β-blockers, and/or calcium channel blockers. Heparin and/or thrombolytic therapy should also be considered during the acute phase.

Despite the ECG showing only 1.5 mm of ST segment depression and no acute changes indicative of MI, the patient should be hospitalized and placed in the CCU. Serial measurements of CK-MB fractions should be performed.

A6. **d.** Prinzmetal's angina (coronary artery vaso-spasm) is angina that occurs in the absence of pre-cipitating factors. It is most common in the early morning, often awakening the patient from sleep. It is usually associated with ST segment elevation rather than ST segment depression. Coronary angiography should be performed to rule out coexisting fixed ste-notic lesions. Calcium channel blockers are probably the drugs of choice for Prinzmetal's angina. Nitrates are also effective. β-Blockers are contraindicated in patients who have vasospasm without fixed, stenotic lesions.

A7. **d.**

A8. **d.** Percutaneous transluminal coronary angio-plasty (PTCA) as a treatment for dilating stenotic coro-nary arterial lesions was introduced in 1977. Today successful dilatation rates per stenosis exceed 90%, complication rates have fallen to 4%, and procedure-related MI and death remain uncommon.

Recent enthusiasm for balloon dilatation has been accompanied by its increasing application to more complex forms of coronary disease and a marked in-crease in the number of procedures performed annu-ally in many American centers. In many centers, PTCA is now the most commonly used invasive therapy for coronary artery disease.

The initial results of PTCA were considered accept-able, but the major concern at present is long-term sta-bility of revascularization. Significant restenosis oc-curs within the first year in up to 40% of lesions, and both symptomatic recurrence and reintervention rates have been high during follow-up. Various strategies—from the use of intravascular stents to concomitant treatment with glycoprotein IIb/IIIa inhibitors—have demonstrated some improvement in acute graft clo-sure and restenosis. In retrospective studies compar-ing the long-term results of PTCA and CABG, it ap-pears that angina recurrence and event-free survival rates are significantly better in CABG despite similar entry criteria. This is particularly true in diabetics, who have two times the reocclusion rates of nondia-betics with PTCA.

In summary, we are currently unsure about the role of PTCA. There is no evidence that it improves mor-tality. It seems appropriate that until long-term data are available, the currently accelerating enthusiasm for PTCA in complex forms of coronary disease should be held in check, reserving its major application for (a) patients with severe symptoms from low-risk obstruc-tions (such as single-vessel and mild double-vessel disease) that do not warrant surgical intervention for prognostic reasons and (b) high-risk patients who would not survive CABG.

The most likely condition of the choices listed for PTCA would be single-vessel disease. Triple-vessel disease and left ventricular aneurysms are definite contraindications to PTCA. Left main stem disease is also a contraindication.

A9. **b.** Of the combinations listed, the least likely combination of drugs to treat angina pectoris would be nitroglycerin-enalapril-nifedipine. Enalapril is an angiotensin-converting enzyme (ACE) inhibitor. Un-less the patient also has congestive heart failure, ACE inhibitors are generally not used as medical therapy for angina pectoris.

A10. **a.** The most effective dilator of those listed is ni-fedipine. Nifedipine and verapamil are both calcium channel blockers; of the two, nifedipine is the more potent vasodilator. Sublingual nifedipine had been used in the treatment of hypertensive crises and emer-gencies, but this is no longer recommended given the risk of reflex tachycardia and the potential unmasking of cardiac ischemia. The other three drugs (metopro-lol, atenolol, and propranolol) are β-blockers.

A11. **d.** CABG may be the treatment of choice in any of the conditions listed: triple-vessel disease, double-vessel disease, or single-vessel disease. Although single-vessel disease may be treated with PTCA, the discussion on PTCA indicates that both angina and event-free survival are better with CABG.

A12. **e.** A patient with both angina pectoris and hy-pertension should be treated with a calcium channel blocker, a β-blocker, or both. In this case the calcium channel blocker verapamil or the β-blocker atenolol would be a reasonable treatment option.

A13. **e.** Patients suspected of having angina pectoris need (a) a CBC; (b) a fasting lipid profile; (c) a chest x-ray film; (d) an ECG; and (e) thyroid function test-ing. Moreover, renal function should be evaluated and electrolyte and blood glucose measurements made. Testing for hyperhomocystinemia may also be war-ranted. If the patient appears to have significant chronic obstructive pulmonary disease (COPD), spi-rometry may also be helpful. Since at this time we are describing an ambulatory patient, it is a better concept to promote spirometry rather than arterial blood gas (ABG) studies. ABG testing is second-line, expensive, painful, and should be reserved for patients with es-tablished COPD.

A14. **c.** The basic pathophysiology in patients with angina pectoris is an imbalance between oxygen sup-ply and oxygen demand resulting from atherosclerotic narrowing of the coronary arteries. Atherosclerosis, the underlying pathophysiologic lesion, can be broken down into two components:

    a. "Atheroma" of the intima—the deposition of cholesterol/fibrin/calcium plaques on the intimal surface

    b. "Sclerosis," or "hardening," of the media. However, many patients with angina pectoris have been found to have a "coronary spasm" component to this "constricting" process. This vasospasm component may be present even in the absence of true Prinzmetal's angina or coronary artery spasm angina.

A15. **e.** Unstable angina pectoris is characterized by:

    a. New-onset angina (>2 months) that is severe and/or frequent (<3 episodes daily)

    b. Patients with accelerating angina

    c. Patients with angina at rest

SOLUTION TO THE SHORT ANSWER MANAGEMENT PROBLEM

Obstructive coronary artery disease, acute MI, and transient myocardial ischemia are frequently asymptomatic. The majority of patients with typical chronic angina pectoris are found to have objective evidence of myocardial ischemia (ST segment depression). However, many of these same patients and some other patients who are always asymptomatic are at high risk for coronary events. Longitudinal studies have demonstrated an increased incidence of coronary events, including sudden death, MI, and angina pectoris, in asymptomatic patients with positive exercise tests. In addition, patients with asymptomatic ischemia after MI are at far greater risk for a secondary coronary event than symptomatic patients.

Patients who are found to have asymptomatic ischemia should be evaluated by both stress ECG and radionuclide scintigraphy.

The management of asymptomatic ischemia must be individualized and depends on the following:

1. The degree of positivity of the exercise test
2. The ECG leads showing a positive response
3. Other factors, such as:
    a. The patient's age
    b. The patient's occupation
    c. The patient's general medical condition

However, it is generally recommended that further testing and treatment be as follows:

1. Patients with severe ischemia on noninvasive testing should be referred for coronary arteriography. This may lead to a CABG procedure.
2. General management at this time favors aspirin and prophylactic β-blockade.

SUMMARY OF THE DIAGNOSIS AND TREATMENT OF ANGINA PECTORIS

1. Definition: Angina pectoris can be defined as an imbalance between myocardial requirements for oxygen and the amount of oxygen delivered through the coronary arteries. This can occur via a mechanism of increased demand, diminished delivery, or both.

2. Symptoms: The patient with angina pectoris frequently describes the pain as either a "retrosternal tightness" or "retrosternal pain." Other descriptions include "retrosternal burning," "retrosternal pressing," "retrosternal choking," "retrosternal aching," "retrosternal gas," and "retrosternal indigestion." These symptoms are typically located in the retrosternal area or the left side of the chest. Usual radiation to the left shoulder, left arm, or jaw occurs. Typical angina is aggravated by exercise and relieved by rest.

3. Signs: Physical examination is often normal, although hypertension is sometimes present.

4. Initial laboratory evaluation: CBC, urinalysis, electrolytes, blood glucose levels, blood lipids, uric acid, thyroid function tests, chest x-ray film, ECG, and stress ECG testing are basic. Radionuclide scintigraphy and coronary angiography may follow.

5. Treatment:
    a. Acute attacks:
        1) Mild: Sublingual nitroglycerin or nitroglycerin spray
        2) Severe: IV nitroglycerin
    b. Long-term prophylaxis and treatment: Long-acting nitroglycerin, long-acting calcium channel blockers, or β-blockers alone or in combination
    c. Intervention/surgery:
        1) PTCA has not demonstrated reduction in morbidity or mortality.
        2) CABG is the preferred method of intervention at this time.

6. Angina variants:
    a. Prinzmetal's angina: Prinzmetal's angina is due to coronary artery spasm with or without fixed stenotic lesions. It is more common in women than in men. ST segment elevation is more common than ST segment depression. Calcium channel blockers are the treatment of choice.
    b. Unstable angina: Unstable angina is an accelerating or "crescendo" pattern of angina. It may represent intermittent incomplete occlusion of coronary arteries. Acute treatment includes IV

nitroglycerin or an IV β-blocker. All patients with unstable angina should be taking one aspirin daily along with a combination of antiangina agents.

SUGGESTED READINGS

Califf RM: Acute ischemic syndromes, *Med Clin North Am* 79:999, 1995.

Glasser S: Angina pectoris. In Rakel R, ed: *Conn's current therapy*, Philadelphia, 1994, WB Saunders.

Solomon AJ, Gersh BJ: Management of chronic stable angina: Medical therapy, PTCA and CABG, *Ann Intern Med* 128:216, 1998.

P R O B L E M · 3

DYSLIPIDEMIA

"Where Can I Get Some of That Good Cholesterol?"

Case 1 ■ A 51-Year-Old Male with a High Blood Cholesterol Level

A 51-year-old male comes to your office for his "yearly work-up." He is a typical type A personality: hard driving and "married to my job and proud of it." He is, however, married to his wife as well, as he points out in retrospect. He has had previous problems with "high blood cholesterol" and wishes to have his cholesterol checked today.

On examination, his blood pressure is 170/100 mm Hg. His pulse is 84 bpm and regular. His body mass index is 31. His abdomen is obese.

His family history is significant for hypertension in both parents. His uncle sustained a myocardial infarction at age 58 years and his older brother had "heart problems" at age 55 years. His spot blood cholesterol level in your office (nonfasting) is 8.2 mmol/L (328 mg/dl).

The patient is asked to return in 1 week for a fasting sample. The results are as follows:

Total cholesterol (TC): 288 mg/dl
Triglycerides: 262 mg/dl
High-density lipoproteins (HDL): 37 mg/dl
Low-density lipoproteins (LDL): 199 mg/dl

SELECT THE BEST ANSWER
TO THE FOLLOWING QUESTIONS

Q1. Regarding this patient's lipid profile, which of the following statements is true?
   a. this is a normal profile given his age and family history
   b. a second fasting lipid profile should be obtained before any conclusions can be drawn

   c. intense dietary therapy and drug therapy should be considered immediately
   d. although this is an abnormal profile, in the absence of known coronary disease, careful observation of the cholesterol level is all that is required at this time
   e. treatment decisions should be based on apoprotein levels

Q2. Which of the following, according to the National Cholesterol Education Program, defines high blood cholesterol?
   a. TC, 200 mg/dl; LDL, 130 mg/dl
   b. TC, 240 mg/dl; LDL, 160 mg/dl
   c. TC, 280 mg/dl; LDL, 190 mg/dl
   d. TC, 320 mg/dl; LDL, 220 mg/dl
   e. TC, 360 mg/dl; LDL, 250 mg/dl

Q3. What is the single most important risk factor for coronary artery disease?
   a. an elevated HDL level
   b. an elevated triglyceride level
   c. an elevated LDL level
   d. a depressed HDL level
   e. an elevated total blood cholesterol level

Q4. An elevated triglyceride level is most closely associated with serum concentration of which of the following?
   a. LDL cholesterol
   b. HDL cholesterol
   c. very low-density lipoprotein (VLDL) cholesterol
   d. total blood cholesterol
   e. apoprotein E

Q5. At what level of LDL cholesterol is treatment definitely indicated?
   a. 4.1 mmol/L (160 mg/dl)
   b. 3.4 mmol/L (130 mg/dl)
   c. 3.8 mmol/L (151 mg/dl)
   d. 5.2 mmol/L (206 mg/dl)
   e. 3.1 mmol/L (123 mg/dl)

Q6. Which of the following is the treatment of choice for hypercholesterolemia?
   a. gemfibrozil
   b. colestipol
   c. nicotinic acid
   d. lovastatin
   e. none of the above

Q7. What is the drug class of choice for the management of mild to moderate elevations of plasma LDL?
   a. the fibric acid derivatives

b. the nicotinic acid derivatives
c. the 3-hydroxy-3-methylglutaryl coenzyme A (HMG CoA) reductase inhibitors
d. the bile acid sequestrants
e. any of the above

Q8. The patient described in Case 1 is taking hydrochlorothiazide and propranolol. Which of the following statements is true concerning the effect of these drugs on plasma lipoproteins?
a. hydrochlorothiazide has no effect on plasma lipoproteins
b. propranolol has no effect on plasma lipoproteins
c. neither hydrochlorothiazide nor propranolol has any effect on plasma lipoproteins
d. both hydrochlorothiazide and propranolol can adversely affect plasma lipoproteins
e. the effects of both drugs are idiosyncratic on plasma lipoproteins, not dose dependent

Q9. A 56-year-old male with hyperlipidemia needs a β-blocker to help control hypertension. Which of the following would be the agent of choice?
a. propranolol
b. metoprolol
c. atenolol
d. nadolol
e. acebutolol

Q10. Which of the following is an (are) independent risk factor(s) for coronary artery disease?
a. increased LDL concentration
b. decreased HDL concentration
c. increased TC concentration
d. increased triglyceride concentration
e. all of the above

Q11. Which of the following antihypertensive drugs does (do) not have an adverse effect on plasma lipids?
a. hydrochlorothiazide
b. fosinopril
c. atenolol
d. nifedipine
e. b and d

Q12. The American Heart Association's Step 1 diet allows how much fat as a percentage of total daily calories?
a. 20%
b. 30%
c. 10%

d. 15%
e. 40%

Q13. The American Heart Association's Step 1 diet allows how much saturated fat as a percentage of total daily calories?
a. 10%
b. 15%
c. 20%
d. 25%
e. 30%

Q14. The American Heart Association's Step 1 diet allows how much TC in the daily intake?
a. 500 mg
b. 400 mg
c. 350 mg
d. 300 mg
e. 200 mg

Q15. Which of the following statements is (are) true regarding fish oil supplements?
a. fish oils have been shown to lower plasma triglyceride levels
b. fish oils inhibit platelet aggregation
c. fish oils have been shown to increase HDL levels
d. fish oils may decrease blood pressure and blood viscosity
e. all of the above are true

Q16. A 56-year-old physician comes to your office for a complete health assessment. When you question him about his alcohol intake, he replies that he simply uses alcohol to favorably affect his apolipoprotein ratio. Which of the following statements regarding alcohol and apolipoproteins is (are) true?
a. ingestion of alcohol decreases apolipoprotein A-1 levels
b. ingestion of alcohol increases apolipoprotein A-1 levels
c. ingestion of alcohol increases apolipoprotein B levels
d. ingestion of alcohol decreases apolipoprotein B levels
e. both b and d

Q17. What is the drug of choice for the treatment of hypertriglyceridemia?
a. nicotinic acid
b. gemfibrozil
c. lovastatin
d. cholestyramine
e. none of the above

Q18. Which of the following is a (are) secondary cause(s) of hyperlipidemia?
   a. diabetes mellitus
   b. alcohol
   c. oral contraceptives
   d. all of the above
   e. none of the above

Q19. Chylomicrons are most closely associated with which of the following?
   a. LDL
   b. HDL
   c. VLDL
   d. medium-density lipoproteins (MDL)
   e. chylomicrons are associated with all of the above

Q20. Regarding the home monitoring of cholesterol, which of the following statements is true?
   a. home monitoring is recommended for patients with very high cholesterol levels
   b. home cholesterol monitoring is sensitive
   c. home cholesterol monitoring is specific
   d. home cholesterol monitoring is both sensitive and specific
   e. none of the above

SHORT ANSWER MANAGEMENT PROBLEM
List the risk factors shown to increase the risk of coronary artery disease in the population.

ANSWERS

A1. **b.** Given this patient's age and risk factors, it was appropriate to proceed directly to a full (fasting) lipid profile. However, before treatment decisions, especially those involving medication, are considered, the results should be verified by a confirmatory test within 8 weeks, with the estimates less than 10% different.

Normal serum cholesterol level is under 5.2 mmol/L (200 mg/dl). Borderline serum cholesterol level is 5.2 to 6.2 mmol/L (200 mg/dl to 240 mg/dl). High serum cholesterol level exceeds 6.2 mmol/L (240 mg/dl).

The question of which patients should be screened for hypercholesterolemia continues to be debated. There are basically two approaches to screening: (a) screen all adult patients at periodic intervals or (b) screen only patients who have a family history of coronary risk factors or who have other coronary risk factors themselves. The cost implications of mass screening and subsequent diagnosis and treatment must be considered in making this decision. The current recommendation is to screen with a nonfasting sample.

A2. **b.** The National Cholesterol Education Program defines high blood cholesterol level as TC, 240 mg/dl (6.2 mmol/L) and LDL, 160 mg/dl (4.1 mmol/L).

A3. **c.** The single most important risk factor for coronary artery disease is an elevated LDL cholesterol level. The second most important risk factor is depressed HDL cholesterol level.

A4. **c.** An elevated triglyceride level is most closely associated with an elevated VLDL level. A triglyceride level greater than 250 mg/dl is considered definitely elevated. A triglyceride level greater than 500 mg/dl is often seen with diabetes mellitus. Although triglycerides were not previously considered an independent risk factor for coronary artery disease, they are now thought to be so.

A5. **a.** An LDL level is considered definitely elevated when it is above 4.1 mmol/L (160 mg/dl). The borderline level is between 3.4 and 4.1 mmol/L (130 mg/dl and 160 mg/dl).

A6. **e.** The treatment of choice for hypercholesterolemia is diet therapy. The American Heart Association has produced Step 1 and Step 2 diets. The Step 1 diet includes less than 30% of total calories from fat, less than 10% of calories from saturated fat, and less than 300 mg/day of cholesterol. The Step 2 diet includes less than 30% of total daily calories as fat, less than 7% of calories from saturated fat, and less than 200 mg/day of cholesterol.

Management of hypercholesterolemia with drugs is indicated only after dietary treatment over a reasonable length of time has failed to reduce the cholesterol level to a sufficiently low level, although there is a newfound sense of more aggressive treatment, even for primary prevention, as the result of studies such as AFCAP/TEXCAP. The current recommendations that diet therapy be continued for 6 months before drug therapy is started are often supplanted, since this study and others have conclusively shown that aggressive treatment of even low-risk middle-aged adults with statin therapy can reduce cardiac morbidity and mortality.

A7. **c.** The drug class of choice for mild to moderate LDL elevation is one of the HMG CoA reductase inhibitors on the market. These include lovastatin (Mevacor), pravastatin (Pravachol), simvastatin (Zocor), atorvastatin (Lipitor), and cerivistatin (Baycol).

All patients who are started on HMG CoA inhibitors should have not only the plasma lipids but also the liver function tests monthly for 3 months, then every 3 months for 6 months, and every 4 to 6 months thereafter. There is a low risk of myositis, so creatinine kinase levels should be measured if patients complain of leg pain or muscle cramps. In patients with mild to moderate isolated LDL elevation (type IIA), plasma lipid levels may be normalized with 10 to 20 mg once daily of any of these agents. Patients with higher LDL levels may require higher doses of single-agent therapy or, alternately, multidrug therapy. With such therapy, LDL cholesterol may be lowered up to 40% and triglyceride levels lowered 10% to 15%. There appears to be little change in the HDL level. All the above drugs have been known to produce hepatic and skeletal muscle toxicity as well as insomnia and weight gain. These side effects, however, are relatively uncommon, are dose related, and occur much more frequently in patients who are on multidrug therapy.

The drug of second choice for type IIA hyperlipoproteinemia is niacin. The total daily dose (500-mg tablets) is up to 3 g. All patients taking niacin require monitoring of liver function tests and creatine phosphokinase monthly for 3 months, then every 3 months for 6 months, and every 4 to 6 months thereafter. Niacin may lower plasma LDL levels by up to 35%, may lower triglyceride levels by up to 75%, and at the same time may raise HDL levels by up to 100%. In addition, the apolipoprotein A level is lowered by up to 50%. In atherosclerosis regression trials, niacin has been the most effective agent in promoting stability and regression of coronary lesions.

Unfortunately, niacin has a considerable number of significant possible side effects, including:

a. Inducing gastric irritation and gastritis
b. Activating long-dormant peptic ulcers
c. Elevating plasma uric acid levels, precipitating an attack of gout
d. Elevating blood glucose levels
e. Exacerbating diabetes
f. Most commonly, causing cutaneous flushing, dry and even scaly skin, and in rare instances acanthosis nigricans

Some of these nuisance side effects can be ameliorated by coadministration of aspirin and/or prescribing the long-acting formulation of niacin. Fortunately, all side effects disappear when the drug is discontinued.

Resins, including cholestyramine (Questran) and colestipol (Colestid), are the drugs of third choice for patients with type IIA hyperlipoproteinemia. The dose ranges are 4 to 8 g once or twice daily for cholestyramine and 5 to 10 g once or twice daily for colestipol. Their advantages include an almost complete lack of absorption and potential for systemic toxicity that goes with it. Their disadvantages include an unpleasant grittiness and multiple gastrointestinal side effects, including abdominal bloating, abdominal pain, some-

times severe constipation, and gastrointestinal bleeding. Because resins may decrease the absorption of other drugs, they and other drugs should be taken 2 hours apart.

A8. **d.** Both hydrochlorothiazide and propranolol can adversely affect plasma lipoproteins, generally in a dose-dependent fashion. Hydrochlorothiazide increases TC and triglyceride concentrations. In addition, VLDL cholesterol levels and LDL levels are increased; HDL cholesterol level changes are variable.

Propranolol increases plasma triglyceride levels but does not alter TC concentrations. However, propranolol does decrease HDL cholesterol levels. LDL cholesterol changes with propranolol are more variable.

The β_1-selective adrenergic blockers, like the nonselective agents, increase triglyceride levels and lower HDL cholesterol levels without altering TC concentration. The adverse effects on lipoproteins tend to be less, however, than the changes observed with the nonselective agents.

A9. **e.** Acebutolol hydrochloride, oxprenolol hydrochloride, and pindolol hydrochloride are β-adrenergic blocking drugs that possess intrinsic sympathomimetic activity (ISA). Acebutolol is β_1-selective, whereas the latter two are not. Oxprenolol may increase triglyceride concentrations and lower HDL cholesterol. Pindolol and acebutolol are lipid neutral.

Acebutolol hydrochloride would be the β-blocker of choice in the patient described in this question because it combines ISA activity, β-selectivity, and a favorable side effect profile.

A10. **e.** Risk factors for coronary artery disease include the following:

a. Increased LDL concentration (most important lipid risk factor)
b. Decreased HDL level (second most important risk factor)
c. Increased TC level
d. Increased triglyceride concentration

A11. **e.** Nifedipine, a calcium channel blocker, and fosinopril, an ACE inhibitor, are the only drugs listed that do not have an adverse affect on plasma lipids (angiotensin receptor blockers are also neutral with respect to plasma lipids, and α-blockers appear to have a beneficial effect on HDL levels). The β-blocker listed, metoprolol, and hydrochlorothiazide also adversely affect plasma lipid levels.

A12. **b.**

A13. **a.**

A14. **d.** As mentioned previously, the treatment of first choice for hyperlipidemia is diet. The American Heart Association's Step 1 diet and Step 2 diet are as follows:

	Step 1	Step 2
Cholesterol	300 mg	200 mg
Saturated fat	10% of calories	7% of calories

A15. **e.** Fish and fish oil supplements may lower plasma lipid levels (especially triglycerides), inhibit platelet aggregation, decrease blood pressure and viscosity, and increase HDL cholesterol levels. However, it is difficult to recommend fish oils for general use.

A16. **e.** There is an inverse relationship between low to moderate alcohol consumption and coronary artery disease. This may result from an inhibitory effect on platelet aggregation or an increased coronary artery diameter. In addition, low doses of alcohol appear to increase the cardioprotective apolipoprotein A-1 and decrease the atherogenic apolipoprotein B.

In this patient, find out how much alcohol this physician actually does use to favorably influence his apolipoprotein ratio. It is a fairly safe bet that it is more than currently recommended.

A17. **b.** The drug of choice for most hypertriglyceridemia is gemfibrozil or another fibric acid derivative. Hypertriglyceridemia may be associated with type IIa, type IIb, type III, or type IV hyperlipoproteinemia. The usual dose of gemfibrozil is 0.6 g bid. Gemfibrozil will decrease hypertriglyceridemia by 40% to 80% and will increase HDL by 10% to 40%.

Until very recently, combining a reductase inhibitor with gemfibrozil was not recommended. This combination should still be used with caution, but may be tolerated if a low dose of one drug is given 12 hours apart from a low dose of the other (e.g., pravastatin, 10 to 20 mg, in the morning with gemfibrozil, 600 mg, in the evening).

A18. **d.** Diabetes mellitus usually produces a very significant elevation of plasma triglyceride and plasma VLDL levels. Triglyceride levels as high as 25,000 mg/dl have been reported in diabetes.

The daily consumption of large amounts of alcohol can produce a mild, asymptomatic elevation in plasma triglycerides caused by an elevation of VLDL. The ingestion of estrogen-containing birth control pills causes an increase in the VLDL secretion rate from the liver and subsequent elevation in the triglyceride level.

A19. **c.** Chylomicrons are usually associated with an elevation of plasma VLDL and thus plasma triglycerides.

A20. **e.** Home cholesterol monitoring is now available. This will likely result in:
a. Increased sales of the products available
b. Increased proportion of the public becoming cholesterol-phobic
c. Increased anxiety regarding "cardiac status"
d. Increased costs to the health care system

The laboratory standardization panel of the National Cholesterol Education Program has recommended that for a method of cholesterol determination to be acceptable, the number of analyses having an error of more than 8.9% compared to the standard chemical method should not exceed 5%. In a recent study of home cholesterol monitoring products, this figure was 11.9%.

It is very likely that the increased sales of home cholesterol monitors will result in more visits to physicians, more tests, and more anxiety. Whether it will result in any significant benefit to the patient population is highly debatable.

SOLUTION TO THE SHORT ANSWER MANAGEMENT PROBLEM

The risk factors for coronary artery disease in the population are as follows:
a. Family history of coronary artery disease
b. Male sex
c. Hypertension
d. Hypercholesterolemia: high LDL levels
e. Hypercholesterolemia: low HDL levels
f. Hypertriglyceridemia: high VLDL levels
g. Cigarette smoking
h. High alcohol intake (via its effect on hypertension)
i. Lack of aerobic exercise
j. Obesity
k. Diabetes mellitus: IDDM
l. Diabetes mellitus: NIDDM
m. Postmenopausal women not taking estrogen or experiencing premature menopause
n. Hyperhomocystinemia

SUMMARY OF THE DIAGNOSIS AND MANAGEMENT OF HYPERLIPOPROTEINEMIA

1. Screening: The U.S. Preventive Services Task Force recommendation is as follows: "Periodic measurement of total serum cholesterol is most important for middle aged men, and it may also be clinically

prudent in young men, women, and the elderly. All patients should receive periodic counseling regarding dietary intake of fat (especially saturated fat) and cholesterol."

2. Normal and high cholesterol values:
   a. TC:
      Normal: 5.2 mmol/L (200 mg/dl)
      Borderline: 5.2 to 6.2 mmol/L (200 to 240 mg/dl)
      Elevated: 6.2 mmol/L (240 mg/dl)
   b. LDL cholesterol:
      Ideal: 3.4 mmol/L (130 mg/dl)
      Borderline: 3.4 to 4.1 mmol/L (130 to 159 mg/dl)
      Elevated: 4.1 mmol/L (159 mg/dl)
   c. VLDL cholesterol (triglycerides):
      Ideal: 1.4 mmol/L (125 mg/dl)
      Borderline: 1.4 to 2.8 mmol/L (125 to 250 mg/dl)
      Elevated: 2.8 mmol/L (250 mg/dl)

3. Treatment of hypercholesterolemia: Treat hypercholesterolemia if LDL cholesterol is greater than 4.1 mmol/L or 3.4 mmol/L with two or more risk factors.
   a. Dietary management is the treatment of first choice. Begin with the American Heart Association's Step 1 diet:
      1) No more than 300 mg cholesterol
      2) No more than 30% total fat
      3) No more than 10% saturated fat
   b. Continue for at least 6 months. If cholesterol levels do not normalize, consider American Heart Association's Step 2 diet:
      1) No more than 200 mg cholesterol
      2) No more than 30% total fat
      3) No more than 7% saturated fat
   c. Drug treatments for hypercholesterolemia:
      1) Drugs of first choice: HMG CoA reductase inhibitors. The Scandinavian Simvastatin Survival Study has shown that cholesterol-lowering drugs reduce deaths from coronary artery disease and sudden cardiac death. In this study the HMG CoA reductase inhibitor simvastatin substantially improved survival, reducing the overall risk of death by 30% and the risk of coronary death by 42%. This adds even more credibility to the recommendation that HMG CoA reductase inhibitors be considered the drugs of first choice for the treatment of hyperlipidemia.
      2) Drug of second choice: niacin
      3) Drug of third choice: bile acid sequestrants

4. Hypertriglyceridemia: Hypertriglyceridemia has been established as an independent risk factor for coronary artery disease. Always look for a second-

ary cause of hypertriglyceridemia, such as diabetes mellitus, alcohol, or oral contraceptives.

Treatments for hypertriglyceridemia include the American Heart Association's Step 1 and Step 2 diets mentioned previously, and the drug of choice for drug treatment of hyperlipoproteinemia that is mainly elevated triglyceride levels is gemfibrozil.

SUGGESTED READINGS

Gaziano JM et al: Cholesterol reduction: weighing the benefits and risks, *Ann Intern Med* 124:914, 1996.

Lees R, Lees A: Hyperlipoproteinemia. In Rakel R, ed: *Conn's current therapy,* Philadelphia, 1994, WB Saunders.

National Heart, Lung and Blood Institute: *National Cholesterol Education Program,* 1999, http://www.NHLBI.NIH.gov.

US Preventive Services Task Force: *Guide to clinical preventive services: an assessment of the effectiveness of 169 interventions,* Baltimore, 1989, Williams & Wilkins.

PROBLEM·4

CONGESTIVE HEART FAILURE

"I Get So Scared. Sometimes in the Middle of the Night I Can't Catch My Breath."

Case 1 ■ A 78-Year-Old Male with Shortness of Breath

A 78-year-old male comes to your office with a 6-month history of shortness of breath that is aggravated by exertion. He has found that he has to get up at night and open the window to get air. There has not been any significant weight gain, nor has there been any swelling of his ankles and legs.

His history reveals a myocardial infarction 8 years ago. Although the shortness of breath has been a significant problem for only 6 months, he does mention having "some problems" for at least 4 years.

On physical examination, the patient's blood pressure is 140/90 mm Hg. Both S_1 and S_2 are normal; there are no extra sounds and no murmurs. The jugulovenous pressure (JVP) does not appear to be elevated. Evaluation of the hepatojugular reflex is negative. Examination of the respiratory system reveals rales in both lung bases. The respiratory rate is 28 breaths/min.

SELECT THE BEST ANSWER
TO THE FOLLOWING QUESTIONS

Q1. Based on the history and physical examination, what is the most likely diagnosis?
   a. left ventricular heart failure
   b. right ventricular heart failure

c. biventricular heart failure

d. cor pulmonale

e. bronchial asthma

Q2. The patient just described is treated with bed rest and the appropriate medication. He returns 1 month later complaining of dyspnea and fatigue as before, but now significant dependent edema has developed. At this time, the JVP has risen to 8 cm above the sternal angle. The hepatojugular reflex is now positive, and there is 3+ pitting edema. He has gained 10 pounds. At this time, what is the most likely diagnosis?

a. left ventricular failure

b. right ventricular failure

c. biventricular heart failure

d. cor pulmonale

e. bronchial asthma

Q3. The nonpharmacologic treatment(s) of choice for this condition may include which of the following?

a. salt restriction

b. fat restriction

c. water restriction

d. all of the above

e. none of the above

Q4. Which of the following is (are) the current indication(s) for the use of digitalis in this condition?

a. a dilated left ventricle

b. an S_3 or S_4 gallop

c. decreased ejection fraction

d. atrial fibrillation with a rapid ventricular rate

e. c and d

f. all of the above

Q5. Physiologically speaking, the condition just described (as illustrated by the second presentation of this patient) has which of the following characteristics?

a. elevated preload

b. elevated afterload

c. reduced preload

d. reduced afterload

e. a and b

f. c and d

Q6. In evaluating a patient for systolic dysfunction, the most important characteristic found on echocardiogram is:

a. myocardial hypertrophy

b. valvular heart disease

c. cor pulmonale

d. low ejection fraction

e. wall motion abnormalities

Q7. Which is the drug of first choice for the management of systolic dysfunction?

a. a thiazide diuretic

b. a loop diuretic

c. a vasodilator

d. a β-blocker

e. an angiotensin-converting enzyme (ACE) inhibitor

Q8. Which is the drug of first choice for moderate to severe cases of diastolic dysfunction?

a. a thiazide diuretic

b. a loop diuretic

c. a vasodilator

d. a β-blocker

e. an ACE inhibitor

Q9. True statements concerning the use of β-blockers in the treatment of diastolic dysfunction include which of the following?

a. β-blockers result in an improved ejection fraction and fewer hospitalizations

b. β-blockers protect the myocardium from adrenergic stimulation

c. all β-blockers are shown to decrease overall mortality

d. all are true

e. only a and b are true

Q10. What is the single most important treatment for increasing both the quality and the quantity of remaining life for patients with severe systolic dysfunction?

a. a β-blocker

b. a loop diuretic

c. an ACE inhibitor

d. a calcium channel blocker

e. any of the above

Q11. Which of the following drugs decrease(s) mortality in the treatment of systolic dysfunction?

a. ACE inhibitors

b. hydralazine and nitrates combined

c. carvedilol (Coreg)

d. diuretics

e. a, b, and c

f. all of the above

SHORT ANSWER MANAGEMENT PROBLEM
A major error in treating heart failure is assuming that all patients who appear to be in heart failure need furosemide. When given furosemide, some patients actually get worse. Provide an example of a practical situation in which this could occur.

ANSWERS

A1. **a.** This patient has left ventricular failure. Dyspnea is the most common sign of left-sided congestive heart failure. Initially, the dyspnea is present only with moderate amounts of exertion, but as the severity of the heart failure increases, the shortness of breath may occur with only minimal exertion or even at rest. Other common symptoms are fatigue and lethargy.

In a patient with left-sided cardiac failure, lying flat is often followed by increasing shortness of breath. Paroxysms of nocturnal dyspnea suggest severe left-sided failure. On careful questioning the patient describes the bouts as marked breathlessness or a "suffocating feeling," and these symptoms are often accompanied by significant anxiety. The patient must sit upright or even stand up to breathe and may have the urge to rush to an open window to relieve the "suffocating feeling." Extra pillows are needed to reduce the number and severity of attacks. Some patients even resort to sleeping upright in a chair at all times.

In severe left-sided congestive heart failure, pulmonary edema occurs and is usually severe and is accompanied by cough, frothy sputum, blood-tinged secretions, and wheezing (the so-called condition of cardiac asthma).

In this patient the absence of (a) peripheral edema, (b) hepatic congestion/absent hepatojugular reflex, and (c) elevated JVP indicates that right-sided heart failure has not yet developed.

A2. **c.** At this time the patient has developed signs of right ventricular failure secondary to left ventricular failure, hence the diagnosis is biventricular failure.

Whereas left ventricular cardiac failure is manifested by symptoms, right ventricular cardiac failure is manifested by signs. As in this patient, enlargement of the liver, a positive hepatojugular reflex, and an elevated JVP occur.

In severe cases of elevated right-sided atrial pressure, splanchnic engorgement may accompany anorexia, nausea, vomiting, ascites, and eventually cachexia.

A3. **d.** Nonpharmacologic therapy for congestive heart failure involves the following in order of importance:
a. Bed rest
b. Salt restriction (2 to 3 g/day)

c. Fluid restriction (related to sodium restriction)
d. Fat restriction (as a reasonable approach to a healthy lifestyle—American Heart Association Step 1 diet: 300 mg cholesterol; 30% total calories from fat; 10% of calories from saturated fat)

A4. **e.** Digoxin has come full circle. This drug, isolated from the foxglove plant, used to be the mainstay of treatment for congestive heart failure. For various reasons, it fell into disfavor to the point where it was virtually never used. The completion of the circle has resulted in digoxin once again being used extensively for specific purposes. Its primary indications are in cases with a reduced ejection fraction and in atrial fibrillation with a rapid ventricular rate. Physicians should be aware of drug interactions that may increase digoxin levels. These include the use of digoxin with verapamil, quinidine, procainamide, nifedipine, or amiodarone, as well as electrolyte abnormalities (hypokalemia and hypomagnesemia) induced by diuretics, and overdosing in the elderly, who may have decreased renal clearance.

A5. **e.** Biventricular congestive cardiac failure is manifested by two components: preload (or venous return) and afterload (vasoconstriction). The afterload is associated with elevated left ventricular end-diastolic volume (left-sided failure); the preload is associated with elevated venous volume (right-sided failure).

A6. **d.** In defining systolic dysfunction the most important characteristic is a low ejection fraction. In diastolic dysfunction the primary characteristic on echocardiogram is a "stiff ventricle," with a normal or elevated ejection fraction.

A7. **e.** For systolic dysfunction, ACE inhibitors are considered the drug of choice. Additional medications include diuretics, digoxin, nitrates, and carvedilol (Coreg)—a medication with nonselective β-blocking and α_1-activity.

A8. **d.** The important goal in treating diastolic dysfunction is to slow the heart rate to allow the stiff ventricles found in diastolic dysfunction enough time for ventricular filling. This is accomplished with β-blockers such as propranolol, metoprolol, timolol, or atenolol. Secondary medications include calcium channel blockers (diltiazem or verapamil).

A9. **e.**

A10. **c.** ACE inhibitor drugs such as captopril, enalapril, or lisinopril have been shown to reduce both morbidity and mortality in patients with severe systolic heart failure.

A11. **e.** Through various studies, ACE inhibitors, the combination of hydralazine and nitrates, and carvedilol have been shown to decrease mortality when treating systolic dysfunction. Diuretics, nitrates (when used alone), digoxin, and β-blockers may improve symptoms and decrease morbidity, but they do not decrease mortality.

SOLUTION TO THE SHORT ANSWER MANAGEMENT PROBLEM

A practical example of a patient becoming worse after being given furosemide is the following:

A 55-year-old uremic male with a history of congestive heart failure manifests an increasing shortness of breath and increasing edema of the extremities. You naturally assume that his condition is worsening, and you administer furosemide. His condition deteriorates rapidly. The cause? Uremic pericarditis. What appeared to be congestive heart failure was not; uremic pericarditis can cause a failure-like syndrome.

Make sure the patient has congestive heart failure before you treat the failure!

SUMMARY OF THE DIAGNOSIS AND TREATMENT OF CONGESTIVE HEART FAILURE

1. Left-sided failure produces mainly symptoms such as increasing shortness of breath (dyspnea), shortness of breath on assuming the recumbent position (orthopnea), and having to wake up at night to catch one's breath (paroxysmal nocturnal dyspnea).

2. Right-sided failure produces mainly signs such as increasing dependent edema and increased JVP and a positive hepatojugular reflex.

3. Biventricular failure: The most common cause of right-sided heart failure is left-sided heart failure.

4. Pathophysiology of heart failure: This is explained best by the Frank-Starling curve: left ventricular end-diastolic volume versus cardiac work. Compensation via the sympathetic nervous system allows normal cardiac output to be maintained to a certain point; following that, decompensation begins.

5. Treatment:
   a. Nonpharmacologic:
      1) Correct reversible causes
      2) Bed rest
      3) Sodium restriction
      4) Water restriction
      5) Avoidance of other risk factors: stop smoking, avoid excessive alcohol intake, avoid high-fat diet
      6) Increased aerobic exercise
   b. Pharmacologic:
      1) Use loop diuretics (furosemide) to decrease preload.
      2) Add other classes of diuretics to increase effectiveness of the loop diuretics if needed.
      3) ACE inhibitors such as captopril, enalapril, or lisinopril decrease both preload and afterload and are the drugs of first choice in moderate to severe heart failure.
      4) Digoxin can be combined with the drugs just listed to improve the contractility (positive inotropic effect).

SUGGESTED READINGS
Heart Failure Guideline Panel: Heart failure: management of patients with left ventricular systolic dysfunction, *Am Fam Physician* 50:603-615, 1994.

Tierney LM, McPhee SJ, Papadakis MA, eds: *Current medical diagnosis and treatment, 2000,* ed 39, Stamford, Conn, 1999, Appleton & Lange.

The US Carvedilol Heart Failure Study Group: The effect of carvedilol on morbidity in patients with chronic heart failure, *N Engl J Med* 334:1349-1355, 1996.

PROBLEM·5

HYPERTENSION

"I Feel Fine, but Those Pills Were Distressing Me, So I Stopped Taking Them."

Case 1 ■ An Obese 47-Year-Old Male with Hypertension

A 47-year-old male comes to your office for a yearly checkup. He is 5'10," weighs 250 pounds, smokes two packs of cigarettes per day, and "slams down" 12 ounces of whiskey each day.

On physical examination you detect a number of extra systoles each minute. His blood pressure is 180/105 mm Hg. His point of maximum impulse (PMI) is detected in the sixth intercostal space in the anterior axillary line. His funduscopic examination is normal.

SELECT THE BEST ANSWER TO THE FOLLOWING QUESTIONS

Q1. Which of the following statements about this patient's blood pressure is false?
   a. a single blood pressure reading of diastolic 105 is satisfactory for a diagnosis of hypertension

b. this patient's alcohol intake may be a significant contributing factor to his elevated blood pressure
c. the patient should have his blood pressure rechecked after a period of rest in the office
d. the patient should return for reassessment of his blood pressure in 1 week
e. the patient's cigarette smoking may be a significant contributing factor to his elevated blood pressure

Q2. A single diastolic reading of what level is considered to be diagnostic of hypertension?
a. 90 mm Hg
b. 95 mm Hg
c. 100 mm Hg
d. 105 mm Hg
e. 110 mm Hg

Q3. The minimum goal in hypertension therapy is to reduce his blood pressure to a level below which of the following?
a. 150/90 mm Hg
b. 140/90 mm Hg
c. 130/90 mm Hg
d. 120/80 mm Hg
e. 110/70 mm Hg

Q4. Assuming secondary causes of hypertension are ruled out, what is the treatment of choice in the patient described (presuming his other blood pressure readings are similar to the one today)?
a. hydrochlorothiazide (a thiazide diuretic)
b. a β-blocker
c. a calcium channel blocker
d. an angiotensin converting enzyme (ACE) inhibitor
e. none of the above

Q5. What is the first-line pharmacologic therapy now recommended for most patients with hypertension?
a. a β-blocker
b. a thiazide diuretic
c. a calcium channel blocker
d. an ACE inhibitor
e. any of the above

Q6. What is the starting dosage of a thiazide diuretic in a patient with hypertension?
a. 25 mg
b. 50 mg
c. 75 mg
d. 100 mg
e. 125 mg

Q7. The *Sixth Report of the Joint National Committee on Detection, Evaluation, and Treatment of High Blood Pressure (JNC VI)* would recommend *against* which of the following as a drug of first choice?
a. atenolol
b. enalapril
c. nifedipine
d. prazosin
e. clonidine

Q8. The initial diagnostic work-up of a patient with hypertension should include which of the following?
a. electrolytes
b. blood urea nitrogen (BUN)
c. creatinine
d. 24-hour urine for vanillylmandelic acid (VMA) and metanephrine
e. a, b, and c
f. all of the above

Q9. Based on the patient's history and physical examination, which of the following statements concerning hypertensive complications is true?
a. the patient is unlikely to have any hypertensive complications
b. this patient likely has hypertensive retinopathy
c. this patient likely has cardiac hypertrophy
d. this patient likely has hypertensive renal failure
e. none of the above is true

Q10. Which of the following statements accurately applies to mild hypertension?
a. the term is no longer considered appropriate in defining hypertension
b. mild hypertension describes a systolic level of 140 to 159 mm Hg
c. mild hypertension describes a diastolic level of 90 to 104 mm Hg
d. b and c
e. none of the above

Q11. Which of the following drugs is (are) useful for the treatment of hypertensive emergencies and urgencies?
a. intravenous labetalol
b. oral clonidine
c. oral or sublingual nifedipine
d. all of the above
e. none of the above

Q12. A 50-year-old male is being treated for hypertension with a low-salt diet, hydrochlorothiazide 25 mg/day, and propranolol 120 mg bid. His blood

pressure at present is 180/100 mm Hg. Which of the following would be a reasonable third-line agent for the treatment of this patient's blood pressure?
a. atenolol
b. metoprolol
c. labetalol
d. furosemide
e. enalapril

Q13. What is the most common side effect of ACE inhibitors?
a. cough
b. constipation
c. headache
d. skin rash
e. depression

Q14. What is the most common side effect of propranolol?
a. cough
b. constipation
c. headache
d. skin rash
e. depression

Q15. Based on the history and physical examination of the patient described in Case 1, which of the following additional investigations should be undertaken?
a. digital subtraction angiography
b. intravenous pyelogram (IVP)
c. echocardiogram
d. retinal ultrasound
e. renal ultrasound

SHORT ANSWER MANAGEMENT PROBLEM

Specify the recommended and contraindicated antihypertensive drugs for the following patients:
Patient 1: A young patient with hyperdynamic circulation
Patient 2: An elderly patient with no particular chronic diseases other than hypertension
Patient 3: An African-American patient
Patient 4: A patient with gout
Patient 5: A patient with ischemic heart disease
Patient 6: A patient with asthma
Patient 7: A patient with peripheral vascular disease
Patient 8: A patient with non-insulin-dependent diabetes
Patient 9: A patient with insulin-dependent diabetes
Patient 10: A patient with hypercholesterolemia
Patient 11: A patient with congestive heart failure
Patient 12: A patient who is pregnant

ANSWERS

A1. **a.** Hypertension should not be diagnosed until a sustained, repetitive elevation of blood pressure has been documented. For diagnosis, at least three readings that average greater than 140 mm Hg systolic or 90 mm Hg diastolic must be documented, preferably by the same observer using the same technique.

A2. **e.** If a single diastolic blood pressure reading of 110 mm Hg is documented, the probability that the blood pressure will return to normal is slight enough that the diagnosis of hypertension usually can be made. If end organ damage consistent with hypertension is detected, these criteria may not apply. In this patient, although his PMI is displaced, we cannot necessarily assume that this is the result of hypertension.

Alcohol abuse is a significant cause of hypertension. Any patient with hypertension should be questioned regarding alcohol intake. Although a low dose of alcohol has been shown to be cardioprotective, the term *low* must be carefully defined. An absolute maximum of two drinks per day may be cardioprotective; any more than that may be harmful and an additional risk factor for coronary artery disease.

The patient described in this case should have his blood pressure taken again after 5 minutes of controlled rest. If his arm circumference is greater than 33 cm, obtain his blood pressure reading with the obese blood pressure cuff. Also instruct this patient to abstain from caffeine and cigarette smoking for at least 2 hours before his pressure is checked on his next visit.

A patient whose blood pressure returns to normal after a period of rest is known as a *labile hypertensive*. About 50% of labile hypertensives eventually develop sustained hypertension.

It has been well established that home blood pressure readings (if done correctly and taken with a blood pressure recording device that has been calibrated against a mercury manometer) are more accurate and a more significant predictor of cardiovascular morbidity and mortality than office blood pressure readings.

The patient should not be given antihypertensive medication at this time. First, the diagnosis must be established. Second, before considering antihypertensive medication you must consider nonpharmacologic therapy and attempt to lower his blood pressure without drugs.

A3. **b.** The minimum goal in antihypertensive therapy is to reduce the blood pressure to a level of 140 mm Hg systolic and 90 mm Hg diastolic.

A4. **e.** The first step in treating this patient's blood pressure is to use nondrug, or nonpharmacologic, therapy. There is no doubt that nonpharmacologic therapy has a major role to play in the management of hypertension. In this patient the following are the non-pharmacologic therapies that have been shown to make a difference:

a. Weight reduction
b. Alcohol elimination (in a person such as this, who "slams down" 12 ounces of whiskey per day, your best bet would be to attempt to eliminate the "slamming" completely)
c. Cigarette smoking cessation
d. Aerobic exercise (4 hrs/week or 1200 kcal); in this patient, after an exercise tolerance test
e. Salt reduction
f. Fat reduction, following the American Heart Association's Step 1 diet (decreasing the fat content of the diet without changing the total caloric intake will automatically begin the weight reduction process) or National Heart Lung and Blood Institute DASH diet (a combination diet rich in fruits, vegetables, and low-fat dairy foods and low in saturated and total fat) that has been shown to lower blood pressure.

You need to decide which of these therapies you are going to begin with; obviously attempting to alter everything at once will not work. An alcohol rehabilitation program or a smoking cessation program would be an excellent first choice.

A5. **e.** The *Sixth Report of the Joint National Committee on Detection, Evaluation, and Treatment of High Blood Pressure (JNC VI)* recommends an individualized approach to the initial drug choice for patients with hypertension. For patients with uncomplicated hypertension, diuretics and β-blockers are still recommended. These are the only drugs shown to reduce both morbidity and mortality. However, in a departure from *JNC V*, the *JNC VI* also recommends the use of other agents as initial drug choices where there are compelling indications. For instance, in diabetes mellitus type 1 with proteinuria, an ACE inhibitor is recommended. In heart failure, ACE inhibitors and diuretics are recommended. In isolated systolic hypertension of older individuals, diuretics are preferred and long-acting dihydropyridine calcium antagonists are also acceptable. In myocardial infarction, β-blockers and ACE inhibitors are recommended.

A6. **a.** The starting dose of a thiazide diuretic (such as hydrochlorothiazide) is 25 mg. A low dose (25 mg) has been shown in many studies to be just as efficacious as a higher dose (50, 75, or 100 mg). The only difference between the low dose and the high dose is the greatly increased incidence of side effects with the high doses. Thiazide diuretics may produce any of six metabolic side effects: hyperglycemia, hyperuricemia, hyperlipidemia, hypomagnesemia, hyponatremia, and hypokalemia.

A7. **e.** Some antihypertensive agents such as direct-acting smooth muscle vessel dilators (e.g., hydralazine), central α_2-agonists, (e.g., clonidine), and peripheral adrenergic antagonists (e.g., guanethidine) are not well suited for initial monotherapy because they provide a variety of annoying adverse side effects.

A8. **e.** The basic (and cost-effective) hypertensive work-up includes:

a. Complete urinalysis
b. Hemoglobin and hematocrit
c. BUN and creatinine levels
d. Serum calcium levels
e. Random cholesterol levels
f. Plasma glucose levels
g. Plasma uric acid
h. Chest x-ray film
i. Electrocardiogram (ECG)

Other tests, including renal ultrasound, IVP, and 24-hour urine for VMA and metanephrine, are indicated only under special circumstances. For example, a patient who is 55 years old and develops hypertension for the first time should be suspected of having a secondary cause. (As a general rule, if essential hypertension is going to develop, it will develop before age 50 years.) In a patient age 50 years the most common secondary cause of hypertension is renal artery stenosis. This would call for investigation with abdominal/renal ultrasound and possibly further with IVP and digital subtraction angiography.

Other secondary causes include pheochromocytoma (hypertension, sweating, and palpitations) and hyperthyroidism (hypertension, sweating, and palpitations).

A9. **c.** This patient probably has cardiac hypertrophy. This is suspected from the physical examination of the heart, when the PMI is found in the sixth intercostal space–anterior axillary line. The normal apical impulse is located at or medial to the midclavicular line in the fourth or fifth intercostal space.

A10. **a.** The term *mild hypertension* is no longer considered appropriate in defining hypertension because it may give some a false sense of security ("I've been told I have hypertension, but I've also been told it is mild; therefore I really don't have to worry about it"). See the table below for the newer Joint National Committee on Detection, Evaluation and Treatment of High Blood Pressure classification.

A11. **d.** A hypertensive emergency is a clinical situation in which blood pressure must be lowered within 1 hour to prevent or limit target organ damage. Examples of hypertensive emergencies are malignant hy-

■ Classification of Blood Pressure for Adults

Classification	Systolic (mm Hg)	Diastolic (mm Hg)
Optimal	≤120	≤80
Normal	<130	<85
High normal	130-139	85-89
Hypertension		
Stage 1 (mild)	140-159	90-99
Stage 2 (moderate)	160-179	100-109
Stage 3 (severe)	>179	>109
Isolated systolic hypertension	≥140	<90

pertension, acute myocardial ischemic syndromes, acute pulmonary edema, acute renal insufficiency, acute intracranial events, postoperative bleeding, eclampsia, and pheochromocytoma. A hypertensive urgency is a clinical situation in which blood pressure should be lowered within a few hours. Examples of hypertensive urgencies are accelerated hypertension, marked hypertension associated with congestive cardiac failure, stable angina pectoris, transient cerebral ischemic attacks, and perioperative hypertension.

Hypertensive emergency/urgency drug selection must be made on a pathophysiologic basis. A summary of current recommendations is as follows:
a. Central nervous system disorder:
1) Drug of choice: Sodium nitroprusside
2) Alternatives: Trimethaphan camsylate, labetalol
b. Intracranial hemorrhage:
1) Drug of choice: Sodium nitroprusside
2) Alternatives: Trimethaphan camsylate, labetalol
c. Acute left ventricular failure:
1) Drug of choice: Enalaprilat
2) Alternative: Trimethaphan camsylate
3) Contraindicated: Labetalol
d. Acute coronary ischemia:
1) Drug of choice: Nitroglycerin
2) Alternatives: Labetalol, sodium nitroprusside
e. Unstable angina:
1) Drug of choice: Nitroglycerin
2) Alternative: Labetalol
f. Aortic dissection:
1) Drug of choice: Esmolol hydrochloride
2) Alternatives: Sodium nitroprusside, propranolol
3) Contraindicated: Hydralazine
g. Eclampsia:
1) Drug of choice: Magnesium sulfate ($MgSO_4$)
2) Alternative: Hydralazine
h. Pheochromocytoma:
1) Drug of choice: Phentolamine
2) Contraindicated: β-Adrenoreceptor blockers

i. Stage 3 or 4 hypertension with imminent or mild target organ damage:
1) Drug of choice: Nicardipine hydrochloride
2) Alternatives: Captopril, clonidine, labetalol

A12. e. This patient is currently taking a thiazide diuretic and a β-blocker. Therefore the most reasonable alternative as a third-line agent would be either an ACE inhibitor or a calcium channel blocker.

Atenolol and metoprolol are also β-blockers and thus would not be reasonable choices.

Labetalol is a combination α-β–blocker and thus would also be a poor choice.

Furosemide is a loop diuretic and would not be a reasonable choice for the management of this patient's hypertension.

Enalapril is an ACE inhibitor and would be an excellent choice for a third-line agent.

A13. a. The most common side effect of ACE inhibitors is cough. The mechanism of the cough appears to be bradykinin induced. It does not appear to be truly allergic in nature. Approximately 15% of patients taking long-term ACE inhibitors develop a chronic cough. Angiotensin II receptor antagonists do not have this side effect.

A14. e. The most common side effect of propranolol is depression. Propranolol is certainly one of the most common depression-causing drugs, if not the most common one.

A15. c. The patient's PMI is in the sixth intercostal space in the anterior axillary line. This suggests left ventricular hypertrophy secondary to hypertension (and perhaps also resulting from the obesity). An echocardiogram is indicated to evaluate the thickness of the left ventricle.

SOLUTION TO THE SHORT ANSWER MANAGEMENT PROBLEM

Patient 1: A young patient with hyperdynamic circulation
Recommended drugs: β-Blockers
Contraindicated drugs: None
Patient 2: An elderly patient with no particular chronic diseases other than hypertension. Such a person is liable to suffer from isolated systolic hypertension due to increased vascular stiffness (decreased compliance).
Recommended drugs:
First-line agents: Diuretics, with reduced drug dose

Second-line agents: ACE inhibitors, long-acting calcium channel blockers
Contraindicated drugs: None

Patient 3: An African-American patient
Recommended drugs: Thiazide diuretics are preferred initial therapy; calcium channel antagonists also effective
Contraindicated drugs: None, but in the absence of concomitant thiazide therapy the effect of ACE inhibitors or β-blockers is blunted

Patient 4: A patient with gout
Recommended drugs: Any drug but diuretics
Contraindicated drugs: Diuretics

Patient 5: A patient with ischemic heart disease
Recommended drugs: β-Blockers, calcium channel blockers
Contraindicated drugs: None

Patient 6: A patient with asthma
Recommended drugs: Calcium channel blockers
Contraindicated drugs: β-Blockers

Patient 7: A patient with peripheral vascular disease
Recommended drugs: Calcium channel blockers or other vasodilators
Contraindicated drugs: β-Blockers

Patient 8: A patient with non-insulin-dependent diabetes
Recommended drugs: ACE inhibitors
Contraindicated drugs: None, although diuretics may raise blood sugar levels

Patient 9: A patient with insulin-dependent diabetes
Recommended drugs: ACE inhibitors
Contraindicated drugs: β-Blockers

Patient 10: A patient with hypercholesterolemia
Recommended drugs: ACE inhibitors, calcium channel blockers, α-blockers, β-blockers with intracarotid sodium amytal (ISA)
Contraindicated drugs: High-dose β-blockers without ISA, high-dose diuretics

Patient 11: A patient with congestive heart failure
Recommended drugs: ACE inhibitors, diuretics
Contraindicated drugs: None, although β-blockers should be used with caution

Patient 12: A patient who is pregnant
Recommended drugs: α-Methyldopa, hydralazine
Contraindicated drugs: Diuretics, ACE inhibitors

SUMMARY OF THE DETECTION, EVALUATION, AND TREATMENT OF PATIENTS WITH HIGH BLOOD PRESSURE

1. Diagnosis: Blood pressure measurement: Three readings, separated by a time of at least 1 week where (a) after 5 minutes of controlled rest and (b) after not consuming caffeine or smoking during the last hour, the average systolic pressure is at least 140 mm Hg and/or the average diastolic pressure is at least 90 mm Hg. A single diastolic reading of 110 mm Hg is probably sufficient for the diagnosis of hypertension.

2. Evaluation: History, physical examination, and laboratory evaluation should include the evaluation of other risk factors, including family history of hypertension and other cardiovascular disease, presence of diabetes mellitus, obesity, alcohol intake, hyperlipidemia, smoking, exercise pattern, and stress.
   a. Look for evidence of end-organ damage: Cardiac hypertrophy (may need echocardiogram); use funduscope; check renal function.
   b. Laboratory evaluation should include complete blood count, urinalysis, electrolytes, BUN, creatinine, calcium, cholesterol, glucose, uric acid, and ECG.

3. Classification: Staging system outlined in Answer 2. Stages have replaced mild, moderate, and severe hypertension.

4. Treatment:
   a. Nonpharmacologic:
      1) Weight reduction
      2) Increased aerobic exercise
      3) Restriction of sodium
      4) Restriction of saturated fat (DASH diet)
      5) Discontinuation of smoking
      6) Decreased stress
   b. Pharmacologic: The *JNC VI* reverses therapy recommendations found in the previous report (*JNC V*). Optimal formulation should be effective for 24 hours, requiring only a once-daily dose, if at all possible. Long-acting formulations are preferred over short-acting agents because adherence to therapy is better, control is consistent and persistent, cost may be lower, and night-time protection from sudden rises in blood pressure is present. Combinations of low doses of two agents from different classes may minimize dose-dependent adverse effects and should be considered.

SUGGESTED READINGS

Hall WD: A rational approach for the treatment of hypertension in special populations, *Am Fam Physician* 60:156-162, 1999.

National Heart, Lung and Blood Institutes of Health: *High Blood Pressure Information for Health Professionals*, 1999, http://www.NHLBI.NIH.gov.

Sixth Report of the Joint National Committee on Detection, Evaluation, and Treatment of High Blood Pressure (JNC VI), NIH Publication #98-4080, November, 1997, US Government Printing Office.

The World Health Association and International Society of Hypertension: Clinical update, 1999 guidelines for hypertension, *Clin Rev* 9(6):123-126, 1999.

PROBLEM · 6

DYSRHYTHMIA

"Sometimes My Heart Forgets a Beat or Two."

Case 1 ■ A 37-Year-Old Male with "Skipping Heart Beats"

A 37-year-old male comes to your office for assessment of "skipping heart beats." These skipped beats have been a concern for the past 8 months. The patient reports no other symptoms accompanying these skipped beats. Specifically, he reports no increased sweating, no palpitations, no weight loss, no chest pain, no pleuritic pain, and no anxiety.

On physical examination, his blood pressure is 100/70 mm Hg. On auscultation of his heart you observe that S_1 and S_2 are normal—there are no extra sounds or murmurs. You hear about 5 premature beats per minute.

SELECT THE BEST ANSWER TO THE FOLLOWING QUESTIONS

Q1. What is the most commonly encountered "premature contraction?"
- a. a ventricular premature beat
- b. an atrial premature beat
- c. atrial flutter
- d. atrial fibrillation
- e. none of the above

Q2. Most atrial premature beats discovered on clinical examination are:
- a. associated with chronic obstructive pulmonary disease (COPD)
- b. completely benign
- c. associated with valvular heart disease
- d. associated with an increase in cardiovascular mortality
- e. none of the above

Q3. Most ventricular premature beats discovered on clinical examination are:
- a. associated with COPD
- b. completely benign
- c. associated with valvular heart disease
- d. associated with an increase in cardiovascular mortality
- e. none of the above

Case 2 ■ A 51-Year-Old Male with Acute Chest Pain

A 51-year-old male comes to the Emergency Department with an acute episode of chest pain. He has a history of atrial fibrillation. On examination, his blood pressure is 80/60 mm Hg and his ventricular rate is approximately 160 bpm. He is in acute distress. His respiratory rate is 32 breaths/min. His electrocardiogram (ECG) shows atrial fibrillation with a rapid ventricular response.

Q4. What should your first step in management be?
- a. digitalize the patient
- b. give the patient intravenous (IV) verapamil
- c. give the patient IV procainamide
- d. cardiovert the patient with a direct current (DC)
- e. start rapid IV hydration

Case 3 ■ A 44-Year-Old White Male with Palpitations

A 44-year-old white male comes to the Emergency Department complaining of palpitations. He denies chest pain and shortness of breath. There is no history of known heart disease or cardiac risk factors except for mild obesity. He does admit to drinking heavily the night before at an office retirement party.

On physical examination, his blood pressure is 120/80 mm Hg and his ventricular rate is again 160 bpm. His ECG confirms atrial fibrillation with a rapid ventricular response.

Q5. What should you do at this time?
- a. digitalize the patient
- b. treat the patient with IV verapamil
- c. treat the patient with IV procainamide
- d. cardiovert the patient
- e. have him perform a Valsalva maneuver by rebreathing into a paper bag

Q6. What is the recommended treatment for paroxysmal supraventricular tachycardia (PSVT) with hemodynamic compromise?
- a. synchronized cardioversion
- b. DC countershock
- c. IV adenosine
- d. IV verapamil
- e. IV digoxin

Q7. Patients with chronic atrial fibrillation are at increased risk for which of the following conditions?
- a. acute myocardial infarction (MI)
- b. ventricular tachycardia

c. sudden cardiac death
d. cerebrovascular accident
e. ventricular fibrillation

Q8. What is the drug of choice for prevention of the complication described in Question 7?
a. prophylactic streptokinase
b. prophylactic warfarin
c. prophylactic heparin
d. prophylactic lidocaine
e. no drug is recommended

Q9. Which of the following statements regarding the medical treatment of atrial premature beats with antiarrhythmic drugs is true?
a. the benefit outweighs the risk
b. the risk outweighs the benefit
c. the risk and the benefit are equal
d. the risk and benefit depend on the patient
e. nobody really knows for sure

Q10. Which of the following statements regarding the medical treatment of ventricular premature beats with antiarrhythmic drugs is true?
a. the benefit outweighs the risk
b. the risk outweighs the benefit
c. the risk and the benefit are equal
d. the risk and the benefit depend on the patient
e. nobody really knows for sure

SHORT ANSWER MANAGEMENT PROBLEM
Discuss the significance of the results of the Cardiac Arrhythmia Suppression Trial (CAST) study with respect to the treatment of ventricular extrasystole.

ANSWERS

A1. **b.** Atrial premature beats are the most common premature beats encountered in the adult population. They are almost always asymptomatic and are often discovered incidentally during a medical examination. Patients with atrial premature beats often complain of "palpitations" or "a feeling of skipped heart beats" during periods of emotional stress or during periods of quiet such as while resting in bed. Atrial premature beats may be associated with tachycardias that, particularly if nonsustained (less than 30 seconds), may not be perceived by the patient.

A2. **b.** Atrial premature beats require no treatment except reassurance of the patient. Reassurance is par-

ticularly important because the more convinced the patient is that something is seriously wrong, the more atrial premature beats he or she will sustain.

There are obviously other causes of palpitations that must be considered, such as thyrotoxicosis, panic disorder, and pheochromocytoma. However, benign premature atrial contractions are much more common than premature atrial contractions due to thyrotoxicosis, panic disorder, or pheochromocytoma.

A3. **b.** Most premature ventricular contractions (PVCs), as with premature atrial contractions (PACs), turn out to be completely benign. As with PACs, most patients simply need reassurance. Also, as with PACs, most PVCs are asymptomatic and are often discovered during a medical examination. Occasionally, PVCs (in contradistinction to PACs) may be symptoms of more serious underlying heart disease. With runs of PVCs (ventricular tachycardia), the patient may develop angina, dyspnea, dizziness, syncope, and even cardiac arrest.

If there is a serious question about the number of ventricular premature beats per minute, a 24-hour Holter monitor is an excellent way to measure. Again, however (and this will be discussed later in more detail), the risk of giving a patient a prophylactic antiarrhythmic drug for ventricular ectopy outweighs the benefit.

A4. **d.** This patient appears to be having an acute attack of atrial fibrillation with rapid ventricular response. The treatment of choice for this patient is synchronized cardioversion at 100 joules of energy. Advanced Cardiac Life Support (ACLS) protocol recommends cardioversion energies of (a) 100 joules, (b) 200 joules, (c) 300 joules, and (d) 360 joules, in that order, and in succession if the previous energy level was not successful.

A5. **b.** In this case the patient has the same condition, atrial fibrillation. However, here he is hemodynamically stable instead of hemodynamically unstable. Therefore a less dramatic intervention than cardioversion can be attempted at this time. The scenario of atrial fibrillation after alcohol ingestion ("holiday heart syndrome") is frequently recognized over holidays and weekends. Generally, the acute cardiac rhythm disturbance occurs in the background of heavy chronic alcohol consumption. Occasionally the arrhythmia may be induced acutely without chronic abuse, especially after a period of prolonged sleeplessness.

ACLS protocol would suggest that, for rate control in this situation, both β-blockers and calcium channel blockers are appropriate. The pharmacologic drug of choice at this time is IV verapamil 2.5 to 5.0 mg.

A6. **c.** A patient who has PSVT should first be treated with vagal maneuvers. The term *vagal maneuvers* is commonly used, yet few people know how many vagal maneuvers there are. Also, the character of these vagal maneuvers varies from the commonplace to the bizarre. The list includes carotid sinus pressure; breath holding; facial immersion in ice water; coughing; nasogastric tube placement; gag reflex stimulation by tongue blades, fingers, and oral ipecac; eyeball pressure; squatting; medical antishock trousers; Trendelenburg position; and a circumferential digital sweep of the anus.

The treatment of choice in this case is adenosine. The dose recommended for PSVT is 6 mg rapid IV push over 1 to 3 seconds.

A7. **d.**

A8. **b.** For some inexplicable reason, patients with chronic atrial fibrillation are often left untreated. Since these patients are at risk for embolic cerebrovascular accidents, it is recommended that they be given warfarin prophylaxis, provided there is no contraindication. All trials to date have shown that chronic warfarin therapy maintained with an international normalized ratio of 2.0 to 4.5 significantly reduces the incidence of strokes (0.5 to 2.0 strokes per year) in patients with chronic atrial fibrillation (whether persistent or intermittent). One trial has shown that the benefit of aspirin, 160 to 325 mg/day, is equivalent to warfarin when risk of stroke or major hemorrhage is considered.

A9. **b.**

A10. **b.** In patients with either PACs or PVCs it is obvious that, unless the circumstances are unusual and have been documented electrophysiologically, the risk of treatment with antiarrhythmic drugs outweighs the benefit. A number of trials have confirmed this.

SOLUTION TO THE SHORT ANSWER MANAGEMENT PROBLEM

Treatment of potentially dangerous dysrhythmias in high-risk populations, especially after MI, has not proven beneficial. The largest study, the CAST, was a multicenter study designed to determine the effects of suppression of ventricular extrasystoles in post-MI patients with decreased left ventricular function and more than six ventricular extrasystoles per hour on a 24-hour Holter recording. After demonstration of suppression of the extrasystole by dysrhythmic therapy, patients were randomly assigned to medical therapy or placebo.

"In CAST, the two most effective drugs with the fewest noncardiac side effects, flecainide and encainide, were used. The CAST study was terminated early due to an increase in mortality in the patients treated with either of these drugs."*

SUMMARY OF THE DIAGNOSIS AND TREATMENT OF PREMATURE BEATS AND CERTAIN SUPRAVENTRICULAR RHYTHMS

1. Atrial premature beats: These are benign and extremely common; reassurance is the only treatment recommended.

2. Ventricular premature beats: The vast majority are benign, they are extremely common, and reassurance is the only treatment recommended after a complete cardiovascular status is determined for the patient. According to the CAST study, with ventricular ectopy, even in patients at high risk (that is, after an MI), the risk of treating this dysrhythmia is greater than the risk of doing nothing.

3. Treatment for paroxysmal supraventricular tachycardia:
   a. Vagal maneuvers
   b. Adenosine 6 mg IV push has replaced verapamil as the treatment of choice

4. Treatment for atrial fibrillation:
   a. Hemodynamically unstable: cardiovert: 100 joules, 200 joules, 300 joules, 360 joules
   b. Hemodynamically stable: IV verapamil is the treatment of choice
   c. Prophylaxis against embolic cerebrovascular accidents should be maintained with warfarin. If warfarin is contraindicated, one aspirin per day is effective.

SUGGESTED READINGS

Emergency Cardiac Care Committee and Subcommittees, American Heart Association: Guidelines for cardiopulmonary resuscitation and emergency cardiac care, *JAMA* 268:2172-2183, 1992.

Goldberg AD: Premature beats. In Rakel R, ed: *Conn's current therapy*, Philadelphia, 1994, WB Saunders.

McAnulty J: Atrial fibrillation. In Rakel R, ed: *Conn's current therapy*, Philadelphia, 1994, WB Saunders.

---

*Goldberg AD: Premature beats. In Rakel R, ed: *Conn's current therapy*, Philadelphia, 1994, WB Saunders.

PROBLEM · 7

OBESITY

"My Doctor Has Me on a Diet. So Please Leave the Nuts and Cherry Off of My Banana Split."

Case 1 ■ A 45-Year-Old, 320-Pound Male Complaining of Fatigue

A 320-pound, 45-year-old male comes to your office complaining of fatigue. He has been obese all his life. He tells you that his obesity has nothing to do with calorie intake and everything to do with his slow metabolic rate. He has been investigated extensively at many major centers specializing in "slow metabolic rates." The result of his encounters has been a conclusion that he is simply "eating too much" (with which he disagrees). He has heard from a friend that "you are different" and he has come to you for "the truth."

On examination, his body mass index (BMI) is off the scale. Although you cannot feel his point of maximal impulse, you believe it is in the region of the anterior axillary line, sixth intercostal space. S_1 and S_2 are distant, as are his breath sounds. His abdomen is obese and covered with striae. His liver and spleen cannot be felt.

You refer him to your local dietician and promise that you will "investigate his slow metabolic rate" if he will agree to adhere to a diet. The dietician puts him on a 1800 kcal/day diet and calculates his ideal weight to be 170 pounds.

SELECT THE BEST ANSWER TO THE FOLLOWING QUESTIONS

Q1. Assuming that his total energy expenditure is 2300 kcal/day and he does, in fact, stick to his 1800 kcal/day diet, how long will it take for him to reach his ideal weight?
   a. 125 days
   b. 225 days
   c. 325 days
   d. 525 days
   e. 1050 days

Q2. How is obesity generally defined?
   a. an increase in the ponderal index of 20% above normal
   b. a decrease in the ponderal index of 30% below normal
   c. an increase in the BMI of 20% above normal
   d. a BMI of 27 kg/m² or greater
   e. none of the above

Q3. Which of the following statements is (are) true regarding obesity?
   a. obesity is associated with increased death rates from cancer
   b. obesity is associated with increased death rates from coronary artery disease
   c. obesity is associated with increased death rates from diabetes mellitus
   d. a and b are both true; c has not been proven
   e. all of the above

Q4. What is the overall prevalence of obesity in the United States?
   a. 5%
   b. 10%
   c. 20%
   d. 34%
   e. 50%

Q5. With which of the following conditions is obesity most commonly associated?
   a. alveolar hypoventilation syndrome
   b. hypertension
   c. hyperlipidemia
   d. diabetes mellitus
   e. angina pectoris

Q6. The use of severe calorie-restricted diets (800 kcal/day) has been responsible for many deaths. What is the most common cause of death in these cases?
   a. sudden cardiac death, secondary to dysrhythmia
   b. congestive cardiac failure, secondary to anemia
   c. hepatic failure
   d. renal failure
   e. septicemia

Q7. Which of the following theories has (have) been postulated to explain the physiology of obesity?
   a. fat-cell theory
   b. lipoprotein-lipase theory
   c. thermogenesis-brown adipose tissue theory
   d. all of the above
   e. none of the above

Q8. Which of the following statements is (are) true regarding the use of anorexic drugs?
   a. short-term studies demonstrate that weight loss is greater with these agents at 1 month than with placebo agents
   b. hypertension is a documented side effect of these agents

c. renal failure is a documented side effect of these agents

d. long-term studies suggest that these agents are not beneficial as part of a weight loss program

e. all of the above

Q9. Which of the following is (are) advocated as part of a weight loss program?

a. a nutritionally balanced diet

b. decreasing the percentage of calories derived from fat

c. an exercise program

d. caloric restriction to approximately 500 kcal/day less than maintenance

e. all of the above

Q10. The practical management of weight loss by the family physician should involve which of the following?

a. multiple office visits over 8 to 12 weeks

b. changes in the act of eating

c. keeping a daily food diary

d. all of the above

e. none of the above

Q11. Which one of the following statements concerning the use of echocardiography in obese patients is true?

a. echocardiography is not indicated in obese patients

b. echocardiography cannot predict future risk in obese patients

c. echocardiography is indicated in obese patients to document the size of the right ventricle; right ventricular hypertrophy is a major predicator of future risk

d. echocardiography may disclose the formation of "obese heart clots"

e. none of the above is true

SHORT ANSWER MANAGEMENT PROBLEM

The vast majority of patients with obesity have essential obesity (analogous to essential hypertension). There are, however, secondary causes. List the potential secondary causes of obesity.

ANSWERS

A1. **e.** One pound of fat is equal to 3500 kcal. Therefore, if his total energy expenditure is 2300 kcal/day and the patient is taking in only 1800 kcal/day (the recommended difference in a weight loss program between energy expenditure and energy intake is 500

kcal), his energy deficit is 500 kcal/day. His excess weight above ideal body weight is 150 pounds. These 150 pounds are equal to 525,000 kcal. The corresponding time to lose this number of calories is 1050 days (2.87 years).

A2. **d.** The National Institutes of Health defines obesity as a relative weight over 120% or BMI greater than 27 kg/m^2. Mild obesity is a relative weight excess of 120% to 140% (BMI 27 to 30 kg/m^2), moderate obesity is a relative weight excess of 140% to 200% (BMI 30 to 40 kg/m^2), and severe or morbid obesity is a relative weight excess of over 200% (BMI > 40 kg/m^2).

A3. **e.** Obesity is a major public health issue. There is a certain stigmatization to the diagnosis of obesity not present in other conditions. Some authorities suggest that we should label obesity as essential obesity in the same way that we label hypertension as essential hypertension. The comparison between hypertension and obesity does not end there. Obesity is a major risk factor for coronary artery disease and other cardiovascular conditions, including hypertension, congestive heart failure, cardiomyopathy, and angina pectoris.

Obesity is associated with an increased incidence of non-insulin-dependent diabetes mellitus, caused by an effective increase in insulin resistance. Obesity has been established indirectly as a risk factor for some cancers. For example, it appears from some studies that the high-fat diet usually associated with obesity is also associated with an increased risk of colon cancer. Other diseases that have been shown to be directly linked to obesity include the following:

a. Thromboembolic disease

b. Endometrial carcinoma

c. Restrictive lung disease

d. Pickwickian syndrome

e. Gout

f. Degenerative arthritis

g. Gallstone formation and gallbladder disease

h. Infertility

i. Hyperlipoproteinemias

j. Hernias and esophageal reflux

k. Psychosocial disabilities

l. Increased risk of obstetrical and surgical morbidity

A4. **d.** The overall prevalence of obesity in the North American population is approximately 34% (relative weight excess of 120%). In certain groups, such as the Pima Indians, the prevalence is 50%. A higher prevalence of obesity appears in those individuals in the lowest socioeconomic groups; the prevalence does, in fact, decrease as socioeconomic status increases.

A5. **b.** Of the conditions already postulated as linked with obesity, the strongest association is between obesity and hypertension. The other conditions listed previously are also linked to obesity.

A6. **a.** The most common cause of death reported among patients who are on severe calorie-restricted diets is sudden cardiac death due to ventricular arrhythmias or dysrhythmias.

A7. **d.** Some of the theories brought forward to explain essential obesity include the following:
   a. The fat-cell theory
   b. The lipoprotein-lipase theory
   c. The thermogenesis-brown fat adipose tissue theory

Studies done on monozygotic twins have established that 70% of the variance in BMI results from genetic factors, with only 30% caused by environmental factors. This puts a different light on the whole question of slow metabolizers versus fast metabolizers. This genetic information suggests that metabolism is very much a function of genetics and genetic endowment.

A8. **e.** Although short-term weight loss is enhanced by these agents, long-term studies demonstrate that most patients suffer a rebound effect and actually may end up even heavier. In addition, hypertension and renal failures have been documented in patients using anorexic drugs. These medications can be classified as catecholaminergic or serotonergic:
   a. Catecholaminergic agents include amphetamines, appetite suppressants such as phentermine, diethylpropion, and mazindol and phenylpropanolamine, which is an over-the-counter agent.
   b. The serotonergic agents fenfluramine and dexfenfluramine were withdrawn from the market in 1997, and although fluoxetine (Prozac) and sertraline are serotonergic, they are not approved for the treatment of obesity. Newer medications, including sibutramine (Meridia), and orlistat, were approved by the Food and Drug Administration in 1999.

Surgical intervention to treat obesity should be limited to those with a BMI exceeding 40. Over 100,000 patients have undergone gastroplasty, with vertical band (Mason) gastroplasty the treatment of choice.

A9. **e.** A structured program is essential for successful long-term weight loss. Most successful weight loss programs are multidisciplinary, concentrating on hypocaloric diets, behavior modification to change eating behaviors, aerobic exercise, and social support.

The weight loss program must contain three essential components: (a) a nutritionally balanced diet, (b) aerobic exercise, and (c) a reduction in the percentage of calories derived from fat. It has now been shown that reducing the percentage of calories derived from fat (compared to carbohydrates and proteins) by itself produces weight loss. Current recommendations suggest that the energy intake should be approximately 500 calories less than energy output in a weight loss program. As also noted in Answer 7, newer research strongly implicates genetic influences. Some believe that 50% to 75% of obesity may be explained by genetic causes.

A10. **d.** The practical management of weight loss in a patient by the patient's family physician should include the following:
   a. Weekly office visits over a period of 8 to 12 weeks and gradual lengthening of time between visits after that
   b. Modification of eating habits
   c. Keeping a food diary
   d. Increasing aerobic exercise activity

Home weighing is not recommended because of the significant fluctuations in body weight resulting from body water. If it is necessary for the patient to weigh himself or herself at home, it should be done no more than once every 2 weeks.

The modification of eating habits is an important and interesting component of the overall plan. First, patients must begin to regard eating as a conscious activity rather than something that happens while thinking of other things. Second, the suggestion of drinking two glasses of water just before the meal to decrease appetite has validity. Third, instructing the patient to eat more slowly and chew food more thoroughly also appears to be valid.

A11. **e.** Echocardiography is an important investigational modality in obese patients. It measures the size of the left, not the right, ventricle and is an indicator of left, not right, ventricular hypertrophy. Left ventricular hypertrophy is a major predictor of morbidity and mortality, and hypertrophy is significantly more common in obese than nonobese patients. The Centers for Disease Control and Prevention recommends an echocardiogram for any patient who took dexfenfluramine or fenfluramine and develops a new-onset murmur or cardiac symptoms.

SOLUTION TO THE SHORT ANSWER MANAGEMENT PROBLEM

The most common causes of secondary obesity include the following:

1. Iatrogenic disease: drugs that produce either
   a. weight gain as a side effect
   b. salt and water retention
2. Depression: many patients gain rather than lose weight
3. Cushing's syndrome
4. Hypothyroidism
5. Diabetes mellitus type 2; but remember that less than 1% of obese patients have an identifiable secondary cause of obesity

SUMMARY OF THE DIAGNOSIS AND MANAGEMENT OF OBESITY

1. Pathophysiology: Evidence suggests that the cause of obesity is at least 70% genetic and only 30% environmental.

2. Definition:
   a. BMI greater than 27 kg/m^2 or, alternatively,
   b. 20% above suggested ideal body weight

3. Prevalence: 34% of those in the United States, up from 25% in 1970

4. Importance:
   a. Obesity is now regarded as the most important public health problem in the United States. Unfortunately, it is often ignored because of the social stigma attached to it.
   b. Even more important is the increase in prevalence in obesity in adolescents. In 1970, 15% of adolescents in the United States were obese; in 1995, 22% of adolescents in the United States were obese (approximately a 7% increase).

5. Complications: This increase in obesity translates into increased prevalence of:
   a. Coronary heart disease
   b. Myocardial infarction
   c. Cerebrovascular disease; obese patients are 250% more likely to develop coronary artery disease than nonobese patients
   d. Left ventricular hypertrophy and congestive heart failure
   e. Hyperlipidemia
   f. Diabetes mellitus type 2 with macrovascular complications
      1) Diabetic nephropathy
      2) Diabetic retinopathy
      3) Diabetic neuropathy
      4) Autonomic neuropathy
      5) Generalized atherosclerotic vascular disease
   g. Osteoarthritis
   h. Cholelithiasis and cholecystitis
   i. Chronic renal failure (Remember, diabetes mellitus type 2 is the most common cause of chronic renal failure in the United States, occurring 10 times more frequently than type 1 diabetes.)
   j. Obstructive sleep apnea and pickwickian syndrome
   k. Restrictive lung disease
   l. Cancer (associated with a high-fat diet)
   m. Gout

6. Treatment:
   a. Avoid all diet fads and diet "revolutions." Also avoid anorexic drugs.
   b. Change the composition of the diet: increase carbohydrate, increase protein, and decrease fat.
   c. Multiple office visits are essential to establish a baseline and to motivate continual weight loss.
   d. Decrease caloric intake to approximately 500 kcal/day less than energy expenditure. This produces a weight loss of approximately 1 pound per week.
   e. Increase aerobic exercise. This is essential to long-term weight loss and maintenance.
   f. Receive positive reinforcement from a support group, the physician, family, and friends.

SUGGESTED READINGS

Garrow JS: Treatment of obesity, *Lancet* 340:409-413, 1992.
Ravussin E, Swinburn B: Pathophysiology of obesity, *Lancet* 340:404-408, 1992.
Rosenbaum M et al: Obesity, *N Engl J Med* 337:396, 1997.
Stevens J et al: The effect of age on the association between body mass index and mortality, *N Engl J Med* 338:1, 1998.
Tierney LM, McPhee SJ, Papadakis MA, eds: *Current medical diagnosis and treatment, 2000*, ed 39, Stamford, Conn, 1999, Appleton & Lange.

PROBLEM·8

PULMONARY EMBOLISM

"A Broken Leg Killed My Wife?"

Case 1 ■ A 65-Year-Old Female with Cyanosis, Shortness of Breath, and Substernal Chest Pain

A 65-year-old female is admitted to the Emergency Department with a 3-hour history of cyanosis, shortness of breath, and substernal chest pain. She had been discharged 5 days earlier after having a total hip replacement for severe osteoarthritis. The hip surgery was uneventful.

On physical examination, the patient is in obvious acute respiratory distress. Her respiratory rate is 40 breaths/min and her breathing is labored. Her blood pressure is 100/70 mm Hg. Cyanosis is present. There appear to be decreased breath sounds in the lower lobe of the right lung, as well as adventitious breath sounds in all lobes.

SELECT THE BEST ANSWER TO THE FOLLOWING QUESTIONS

Q1. Based on the information provided, what is the most likely diagnosis in this patient?
a. fat embolus
b. acute myocardial infarction
c. dissecting aortic aneurysm
d. acute pulmonary embolism
e. cholesterol emboli syndrome

Q2. Which of the following scintigraphic findings is most sensitive in diagnosing the condition just described?
a. no perfusion defects
b. two or more medium to large perfusion defects with no V/Q mismatch
c. two or more medium to large perfusion defects with V/Q mismatch
d. a single medium or large perfusion defect with V/Q mismatch
e. none of the above

Q3. On clinical examination of a patient with the precursor condition leading to the ultimate diagnosis as just described, which of the following statements is true?
a. clinical examination is diagnostic in every case
b. clinical examination is, in most cases, diagnostic
c. clinical examination is of some value but has low sensitivity and low specificity
d. clinical examination is of no value
e. nobody really knows for sure

Q4. Which of the following blood gas combinations occurs most commonly in the condition just described?
a. decreased Po_2 and decreased Pco_2
b. decreased Po_2 and increased Pco_2
c. increased Po_2 and increased Pco_2
d. increased Po_2 and decreased Pco_2
e. none of the above

Q5. What is the most common cause of morbidity and mortality among hospitalized immobile patients?
a. myocardial infarction
b. cerebrovascular accident
c. deep venous thrombosis (DVT)/pulmonary embolism (PE)
d. nosocomial infection
e. none of the above

Q6. What is (are) the drug(s) of choice for patients with a documented pulmonary embolus?
a. continuous intravenous (IV) heparin
b. intermittent IV heparin
c. intermittent subcutaneous heparin
d. any of the above
e. none of the above

Q7. Which of the following is evidence of adequate anticoagulation with heparin in patients with DVT/PE?
a. partial thromboplastin time (PTT) 1.2 times that of the control
b. PTT 1.4 times that of the control
c. PTT 1.5 to 2.0 times that of the control
d. PTT 2.0 to 3.0 times that of the control
e. none of the above

Q8. Which of the following is a (are) risk factor(s) for the condition just described?
a. prolonged immobilization
b. long leg fractures
c. pregnancy
d. malignancy
e. all of the above

Q9. What would be the diagnostic procedure of choice for this patient in the outpatient setting?
a. pulmonary angiography
b. pelvic vein ultrasound
c. impedance plethysmography
d. V/Q scan
e. magnetic resonance imaging (MRI) scan

Q10. What is the diagnostic procedure of choice for a patient who comes to the Emergency Department with "a swollen leg" and has one or more of the risk factors described in Question 8?
a. pulmonary angiography
b. pelvic vein ultrasound
c. impedance plethysmography
d. V/Q scan
e. MRI scan

Q11. Which of the following is a (are) specific recommendation(s) regarding DVT prophylaxis?
 a. patients at moderate risk for any reason should receive low-dose heparin or intermittent pneumatic compression
 b. patients undergoing neurosurgical procedures should be treated with pneumatic compression
 c. patients undergoing urologic procedures should be treated with pneumatic compression
 d. patients undergoing surgery for hip fracture should receive warfarin to a PTT of 1.2 to 1.5 times that of the control
 e. all of the above

SHORT ANSWER MANAGEMENT PROBLEM

The management of the condition described in this problem has changed significantly over the last 2 years. Describe the treatment of the following: (1) a patient with this condition but without "severe disease" or hypotension and (2) a patient with this condition but with either "severe disease" or hypotension.

ANSWERS

A1. **d.** This patient most likely has a PE. Hip surgery is a common predisposing factor for PE. Symptoms of PE are often subtle, and it is often impossible to distinguish PE from myocardial infarction on the basis of the symptoms alone. Chest pain, dyspnea, anxiety, hyperventilation, and syncope are common to both conditions. Signs of PE include adventitious breath sounds, fever, and cyanosis. PE is suggested by the triad of cough, hemoptysis, and pleuritic chest pain.

PE may lead to acute cor pulmonale. This complication produces the following:
 a. Distended neck veins
 b. Tachycardia
 c. An accentuated and split pneumonic heart sound
 d. Kussmaul's sign (distention of the jugular veins on inspiration)
 e. Pulsus paradoxus (exaggerated fall in blood pressure on inspiration); systemic hypotension and shock suggest massive PE

In the postoperative setting, fat and cholesterol emboli syndromes always need to be considered. A hallmark of both of these disorders is the presence of purpura. Fat embolism typically occurs on the upper body 2 to 3 days after a major injury. Through the use of special fixatives the emboli can be demonstrated in biopsy specimens of the petechiae. Cholesterol emboli are usually seen on the lower extremities of patients with atherosclerotic vascular disease. They often follow anticoagulant therapy or an invasive vascular procedure such as an arteriogram. Associated findings include livedo reticularis, gangrene, cyanosis, subcutaneous nodules, and ischemic ulcerations.

A2. **c.** If two or more medium or large perfusion defects on V/Q scan mismatch, there is a 90% probability of PE. Although a negative V/Q scan virtually excludes PE (high sensitivity), a positive scan does not confirm the diagnosis (low specificity). If only a single medium or large defect with mismatch is present, the probability of PE drops to less than 50%. Small perfusion defects with V/Q mismatch confer a low probability of PE.

A3. **c.** The clinical diagnosis of DVT is difficult and unreliable. DVT is frequently present in the absence of clinical signs (such as pain, heat, or swelling), and it is absent in 50% of patients in whom clinical signs or symptoms suggest its presence.

A4. **a.** Massive embolism is commonly associated with arterial hypoxemia, hypocapnia, and respiratory alkalosis. In addition, the difference between the alveolar Po_2 and the arterial Po_2 ($PAco_2 - Paco_2$) may be widened because of the increase in alveolar dead space. However, a normal PAo_2 does not exclude the diagnosis.

A5. **c.** The most common causes of morbidity and mortality among hospitalized immobile patients are DVT and PE. These are directly related to the immobile state.

In the United States the incidence of fatal plus nonfatal PE exceeds 500,000 annually. This overall incidence is verified by autopsy statistics. Evidence of recent or old embolism is detected in 25% to 30% of routine autopsies.

A6. **d.** In DVT and PE, three methods of heparin administration have been advocated by various investigators:
 a. Continuous IV heparin
 b. Intermittent IV heparin
 c. Intermittent subcutaneous heparin

Continuous IV heparin is usually given in a dose of approximately 1000 units/hr. Intermittent IV heparin is commonly given in a dose of 5000 units q4h or 7500 units q6h. Subcutaneous heparin has been recommended in a dose of 5000 units q4h, 10,000 units q8h, or 20,000 units q12h. Currently, it is unclear which method is best. Intramuscular injection of heparin should be avoided because of hematoma development.

A7. **c.** The value of PTT or clotting time in monitoring the safety and efficacy of heparin administration remains controversial. With respect to safety, the risk of hemorrhage (the principal complication of heparin therapy) is not clearly related to coagulation test alterations; rather, it appears related to factors such as the coexistence of other diseases associated with bleeding risk (gastric or duodenal ulcer, coagulopathies, uremia) and advanced age. Similarly, achievement of the desired effect of heparin (cessation of thrombus growth in vivo) has not been related consistently to coagulation tests.

Current recommendations suggest keeping the PTT measured just before the next intermittent dose at or above 1.5 times the control, and at 1.5 to 2.0 times the control with the continuous infusion regimen.

A8. **e.** The risk of DVT and PE is increased by the following factors:
   a. Immobility (both posttraumatic and postoperative)
   b. Long leg fractures
   c. A history of DVT
   d. Oral contraceptive or estrogen use
   e. Cerebrovascular accident (CVA) or a history of CVA
   f. Pregnancy
   g. Malignancy
   h. Autoimmune disease
   i. Nephrotic syndrome
   j. Polycythemia
   k. Inflammatory bowel disease
   l. Congestive heart failure
   m. Obesity

A9. **c.** In the outpatient setting, impedance plethysmography would be the most useful and available investigational tool. Impedance plethysmography can be performed by a physician in the office and offers a fair sensitivity in the diagnosis of DVT.

A10. **d.** For the patient who comes to the Emergency Department with a swollen leg and one or more risk factors, the diagnostic modality of choice would be the V/Q scan.

The current investigational modalities for DVT and PE include the following:
   a. The chest x-ray: may show a parenchymal infiltrate and evidence of a pleural effusion if pulmonary infarction has occurred.
   b. Transthoracic echo-Doppler studies: standard transthoracic echo-Doppler studies may suggest the diagnosis of PE by demonstrating right ventricular enlargement, thrombi "trapped" in the right atrium or ventricle; an elevated pulmonary

artery pressure; or echogenic densities in the right main pulmonary artery.
   c. Computed tomography (CT)/MRI scanning: the value of CT scanning with contrast and MRI scanning in the diagnosis of PE remains to be determined.
   d. Arterial blood gases: blood gas results in PE show arterial hypoxemia, hypocapnia, and respiratory alkalosis. Blood gas results are most useful when combined with other information.
   e. The V/Q scan: the diagnostic modality of choice in the acute care facility setting. The diagnosis of PE is made when there are two or more perfusion defects with no matching ventilation defects.
   f. Impedance plethysmography (IPG): an excellent screening tool for DVT that can be used by the physician in the office either to establish the diagnosis of DVT or to increase the index of suspicion regarding the diagnosis of DVT. IPG is highly sensitive for detecting proximal DVT but not for detecting thrombi in the calves.
   g. Pelvic vein ultrasound: presently used in some centers, this technique will evolve as time and experience are gained.
   h. Radionuclide scanning: sensitive for detecting thrombi in the calves.
   i. Pulmonary angiography: the "gold standard" for the diagnosis of PE in the presence of an equivocal V/Q scan.
   j. Venography: ascending venography is the "gold standard" for the diagnosis of DVT.

A11. **e.** Recommendations for the prevention of venous thromboembolism include the following:
   a. Patients at moderate risk of venous thromboembolism for any reason should receive preventive therapy with low-dose heparin (5000 units q12h) or with intermittent pneumatic compression.
   b. Patients undergoing neurosurgical procedures, urologic procedures, and major knee surgery should be treated with intermittent pneumatic compression.
   c. Patients undergoing elective hip surgery should receive prophylaxis with adjusted-dose heparin therapy or moderate-dose warfarin therapy.
   d. Patients who are undergoing repair of a hip fracture should receive prophylactic therapy with moderate-dose warfarin therapy.

SOLUTION TO THE SHORT ANSWER MANAGEMENT PROBLEM

1. Treatment of DVT/PE without severe cardiovascular compromise:
   a. Full anticoagulation is advised for 7 to 10 days.

b. Supplementary oxygen is given in the acute phase at a rate of 3 L/min.

c. With heparin, three treatment regimens are acceptable:

   1) Continuous infusion IV heparin: 1000 units/hr

   2) Intermittent IV infusion: 5000 units q4h or 7500 units q6h

   3) Subcutaneous heparin: 5000 units q4h, 10,000 units q8h, or 20,000 units q12h

d. Warfarin should be initiated on day 2 or 3 of heparin therapy. Do not discontinue heparin until the prothrombin time is 1.5 to 1.8 times that of the control for at least 3 days.

e. An option for prophylactic warfarin is self-injected subcutaneous heparin.

f. Prophylactic treatment time is at least 3 months; 6 months is probably wiser.

g. The progress of therapy is noted by a PTT for heparin that is 1.5 to 2.0 that of the control and a PTT for warfarin that is 1.5 to 1.8 that of the control.

h. Currently, the use of low molecular weight heparin (LMWH) is gaining in popularity. A growing body of evidence shows LMWH to be as safe or safer than conventional IV heparin for the acute management of DVT and, in carefully identified patients, for PE.

2. The treatment of DVT/PE with severe cardiovascular compromise is the same as the treatment regimen just described plus a first- or second-generation thrombolytic agent (first generation, streptokinase; second generation, t-PA).

3. Recommended dosages are as follows:

   a. Streptokinase: 250,000 IV loading with 100,000 units/hr for 24 hours

   b. t-PA: 100 mg as a peripheral infusion over 2 hours

SUMMARY OF THE DIAGNOSIS AND TREATMENT OF DEEP VENOUS THROMBOSIS AND PULMONARY THROMBOEMBOLISM

1. Diagnosis: Most patients who develop DVT and subsequent PE have one of the previously described risk factors. Remember that DVT is often clinically silent, and the clinical diagnosis is notoriously inaccurate. PE, however, is often heralded by the abrupt onset of dyspnea, chest pain, apprehension, hemoptysis, or syncope. When massive PE is present, the signs of acute cor pulmonale are evident. With PE, rhonchi are frequently heard in the chest.

2. Laboratory diagnosis: Obtain a blood sample and check arterial blood gases; finding a low P_{O_2}, low P_{CO_2}, and respiratory alkalosis is diagnostic.

3. Diagnostic imaging:

   a. For DVT: IPG is very sensitive in the diagnosis of proximal thrombi but lacks sensitivity with more distal thrombi. Consider radionuclide scanning in more distal thrombi. Venography is the "gold standard" for the diagnosis of DVT.

   b. For pulmonary thromboembolism: V/Q scan is 90% sensitive when there are at least two perfusion defects with no matching ventilation defects (V/Q mismatch).

4. Treatment:

   a. Give supplemental oxygen.

   b. Heparin: Continuous IV, intermittent IV, or subcutaneous.

   c. Warfarin: Begin warfarin on second or third day.

   d. Thrombolytic therapy: Consider streptokinase or t-PA when the patient has significant cardiovascular compromise.

5. Length of treatment time and prophylaxis:

   a. Treat for at least 3 months and possibly up to 6 months with warfarin.

   b. Consider prophylaxis for those surgical procedures just described.

SUGGESTED READINGS

Goldhaber SZ: Pulmonary thromboembolism. In Fauci AS et al, eds: *Harrison's principles of internal medicine,* ed 14, New York, 1998, McGraw-Hill.

Levine M et al: A comparison of low-molecular weight heparin administered primarily at home with unfractionated heparin administered in the hospital for proximal deep vein thrombosis, *N Engl J Med* 334:667-681, 1996.

PROBLEM · 9

CHRONIC OBSTRUCTIVE PULMONARY DISEASE

"I Quit Smoking, So Why Am I Still Coughing?"

Case 1 ■ A 55-Year-Old Male with a Chronic Cough

A 55-year-old male comes to your office for assessment of a chronic cough. He complains of "coughing for the last 10 years"; the cough has become more bothersome lately. The cough is productive of sputum that is usually mucoid; occasionally it becomes purulent.

He has a 35-year history of smoking two packs of cigarettes a day (70 pack/year history). He quit smoking approximately 2 years ago.

On physical examination, his blood pressure is 160/85 mm Hg. His pulse is 96 bpm and regular. He has a body mass index of 34, and he weighs 280 pounds. He wheezes while he talks. On auscultation, adventitious breath sounds are heard in all lobes. His chest x-ray reveals significant bronchial wall thickening. There are increased markings at both lung bases.

SELECT THE BEST ANSWER TO THE FOLLOWING QUESTIONS

Q1. What is the most likely diagnosis in this patient?
   a. smoker's cough
   b. subacute bronchitis
   c. emphysema
   d. chronic bronchitis
   e. allergic bronchitis

Q2. What is the most likely cause of this condition?
   a. right-sided heart failure
   b. cor pulmonale
   c. cigarette smoking
   d. obstructive sleep apnea
   e. hypercarbia

Q3. Which of the following statements regarding this condition is (are) true?
   a. the disease develops in 10% to 15% of cigarette smokers
   b. cigarette smokers in whom this disease develops usually report the onset of cough with expectoration 10 to 12 years after smoking began
   c. dyspnea is noted initially only on extreme exertion; as the condition progresses, it becomes more severe and occurs with mild activity
   d. pneumonia, pulmonary hypertension, cor pulmonale, and chronic respiratory failure characterize the late stages of the disease
   e. all of the above are true

Q4. Which of the following regarding the patient in Case 1 is (are) true?
   a. this patient is a "pink puffer"
   b. this patient's blood gas measurements will likely show a decreased P_{CO_2}
   c. this patient's chest x-ray will demonstrate normal or increased lung markings
   d. this patient's disease is a disorder of the terminal bronchi
   e. all of the above are true

Q5. Which of the following pulmonary function results is not associated with the condition just described?
   a. decreased forced expiratory volume in 1 second (FEV_1)
   b. decreased forced expiratory volume in 1 second/forced vital capacity (FEV_1/FVC)
   c. decreased forced expiratory flow during the middle 50% of the FVC (FEF_{25-75})
   d. decreased residual volume
   e. none of the above is associated with this disease state

Q6. Regarding the pathophysiology of chronic bronchitis, which of the following statements is false?
   a. most histologic studies in patients with chronic bronchitis have shown an increase in the size of mucus-secreting glands as measured by the Reid index (a ratio of gland to bronchial wall thickness)
   b. smooth muscle hyperplasia occurs in patients with chronic bronchitis
   c. chronic bronchitis is characterized by chronic, excessive secretion of mucus
   d. in chronic bronchitis, there is a clear relationship between smooth muscle hyperplasia and bronchodilator responsiveness or methacholine sensitivity
   e. none of the above is false

Q7. Which of the following is an (are) established risk factor(s) for chronic obstructive pulmonary disease (COPD)?
   a. smoking
   b. atopy
   c. elevated levels of immunoglobulin E (IgE)
   d. bronchial hyperresponsiveness
   e. all of the above

Q8. Which of the following is an (are) accurate statement(s) regarding the role of bacteria in chronic bronchitis?
   a. the delay in mucociliary clearance allows inhaled bacteria to colonize the normally sterile airways and to multiply, leading to further infectious exacerbations
   b. *Haemophilus influenzae, Streptococcus pneumoniae,* and *Moraxella catarrhalis* account for 75% of all exacerbations of chronic bronchitis
   c. bacteria may act synergistically with tobacco smoke to impede mucociliary clearance and allow organisms to colonize the airways further

d. nicotine stimulates the growth of *H. influenzae*
e. a, b, and c
f. all of the above

Q9. Which of the following is a (are) consideration(s) in the diagnosis of chronic bronchitis?
a. asthma
b. postnasal drip from sinusitis
c. chronic angiotensin-converting enzyme (ACE) inhibitor therapy
d. a and b
e. all of the above

Q10. Which of the following statements regarding smoking cessation and COPD is (are) true?
a. cessation of smoking dramatically reduces symptoms in established COPD patients
b. coughing stops in 80% of patients with COPD who stop smoking
c. coughing stops in over 50% of patients with COPD within 4 weeks
d. all of the above
e. none of the above

Q11. Which of the following drugs is (are) the most effective for long-term pharmacologic management in a patient with chronic bronchitis?
a. an inhaled β-agonist
b. an inhaled anticholinergic agent
c. an inhaled corticosteroid
d. oral prednisone
e. a, b, and c are considered to be equally efficacious

Q12. Which of the following drugs is (are) recommended as routine symptomatic management for a patient with chronic bronchitis?
a. an inhaled β-agonist
b. an inhaled anticholinergic agent
c. an inhaled corticosteroid
d. a and b
e. all of the above

Q13. Long-term home oxygen therapy is indicated in which patients with chronic bronchitis?
a. all patients who have established chronic bronchitis and who have met the criteria of symptoms for at least 5 years
b. all patients who have a resting arterial partial pressure of oxygen (PaO_2) of 55 mm Hg or less
c. all patients who have a resting PaO_2 of 60 mm Hg or less with evidence of chronic tissue hypoxia as demonstrated by cor pulmonale or polycythemia

d. b and c
e. all of the above

Case 2 ■ Second-Hand Smoke Is Less Than Beneficial

The patient described in Case 1 is stabilized on long-term therapy. Unfortunately, during winter holidays, he travels to his son's home in a distant state and finds himself in an environment where six packs of cigarettes a day are being smoked by his son and his son's wife (four packs for the son and two packs for his wife). There is a layer of definite haze that hangs approximately 1 foot below all the ceilings in the house. As he sits around the house one day (unable to go outside or walk any distance at all because of significantly increased shortness of breath since arriving) he counts the number of ashtrays (47). His son, through the haze of smoke, finally notices that his dad is out of breath and his lips appear very blue. He takes him to the nearest Emergency Department.

The Emergency Department doctor diagnoses his condition as an acute exacerbation of chronic bronchitis. His major symptoms at this time include dyspnea, increased sputum production, and purulence. The patient's PaO_2 when measured in the Emergency Department is 44 mm Hg.

Q14. Which of the following should be instituted as therapy for this condition?
a. low-flow oxygen
b. intravenous (IV) corticosteroids
c. oral ciprofloxacin
d. a and b only
e. all of the above

Q15. Which of the following organisms has (have) been implicated in the pathogenesis of acute exacerbations of chronic bronchitis and has exhibited resistance in vivo to ampicillin?
a. *H. influenzae*
b. *S. pneumoniae*
c. *M. catarrhalis*
d. a and b only
e. all of the above

Case 3 ■ A 23-Year-Old Male with a 10-Day Cough

A 23-year-old male comes to your office for assessment of a 10-day cough that has "now gone into my lungs." He complains of sputum production, which was initially clear but has now turned "yellow." He said that he called your partner last night and your partner told him to "get in here today and we will prescribe an antibiotic and clear this thing up quick." This patient has no history of other respiratory illnesses. On examination, the patient's lungs are clear. His temperature is normal (37° C). No other positive physical findings are present.

Q16. What would you do?
a. reach for the "good old prescription pad" and scribble down the first reasonable thing that comes to mind
b. reach for the "good old prescription pad," but think briefly about which antibiotic you wish to prescribe before you prescribe it
c. reach for the "good old prescription pad," but think quite a bit before deciding which antibiotic you wish to prescribe
d. auscultate the patient's lung through his shirt, sweater, and winter jacket, and then reach for the prescription pad
e. take the Fifth Amendment on this question
f. none of the above

SHORT ANSWER MANAGEMENT PROBLEM
Describe the difference between the two major types of COPD in terms of (1) part of airway affected, (2) color of lips in a severely affected individual, (3) definition of both types, (4) pathophysiology, and (5) the causes.

ANSWERS

A1. **d.** This patient has chronic bronchitis. Chronic bronchitis is defined as cough and sputum production on most days for at least 3 months of the year over a period of at least 2 years. Chronic bronchitis and emphysema are the two underlying conditions in COPD.

Emphysema is a destructive process involving the lung parenchyma. It is defined as abnormal permanent enlargement of air spaces distal to the terminal bronchioles accompanied by destruction of alveolar walls.

Acute bronchitis is an inflammation of the bronchi caused by an infectious agent or acute exposure to a nonspecific irritant. Acute bronchitis is most often caused by a viral infection. Acute bronchitis may occur as a complication of chronic bronchitis.

A2. **c.** Chronic bronchitis is most commonly caused by cigarette smoking. Right-sided heart failure and cor pulmonale may result from chronic bronchitis and/or emphysema. Obstructive sleep apnea is often a complication of COPD. Hypercarbia (increased P_{CO_2} level) is a valuable prognostic sign in chronic bronchitis and allows the prediction (along with decreased P_{O_2}) of

when certain therapies, especially home oxygen, should be used.

A3. **e.** Chronic bronchitis usually develops in cigarette smokers about 10 to 12 years after smoking initiation. Patients with chronic bronchitis have an increased susceptibility to recurrent respiratory tract infections.

COPD develops in 10% to 15% of patients who are cigarette smokers. In these patients, airflow obstruction worsens over time if cigarette smoking is continued.

Dyspnea is initially noted only on extreme exertion, but as the COPD progresses, it becomes more severe and occurs with mild activity. In severe disease, dyspnea may occur at rest.

Complications of COPD include pneumonia, pulmonary hypertension, cor pulmonale, and chronic respiratory failure.

A4. **c.** COPD patients can be classified into two basic types: type A COPD patients with obstructive disease, or "pink puffers," and type B COPD patients with restrictive disease, or "blue bloaters." The patient described in this question is a typical blue bloater.
Blue bloaters:
a. Are often stocky or obese
b. Often have cough and sputum production
c. Have normal or increased lung markings
d. Usually have a markedly reduced P_{O_2} and an elevated P_{CO_2}
e. Often develop pulmonary hypertension and/or cor pulmonale
Blue bloaters have chronic bronchitis.
Pink puffers:
a. Are usually thin
b. Usually have dyspnea
c. Have hyperinflated lungs on chest x-ray films
d. Have a slightly decreased P_{O_2} and a normal or slightly decreased P_{CO_2}
Pink puffers have emphysema.

A5. **d.** Chronic bronchitis is characterized by several abnormalities observed on pulmonary function testing. Abnormalities noted most frequently include the following:
a. An increased (not decreased) residual volume
b. A decrease in FEV_1
c. A decrease in FEV_1/FVC
d. A decrease in FEF_{25-75}

A6. **d.** Most mucus is secreted by subepithelial glands in the large airways. It follows that chronic bronchitis, a disorder characterized by chronic, excessive secretion of mucus, is a disease of the large airways. Most histologic studies of chronic bronchitis have shown an increase in the size of the mucus-secreting glands as measured by the Reid index, although no clear-cut relation between this index and the degree of airflow obstruction has been established. Patients with chronic bronchitis also have smooth muscle hyperplasia; however, unlike the situation in asthma, there is no clear-cut relationship between their responsiveness and methacholine sensitivity. Bronchial hyperresponsiveness, which is present in at least 50% of patients with COPD, may lead to dyspnea and hypoxemia.

A7. **e.** It is commonly thought that cigarette smoking is the only risk factor for COPD. In fact, a number of other risk factors are implicated, including the following:

    a. Exposure to tobacco smoke
    b. Domestic and occupational pollutants and recurrent respiratory tract infections, particularly in infancy
    c. Atopy, which is characterized by eosinophilia or an increased level of serum IgE
    d. The presence of bronchial hyperresponsiveness
    e. A family history of COPD
    f. Certain protease deficiencies such as α_1-antitrypsin deficiency

A8. **f.** Cigarette smoking, as the most common cause of chronic bronchitis, leads to loss of ciliated epithelium and more viscous secretions, compromising the local defenses of the respiratory tract. The delay in mucociliary clearance allows inhaled bacteria to colonize the normally sterile airways and to multiply, leading to further infectious exacerbations. *H. influenzae* is present in the sputum of about 60% of patients with stable chronic bronchitis. *H. influenzae, S. pneumoniae,* and *M. catarrhalis* account for 75% of all exacerbations of chronic bronchitis and 85% to 95% of bacterial exacerbations. *H. influenzae* may act synergistically with tobacco smoke to impede mucociliary clearance and allow further multiplication and colonization of the airway. By-products of *H. influenzae* metabolism have been shown to cause further impairment of ciliated cells in vitro, stimulate mucus production, and secrete IgA protease, which may further impair host defenses. In addition, nicotine has been shown to stimulate the growth of this organism, and *H. influenzae* has been shown to engender an immune reaction in the airways.

A9. **e.** The diagnosis of chronic bronchitis rests on clinical criteria that have already been described. There are no characteristic physical findings and no specific radiographic changes or laboratory features diagnostic of this disease.

The differential diagnosis of chronic cough, however, must be considered. This includes the following:

    a. Asthma
    b. Postnasal drip
    c. Gastroesophageal reflux
    d. Foreign body aspiration
    e. Congestive heart failure
    f. Bronchiectasis
    g. Chronic ACE inhibitor therapy (15% of patients taking ACE inhibitors develop a chronic cough)

A10. **d.** The cessation of smoking produces dramatic symptomatic benefits for patients with chronic bronchitis. Coughing stops in up to 77% of quitters and improves in another 17%. When coughing stops, it does so within 4 weeks in 54% of patients.

Influenza virus can worsen the epithelial damage induced by cigarette smoke and predispose the airways to subsequent bacterial proliferation, leading to excessive mucus hypersecretion and greater airflow obstruction. Annual influenza vaccination reduces morbidity and mortality caused by influenza in patients with COPD, although its role in this disease has not been assessed in large-scale clinical trials. COPD patients should also receive pneumococcal vaccine.

A11. **b.** Ipratropium bromide is the most effective long-term pharmacologic agent used in chronic bronchitis and COPD.

A12. **d.**

A13. **d.** Symptomatic therapy for patients with chronic bronchitis includes the use of the following:

    a. Inhaled bronchodilators
    b. Oral bronchodilators
    c. Inhaled corticosteroids
    d. Oral corticosteroids
    e. Inhaled anticholinergics
    f. Home oxygen therapy
    g. Rehabilitation programs

The use of inhaled bronchodilators by patients with airflow obstruction may increase flow rates and reduce dyspnea. Inhaled anticholinergic agents appear to produce greater bronchodilatation with fewer side effects than inhaled β_2-agonists in COPD. This may be related to increased cholinergic tone in the airways as the degree of obstruction progresses. Combination therapy with agents from both groups may have an additive effect in some patients. Patients who demonstrate symptomatic or physiologic improvement, or both, with these medications should be maintained on the inhaled drugs indefinitely. In patients who remain symptomatic on inhaled bronchodilators, a trial of an oral theophylline medication is warranted. These medications are weaker bronchodilators than inhaled anticholinergics or β-agonist drugs but may have additional beneficial effects in chronic bronchitis by increasing respiratory muscle strength and endurance, improving mucociliary clearance, and increasing central respiratory drive, all of which may lead to a symptomatic improvement in patients with the disease.

At present, regular use of oral or inhaled corticosteroids cannot be recommended as routine therapy for all patients with chronic bronchitis. Although steroids have clear anti-inflammatory effects and decrease mucus hypersecretion, a beneficial effect can be shown in only 10% to 20% of patients.

The benefits of home oxygen therapy have been clearly demonstrated in major clinical trials. To be considered candidates for treatment, patients must (a) be in a stable clinical state, (b) have a resting PaO_2 of 55 mm Hg or less, or (c) have a PaO_2 of 60 mm Hg with evidence of chronic tissue hypoxia as demonstrated by cor pulmonale or polycythemia. In properly selected patients the use of home oxygen for more than 18 hr/day may increase the life span of the COPD patient by 6 or 7 years.

A14. **e.** Treatment of an acute exacerbation of chronic bronchitis provides symptomatic relief and prevents any transient decline in pulmonary function. Low-flow oxygen should be instituted if hypoxemia is present (as in this case). The goal of oxygen therapy in this case is to get the PaO_2 above 60 mm Hg. In addition, oral or IV corticosteroids should be given, as they have been shown to hasten resolution in the acute exacerbation phase of chronic bronchitis.

Patients with all three of the following "acute exacerbative symptoms" have been shown to benefit from antibiotic therapy:
 a. Increasing dyspnea
 b. Increased sputum production
 c. Purulence of sputum

In patients with one or two of the three symptoms, the case is less clear.

A15. **e.** Antibiotic choices should obviously be based on both host and pathogen factors. The latter relate to resistance problems. The three most common isolates associated with acute exacerbations of chronic bronchitis are as follows:
 a. *H. influenzae*
 b. *S. pneumoniae*
 c. *M. catarrhalis*

All have exhibited resistance in vivo to ampicillin and other first-line agents. Nevertheless, most U.S. and international guidelines recommend initial treatment of acute exacerbations of chronic bronchitis with amoxicillin or tetracycline derivatives. Other potential

first-line agents include trimethoprim-sulfamethoxazole (TMP-SMX) and cefaclor. In most complicated cases of acute exacerbation of chronic bronchitis, guidelines generally recommend quinolones, newer macrolides, and a second- or third-generation cephalosporin as the initial agent.

A16. **f.** This patient has acute bronchitis and is a healthy young man with no concomitant illnesses. The cause of acute bronchitis in a patient like this is almost always a viral infection (adenovirus, influenza virus, or rhinovirus). It has only been present for 24 hours, and at this time there is no good reason for prescribing an antibiotic. What your partner says and what your patient expects are not satisfactory reasons for doing something that, on the basis of probability, is likely to do no good whatsoever.

A reasonable treatment protocol to follow for the treatment of acute bronchitis is as follows:
 a. Healthy middle-aged adult, no other respiratory problems, cough and purulent sputum production of short duration: no culture and no antibiotic
 b. Healthy middle-aged adult, no other respiratory problems, cough and purulent sputum production persists for longer than 1 week: no culture, macrolide antibiotic (to cover *Mycoplasma*)
 c. Healthy elderly adult, no other respiratory problems, cough and purulent sputum production of short duration: no culture, no antibiotic
 d. Healthy elderly adult, no other respiratory problems, cough and purulent sputum production for greater than 1 week: no culture, give TMP-SMX (Septra) or amoxicillin
 e. Elderly adult with chronic disease, cough, and sputum production: no culture initially, give macrolide no matter how long symptoms have persisted

SOLUTION TO THE SHORT ANSWER MANAGEMENT PROBLEM

1. The two forms of COPD are chronic bronchitis and emphysema.
   a. Chronic bronchitis affects the large airways of the lung
   b. Emphysema affects the terminal bronchi
2. The color of lips in severely affected individuals is either:
   a. Blue: Is a "blue bloater," indicating chronic bronchitis
   b. Pink: Is a "pink puffer," indicating emphysema

3. Definitions:
   a. Chronic bronchitis: Excessive cough, productive of sputum on most days, extends for at least 3 months a year, occurs at least 2 consecutive years
   b. Emphysema: Defined histologically by abnormal permanent enlargement, without obvious fibrosis, of the air spaces distal to the terminal bronchi, accompanied by destruction of their walls
4. Pathophysiology:
   a. Chronic bronchitis:
      1) Chronic, excessive secretion of mucus
      2) Increase in the size of the mucus-secreting cells
      3) Smooth muscle hyperplasia
      4) Bronchial airway hyperresponsiveness
   b. Emphysema:
      1) Distal airspace enlargement
      2) No significant fibrosis
      3) Loss of alveolar attachments
      4) Decrease in elastic recoil
      5) Increase in lung compliance
      6) Hyperinflation
      7) Ventilation-perfusion mismatching
5. Causes: Most cases of both chronic bronchitis and emphysema are caused by cigarette smoking; α_1-antitrypsin deficiency is a factor in some cases of emphysema.

SUMMARY OF THE DIAGNOSIS AND MANAGEMENT OF CHRONIC OBSTRUCTIVE PULMONARY DISEASE

1. Definitions: See the Short Answer Management Problem.

2. Pathophysiology: See the Short Answer Management Problem.

3. Differentiation of disease entities in COPD: See the Short Answer Management Problem.

4. Signs and symptoms:
   a. Symptoms: Dyspnea, cough, sputum production, and sputum purulence. When cor pulmonale and right-sided heart failure are present—extremity swelling
   b. Signs: Increased respiratory rate, respiratory distress, cyanosis, barrel chest, distant heart sounds, increased jugular venous pressure
   c. Three most important signs/symptoms indicating deterioration:
      1) Increasing dyspnea
      2) Increased sputum volume
      3) Increased purulence

5. Pulmonary function test abnormalities:
   a. Decreased FEV_1
   b. Decreased ratio of FEV_1/FVC
   c. Decreased FEF_{25-75}
   d. Increased residual volume
   e. Normal to increased functional residual capacity
   f. Decreased diffusion capacity

6. Pathologic organisms associated with infection in COPD:
   a. *H. influenzae*
   b. *S. pneumoniae*
   c. *M. catarrhalis*

7. Treatment:
   a. Bronchodilators:
      1) Best single agent for long-term treatment in chronic bronchitis is an inhaled anticholinergic-ipratropium (Atrovent).
      2) β-Agonists should be combined with an inhaled anticholinergic-ipratropium (Atrovent).
   b. Corticosteroids: Routine use of inhaled corticosteroids cannot be recommended in chronic care. Corticosteroids (both inhaled and IV/oral) are most helpful in acute exacerbations.
   c. Antibiotics: Routine prophylactic use of antibiotics cannot be recommended. They are most useful in acute exacerbations if all three of the following are present:
      1) Increasing dyspnea
      2) Increasing sputum production
      3) Increasing sputum purulence
   Antibiotics of choice include ampicillin, TMP-SMX, amoxicillin, and doxycycline or cefaclor; ofloxacin (Floxin) is given for severe exacerbations.
   d. Home oxygen: Home oxygen is indicated if the Pa_{O_2} is 55 mm Hg or less at rest or if the Pa_{O_2} is 60 mm Hg with evidence of chronic tissue hypoxia as demonstrated by cor pulmonale or polycythemia.
   e. Diuretics: Use is indicated only for treatment of cor pulmonale and right-sided heart failure.
   f. Smoking cessation: At any time in the course of COPD, smoking cessation can be and is of benefit. Do not accept the excuse "I've smoked too long and I am too old to quit."
   g. Counseling/support groups: Group therapy with other COPD patients is often of aid in helping the patient come to terms with the disease.

SUGGESTED READINGS

Liu HH: Overuse of antimicrobial therapy for upper respiratory infections and acute bronchitis: who, why, and what can be done, *Pharmacotherapy* 19(4):371-373, 1999.

Nelson HS: Beta-adrenergic bronchodilators, *N Engl J Med* 333(8):499-506, 1995.

Petty TL, Weinmann GG: Building a national strategy for the prevention and management of and research in chronic obstructive pulmonary disease, *JAMA* 277(3):246-253, 1997.

Saint S et al: Antibiotics in chronic obstructive pulmonary disease exacerbations, a meta-analysis, *JAMA* 273(12):957-960, 1995.

Van Schayck C et al: Periodic treatment regimens with inhaled steroids in asthma or chronic obstructive pulmonary disease, *JAMA* 274(2):161-164, 1995.

PROBLEM·10

ASTHMA

Some Wheeze, Some Don't, but It's Still Serious.

Case 1 ■ A 22-Year-Old Male with a Chronic Cough

A 22-year-old male comes to your office for assessment of a chronic cough. He has just moved to your city and will be attending the university there. He has moved into a bachelor apartment in the basement of a house.

As soon as he moved in, he began to notice a chronic, nonproductive cough associated with shortness of breath. He has never had these symptoms before, and he has no known allergies. When he leaves for school for the day, the symptoms disappear. The symptoms are definitely worse at night.

His landlady has three cats. He didn't think he was allergic to cats, but now he thinks that might be the case.

On examination, his respiratory rate is 16 breaths/min and regular. He is in no distress at the present time. There are a few expiratory rhonchi heard in all lobes. His blood pressure is 120/70 mm Hg, and his pulse is 72 bpm and regular.

SELECT THE BEST ANSWER TO THE FOLLOWING QUESTIONS

Q1. What is the most likely diagnosis in this patient?
   a. paroxysmal nocturnal cough syndrome
   b. hyporesponsive airways disease
   c. cough variant asthma
   d. bronchial asthma: nonwheezing variant
   e. allergic bronchitis

Q2. In children, which of the following statements is (are) true?
   a. it is often difficult to differentiate asthma from bronchiolitis
   b. children with bronchiolitis who do not develop asthma may be inappropriately labeled with the "stigma" of asthma

   c. the relationship between bronchiolitis, ongoing bronchial hyperactivity, and bronchial asthma is unclear; it appears that bronchiolitis may precipitate bronchial asthma
   d. all of the above
   e. none of the above

Q3. Which of the following is (are) included in the working definition of asthma?
   a. reversible airway obstruction
   b. bronchial airway inflammation
   c. bronchial airway hyperresponsiveness to various stimuli
   d. expiratory rhonchi
   e. a, b, and c
   f. all of the above

Q4. Which of the following statements regarding health care costs and mortality with respect to asthma is (are) false?
   a. the mortality from asthma is decreasing (presumably because of improved therapies)
   b. more cases of asthma are being associated with environmental pollutants than was previously the case
   c. in the United States in 1990 the estimated health care costs associated with asthma were approximately $3.4 billion
   d. all of the above statements are false
   e. none of the above statements is false

Q5. On a pathophysiologic basis, asthma is primarily:
   a. a bronchoconstricting process
   b. an allergenic stimulus process
   c. an inflammatory process
   d. a bronchial hyperreactivity process
   e. an immunoglobulin E (IgE)-mediated antigen-antibody reaction

Q6. Following antigenic stimulation of the bronchial airway, which cell is most responsible for the beginning of the airway's response?
   a. the basophil
   b. the mast cell
   c. the eosinophil
   d. the bronchial epithelial cell
   e. the bronchial mucus-producing goblet cells

Q7. Of the following, what is the substance released by the cell that is most responsible for the beginning of the airway's response?
   a. histamine
   b. proteolytic enzymes
   c. heparin

d. chemotactic factors

e. all of the above

Q8. The substance released by the cell that is most responsible for the beginning of the airway's response induces which of the following responses?

a. bronchoconstriction of the airway

b. edema of the airway

c. increased mucus secretion in the airway

d. all of the above

e. none of the above

Q9. Triggering the release of substances from the cell most responsible for the beginning of the airway's response leads to activation of which of the following?

a. neutrophils

b. eosinophils

c. mononuclear cells

d. b and c

e. all of the above

Q10. The reversible airflow obstruction seen in asthma results from which of the following?

a. bronchoconstriction

b. mucous plug formation

c. edema

d. a and b

e. all of the above

Q11. Which of the following is (are) a clinical hallmark of asthma?

a. cough

b. nocturnal dyspnea

c. wheezing

d. shortness of breath

e. a, c, and d

Case 2 ■ A 24-Year-Old Woman Develops Wheezing and Shortness of Breath

A 24-year-old woman develops wheezing and shortness of breath when she is exposed to cold air or when she is exercising. These symptoms are becoming worse.

Q12. Which of the following is the prophylactic agent of choice for the treatment of asthma in these circumstances?

a. inhaled β_2-agonists

b. oral aminophylline

c. inhaled anticholinergics

d. inhaled sodium cromoglycate

e. oral corticosteroids

Q13. What is the mechanism of action of the agent of choice in Question 12?

a. mast cell stabilizer

b. inhibitor of early-phase reaction

c. inhibitor of late-phase reaction

d. bronchodilator

e. none of the above

Q14. What is the treatment of choice for long-term stabilization?

a. long-acting β_2-agonists

b. leukotriene modifiers

c. an inhaled anticholinergic

d. an inhaled steroid

e. a and b

Q15. Which of the following stepped-care classifications used to guide pharmacotherapy in asthma requires environmental control as the necessary first step for treatment?

a. mild intermittent asthma

b. mild persistent asthma

c. moderate persistent asthma

d. severe persistent asthma

e. all of the above

Q16. All the following except which is (are) characteristic of mild persistent asthma?

a. symptoms occurring more than twice a week but less than once a day

b. exacerbations that affect activity

c. peak expiratory flow greater than 80% of personal best

d. peak expiratory flow variability of 20% to 30%

e. nocturnal symptoms two to three times per week

Q17. Which of the following most accurately describes the preferred pharmacologic treatment of moderate persistent asthma in adults?

a. inhaled sodium cromoglycate alone

b. inhaled β_2-agonists alone

c. inhaled corticosteroids alone

d. daily-inhaled corticosteroids and long-acting, inhaled β_2-agonists, if needed

e. inhaled sodium cromoglycate continually and intermittent inhaled β_2-agonists

Q18. All the following are characteristics of severe persistent asthma except:

a. continual symptoms

b. frequent exacerbations that may last days

c. infrequent nighttime symptoms

d. peak expiratory flow rates less than 60% of personal best

e. peak expiratory flow variability of more than 30%

Q19. Pharmacotherapy of severe persistent asthma in children less than age 5 years includes:
a. high-dose steroids via mask
b. if needed, systemic corticosteroids 2 mg/kg/day
c. switching to cromolyn if possible
d. quick relief with a bronchodilator up to 3 times per day
e. all of the above

Q20. In a patient whose peak expiratory flow rate is below 50% of personal best, suggesting a severe exacerbation, the initial home treatment includes which of the following?
a. an inhaled short-acting β_2-agonist administered three times via metered dose inhaler or once via nebulizer
b. inhaled cromolyn, three times via metered dose inhaler or once via nebulizer
c. an inhaled corticosteroid, administered three times via metered dose inhaler or once via nebulizer
d. subcutaneous self-administered epinephrine
e. none of the above

Q21. Which of the following pulmonary function tests is the most useful for the diagnosis of asthma?
a. decreased forced vital capacity (FVC)
b. increased residual volume
c. a ratio of 1 second forced expiratory volume (FEV_1)/75% of the forced vital capacity ($FVC_{75\%}$)
d. increased functional residual capacity
e. increased total lung capacity

Q22. Which of the following pulmonary function tests is most easily carried out at home?
a. FEV_1/FVC ratio
b. FVC
c. mid-expiratory flow rate
d. peak expiratory flow rate
e. residual volume

Q23. Which of the following is the most common abnormality observed on the chest x-ray in a patient with asthma?
a. hyperinflation
b. increased bronchial markings
c. atelectasis
d. flattening of the diaphragm
e. all of the above are equally common

Q24. What is the most common abnormality seen on physical examination of an asthmatic patient?
a. increased respiratory rate
b. inspiratory rales
c. inspiratory rhonchi
d. expiratory rales
e. expiratory wheezes

Q25. Environmental control as a part of the therapeutic intervention involves a search for and elimination of which of the following agents from the patient's environment?
a. air pollution
b. pollens, molds, mites, cockroaches, and pets
c. tobacco smoke, wood stoves, and fumes
d. work place exposures
e. sulfates, aspirin, other nonsteroidal antiinflammatory drugs (NSAIDs), and other potentially offending drugs
f. all of the above

Q26. Pure cough variant asthma has which of the following characteristics?
a. patients often have to go from doctor to doctor until someone makes the diagnosis
b. patients are treated in the same manner as noncough variant asthma
c. cough variant asthma is very uncommon
d. a and b
e. all of the above

Q27. A patient who comes to the Emergency Department in acute respiratory distress caused by a severe attack of asthma should be treated with all of the following except:
a. warm, humidified, high-flow-rate oxygen
b. constant bedside monitoring
c. intravenous (IV) corticosteroids
d. IV fluids
e. IV antibiotics

Q28. Which of the following statements regarding childhood asthma is false?
a. there is a very significant hereditary component to the probability of a child acquiring asthma
b. asthma in children is often associated with parental smoking
c. asthmatic children are often allergic to aspirin
d. inhaled corticosteroids administered properly do not pose a major risk or hazard to childhood growth
e. many children who are asthmatic go on to outgrow it

Q29. Which of the following viral agents has been implicated as a cause of asthma?
   a. respiratory syncytial virus
   b. parainfluenza virus
   c. adenovirus
   d. rhinovirus
   e. influenza virus

SHORT ANSWER MANAGEMENT PROBLEM
A rural family physician has noticed an interesting phenomenon. This summer, there have been two very severe lightning storms. In the first instance, approximately 1 hour after the storm subsided, six children displayed signs and symptoms of bronchial asthma. In the second instance, eight children displayed signs and symptoms of bronchial asthma an hour after the storm. (Only three children appeared on both occasions.) Can you explain this?

ANSWERS

A1. **c.** This patient has cough variant asthma. Physicians should be aware that cough variant asthma is particularly common in children but can occur, as in this case, in adults as well. The diagnosis is often missed because in many cases there is no wheezing.

A2. **d.** First, it is sometimes difficult to differentiate on the basis of symptoms, signs, and laboratory findings between bronchial asthma and bronchiolitis. Second, a physician may, in fact, make an inappropriate diagnosis of bronchial asthma that may "stick for life." Third, the relationship between bronchiolitis and bronchial asthma is unclear. There is good evidence at this time that bronchiolitis may be a risk factor for bronchial asthma and may predispose to bronchial asthma.

A3. **e.** The current working definition of bronchial asthma is as follows:
   a. A lung disease with airway obstruction that is usually reversible
   b. A lung disease that is characterized by airway inflammation
   c. A lung disease that is characterized by increased bronchial hyperresponsiveness to various stimuli

A4. **a.** The morbidity and mortality from bronchial asthma are increasing, not decreasing. It is associated with staggering health care costs. Last year the estimated direct cost in health expenditure for asthma was approximately $3.4 billion, and the indirect costs were estimated to be another $2.5 billion. These costs are increasing. Despite the vast sums of money invested in both direct and indirect health care for asthma prevention and management, the mortality from asthma continues to rise.

A5. **c.** Our understanding of the pathophysiology of asthma has undergone considerable change in the past few years. This has had a substantial impact on treatment. Asthma is now recognized as an inflammatory disorder. Although bronchoconstriction and bronchial hyperreactivity are characteristics of asthma, the basic underlying pathophysiologic process is inflammation in the bronchial wall.

A6. **b.** See Answer 11.

A7. **e.** See Answer 11.

A8. **e.** See Answer 11.

A9. **e.** See Answer 11.

A10. **b.** See Answer 11.

A11. **e.** Questions 6 to 11 describe the pathophysiology of bronchial asthma. The order of events is as follows:
   Event 1: Beginning of the response of the bronchial wall to the particular antigenic stimulation
   Event 2: Antigenic stimulation leads to mast cell degranulation
   Event 3: Mast cell degranulation leads to:
      a. Immediate release of preformed mediators from granules
      b. Release of secondary mediators, including:
         1) Histamine
         2) Chemotactic factors
         3) Proteolytic enzymes
         4) Heparin
   Event 4: The release of secondary mediators leads to significant smooth muscle bronchoconstriction
   Event 5: The initial bronchial constriction leads to recruitment of other inflammatory cells, including the following:
      a. Neutrophils
      b. Eosinophils
      c. Mononuclear cells
   Event 6: The recruitment of these "secondary mediator cells" has demonstrated the release of the following:
      a. Cytokines
      b. Vasoactive factors
      c. Arachidonic acid metabolites

Event 7: Activation of epithelial and endothelial cells occurs, enhancing inflammatory responses

Event 8: Release of interleukins 3 to 6, tumor necrosis factor, and interferon-γ has been demonstrated in the inflammatory response

Important summary points:

a. Asthma is a chronic inflammatory disorder of the lower airways characterized by episodes of acute symptomatic exacerbations overlying chronic inflammation. Inflammation results in:
1) Increased bronchial hyperresponsiveness to stimuli
2) Reversible airflow obstruction by:
 a) Bronchoconstriction
 b) Mucous plug formation
 c) Edema
b. The early-phase reaction of asthma is mediated by the "primary mediators": Neutrophils, eosinophils, and mononuclear cells
c. The late-phase reaction of asthma is mediated by the "secondary mediators": Cytokines, vasoactive factors, and arachidonic acid metabolites
d. Atopy is a predisposing factor in many patients

A12. **a.** The prophylactic agent of choice for exercise-induced or cold-air–induced bronchial asthma is a β₂-agonist, short-acting form, namely albuterol.

A13. **d.** Albuterol works as a bronchodilator.

A14. **e.** Both prophylactic daily leukotriene modifiers and long-acting β₂-agonists have been used successfully for long-term stabilization of competitive athletes' exercise-induced asthma.

A15. **e.**

A16. **e.**

A17. **d.** The pharmacotherapy for moderate persistent asthma in adults and children age 5 years and older includes the use of a daily medium-dose inhaled corticosteroid and a long-acting inhaled β₂-agonist or sustained-released theophylline, if needed.

A18. **c.**

A19. **e.**

A20. **a.** A peak expiratory flow measuring less than 50% of personal best suggests a severe exacerbation. Initial treatment should include an inhaled short-acting β₂-agonist administered three times via metered dose inhaler or once via nebulizer. If the peak ex-

piratory flow rate remains less than 50% of personal best or wheezing and shortness of breath persist, the patient should repeat the β₂-agonist and proceed to the nearest Emergency Department.

A21. **c.**

A22. **d.** The peak expiratory flow rate is a useful tool for clinician assessment and patient self-assessment of asthma. It is also useful to monitor and change therapy and to diagnose exacerbations. Patients should establish their personal best peak expiratory flow rate. This is established after therapy extinguishes symptoms. The patient records daily, for 2 to 3 weeks, his/her peak expiratory flow rate in the early afternoon with the same meter. An average is obtained. Peak expiratory flow rate should be recalculated every 6 months to account for growth in children or disease progression.

A23. **b.**

A24. **a.** Following is an overview of the clinical findings and their importance in asthma.

a. Physical examination signs and symptoms:
1) Increased respiratory rate
2) Use of accessory muscles of respiration (intercostals, sternocleidomastoid, scalene muscles)
3) Dyspnea and anxiety
4) The most characteristic lung finding on auscultation is expiratory rhonchi (wheezes); rhonchi are high-pitched sounds that occur when air has to travel through a constricted or inflamed passageway
5) Nasal flaring
6) Cyanosis in severe cases (lips)
7) Paroxysmal cough
b. Chest x-ray findings:
1) The most characteristic chest x-ray abnormality in bronchial asthma is the presence of increased bronchial wall markings. This is most prominent when viewed from the end-on position. This finding results from increase in the thickness of the bronchial wall and changes in the epithelium that are associated with inflammation. These changes are translated into increased radiopacity.
2) There is also flattening of the diaphragm in some cases because of chronic inflammation and use of the accessory muscles of respiration.
c. Most useful pulmonary function tests:
1) Peak expiratory flow rate: Discussed above
2) FEV_1/FVC in percentage (normal 80%): This measures the amount of air volume that can be

expressed in 1 second over the total amount of lung air volume that can be expressed. It is by far the most important test done in a spirometry laboratory for the diagnosis and management of bronchial asthma.

3) The maximum expiratory flow that occurs between 25% and 75% of the vital capacity (normal 75%).

A25. **f.**

A26. **d.** The following features of cough variant asthma should be borne in mind:
  a. Cough variant asthma is very common. At least 33% of children with asthma will have only the cough, no wheezing.
  b. Adults, as with the patient described, may also present with cough variant asthma.

A27. **e.** An acute, severe asthmatic attack is an emergency. The basic elements of treatment are as follows:
  a. Agonist via nebulizer-inhaled β_2.
  b. The patient should be sitting up.
  c. Immediately give the patient warm, humidified 100% oxygen via a Venturi mask.
  d. Start two IV lines.
  e. Begin an IV corticosteroid immediately.
  f. Draw blood gases and electrolytes.
  g. Monitor vital signs continuously (with an electrocardiogram hooked into the main computer at the nurses' desk).
  h. Once the patient is stable, transfer him/her to an observation unit ward: if this has been a severe attack and you have had trouble controlling it, do not discharge the patient.

A28. **e.** First, there is a very significant heredity component to bronchial asthma. If one parent has it, the child may have up to a 25% risk. If two parents have it, the child's risk may be up to 50%. Second, there is a very strong association between parental smoking and bronchial asthma in children. Third, many children who have bronchial asthma are allergic to aspirin and other NSAIDs.

Remember that asthma, nasal polyps, and aspirin allergy constitute a recognized triad.

Finally, patients do not "outgrow" asthma. Children who have asthma may experience less severe attacks as adults, or they may never experience problems. However, they have not outgrown it.

A29. **a.** There appears to be a very strong association between respiratory syncytial virus (the main virus-causing bronchiolitis) and asthma. Although it is difficult to say that the relationship is cause and effect, there is enough good evidence to suggest that it might be.

SOLUTION TO THE SHORT ANSWER MANAGEMENT PROBLEM

Indeed, this is a fascinating situation. The town in which the physician practices is, by the way, very small, having a population of only 3200 people. An environmentalist she knew suggested the possibility of ozone production as a side effect of the lightning strikes. In fact, ozone has been shown to be associated with asthma, and it appears that this is the most probable explanation.

SUMMARY OF THE DIAGNOSIS AND TREATMENT OF ASTHMA

1. All that wheezes is not asthma, and all asthma does not wheeze.

2. A moderately severe to a severe attack of asthma is an emergency. Do not discharge the patient unless you are sure that the asthma attack is completely resolved.

3. Asthma is an inflammatory disease.

4. The mortality from asthma is rising, not falling.

5. There is effective prophylaxis for exercise-induced asthma.

6. Cough variant asthma is very common.

7. There is nothing wrong with a short course of oral steroids (prednisone 20 to 30 mg/day) for a severe case of asthma. It works, and it will keep the patient out of the hospital and out of danger.

8. Suggest peak flow meters to all of your asthmatic patients for home monitoring.

9. Stepped care provides a rational rubric for pharmacotherapy.

SUGGESTED READINGS

Barnes PJ: Inhaled glucocorticoids for asthma, *N Engl J Med* 332(13):868-875, 1995.

Bernstein DI: Allergic reactions to workplace allergens, *JAMA* 278(22):1907-1913, 1997.

Chan-Yeung M, Malo JL: Occupational asthma, *N Engl J Med* 333(2):107-112, 1995.

Donahue JG et al: Inhaled steroids and the risk of hospitalization for asthma, *JAMA* 277(11):887-891, 1997.

Drugs for asthma, *Med Lett* 37(939):1-4, 1995.

Fluticasone propionate for chronic asthma, *Med Lett* 38(983):83-84, 1996.

Lemanske RF, Busse WW: Asthma, *JAMA* 278(22):1855-1873, 1997.

National Heart, Lung, and Blood Institute (NIH) Expert Panel Report #2: *Guidelines for the Diagnosis and Management of Asthma*, 1999, http://www.nhlbi.nih.gov.

Weinberger M, Hendeles L: Theophylline in asthma, *N Engl J Med* 334(21):1380-1388, 1996.

Zafirlukast for asthma, *Med Lett* 38(990):111-112, 1996.

Zileuton for asthma, *Med Lett* 39(995):18-19, 1997.

PROBLEM · 11

PNEUMONIA

"You Gave Mrs. Jones a Shot. Why Can't I Have One, Too?"

Case 1 ■ A 24-Year-Old University Student with Pneumonia

A 24-year-old university student comes to the Student Health Service with a 3-day history of a dry hacking cough that was initially nonproductive but has become productive of scant, white sputum. The patient also complains of malaise, headache, fever, muscle aches, and pains. The patient did not have any other upper respiratory tract symptoms before this illness began (no rhinorrhea, no sore throat, and no conjunctivitis).

The patient has had no episodes like this in the past; however, her roommate developed the same symptoms 2 days ago.

On examination, the patient has a temperature of 39° C. You hear a few scattered rales in the left lung base. No other abnormalities are found.

SELECT THE BEST ANSWER TO THE FOLLOWING QUESTIONS

Q1. Which of the following is the most cost-effective strategy at the present time?
  a. order no laboratory tests or imaging investigations; assume that it is viral and will clear up on its own
  b. order no laboratory tests or imaging investigations; treat with ampicillin just to be on the safe side
  c. order the complete work-up, every possible test; no matter what the patient has, you are not the one who is going to get sued
  d. order a chest x-ray on the basis of your clinical findings
  e. forget the tests; just treat her with "big gun therapy"

Q2. What is the most likely diagnosis in this patient?
  a. viral pneumonia
  b. *Mycoplasma pneumoniae* pneumonia
  c. *Streptococcus pneumoniae* pneumonia
  d. *Klebsiella pneumoniae* pneumonia
  e. no pneumonia of any kind; a case of simple acute bronchitis

Q3. If you ordered a chest x-ray, what would be the most likely finding?
  a. nothing (clear and normal)
  b. left lower lobe pneumonia
  c. left lower lobe interstitial pneumonia
  d. bilateral lower lobe infiltrates
  e. bilateral upper lobe infiltrates

Q4. What is the treatment of choice for the patient described in Case 1?
  a. symptomatic treatment only
  b. ribavirin for respiratory syncytial virus
  c. erythromycin (EES)
  d. ampicillin
  e. penicillin G

Case 2 ■ A 55-Year-Old Female Who Takes a Turn for the Worse

A 55-year-old female, previously healthy and recovering from an episode of bronchitis, suddenly develops a "shaking chill" followed by the onset of a high fever (40° C), pleuritic chest pain, and cough productive of purulent, rust-colored sputum.

On examination, the patient appears ill. Her respiratory rate is 30 breaths/min, and chest splinting is heard. Bronchial breath sounds are heard in the left lower lobe. Chest x-ray reveals consolidation present in the left lower lobe.

Q5. On the basis of the history, the physical examination, and the chest x-ray, what is the most likely organism responsible for this patient's illness?
  a. gram-negative bacillus
  b. gram-negative cocci
  c. gram-positive bacillus
  d. gram-positive cocci (lancet-shaped)
  e. no growth on aerobic growth media

Q6. What is the most likely organism responsible for this patient's illness?
  a. *S. pneumoniae*
  b. *K. pneumoniae*
  c. *M. pneumoniae*
  d. influenza A
  e. *Haemophilus influenzae*

Q7. What is the treatment of choice for the patient described in Case 2?
   a. penicillin
   b. ciprofloxacin
   c. gentamicin
   d. cephalexin
   e. a and c

Case 3 ■ A 35-Year-Old Renal Transplant Patient with Fever, Dyspnea, and 2 Days of Diarrhea

A 35-year-old male patient has chronic renal failure. He had a renal transplant 6 months ago and is being treated with corticosteroids and cyclosporine. He came to the Emergency Department 4 days ago with fever, dyspnea, and 2 days of diarrhea. The chest x-ray showed an area of consolidation in the right middle lobe and a diffuse interstitial infiltrate. He has failed to respond to ceftriaxone and continues with a fever and a cough. Today he is lethargic and confused.

Q8. What is the most likely organism causing his pneumonia?
   a. *Pneumocystis carinii*
   b. *Legionella pneumoniae*
   c. *Mycobacterium tuberculosis*
   d. *Mycobacterium avium intracellulare*
   e. *Cytomegalovirus*

Q9. What is the drug of first choice for the patient described in Case 3?
   a. EES
   b. ceftriaxone
   c. ciprofloxacin
   d. trimethoprim-sulfamethoxazole (TMP-SMX)
   e. doxycycline

Case 4 ■ A 75-Year-Old Alcoholic with Fever, Shortness of Breath, Chest Pain, and Cough Productive of Purulent Sputum and Blood

A 75-year-old alcoholic with a history of congestive heart failure is admitted to the hospital suffering from fever, shortness of breath, chest pain, and cough productive of purulent sputum and blood. On physical examination, the patient has a temperature of 39° C, a respiratory rate of 28 breaths/min, and bronchial breath sounds in the right upper lobe.

A chest x-ray confirms the diagnosis of a right upper lobe pneumonia, with a small cavitary lesion.

Q10. What is the most likely organism responsible for this patient's illness?

   a. *S. pneumoniae*
   b. *K. pneumoniae*
   c. *M. pneumoniae*
   d. influenza A
   e. *H. influenzae*

Q11. What is the treatment of choice for the patient described in Case 4?
   a. EES
   b. ceftriaxone and azithromycin
   c. penicillin G
   d. ampicillin
   e. ampicillin and gentamicin

Case 5 ■ A 55-Year-Old Male Smoker with Chronic Obstructive Pulmonary Disease (COPD), High Fever, Chills, Cough, and Shortness of Breath

A 55-year-old male with a 60-pack/year history of smoking and documented COPD comes to your office with a high fever, chills, a productive cough (yellowish green sputum), and shortness of breath. On examination, the patient has decreased breath sounds in the right middle lobe and right lower lobe. You suspect pneumonia.

A chest x-ray confirms right middle lobe and right lower lobe pneumonia. A Gram stain reveals gram-negative rods in abundance.

Q12. Based on his 60-pack/year history of smoking, the Gram stain result, and his history of chronic bronchitis, what is the most likely organism in this patient?
   a. *Moraxella catarrhalis*
   b. *M. pneumoniae*
   c. *H. influenzae*
   d. a or b
   e. a or c

Q13. What is the treatment of choice for this patient?
   a. EES
   b. cefuroxime and azithromycin
   c. penicillin G
   d. ampicillin
   e. ampicillin and gentamicin

Q14. An elderly patient in a long-term care facility develops influenza A pneumonia despite both vaccination and amantadine prophylaxis. What is the organism most likely to complicate influenza pneumonia?
   a. *S. pneumoniae*
   b. *H. influenzae*
   c. *Chlamydia trachomatis*

d. *Chlamydia pneumoniae*
e. *M. pneumoniae*

Q15. What is the most common cause of community-acquired pneumonia?
a. *M. pneumoniae*
b. *H. influenzae*
c. *S. pneumoniae*
d. *Staphylococcus aureus*
e. viral pneumonia

Q16. What is the most common cause of nosocomial pneumonia?
a. *M. pneumoniae*
b. aerobic gram-negative bacteria
c. *S. pneumoniae*
d. *H. influenzae*
e. viral pneumonia

SHORT ANSWER MANAGEMENT PROBLEM
Discuss the characteristics of a satisfactory sputum specimen (satisfactory for Gram stain and for culture).

ANSWERS

A1. **d.**

A2. **b.** This patient most likely has a *Mycoplasma* pneumonia. *M. pneumoniae* is a common respiratory tract pathogen in young adults. The most common respiratory symptom is a dry, hacking, usually nonproductive cough. Systemic symptoms include malaise, headache, and fever. Rash, serous otitis media, and joint symptoms occasionally accompany the respiratory symptoms.

A3. **d.** Physical findings are usually either minimal or unremarkable. Auscultation of the chest usually reveals only scattered rhonchi or fine, localized rales. The chest x-ray, on the other hand, often reveals fine or patchy lower lobe or perihilar infiltrates. The white blood cell (WBC) count is often elevated (10,000 to 15,000/mm^3). Cold agglutinins are nonspecific and found in only 30% to 50% of cases. The diagnosis can be confirmed by acute and convalescent mycoplasma complement fixation or enzyme immunoassay titers.

Clinically and radiographically, pneumonia caused by adenovirus is often difficult to differentiate from a *Mycoplasma* pneumonia. The clinical picture does not fit that of a *Streptococcus* pneumonia, and the patient has no risk factors that should produce a *Klebsiella* pneumonia.

Mycoplasma pneumonia is the favored diagnosis

over viral pneumonia (adenovirus) because of age, the absence of other upper respiratory tract symptoms, the prevalence of a *Mycoplasma* pneumonia in students of colleges and universities, and the disparity of findings on auscultation relative to the findings on chest x-ray.

A4. **c.** Certainly the most reasonable course of action following the history and physical examination is to perform a chest x-ray. The treatment of choice is either EES (or one of the newer macrolides such as azithromycin or clarithromycin) or tetracycline for 10 days.

A5. **d.**

A6. **a.** This patient has a classic history of pneumococcal pneumonia. *S. pneumoniae* (pneumococcus) is the most common cause of bacterial pneumonia in adults.

Pneumococcal pneumonia often presents with a "shaking rigor" (as in this patient), followed by fever, pleuritic chest pain, and cough with purulent or rust-colored sputum. Viral upper or lower respiratory tract infections may precede pneumococcal pneumonia.

In elderly or debilitated patients the presentation may be atypical. Fever may be low grade, behavior disturbances may seem more significant than respiratory symptoms, and cough may not be prominent. Patients appear acutely ill, frequently with dyspnea and chest splinting. Signs of consolidation are frequently present.

An elevated WBC count with left shift is common. Chest x-ray usually shows disease confined to one lobe (frequently a lower lobe), but several lobes may be involved with either consolidation or bronchopneumonia. Gram stain of the sputum shows polymorphonuclear leukocytes and lancet-shaped gram-positive diplococci.

Sputum cultures should be obtained, but up to 40% of patients with bacteremic pneumococcal pneumonia have negative sputum cultures. Therefore blood cultures should be obtained in these patients.

A7. **a.** The treatment of choice for a *Streptococcus* pneumonia is penicillin G. However, there has been a significant increase in resistance to penicillin among the pneumococci, with reported rates of resistance as high as 36%. For that reason, many authorities recommend initial treatment with a cephalosporin (such as ceftriaxone) or a new-generation quinolone (such as levofloxacin) until the sensitivity test results are available. Ciprofloxacin should not be used because of its poor activity against *S. pneumoniae*. Because it is impossible to exclude *Legionella* given these clinical findings, a macrolide should be added to the cephalosporin, or the quinolone could be used alone. With the patient's clinical picture including a respiratory rate of 30 breaths/min and chest splinting, hospitalization with intravenous therapy is indicated.

A8. **b.** The combination of a pneumonia in an immunocompromised host and failure to respond to standard antibiotics such as ceftriaxone points to the diagnosis of *Legionella*.

A9. **a.** *Legionella* is best treated by EES with or without rifampin. Second-line choices include azithromycin, clarithromycin, quinolones (ciprofloxacin or levofloxacin), doxycycline with or without rifampin, or TMP-SMX.

A10. **b.** The most likely cause of pneumonia in an elderly, debilitated alcoholic is *S. pneumoniae*, but you would also be concerned about a gram-negative organism and most commonly in alcoholics the organism *K. pneumoniae*, which is frequently seen in nosocomial pneumonias.

Although the presentation may be similar to pneumococcal pneumonia, the upper lobes are more frequently involved than the lower lobes. Sudden onset is common. Pleuritic chest pain and hemoptysis are common features. Sputum is thick and often bloody. Since this is a necrotizing pneumonia, cavitary lesions may be found, which do not occur with *S. pneumoniae*. Other important causes of pneumonia in elderly patients include other gram-negative organisms such as *Escherichia coli*, *H. influenzae*, and gram-positive organisms such as *S. pneumoniae* and *S. aureus*.

A11. **b.** The treatment of first choice for this patient is the cephalosporin cefuroxime (or ceftriaxone) and azithromycin. This drug combination is effective against all the pathogens listed. An alternative is to use one of the newer quinolones (such as levofloxacin) alone.

A12. **e.** In a patient with a pneumonia complicating chronic bronchitis, likely organisms include *H. influenzae* and *M. catarrhalis*.

A13. **b.** The treatment of choice is the same as for the patient in Case 4: a cephalosporin (such as cefuroxime or ceftriaxone) and a new macrolide (such as azithromycin [Zithromax] or clarithromycin [Biaxin]).

A14. **a.** The most likely organism to complicate influenza pneumonia is *S. pneumoniae*.

A15. **c.** The most common cause of community-acquired pneumonia is *S. pneumoniae*.

A16. **b.** The most common cause of nosocomial pneumonia is aerobic gram-negative bacteria, although recent studies have shown that *S. aureus* now occurs with almost equal frequency.

SOLUTION TO THE SHORT ANSWER MANAGEMENT PROBLEM

Sputum cytology is essential to make an accurate diagnosis of pneumonia. Saliva or nasopharyngeal secretions are of little value in determining the cause of pneumonia because colonization with gram-negative bacilli and other organisms is frequent.

If more than 25 squamous epithelial cells are seen per low-power field (LPF), the specimen is considered inadequate for culture. The ideal sputum specimen contains fewer than 10 squamous epithelial cells per LPF and many polymorphonuclear leukocytes.

SUMMARY OF THE DIAGNOSIS AND MANAGEMENT OF PNEUMONIA IN ADULTS

1. Community-acquired pneumonia: In all age groups the most common cause is *S. pneumoniae*. Another common cause is *C. pneumoniae*, which causes around 15% of all pneumonias. Certain risk factors (e.g., age, underlying illness) can suggest other possible causes.

2. Young adults with *Mycoplasma* pneumonia:
   a. *Mycoplasma* pneumonia is common. In *Mycoplasma* pneumonia, there is often a difference between the signs and symptoms as elicited on history and physical examination and the findings on chest x-ray.
   b. Diagnostic clues to *Mycoplasma* pneumonia are a harsh, nonproductive, constant cough with little evidence of the shaking chills and high fever seen in streptococcal pneumonia. The major differential diagnosis is adenoviral pneumonia.

3. Middle-aged adults with COPD:
   a. *H. influenzae*: *H. influenzae* pneumonia is a common pneumonia complicating COPD.
   b. Another common cause is *M. catarrhalis*, which is seen primarily in patients with underlying cardiopulmonary disease.

4. Immunocompromised individuals or individuals with COPD who fail to respond to conventional therapy: Suspect *Legionella* pneumonia. The signs

and symptom of *Legionella* pneumonia include the following:
a. Malaise
b. Headache
c. Myalgia
d. Weakness
e. Fever and intermittent rigors 24 hours after malaise, headache, myalgia, and weakness
f. Nonproductive or minimally productive cough
g. Scant hemoptysis and pleuritic chest pain are common

5. Elderly patients with immune compromise secondary to alcohol: Suspect *K. pneumoniae. Klebsiella* pneumonia has much the same signs and symptoms as other bacterial pneumonias (see the following section).

6. Bacterial versus viral pneumonia:
a. Bacterial pneumonia: Fever, chills (sudden onset of shaking chills in pneumococcal pneumonia), pleuritic chest pain, productive cough, purulent sputum, tachycardia, tachypnea, bronchial breath sounds.
b. Viral pneumonia: Gradual onset, general malaise, headache, prominent cough (often nonproductive), sometimes few abnormalities on examination of the lungs (auscultation). Chest x-ray findings are more prominent.
c. *Mycoplasma* pneumonia: As in viral pneumonia, except cough can be almost constant, harsh, nonproductive, and irritative.

7. Treatment:
a. For patients with community-acquired pneumonia who do not require hospital admission, the treatment of choice is either a macrolide (EES, azithromycin, or clarithromycin) or one of the newer quinolones (such as levofloxacin).
b. For patients who require hospital admission, the treatment of choice is either a cephalosporin (such as cefuroxime or ceftriaxone) and a macrolide (EES or azithromycin) or one of the newer quinolones (levofloxacin) alone.

8. Prevention:
a. Pneumococcal vaccine: All patients at high risk
b. Influenza vaccine (annually): All patients and health care workers at high risk

SUGGESTED READINGS

Bartlett JG et al: Community-acquired pneumonia in adults: Guidelines for management, *Clin Infect Dis* 26:811-838, 1998.
Fauci AL et al, eds: *Harrison's principles of internal medicine,* ed 14, New York, 1998, McGraw-Hill.

PROBLEM · 12

ESOPHAGEAL MOTILITY DISORDER

"It Is My Heart, Isn't It?"

Case 1 ■ A 53-Year-Old Male with Burning Substernal and Retrosternal Pain

A 53-year-old male comes to your office with a 3-month history of intermittent burning substernal and retrosternal pain radiating to his neck. The burning is usually relieved quickly with antacids. There is no relationship of these symptoms to exercise or exertion.

On physical examination, his blood pressure is 140/85 mm Hg and his pulse is 96 bpm and regular. His heart sounds are normal. His lungs are clear. His abdomen is soft; no masses and no tenderness are felt.

SELECT THE BEST ANSWER TO THE FOLLOWING QUESTIONS

Q1. Which of the following must be considered in the differential diagnosis of this patient's problem?
a. acid reflux disease
b. myocardial ischemia
c. peptic ulcer disease
d. panic disorder
e. a, b, and c only
f. all of the above

Q2. Given the history and physical examination, which one of the following conditions is the most likely diagnosis?
a. acid reflux disease
b. peptic ulcer disease
c. myocardial ischemia
d. panic disorder
e. it is difficult to say

Q3. What is the major pathophysiologic mechanism involved in the condition described?
a. transient relaxation of the lower esophageal sphincter
b. decreased resting pressure of the lower esophageal sphincter
c. coronary artery thrombosis
d. excess production of hydrogen ions (H^+) in the stomach
e. decreased levels of serotonin in the brain

Q4. At this time, what would you do?
a. send the patient as soon as possible to a psychiatrist and end the consultation

b. obtain an electrocardiogram (ECG)

c. perform an ECG and, if normal, prescribe definitive therapy

d. perform an ECG and serial creatine phosphokinase enzyme levels

e. call the cardiologist and have a thrombolytic agent injected as quickly as possible

Q5. What are the drugs of first and second choice (in order) in this patient?

a. calcium carbonate (Tums) and Maalox

b. streptokinase and heparin

c. imipramine and fluoxetine

d. an H2 receptor blocker and omeprazole

e. omeprazole and an H2 receptor blocker

Q6. What is the most common cause of dysphagia?

a. achalasia

b. esophageal spasm

c. a lower esophageal ring (Schatzki ring)

d. nonspecific motor disorders

e. an esophageal stricture

Q7. What is malignant dysphagia usually related to?

a. a squamous cell carcinoma related to Barrett's esophagus

b. an adenocarcinoma related to Barrett's esophagus

c. a squamous cell carcinoma unrelated to Barrett's esophagus

d. an adenocarcinoma unrelated to Barrett's esophagus

e. none of the above

Q8. What is the drug of choice in the treatment of achalasia?

a. a nitroglycerin derivative

b. a calcium channel blocker

c. a benzodiazepine

d. an antacid

e. any of the above

Q9. Achalasia is characterized by which of the following?

a. transient relaxation of the lower esophageal sphincter

b. decreased resting pressure of the lower esophageal sphincter

c. abnormal production of H^+ in the stomach leading to acid-induced damage in the lower and middle esophagus

d. loss of peristalsis and relaxation of the lower esophageal sphincter

e. none of the above

Q10. Esophageal spasm is best characterized by which of the following?

a. a loss of peristalsis and relaxation of the lower esophageal sphincter

b. increased resting pressure of the lower esophageal sphincter

c. an increased percentage of simultaneous waves with some discoordinated peristalsis

d. transient contraction of the lower esophageal sphincter

e. none of the above

SHORT ANSWER MANAGEMENT PROBLEM
Provide:
1. A differential diagnosis of the common causes of dysphagia
2. The definition of each
3. The treatment of each
(This will serve as the summary of the diagnosis and treatment of dysphagia.)

ANSWERS

A1. **e.** The differential diagnosis in this patient lies between:

a. Acid reflux disease (or heartburn)

b. Peptic ulcer disease with associated acid reflux disease

c. Esophageal motility disorders

d. Myocardial ischemia, injury, or infarction

A2. **a.** The most likely diagnosis is acid reflux disease. Although it is often difficult to differentiate acid reflux disease from myocardial ischemia, there are two clues in this patient that point to acid reflux disease:

a. No relationship of the symptoms to exercise

b. Relief of the symptoms quickly with the administration of calcium carbonate

Esophageal motility disease is subdivided into achalasia, esophageal spasm, nonspecific motor disorders, and systemic sclerosis. The two most common disorders are achalasia and esophageal spasm. The pain of esophageal motility disease is much more likely to produce a spasmodic type of pain rather than a heartburnlike type of pain.

Although chest discomfort is often present in panic disorder, the absence of other symptoms makes the diagnosis unlikely.

A3. **a.** For many years, it has been assumed that decreased pressure in the lower esophageal sphincter was the primary determinant of acid reflux. It is now recognized, however, that transient relaxation as opposed to decreased pressure of the lower esophageal sphincter is the most important determinant of reflux.

A4. **c.**

A5. **d.** At this time you should:
   a. Perform an ECG to rule out myocardial ischemia or injury.
   b. Prescribe a mixture of (1) magnesium and aluminum hydroxide and (2) viscous lidocaine (known as the "pink lady") as an acute diagnostic and therapeutic test.
   c. Prescribe an H2 receptor blocker such as cimetidine or ranitidine. Omeprazole may also be considered as a therapeutic alternative.

   If after a few weeks the therapy is ineffective, endoscopy should be considered.

   Cisapride (a prokinetic motility agent) is now the drug of choice to prevent relapse of the disorder.

A6. **c.** The most common cause of dysphagia is an esophageal, or Schatzki, ring at the border of the esophagus and stomach. It is almost always associated with a hiatal hernia because the ring is just proximal to the hernia. Most commonly the dysphagia is intermittent and applies to solid foods only. Once the diagnosis is confirmed by radiographic or endoscopic means (or both), the treatment of choice is rupture of the ring by dilatation.

A7. **b.** Malignant dysphagia is usually related to squamous cell carcinoma or adenocarcinoma, the latter of which is often secondary to Barrett's esophagus. Barrett's esophagus is an acquired metaphasia that replaces the normal squamous epithelium of the distal esophagus. The change is thought to be induced by chronic gastroesophageal reflux and is of major clinical significance because of its unequivocal association with adenocarcinoma. Adenocarcinoma of the esophagus is found in 10% of patients with Barrett's esophagus at first endoscopic examination.

A8. **b.**

A9. **d.** Achalasia is characterized by a loss of normal peristalsis and by relaxation of the lower esophageal sphincter in response to swallowing. All treatments are designed to reduce the functional obstruction of the sphincter.

   The treatment of first choice is a calcium channel blocker, especially nifedipine. This agent reduces the resting lower esophageal sphincter pressure. The usual recommendation is to bite a 10-mg nifedipine capsule and then swallow the capsule (approximately 30 minutes before meals).

   Most patients with achalasia should undergo pneumatic dilatation of the esophagus. Various dilators have been used, including the Microvasive Rigiflex achalasia dilator.

A10. **c.** Esophageal spasm is a disorder in which there is an increased percentage of simultaneous waves, with some preserved peristalsis. No drug has been found to be effective. However, sublingual or oral nitrates, sublingual or oral anxiolytics, and calcium channel blockers have been used with some success. The other treatment that appears to many experts to be the treatment of choice is dilatation of the esophagus with a bougienage.

SOLUTION TO THE SHORT ANSWER MANAGEMENT PROBLEM AND SUMMARY

A differential diagnosis of the common causes of dysphagia is as follows:
1. Achalasia: Characterized by the loss of peristalsis and constriction of the lower esophageal sphincter
   a. Diagnosis:
      1) Esophageal manometry: Measures intraluminal pressure, pH, and transit time
      2) Pneumatic dilatation of the esophagus with the Microvasive Rigiflex achalasia dilator
   b. Treatment: Nifedipine (sublingual)
2. Esophageal spasm: A disorder in which there is an increased percentage of simultaneous waves with some preserved peristalsis
   a. Diagnosis:
      1) Esophageal manometry
      2) Treatment with bougienage
   b. Treatment:
      1) Calcium channel blockers
      2) Nitrates
      3) Anxiolytics
3. Systemic sclerosis: Characterized by progressive muscle atrophy and fibrosis, leading to loss of peristalsis as well as reduction of sphincter pressure
   a. Potential complications: May lead to substantial gastroesophageal reflux disease and its complications.
   b. Treatment:
      1) Chew food well and drink adequate liquids with food.
      2) Use H2 receptor blockers or proton pump inhibitors.
4. Mechanical obstruction: Esophageal rings—constriction of the lower esophageal sphincter that leads to dysphagia for solids only; almost always associated with a hiatal hernia. Because of the pathophysiology, the dysphagia is intermittent and for solid food only.
   a. Diagnosis: Confirmation of diagnosis by barium swallow or endoscopy
   b. Treatment of choice: Dilatation of the ring
5. Mechanical obstruction: Esophageal stricture—narrowing in one or more parts of the esophagus,

most often caused by ingestion of toxic liquids or solids
  a. Diagnosis: Barium swallow or endoscopy
  b. Treatment of choice: Progressive dilatation
6. Neoplasms, malignant:
  a. Adenocarcinoma of the esophagus is the most common cancer. It usually occurs secondary to Barrett's esophagus.
  b. Squamous cell carcinoma can also occur.
    1) Diagnosis: Endoscopy with biopsy is preferable.
    2) Treatment: Surgical resection is the procedure of choice. Radiotherapy can be used for palliation.
7. Gastroesophageal reflux: A transient relaxation of the lower esophageal sphincter
  a. Diagnosis:
    1) Therapeutic challenge: Magnesium and aluminum hydroxide and viscous lidocaine; if symptoms improve, the diagnosis is probable
    2) Endoscopy to rule out Barrett's esophagus in chronic reflux
  b. Treatment:
    1) H2 blockers and omeprazole (in that order)
    2) Cisapride (motility prokinetic agent) considered as long-term prophylactic therapy.
8. Miscellaneous disorders:
  a. Acquired immunodeficiency syndrome (AIDS) candidal esophagitis
  b. AIDS herpes simplex esophagitis
  c. Acute obstruction and foreign body (especially in children)
  d. Cerebrovascular accidents and other neurologic disorders

SUGGESTED READING

Traube M: Dysphagia and esophageal obstruction. In Rakel R, ed: *Conn's current therapy*, Philadelphia, 1995, WB Saunders.

PROBLEM·13

INFLAMMATORY BOWEL DISEASE

"I Must Have Picked Up a Bug; It's Tearing My Gut Out!"

Case 1 ■ A 32-Year-Old Female with Fever, Weight Loss, and Chronic Diarrhea

A 32-year-old female comes to your office with a 6-month history of loose bowel movements, approximately eight per day. Blood has been present in many of them. She has lost 30 pounds. For the past 6 weeks she has had an intermittent fever. She has had no previous gastrointestinal (GI) problems, nor is there any family history of GI problems.

On examination, the patient looks ill. Her blood pressure is 130/70 mm Hg. Her pulse is 108 bpm and regular. There is generalized abdominal tenderness with no rebound. A sigmoidoscopy reveals a friable rectal mucosa with multiple bleeding points.

SELECT THE BEST ANSWER TO THE FOLLOWING QUESTIONS

Q1. What is the most likely diagnosis in this patient?
  a. irritable bowel syndrome
  b. Crohn's disease
  c. ulcerative colitis
  d. Crohn's colitis
  e. bacterial dysentery

Q2. The investigations at this time should include which of the following?
  a. colonoscopy
  b. barium enema
  c. upper GI series and follow-through
  d. a and c
  e. all of the above

Q3. Which of the following may be indicated in the management of the acute phase of the condition described?
  a. steroid enemas
  b. oral corticosteroids
  c. parenteral corticosteroids
  d. a and b
  e. all of the above

Q4. Which of the following statements regarding the use of sulfasalazine in the condition described is false?
  a. sulfasalazine is structurally related to both aspirin and to sulfa drugs
  b. sulfasalazine is effective in maintaining remission in this condition as well as in the acute treatment of mild disease
  c. sulfasalazine may impair folic acid metabolism
  d. all of the above are false
  e. none of the above statements is false

Q5. Which of the following statements regarding the long-term prognosis of the patient described in Case 1 is false?
  a. after an initial attack, 10% of patients go into remission lasting up to 15 years
  b. after an initial attack, 75/% of patients experience intermittent exacerbations for many years

c. after an initial attack, 10% of patients continue to have active disease until surgical intervention is undertaken

d. after an initial attack, 5% of patients die within a year

e. none of the above is false

Q6. Which of the following is a (are) complication(s) of the disease described?
a. toxic megacolon
b. colonic cancer
c. colonic strictures
d. iritis
e. a, b, and c
f. all of the above

Case 2 ■ A 25-Year-Old Male with an 18-Month History of Chronic Abdominal Pain

A 25-year-old male comes to your office with an 18-month history of chronic abdominal pain. The patient has seen several physicians and has been diagnosed as having a "nervous stomach," irritable bowel syndrome, and "depression." Associated with this abdominal pain for the last 3 months has been nonbloody diarrhea, anorexia, and a weight loss of 20 pounds. He has developed a painful area around the anus.

On examination, the patient has diffuse abdominal tenderness. He looks thin and unwell. He has a tender, erythematous area in the right perirectal area.

Q7. What is the most likely diagnosis?
a. irritable bowel syndrome
b. Crohn's disease
c. ulcerative colitis
d. bacterial dysentery
e. amebiasis

Q8. Pathologically, what is the difference between the patient in Case 2 and the patient in Case 1?
a. inflammation in Case 2 involves all layers of the bowel; Case 1 involves only the mucosa
b. inflammation in Case 1 involves all layers of the bowel; Case 2 involves only the mucosa
c. inflammation in Case 1 involves the first two layers of the bowel (mucosa and submucosa); Case 2 involves only the mucosa
d. inflammation in Case 2 involves the first two layers of the bowel (mucosa and submucosa); Case 1 involves only the mucosa
e. the two diseases are identical on a pathophysiologic basis

Q9. Which of the following investigations is the most sensitive test for confirming the diagnosis in this patient?
a. sigmoidoscopy
b. colonoscopy
c. barium enema
d. Computed tomography (CT) scan of the abdomen
e. Magnetic resonance imaging (MRI) scan of the abdomen

Q10. Which of the following drugs is the most appropriate initial therapy in the acute phase of the condition described in Case 2?
a. prednisone
b. sulfasalazine
c. metronidazole
d. 6-mercaptopurine
e. azathioprine

Q11. Sulfasalazine is effective in which of the following subtypes of Crohn's disease?
a. Crohn's colitis
b. Crohn's ileocolitis
c. Crohn's disease of the small bowel
d. a and b
e. all of the above

Q12. Which of the following is (are) associated with Crohn's disease?
a. skip lesions on x-ray
b. thumbprinting on x-ray
c. ineffective surgical treatment
d. none of the above
e. a, b, and c

Q13. Which of the following statements regarding complications of the condition described in Case 2 is false?
a. rectal fissures, rectocutaneous fistulas, and perirectal abscesses are common complications of this condition
b. arthritis is sometimes seen as a complication of this condition
c. erythema nodosum and pyoderma gangrenosum are sometimes found with this condition
d. patients with this condition are not at increased risk of colorectal cancer
e. none of the above statements is false

Case 3 ■ A 31-Year-Old Female with a 6-Month History of Gastrointestinal Complaints

A 31-year-old female comes to your office with a 6-month history of GI complaints that include abdominal distention, excessive flatus, foul-smelling stools, weight loss, and nonspecific complaints of weakness and fatigue. The patient describes the symptoms as being especially severe after the intake of cereal grains and bread of any kind.

The patient has not traveled to any specific area in the recent past. She has not left the country.

Examination of the patient reveals that she is in semiacute distress. She is thin and looks anemic.

Q14. On the basis of this information, what is the most likely diagnosis in this patient?
a. lactase deficiency
b. acute pancreatitis
c. celiac sprue
d. tropical sprue
e. bacterial overgrowth syndrome

Q15. What is the pathophysiology of this disease?
a. an immunologic disorder of the small bowel mucosa
b. a disaccharide deficiency of the small intestinal mucosa
c. a deficiency of pancreatic exocrine
d. secondary contamination of the small intestine by coliform bacteria
e. none of the above

Case 4 ■ A 15-Year-Old Female with a 1-Month History of Abdominal Cramping, Abdominal Bloating, and Increased Flatulence

A 15-year-old female comes to your office with a 1-month history of abdominal cramping, abdominal bloating, and increased flatulence after the ingestion of milk or milk products. The patient drank three glasses of milk 2 hours ago.

On examination, the abdomen is tympanic and appears to be slightly distended. No other abnormalities are found on examination.

Q16. What is the most likely diagnosis in this patient?
a. tropical sprue
b. celiac sprue
c. lactase deficiency
d. regional enteritis
e. chronic pancreatitis

SHORT ANSWER MANAGEMENT PROBLEM
Discuss the relationship between inflammatory bowel disease (ulcerative colitis and Crohn's disease) and the risk of acquiring carcinoma of the colon.

ANSWERS

A1. **c.** This patient almost certainly has ulcerative colitis. Ulcerative colitis usually presents with the following:
a. Abdominal pain
b. Diarrhea
c. Passage of blood via the rectum
d. Tenesmus
e. Fever
f. Chills
g. Malaise and fatigue
h. Weight loss
Sigmoidoscopy usually reveals friability (with easy bleeding) and granularity.

Crohn's disease (regional enteritis) is usually not associated with rectal bleeding, although it may be. Crohn's disease will be discussed in Answer 8 below.

Bacterial dysentery would not be as long-lasting as this illness.

Irritable bowel syndrome is a diagnosis of exclusion and does not present with systemic symptoms.

A2. **a.** Barium enema or colonoscopy may be performed in this patient. However, colonoscopy is preferable because it identifies the extent of disease and at the same time allows biopsies to be taken. Sigmoidoscopy has already been done. Findings in ulcerative colitis include the following:
a. Loss of haustral pattern
b. Foreshortening of the colon in certain places
c. The presence of gross ulcers at the mucosal margin

Although the rectum and the distal colon are the most common sites of involvement, patients with more severe disease may have involvement of the entire colon.

A GI series and follow-through would not add any useful information to the investigation of a patient strongly suspected of having ulcerative colitis.

A3. **e.** The initial therapy of ulcerative colitis depends on the severity of the disease and the site of the disease.
a. Mild to moderate disease:
1) Sulfasalazine remains the initial therapy of choice in the treatment of patients with mild to moderate disease and in the maintenance of remission.
2) Mesalamine and olsalazine may be used as the drugs of first choice in some patients. In addition, mesalamine can be given in an enema preparation or suppository and achieves a high local concentration.
b. Moderate to severe disease:
1) Corticosteroids remain the cornerstone of management of patients with acute ulcerative

colitis. They are not, however, efficacious in the maintenance of remission.

2) Topical corticosteroids: Local corticosteroid therapy may be useful in the treatment of patients with active left-sided disease. Corticosteroids can be given as a retention enema, hydrocortisone 100 mg once or twice daily.

3) Oral corticosteroids: For moderate to severe acute ulcerative colitis, oral corticosteroids are indicated. They are usually given as prednisone in the range of 20 to 60 mg/day as a single oral dose for 2 to 4 weeks. When the relief of symptoms has been attained, the dose can be tapered gradually.

4) Parenteral corticosteroids: IV corticosteroids should be considered in patients with severe to fulminant ulcerative colitis. These patients are usually severely ill and require hospitalization. They also need to be closely monitored for the development of toxic megacolon and silent perforation.

5) Refractory ulcerative colitis: The purine analogues, azathioprine (Imuran) and 6-mercaptopurine, have corticosteroid-sparing effects and may be useful in the induction and maintenance of remission in patients with refractory ulcerative colitis.

6) Cyclosporine: A preliminary report suggests that this drug, an immunosuppressant that acts by inhibiting the production of cytokine by helper T cells, may have a role in patients who have very severe disease refractory to IV corticosteroids.

7) Methotrexate: This, along with other immunosuppressive agents, has been used in the treatment of ulcerative colitis. Data are limited regarding control trials that have shown evidence of disease remission.

A4. **e.** Sulfasalazine has a proven efficacy in the management of patients with ulcerative colitis. It is the therapy of choice in the treatment of patients with mild to moderately severe active disease as well as for the maintenance of remission in patients with established ulcerative colitis.

Sulfasalazine is structurally related both to aspirin and to sulfa drugs. It inhibits folic acid, and patients taking it thus need a supplement of at least 1 mg of folic acid per day.

A5. **e.** All of the statements are true. Following an initial attack of ulcerative colitis, 10% of patients go into remission lasting up to 15 years. Of patients, 75% have intermittent exacerbation, 10% have continually active disease, and 5% die within 1 year of the initial attack.

Of all the patients with ulcerative colitis of any severity, 25% will undergo total proctocolectomy within 5 years of the first attack. The risk of colonic cancer increases with time. By 15 years after the initial diagnosis, patients with colonic disease are at a risk significant enough to consider prophylactic hemicolectomy.

A6. **f.** Complications of ulcerative colitis include the following:
   a. Toxic megacolon
   b. Perforation
   c. Colorectal carcinoma
   d. Colonic stricture
   e. Hemorrhage
Extracolonic complications include the following:
   a. Skin disease: Erythema nodosum and pyoderma gangrenosum
   b. Aphthous ulcers
   c. Iritis
   d. Arthritis
   e. Hepatic disease

A7. **b.** This patient has Crohn's disease (regional enteritis).

A8. **a.** Pathologically, Crohn's disease involves an inflammation of all layers of the bowel, in contradistinction to ulcerative colitis, which involves just the mucosa.

Associated anorectal complications include the following:
   a. Fistulas
   b. Fissures
   c. Perirectal abscesses
The peak incidence of Crohn's disease is at age 30 years; most cases occur between ages 20 and 40 years. Crohn's disease may follow an indolent course, resulting in diagnostic delay. The signs and symptoms include the following:
   a. Mild chronic abdominal pain
   b. Mild nonbloody diarrhea
   c. Anorexia
   d. Weight loss
   e. Fatigue
Pain is often confined to the lower abdomen and is "aching" or "cramping." A misdiagnosis of irritable bowel syndrome is often made.

A9. **c.** An air-contrast barium enema is the most important single diagnostic procedure in the confirmation of the diagnosis of Crohn's disease in this patient. Crohn's disease often presents as segmental involvement of two or more colonic areas; between these areas the colon is normal. The transmural involvement is often suggested by radiologic features including the protrusion of a defect into the lumen (thumbprinting).

Sigmoidoscopy will miss Crohn's disease in 30% to 50% of patients. Colonoscopy is more sensitive than sigmoidoscopy but will not show the transmural involvement.

CT and MRI scans are not commonly employed in Crohn's disease.

A10. **a.** The drug of choice for the induction of remission in patients with Crohn's disease is prednisone. The initial dose is between 20 and 40 mg/day. As in ulcerative colitis, this dosage can often be tapered after a few weeks of therapy. Metronidazole, azathioprine, and 6-mercaptopurine are used when prednisone is not effective or is contraindicated. The use of sulfasalazine is discussed in Answer 11. Infliximab (Remicade), a monoclonal antibody that inhibits tumor necrosis factor, is effective as an IV therapy in moderate to severe refractory cases.

A11. **d.** Sulfasalazine is effective in the management of Crohn's colitis and Crohn's ileocolitis. It is not, however, effective in the treatment of Crohn's disease of the small bowel.

A12. **e.** Radiographic manifestations of Crohn's disease include skip lesions on x-ray (normal and abnormal alternating sections of bowel) and thumbprinting. In addition, surgical treatment appears to be relatively ineffective. If an area of bowel affected by Crohn's disease is removed, the disease often recurs in other unaffected segments.

A13. **d.** Rectal fissures, rectocutaneous fistulas, or perirectal abscesses occur in up to 50% of patients with Crohn's disease at some time during their illness. Extracolonic manifestations of Crohn's disease occur in 10% of patients with the disease. These include arthritis (which in fact may precede the GI symptoms), iritis, erythema nodosum, pyoderma gangrenosum, and aphthous ulcers.

The risk of colorectal cancer is less in patients with Crohn's disease than in patients with ulcerative colitis. Patients who have had the disease for more than 15 years are still, however, at increased risk of a malignancy.

A14. **c.** This patient has celiac sprue (gluten enteropathy).

A15. **a.** Gluten enteropathy is an immunologic disorder of the small bowel observed in both children and adults. Exposure of the small intestine to antigenic components of certain cereal grains in susceptible persons causes subtotal or total villous atrophy with reactive crypt hyperplasia.

Common GI complaints include the following:
a. Abdominal distention
b. Excessive flatus
c. Large, bulky, foul-smelling stools
d. Weight loss

Other nonspecific complaints that commonly occur are weakness or fatigue. Patients may have anemia, either an iron deficiency anemia or a megaloblastic anemia (folic acid deficiency). Other patients suffer from deficiency of a fat-soluble vitamin or vitamin B_{12}.

Therapy consists of a gluten-free diet (avoiding any products containing wheat, rye, barley, or oats). Cereals such as corn, rice, buckwheat, sorghum, and millet are not pathogenic and may be substituted. Clinical improvement is generally seen after several days on a gluten-free diet. Restoration of normal histologic architecture takes weeks to months.

A16. **c.** This patient has a lactase deficiency in the small intestine. Thus symptoms characteristic of malabsorption (i.e., bloating, diarrhea, crampy abdominal pain, and foul-smelling stools) occur when milk or milk products are ingested. The treatment of choice for these patients is replacement of the deficient enzyme with an enzyme supplement such as Lactaid tablets and/or replacement of lactose-rich dairy products with low-lactose products, such as yogurt, lactose-reduced milk, and most hard (fermented) cheeses.

SOLUTION TO THE SHORT ANSWER MANAGEMENT PROBLEM

Inflammatory bowel disease, which includes ulcerative colitis and Crohn's disease, is directly related to the risk of acquiring carcinoma of the colon. The risk is related to the following:
1. Disease: Ulcerative colitis has a greater risk than Crohn's disease.
2. Severity of the disease: The more severe the disease, the greater is the risk of carcinoma of the colon.
3. The length of the disease: The longer the patient has had the disease, the greater the risk.
4. The site of the disease: The risk of cancer of the colon is much higher in patients who have ulcerative colitis than in those with ulcerative proctitis.

Patients with ulcerative proctitis, ulcerative colitis, and Crohn's colitis should be screened by endoscopy (colonoscopy) every 1 to 2 years depending on the factors just listed. For ulcerative colitis the screening process may indicate the appropriate time for a prophylactic hemicolectomy (average 15 years since disease onset).

SUMMARY OF THE DIAGNOSIS AND TREATMENT OF INFLAMMATORY BOWEL DISEASE

1. Ulcerative colitis:
   a. Pathophysiology involves the mucosa only.
   b. Local symptoms include the following:
      1) Diarrhea (bloody)
      2) Mucus from the rectum
      3) Tenesmus
      4) Constipation (may alternate with diarrhea)
      5) Abdominal pain
   c. Complications such as toxic megacolon and perforation are uncommon.
   d. Systemic symptoms include fever, chills, anorexia, weight loss, malaise, fatigue, erythema nodosum, pyoderma gangrenosum, aphthous ulcers, iritis, arthritis, and hepatic disease.
   e. Investigations include sigmoidoscopy, colonoscopy, and air-contrast barium enema. If there is danger of perforation (megacolon), barium enema is contraindicated.
   f. Treatment of acute disease:
      1) Mild disease: Sulfasalazine or mesalamine
      2) Local disease (proctitis): Hydrocortisone enemas
      3) Moderate to severe disease: Oral corticosteroids (prednisone 40 to 60 mg/day), parenteral corticosteroids, azathioprine, 6-mercaptopurine
      4) Nutritional support: Total parenteral nutrition may be necessary for some very ill patients
   g. Treatment for maintenance of remission:
      1) Sulfasalazine
      2) Mesalamine

2. Crohn's disease:
   a. Pathophysiology: Involves all layers of the bowel wall
   b. Local symptoms: Abdominal pain, nonbloody diarrhea, mucus from the rectum
   c. Systemic symptoms: Fever, chills, anorexia, malaise, fatigue, weight loss, erythema nodosum, pyoderma gangrenosum, aphthous ulcers, arthritis, and iritis
   d. Other features: Rectal fistulas, rectal fissures, and perirectal abscesses
   e. Investigations: Barium enema and GI series and follow-through
   f. Treatment of acute disease:
      1) Oral corticosteroids (prednisone 20 to 40 mg/day)
      2) Azathioprine, 6-mercaptopurine
      3) Nutritional support with total parenteral nutrition in severe cases

      4) Metronidazole or IV infliximab when other treatments are ineffective
   g. Treatment to maintain remissions:
      1) Sulfasalazine and mesalamine are useful for Crohn's colitis and Crohn's ileocolitis only, not for Crohn's disease of the small bowel
      2) Metronidazole
      3) Surgery: Results are disappointing; when the diseased area is removed, other areas assume disease profile

3. Other diseases that may resemble inflammatory bowel disease:
   a. Celiac sprue:
      1) Pathophysiology: Gluten-sensitive enteropathy. It is an immunologic reaction of the small bowel wall that causes villous atrophy and crypt hyperplasia.
      2) Symptoms: Bloating, diarrhea, foul-smelling stools, and weight loss, especially after eating gluten-containing products (breads, etc.)
      3) Treatment: Elimination of gluten from the diet
   b. Lactase deficiency:
      1) Pathophysiology: Deficiency of the disaccharide enzyme lactase
      2) Symptoms: Crampy abdominal pain, bloating, foul-smelling stools, and diarrhea after the ingestion of milk or dairy products
      3) Treatment: Replacement enzymes, such as lactase supplements before ingesting milk and milk products

SUGGESTED READINGS

Bickston SJ, Cominelli F: Inflammatory bowel disease: Short- and long- term treatments, *Adv Intern Med* 43(5):143-174, 1998.

D'haens G et al: Endoscopic and histological healing with Infliximab anti-tumor necrosis factor antibodies in Crohn's disease: A European multicenter trial, *Gastroenterology* 116(5):1029-1034, 1999.

Hanauer SB, Meyers S: Management of Crohn's disease in adults, *Am J Gastroenterol* 92(4):559-566, 1997.

Moses PL et al: Inflammatory bowel disease, *Postgrad Med* 103(5):77-84, 1998.

Roy MA: Inflammatory bowel disease, *Surg Clin North Am* 77(6):1419-1431, 1997.

PROBLEM·14

PEPTIC ULCER DISEASE

"You Mean I Have Bacteria Eating Holes in My Intestines?"

Case 1 ■ A 51-Year-Old Male with Epigastric Pain

A 51-year-old male with a 4-month history of epigastric pain comes to your office. The characterization of the pain is as follows: (1) *location:* epigastrium; (2) *quality:* dull ache; (3) *quantity:* baseline 6/10, intermittent increases of 8/10, intermittent decreases to 0/10; (4) *constant/intermittent:* intermittent; (5) *radiation:* none; (6) *aggravating factors:* coffee only; (7) *relieving factors:* milk, most meals; (8) *chronology:* began 4 months ago; intensity, location, and other factors have stayed the same; (9) *previous pain history:* no significant pain syndromes in the past, including no history of this type of pain; (10) *provocative maneuver:* palpation in the epigastric area; (11) *associated manifestations:* heartburn; (11) *quality of life:* some effect, although not marked.

In terms of other important history, the patient has not been taking any medication (specifically aspirin or nonsteroidal antiinflammatory drugs [NSAIDs]). He describes his profession as a "high-powered executive." He admits to being a "workaholic."

On examination, the patient has epigastric tenderness. No other abnormalities are found.

SELECT THE BEST ANSWER TO THE FOLLOWING QUESTIONS

Q1. What is the most likely diagnosis in this patient?
a. gastric carcinoma
b. gastric ulcer
c. duodenal ulcer
d. cholecystitis/cholelithiasis
e. irritable bowel syndrome

Q2. Which of the following statements regarding the patient described is false?
a. if you are going to investigate this patient, an upper endoscopy with antral biopsy for *Helicobacter pylori* is the diagnostic procedure of choice
b. cigarette smoking may aggravate the condition
c. drinking alcohol aggravates the condition
d. this patient should be treated with a bland diet
e. this condition may be aggravated by the ingestion of certain medications

Q3. The patient is given a combination of bismuth, metronidazole, and amoxicillin for his condition. His symptoms improve rapidly, and he is essentially free of pain in 2 weeks. Which of the following statements is (are) true about this treatment?
a. amoxicillin was prescribed because of a high probability of sepsis in his condition
b. amoxicillin and metronidazole were prescribed because of the association between this condition and *H. pylori*
c. the addition of omeprazole to the regime of bismuth, metronidazole, and amoxicillin in-creases the cure rate of *H. pylori*-induced peptic ulcer disease
d. b and c
e. a and c

Q4. Which of the following drugs show(s) effectiveness against *H. pylori*?
a. bismuth subsalicylate
b. metronidazole
c. amoxicillin
d. b and c
e. all of the above

Q5. What is the mode of action of omeprazole?
a. an H1 receptor antagonist
b. an H2 receptor antagonist
c. a proton pump inhibitor
d. a cytoprotective agent
e. an anticholinergic agent

Q6. The condition described should respond to treatment with complete healing within a maximum of how many weeks?
a. 1 to 2
b. 3 to 6
c. 8 to 12
d. 16 to 20
e. 26 to 52

Q7. Which of the following drugs is classified as an H2 receptor antagonist?
a. cimetidine
b. ranitidine
c. famotidine
d. a and b
e. all of the above

Q8. Which of the following statements regarding the role of drugs in the condition just described is (are) true?
a. the incidence of this condition in patients taking indomethacin or other NSAIDs is increased
b. the use of dexamethasone is a risk factor for this condition
c. aspirin may precipitate this condition
d. some NSAIDs seem more likely to precipitate this condition than others
e. all of the above are true

Q9. Which of the following statements regarding cimetidine is (are) true?
a. cimetidine is an H2 receptor antagonist
b. cimetidine and antacids are no more effective than cimetidine alone in the treatment of the condition just described

c. recurrence of the condition described is common
d. cimetidine may interfere with warfarin metabolism
e. all of the above are true

Q10. Which of the following statements regarding the diagnosis and treatment of gastric ulcers is (are) true?
a. the pain of gastric ulcers in contrast with duodenal ulcers is sometimes aggravated rather than relieved by food
b. anorexia, nausea, and vomiting are more common in patients with a gastric ulcer than in those with a duodenal ulcer
c. endoscopy should follow the identification of a gastric ulcer on a gastrointestinal (GI) series
d. the healing rate and the time to heal for gastric ulcers are generally longer than for duodenal ulcers
e. all of the above

SHORT ANSWER MANAGEMENT PROBLEM
Describe the pathophysiologic differences between a peptic ulcer related to NSAIDs and a peptic ulcer not related to NSAIDs.

ANSWERS

A1. **c.** This patient has a duodenal ulcer. Duodenal ulcer pain is characterized by a deep, aching, recurrent pain located in the mid-epigastrium. It is often relieved by food or antacids and aggravated by aspirin, coffee, or other irritants. Nocturnal pain is common and may awaken the patient at night.

Anorexia, weight loss, and vomiting are infrequently associated symptoms of duodenal ulcer. The occurrence of these symptoms should lead one to suspect a gastric ulcer, which may be worse with food.

A2. **d.** The diagnostic procedures of choice in this patient is an upper endoscopy with an antral biopsy for *H. pylori*. It is reasonable and safe, however, to treat patients with typical duodenal ulcer symptoms for 6 weeks before investigating. If the symptoms improve during that time, no investigation is needed. If they do not, investigation with a gastroscopy should proceed. Blood work for *H. pylori* may also be helpful.

Cigarette smoking aggravates peptic ulcer disease and delays healing of peptic ulcers. Patients who smoke also have an increased probability of recurrence.

Aspirin and other NSAIDs may aggravate or produce a peptic ulcer. Alcohol is a strong stimulant of acid secretion.

Bland diets or other special diets should not be prescribed; they may actually increase acid production.

A3. **d.** *H. pylori* is a cofactor in 95% of patients with a duodenal ulcer and 80% of patients with a gastric ulcer. After standard acid-blocking therapies, 70% to 85% of patients have an endoscopically documented recurrence within 1 year. With the successful eradication of *H. pylori*, the recurrence rate is less. The addition of omeprazole to the regimen of metronidazole, bismuth, and amoxicillin increases the cure rate from 88% to between 94% and 98%. The use of amoxicillin in the treatment of peptic ulcer disease has nothing to do with sepsis.

A4. **e.** Amoxicillin is often prescribed because of the association between active peptic ulcers (not related to NSAIDs) and infection with *H. pylori*.

The eradication of *H. pylori* is quite difficult, and multiple drugs are required. Quadruple therapy with bismuth 120 mg qid, tetracycline 500 mg qid, metronidazole 500 mg tid, and omeprazole 20 mg bid has an eradication rate of 98%. Triple therapy with omeprazole 20 mg twice a day, amoxicillin 1 gram twice a day, and clarithromycin 500 mg twice a day has an eradication rate of 96%. Treatment regimens should be for at least 7 to 14 days. Administration of proton pump inhibitors should be continued 4 to 6 weeks after the antibiotics to promote ulcer healing. A recent concern in the treatment of *H. pylori* ulcer disease is the development of antibiotic resistance associated with the increased use of antibiotics. As a result, antibiotic sensitivity will play a greater role in future eradication therapy.

A5. **c.** Omeprazole binds to the proton pump of the parietal cell, inhibiting secretion of hydrogen ions into the gastric lumen. In doses of 20 to 40 mg/day, it inhibits more than 90% of total 24-hour gastric acid secretion, a significant improvement when compared with the 50% to 80% inhibition achieved with an H2 blocker. This greater inhibition of gastric acid secretion results in greater pain relief and a decrease in healing time for the peptic ulcer.

A6. **b.** A duodenal ulcer treated appropriately should respond to treatment and heal completely within 3 to 6 weeks. Although treatment time for *H. pylori* is 10 to 14 days, either a proton pump inhibitor or an H2 receptor antagonist should be continued for an additional 4 to 6 weeks to promote ulcer healing.

A7. **e.** Ranitidine, famotidine, cimetidine, and nizatidine, are all H2 receptor antagonists. H2 receptor antagonists inhibit the action of histamine at the histamine H2 receptor of the parietal cell, decreasing both basal- and food-stimulated acid secretion. All H2 receptor antagonists are equally efficacious.

At this time the treatment of choice for peptic ulcer disease not associated with *H. pylori* is either a proton pump inhibitor or an H2 receptor antagonists. The proton pump inhibitors omeprazole and lansoprazole have the advantage of inducing a shorter healing time with a lower chance of recurrence.

A8. **e.** NSAIDs, including indomethacin, are well known to be causative agents in both gastritis and peptic ulcer disease. There is a 10% to 20% prevalence of gastric ulcers and a 25% prevalence of duodenal ulcers in chronic NSAID users.

Dexamethasone (a potent corticosteroid) is extensively used in palliative care to reduce cerebral edema and inhibit centrally mediated nausea and/or vomiting. It is, however, a potent stimulator of gastric acid secretion and must be used with an H2 receptor antagonist or a proton pump inhibitor to prevent gastritis or peptic ulcer formation. Aspirin is the most ulcerogenic NSAID. The risk appears to be dose related and is present even at doses of 325 mg every other day.

Risks of peptic ulcer disease/gastritis with NSAIDs increase with age, prior GI disease, steroid use, anticoagulant use, female sex, and increased dose.

A9. **e.** Cimetidine is an H2 receptor antagonist. Other H2 receptor antagonists such as famotidine, nizatidine, or ranitidine have fewer side effects and thus have become the H2 receptor antagonists of choice. Cimetidine can cause confusion in the elderly, and, when given with warfarin, it increases the international normalized ratio (increases anticoagulation).

An H2 receptor antagonist used in combination with an antacid is no more effective than an H2 receptor antagonist alone for either treatment or maintenance.

The 1-year recurrence rate for duodenal ulcer is at least 60% in nonsmokers and greater than 75% in smokers. The endoscopic recurrence rate is 20% higher in both cases. Controversy exists regarding which patients should be offered prophylactic therapy. A reasonable approach appears to be the offering of prophylactic therapy to those with frequent recurrences. Omeprazole has lowered this 1-year recurrence rate substantially.

A10. **e.** A gastric ulcer identified endoscopically must be followed by another endoscopy to confirm that healing has occurred. The pain of gastric ulcer disease is aggravated rather than relieved by food. Anorexia, nausea, and vomiting are more common in patients with gastric ulcers than in patients with duodenal ulcers. Also, the healing rate for gastric ulcers generally is slower than for duodenal ulcers.

SOLUTION TO THE SHORT ANSWER MANAGEMENT PROBLEM

The pathophysiologic difference between NSAID-related peptic ulcer and non-NSAID-related peptic ulcer reflects the direct gastric irritative effect of NSAID drugs. NSAIDs may produce an acute or chronic gastritis, a reflux esophagitis, or a peptic ulcer. NSAID-related peptic ulcer is not associated with *H. pylori*, whereas non-NSAID-related ulcers are.

The significance of this pathologic difference is reflected in treatment. Patients with non-NSAID-related peptic ulcer must receive a treatment protocol that includes treatment for *H. pylori*; NSAID-related peptic ulcer patients should not.

SUMMARY OF THE DIAGNOSIS AND MANAGEMENT OF DUODENAL AND PEPTIC ULCER DISEASES

1. Symptoms:
   a. Duodenal ulcer: Midepigastric pain relieved by ingestion of food or antacids. Nocturnal pain is present.
   b. Gastric ulcer: Midepigastric pain, relieved by antacids but often aggravated by food. Anorexia, weight loss, nausea, and vomiting are frequently associated.

2. Differential diagnosis: Cholecystitis, pancreatitis, appendicitis, carcinoma of the stomach, ischemic bowel disease in the elderly, and inflammatory bowel disease

3. Investigations:
   a. No investigation may be appropriate if the symptoms suggest duodenal ulcer and healing takes place within a maximum of 6 weeks.
   b. Gastroscopy must be used for both the assessment and the reassessment of gastric ulcers; a GI series and follow-through may be sufficient for duodenal ulcers.

4. Treatment:
   a. NSAID-associated peptic ulcer:
      1) H2 receptor antagonist
      2) proton pump inhibitor (omeprazole)
   b. Non-NSAID-associated peptic ulcer associated with *H. pylori*; see treatment protocols
   c. Limited role at this time for antacid therapy, sucralfate, and misoprostol, which has as its chief function the possible prevention of gastric ulcers

SUGGESTED READINGS

Achord J: Peptic ulcer disease. In Rakel R, ed: *Conn's current therapy*, Philadelphia, 1997, WB Saunders.

Neides D, Katz PO: Peptic ulcer disease In Barker LR et al, eds: *Principles of ambulatory medicine*, ed 5, Baltimore, 1998, JB Lippincott.

Salcedo JA, Al-Kawas F: Treatment of *Helicobacter pylori* infection, *Arch Intern Med* 158(8):842-851, 1998.

Tierney LM, McPhee SJ, Papadakis MA, eds: *Current medical diagnosis and treatment 2000*, ed 39, Stamford, Conn, 1999, Appleton & Lange.

PROBLEM · 15

MONONUCLEOSIS

"Oh, Doctor, You Mean I Have the Kissing Disease? What Will People Think?"

Case 1 ■ A 20-Year-Old College Student with a Fever and a Sore Throat

A 20-year-old college student comes to your office with a 3-week history of fatigue, malaise, fever, chills, and a sore throat. She was well before the onset of this illness and was taking part in many activities. She finds at this time that she has no energy and is barely able to make her university classes in the mornings. She also describes aches and pains all over.

On physical examination, the patient's temperature is 39° C. There is pharyngeal hyperemia and edema, and marked exudates are present in both tonsillar areas. There is significant cervical lymphadenopathy present.

On abdominal examination, there is dullness over the left upper quadrant, and you can just feel the tip of the spleen. There is no hepatic enlargement.

SELECT THE BEST ANSWER TO THE FOLLOWING QUESTIONS

Q1. Based on the history and the physical examination described, what is the most likely diagnosis in this patient?
a. infectious hepatitis
b. infectious mononucleosis
c. chronic fatigue syndrome
d. fibromyalgia
e. acute lymphoblastic leukemia

Q2. Of the following clinical features of the disorder, what is the least common?
a. splenomegaly
b. hepatomegaly
c. fever
d. exudative tonsillitis
e. lymphadenopathy

Q3. Which of the following statements regarding this condition is false?
a. this condition is caused by the Epstein-Barr virus
b. kissing is thought to be the most common mode of transmission
c. greater than 90% of all adults are carriers of the virus that causes the disease
d. in young children, fever and pharyngitis may be clinically indistinguishable from upper respiratory tract infections caused by other viral agents
e. a bacterial throat culture is unnecessary in patients suspected of having this disease

Q4. Which of the following statements concerning the serologic testing for the condition described is false?
a. the heterophile antibody test is negative in up to 20% of adults
b. the heterophile antibody test will be negative 12 months after onset of symptoms
c. in acute primary infections, anti-early antigen (EA) titers are usually low
d. in acute primary infections, IgM viral capsid antigen (IgM-VCA) titers are high
e. after several months the anti-Epstein-Barr nuclear antigen (EBNA) titers become high

Q5. The infectious agent that causes most of the cases of this disease has been associated with another condition. In fact, infection with the condition described could lead to this complication. What is this complication?
a. fibromyalgia
b. fifth disease
c. chronic fatigue syndrome
d. acute lymphocytic leukemia
e. none of the above

Q6. Of the following clinical features of the acute infection described, which is most common?
a. fever
b. hepatomegaly
c. eyelid edema
d. palatal petechiae
e. splenomegaly

Q7. What is the treatment of choice for an uncomplicated episode of this condition?
a. penicillin
b. prednisone
c. penicillin and prednisone
d. strict bed rest
e. none of the above

Q8. Which of the following is (are) a complication of this condition?
  a. splenic rupture
  b. myocarditis
  c. meningoencephalitis
  d. Bell's palsy
  e. all of the above

Q9. In patients with this condition and splenomegaly, which of the following is recommended?
  a. stool softeners
  b. prednisone
  c. acyclovir
  d. ampicillin
  e. splenectomy

Q10. The patient described comes to your office 1 week later with great difficulty swallowing solids or liquids. You notice a significant increase in the erythema of the pharynx, an increase in tonsillar hypertrophy, and increased exudates on the tonsils. What should you do at this time?
  a. repeat the throat culture
  b. start the patient on ampicillin
  c. start the patient on penicillin
  d. start the patient on prednisone
  e. start the patient on high-dose acetylsalicylic acid

Q11. The disease is an infection of which of the following?
  a. T-cell lymphocytes
  b. B-cell lymphocytes
  c. neutrophils
  d. basophils
  e. none of the above

SHORT ANSWER MANAGEMENT PROBLEM
What is the relationship between acute infectious mononucleosis and chronic fatigue syndrome?

ANSWERS

A1. **b.** This patient has infectious mononucleosis. Infectious mononucleosis is caused by the Epstein-Barr virus and is most commonly seen in children and young adults, particularly college students and military recruits.

The major symptoms of infectious mononucleosis are a sore throat, fatigue, and malaise; the major signs include fever, pharyngeal erythema, pharyngeal edema, tonsillar exudates, lymphadenopathy, splenomegaly, palatal petechiae, eyelid edema, and hepatomegaly.

Fibromyalgia, although most characteristic for its description of "pain all over" is characterized by multiple trigger points on examination.

Infectious hepatitis, although it presents with fatigue and malaise, also presents with abdominal pain, jaundice, an aversion to cigarettes, and significantly elevated liver function test values.

Chronic fatigue syndrome shares certain characteristics with infectious mononucleosis. However, patients with chronic fatigue syndrome must meet specific criteria defined by the Centers for Disease Control and Prevention to be classified as such. These criteria are as follows:
  a. Unexplained fatigue for more than 6 months' time
  b. Four or more of the following:
    1) Memory/concentration problems
    2) Sore throat
    3) Cervical or axillary nodes
    4) Myalgias
    5) Multijoint pain
    6) New headaches
    7) Unrefreshing sleep
    8) Postexertion malaise

Also, chronic fatigue syndrome occurs predominately in middle-aged individuals, whereas infectious mononucleosis is primarily a disease of young adults.

Although acute lymphoblastic leukemia can have very similar signs and symptoms, it is more commonly seen in children and is not the most likely diagnosis.

A2. **b.** The least common clinical feature is hepatomegaly. It occurs in about 30% to 50% of cases. Splenomegaly occurs in more than 50% of cases. Fever, exudative tonsillitis, and lymphadenopathy are most common.

A3. **e.** Infectious mononucleosis is caused by the Epstein-Barr virus. The usual mode of transmission of the virus is through infected saliva (kissing). Most adults (90%) have been infected with Epstein-Barr virus and are carriers.

Infectious mononucleosis is usually distinguishable from other viral infections in older children and young adults. In younger children and older adults, however, it may be difficult to distinguish from other respiratory tract infections, including those caused by other viruses, mycoplasma, or streptococci. Bacterial throat culture should be done in patients with significant pharyngitis to exclude coexisting group A β-hemolytic streptococcal infection.

A4. **c.** The heterophil antibody test can be negative in up to 20% of adults with Epstein-Barr virus-associated infectious mononucleosis. Persistence of heterophile antibody for 3 to 12 months after onset symptoms occurs in about 30% of patients. After 12 months the test is negative.

Serologic testing for Epstein-Barr virus infection includes determining antibody titers to latently infected (anti-EBNA) viral proteins and determining antibody titers to early-replication-cycle (anti-EA) viral proteins, or determining antibody titers to late-replication-cycle (anti-VCA) viral proteins.

Acute infectious mononucleosis produces high anti-EA and anti-IgM-VCA titers and low anti-IgG-VCA and anti-EBNA titers. In recovering patients the anti-IgG-VCA titer is high and the anti-EA, anti-IgM, and anti-EBNA titers are low. With time the anti-EBNA titer also becomes high.

A5. e. The Epstein-Barr virus has been associated with Burkitt's lymphoma. Studies have not supported any association with chronic fatigue syndrome.

A6. a. The following are the major clinical features of acute symptomatic infectious mononucleosis:

Symptom	Percentage of Patients
Fever	98-100
Lymphadenopathy	98-100
Tonsillopharyngitis	80-90
Splenomegaly	50
Eyelid edema	35
Hepatomegaly	30
Palatal petechiae	25

A7. e. Supportive care, including rest, avoidance of strenuous exercise due to the potential complication of splenic rupture, and analgesics, is the only treatment necessary in acute uncomplicated infectious mononucleosis. There is no evidence that bed rest hastens recovery.

Antibiotics are unnecessary unless a streptococcal pharyngitis coexists. Ampicillin should be avoided because it produces a skin rash in approximately 90% of patients with infectious mononucleosis.

A8. e. The complications of acute infectious mononucleosis include meningoencephalitis, Guillain-Barré syndrome, Bell's palsy, pneumonitis, pericarditis, myocarditis, and splenic rupture.

A9. a. To decrease the risk of splenic rupture, straining with bowel movements is to be avoided. Therefore increased fluids and/or stool softeners should be rec-

ommended. Prednisone, acyclovir, and ampicillin have no effect on the incidence of splenic rupture. There is no medical indication for splenectomy.

A10. d. At this time the single most important maneuver is to begin the patient on a corticosteroid to decrease the swelling and inflammation present in the airway. In severe cases of infectious mononucleosis the swelling and inflammation of the airway may be so significant that airway compromise and respiratory distress may occur. A reasonable starting dose would be 40 to 60 mg of prednisone per day with gradual tapering of the dose over 10 to 14 days.

A11. b. The Epstein-Barr virus, which causes infectious mononucleosis, is a B-cell lymphotropic human herpes virus. Epstein-Barr virus is a ubiquitous agent found in all population groups surveyed to date.

SOLUTION TO THE SHORT ANSWER MANAGEMENT PROBLEM

Acute mononucleosis and chronic fatigue syndrome share symptomatology. However, no link has been established between the causative agent in mononucleosis and that in chronic fatigue syndrome. As yet, no causative agent or agents have been established for chronic fatigue syndrome. Serologic antibody levels against Epstein-Barr virus are no more common in patients with chronic fatigue syndrome than in the general population.

SUMMARY OF THE DIAGNOSIS AND MANAGEMENT OF INFECTIOUS MONONUCLEOSIS

1. Identification: Epstein-Barr virus is the causative agent.

2. Incubation period: 2 to 5 weeks

3. Symptoms: Malaise, fatigue, fever, chills, myalgias, and severe sore throat

4. Signs: Pharyngeal erythema and edema, exudative tonsillitis, lymphadenopathy, splenomegaly, and hepatomegaly

5. Laboratory diagnosis: Lymphocyte atypia, positive heterophil antibody titer, and antibodies to Epstein-Barr viral antigens:
   a. Acute phase antibodies: Anti-EA, anti-IgM-VCA
   b. Convalescent antibody: Anti-IgG-VCA
   c. Recovered state: Anti-IgG-VCA, anti-EBNA

6. Treatment:
   a. Symptomatic treatment: Rest, fluids, mild analgesics
   b. Treatment of severe odynophagia and airway compromise: Oral prednisone

SUGGESTED READINGS

Bailey RE: Diagnosis and treatment of infectious mononucleosis, *Am Fam Physician* 49:879-888, 1994.

D'Angelo L: Infectious mononucleosis. In Rakel R, ed: *Conn's current therapy*, Philadelphia, 1994, WB Saunders.

Hickey SM et al: What every pediatrician should know about infectious mononucleosis in adolescents, *Pediatr Clin North Am* 44(6):1541-1546, 1997.

Komaroff AL, Buchwald DS: Chronic fatigue syndrome: an update, *Annu Rev Med* 49:1-13, 1998.

Okano M: Epstein-Barr virus infection and its role in the expanding spectrum of human disease, *Acta Paediatr* 87(1):11-18, 1998.

Peter J, Ray CG: Infectious mononucleosis, *Pediatr Rev* 19(8):276-279, 1998.

Sever TL: Infectious disease in athletes, *Med Clin North Am* 78(2):389-412, 1994.

PROBLEM·16

HEPATITIS AND CIRRHOSIS

"My Husband's Beer Belly Is Ballooning."

Case 1 ■ A 50-Year-Old Male with Ascites

A 50-year-old male is brought to your office by his wife. His wife states that for the past several months he has experienced extreme weakness and fatigue. In addition, he has gained 20 pounds in the past 3 weeks. During the last few weeks the patient has eaten nothing. When you question the patient, he states that his wife is overreacting. The patient's wife is extremely concerned about his alcohol intake. When you question the patient, he states that he is a social drinker. When you pursue this line of questioning further and ask him what he means by being a social drinker, you find out that he means that he drinks a few drinks before and after most meals plus a few drinks before he goes to bed.

You decide to pursue the question of drinking even further. When you ask him what he drinks, he says vodka. When you ask him if he drinks two 26-ounce bottles a day he says, "Heck, no! I would never put away more than a bottle a day."

On physical examination, the patient has a significantly enlarged abdominal girth. There is a level of shifting dullness present. The patient's liver edge is felt 6 cm below the right costal margin. It has a nodular edge. In addition, spider nevi are present over the upper part of the patient's body. Palmar erythema is noted, and a flapping tremor is elicited.

SELECT THE BEST ANSWER TO THE FOLLOWING QUESTIONS

Q1. Which of the following statements regarding this patient's condition is false?
   a. the most likely diagnosis is cirrhosis of the liver
   b. this condition is probably associated with alcohol abuse
   c. jaundice is an uncommon sign in the disorder described
   d. approximately 33% of patients with a history of alcohol abuse will develop alcoholic hepatitis
   e. approximately 50% of patients with this condition (in an advanced stage) will die within 2 years

Case 2 ■ A 25-Year-Old Male with Abdominal Pain for the Past 3 Weeks

A 25-year-old male with a history of heavy alcohol intake comes to your office for a periodic health assessment. He states that his appetite has been "off" and he has had generalized abdominal pain for the past 3 weeks.

On examination, there is no clinical jaundice. There is tenderness present in the right upper quadrant of the abdomen. The liver edge is palpable 5 cm below the right costal margin. You suspect alcoholic hepatitis.

Q2. Which of the following statements regarding alcoholic hepatitis is false?
   a. alcoholic cirrhosis develops in approximately 10% of patients with alcoholic hepatitis
   b. serum bilirubin is often 10 to 20 times normal in this condition
   c. serum alanine aminotransferase (ALT) is almost always lower than serum aspartate aminotransferase (AST)
   d. hepatomegaly is seen in 80% to 90% of patients with alcoholic hepatitis
   e. a mortality of 10% to 15% is seen in acute alcoholic hepatitis

Q3. What is the most common cause of cirrhosis in the United States?
   a. hepatitis A
   b. hepatitis B
   c. hepatitis C
   d. alcoholism
   e. cytomegalovirus hepatitis

Q4. The ascites associated with cirrhosis should generally be treated by which of the following?
a. sodium restriction
b. water restriction
c. spironolactone
d. a and c
e. a, b, and c

Case 3 ■ A 25-Year-Old Schoolteacher with Icteric
Sclera and Right Upper Quadrant Pain

A 25-year-old schoolteacher comes to a walk-in clinic with nausea, vomiting, anorexia, aversion to her usual two-pack-a-day tobacco habit, and right upper quadrant pain. She has been sick for the past 3 days. Two of the students in her class have come down with similar symptoms. She has had no exposure to blood products and has no other significant risk factors for sexually transmitted disease.

On examination, her sclerae are icteric and her liver edge is tender. She looks acutely ill.

Q5. What is the most likely diagnosis in this patient?
a. hepatitis A
b. hepatitis B
c. hepatitis C
d. atypical infectious mononucleosis
e. none of the above

Q6. Which of the following tests is the most sensitive in confirming the diagnosis suspected in this patient?
a. anti-hepatitis A virus (HAV)-immunoglobulin G (IgG)
b. anti-HAV-immunoglobulin M (IgM)
c. HAV core antigen
d. anti-hepatitis B core antigen (HBcAg)
e. anti-hepatitis C virus (HCV)

Q7. Initial screening for hepatitis B should include which of the following?
a. anti-hepatitis B surface antigen (HBsAg) and anti-HBc
b. hepatitis B early antigen (HBeAg) and anti-HBe
c. HBsAg and anti-HBs
d. HBsAg and anti-HBc
e. anti-HBe and anti-HBc

Q8. Which of the following laboratory tests is (are) usually abnormal in a patient with acute viral hepatitis?
a. serum AST
b. serum bilirubin
c. serum ALT
d. serum alkaline phosphatase
e. all of the above

Q9. Clinical manifestations of cirrhosis include which of the following?
a. fatigue
b. jaundice
c. splenomegaly
d. hypoalbuminemia
e. all of the above

Q10. Indications for the use of hepatitis B vaccine include which of the following?
a. health care personnel
b. hemodialysis patients
c. all children
d. a and b only
e. all of the above

Q11. Which of the following types of viral hepatitis is (are) associated with the development of chronic active hepatitis?
a. hepatitis B
b. hepatitis C
c. hepatitis A
d. a and b only
e. all of the above

Q12. The pathophysiology of alcoholic cirrhosis includes which of the following?
a. macronodular and micronodular fibrosis
b. nodular regeneration
c. increased portal vein pressure
d. increase in hepatic size followed by a decrease
e. all of the above

Q13. Which of the following has (have) been suggested as treatment for complications of cirrhosis of the liver?
a. prednisone
b. propranolol
c. colchicine
d. propylthiouracil
e. all of the above

Q14. Which of the following is (are) a complication of alcoholic cirrhosis?
a. hypersplenism
b. hepatic encephalopathy
c. congestive gastropathy
d. spontaneous bacterial peritonitis
e. all of the above

Q15. Treatment of the ascites accompanying cirrhosis may include which of the following?
a. spironolactone
b. hydrochlorothiazide
c. furosemide
d. all of the above
e. a and b only

SHORT ANSWER MANAGEMENT PROBLEM
Describe the pathophysiology of cirrhosis of the liver and the relationship between cirrhosis of the liver and right-sided heart failure.

ANSWERS

A1. **c.** This patient has cirrhosis of the liver and alcoholism. Most cases of cirrhosis of the liver are directly attributable to alcohol abuse.

Cirrhosis is an irreversible inflammatory disease that disrupts liver structure and function. It is the fifth leading cause of death in the United States. Cirrhosis is the disorganization of hepatic tissues caused by diffuse fibrosis and nodular regeneration. Nodules of regenerated tissue form between fibrous bands, giving the liver a cobbled appearance.

Symptoms of early cirrhotic liver disease include weakness, fatigue, and weight loss. In advanced disease the patient develops anorexia, nausea and vomiting, swelling of the abdomen and lower extremities, and central nervous system symptoms related to the cirrhotic liver disease. Other symptoms that may occur include loss of libido, gynecomastia, and menstrual irregularities in women.

The liver is usually enlarged, palpable, and firm. In advanced cirrhosis the liver may actually shrink. Dermatologic manifestations include spider nevi, palmar erythema, telangiectases on exposed areas, and occasional evidence of vitamin deficiencies. Although jaundice is rarely an initial sign, it usually develops later. Other later-developing signs include ascites, lower extremity edema, pleural effusion, purpuric lesions, asterixis, tremor, delirium, coma, fever, splenomegaly, and superficial venous dilatation of the abdomen and thorax.

Approximately 33% of chronic alcoholics develop alcoholic hepatitis. Many of these then develop cirrhosis of the liver. There appears to be a genetic predisposition to the development of these complications.

Of patients with advanced cirrhosis, 50% will be dead in a period of 2 years and 65% will be dead in 5 years. Hematemesis, jaundice, and ascites are unfavorable signs.

A2. **a.** The first clinical stage of alcoholic liver disease is termed *alcoholic hepatitis*. Alcoholic hepatitis is a precursor of cirrhosis that is characterized by inflammation, degeneration, necrosis of hepatocytes, and infiltration of polymorphonuclear leukocytes and lymphocytes.

Over the last 10 years in the United States deaths from alcohol-related liver disease have increased. The incidence is greatest in middle-aged males, and mortality from cirrhosis is higher in blacks than in whites. Although alcoholic cirrhosis is the most prevalent type of cirrhosis, only about 15% of alcoholics actually develop the disease. There appears to be a genetic predisposition to its development. The amount and duration of alcohol consumption are correlated directly with the extent of damage to the liver.

The symptoms of alcoholic hepatitis include anorexia, nausea, vomiting, weight loss, emesis, fever, and generalized abdominal pain.

Hepatomegaly is found in 80% to 90% of these patients. Other signs include jaundice, ascites, splenomegaly, and spider angiomas.

Laboratory abnormalities in alcoholic hepatitis include hyperbilirubinemia and elevated serum transaminase levels. The ratio of serum AST to serum ALT is often 2:1 or greater. This can help differentiate alcoholic hepatitis from viral hepatitis. Other laboratory abnormalities include elevated alkaline phosphatase levels, hypoalbuminemia, and a prolonged prothrombin time.

The prognosis of alcoholic hepatitis is variable; many patients develop only a mild illness. There is, however, a 10% to 15% mortality from the acute event.

The treatment of alcoholic hepatitis involves cessation of alcohol consumption, increased caloric and protein intake, and vitamin supplementation (especially thiamine). Alcoholic cirrhosis develops in approximately 50% of patients surviving alcoholic hepatitis. In the other 50%, various degrees of hepatic fibrosis develop.

A3. **d.** The most common cause of cirrhosis in the United States is alcoholism. Hepatitis A does not progress to chronic active hepatitis. Hepatitis B progresses to chronic active hepatitis and subsequently to cirrhosis in approximately 10% of cases. Patients with hepatitis C go on to develop chronic active hepatitis and subsequent cirrhosis in approximately 20% to 40% of cases. Cytomegalovirus infection does not produce cirrhosis.

A4. **d.** The treatment of ascites and the edema associated with ascites includes the following:
a. Sodium restriction to 800 mg/day (or 2 g of NaCl)

b. Spironolactone (Aldactone) 25 to 100 mg qid (effective in 40% to 75% of cases)
c. Paracentesis
d. Combination diuretic therapy in those patients who do not respond: (1) spironolactone and hydrochlorothiazide; (2) spironolactone and furosemide
e. Paracentesis with albumin (or dextran) infusion in refractory cases

Fluid restriction is not used to treat ascites.

A5. **a.** This patient most likely has hepatitis A, which is caused by the HAV, an ether-resistant RNA virus in the hepatovirus genus of the picornavirus family. Hepatitis A occurs either spontaneously or in epidemics. Transmission is via the oral-fecal route. The presenting signs and symptoms of hepatitis A include the following:
a. General malaise and fatigue
b. General myalgias
c. Arthralgias
d. Abdominal pain
e. Nausea and vomiting
f. Severe anorexia out of proportion to the degree of illness
g. Aversion to smoking

Hepatitis B and hepatitis C are unlikely in this case because risk factors are absent. Although infectious mononucleosis may involve the liver and may occur with some of the same signs and symptoms, hepatitis A is much more likely.

A6. **b.** Acute infection with hepatitis A is confirmed by the demonstration of IgM antibodies to HAV (IgM-anti-HAV). These antibodies persist for approximately 12 weeks after appearance. IgG antibodies to HAV follow and simply indicate exposure at some time in the past.

Hepatitis A does not possess a recognizable core or surface antigen; these tests apply to hepatitis B only. The hepatitis B virus has a compact DNA core and belongs to the hepatotropic DNA virus family. Antibodies to HBcAg have nothing to do with hepatitis A. Anti-non-A, non-B hepatitis antigen does not exist.

A7. **d.** There are so many antigens and antibodies associated with hepatitis virology that it is difficult to figure out what is what. However, it can be simplified considerably.

Initial screening for hepatitis B should include HBsAg and anti-HBc (the antibody to the core antigen). These two tests will identify most cases of acute hepatitis B.

There is a window period between the clearance of HBsAg and the appearance of anti-HBs. This period

lasts 4 to 6 weeks, and during this time the only marker for hepatitis B that can detect the infection with any certainty is anti-HBc. If acute hepatitis B is suggested from the initial screening, further laboratory tests should be ordered, including the following:
a. HBeAg: The e antigen indicates the presence of a highly infectious or contagious state or a chronic infection.
b. anti-HBe (the antibody to the antigen above): The presence of this antibody indicates low infectivity and predicts the later seroconversion or resolution of hepatitis B.
c. anti-HBs: The presence of this antibody indicates past hepatitis B infection and current immunity.

A8. **e.** In acute viral hepatitis the serum AST and serum ALT levels are elevated, along with serum bilirubin and serum alkaline phosphatase levels.

A9. **e.** The clinical manifestations of cirrhosis were discussed earlier. Another common finding in cirrhosis is hypoalbuminemia as a result of the accumulation of ascitic fluid in the abdomen.

A10. **e.** Hepatitis B vaccine should be offered to persons at high risk and those with continued exposure to hepatitis B infection. Persons at high risk for acquiring hepatitis B include the following:
a. All health care personnel
b. Hemodialysis patients
c. Patients requiring frequent blood transfusions
d. Employees and residents of institutions for people with developmental disabilities
e. Male homosexuals and all of their contacts
f. Intravenous drug users
g. Sexual contacts of chronic HBsAg carriers
h. Children born to mothers who have chronic hepatitis B

In addition, the Centers for Disease Control and Prevention now recommends that all children be immunized with hepatitis B vaccine (see Problem 81).

A11. **d.** Chronic active hepatitis (which may lead to cirrhosis of the liver, liver failure, and hepatocellular carcinoma) is associated with hepatitis B, hepatitis C, and hepatitis D (delta virus hepatitis, which occurs only in patients who are also chronically infected with hepatitis B). Chronic active hepatitis is not associated with hepatitis A or hepatitis E.

A12. **e.** Cirrhosis is an irreversible inflammatory condition of disordered and disrupted liver structure and function. Cirrhosis results from the disorganization of hepatic tissues caused by diffuse fibrosis and nodular regeneration. Micronodular and macronodular fibrosis occurs. Nodules of regenerated tissue form between the fibrous bands, giving the liver a cobbled appearance. The liver is initially larger than normal in size and then usually becomes smaller than normal. The changes in the liver result in increased portal vein pressure, which leads to the formation of ascites as well as to esophageal varices.

A13. **e.** Treatments suggested as possibly beneficial for cirrhosis of the liver include the following:

    a. Colchicine, which was shown in one long-term study to slow disease progression and increase longevity

    b. β-Blockers, which may reduce the risk of variceal bleeding

Other treatments for cirrhosis include lactulose or neomycin for hepatic encephalopathy and shunt placement to reduce portal hypertension.

A14. **e.** Complications of cirrhosis include the following:

    a. Portal hypertension, leading to esophageal varices, congestive gastropathy, and hypersplenism

    b. Hepatic encephalopathy

    c. Ascites, leading to spontaneous bacterial peritonitis and umbilical hernia (spontaneous rupture)

    d. Hepatorenal syndrome

    e. Coagulation abnormalities

    f. Hepatocellular carcinoma

    g. Pulmonary dysfunction

    h. Hepatic osteodystrophy

    i. Cholelithiasis

    j. Pericardial effusion

    k. Impaired reticuloendothelial system function

A15. **d.** The management of ascites in cirrhotic patients is complicated. Diagnostic paracentesis should be performed in any cirrhotic patient who undergoes clinical deterioration. Defined indications for the treatment of ascites include significant patient discomfort, respiratory compromise, a large umbilical hernia, and recurrent bacterial peritonitis.

Sodium restriction is considered the cornerstone of therapy for ascites. Cirrhotic patients require significant curtailment of sodium intake (800 mg/day) to obtain clinical benefit. Approximately 10% to 20% of patients who maintain a strict low-salt diet achieve complete resolution of ascites without additional therapy.

Spironolactone (Aldactone), an aldosterone antagonist, is the first-line diuretic of choice in the treatment of cirrhotic ascites. It is effective in controlling 40% to 75% of patients with cirrhosis. Other potassium-sparing diuretics may be substituted for spironolactone, including triamterene (Dyrenium) and amiloride

(Midamor). Sometimes either a thiazide diuretic (such as hydrochlorothiazide) or a loop diuretic (such as furosemide) must be added to achieve maximum benefit.

SOLUTION TO THE SHORT ANSWER MANAGEMENT PROBLEM

The pathophysiology of cirrhosis has already been discussed. Briefly, micronodular fibrosis, macronodular fibrosis, and nodular regeneration eventually lead to portal hypertension with all of its complications.

SUMMARY OF THE DIAGNOSIS AND TREATMENT OF HEPATITIS AND CIRRHOSIS

1. Infectious forms of hepatitis:

    a. Hepatitis A:

        1) Etiologic agent: RNA hepatovirus

        2) Epidemiology: Sporadic infection or epidemic, spread by oral-fecal route

        3) Symptoms: Anorexia, nausea, vomiting, malaise, aversion to smoking

        4) Signs: Fever, enlarged tender liver, jaundice

        5) Laboratory findings: Normal to low white blood cell count; abnormal ALT, AST, bilirubin, and alkaline phosphatase levels

        6) Diagnostic clues: Transaminase elevations, IgM anti-HAV

        7) Treatment: Symptomatic; rest; condition is rarely fulminating and does not become chronic.

        8) Prevention: Because oral-fecal route is the main route of spread, meticulous hand washing is essential. Hepatitis A vaccine is available for patients who are traveling to endemic areas.

    b. Hepatitis B:

        1) Etiologic agent: DNA hepadnavirus

        2) Epidemiology: Usually transmitted by blood or blood products; particularly common in intravenous drug users and in patients with acquired immunodeficiency syndrome. Up to 30% of infected individuals may be carriers.

        3) Treatment: Symptomatic unless it becomes fulminating, as it will in 0.1% to 1%, or chronic, as it will in 1% to 10% of adults and 90% of neonates. Treat symptoms with interferon; 40% success rate.

        4) Diagnosis: Transaminase elevation, HBsAg, anti-HBc

        5) Prevention: Hepatitis B hyperimmunoglobulin after exposure, hepatitis B vaccine now

recommended for all children by the Centers for Disease Control and Prevention.
  c. Hepatitis C:
    1) Etiologic agent: A single-stranded RNA virus belonging to the *Flaviviridae* family. More than 100 strains belong to six major "genotypes."
    2) Epidemiology: Usually transmitted by blood or blood products. Sexual transmission is also suspect. The development of a screening test in 1990 virtually eliminated spread via transfusions, and it is thought that sharing of contaminated needles is the main route of transfer.
    3) Disease course: Very variable. From 15% to 25% of infected individuals recover spontaneously. The remaining individuals become chronically infected, of whom 10% to 20% will develop cirrhosis and another 1% to 5% will develop hepatocellular cancer.
    4) Prevalence: The October 16, 1998 *CDC Morbidity and Mortality Weekly Report* states that hepatitis C is the most common chronic blood-borne infection in the United States. Some 3.9 million, or about 1.8%, of the U.S. population is infected, and as the population ages, hepatitis C–related deaths, now about 8000 to 10,000 per year, will increase. The prevalence in some other countries is much higher. The hardest hit country is probably Egypt, where it is estimated that 25% of the population carry the hepatis C virus. In industrialized countries hepatitis C causes 20% of the cases of acute hepatitis, 70% of the cases of chronic hepatitis, 40% of the cases of end-stage cirrhosis, 60% of the cases of hepatocellular carcinoma, and 30% of the cases of liver transplants.
    5) Treatment: Symptomatic; often progresses to chronic infection. Chronic disease can be treated with three interferon injections per week for as long as a year. This eliminates the virus in about 20% of the patients. Recent trials suggest that combining interferon with the antiviral ribavirin doubles the chances of success. However, a 48-week treatment costs $20,000 and causes debilitating flulike symptoms.
  d. Delta hepatitis (hepatitis D) is caused by a defective RNA virus and requires the hepatitis B virus for replication and expression. Therefore, clinically speaking, it is found only in association with chronic hepatitis B. This combination is particularly likely to lead to chronic active hepatitis and its complications, including cirrhosis, liver cell failure, and hepatocellular carcinoma.
  e. Hepatitis E is caused by an RNA virus somewhat similar to the HAV. It, too, is an enterically transmitted form of hepatitis. Like hepatitis A, it never leads to chronic infection.
  f. Hepatitis G, or GB virus C, has recently been characterized. It is an RNA virus distinct from but similar to the hepatitis C virus, and the two are often found in conjunction with each other. Although transmitted by transfusion and sexual contact, hepatitis G appears to lack clinical significance.
  g. Alcoholic hepatitis:
    1) Signs and symptoms: The symptoms of alcoholic hepatitis closely resemble those of viral hepatitis. In alcoholic hepatitis the ratio of AST to ALT is usually 2:1.
    2) Patients who develop alcoholic hepatitis are at high risk for developing cirrhosis of the liver.
  h. Cirrhosis of the liver:
    1) Symptoms and signs: Weakness, fatigue, weight loss, anorexia, hepatomegaly, spider nevi, palmar erythema, asterixis, tremor, and ascites. Patients often develop portal hypertension with its complications and hepatic encephalopathy.
    2) Treatment: Supportive. Use of glucocorticoids in acute alcoholic hepatitis is controversial. Colchicine may slow disease progression. Treatments for ascites include sodium restriction, diuretics (especially spironolactone) with or without thiazides or loop diuretics, paracentesis, and shunts.
    3) Complications: Upper gastrointestinal bleeding from varices, hemorrhagic gastritis, or gastroduodenal ulcers; liver failure, hepatic encephalopathy, hepatorenal syndrome, and hepatocellular carcinoma.

SUGGESTED READINGS

Cohen J: The scientific challenge of hepatitis C, *Science* 285(5424):26-30, 1999.

Dienstag JL, Isselbacher KJ: Acute viral hepatitis. In Fauci AS et al, eds: *Harrison's principles of internal medicine,* ed 14, New York, 1998, McGraw-Hill.

Lefrère JJ et al: Carriage of GB virus C/hepatitis G virus RNA is associated with a slower immunologic, virologic, and clinical progression of human immunodeficiency virus disease in coinfected persons, *J Infect Dis* 179(4):783-789, 1999.

Rose VL: CDC issues new recommendations for the prevention and control of hepatitis C virus infection, *Am Fam Physician* 59(5): 1321-1323, 1999.

Sievert W: Acute and chronic hepatitis. In Rakel R, ed: *Conn's current therapy,* Philadelphia, 1994, WB Saunders.

Zucker S, Gollan J: Cirrhosis. In Rakel R, ed: *Conn's current therapy,* Philadelphia, 1994, WB Saunders.

PROBLEM · 17

IRRITABLE BOWEL DISEASE

"I Strain So Hard and I Find Mucus on the Toilet Paper."

Case 1 ■ A 38-Year-Old Female with Lower Abdominal Pain and Constipation

A 38-year-old female comes to your office with a 1-year history of lower abdominal pain associated with constipation (one hard bowel movement every 3 days) and the passage of mucus per rectum on a regular basis. She has never passed blood per rectum to her knowledge. She describes no fever, chills, weight loss, jaundice, or other symptoms. There is no relationship between the abdominal pain and food intake.

On physical examination, the abdomen is scaphoid and no hepatosplenomegaly or other masses are palpated. There is a very mild generalized abdominal tenderness, but it does not localize.

SELECT THE BEST ANSWER
TO THE FOLLOWING QUESTIONS

Q1. What is the most likely diagnosis in this patient?
   a. *Yersinia* enterocolitis
   b. Crohn's disease
   c. ulcerative colitis
   d. lactose intolerance
   e. none of the above

Q2. Which of the following statements regarding the condition described is false?
   a. the typical location of the abdominal pain is the lower abdomen
   b. defecation frequently relieves the pain
   c. there is often a perception of incomplete emptying of the rectum
   d. bowel action is often irregular
   e. very severe abdominal tenderness is a hallmark of the disease

Q3. What is the most likely cause of the disorder described?
   a. a mass lesion in the area of the sigmoid colon
   b. a low-grade chronic inflammation of the entire small and large bowel
   c. an autoimmune phenomenon
   d. a decreased ability to digest certain foods
   e. none of the above

Q4. Which of the following would be most unlikely in a patient with the above condition?

a. alternating diarrhea and constipation
b. increased pain at times of stress
c. pain on awakening from sleep
d. abdominal bloating
e. increased passage of flatus

Q5. Which of the following investigations is not indicated in the condition described?
   a. a complete blood count (CBC)
   b. an erythrocyte sedimentation rate (ESR)
   c. electrolytes
   d. abdominal ultrasound
   e. thyroid function studies

Q6. Which of the following may have to be considered in the differential diagnosis of the condition just described?
   a. colonic adenocarcinoma
   b. fecal impaction
   c. celiac disease
   d. endometriosis
   e. all of the above

Q7. Which of the following conditions (symptoms) is not associated with the condition?
   a. gastroesophageal reflux disease
   b. cholelithiasis
   c. noncardiac chest pain
   d. depression
   e. fatigue

Q8. Which of the following statements concerning the condition described is (are) true?
   a. this condition is the most common reason for referral from a family physician to a gastroenterologist
   b. this condition is slightly more common in men
   c. the symptoms associated with this condition are more common in young adults than in older adults
   d. this condition has been associated with a specific biochemical abnormality in some patients
   e. all of the above statements are true

Q9. Which of the following is the most important component of management for the condition described?
   a. single-agent pharmacologic therapy
   b. multiple-agent pharmacologic therapy
   c. a therapeutic physician-patient relationship
   d. a focused diet
   e. a diet elimination trial: eliminating one food at a time until the responsible food is found

Q10. Which of the following medications should not be used in the treatment of this condition?
 a. psyllium
 b. loperamide
 c. cholestyramine
 d. codeine phosphate
 e. desipramine

Q11. Recent initial research suggests a significant correlation between the disorder described in Case 1 and which of the following?
 a. hypochondriasis
 b. history of sexual abuse
 c. somatoform disease
 d. early ulcerative colitis
 e. none of the above

SHORT ANSWER MANAGEMENT PROBLEM

A 32-year-old female with chronic abdominal pain that has been fully investigated and diagnosed with irritable bowel syndrome (IBS) comes to your office as a new patient. She has seen two family physicians and two gastroenterologists. Although she has been told the same thing by all physicians, she seeks another opinion from you. Discuss what you would and would not do in your consultation with this patient.

ANSWERS

A1. **e.** The most likely diagnosis is IBS, which is characterized by:
 a. Abdominal pain or discomfort, relieved with defecation or associated with a change in frequency or consistency of stools
 b. An irregular pattern of defecation at least 25% of the time, consisting of three or more of the following:
  1) Altered stool frequency
  2) Altered stool form (hard or loose and watery)
  3) Altered stool passage (straining or urgency), feeling of incomplete evacuation
  4) Passage of mucus
  5) Bloating or a feeling of abdominal distention

Yersinia is one of several bacteria (others include *Campylobacter, Shigella,* and *Salmonella*) that can produce a diarrheal syndrome. *Yersinia* has been associated with a more chronic enterocolitis, but this is usually seen in children age 1 to 4 years and can mimic appendicitis. Occasionally, young adults can present with a syndrome that includes low-grade fever, crampy abdominal pain, nausea and vomiting, hematochezia, and a generalized maculopapular rash.

Crohn's disease is unlikely in the absence of systemic symptoms including nonbloody diarrhea, anorexia, weight loss, fever, and fatigue.

Ulcerative colitis is unlikely in the absence of weight loss, tenesmus, and the passage of bright red blood per rectum.

Lactose intolerance is specifically linked to the intake of milk and milk products.

Although many consider IBS to be a diagnosis of exclusion, the diagnostic criteria given in this answer suggest very specific inclusive clues. This suggests that in a field as complicated as medicine and oriented toward the biopsychosocial model of illness, it is rather dangerous to suggest the following: if not (A), if not (B), and if not (C), then (D).

A2. **e.** The perception of incomplete emptying of the rectum, the irregular bowel action, and the relief of the abdominal pain with defecation have already been discussed. In IBS the abdominal pain is confined to the lower abdomen, with the most common location being in the area of the sigmoid colon. Although abdominal tenderness may be present, it is usually not very severe, and it certainly is not a hallmark of the disease.

A3. **e.** The cause of IBS is unknown, except for a likely association with either altered motility or altered visceral sensation. IBS may be associated with significant psychosocial dysfunction or psychologic (psychiatric) disorders. Spousal abuse, a history of sexual abuse, or depression should be considered.

A4. **c.** Pain on awakening from sleep is suggestive of an organic cause. In addition to this symptom, pain that interferes with normal sleep patterns, diarrhea that awakens the patient from sleep, visible or occult blood in the stool, weight loss, and fever also suggest organic disease.

A5. **d.** The investigations recommended in a patient with IBS include CBC; ESR; a chemistry panel; a flexible sigmoidoscopy; a stool for ova, parasites, and fecal leukocytes; and thyroid function studies.

A6. **e.** Diagnoses that may need to be considered in patients with symptoms of IBS include colonic adenocarcinoma, ulcerative colitis, Crohn's disease, abdominal angina, ischemic colitis, drugs, pseudo-obstruction, intermittent sigmoid volvulus, megacolon, celiac disease, bacterial overgrowth syndrome, giardiasis, endometriosis, depression, somatization, and panic disorder.

A7. **b.** Conditions that are more common in patients with IBS include gastroesophageal reflux disease with heartburn, dysphagia, globus hystericus, noncardiac chest pain, urologic dysfunction, fatigue, and gynecologic problems. Cholelithiasis is not associated with IBS.

A8. **a.** IBS is the most common reason for referral by a family physician to a gastrointestinal specialist.

IBS is slightly more common in women than in men. Although symptoms typically begin in young adulthood, the prevalence is similar in elderly and younger adults.

IBS is one of a group of disorders that includes chest pain of unexplained origin, nonulcer dyspepsia, and biliary dyskinesia. These chronic disorders are frequently considered functional because no specific structural or biochemical causes have been found.

A9. **c.** The most important component of treatment in IBS is establishing a therapeutic, communicative, and trusting physician-patient relationship and educating the patient regarding the benign nature of the condition and favorable long-term prognosis.

The important components of the physician-patient relationship to emphasize include a nonjudgmental attitude, concern regarding the patient's understanding of the illness, expectations and consistent limits, and involvement of the patient in treatment decisions. Because of the long-term nature of IBS, primary management by a family physician is essential. Although consultants may be needed in some cases for both patient and family physician reassurance, this should be the exception rather than the rule.

Diet therapy and pharmacologic therapy are discussed in Answer 10.

A10. **d.** Treatment of IBS includes the following:
   a. The elimination of certain foods, including gas-forming foods such as legumes or dairy products
   b. The consumption of supplements with high-fiber foods such as bran
Other agents recommended in the treatment of IBS are as follows:
   a. Psyllium (another bulking agent)
   b. Antispasmodic or anticholinergic agents such as belladonna and dicyclomine when abdominal spasm is the predominant symptom
   c. Antidiarrheal agents such as diphenoxylate, loperamide, or cholestyramine when diarrhea is the predominant symptom
   d. Tricyclic antidepressants such as amitriptyline or desipramine when pain (or a chronic pain syndrome) is the predominant symptom
   e. Prokinetic agents such as cisapride for patients when constipation is the predominant symptom
Long-term benzodiazepines are not recommended,

although treatment for short periods may be indicated. Codeine phosphate or other narcotic agents are contraindicated in the treatment of IBS because of the potential for abuse or tolerance.

A11. **b.** A disturbing correlation between IBS and a previous history of sexual abuse in the patient has recently been established. Although the results need to be verified, this should alert the clinician to ask about sexual abuse in anyone who comes with or is diagnosed as having IBS. Thus a history of sexual abuse joins the questions associated with depression as lead questions required to be asked by the family physician.

SOLUTION TO THE SHORT ANSWER MANAGEMENT PROBLEM

In the management of this patient, you, the new family physician, should consider doing and not doing the following:
   1. You should:
      a. Perform a complete history including a psychosocial history, a family history, and a marital history.
      b. Attempt to ascertain the patient's understanding and concerns about the condition.
      c. Establish a strong, trusting family physician-patient relationship. This forms the basis for the therapy (supportive psychotherapy) that follows.
      d. Have the patient ask all of his or her questions in an unhurried atmosphere.
      e. Perform a complete or relatively complete physical examination for two reasons: to reassure yourself that nothing significant has been missed and to reassure the patient that you are truly interested in the problem.
      f. Ascertain what dietary and drug therapies have been tried, and decide on those therapies that may be indicated at this time.
   2. You should not:
      a. Repeat investigations, nor should you order other, more costly investigations.
      b. Criticize your colleagues for failure to completely investigate this problem until a cause was found; you will find yourself in the same situation someday.
      c. Promise what you cannot deliver: a cure for IBS. Also, do not let the patient transfer ownership of the problem to you. It is the patient's problem, and your job is not to solve it; your job is to provide the empathic support necessary to help the patient understand and deal with the illness.

d. Rely on a polypharmacy approach to achieve a better result. Use the suggested drugs with prudence and caution.

e. Use narcotic analgesics as a treatment for IBS.

SUMMARY OF SYMPTOMS, PREVALENCE, AND MANAGEMENT OF IRRITABLE BOWEL SYNDROME

1. IBS is extremely common; prevalence estimates suggest that 10% to 22% of the population have symptoms compatible with this diagnosis at some time in their lives.

2. IBS is the most common condition that gastroenterologists see in referral or consultation practice.

3. Consider IBS as a diagnosis of inclusion rather than exclusion. Base your diagnosis on the positive criteria discussed previously.

4. Consider the minimal investigations that have been suggested as sufficient; do not over-investigate. Remember the definition of a "normal" person is someone who has not been sufficiently investigated.

5. After establishing a strong physician-patient relationship, consider dietary manipulation as primary therapy.

6. Antispasmodics, anticholinergics, tricyclic antidepressants, antidiarrheal agents, and prokinetic agents can be used for the treatment of IBS. Use caution combining them.

7. Reassurance regarding the benign nature of the condition and the provision of hope for eventual resolution of the symptoms are likely the most important therapy for this condition (supportive psychotherapy).

8. Identification and treatment of psychosocial stressors (stressors of some kind are almost invariably associated with this condition) are paramount.

9. Recent research suggests a strong correlation between IBS and a history of sexual abuse.

SUGGESTED READINGS

Cover TL, Aber RC: *Yersinia enterocolitica*, *N Engl J Med* 321:16, 1989.

Gwyther RE et al: Validity of the family APGAR in patients with irritable bowel syndrome, *Fam Med* 25:21-25, 1993.

Lynn RB, Friedman LS: Irritable bowel syndrome, *N Engl J Med* 329(26):1940-1945, 1993.

PROBLEM · 18

CANCER PAIN MANAGEMENT

When Not to Say No to Drugs

Case 1 ■ A 75-Year-Old Male with Metastatic Bone Pain Secondary to Advanced Prostate Cancer

A 75-year-old male diagnosed with stage D cancer of the prostate 6 months ago comes to your office. He has been asymptomatic for the past 6 months, but last week he began to develop severe pain in the lower lumbar spine. He also appears quite pale.

On examination his prostate is rock-hard. He has tender lumbar vertebrae L2 to L5. Your suspicions of metastatic bone disease are confirmed when a technetium-99 bone scan shows increased uptake of radionuclide in L2-L5 and in both femurs, both tibias, and both humeri.

SELECT THE BEST ANSWER TO THE FOLLOWING QUESTIONS

Q1. What is the treatment of first choice at this time?
a. high-dose morphine sulfate
b. high-dose hydromorphone
c. transdermal fentanyl
d. palliative radiotherapy to the lumbar spine
e. acetaminophen-hydrocodone

Q2. You institute appropriate therapy for this patient. He quickly becomes pain free and remains that way for 6 months. He then returns with cervical, thoracic, and lumbar back pain; bilateral thigh pain; bilateral knee and leg pain; and pain in both shoulders and both arms (diffuse). Therapeutic options at this time include which of the following?
a. intravenous (IV) chlodrinate
b. IV radioactive strontium
c. morphine sulfate
d. hydromorphone
e. naproxen
f. all of the above

Q3. Which of the following pharmacologic agents is the drug of first choice for the treatment of mild metastatic bone pain?
a. morphine sulfate
b. hydromorphone
c. fentanyl
d. nonsteroidal antiinflammatory drug (NSAID)
e. carbamazepine

Q4. Which of the following drugs should not be used in the management of chronic pain?
   a. codeine
   b. meperidine
   c. levorphanol
   d. methadone
   e. a and b
   f. b and d

Case 2 ■ A 52-Year-Old Male with Metastatic Renal Cell Carcinoma

A 52-year-old male with metastatic renal cell carcinoma comes to your office for assessment of a pain beginning in the buttocks and traveling down the left leg. It has a sharp, stabbing, burning, or "zingerlike" quality, according to the patient. The patient indicates that the baseline pain is 5 on a 10-point scale, increasing up to 7/10 and decreasing down to 3/10.

Q5. What is the drug of first choice for the management of this patient's cancer pain?
   a. carbamazepine
   b. hydromorphone
   c. morphine sulfate
   d. amitriptyline
   e. desipramine

Case 3 ■ A 66-Year-Old Female with Metastatic Renal Cell Carcinoma

A 66-year-old female patient with metastatic renal cell carcinoma comes to your office for assessment of a pain beginning in the buttocks and traveling down the left leg. The only difference between this patient's pain and that of the patient in Case 2 is that this patient describes her pain as dull and throbbing. The baseline level is 4/10, increasing up to 8/10 and decreasing down to 2/10.

Q6. What is the drug of first choice for the management of this patient's cancer pain?
   a. carbamazepine
   b. hydromorphone
   c. morphine sulfate
   d. desipramine
   e. valproic acid

Q7. The location of the lesions described in the two patients presented in Cases 2 and 3 is best portrayed as which of the following?
   a. retroperitoneal
   b. lumbar-sacral plexopathy
   c. intraabdominal-visceral

   d. a and b
   e. b and c

Q8. What percentage of patients with cancer pain respond well to first-line analgesic therapy, such as acetaminophen or NSAIDs?
   a. 1%
   b. 5%
   c. 10%
   d. 15%
   e. 20%

Q9. Which of the following agents would be classified as second-line analgesic therapy for the management of cancer pain?
   a. hydrocodone
   b. acetaminophen
   c. morphine sulfate
   d. levorphanol
   e. hydromorphone

Q10. Which of the following agents is not classified as a third-line pharmacologic agent in the management of cancer pain?
   a. methadone
   b. morphine sulfate
   c. hydromorphone
   d. fentanyl
   e. codeine

Q11. A patient comes to your office with moderately severe cancer pain. You prescribe the third-line agent (since the patient describes the pain as moderately severe). Which of the following best describes the preferred approach to managing this patient's cancer pain?
   a. begin with a twice daily oral (PO) dose of long-acting morphine
   b. begin with a twice daily PO dose of long-acting morphine and short-acting PO morphine for breakthrough pain
   c. begin with a q4h dose of short-acting PO morphine
   d. begin with a transdermal fentanyl analgesic patch
   e. begin with a morphine dose of 200 mg/day in any form

Q12. A patient who is maintained on long-acting morphine with short-acting morphine for breakthrough pain comes to your office with a 1-week history of an increasing need for short-acting morphine. He is now taking three times the number of short-acting tablets as he was previously. What should you do at this time?

a. prescribe more short-acting morphine; keep the amount of long-acting morphine the same

b. transfer the increased requirement into long-acting morphine and maintain a supply of short-acting morphine

c. transfer the increased requirement into both increasing amounts of long-acting morphine and increased amounts of short-acting morphine

d. switch to another third-line oral agent

e. switch to a transdermal delivery system

Q13. What is the average starting daily dose of morphine sulfate in the treatment of a patient with moderately severe cancer pain?
a. 10 to 15 mg
b. 15 to 30 mg
c. 30 to 60 mg
d. 60 to 120 mg
e. 120 to 240 mg

Q14. Which of the following statements regarding the use of morphine in the treatment of a terminal cancer pain is (are) true?
a. morphine produces rapid tolerance
b. morphine produces euphoria
c. morphine produces respiratory depression
d. none of the above
e. all of the above

Q15. When starting a patient on a narcotic analgesic, what is the single most important agent that should be started at the same time?
a. an agent to prevent constipation
b. an agent to prevent nausea and vomiting
c. an agent to enhance sedation
d. an agent to prevent drowsiness
e. an antidepressant

Q16. Which of the following is (are) an essential element of cancer pain management?
a. a collaborative, interdisciplinary approach to care
b. an individualized pain control plan developed and agreed on by the patient
c. ongoing assessment and reassessment of the patient's pain
d. the use of both pharmacologic and nonpharmacologic therapies to prevent or control pain
e. all of the above

Q17. Which of the following is (are) an aim of pain management in palliative care?

a. to identify the cause of the pain
b. to prevent the pain from recurring
c. to maintain a clear sensorium
d. to maintain a normal effect
e. all of the above

Q18. Which of the following factors modify(ies) the pain threshold in patients with cancer pain?
a. insomnia
b. fear
c. anxiety
d. sadness
e. all of the above

Q19. Which of the following statements concerning the use of narcotic analgesics in the treatment of cancer pain is (are) true?
a. most patients with cancer pain can be effectively treated with oral agents
b. narcotic analgesics may be effectively administered by the rectal route
c. the subcutaneous infusion of narcotic analgesics has become the delivery method of choice in patients who cannot, for whatever reason, tolerate oral analgesics any longer
d. intramuscular narcotic administration on a regular basis is a reasonable alternative for pain control in terminally ill cancer patients
e. all of the above
f. a, b, and c only

Q20. A patient develops severe nausea and vomiting as the dose of morphine being used for terminal cancer pain (endometrial) is increased. The patient is on triple antinauseant therapy. Triple antinauseant therapy includes dimenhydrinate, metoclopramide, and prochlorperazine. Which of the following statements regarding this situation is true?
a. you should add a fourth antinauseant to the regimen at this time, preferably a corticosteroid or ondansetron
b. you should put an IV in place and make sure the input equals the output; do not change drugs
c. decrease the dose of the morphine by 10% for 24 hours
d. switch to another narcotic analgesic; no further investigations are necessary or desired
e. none of the above

Q21. A patient is switched from morphine sulfate to hydromorphone. You are aware that the oral

equianalgesic equivalent dose is 6/1 (6 parts morphine to 1 part hydromorphone). What should you do at this time?
a. start PO hydromorphone at the equianalgesic dose
b. start PO hydromorphone at 1/5 of the equianalgesic dose
c. start PO hydromorphone at twice the equianalgesic dose
d. start PO hydromorphone at 1/2 the equianalgesic dose
e. start PO hydromorphone at 1/3 the equianalgesic dose

Q22. A patient who is being treated for terminal cancer pain (esophageal adenocarcinoma) with PO morphine is requiring increased morphine doses daily. His morphine dose was 180 mg/day 6 weeks ago; it is 600 mg/day now. Which of the following statements regarding this increased dose of morphine is (are) true?
a. the dosage increase most likely represents tolerance to the morphine
b. the dosage increase most likely represents increased requirements because of tumor growth
c. both of the above statements are true
d. either a or b could be true, but not both
e. neither a nor b

Q23. A patient is being treated for breast cancer with adjuvant chemotherapy after a lumpectomy. One of the drugs she is taking is cisplatin. She develops intractable nausea and vomiting while on this drug. Which of the following antiemetics is the drug of first choice for this patient?
a. prochlorperazine
b. ondansetron
c. dimenhydrinate
d. metoclopramide
e. dexamethasone

Q24. A patient develops intractable nausea and vomiting secondary to carcinoma of the colon with partial bowel obstruction. She has taken both morphine and hydromorphone by mouth but is having great difficulty keeping anything down. What would you do at this time?
a. switch to levorphanol for the pain
b. switch to methadone for the pain
c. switch from the oral medication route to a subcutaneous infusion
d. switch from the oral route to the suppository route
e. switch from the oral route to the IV route

SHORT ANSWER MANAGEMENT PROBLEM

Discuss the following statement: "Overdosing cancer patients with narcotic analgesics is much more of a problem than underdosing cancer patients with narcotic analgesics."

ANSWERS

A1. **d.** This patient, who was diagnosed as having stage D cancer of the prostate 6 months ago, was treated in a responsible way. When a man with metastatic cancer has no symptoms, it is probably better to wait and save the limited weapons available until needed.

A very important point in this case is that although his bone scan shows more diffuse skeletal disease, his clinical status suggests symptoms only in the lumbar spine. Thus radiation therapy to the lumbar spine is the most reasonable course of action. Again, the reasoning is that local symptoms should receive local therapy. (This applies to palliative situations only.)

Although it would not be wrong to start with morphine sulfate or hydromorphone, it would be wrong to start high-dose morphine sulfate or high-dose hydromorphone. These narcotics will be discussed at great length in subsequent answers.

A2. **f.** The therapeutic options for the treatment of metastatic bone disease are rapidly increasing. The following treatment options have been shown to be effective: Bisphosphonates, radioactive strontium, NSAIDs, and narcotic analgesics.

A reasonable treatment plan at this time would be the following: Begin with an NSAID (naproxen) and short-acting morphine sulfate or short-acting hydromorphone for breakthrough pain. Ask the patient to call you within 24 hours to ensure the pain begins to decrease. On his next visit (in perhaps a week if you are beginning to get his pain under control) you could (a) switch him to a long-acting morphine preparation or a longer-acting hydromorphone preparation, (b) continue the NSAID, (c) continue to supply him with short-acting narcotics for breakthrough pain, (d) decide on either clodrinate or radioactive strontium as adjuvant therapy.

A3. **d.** The drug class of first choice for the management of mild to moderate metastatic bone pain is the NSAID agents. If these do not work, opioids can be added to NSAIDs for mild to moderate pain.

A4. **b.** Meperidine (Demerol) is contraindicated in the management of chronic pain (both malignant and nonmalignant) because of its relatively short half-life and its lack of efficacy.

The other drugs, levorphanol (PO) and methadone (PO), are very reasonable agents to use in the management of chronic cancer pain, as is fentanyl (transdermally, subcutaneously, or IV). Note the words "cancer pain." From experience and the opinions of world authorities on this issue, it is best (in almost all cases) not to use narcotic analgesics to manage chronic nonmalignant pain.

A5. **a.** See Answer 6.

A6. **d.** These two cases illustrate the use of adjuvant analgesics in the treatment of neuropathic pain. Neuropathic pain is the most common type of cancer pain and presents diagnostic and therapeutic challenges. It is basically described as being either a sharp, stabbing, burning, or "zingerlike" pain or a dull, aching pain. With respect to the two types of neuropathic pain:
   a. Both types respond better to adjuvant analgesics than to narcotic analgesics.
   b. Differences in response of the two pain types to typical adjuvant agents are as follows:
      1) The sharp, stabbing, burning pain responds better to anticonvulsant medications.
         a) The first choice is carbamazepine
         b) The second choice is valproic acid
      2) The dull, "aching" pain responds better to two tricyclic antidepressants:
         a) The first choice is desipramine
         b) The second choice is amitriptyline (unless sedation also would be of benefit to the patient)

A7. **d.** The greatest number of neuropathic pains seen in cancer pain management result from retroperitoneal lesions either infiltrating or pressing on the lumbosacral plexus.

A8. **e.**

A9. **a.**

A10. **e.** The World Health Organization (WHO) has developed an analgesic ladder for the treatment of cancer pain. Although it is not necessarily always in the patient's best interest to start with a first-line agent (the pain may be too severe), many patients can be managed with first-line agents such as acetaminophen or NSAIDs. In fact, 20% to 25% of patients with cancer pain can have their pain totally or almost totally controlled with these agents.

The WHO's analgesic ladder is summarized as follows:
   a. First-line agents:
      1) acetylsalicylic acid (ASA)
      2) Other NSAIDs
      3) Acetaminophen
   b. Second-line agents:
      1) Hydrocodone
      2) Codeine
   c. Third-line agents:
      1) Morphine sulfate
      2) Hydromorphone
      3) Fentanyl
      4) Levorphanol
      5) Methadone

A11. **c.** The best approach to the management of moderately severe cancer pain is to begin with an every-4-hour dose of short-acting morphine sulfate (the drug of first choice in the third-line group) and have the patient use the analgesic as needed to attain complete pain control. Once the dose is established, you may switch to a longer-acting preparation (twice daily) and maintain for the patient a supply of short-acting morphine for breakthrough pain.

A12. **b.** What the patient needs at this time is an increased supply of long-acting morphine as well as the maintenance of a supply of short-acting morphine for breakthrough pain.

A13. **c.** The average daily starting dose of morphine sulfate (PO) in a patient with moderately severe cancer pain is 30 to 60 mg.

A14. **d.** Although the use of morphine may cause tolerance, euphoria, and respiratory depression, these statements do not apply to patients who are in the terminal or palliative phase of their illness.

There is no maximum morphine or other analgesic equivalent dose. Each patient requires the dose to be individualized. This should be done by starting at lower doses and increasing the dose until you have achieved total pain control and are able to prevent further pain.

A15. **a.** Any patient who is started on a narcotic analgesic should also be started on a regimen to prevent constipation. The drugs most commonly used at this time include lactulose, an osmotic agent, and a combination of a stool softener and a peristaltic stimulant (such as docusate sodium and senna). An antiemetic such as dimenhydrinate, prochlorperazine, or metoclopramide may be indicated for the first 2 or 3 weeks to prevent nausea and vomiting that sometimes accompanies the initiation of a narcotic.

A16. **e.** New clinical practice guidelines have been issued by the Agency for Health Care Policy and Research, a branch of the Department of Health and Human Services. The purpose of these guidelines is to correct the problem of inadequate treatment (or underdosing) pain treatment for cancer. These guidelines call for the following:

a. A collaborative, interdisciplinary approach to the care of patients with cancer pain.
b. An individualized pain control plan developed and agreed on by the patient. The patient must be regarded as the head of the health care team.
c. Ongoing assessment and reassessment of the patient's pain.
d. The use of both nonpharmacologic and pharmacologic therapies to prevent or control pain.
e. Explicit institutional policies on the management of cancer pain, with clear lines of responsibility for pain management and for monitoring its effectiveness.

A17. **e.** The aims of pain management in palliative care are as follows:

a. To identify the cause of the pain
b. To prevent the pain from occurring again
c. To erase the memory of the pain
d. To maintain a clear sensorium and a normal effect

Remember that palliative care is active treatment, not passive treatment.

A18. **e.** Cancer pain is a complex entity that requires treatment of not only the somatic source(s) but also the other aspects, including depression, anxiety, anger, and isolation. Pain threshold is raised by relief of symptoms, sleep, rest, empathy, understanding, diversion, elevation of mood, effective analgesic therapy, anxiolytic therapy, and antidepressant therapy.

Pain threshold is lowered by discomfort, insomnia, fatigue, anxiety, fear, anger, sadness, depression, mental isolation, introversion, and past painful experiences.

Cancer pain should be considered as a complex consisting of a physical component, a psychologic component, a social component, and a spiritual component. Unless each one of these areas is addressed in the overall cancer pain management strategy, therapy will not be effective.

A19. **f.** The following facts and treatments should be considered in cancer pain management:

a. Cancer pain can be controlled in 90% of patients with oral medication.
b. The subcutaneous infusion of opioid analgesics by a programmed subcutaneous pump is the treatment of choice in patients who, for whatever reason, cannot tolerate the oral route.
c. The rectal route is an acceptable alternative for patients who cannot tolerate the oral route.

Regular intramuscular injections to control cancer pain should be discouraged because of pain, inconvenience, and unreliable drug absorption.

A20. **e.** At this time the first priority is to determine the cause of the nausea. The narcotic analgesic may not be the cause. A thorough search for all other serious and potential causes of the nausea must be undertaken. In this case a likely cause is hypercalcemia. Another common cause is the production by the tumor of emetic substances. Once causes such as these are ruled out, it is then reasonable to switch to another narcotic analgesic (such as hydromorphone) and/or to institute effective antiemetic therapy.

A21. **b.** When a patient is switched from one narcotic analgesic to another, a major adjustment must be made in equianalgesic dose. A common mistake made is to begin the patient on the exact equivalent (in milligrams) of the previously used narcotic. An equianalgesic dose no greater than 1/5 should be the starting dose of the next opioid. This is due to different types of opioid receptors in the brain.

For example, the switch from PO morphine to PO hydromorphone should be as follows:

a. The patient is currently taking 120 mg of PO morphine per day.
b. The equianalgesic dose is 120 mg/6 = 20 mg hydromorphone.
c. Starting the patient at 1/5 of the equianalgesic dose will be 20 mg/5 = 4 mg hydromorphone.

The pain control should be assessed frequently and the dose increased as needed.

A22. **c.** The increase in dose of morphine over the 6-week period most likely represents a combination of tolerance to morphine and increased requirements due to growth of the tumor. As pointed out earlier, rapid tolerance is not usually seen when the patient is being given a narcotic for cancer pain. However, tolerance can be developed over time and must be considered.

A23. **b.** Chemotherapy that includes the drug cisplatin is very likely to produce very severe nausea and vomiting. It is mandatory, therefore, to treat this aggressively. Ondansetron, a new serotonin antagonist, has been found extremely useful for the control of chemotherapy-induced nausea and is recommended. In other cases in which control is difficult despite combination antinauseant therapy, ondansetron should also be used.

A24. **c.** Cancer pain can be controlled by oral medications in the vast majority of cases (90%). When control with oral medications becomes impossible, however, it is necessary to switch to another route. Four possible routes are available: the suppository route, the IV route, the subcutaneous route, and the transdermal route.

With a patient in severe discomfort, the subcutaneous route is the route of choice. This is best accomplished using a computer-controlled subcutaneous infusion pump. This provides a constant infusion rate and boluses whenever needed.

SOLUTION TO THE SHORT ANSWER MANAGEMENT PROBLEM

This statement is completely false. Exactly the opposite is true. Patients with cancer pain are often very ineffectively treated. The ineffectiveness of treatment equates to significant undertreatment. It is estimated that 50% of patients with cancer pain die in significant pain. The major reasons for this appear to be as follows:

1. Fear on the part of physicians of using "too much" narcotic.
2. Fear on the part of physicians that the cancer patients will become addicted to the narcotics.
3. Fear on the part of physicians that they will personally get in trouble with their state medical board for prescribing strong narcotics to anyone.
4. A lack of knowledge regarding cancer pain management, the drugs that need to be used, and the doses of those drugs.

All of these contribute to the significant undertreatment described. Consequently, many patients suffer needless pain in the final stages of life.

SUMMARY OF THE DIAGNOSIS AND TREATMENT OF CANCER PAIN

The 10 commandments of cancer pain management:

1. Thou shalt not assume that the patient's pain is due to the malignant process. Always begin with steps aimed at making a specific, anatomic, and pathologic diagnosis.

2. Thou shalt consider the patient's feelings. Pain threshold varies with mood and morale. Given the opportunity to express fears, the patient should experience less pain.

3. Thou shalt not use the abbreviation *PRN (as needed)*. Achieving balanced pain control means avoiding the return of pain due to gaps in medication administration. Less medication will be required if given around the clock.

4. Thou shalt prescribe adequate amounts of medication. The right dose of medication is not dictated by recommendations from a book, but rather by the patient's level of pain. Use what it takes to relieve the pain, titrating for effect.

5. Thou shalt always try nonnarcotic medications as the first step unless your clinical judgment deems the patient to be in moderately severe or severe pain. Mild to moderate pain in many cases will respond to acetaminophen or NSAIDs. NSAIDs are particularly useful for bony metastases.

6. Thou shalt not be afraid of narcotic analgesics. When nonnarcotic agents fail, move to a narcotic agent quickly.

7. Thou shalt not limit thyself to using only drug therapies. Nondrug therapies such as hypnosis, imagery techniques, biofeedback, physiotherapy, individual psychotherapy, group psychotherapy, and family psychotherapy are very beneficial.

8. Thou shalt not be reluctant to seek a colleague's advice. When you have exhausted your skills or run out of ideas, ask someone else to evaluate your patient.

9. Thou shalt provide support for the entire family. Treatment of anticipatory grief experienced by the family will help to prevent isolation and loneliness. Be able to intervene quickly when a crisis arises.

10. Thou shalt maintain an air of quiet confidence and cautious optimism. Aim for "graded relief," choosing small goals that can be accomplished to build the patient's trust and hope. Exhibit a determination to succeed.

The WHO Analgesic Ladder is as follows:

1. Step 3:
   a. Morphine sulfate
   b. Hydromorphone
   c. Fentanyl
   d. Levorphanol
   e. Methadone

2. Step 2:
   a. Codeine (with or without acetaminophen)

b. Hydrocodone (with or without acetaminophen or ASA)

3. Step 1:
   a. Acetaminophen
   b. ASA
   c. NSAIDs

Classification of cancer pain is as follows:

1. Somatic pain (including bone pain)

2. Neuropathic pain:
   a. Sharp, stabbing, burning, "zingerlike"= type I
   b. Dull, aching = type II

3. Visceral pain

Adjuvant analgesics:

1. Corticosteroids: Used especially in visceral pain where there is swelling around a visceral capsule (e.g., the hepatic capsule); can also provide antiinflammatory activity, stimulate appetite, and decrease cerebral or spinal cord swelling.

2. Tricyclic antidepressants: Used for neuropathic pain of the dull, aching pain (amitriptyline, desipramine).

3. Anticonvulsant medications: Used for neuropathic pain of the sharp, stabbing, burning, "zingerlike" type.

4. NSAIDs: Used for somatic pain (metastatic bone).

Pathophysiology of cancer pain:

1. Physical (biologic) component: 25%

2. Psychologic (emotional) component: 25%

3. Social component: 25%

4. Spiritual component: 25%
   Unless all four components are addressed, the treatment of cancer pain will be unsuccessful.

Routes of administration:

1. Oral (90% of cancer cases)

2. Subcutaneous (5% of cancer cases)

3. Rectal (5% of cancer cases)

Conversion of one narcotic analgesic to another:

1. Calculate equianalgesic doses between drug 1 (the drug about to be discontinued) and drug 2 (the drug to be started).

2. Begin drug 2 at no more than 20% of equianalgesic dose. The reasons for this are that there is tolerance built up to the first drug and that different narcotics react on different receptors in the brain.

Method of beginning narcotic analgesic for moderate to severe cancer pain:

1. Choice drug: Usually morphine sulfate

2. Begin morphine sulfate with short-acting morphine (morphine, 5- or 10-mg tablets)

3. Daily starting dose: 30 to 60 mg/day

4. In 1 week switch total daily dose to long-acting morphine; continue short-acting morphine for breakthrough pain

5. Begin bowel regimen at same time as narcotic is begun: (1) lactulose or (2) stool softener (Colace) and peristaltic stimulant (senna alkaloid)

6. Consider antiemetic therapy for the first few weeks of narcotic therapy (prochlorperazine, dimenhydrinate, metoclopramide)

Cancer pain: Optimal management combines pharmacologic management with nonpharmacologic management:

1. Nonpharmacologic therapies:
   a. Relaxation techniques
   b. Support groups
   c. Biofeedback
   d. Mental imagery
   e. Physiotherapy
   f. Transcutaneous electrical nerve stimulation
   g. Physical activity
   h. Individual psychotherapy
   i. Group psychotherapy
   j. Family psychotherapy

Other forms of palliative cancer pain therapy include the following:

1. Palliative radiotherapy: Especially useful for metastatic bone pain and neuropathic pain (lumbosacral plexopathy and brachial plexopathy)

2. Palliative surgery

3. Palliative chemotherapy

SUGGESTED READINGS

Agency for Health Care Policy and Research: Management of cancer pain, *Clinical Practice Guideline #9*,1994; *http://www.AHCPR.gov.*

Doyle D et al, eds: *Oxford textbook of palliative medicine*, Oxford, 1993, Oxford University Press.

Ferri F et al: *Practical guide to the care of the geriatric patient*, St Louis, 1997, Mosby.

Tierney LM, McPhee SJ, Papadakis MA, eds: *Current medical diagnosis and treatment 2000*, ed 39, Stamford, Conn, 1999, Appleton & Lange.

Twycross R: Principles and practice of pain relief in terminal cancer. In Corr C, Corr D, eds: *Hospice care: Principles and practice*, New York, 1983, Springer.

PROBLEM · 19

MANAGEMENT IN PALLIATIVE CARE

"Oh Doctor, That Shot Gave Me a New Lease on Life."

Case 1 ■ A 51-Year-Old Female with Severe Nausea, Vomiting, and Anorexia with Advanced Ovarian Cancer

A 51-year-old female patient with advanced ovarian cancer has terminal disease. She is constantly nauseated, vomiting, and anorexic. You are called to see her at home. In addition to the symptoms mentioned, the patient complains of a "sore abdomen" and is having significant difficulty breathing. She also has a "sore mouth."

The patient has gone through chemotherapy with cisplatinum. This therapy ended 8 months ago. Her ovarian cancer was first discovered 12 months ago. Since that time her condition has deteriorated to the point where she has lost 40 pounds and is feeling "weaker and weaker" every day.

On examination, the patient's breathing is labored. Her respiratory rate is 28 breaths/min. The breath sounds heard in both lungs are normal. Her mouth is dry, and there are whitish lesions that rub off with a tongue depressor. She looks significantly cachectic. Her abdomen is significantly enlarged. There is a level of shifting dullness as well as the presence of a large abdominal mass that is approximately 8 cm × 35 cm.

SELECT THE BEST ANSWER TO THE FOLLOWING QUESTIONS

Q1. What is the drug of choice for the management of cancer-associated cachexia and anorexia?
   a. prednisone
   b. prochlorperazine
   c. megestrol acetate
   d. cyproheptadine
   e. a or c

Q2. The nausea and vomiting that this patient has developed may be treated with various measures or drugs. Which of the following could be recommended as first-line agents for this patient's nausea and vomiting?
   a. prochlorperazine
   b. dimenhydrinate
   c. metoclopramide
   d. all of the above
   e. none of the above

Q3. The drug that you selected for the treatment of the nausea and vomiting unfortunately was not effective. What would you do at this time?
   a. forget drugs and use a nasogastric (NG) tube
   b. combine two or three of the previously mentioned drugs
   c. forget treatment and attempt hydration with intravenous (IV) fluids
   d. select ondansetron as an antiemetic
   e. b or d

Q4. Based on the history of her "sore mouth" and white lesions that scrape off with a tongue depressor, what would you recommend treatment with?
   a. ketoconazole
   b. penicillin
   c. amphotericin B
   d. chloramphenicol
   e. methotrexate

Q5. The patient described undergoes palliative radiotherapy for severe bone pain that develops 1 month after the problems described. After this, significant diarrhea develops. Which of the following agents may be helpful in the treatment of this problem?
   a. diphenoxylate hydrochloride
   b. loperamide
   c. codeine
   d. all of the above
   e. none of the above

Q6. What is the most prevalent symptom in patients with cancer?
   a. anorexia
   b. asthenia
   c. pain
   d. nausea
   e. constipation

Q7. What is the most frequent cause of chronic nausea and vomiting in advanced cancer?
   a. bowel obstruction
   b. raised intracranial pressure
   c. narcotic bowel syndrome
   d. hypercalcemia
   e. autonomic failure

Q8. The patient described becomes increasingly short of breath. You suspect a pleural effusion. A chest x-ray confirms the diagnosis of a left pleural effusion. Which of the following is the treatment of first choice for this complication?
   a. a thoracocentesis
   b. home oxygen
   c. a hospital bed that is elevated at the head
   d. decreased fluid intake
   e. prochlorperazine

Q9. Which of the following treatments may also be useful for this symptom?
   a. palliative radiotherapy
   b. prednisone
   c. morphine sulfate
   d. dexamethasone
   e. all of the above

Q10. You treat the patient's pleural effusion effectively. She develops increasing abdominal distention, nausea, and vomiting 1 week later. You suspect a partial bowel obstruction. On examination, there are increased bowel sounds. A plain film of the abdomen confirms a diagnosis of partial bowel obstruction. Which of the following is (are) generally recommended as a palliative measure for this symptom?
   a. decreased fluid intake
   b. metoclopramide
   c. chlorpromazine
   d. all of the above
   e. none of the above

Case 2 ■ A 53-Year-Old Male with Sudden-Onset Left-Sided Weakness

A 53-year-old male comes to the Emergency Department with the sudden onset of left-sided weakness. He has a history of chronic obstructive pulmonary disease from chronic bronchitis. He describes himself as "healthy as a horse" even though he smokes three packs of cigarettes per day.

On examination, the patient has a left-sided hemiplegia. A chest x-ray shows a left-sided mass lesion and prominent hilar lymphadenopathy. You suspect a bronchogenic carcinoma.

Q11. Which of the following statements regarding this patient is true?
   a. there is likely no relationship between the hemiplegia and the chest x-ray findings
   b. the chances of recovery from the hemiplegia are essentially zero
   c. the cause of the hemiplegia is likely a cerebral embolus
   d. dexamethasone may be used both as a diagnostic test and as a therapeutic maneuver in this patient
   e. none of the above is true

Case 3 ■ A 42-Year-Old Female with Disseminated Breast Cancer

You are called to the home of a 42-year-old female with disseminated breast cancer. She has a fungating breast carcinoma that is emitting a very offensive odor. Her friends have stopped coming to see her because of the odor. The patient and her family have tried numerous remedies without success.

Q12. Which of the following may be useful in the treatment of the odor associated with this fungating growth?
   a. frequent cleansings with saline solution
   b. application of yogurt dressings
   c. application of buttermilk dressings
   d. charcoal briquettes strategically placed throughout the house
   e. all of the above

Case 4 ■ A 51-Year-Old Patient with Terminal Colon Cancer

You are called to the home of a 51-year-old patient with terminal colon cancer. He has become increasingly depressed and agitated and now is unable to sleep at night. As you talk to the patient and review in your head the DSM-IV criteria for depression, you realize that this patient has an agitated depression.

Q13. Which of the following may be indicated in the treatment of this patient's condition?
   a. a sedating tricyclic antidepressant in the evening
   b. an anxiolytic agent given on an as-needed (PRN) basis
   c. fluoxetine

d. a and/or b
e. all of the above

Q14. With regard to narcotic-induced nausea and vomiting, which of the following statements is (are) true?
a. nausea and/or vomiting is common in the initial narcotic administration period
b. nausea and/or vomiting associated with narcotic analgesics usually subsides within 2 weeks of beginning therapy
c. nausea and/or vomiting associated with narcotic administration can usually be prevented by the prophylactic use of medication
d. all of the above are true
e. none of the above is true

Q15. What is the drug of choice for the medical management of malignant ascites?
a. hydrochlorothiazide
b. spironolactone
c. prednisone
d. dexamethasone
e. none of the above

Q16. What is the most common metabolic derangement associated with advanced malignancy?
a. hyponatremia
b. hypokalemia
c. hypercalcemia
d. hypomagnesemia
e. hyperkalemia

Q17. What is the drug of choice for the management of narcotic-induced constipation?
a. a senna preparation
b. a psyllium compound
c. sodium docusate
d. lactulose
e. Metamucil

Q18. Which of the following statements regarding the use of combination antinauseant therapy in cancer is true?
a. combination antinauseants should not be used
b. the combination of any two drugs is just as effective as the combination of any other two
c. combination drugs should have affinity for different therapeutic receptors
d. oral antinauseants, especially when given together, are rarely effective for resistant nausea and/or vomiting
e. none of the above is true

SHORT ANSWER MANAGEMENT PROBLEM

Asthenia is the most commonly encountered symptom in terminally ill patients. Describe what the term *asthenia* means to you.

ANSWERS

A1. **e.** Prednisone (a corticosteroid) and megestrol acetate (a progestational agent) are the pharmacologic treatments of choice in patients with advanced cancer who have significant anorexia.

In patients with anorexia, oral nutrition should be the first priority, with particular attention paid to the timing of meals in relation to medical and nursing procedures and to the administration of drugs. Selected patients in whom oral nutrition or hydration is impossible may benefit from enteral nutrition or hypodermoclysis. Parenteral nutrition has shown no significant benefit in terms of improving survival or comfort, and its routine use is not indicated in palliative care.

Megestrol acetate in a dosage of 460 mg/day is rapidly becoming the pharmacologic agent of choice in the treatment of anorexia. An alternative to progestational agents is prednisone. Prednisone may be given in doses of approximately 10 to 15 mg/day. This may be increased if necessary.

With anorexia, particular attention must be paid to the mouth to prevent candidiasis and other problems.

Other potential choices for the pharmacologic treatment of anorexia include cyproheptadine, hydrazine sulfate, and cannabinoids.

A2. **d.** The nonpharmacologic treatment of nausea and vomiting should include (a) attempting to find the cause; (b) the avoidance of a supine position to prevent the dangers of aspiration of vomit; (c) a general assessment of the environment of the patient and how it could be improved; (d) attention to body odors; (e) small, frequent meals that the patient likes (not a bland diet); and (f) attractive food presentation.

Antiemetics can be divided into several classes, as follows:
a. Anticholinergics such as hyoscine and atropine
b. Phenothiazines such as prochlorperazine and chlorpromazine
c. Butyrophenones such as haloperidol and droperidol
d. Antihistamines such as cyclizine and promethazine
e. Gastrokinetic agents such as domperidone and metoclopramide
f. 5-HT_3 receptor antagonists such as ondansetron
g. Corticosteroids such as prednisone and dexamethasone

h. Miscellaneous agents such as ibuprofen, tricyclic antidepressants, benzodiazepines, and nabilone

There are some specific indications for certain antinauseants, such as the treatment of a partial bowel obstruction with a gastrokinetic agent, cyclizine for vestibular-associated emesis, and ondansetron for chemotherapy-induced emesis. In most cases, however, an antinauseant from any of the classes can be tried for any cancer-associated nausea.

Three general rules should be followed when prescribing antinauseants in cancer and palliative care management:

a. Before prescribing an antinauseant on a long-term basis, conduct a vigorous search for the underlying cause of the nausea.
b. If you are using combination antinauseant therapy, do not combine antinauseants from the same class of drugs.
c. If you are using combination antinauseant therapy, remember that antinauseants that work on the same neurotransmitter (dopamine, muscarinic/cholinergic, histamine) tend to be less effective when combined than antinauseants that work on different receptors.

Although a discussion of the receptors involved in each antinauseant is too detailed for this book, the following approach to treating the nausea and vomiting associated with cancer and palliative care is suggested:

a. Always consider nonpharmacologic therapy first plus small, frequent meals; appropriate food presentation; and foods that the patient likes.
b. Begin with prochlorperazine, dimenhydrinate, or metoclopramide.
c. Combine any two of the above or all three for resistant nausea.
d. Consider adding a corticosteroid such as prednisone or dexamethasone to the treatment regimen.
e. Consider ondansetron for chemotherapy-induced nausea and vomiting.
f. If emesis continues despite the above, try the rectal, subcutaneous, or suppository route.

A3. **e.** As mentioned, a combination of two or three of the antinauseants discussed in the choices in Question 2 would be very appropriate. Surprisingly, few significant problems with extrapyramidal side effects occur with combination therapy.

Ondansetron, the newest antiemetic, is a 5-HT receptor antagonist. However, it is very expensive ($15.00 per tablet), and this should certainly be considered when selecting between this and a combination of older agents.

Try to avoid an NG tube in palliative care patients whenever possible. NG tubes are uncomfortable and thus tend to have a negative, rather than a positive, impact on symptom control in cancer patients.

A4. **a.** White lesions that scrape off with a tongue depressor are almost certainly oral thrush. Oral thrush is extremely common in palliative cancer patients, even with good mouth care. Treatment with mycostatin, nystatin, or a newer agent such as ketoconazole is recommended.

A5. **d.** The diarrhea in this case is likely due to the effect of the radiotherapy on the bowel. Diphenoxylate, loperamide, and codeine are all good treatment choices. In most patients the diarrhea will settle down 1 to 2 weeks after the completion of the course of radiotherapy.

A6. **b.** Asthenia (fatigue) is the most prevalent symptom in advanced cancer patients. The prevalence of symptoms in advanced cancer patients is as follows: (a) asthenia, 90%; (b) anorexia, 85%; (c) pain, 76%; (d) nausea, 68%; (e) constipation, 65%; (f) sedation, 60%; (g) confusion, 60%; and (h) dyspnea, 12%.

A7. **a.** Although autonomic failure, hypercalcemia, narcotic bowel syndrome, and raised intracranial pressure can cause nausea and vomiting, the most frequent cause is bowel obstruction resulting from pressure caused by an intraabdominal tumor on the bowel itself, involvement of the bowel in the tumor process, associated gastric stasis, or other causes.

A8. **a.** A large pleural effusion should initially be treated by thoracentesis. If it recurs at infrequent intervals, this technique can be used repeatedly and with a sclerosing agent, such as talc infused. This can reduce the recurrence of a malignant effusion but is often irritating to the patient.

A9. **e.** However, if it recurs frequently, you may decide to use other symptom-relieving measures, including elevating the head of the bed, oxygen, fresh air, decreased fluid intake, prednisone or dexamethasone, morphine, and palliative radiotherapy.

A10. **d.** A partial bowel obstruction may be treated effectively by any of the following: gastrokinetic agents such as metoclopramide or domperidone; decreased fluid intake; antiemetic agents such as prochlorperazine, dimenhydrinate, metoclopramide, or ondansetron; or corticosteroids such as prednisone.

A11. **d.** This patient most likely has a primary lung carcinoma with metastatic disease to the brain. The metastatic disease has produced increased intracranial pressure, which has resulted in the neurologic symptoms.

The use of dexamethasone in this case can be both diagnostic and therapeutic. If the symptoms improve with dexamethasone, your suspicion of increased intracranial pressure as a cause of the symptoms is confirmed. An H2 receptor antagonist such as ranitidine should always be used when a palliative care patient is being treated with dexamethasone.

A12. **e.** Fungating growths, particularly carcinomas of the breast, can produce very unsightly lesions, as well as very offensive odors that have psychologic and social as well as medical implications. Often friends of the patient will stop coming because of the odor.

The most important aspects of treatment include proper cleaning of the fungating growth with saline compresses (not Dakin's solution or other solutions that may actually make it worse, not better), the application of yogurt (not fruit flavored) or buttermilk dressings, and the placement of charcoal briquettes strategically throughout the patient's room. The latter are very effective in weakening the odor of the fungating growth.

A13. **d.** An agitated depression is best treated by a combination of a sedating tricyclic antidepressant and/or an anxiolytic agent given on a PRN basis. Fluoxetine, in this case, may actually make the situation worse. Although fluoxetine and other selective serotonin reuptake inhibitors (SSRIs) have turned out to be a very important advance in the treatment of depressive disorders, fluoxetine can make an agitated depression worse. Thus, in this case, it is safer to stick to the older, proven reliable tricyclic antidepressants, especially one with sedating properties.

A14. **d.** When starting a patient on a narcotic analgesic, it is wise also to begin the patient on an antiemetic agent. Nausea and/or vomiting is an extremely common initial side effect that quickly (within 2 to 3 weeks) disappears. The antiemetic can then be discontinued. A good initial choice is prochlorperazine or dimenhydrinate.

A15. **b.** The drug of choice for the management of malignant ascites is the aldosterone antagonist spironolactone. Spironolactone has been shown to be effective in both malignant ascites and in the ascites associated with cirrhotic liver disease. Paracentesis may provide significant relief from malignant ascites and should be considered a method of first choice for acute relief.

A16. **c.** Hypercalcemia is the most common life-threatening metabolic disorder associated with cancer. It usually occurs in the context of advanced disseminated malignancy and produces a number of distressing symptoms. These include general symptoms such as dehydration, polydipsia, polyuria, and pruritus; gastrointestinal symptoms such as anorexia, weight loss, nausea, vomiting, constipation, and ileus; neurologic symptoms such as fatigue, lethargy, confusion, myopathy, hyporeflexia, seizures, psychosis, and coma; and cardiovascular symptoms such as bradycardia, atrial dysrhythmias, ventricular dysrhythmias, prolonged PR intervals, QT interval reductions, and wide T waves.

The primary treatment of hypercalcemia is IV fluid therapy. Other important treatments include corticosteroids, bisphosphonates, and calcitonin.

A17. **d.** The treatment of choice for narcotic-induced constipation is lactulose. Lactulose is an osmotic agent shown to be extremely useful in the management of hepatic encephalopathy. A very reasonable alternative would be a combination of a stool softener such as docusate sodium and a peristaltic stimulant such as senna.

The advantages of lactulose appear to be greater efficacy, especially in patients who are on high-dose narcotics, and the fact that it is a liquid rather than a pill.

Metamucil is contraindicated in the treatment of constipation in patients taking narcotic analgesics. Metamucil appears, in many cases, to make things worse by absorbing water and actually increasing the mass of stool that has to be evacuated.

Always attempt to find out why the patient is constipated; do not assume that it is due to narcotic analgesics.

A18. **c.** Antinauseants have been discussed previously. It was also mentioned that there are various neurotransmitter receptor sites that have been identified for antiemetic drugs. These neurotransmitters include dopamine, muscarinic/cholinergic receptors, and histamine receptors. In brief, some of the common antiemetics and their predominant neurotransmitter receptor sites include the following:

Antiemetic	Receptor Site
Dimenhydrinate	Dopamine
Prochlorperazine	Muscarinic/cholinergic
Chlorpromazine	Muscarinic/cholinergic
Metoclopramide	Muscarinic/cholinergic
Hyoscine	Dopamine/muscarinic/cholinergic

SOLUTION TO THE SHORT ANSWER MANAGEMENT PROBLEM

Asthenia is the most prevalent symptom in patients with advanced cancer. Two symptoms are usually included in the term *asthenia*: (1) fatigue or lassitude, defined as easy tiring and decreased capacity to maintain adequate performance, and (2) generalized weakness, defined as the anticipatory subjective sensation of difficulty in initiating a certain activity.

SUMMARY OF SYMPTOM MANAGEMENT IN PALLIATIVE CARE

1. Nausea and vomiting:
   a. Small, frequent meals
   b. Avoid bland foods. Give the patient what he/she wants to eat.
   c. Antiemetics:
      1) Prochlorperazine
      2) Dimenhydrinate
      3) Metoclopramide
      4) Prednisone
      5) Hycosin/atropine
      6) Ondansetron
   d. Consider a combination of antiemetics if one is not sufficient.
   e. If vomiting continues, consider the suppository or subcutaneous routes.

2. Constipation:
   a. Attempt to find the cause. Do not automatically assume it is due to narcotics.
   b. Lactulose appears to be the agent of choice for the treatment of constipation in palliative care. A combination of a stool softener and a peristaltic stimulant is a good alternative.

3. Anorexia:
   a. Small, frequent meals
   b. Avoid blended, pulverized foods; give the patient what he/she wants to eat.
   c. Megestrol acetate is the most effective agent for treating anorexia and cachexia in terminally ill patients. Prednisone is a good alternative.

4. Dry mouth/oral thrush:
   a. Mouth care is very important.
   b. Avoid drying agents such as lemon-glycerine swabs.
   c. Hydrogen peroxide at one-quarter strength, lemon drops, pineapple chunks, and tart juices.
   d. Look for oral thrush every day; treat with nystatin, mycostatin, or, if treatment-resistant, ketoconazole.

5. Dehydration: Dehydration is usually not symptomatic, that is, it usually does not have to be treated. Always base your decision to use fluids on whether or not you think it will make the patient feel better and improve the patient's quality of life. Remember, the most common occurrence from treating palliative care patients with IV fluids is iatrogenic pulmonary edema.

6. Diarrhea:
   a. Try to identify the cause.
   b. Diphenoxylate, loperamide, and codeine are equally effective.

7. Dyspnea and pleural effusion: Open windows, supplementary oxygen, semi-Fowler's position, bronchodilators, prednisone, narcotic analgesics, anxiolytics, diuretics, and palliative radiotherapy may all be of help with recurrent pleural effusions. Treat the first occurrence with thoracocentesis. How often you repeat this procedure depends on the patient's comfort level and how quickly the fluid reaccumulates.

8. Partial bowel obstruction:
   a. Restrict fluids.
   b. Antiemetics: Consider prokinetic agents such as metoclopramide first.
   c. Corticosteroids: Prednisone.
   d. Narcotic analgesics.
   e. Try to avoid using an NG tube if possible.

9. Malignant ascites:
   a. Paracentesis is often effective: How often you perform this procedure is dependent on the reaccumulation of fluid.
   b. Spironolactone alone or with thiazide and/or loop diuretics may be helpful.

10. Cerebral edema: Dexamethasone with an H2 receptor antagonist is both diagnostic and therapeutic.

11. Fungating growths:
    a. Frequent dressing changes; normal saline solution or hydrogen peroxide
    b. Yogurt or buttermilk dressings
    c. Charcoal briquettes around the house
    d. Fresh air

12. Depression and anxiety:
    a. Remember the bio-psycho-social-spiritual model of pain and symptom control.
    b. Psychotherapy: "be there, be sensitive, be silent."
    c. Tricyclic antidepressants/SSRIs.
    d. Anxiolytics (sublingual especially effective).

13. Hypercalcemia:
    a. Most common serious metabolic abnormality in palliative care.
    b. Think about the diagnosis: Otherwise, you will not make it.
    c. Fluids will effectively treat hypercalcemia in most cases.

SUGGESTED READINGS

Doyle D et al: *Oxford textbook of palliative medicine,* Oxford, 1993, Oxford University Press.

National Cancer Institute. *Pain management,* 1999, Cancer Net; http://www.nci.nih.gov.

PROBLEM·20

DIABETES MELLITUS

"I Must'a Gotten Up 10 Times Last Night To Go Potty."

Case 1 ■ A 17-Year-Old Female with Weight Loss, Polyuria, and Polydipsia

A 17-year-old female comes to your office with her mother. Her mother tells you that her daughter has lost 20 pounds in the last 6 months. In addition, she has been increasingly thirsty and has been experiencing a significantly increased frequency of urination. The patient has been feeling generally well, but she complains that her breath smells "funny."

On examination, the patient is well below the fifth percentile for weight. She looks thin and pale. Her blood pressure is 100/70 mm Hg. She has a few anterior cervical and axillary nodes measuring 1.0 cm. Her abdomen is slightly tender. No other abnormalities are found.

SELECT THE BEST ANSWER TO THE FOLLOWING QUESTIONS

Q1. If you could order only one test, which would it be?
    a. urine for protein and glucose
    b. fingerstick blood sugar level
    c. serum electrolytes
    d. blood gases
    e. complete blood count

Q2. You perform your one test. The result is 250 mg/dl. Which of the following statements is false?
    a. the diagnosis of the above disorder should be confirmed with a 3-hour test
    b. the diet used to manage this condition is based on exchanges
    c. a special diet is an essential component of treatment of this disorder
    d. insulin will likely be required to manage this patient's illness
    e. hospital inpatient management may not be necessary to begin treatment of this disorder

Q3. Which of the following statements regarding the diagnosis of the above disorder is (are) true?
    a. this disorder is confirmed if the fasting level of the particular substance exceeds 125 mg/dl on two occasions
    b. this disorder is confirmed if the venous plasma level of the particular substance exceeds 200 mg/dl on one occasion in the presence of symptoms
    c. this disorder is confirmed if, following a 3-hour test, two values measuring the particular substance exceed 200 mg/dl
    d. all of the above
    e. none of the above

Q4. Which of the following conditions is most closely associated with the described disorder?
    a. hypercholesterolemia
    b. hypothyroidism
    c. hypertriglyceridemia
    d. obesity
    e. cholelithiasis

Q5. What is the best measure of long-term control of the disease described?
    a. urine sugar levels
    b. daily blood sugar levels (3 or 4 times per day)
    c. hemoglobin A_{1C}
    d. hemoglobin F
    e. no microvascular or macrovascular complications

Q6. The hemoglobin A_{1C} should be below what value to be of use in predicting the development of microvascular and macrovascular complications?
    a. 3.5%
    b. 5.0%
    c. 7.2%
    d. 9.0%
    e. 10.0%

Q7. Which of the following statements is true?
a. microvascular complications are associated with type 1 diabetes; macrovascular complications are associated with type 2 diabetes
b. macrovascular complications are associated with type 1 diabetes; microvascular complications are associated with type 2 diabetes
c. microvascular and macrovascular complications are associated with type 1 diabetes; neither is associated with type 2 diabetes
d. microvascular and macrovascular complications are associated with both type 1 and type 2 diabetes
e. none of the above

Q8. Type 2 diabetics develop diabetic retinopathy in what percentage of cases?
a. 80%
b. 60%
c. 40%
d. 20%
e. 5%

Q9. Type 1 diabetics develop diabetic retinopathy in what percentage of cases?
a. 80%
b. 60%
c. 40%
d. 20%
e. 10%

Q10. Type 2 diabetics develop diabetic nephropathy in what percentage of cases?
a. 80%
b. 60%
c. 40%
d. 20%
e. 5%

Q11. Type 1 diabetics develop diabetic nephropathy in what percentage of cases?
a. 80%
b. 60%
c. 40%
d. 20%
e. 5%

Q12. Which one of the following statements is (are) true regarding diabetic nephropathy in the United States?
a. the prevalence of diabetic nephropathy is mainly contributed to by type 1 diabetics
b. the prevalence of diabetic nephropathy is mainly contributed to by type 2 diabetics

c. the ratio of type 2 diabetics to type 1 diabetics in the United States is 10:1
d. the ratio of type 1 diabetics to type 2 diabetics in the United States is 2:1
e. a and d
f. b and c

Case 2 ■ A 27-Year-Old Type 1 Diabetic with Protein in Her Urine

A 27-year-old type 1 diabetic comes to your office for her regular 3-month checkup. Your urine dipstick shows proteinuria 11. A 24-hour urine measurement produces a protein reading of 150 mg.

Q13. What should your next management step be?
a. do nothing; this is microalbuminuria
b. do nothing; this is still considered normal
c. start the patient on an angiotensin-converting enzyme (ACE) inhibitor
d. change the patient's diet—decrease protein by 10% a day
e. refer the patient to a diabetologist

Q14. Which one of the following statements regarding diet and diabetes is false?
a. diet is basic in the treatment of all diabetics
b. new evidence suggests that diabetics do not have to avoid foods that contain simple carbohydrates
c. the diabetic on insulin therapy must have three meals plus a bedtime snack at fixed times each day
d. the diabetic on insulin therapy should have frequent snacks
e. the diabetic on insulin should have a fixed caloric distribution

Q15. What is the average starting insulin dose for a newly diagnosed diabetic?
a. 2 to 4 units
b. 6 to 8 units
c. 10 to 12 units
d. 15 to 20 units
e. 20 to 30 units

Q16. Which of the following best explain(s) the Somogyi effect?
a. the Somogyi effect results from rebound hyperglycemia
b. the Somogyi effect results from relative insulin deficiency in the morning
c. the Somogyi effect results from rebound hypoglycemia

d. the Somogyi effect results from relative insulin excess resulting from administration of excessive insulin in the evening

e. a and d

Q17. Which of the following best explains the dawn phenomenon?

a. the dawn phenomenon results from relative insulin deficiency in the morning

b. the dawn phenomenon results from rebound hyperglycemia

c. the dawn phenomenon results from rebound hypoglycemia

d. the dawn phenomenon results from the wrong mixture of insulins

e. none of the above

Q18. A newly diagnosed type 1 diabetic is given a total insulin dose of 18 units. Which of the following is likely to be the correct morning/evening (AM/PM), regular/intermediate insulin dose?

a. morning: total 12 units: regular 6 units, intermediate 6 units; evening: total 6 units: regular 3 units, intermediate 3 units

b. morning: total 9 units: regular 6 units, intermediate 3 units; evening: total 9 units: regular 6 units, intermediate 3 units

c. morning: total 12 units: regular 4 units, intermediate 8 units; evening: total 6 units: regular 2 units, intermediate 4 units

d. morning: total 6 units: regular 4 units, intermediate 2 units; evening: total 12 units: regular 4 units, intermediate 8 units

e. morning: total 6 units: regular 3 units, intermediate 3 units; evening: total 12 units: regular 8 units, intermediate 4 units

Q19. What is the most likely explanation for the "abnormal gas in the stomach" seen in upright abdominal radiographs of many diabetics?

a. gastroparesis resulting from diabetic autonomic neuropathy

b. gastroparesis caused by sympathetic dysfunction

c. associated with diabetic ketoacidosis

d. associated with hyperosmolar coma

e. none of the above

Q20. Regarding the pathophysiology of the disorder described in Case 1, which of the following statements is (are) true?

a. environmental factors are likely involved in the pathology of this condition

b. human leukocyte antigen (HLA-DR4) is strongly associated with this condition

c. this disorder may be associated with other autoimmune disorders

d. all of the above

e. none of the above

Case 3 ■ A 65-Year-Old Female with a Fasting Sugar Level of 240 mg/dl

A 65-year-old asymptomatic obese female has a routine fasting sugar level drawn at the time of her annual physical examination. The level comes back at 240 mg/dl. Her urine is negative for ketones. The test is repeated the following day and comes back at the same level.

Q21. Which of the following statements about this patient is incorrect?

a. the patient has type 2 diabetes mellitus

b. insulin is the agent of first choice in the management of this condition

c. a diabetic diet forms the cornerstone of therapy in this condition

d. insulin and an oral hypoglycemic agent may be used together in the treatment of this condition

e. monitoring of this condition is best done by home glucose monitoring

Q22. The pathophysiology of type 2 diabetes is associated with all of the following except:

a. increased insulin resistance

b. decreased serum insulin levels

c. abnormal glucagon secretion

d. a decrease in beta-cell mass, abnormal function of beta-cells, or both

e. amyloid of the islet cells

Q23. Gestational diabetes mellitus of pregnancy is screened by a 50-g glucose load, with blood drawn 1 hour after administration of the load. What is the usual value considered the upper limit of normal for this test?

a. 110 mg/dl

b. 140 mg/dl

c. 160 mg/dl

d. 180 mg/dl

e. 200 mg/dl

Q24. Which of the following statements regarding type 2 diabetes mellitus is true?

a. most patients come to their physicians with symptoms

b. most patients are essentially asymptomatic at diagnosis (apart from being obese)

c. most patients can control the diabetes by diet and exercise

d. most patients will not manifest complications

e. most patients are under age 40 years

Q25. Which of the following statements regarding individuals with type 2 diabetes of onset during youth (maturity-onset diabetes of the young [MODY]) is (are) true?

a. these patients are usually normal weight to underweight

b. this is an autosomal dominant condition

c. this type of diabetes is present in 50% of the siblings of the parents with this disease

d. all of the above

e. none of the above

SHORT ANSWER MANAGEMENT PROBLEM
Describe macrovascular and microvascular complications associated with diabetes mellitus.

ANSWERS

A1. **b.**

A2. **a.**

A3. **d.** This patient has diabetes mellitus type 1. Diabetes mellitus type 1 is also known as insulin-dependent diabetes and must be managed with a combination of a diabetic diet using "exchanges," human insulin, and exercise. Unless the patient has diabetic ketoacidosis, there is no reason that both diagnosis and initial management cannot take place on an outpatient basis.

The diagnosis of diabetes mellitus type 1 is very important. The criteria that have been adopted by the American Diabetes Association are as follows:

a. One fasting plasma glucose value exceeding 125 mg/dl

b. One random plasma glucose value exceeding 199 mg/dl in the presence of symptoms

c. Two-hour post-glucose value values exceeding 199 mg/dl in an oral glucose tolerance test (GTT)

Each must be confirmed on a subsequent day by a different method for diagnosis to occur. In the patient described, the second criterion can be used to make the diagnosis of diabetes mellitus. A random nonfasting glucose value of 160 mg/dl or greater is considered a positive screen and warrants further testing to determine if the diagnostic criteria can be met.

A4. **c.** The disease of those listed that is most closely associated with diabetes mellitus is hypertriglyceridemia. Triglyceride levels of two to three times normal

are often the first sign of undiagnosed diabetes mellitus. All individuals with a significantly elevated serum triglyceride level should be screened for diabetes mellitus.

A5. **c.** The best measure of long-term control of diabetes mellitus (type 1 and type 2) is hemoglobin A_{1c}.

A6. **c.** Recent studies have shown that "tight control"(that is, maintenance of the mean plasma glucose level at less than 155 mg/dl and hemoglobin A_{1c} at 7.2% or less) produces at least a 60% reduction in microvascular and macrovascular complications.

A7. **d.** One very important and underappreciated fact is that both macrovascular (atherosclerotic heart disease, coronary artery disease, peripheral vascular disease, cerebrovascular disease) and microvascular (retinopathy, nephropathy, peripheral neuropathy) diseases are associated with both types of diabetes. Type 2 diabetics are not immune to diabetic complications; quite the contrary is true.

A8. **d.**

A9. **d.**

A10. **d.**

A11. **c.** The percentage of complications (macrovascular and microvascular) in type 1 diabetes and type 2 diabetes are as follows:

a. Type 1 diabetes:
1) Retinopathy: 20% of patients
2) Nephropathy: 40% of patients
b. Type 2 diabetes:
1) Retinopathy: 20% of patients
2) Nephropathy: 20% of patients

A12. **f.** Since there are at least 10 type 2 diabetics for each type 1 diabetic patient, the prevalence of complications resulting from type 2 diabetes is higher than for type 1 diabetes.

A13. **c.** The diabetic patient who comes with microalbuminuria already has a problem. The probability of this individual's going on to develop overt nephropathy is quite high. It has now been demonstrated that progression to overt nephropathy can be prevented by the prophylactic administration of an ACE inhibitor. The drugs of choice are captopril or enalapril.

A14. **b.** Diet is an essential component of treatment in all diabetic patients. It is especially important, however, for the insulin-dependent type 1 diabetic. In the diabetic the rate at which insulin enters the blood from an injection site is fixed, and the diabetic must match meals to the pattern of insulin absorption. The diabetic's diet should be the same as the diet suggested for a nondiabetic of the same age.

During the past several years the avoidance of sweets and foods that contain simple carbohydrates has been challenged, but until further information is presented it seems reasonable to instruct diabetics to avoid beverages with sucrose and desserts that are highly sweetened.

The diabetic on insulin therapy must have three meals at fixed times each day, with a fixed distribution of calories. Frequent snacks, also with a fixed distribution of calories, are also recommended.

If a diabetic patient is overweight, a weight-reducing program should be initiated. This may be facilitated by substituting complex carbohydrates with high residue for simple sugars. In addition, saturated animal fats should be replaced with polyunsaturated vegetable fats. One fifth of the daily caloric intake should be consumed at breakfast and about two fifths at each of lunch and supper. These percentages may be reduced to allow for small snacks, such as crackers or fruit, in mid-afternoon and bedtime. A reasonable exercise program is fundamental to the treatment of all diabetics.

A15. d. The average starting dose of insulin is 15 to 20 units. The obese individual may need 25 to 30 units/day. The dose, however, must be individualized; some persons require more, some persons require less. In addition, patients who are initially given insulin in the hospital may end up with very different insulin requirements when they are at home and more active; usually the insulin requirement will be significantly less.

A16. e.

A17. a. Morning hyperglycemia in a diabetic on insulin may result from relative insulin deficiency (the dawn phenomenon) or to rebound hyperglycemia (the Somogyi phenomenon). Because the treatment of these two conditions is completely opposite, they must be distinguished.

The dawn phenomenon, a relative insulin deficiency caused by waning-off of insulin action in the early morning hours, is most likely mediated by an increased nocturnal output of growth hormone (which has antiinsulin activity). It is treated by increasing the dose of evening insulin.

The Somogyi effect, a rebound hyperglycemia after a hypoglycemic reaction, is treated by decreasing, not increasing, the dosage of evening insulin.

The dawn phenomenon can be distinguished from the Somogyi effect by determination of the 3:00 AM glucose. Therefore all diabetic patients should periodically measure their 3:00 AM blood sugar in addition to regularly measuring their blood sugars three or four times a day.

A18. c. The starting dose of insulin is usually as follows:
   a. Morning: two thirds of total daily dose
   b. Evening: one third of total daily dose
   c. Morning: two thirds intermediate, one third regular
   d. Evening: two thirds intermediate, one third regular

A19. a. The "abnormal gas in the stomach" most likely results from diabetic gastroparesis. This is a very common complaint, and it is best treated by a prokinetic agent such as metoclopramide, domperidone, cisapride, or macrolide antibiotics.

A20. d. Two distinct types of type 1 diabetes have been identified. In type 1A, the environmental factors combined with genetic factors are thought to result in cell-mediated destruction of pancreatic beta cells. Human leukocyte antigen (HLA-DR4) is strongly associated with this phenomenon.

Type 1B is an uncommon primary autoimmune condition that occurs in individuals with other autoimmune conditions, such as Hashimoto's disease, Graves' disease, pernicious anemia, and myasthenia gravis. This condition is associated with histocompatibility antigen HLA-DR3 and occurs later in life, typically between ages 30 and 50 years.

Specific environmental factors linked to type 1 diabetes mellitus are the following:
   a. Drugs and chemicals: Streptozocin and pentamidine
   b. Viruses: Mumps, coxsackie, rubella (40% of patients with congenital rubella develop type 1 diabetes later), and cytomegalovirus

A21. b. This patient has type 2 diabetes mellitus. Type 2 diabetes accounts for 90% of all cases of diabetes. Type 2 diabetes is characterized by both an impairment of beta-cell function and a decreased sensitivity to insulin in the cells of the body.

Type 2 diabetes mellitus is often discovered in asymptomatic patients by finding an elevated blood sugar level. It may also present with nonspecific symptoms including fatigue, weakness, blurred vision, vaginal and perineal pruritus and candidiasis, impotence, and paresthesias. Weight loss is uncommon in these patients. The majority of patients with type 2 diabetes mellitus are obese; many have a strong family history of obesity and diabetes.

A diabetic diet, weight management, and exercise should be pushed to the maximum. If these are not effective, an oral hypoglycemic agent should be the next step.

Oral hypoglycemic agents currently available include sulfonylureas, α-glucosidase inhibitors, biguanides, meglitinides, and thiazolidinediones. The first-generation sulfonylurea agents include tolbutamide, chlorpropramide, acetohexamide, and tolazamide. The second-generation agents include glyburide, glipizide, and glimepiride.

Sulfonylureas work by stimulating the secretion of insulin in the pancreas and by increasing insulin sensitivity in the peripheral tissue. Biguanides work by decreasing the production of glucose and increasing its uptake in the periphery. Because of the rare complication of lactic acidosis, biguanides should be used with caution, particularly in patients with renal insufficiency. Meglitinides work by stimulating insulin release from the pancreas. Thiazolidinedione derivatives such as rosiglitazone decrease insulin resistance. Troglitazone, the first agent in this class, caused elevations in hepatic enzymes, jaundice, and, liver failure and was removed from the market. The α-glucosidase inhibitor acarbose works by reduction of the absorption of glucose, but has been associated with gastrointestinal discomfort.

Oral hypoglycemic therapy should begin with the lowest effective dose; this should then be increased every few days to achieve maximal control. Self-monitoring of blood glucose levels is the key to evaluating the efficacy of an oral hypoglycemic-mediated treatment program. The table below summarizes the classes of oral hypoglycemic drugs available.

■ Classes of Oral Agents

Class	Examples	Mechanism of Action
Sulfonylureas	Glyburide	Increased secretion of insulin
Alpha glucosidase inhibitors	Acarbose	Delayed carbohydrate absorption
Biguanides	Metformin	Decreased insulin resistance and gluconeogenesis
Meglitinides	Repaglinide	Increased secretion of insulin
Thiazolindinediones	Rosiglitazone	Decreased insulin resistance

About 25% to 30% of type 2 diabetes mellitus patients fail to respond to sulfonylurea drugs. These patients are called *primary failures*. In addition, about 5% of patients who initially responded to these drugs will lose their responsiveness. These patients are termed *secondary failures*. Sometimes a combination of a morning oral hypoglycemic and an evening intermediate-acting insulin can be beneficial in lowering blood sugar levels to normal.

With the several classes of agents now available, other combination therapies can be used besides combination with insulin. Sulfonylureas may be combined with several different classes of agents, such as with metformin, acarbose, and troglitazone. Sulfonylureas may also be combined with the new class of agents, meglitinides, the first of which was approved by the Food and Drug Administration and is known as repaglinide. Repaglinide is a nonsulfonylurea benzoic acid derivative that stimulates insulin release from the pancreas. Repaglinide may be used in combination with metformin. All combination therapies require the same careful attention to side effect profiles and outcomes that monotherapies do. Nevertheless, with the increased variety and range of agents available, patients with type 2 diabetes now have more options for effective pharmacotherapy.

A22. **b.** The cause of type 2 diabetes mellitus is unknown. Although it is thought to be autosomal recessive, it mainly affects obese people over age 40 years. Subsequent insulin resistance (secondary to obesity) is a factor in 60% to 80% of type 2 diabetics. Decreased beta-cell responsiveness to glucose is noted; abnormal glucagon secretion accompanies this. The islet cell dysfunction may be caused by a decrease in beta-cell mass, abnormal function of the beta-cells, or some other combination.

Amyloid of the islet cells occurs in up to 40% of type 2 diabetics. Fatty infiltration, ischemia caused by vascular sclerosis, and pancreatic fibrosis occur in up to 66% of type 2 diabetics; this contributes to pancreatic atrophy.

A23. **b.** The screening test for gestational diabetes mellitus is as follows:
   a. Time: 24 to 28 weeks
   b. Glucose load: 50 g
   c. Time sample drawn: 1 hour
   d. Screening cut-off: 140 mg/dl

A24. **b.** Patients with type 2 diabetes demonstrate the following:
   a. Most patients are asymptomatic; identification most often occurs by screening.
   b. Most patients are over age 40 years.
   c. Most patients develop the same complications (microvascular and macrovascular complications) as in type 1 diabetics.
   d. Most patients have motivational difficulties in relation to diet and exercise.

A25. **d.** Type 2 diabetes of youth (MODY) has the following characteristics:

  a. Most patients are normal weight to underweight.
  b. Most patients are younger than age 40 years.
  c. Of all patients, 50% have parents with the disorder.
  d. The disorder is autosomal dominant.

SOLUTION TO THE SHORT ANSWER MANAGEMENT PROBLEM

Macrovascular complications:
  1. Atherosclerotic vascular disease:
     a. Coronary artery disease
     b. Myocardial infarction: sudden cardiac death
     c. Cerebrovascular disease and stroke
     d. Peripheral vascular disease
     e. Intestinal ischemia
     f. Renal artery stenosis
Microvascular complications:
  1. Renal disease: Diabetic nephropathy
  2. Peripheral neuropathy:
     a. Paresthesias
     b. "Glove and stocking" neuropathy
  3. Autonomic neuropathy:
     a. Gastroparesis
     b. Impotence
  4. Diabetic retinopathy:
     a. Cotton-wool exudates
     b. Neovascularization

SUMMARY OF THE DIAGNOSIS AND TREATMENT OF DIABETES MELLITUS:

1. Type 1 diabetes:
   a. Epidemiology: 10% of all cases of diabetes
   b. Signs and symptoms: Polyuria, polydipsia, nocturia, weight loss
   c. Etiology: Genetics and environment
      1) Most common: HLA-DR4 and viral exposure
      2) Less common: Associated with other autoimmune diseases
   d. Diagnosis:
      1) Two values of 126 mg/dl or greater
      2) One random blood sugar level ≥200 mg/dl and symptoms
      3) Two blood sugar levels ≥200 mg/dl in a 3-hour 75-g GTT (one value at 2 hours)
   e. Self-monitoring: Home blood sugar monitoring
      1) four values 3 times/week
      2) Strict control reduces complications
   f. Long-term control: Hemoglobin A_{1c}, less than 7.2%

   g. Treatment:
      1) Diet (based on exchanges)
      2) Exercise
      3) Insulin (regular intermediate)
      4) Total initial dose: 15 to 20 units
         a) "The rule of two-thirds": Two thirds of total AM dose (split 2:1, regular:intermediate)
         b) One third of total PM dose (split 2:1, regular:intermediate)
   h. Complications:
      1) Macrovascular
      2) Microvascular
Both type 1 and type 2 diabetes mellitus have macrovascular and microvascular complications. Because the ratio of type 2 to type 1 is 10:1, 80% of the cases of diabetic nephropathy are due to type 2 diabetes.

2. Type 2 diabetes mellitus:
   a. Epidemiology: 90% of all cases of diabetes mellitus are type 2.
   b. Signs and symptoms:
      1) Most patients are discovered when undergoing screening in a medical setting.
      2) The minority of type 2 diabetes present symptoms.
   c. Etiology:
      1) Race (such as North American Indian)
      2) Genetic factor
      3) Obesity
   d. Diagnosis: Diagnosis of type 2 diabetes is the same as type 1.
   e. Self-monitoring: Same as type 1
   f. Long-term control: Same as type 1
   g. Treatment:
      1) Weight control absolutely essential
      2) Exercise (regular: 3 times/week)
      3) Oral hypoglycemics: Second- or first-degree oral agents
      4) A small percentage (15% to 20%) of type 1 diabetics need insulin in the evening in addition to oral hypoglycemics (glyburide/glipizide) in the morning.
   h. Complications: Same as type 1 diabetes mellitus

SUGGESTED READINGS

American Diabetes Association at *http://www.diabetes.org*, 2000.
Bailey CJ, Turner RC: Metformin, *N Engl J Med* 334(9):574-579, 1996.
Beaser RS, White RD: *Strategies for the prevention and treatment of macrovascular complications of type 2 diabetes*, Kansas City, Mo, 1998, AAFP.
Clark CM, Lee DA: Prevention and treatment of the complications of diabetes mellitus, *N Engl J Med* 332(18):1210-1217, 1995.
Curry RW, Horton ES: *Current therapies for the treatment of type 2 diabetes mellitus*, Kansas City, Mo, 1997, AAFP.

Holleman F, Hoekstra JBL: Insulin lispro, *N Engl J Med* 337(3):176-183, 1997.

Reaven GM et al: Hypertension and associated metabolic abnormalities: the role of insulin resistance and the sympathoadrenal system, *N Engl J Med* 334(6):374-381, 1996.

Spann S, Woolf S: *Preventing the microvascular complications of diabetes*, Kansas City, Mo, 1998, AAFP.

Troglitazone for non-insulin-dependent diabetes mellitus, *Med Lett* 39(1001):49-52, 1997.

White JR: The pharmacological reduction of blood glucose in patients with type 2 diabetes mellitus, *Clin Diabetes* 16(2):58-72, 1998.

PROBLEM·21

MISCELLANEOUS ENDOCRINE DISEASE

Too Much or Too Little Messenger or, Perhaps,
Poor Reception.

Case 1 ■ A 45-Year-Old Male with "Visual Problems," Headaches, Weight Gain, Sweating, and "Hands and Feet That Are Changing"

A 45-year-old male comes to your office with his wife. He is very concerned about some "bizarre symptoms" that he has been experiencing. He is the CEO of a major manufacturing company and is "really embarrassed to go out in public any longer." He tells you that about 6 months ago he began to experience the following symptoms: headaches, visual spots or defects, weight gain, an appearance of his forehead growing, enlarging hands and feet (he could no longer get his gloves and shoes on), and increased sweating.

On examination, the apical impulse is felt in the fifth intercostal space, midclavicular line. His blood pressure is 170/105 mm Hg. He does have a protruding brow, and three discrete visual field defects are noted (two in the left eye and one in the right eye). His tongue appears enlarged, and he is sweating profusely.

SELECT THE BEST ANSWER
TO THE FOLLOWING QUESTIONS

Q1. What is the most likely diagnosis in this patient?
a. adrenocorticotropic hormone (ACTH) excess
b. acromegaly
c. prolactinoma
d. primary hypopituitarism
e. primary hyperparathyroidism

Q2. The pathophysiologic lesion resides in which of the following?
a. adrenal gland: adenoma
b. hyperparathyroid glands: adenoma in one or more of the four glands
c. pituitary gland: adenoma
d. gastrointestinal ectopic tumor: adenoma
e. none of the above

Q3. The treatment for this patient may include which of the following?
a. surgery: transsphenoidal
b. radiation
c. bromocriptine
d. heavy-particle pituitary radiation
e. all of the above
f. none of the above

Case 2 ■ A 24-Year-Old Male with Weakness and Hyperpigmentation

A 24-year-old male comes to your office with an extreme feeling of weakness, a 20-pound weight loss, a change in the color of his skin (his skin has become very hyperpigmented), lightheadedness, and dizziness.

On examination, the patient has a definite change in skin color since you last saw him 9 months ago. His blood pressure is 90/70 mm Hg and he looks acutely ill.

On laboratory examination, his serum Na^+ level is low (115 mEq/L); his serum potassium level is high (6.2 mEq/L); his urea level is elevated at 9.0 mg/dl; and his serum calcium level is elevated (12.0 mg/dl).

Q4. On the basis of this history, physical examination, and laboratory findings, what is the most likely diagnosis of this patient?
a. Conn's syndrome
b. Cushing's syndrome
c. Addison's syndrome
d. primary hyperparathyroidism
e. primary pituitary failure

Q5. What is the most likely cause for this patient's symptoms?
a. overstimulation of the adrenal gland
b. an adrenal adenoma
c. autoimmune destruction of the hyperparathyroid glands
d. autoimmune destruction of the adrenal gland
e. a pituitary adenoma

Q6. What is the acute treatment of choice for this patient?
a. prednisone orally
b. dexamethasone orally
c. intravenous (IV) cortisol
d. IV ACTH
e. intramuscular (IM) depo-provera

Q7. This patient will need chronic treatment with which of the following?
    a. hydrocortisone
    b. fludrocortisone acetate
    c. a or b
    d. a and b
    e. none of the above

Case 3 ■ A 25-Year-Old Female with Increased Thirst and Urination

A 25-year-old female comes with reports of a sudden onset of increased thirst and urination. This began abruptly 1 week ago and has not abated since. She states that since that time she has been thirsty all the time. The only significant illness in her life has been the recent diagnosis of bipolar affective illness subtype I that was made 6 weeks ago. She was started on lithium carbonate and is currently taking 1200 mg/day. Her serum lithium levels have been normal since the beginning.

On examination, her blood pressure is 110/70 mm Hg. She has lost 5 pounds during the last week and looks somewhat dehydrated.

Q8. What is the most likely diagnosis in this patient?
    a. psychogenic polydipsia
    b. type I diabetes mellitus
    c. central diabetes insipidus
    d. nephrogenic diabetes insipidus
    e. adverse drug reaction to lithium

Q9. What is the treatment of choice in this patient?
    a. hospitalization and complete psychiatric assessment
    b. insulin: beginning at 10 to 20 units/day
    c. glyburide
    d. discontinuation of lithium carbonate
    e. substitution of carbamazepine for lithium carbonate

Case 4 ■ A 37-Year-Old Overly Tired Hypertensive Female

A 37-year-old female comes to your office because she was found to be "hypertensive" by a nurse in a shopping mall screening program. She tells you that when she thinks about it, she really has not felt well for a couple of months. Her major complaint has been profound generalized fatigue and weakness. She has also been increasingly thirsty, urinating more frequently, and having to urinate frequently at night.

On physical examination, her blood pressure is 190/110 mm Hg. Laboratory abnormalities include a mildly increased serum Na^+ level (150 mEq/L), hy-pokalemic metabolic alkalosis, a low renin level, and increased urine potassium level.

Q10. What is the most likely diagnosis based on the information presented in Case 4?
    a. Conn's syndrome
    b. Cushing's syndrome
    c. Addison's syndrome
    d. Bartter's syndrome
    e. diabetes insipidus

Q11. What is the most likely pathophysiologic cause of this syndrome?
    a. benign adenoma of the adrenal gland
    b. malignant adenoma of the adrenal gland
    c. pituitary adenoma
    d. bilateral hyperplasia of the adrenal gland
    e. none of the above

Q12. What is the treatment of choice for the condition described in Case 4?
    a. bromocriptine
    b. transsphenoidal surgery
    c. clomiphene
    d. spironolactone
    e. surgical removal of the adenoma

Case 5 ■ A 22-Year-Old Female with Breast Secretions, Amenorrhea, and Decreased Libido

A 22-year-old female, married for 18 months, has been trying to get pregnant without success. Approximately 9 months ago, she developed breast secretions, amenorrhea, and decreased libido. No other symptoms are present.

On examination, there is definite galactorrhea present. Her blood pressure is 140/80 mm Hg. No abnormalities are found on physical examination.

Q13. From the information provided, what is the most likely diagnosis?
    a. anorexia nervosa
    b. stress-induced amenorrhea
    c. "I want to have a baby but can't" syndrome
    d. prolactinoma
    e. hypopituitarism

Q14. If you could order only one test, what would that test be?
    a. serum estrogen level
    b. serum progesterone level
    c. serum luteinizing hormone level
    d. serum follicle-stimulating hormone level
    e. serum prolactin level

Q15. What is the treatment of choice for this condition?
- a. transsphenoidal resection
- b. bromocriptine
- c. clomiphene
- d. lithium carbonate
- e. thyroxine

Case 6 ■ A 42-Year-Old Female with Increased Body Hair and Purple Streaks on Her Abdomen

A 42-year-old female comes to your office with the following signs and symptoms: obesity (she has gained 40 pounds in the last 6 months), elevated blood pressure at her last walk-in clinic visit, increased body hair, purple streaks on her abdomen, "a fat face" (her description), and pains in her bones and joints.

She is on no medication at present, nor has she been on any medication for the past year.

On examination, her body mass index is 35. Her blood pressure is 160/110 mm Hg; she has obvious hirsutism over her entire body, and her abdomen (which is obese) has purple striae. Her face is not only plethoric but also demonstrates a double chin. Her thoracic spine shows evidence of what is known as a buffalo hump.

Q16. Based on the information provided, what is the most likely diagnosis in this patient?
- a. Conn's syndrome
- b. Cushing's syndrome
- c. Addison's syndrome
- d. primary hyperparathyroidism
- e. prolactinoma

Q17. Of all the possible causes for the condition in this patient, which of the following is the most common?
- a. adenoma of the adrenal gland
- b. adenoma of the pituitary gland
- c. hyperplasia of the adrenal gland
- d. corticosteroid therapy for suppression of inflammation
- e. small cell carcinoma of the lung

Q18. Which of the following tests is (are) appropriate for screening the patient in Case 6?
- a. serum cortisol level
- b. low-dose dexamethasone (cortisol analogue) suppression test
- c. 24-hour urine for free cortisol
- d. all of the above
- e. none of the above

Q19. Because of the likely pathophysiology of the condition described in the patient in Case 6, which of the following is the recommended treatment?
- a. surgery to remove the adenoma of the pituitary gland
- b. surgery to remove the adenoma of the adrenal gland
- c. surgery to remove the carcinoma of the adrenal gland
- d. chemotherapy to kill as much abnormal tissue as possible
- e. none of the above

Q20. Which of the following conditions is metastatic malignancy most likely to mimic?
- a. Cushing's syndrome
- b. primary hyperparathyroidism
- c. Conn's syndrome
- d. Addison's syndrome
- e. Nelson's syndrome

SHORT ANSWER MANAGEMENT PROBLEM

For the condition hyperparathyroidism:
1. Define the condition.
2. Provide the sex predilection.
3. Provide the age predilection.
4. Explain the pathogenesis.
5. Provide the clinical symptoms.
6. Explain the mnemonic "stones, bones, abdominal groans, and psychic moans."
7. Explain the changes in blood and serum levels that characterize the condition.
8. Discuss treatment.
9. Identify the most characteristic laboratory abnormality.

ANSWERS

A1. **b.** The condition is acromegaly, which often goes undiagnosed for many years. Acromegaly produces many signs and symptoms, including the following:
- a. General symptoms:
  - 1) Fatigue
  - 2) Increased sweating
  - 3) Heat intolerance
  - 4) Weight gain
- b. Changes in peripheral and general appearance:
  - 1) Enlarging hands and feet
  - 2) Coarsening facial features
  - 3) Oily skin
  - 4) Hypertrichosis
- c. Head:
  - 1) Headaches

2) Parotid enlargement
3) Frontal bossing
d. Nose/throat:
1) Sinus congestion
2) Voice change
3) Obstructive sleep apnea
4) Goiter
e. Cardiovascular system:
1) Hypertension
2) Congestive cardiac failure
3) Left ventricular hypertrophy
f. Genitourinary system:
1) Kidney stones
2) Decreased libido/impotence
3) Infertility
4) Oligomenorrhea
g. Neurologic system:
1) Paresthesias
2) Hypersomnolence
3) Carpel tunnel syndrome
h. Muscular system:
1) Weakness
2) Proximal myopathy
i. Skeletal system:
1) Joint pains
2) Osteoarthritis

A2. **c.** Acromegaly results from a growth hormone excess caused by a pituitary adenoma.

A3. **e.** Treatments include transsphenoidal surgery, heavy-particle pituitary radiation, conventional pituitary radiation, bromocriptine, and the somatostatin analogue octreotide.

A4. **c.** This patient has Addison's disease or primary adrenocortical insufficiency. The prominent clinical features of Addison's disease include weakness (100%), weight loss (100%), hyperpigmentation (95%), and hypotension.

The pertinent laboratory findings include hyponatremia, hyperkalemia, increased blood urea nitrogen, hypercalcemia, increased plasma ACTH, and decreased serum cortisol level.

In Addison's disease both the short ACTH stimulation test and the prolonged ACTH stimulation test yield no cortical response.

A5. **d.** Most commonly, Addison's disease results from an autoimmune destruction of the adrenal gland. At least 50% of patients with Addison's disease have antiadrenal antibodies. Other potential causes of adrenocortical insufficiency include tuberculosis, disseminated meningococcemia, and metastatic cancer.

A6. **c.** Because of the patient's acutely ill state, cortisol as a phosphate or succinate ester should be given in a 100-mg bolus IV and infused at a rate of 50 mg/hr until physiologic parameters are restored (especially normotension).

A7. **d.** The chronic treatment of Addison's disease is a combination of hydrocortisone (10 to 30 mg/day) and 9-α-fluorocortisol (50 to 100 mg/day). This combination is based on the need for a combination of glucocorticoid replacement and mineralocorticoid replacement.

A8. **d.** This patient has nephrogenic diabetes insipidus. This has resulted from the lack of renal response to antidiuretic hormone (ADH); in this case the diabetes insipidus is of the nephrogenic subtype and caused by the drug lithium carbonate.

There are two basic types of diabetes insipidus:
a. Central: The central type is usually idiopathic.
b. Nephrogenic: The collecting tubules of the kidney are not responsive to the ADH that is produced.

The nephrogenic type of diabetes is usually caused by either a drug (lithium carbonate, amphotericin B) or severe hypokalemia (which makes the renal tubules resistant to ADH).

A9. **e.** The treatment for central diabetes insipidus is IM ADH; nephrogenic diabetes insipidus is best treated by discontinuation of the offending drug (if the drug is the cause, as is the most common scenario). In the case of this patient, who was given lithium carbonate to treat bipolar affective disorder, a switch to carbamazepine would be most appropriate.

A10. **a.** This patient has Conn's syndrome.

A11. **a.** Conn's syndrome is primary aldosteronism that results from an excess mineralocorticoid production from (in most cases) an adenoma of the adrenal cortex. If not caused by an adenoma, hyperplasia of the adrenal cortex is found. The benign adenoma is usually present in the zona glomerulosa.

The clinical signs and symptoms of Conn's syndrome are weakness (resulting from the effect of hypokalemia); hypertension; carbohydrate intolerance (the result of increased insulin release from hypokalemia); and polyuria, polydipsia, and nocturia caused by either hypokalemic nephropathy or nephrogenic diabetes insipidus.

Laboratory abnormalities include mild hypernatremia, hypokalemic metabolic alkalosis, low renin levels, increased urine potassium level, and an inability to suppress aldosterone with isotonic saline load, captopril, or use of another mineralocorticoid.

A12. **e.** The treatment of choice for the patient described in Case 4 who most probably has a benign adenoma is surgical removal of the adenoma. If a case of Conn's syndrome were caused by a bilateral hyperplasia of the adrenal glands, spironolactone would be the treatment of choice.

A13. **d.** This patient has hyperprolactinemia, most likely the result of a pituitary adenoma. The combination of galactorrhea, amenorrhea, infertility, and decreased libido is almost certainly caused by a prolactinoma.

A14. **e.** A prolactinoma can be confirmed by measuring serum prolactin level. A serum prolactin level of 300 ng/ml or greater is always caused (in the absence of pregnancy) by a pituitary adenoma.

A magnetic resonance imaging (MRI) scan of the pituitary gland will confirm the diagnosis. It should be mentioned that a prolactinoma is the most common overall pituitary tumor in women.

A15. **b.** Treatment is controversial, but because of a high rate of recurrence with surgery, initial therapy with bromocriptine is the best choice. Treatment with bromocriptine is not curative; it does, however, reduce the prolactin level, reduce the tumor mass, and increase fertility. Side effects include nausea and vomiting, increase in liver enzymes, and increase in serum uric acid level.

A16. **b.** This patient has Cushing's syndrome. The definition of Cushing's syndrome is "a manifestation of hypercorticalism due to any cause."

A17. **b.** The most common cause of Cushing's syndrome is corticosteroid therapy. If steroids are excluded, the three major causes are as follows:
  a. Pituitary Cushing's (60% to 70%): an adenoma
  b. Adrenal Cushing's (15%): adenoma, hyperplasia, or malignancy
  c. Ectopic Cushing's (15%): malignancy (small cell carcinoma of the lung)

Thus the most likely cause of Cushing's syndrome in the patient described, who has not been taking any medication for over a year, is a pituitary adenoma. The most common cause, as mentioned, is exogenous steroids.

A18. **d.** The clinical features of Cushing's syndrome consist of the following:
  a. Truncal obesity (90%)
  b. Hypertension (85%)
  c. Decreased glucose tolerance (80%)
  d. Hirsutism (70%)
  e. Wide, purple abdominal striae (65%)
  f. Osteoporosis (55%)
  g. Plethoric face
  h. Easy bruising
  i. Mental aberrations
  j. Myopathy

In terms of laboratory tests, the best overall screening tests are serum cortisol level, low-dose (1 mg) dexamethasone suppression test (in Cushing's syndrome there is no suppression), and 24-hour urine test for free cortisol. Confirmation tests include high-dose (8 mg) dexamethasone suppression test (suppresses pituitary Cushing's but will not suppress adrenal or ectopic Cushing's syndrome), and plasma ACTH (normal to slightly increased in pituitary Cushing's syndrome, markedly increased in ectopic Cushing's syndrome, and very low in adrenal Cushing's syndrome; suppressed by cortisol).

A19. **a.** Because of the very high possibility that this is a pituitary Cushing's syndrome, the correct answer is surgery to remove the pituitary adenoma.

A20. **b.** Metastatic malignancy is most likely to produce hypercalcemia. Hypercalcemia is most likely to mimic primary hyperparathyroidism. (Hyperparathyroidism is discussed in the Short Answer Management Problem.)

SOLUTION TO THE SHORT ANSWER MANAGEMENT PROBLEM

Hyperparathyroidism:
1. Definition: Overactivity of the parathyroid glands (one or more of the four glands)
2. Sex predilection: Females >males
3. Age predilection: Age 40 to 70 years
4. Pathology:
   a. 82% of cases of hyperparathyroidism are caused by adenomas
   b. 15% of cases of hyperparathyroidism are caused by hyperplasia of the glands
   c. 3% are malignant
5. Clinical symptoms:
   a. Renal stones (calcium oxalate): Most common symptomatic presentation
   b. Peptic ulcer disease: Calcium stimulates gastrin release
   c. Acute pancreatitis: Calcium activates phospholipases
   d. Constipation: Most common gastrointestinal complaint
   e. Band keratopathy: Metastatic calcification in the limbus of the eye

f. Nephrocalcinosis: Polyuria, loss of concentrating ability, and diluting capability as a result of metastatic calcification of the renal tubules

g. Pruritus: Metastatic calcification in the skin

h. Short QT interval: Bradycardia

i. Hypertension: Calcium increases muscular contraction in the resistance vessels

j. Osteitis fibrosa cystica: Late finding, commonly found in jaw, called "brown tumor" caused by hemorrhage into cysts

k. Pseudogout: Calcium pyrophosphate; positively birefringement crystals

l. Mental changes: Personality changes, psychosis, depression

m. X-ray changes:
   1) "Salt and pepper skull" on x-ray scan
   2) Subperiosteal resorption of bone from the second and third middle phalanges and lamina dura around the teeth
   3) Distal resorption of clavicle

6. The mnemonic "stones, bones, abdominal groans, and psychic moans"
   a. Stones: Calcium oxalate renal stones
   b. Bones: Osteitis fibrosa cystica, salt and pepper skull, resorption of clavicle, subperiosteal resorption of bone from the second and third phalanges and the lamina dura around the teeth
   c. Abdominal pain: Result of acute pancreatitis
   d. Psychic moans: Psychosis, depression

7. Changes in blood and serum:
   a. Hypercalcemia (most common characteristic)
   b. Hypercalciuria
   c. Hypophosphatemia
   d. Hyperphosphaturia
   e. Normal anion gap metabolic acidosis

8. Treatment:
   a. Adenoma: Surgery to locate and remove adenoma (biopsy second gland to see if atrophic)
   b. Hyperplasia: Subtotal parathyroidectomy, monitor for tetany postoperatively

9. Most common laboratory abnormality: Hypercalcemia

SUMMARY OF THE DIAGNOSIS AND SOME FEATURES OF CERTAIN ENDOCRINE DISEASES

1. Acromegaly:
   a. Signs and symptoms: Enlarged hands, feet, and head; hypertension; cardiomegaly; weight gain
   b. Pathology: Due to pituitary adenoma, growth hormone

c. Treatment: Transsphenoidal surgery, radiation, bromocriptine

2. Addison's disease:
   a. Signs and symptoms: Weakness, hypotension, hyperpigmentation
   b. Pathology: Autoimmune destruction of adrenal glands
   c. Acute treatment: Acutely ill: IV cortisol
   d. Chronic treatment: Replacement with glucocorticoid (hydrocortisone) and mineralocorticoid (9-α-fluorocortisol)
   e. Results: Adrenocortical insufficiency

3. Diabetes insipidus:
   a. Signs and symptoms: Polyuria, polydypsia resulting from a deficiency of ADH
   b. Subtypes: Central and nephrogenic
   c. Differential diagnosis: Psychogenic polydipsia
   d. Most common cause: Nephrogenic subtype most commonly caused by lithium
   e. Treatment: IM ADH for treatment of central subtype

4. Prolactinoma:
   a. Signs/symptoms: Galactorrhea, amenorrhea, infertility, decreased libido
   b. Frequency: Most common pituitary tumor in women
   c. Investigation and confirmation: Serum prolactin ≥ to 300; MRI of pituitary
   d. Differential diagnosis: Rule out pregnancy, drugs (major tranquilizers, oral contraceptive pills, hypothyroidism, IV cimetidine, opiates)
   e. Treatment: Transsphenoidal surgery, bromocriptine

5. Conn's syndrome:
   a. Signs and symptoms: Weakness (caused by hypokalemia), hypertension, carbohydrate intolerance (polyuria, polydipsia)
   b. Most common cause: Adenoma of the adrenal
   c. Pathology: Excess mineralocorticoid production
   d. Laboratory investigations: Mild hypernatremia, hypokalemic metabolic alkalosis
   e. Treatment: Adenoma removal; hyperplasia-spironolactone

6. Cushing's syndrome:
   a. Signs and symptoms: Truncal obesity, carbohydrate intolerance, moon face, buffalo hump, abdominal stria, osteoporosis, psychic changes (depression and euphoria), easy bruising, myopathy, plethoric face
   b. Pathology: Pituitary adenoma, adrenal adenoma, steroid therapy

c. Most common cause: Corticosteroid therapy

d. Laboratory investigation: laboratory screening tests: Serum cortisol level; 24-hour urine for cortisol; dexamethasone suppression test (1 mg). Confirmation and differentiation between pituitary Cushing's, adrenal Cushing's, and ectopic Cushing's; plasma ACTH; high-dose dexamethasone (8 mg) suppression test

e. Treatment:
1) Exogenous Cushing's: Stop steroids, decrease dose, or give every other day steroids with a drug holiday
2) Endogenous Cushing's: Removal of adenoma in pituitary and adrenal Cushing's syndrome

7. Primary hyperparathyroidism:
a. Signs and symptoms: Mnemonic: stones, bones, abdominal groans, psychic moans; renal colic (calcium oxalate); acute pancreatitis; constipation; x-ray: bone resorption, salt and pepper skull

b. Pathology: Most commonly adenoma of the parathyroid gland

c. Laboratory abnormalities: Hypercalcemia, hypophosphatemia, hypocalciuria, hyperphosphaturia. Hypercalcemia is most common metabolic abnormality; may also occur in metastatic carcinoma.

d. Treatment: Adenoma: removal; hyperplasia: subtotal parathyroidectomy

SUGGESTED READINGS

Allerheiligen DA et al: Hyperparathyroidism, *Am Fam Physician* 57(8):1795-1802, 1807-1808, 1998.

Baker JR Jr: Autoimmune endocrine disease, *JAMA* 278(22):1931-1937, 1997.

Ciccarelli E, Camanni F: Diagnosis and drug therapy of prolactinoma, *Drugs* 51(6):954-965, 1996.

Melmed S et al: Current treatment guidelines of acromegaly, *J Clin Endocrinol Metab* 83(8):2646-2652, 1998.

Singer I, Oster JR, Fishman LM: The management of diabetes insipidus in adults, *Arch Intern Med* 157(12):1293-1301, 1997.

Soule SG, Jacobs HS: The evaluation and management of subclinical pituitary disease, *Postgrad Med J* 72(847):258-262, 1996.

PROBLEM·22

THYROID DISEASE

"What Is It, Doc? Tee 4, Tee 3, or Tea to Stay Awake?"

Case 1 ■ A 38-Year-Old Female with Sweating, Palpitations, Nervousness, Irritability, and Tremor

A 38-year-old female comes to your office with a 3-month history of sweating, palpitations, weight loss, nervousness, irritability, insomnia, hand tremors, and diarrhea. She has had no significant past personal illnesses. One of her sisters has rheumatoid arthritis. The patient, a teacher, is finding it harder and harder to perform her job because of profound fatigue and inability to concentrate.

On examination, her blood pressure is 160/70 mm Hg. Her pulse is 120 bpm and regular. She demonstrates mild proptosis. You feel a smooth, diffusely enlarged, and nontender thyroid gland. Cardiovascular examination reveals a loud S_1 and a loud S_2 with an ejection systolic murmur heard loudest along the left sternal edge. This murmur does not radiate. No other abnormalities are noted.

SELECT THE BEST ANSWER TO THE FOLLOWING QUESTIONS

Q1. What is the most likely diagnosis in this patient?
a. toxic multinodular goiter
b. Graves' disease
c. Hashimoto's thyroiditis
d. pheochromocytoma
e. panic disorder

Q2. What is the cause of the disorder just described?
a. idiopathic
b. an autoimmune disease
c. a hereditary disease
d. caused by an as-yet-undetermined interaction between genetic and environmental factors
e. iatrogenic in most cases

Q3. The laboratory test of choice in this patient at this time is which of the following?
a. 24-hour radioiodine uptake test
b. thyroid scan
c. free serum T_4
d. serum thyroid-stimulating hormone (TSH)
e. c and d
f. b and c

Q4. What is the treatment of choice for this patient?
a. propylthiouracil
b. methimazole
c. radioactive iodine
d. subtotal thyroidectomy
e. a or b

Q5. The recommended treatment of choice is undertaken in this patient. Which of the following will be the end result of this treatment?
a. complete cure: no further medication or other treatments necessary

b. complete cure: hyperthyroid medication should be started immediately and continued for life

c. complete cure: patient should be monitored every 6 months for the development of hypothyroidism

d. partial cure: hypothyroid medication needed for 5 years

e. partial cure: hyperthyroid medication needed for 5 years

Case 2 ■ A 25-Year-Old Female with a Higher-Than-Normal T_4 Level

A 25-year-old female is seen for her periodic health examination. Her history is unremarkable; she is feeling well at present and is currently taking oral contraceptive pills. On physical examination, her blood pressure is 130/75 mm Hg. Examination reveals that her head and neck are completely normal; specifically, no abnormalities of the thyroid gland are noted. However, a routine serum T_4 level is elevated at 13 mg/dl (169 mmol/L).

Q6. What is the most likely explanation for the elevated T_4 level in this patient?
a. Graves' disease
b. thyrotoxicosis
c. toxic nodular goiter
d. an elevated thyroid-binding globulin (TBG) secondary to the oral contraceptive pill
e. laboratory error

Q7. To confirm your diagnosis in the patient just described, which of the following would you order?
a. all-out, all-inclusive, miss nothing work-up
b. serum T_3
c. serum TBG
d. serum free T_4
e. serum TSH
f. d or e

Q8. Which of the following statements about the category of disorders labeled as thyroiditis is (are) true?
a. thyroiditis represents a diverse group of conditions
b. inflammation of the thyroid gland is the prominent clinical feature in thyroiditis
c. thyroiditis can be acute, subacute, or chronic
d. thyroiditis may be either symptomatic or asymptomatic
e. all of the above

Case 3 ■ A 28-Year-Old Female Who Is Wonderfully Healthy

A 28-year-old female is seen in your office for a complete baseline health assessment. You have never seen this patient before. She feels well and tells you that she is "wonderfully healthy." She has had no weight loss or gain; no sweating, no tremors, no diarrhea or constipation; no anxiety or depression; no irritability; and no other symptoms.

On examination, she is found to have a 3-cm nodule in the left lobe of the thyroid gland. Her blood pressure is 130/70 mm Hg. Her pulse is 96 bpm and regular.

Q9. What is the most important investigation to be carried out on a patient with this finding?
a. a serum T_4 test
b. a thyroid radionuclide scan
c. a fine needle aspiration of the nodule
d. a thyroid ultrasound
e. a computed tomography scan of the thyroid

Q10. Which of the following statements regarding "warm (hot) nodules" and "cold nodules" found on radionuclide scan is true?
a. cold nodules are more likely to be benign than warm nodules
b. cold nodules need not be investigated any further
c. cold nodules are more likely to be associated with signs and symptoms of hyperthyroidism than warm nodules
d. cold nodules require further investigation to differentiate benign from malignant status
e. none of the above statements is true

Q11. A fine needle aspiration showed that the mass is benign. What would you do now?
a. perform a radionuclide thyroid scan
b. refer the patient to a surgeon for excision
c. give a trial of suppressive levothyroxine and reevaluate in 6 months
d. reassure the patient and give no further therapy
e. obtain a magnetic resonance imaging scan of the head and neck to look for further disease

Q12. What is the most common cause of hypothyroidism in the United States?
a. autoimmune thyroiditis
b. post-^{131}I hypothyroidism
c. iodine deficiency

d. idiopathic hypothyroidism
e. postthyroidectomy hypothyroidism

Q13. Which of the following statements is (are) true regarding Hashimoto's thyroiditis?
a. Hashimoto's thyroiditis is more common in females than in males
b. antithyroid antibodies are found in 80% of individuals with this condition
c. this condition is also known as chronic lymphocytic thyroiditis
d. symptoms of hyperthyroidism often precede symptoms of hypothyroidism
e. a, b, and c
f. all of the above

Case 4 ■ A 65-Year-Old Lethargic Male

A 65-year-old male comes to your office with a 6-month history of lethargy, weakness, psychomotor retardation, cold intolerance, constipation, hair loss, and weight gain. You suspect hypothyroidism.

Q14. Which of the following investigations will provide the most useful information for diagnosing hypothyroidism in this patient?
a. serum T_4 test
b. serum T_3 test
c. free serum T_4 test
d. serum TSH
e. serum TBG

Q15. Which of the following statements regarding the treatment of the patient described in Case 4 is false?
a. optimal therapy for this condition can be determined by measurement of the serum TSH level
b. until the serum TSH is normal, full replacement has not been established
c. patients with significant cardiac disease and elderly patients should be treated cautiously
d. desiccated thyroid is the treatment of choice
e. none of the above statements is false

Q16. Which of the following statements concerning thyroid carcinoma is (are) true?
a. papillary carcinoma is the most common type of thyroid cancer
b. papillary carcinoma is the thyroid cancer with the best prognosis
c. papillary carcinoma, even when metastatic to lymph nodes, may not adversely influence prognosis

d. a and b
e. all of the above

SHORT ANSWER MANAGEMENT PROBLEM
List the most common causes of each of the following thyroid conditions:
1. Hyperthyroidism
2. Hypothyroidism
3. Thyroid antibody-associated condition
4. Thyroid carcinoma
5. Elevated total serum T_4 and elevated TBG levels

ANSWERS

A1. **b.** This patient has Graves' disease, which is the most common cause of hyperthyroidism in the United States. Its usual presenting symptoms are sweating, palpitations, nervousness, irritability, tremor, diarrhea, heat intolerance, and weight loss. The physical signs of Graves' disease include a diffuse, nontender thyroid gland enlargement (goiter), tachycardia, systolic hypertension, loud heart sounds, and a cardiac murmur. A bruit is sometimes heard over the thyroid gland itself. Proptosis, with a straight-ahead stare and lid lag, is frequently seen. Occasionally patients have severe exophthalmos accompanied by ophthalmoplegia, follicular conjunctivitis, chemosis, and even loss of vision.

A2. **b.** Graves' disease is thought to result from an autoimmune process, and antibodies are present in the serum.

Toxic nodular goiter and toxic adenoma are other causes of hyperthyroidism. Their presentation, however, is usually significantly more subtle than the presentation of Graves' disease, and they are generally not confused with this condition.

Hashimoto's thyroiditis is a cause of hypothyroidism rather than hyperthyroidism. Its presentation is discussed in Answers 12 and 13.

Pheochromocytoma and panic disorder are not really serious considerations with this history.

A3. **e.** The methods of measuring thyroid hormone have changed considerably in the last few years, and the serum TSH level is now being used to measure and detect hyperthyroidism as well as hypothyroidism. Indeed, the sine qua non of hyperthyroidism at this time is a low serum TSH level, so this is the screening test that should be used. The T_4 level should be measured; the laboratory will measure total T_4 and calculate a free T_4. If the free T_4 level is normal, then a serum T_3 test should be ordered; 10% to 15% of the cases of hyperthyroidism are actually caused by a T_3 toxicosis rather than a T_4 problem.

A4. **c.** The two basic treatments for Graves' disease are antithyroid drugs (propylthiouracil or methimazole) and radioiodine therapy.
  a. Antithyroid drugs:
    1) Advantage: These drugs provide the opportunity for the patient to experience a spontaneous remission and avoid lifelong medication (e.g., with levothyroxine).
    2) Disadvantages:
      a) Remissions are attained in fewer than 50% of patients.
      b) Continuous or repeated courses of drug therapy are usually necessary.
  b. Radioiodine therapy
    1) Advantages:
      a) Radioiodine is curative.
      b) Managing postradiation hypothyroidism is simpler than managing most patients on long-term antithyroid drug therapy.
    2) Disadvantage: Iatrogenic hypothyroidism is produced in the majority of patients within 10 years.
On the basis of weighing advantages versus disadvantages for both, the recommendation has been made that radioiodine is the treatment of choice for adult patients. In children and adolescents the antithyroid drug therapy remains first-line treatment, with radioiodine being second-line treatment. Radioiodine is contraindicated in pregnant women.

A5. **c.**

A6. **d.** The most likely explanation for the elevated serum T_4 level in this patient is an elevated TBG level secondary to the estrogen component of the oral contraceptive pill.
  a. TBG is increased in the following patients:
    1) Those who are taking oral contraceptive pills
    2) Those who are taking estrogen supplementation
    3) Those with infectious hepatitis
  b. TBG is decreased in the following patients:
    1) Those with chronic liver disease
    2) Patients with nephrotic syndrome
    3) Patients with hypoproteinemia from other causes
    4) Patients on androgen therapy

A7. **f.** To confirm your diagnosis of the patient described in Case 2, you would order either a serum free T_4 level or a TSH level. As stated before, the serum TSH level is now being used to diagnose hyperthyroidism as well as hypothyroidism. Thus, in this patient, you would expect to find a normal TSH level as opposed to a low TSH level.

A8. **e.** The group of disorders labeled as thyroiditis encompasses a diverse group of thyroid disorders of various causes; inflammation of the thyroid gland is a prominent and consistent histologic feature. These may be relatively asymptomatic or self-limited disorders, or they can be accompanied by long-term abnormalities of thyroid growth, including goiter formation and nodularity. Thyroiditis can also be classified as acute, subacute, or chronic.

A9. **c.** The initial procedure of choice in most patients is fine needle aspiration for cytology.

A10. **d.**

A11. **c.**

A12. **a.** The most common cause of hypothyroidism is autoimmune thyroiditis or Hashimoto's thyroiditis. The patient with Hashimoto's thyroiditis may be initially hyperthyroid but always progresses to a hypothyroid state. Symptoms of hypothyroidism include fatigue, lethargy, constipation, cold intolerance, dry skin, hair loss, weight gain, edema, headache, arthralgias, hoarseness, amenorrhea, bradycardia, and hypotension.

A13. **f.** Hashimoto's thyroiditis is also known as chronic lymphocytic thyroiditis. It is much more common in females than in males. Antithyroid antibodies are present in up to 80% of patients. In the acute thyroiditis stage of the disease, symptoms of hyperthyroidism precede symptoms of hypothyroidism.

A14. **d.** The most useful test for diagnosing hypothyroidism is the serum TSH level. Serum TSH levels are elevated in almost all cases of primary hypothyroidism. If hypothyroidism is suspected, the serum TSH measurement will provide definite proof for or against the condition.

A15. **d.** The serum TSH level will determine optimal thyroid replacement therapy. With adequate replacement, the serum TSH level should return to normal.
  Levothyroxine is the preferred therapeutic agent, although both desiccated thyroid and triiodothyronine can return the TSH level to normal.

A16. **e.** The following features of thyroid papillary carcinoma have been found to be true:
  a. It is the most common type of thyroid cancer.
  b. It is the thyroid cancer with the best prognosis.
  c. Spread to regional lymph nodes does not necessarily influence the prognosis.

SOLUTION TO THE SHORT ANSWER MANAGEMENT PROBLEM

The most common causes of thyroid conditions are as follows:

1. Hyperthyroidism: Graves' disease
2. Hypothyroidism: Hashimoto's thyroiditis
3. Thyroid antibody-associated condition: Hashimoto's thyroiditis
4. Thyroid carcinoma: papillary carcinoma
5. Elevated total serum T_4 and elevated TBG levels: oral contraceptive pill

SUMMARY OF THE DIAGNOSIS AND TREATMENT OF THYROID DISORDERS

1. Important epidemiology:
   a. Hypothyroidism is one of the most commonly underdiagnosed conditions, particularly in the elderly.
   b. Hypothyroidism is significantly more common than hyperthyroidism. All elderly patients admitted to a long-term care facility or nursing home should probably have a serum TSH test performed.

2. Hyperthyroidism:
   a. Causes:
      1) Graves' disease: Most common cause
      2) Toxic nodular goiter
      3) Toxic adenoma
   b. Signs and symptoms: Most common signs and symptoms include the following:
      1) Tremor
      2) Anxiety, nervousness, irritability
      3) Diarrhea
      4) Weight loss
      5) Sweating
      6) Palpitations
      7) Insomnia
      8) Proptosis, exophthalmos
      9) Systolic hypertension
      10) Loud cardiac sounds, cardiac murmur
   c. Investigations: A simplified initial investigation approach would be the following:
      1) Directly measured free serum T_4 level
      2) Serum TSH (NOTE: This is becoming more important in the diagnosis of hyperthyroidism as well as hypothyroidism.)
      3) If directly measured free serum T_4 level is normal, measure serum T_3 level
      4) A thyroid scan followed by a thyroid ultrasound to identify and categorize thyroid nodules (cold, warm)

   d. Treatment:
      1) Radiation is the treatment of choice for Graves' disease in adults.
      2) Antithyroid drugs are the treatment of choice in children and adolescents.
      3) Surgery: Subtotal thyroidectomy may be the most appropriate treatment for a toxic or solitary adenoma (nonmalignant). Radiation may sometimes be a reasonable alternative.
      4) Antithyroid drugs of choice are propylthiouracil and methimazole.

3. Hypothyroidism:
   a. Most common cause:
      1) Hashimoto's thyroiditis, or chronic lymphocytic thyroiditis, is the most common cause.
      2) Other common causes include hypothyroidism induced by thyroid surgery or radiation ablation.
   b. Investigations: Serum TSH is the most sensitive test in diagnosing primary hypothyroidism. For the elderly patient who has become depressed and is losing interest in life in general, consider hypothyroidism and screen for it. Screen all elderly patients entering a long-term care facility for clinical hypothyroidism.
   c. Treatment: Levothyroxine 50 to 200 mg/day (start at 50 mg and work up)

4. Thyroid carcinoma: Most common type: papillary carcinoma. Minimally invasive even after it has spread to regional lymph nodes.

SUGGESTED READINGS
Cooper DS: Hyperthyroidism. In Rakel R, ed: *Conn's current therapy,* Philadelphia, 1994, WB Saunders.
Kinder BK: Thyroid cancer. In Rakel R, ed: *Conn's current therapy,* Philadelphia, 1994, WB Saunders.
Magner JA: Hypothyroidism. In Rakel R, ed: *Conn's current therapy,* Philadelphia, 1994, WB Saunders.

PROBLEM·23

MULTIPLE SCLEROSIS

"I'm So Clumsy and I Can Hardly See Out of My Left Eye. What Could Be Happening?"

Case 1 ■ A 27-Year-Old Female with Weakness, Visual Loss, Ataxia, and Sensory Loss

A 27-year-old female comes to your office for assessment of symptoms that include weakness, visual loss, bladder incontinence, sharp, shooting pain in the lower back, clumsiness when walking, and sensory loss. These symptoms have occurred during three episodes (different combinations of symptoms each time) approximately 3 months apart, and each episode lasted approximately 3 days.

The first episode consisted of weakness, bladder incontinence, and sharp shooting pains in the lower back (in both hip girdles). The second episode consisted of visual loss, clumsiness when walking, and sensory loss. The third episode (last week) consisted of sharp, shooting pains in the lower back and sensory loss (bilateral) in the upper extremities.

On neurologic examination, you find swelling of the optic disc on funduscopy, the patient's inability to walk heel to toe, and slight objective weakness of both hip girdles. She has no symptoms today.

SELECT THE BEST ANSWER TO THE FOLLOWING QUESTIONS

Q1. Given this information, what is the most likely diagnosis in this patient?
    a. amyotrophic lateral sclerosis
    b. multiple sclerosis (MS)
    c. vitamin B_{12} deficiency
    d. hysterical conversion reaction
    e. tertiary syphilis

Q2. There are four clinical categories of this disease. Which of the following subtypes does the patient presented fit into?
    a. relapsing-remitting
    b. secondary progressive
    c. primary progressive
    d. progressive relapsing
    e. none of the above

Q3. If you had the opportunity to do only one diagnostic test, which of the following would you choose?
    a. computed tomography scan of the head and spinal cord
    b. magnetic resonance imaging (MRI) scan of the brain and spinal cord
    c. serum vitamin B_{12} levels
    d. Beck's depression scale
    e. Venereal Disease Research Laboratory test for syphilis

Q4. The disease is most correctly described as which of the following?
    a. an uncommon neurologic disease that can be corrected by the administration of subcutaneous vitamin B_{12}
    b. the number one cause of disabling disease in young adults in the United States

c. a very common psychiatric condition in which psychologic symptoms are manifested by physical symptoms
    d. a fatal neurologic condition that results in continual deterioration to the point of respiratory depression and the cessation of respiration
    e. none of the above

Q5. The disease described is associated with which of the following?
    a. racial predilection: whites > blacks
    b. sex predilection: females > males
    c. high socioeconomic status
    d. environmental exposure
    e. all of the above

Q6. Which of the following statements regarding the behavior of the disease described above is (are) true?
    a. in 80% to 90% of all cases the first episode is followed by a cycle of relapses and remissions in 50% of the group labeled "relapsing-remitting"; the relapsing-remitting pattern converts to a progressive course after 5 years
    b. 10% of patients have progressive disease from the onset of symptoms
    c. up to 10% of patients with this disease have a relatively "benign" course
    d. all of the above

Q7. The disease, if diagnosed as a central nervous system (CNS) disease, must involve how many different areas of the CNS?
    a. one
    b. two
    c. three
    d. four
    e. not applicable: not primarily a neurologic disease

Q8. Which of the following clinical findings support(s) the diagnosis made above?
    a. a cerebrospinal fluid (CSF) mononuclear cell pleocytosis
    b. an increase in CSF immunoglobulin G (IgG)
    c. oligoclonal banding of CSF IgG (two or more bands)
    d. abnormalities in evoked response testing (any type)
    e. all of the above

Q9. The target of this disease process is an attack on which of the following?
    a. the neurotransmitter balance in the CNS
    b. the "oligodendrocytes" of the CNS

c. the peripheral nerves in the posterior columns of the spinal cord
d. the cerebral hemispheres
e. the cerebellum

Q10. What is (are) the treatment(s) of choice for the disease process described?
a. adrenocorticotropic hormone (ACTH)
b. corticosteroids
c. cytotoxic immunosuppressive agents
d. interferon-β
e. all of the above

Q11. Which of the following symptoms is the most common in this disorder?
a. optic neuritis
b. ataxia
c. vertigo
d. loss of bladder control
e. impotence

Q12. Which of the following symptoms is the least common?
a. optic neuritis
b. ataxia
c. vertigo
d. loss of bladder control
e. impotence

SHORT ANSWER MANAGEMENT PROBLEM
What causes MS and what cell is the primary target?

ANSWERS

A1. **b.** This patient has MS. Although no laboratory test, symptom, or physical finding necessarily means a person has MS, the diagnosis relies on the following two broad criteria:
a. There must have been two attacks that were defined as the sudden appearance or worsening of an MS symptom or symptoms that last at least 24 hours, at least 1 month apart.
b. There must be more than one area of damage to CNS myelin, the damage having occurred at more than one point in time and not being attributed to any other disease process.

A2. **a.** The most common pattern or clinical category of MS is the relapsing-remitting category. In relapsing-remitting MS, episodes of acute worsening are followed by recovery and a stable course between relapses. In the secondary progressive category, gradual neurologic deterioration occurs with or without superimposed acute relapses in patients who previously have relapsing-remitting MS. In primary progressive MS, gradual continuous deterioration occurs from the onset of symptoms. In progressive relapsing MS, gradual neurologic deterioration occurs from the onset of symptoms, but with subsequent superimposed relapses. This patient most likely has relapsing-remitting MS.

A3. **b.** The most sensitive and specific investigation for this disorder is an MRI scan of the brain and/or spinal cord. The MRI scan will reveal the following abnormalities in a patient with MS:
a. Plaque formation (a subsequent stage that results from the loss of the myelin sheath in different parts of the CNS)
b. Spotty and irregular demyelination in the affected areas

A4. **b.** MS is the number one disabling disease of young adults, primarily women. It is more common at northern than southern latitudes. Other risk factors will be addressed in Answer 5 below.

A5. **e.** The documented risk factors for MS are as follows:
a. White race > African-American race
b. Female > male (2:1)
c. Environmental influence
1) Latitude (north > south)
2) Other unidentified environmental toxins (suspected)
d. Genetic: histocompatibility leukocyte antigens (HLAs)
e. Viral infections: No specific virus has been identified, but suspicion exists
f. High socioeconomic status

A6. **e.** The clinical categories are described above. All of the following are correct:
a. From 80% to 90% of all cases after the first symptom have relapses followed by remissions.
b. Fifty percent of relapsing-remitting cases switch to a progressive course approximately 5 years after the onset of the first symptoms.
c. Ten percent have progressive disease from the onset.
d. Ten percent have clinical courses that are benign. These patients have one or two relapses and then recover. These individuals have multifocal plaques at autopsy without evidence of an inflammatory demyelinating reaction.
There is also a very rare type termed acute MS of the Marburg type with rapid progression of symptoms.

A7. **b.** For a patient to be diagnosed as having MS, two separate areas of the CNS must be involved.

A8. **e.** The following are laboratory findings that support the diagnosis of MS:
   a. CSF mononuclear cell pleocytosis (5 cells/μL).
   b. CSF IgG is increased in the absence of a normal concentration of total protein.
   c. Oligoclonal banding of CSF IgG is detected by agarose gel electrophoresis techniques. Two or more oligoclonal bands are found in 75% to 90% of MS patients.
   d. Metabolites from myelin breakdown may be detected in the CSF.
   e. Evoked response testing may detect slowed or abnormal conduction in visual, auditory, somatosensory, or motor pathways. One or more evoked potentials are abnormal in 80% to 90% of patients with MS.

MRI of the brain is abnormal in a proportion of patients with MS at presentation and is associated with more severe disease.

MRI scan of the brain and spinal cord is the most useful imaging method available, and abnormal MRI scans are seen in 90% of patients with definite MS.

A9. **b.** The targets of the MS disease process are the oligodendrocytes of the CNS. These cells fabricate and maintain the myelin sheaths, the material covering the axons that is necessary for the normal conduction of nerve impulses. Destruction of oligodendrocytes occurs in clusters and is accompanied by loss of oligodendrocytes as well as their myelin sheath appendages with axon sparing (primary demyelination).

The cluster destruction of oligodendrocytes-myelin sheaths forms multifocal plaques, the pathologic hallmark of the disease. The majority of these plaques are in the white matter.

A10. **d.** The treatments of choice for acute attacks of MS are as follows:
   a. Corticosteroids are the mainstay of treatment for acute relapses of MS. While corticosteroid therapy can shorten the duration of the relapse, it is uncertain whether the long-term course of the disease will be altered with their use. ACTH has been replaced by high-dose intravenous methylprednisolone.
   b. Interferon-β remains the treatment of choice for patients with relapsing-remitting MS. Interferon-β is available in two forms, 1A and 1B. Both types are generally well tolerated by most patients. Flulike symptoms are common after each injection, and questions about different responses in different people remain. Therefore interferon-β doses should be individualized.

Glatiramer acetate is an alternative to interferon-β for those who have failed the latter therapy.

Azathioprine and other cytotoxic immunosuppressant agents may reduce the rate of relapse in MS, but have no effect on the progression of the disability. Nevertheless, in progressive MS, cytotoxic immunosuppressant agents have been shown to be of moderate benefit.

A11. **a.**

A12. **e.** The initial symptoms of MS and their frequency are as follows:

Symptom	Percentage of Cases
Optic neuritis	36%
Weakness	35%
Paresthesias	24%
Diplopia	15%
Ataxia	11%
Vertigo	6%
Paroxysmal symptoms	4%
Bladder disorders	4%
Lhermitte's sign	3%
Pain	3%
Dementia	2%
Visual loss	2%
Facial palsy	1%
Impotence	1%
Myokymia	1%
Epilepsy	1%
Falling	1%

Thus, of the symptoms listed in this question, the most common is optic neuritis, and the least common is impotence, along with other sexual dysfunction.

SOLUTION TO THE SHORT ANSWER MANAGEMENT PROBLEM

The etiologic agent(s) producing MS is (are) unknown. There is reasonable evidence that the disease results from an interaction between the individual (immunology) and his/her environment. The basic target of MS is the oligodendrocyte, the cell that fabricates and maintains myelin. Destruction of oligodendrocytes occurs in clusters and is accompanied by loss of not only the oligodendrocyte but, more importantly, their myelin sheaths. The cluster destruction of oligodendro-cytes-myelin sheaths produces plaques, the pathologic hallmark of MS. This destruction of oligodendrocytes and myelin is patchy, leaving more areas unaffected. The axons are invariably spared.

SUMMARY OF THE DIAGNOSIS AND TREATMENT OF MULTIPLE SCLEROSIS

1. Prevalence: Number one disabling condition of young adults in the United States; 250,000 to 350,000 persons in the United States in 1990 had physician-diagnosed MS.

2. Epidemiology:
   a. Almost all patients fit into one or more of the following categories:
      1) After their first symptom, 80% to 90% of patients have a cycle of relapses and re-missions.
      2) Of the 80% to 90%, 50% switch to a pro-gressive course about 5 years after the first symptom.
      3) Of all patients, 10% have progressive disease from the onset.
      4) Up to 10% of patients have a benign course, with one or two relapses and then a good recovery.
   b. Risk factors for MS:
      1) Race: White > African-American
      2) Sex: Females > males (2:1)
      3) High socioeconomic status
      4) Northern latitudes
      5) Other environmental factors as yet not iden-tified, such as toxins and viruses
      6) HLAs

3. Symptoms: Most common symptoms are the following:
   a. Sensory loss
   b. Optic neuritis
   c. Weakness
   d. Paraesthesias

4. Diagnosis: Criteria given previously:
   a. Two episodes, or attacks, of symptoms
   b. Two different areas of the CNS involved

5. Testing for MS:
   a. MRI scan of the brain: This will show the areas of demyelination better than any other test.
   b. CSF pleocytosis
   c. Increased CSF IgG
   d. Oligoclonal banding of IgG in the CSF
   e. Evoked potentials: Visual, auditory, somatosen-sory, and motor

6. Treatment:
   a. Acute attacks:
      1) Methylprednisolone for acute attacks
      2) Interferon-β for long-term treatment
   b. General supportive treatments:
      1) A regular exercise program
      2) The pursuit of wellness and a positive attitude
      3) Education regarding the disease
      4) Support: Family and support groups

SUGGESTED READINGS

National Multiple Sclerosis Society at: *http://www.nmss.org,* 2000
Rudick RA et al: Management of multiple sclerosis, *N Engl J Med* 332(22):1604-1611, 1997.

PROBLEM·24

DIAGNOSIS AND TREATMENT OF HEADACHES

"Acetaminophen Is Just Not Strong Enough!"

Case 1 ■ A 45-Year-Old Male with a Headache

A 45-year-old male comes with a 4-week history of re-current headaches that wake him up in the middle of the night. The headaches have been occurring every night and have been lasting approximately 1 hour. The headaches are described as a deep burning sensation centered behind the left orbit. The headaches are ex-cruciating (he rates them as a 15 on a 10-point scale) and are associated with watery eyes, "a sensation of heat and warmth in my face," nasal discharge, and redness of the left eye.

Before the onset of these headaches 4 weeks ago, the patient describes no more than the occasional tension headache. Headaches were certainly never a problem. The patient describes no recent life changes and no major life stresses. He is happily married, has three children, and has a secure job that he enjoys.

On examination, his blood pressure is 120/70 mm Hg. His pulse is 96 bpm and regular.

SELECT THE BEST ANSWER TO THE FOLLOWING QUESTIONS

Q1. What is the most likely cause of this patient's headache?
   a. subarachnoid hemorrhage
   b. tension-migraine syndrome
   c. atypical migraine headache
   d. cluster headache
   e. classic migraine headache

Q2. Which of the following statements concerning this patient's headaches is false?
   a. oxygen may be useful in treating the acute attack
   b. ergotamine may be used as a prophylactic agent
   c. methysergide may be used as a prophylactic agent
   d. lithium carbonate may be used as a prophylactic agent
   e. none of the above statements is false

Case 2 ■ A 32-Year-Old Female with a 2-Year History of Recurrent Headaches

A 32-year-old female comes to your office with a 2-year history of recurrent headaches. These headaches occur between three and four times per month and last 12 to 24 hours. The headaches are almost always confined to the left side of the head and are associated with malaise, nausea, vomiting, photophobia, and phonophobia.

The patient has been using acetaminophen (up to 6 g in a 12-hour period) without significant relief.

On examination, the patient's blood pressure is 100/70 mm Hg. The optic fundi are normal, as is the rest of the neurologic examination.

Q3. This patient's headache is most likely a:
   a. migraine headache without aura (common migraine)
   b. migraine headache with aura (classic migraine)
   c. complicated migraine
   d. tension-migraine syndrome
   e. nervous headache

Case 3 ■ A 38-Year-Old Female with a 6-Year History of Recurrent Headaches

A 38-year-old female comes to your office complaining about a 6-year history of recurrent headaches. These headaches occur approximately once per week. In contradistinction to the patient in Case 2, this patient has an unusual set of symptoms before both the prodromal phase and the headache itself. The symptoms are actually a "type of odd visual feeling or sight—flashing lights, almost like a pattern in front of my eyes." With respect to the headache itself, it usually lasts 24 to 36 hours. It is throbbing in nature and often "switches from one side to the other" during the acute attack.

On physical examination, the patient's blood pressure is 140/70 mm Hg. Examination of the optic fundi is completely normal, as is the rest of the neurologic examination.

Q4. What is the most likely type of headache in this patient?
   a. migraine headache without aura (common migraine)
   b. migraine headache with aura (classic migraine)
   c. basilar migraine
   d. tension-migraine syndrome
   e. complicated migraine headache

Case 4 ■ A 24-Year-Old Female with Chronic Headaches Preceded by Nausea and Vomiting

A 24-year-old patient comes to your office for assessment of headache. She describes the onset, characteristics, duration, and associated features of a migraine headache that is preceded by nausea and vomiting. It is confined to the left side of the head and is characterized by a throbbing pain lasting approximately 48 hours. The unusual feature of this headache is that it always begins approximately 2 days before menstruation, and it always ends with the onset of menstruation.

On physical examination, the patient's blood pressure is 120/70 mm Hg. Her optic fundi are clear, and her neurologic examination is completely normal.

Q5. What is the most likely type of headache in this patient?
   a. migraine without aura: premenstrual syndrome
   b. menstrual migraine
   c. migraine without aura: premenstrual dysphoric disorder
   d. migraine-tension syndrome: premenstrual symptom complex
   e. complicated migraine syndrome

Q6. Which of the following statements regarding migraine headaches is (are) true?
   a. migraine headache is more common in men than in women
   b. migraine headache is more common in patients who have a family history of migraine headache
   c. migraine headache is more common in patients in lower socioeconomic groups than in those in higher socioeconomic groups
   d. migraine headache is more common in urban dwellers than in rural dwellers
   e. all of the above

Q7. What is the prevalence of migraine headache in adult women?
   a. 1%
   b. 4%

c. 14%
d. 19%
e. 31%

Q8. Regarding the pathogenesis of migraine headache, which of the following theories best explains the symptomatology? Migraine headache is:
a. produced by spasm of the cerebral blood vessels (the aura and the prodrome) followed by spasmodic rebound, producing vasodilatation and the accompanying headache
b. produced by spasmodic rebound of the cerebral blood vessels (the aura and the prodrome) followed by spasm, producing vasodilatation and the accompanying headache
c. produced by an imbalance of the neurotransmitters dopamine and acetylcholine, producing first spasm and then relaxation
d. produced by a complex physiologic process involving platelet aggregation and the release of serotonin in the brain that is accompanied by a cycle of increase/decrease in blood-brain catecholamines
e. produced by a complex physiologic process involving platelet decrease, the depletion of serotonin, and a cycle of increase/decrease in blood-brain catecholamines

Q9. Which of the following is a recognized trigger of migraine headache?
a. stress, worry, and anxiety
b. excessive sleep
c. certain foods and alcohol
d. weather changes
e. all of the above

Q10. What is (are) the drug(s) of first choice for the abortive treatment of moderately severe to very severe migraine headache?
a. sumatriptan
b. dihydroergotamine (DHE) mesylate
c. ergotamine
d. chlorpromazine
e. all of the above

Q11. Which of the following has not been recommended as a prophylactic agent for the prevention of migraine headache?
a. naproxen
b. propranolol
c. amitriptyline
d. fluoxetine
e. methysergide

Case 5 ■ A 35-Year-Old Male with a 6-Month History of Recurrent, Steady, Aching, "Viselike" Headaches

A 35-year-old male comes to your office with a 6-month history of recurrent daily headaches, usually in the late afternoon. The headaches are described by the patient as "a vise around my head."

The headaches are not associated with nausea, vomiting, or malaise. The patient does, however, describe some dizziness and lightheadedness with these headaches.

On examination, the patient's blood pressure is 100/70 mm Hg. His optic fundi are normal. There are no neurologic abnormalities.

Q12. What is the likely type of headache in this patient?
a. chronic daily headache: tension type
b. episodic tension-type headache
c. migraine without aura
d. migraine tension-type headache complex (mixed or combined headache)
e. cluster headache

Q13. What is the treatment of first choice for this patient?
a. a prostaglandin synthetase inhibitor
b. acetaminophen
c. codeine
d. a tricyclic antidepressant
e. all of the above
f. a, b, and/or d

Q14. Consider the patient described in Case 2. You note that the patient is taking 6 g of acetaminophen within a 12-hour period when the acute headache is present. Which of the following statements best represent(s) the recommendation about this drug and this dose?
a. given that this is an infrequent occurrence (once per week to once every 2 weeks), it is unlikely to produce any serious pathologic condition
b. given that this is an infrequent occurrence (once per week to once every 2 weeks) and the dose used is 6 g in 12 hours, it would be prudent to allow the patient to continue this dose under careful monitoring
c. given the dose of acetaminophen used in the very short time interval, it would be wise to check her liver function and suggest a decrease in the dose
d. given the dose of acetaminophen used, the syndrome of analgesic rebound is a definite consideration

e. b and d

f. c and d

Case 6 ■ A 75-Year-Old Female with a Severe Left-Sided Temporal Headache

A 75-year-old female comes to your office with a severe left-sided temporal headache. She describes a tender area in the left temple. She also describes pain in the area of the jaw while chewing her food. This headache has been present for the past 3 days.

On physical examination, the patient's blood pressure is 170/100 mm Hg. Her neurologic examination is normal. There is moderate tenderness in the area of the left temple.

Q15. Which of the following statements regarding this patient's symptoms is (are) true?
  a. this probably represents a late-onset migraine syndrome
  b. simple analgesics should be prescribed before embarking on any extensive investigation of these symptoms
  c. this headache is unlikely to be associated with any significant complications
  d. an erythrocyte sedimentation rate (ESR) should be ordered on this patient
  e. all of the above

Q16. Which of the following statements regarding the investigation of headaches is (are) true?
  a. patients with migraine with aura or migraine without aura rarely require more than a careful history and physical examination
  b. patients with episodic tension-type headaches rarely require more than a careful history and physical examination
  c. the electroencephalogram (EEG) is rarely useful in the diagnosis of headache (other than when headache may indicate a central nervous system brain tumor)
  d. radioisotope brain scanning is no longer indicated in the investigation of a patient with a headache syndrome
  e. all of the above

Case 7 ■ A 35-Year-Old Female with Almost-Constant Migraine Headaches

A 35-year-old female comes to the Emergency Department with another "migraine headache." She has had migraine headaches for the past 20 years, and during the last 4 years they have been almost constant.

Her headaches have required intramuscular me-

peridine (Demerol) and hydromorphone (Dilaudid) injections approximately twice per week for the last 3 years. She has made 157 trips to the Emergency Department with the same symptoms during the past year.

This patient categorically tells you that she has "tried every abortive agent and every prophylactic agent and nothing has worked."

Q17. Which of the following statements regarding this patient's headaches is (are) true?
  a. this headache most likely is an example of status migrainous
  b. the major component of this headache is likely analgesic rebound
  c. the scenario presented here is uncommon
  d. the majority of the patients with this headache type are female
  e. all of the above

Q18. What is the treatment of choice for the headache described in Case 7?
  a. continue the present treatment plan: repeated injections of Demerol and Dilaudid
  b. change the treatment plan to regular injections of DHE and metoclopramide
  c. seek immediate psychiatric consultation
  d. change the treatment plan to one that employs nonnarcotic analgesics (in fairly large doses) in place of the narcotic analgesics
  e. none of the above

Case 8 ■ A 62-Year-Old Male with Headaches That Have Been Getting Progressively Worse

A 62-year-old patient comes to the Emergency Department with headaches that have been getting progressively worse over the last 7 days. He has not had previous problems with headache, and his only significant illness was a lobectomy and radiation therapy for carcinoma of the lung 3 years ago. He has not had any recurrence and is feeling well.

The significant features of this headache include the following: the headache appears to be significantly worse every day; the headache is absolutely constant: it never goes away and never decreases in severity to any extent; and the headache is described as a "terrible pressure within my head."

Q19. What is the most likely cause of this patient's headache?
  a. migraine without aura: status migrainous type
  b. migraine without aura: complex etiology
  c. secondary headache: cerebral edema

d. secondary headache: primary brain tumor resulting from previous radiation therapy

e. none of the above

Q20. What is the drug of choice for this patient at this time?

a. sumatriptan

b. ergotamine

c. meperidine and Dilaudid

d. dexamethasone

e. chlorpromazine

Case 9 ■ A 17-Year-Old Male with a Headache from Hell

A 17-year-old male is brought to the Emergency Department by his mother and has "a headache like I've never had before." The patient has been completely well, healthy, and active before this episode (which began last night). Nausea and vomiting began shortly after the headache's onset.

On examination, there is significant neck stiffness. The patient cannot move his neck without extreme pain. You are about to continue the neurologic examination when a patient with cardiac arrest is wheeled through the Emergency Department doors.

Q21. At this time, with the information you have now, what is the most likely diagnosis?

a. acute subdural hematoma

b. acute epidural hematoma

c. subarachnoid hemorrhage

d. severe migraine headache without aura

e. glioblastoma multiforme

Q22. With the provisional diagnosis you have made for this patient, what should you do?

a. perform a lumbar puncture

b. perform a computed tomography (CT) or magnetic resonance imaging (MRI) scan of the brain

c. observe the patient for 12 hours before doing anything

d. sedate and medicate the patient in an effort to alleviate the headache and sort things out later

e. none of the above

SHORT ANSWER MANAGEMENT PROBLEM
Discuss the classification of primary headache disorders that has recently been proposed by the International Headache Society. Distinguish between primary headache and secondary headache.

ANSWERS

A1. **d.** This patient has developed a typical cluster headache. Although we can diagnose with considerable confidence, it is too early to predict which of the two subtypes of cluster headache the patient will ultimately develop. These subtypes are episodic cluster headache and chronic cluster headache.

The typical cluster headache awakens a patient from sleep, although both daytime clusters and nighttime clusters are well described. Multiple daily episodes, usually lasting between 45 minutes and 1 hour, may occur on a regular basis for periods of 2 to 3 weeks. Remissions may last from several months to several years. Episodic cluster headaches constitute 90% of cases. In the other 10% of patients the headaches do not remit (chronic cluster headache). The typical description of cluster headache is a headache that has the properties of a "deep, burning, or stabbing pain." It is very often described by the patient as "excruciating" or "the worst pain I have ever had." It is almost exclusively unilateral in nature. The pain may become so bad that the patient actually becomes suicidal. Cluster headache is associated with lacrimation, facial flushing, and nasal discharge. The affected eye often becomes red, conjunctival vessels become dilated, and a Horner's-type syndrome, including both ptosis and pupillary constriction, develops.

A2. **e.** Cluster headache is thought by many authorities to be a migraine variant. Sumatriptan (Imitrex) is the drug of choice for acute episodes of cluster headache. In addition, oxygen inhalation is very beneficial in an acute cluster attack. Ergotamine preparations have also been effective. Prophylactic medications indicated in the treatment of cluster headache include verapamil, ergotamine, lithium, methysergide, prednisone and other corticosteroids, indomethacin, β-blockers, tricyclic antidepressants, and selective serotonin reuptake inhibitors (SSRIs).

A3. **a.** This patient has migraine headache without aura (common migraine headache). Migraine headache is a type of headache that is typically episodic, usually occurring 1 or 2 times a month. More frequent episodes of migraine, such as migraine headache every day, every second day, or every third day, should make you suspicious regarding the true diagnosis. The most common alternative diagnosis would be rebound analgesic headaches, and many patients who are labeled as having migraine headaches actually have analgesic rebound headaches.

The prodromal phase of migraine consists of symptoms of excitation or inhibition of the central nervous system, including elation; excitability; irritability; increased appetite and craving for certain foods, especially sweets; depression; sleepiness; and fatigue. This phase occurs in approximately 30% of patients. These symptoms may precede the migraine attack by up to 24 hours. The headache phase of the cycle is certainly the most prominent. Migraine headache is unilateral in more than 50% of patients, but bilateral migraine is more common than previously thought. In addition, it is not uncommon for a migraine headache to begin on one side and switch to the other. The character of the pain is also much more variable than previously thought: "pulsating or throbbing" in only 50% of cases, and a "dull, achy" pain in the other 50%. The headache phase itself usually lasts between 4 and 72 hours but is occasionally longer. Migraine headache is almost invariably associated with other symptoms, including nausea, vomiting, and diarrhea. Heightened sensory perceptions such as photophobia, phonophobia, and increased sensitivity to smell occur during the attacks.

Although a mixed headache syndrome (mixed migraine and tension headaches) and tension headaches themselves are often confused with migraine, pure migraine headache can usually be distinguished by moderate to severe intensity and aggravation by activities such as coughing, running, or bending down. Those two characteristics, and one of nausea, vomiting, photophobia, or phonophobia establish the diagnosis as migraine headache.

A4. **b.** This patient has migraine headache with aura. The visual symptoms that this patient describes follow the classic description for what is called an aura. An aura is usually visual, although neurologic auras consisting of hemisensory disturbances, hemiparesis, dysphasia, and change in memory or state of consciousness can occasionally occur. Only approximately 20% of migraine headaches can be classified as migraine with aura. Also, it is quite frequent for a patient to alternate between migraine with aura and migraine without aura. Migraine with aura and migraine without aura are, other than the aura itself, quite similar in characteristic features.

A5. **b.** Although migraine headache without aura can occur at any time during the menstrual cycle, this patient's description of a cyclic, repeatable headache that occurs between 2 days before menstruation and the last day of menses clearly establishes this headache as menstrual migraine. Estrogen withdrawal is likely the trigger for migrainous attacks.

Therapy for a menstrual headache is similar to that for a nonmenstrual migraine. Prophylaxis for menstrual migraine includes estrogen supplementation, nonsteroidal antiinflammatory drugs (NSAIDs), and 5-HT$_1$ agonists (i.e., sumatriptan).

A6. **b.** Migraine headache is significantly more common in individuals who have a family history of migraine headache, particularly women who had a mother with migraine headache.

Migraine headache prevalence does not vary among the populations of the world; the prevalence is the same in rural Nigeria as it is in cosmopolitan Los Angeles. Moreover, contrary to what is commonly believed, migraine headache is not more common among lower socioeconomic groups than among higher socioeconomic groups unless there are triggering factors (see Answer 9) that may be more common in a certain segment of the population.

A7. **d.** Migraine headache is more common in women than in men. In the general population the prevalence of migraine headache is approximately 19% in women.

A8. **d.** The pathophysiology is best summarized as an orderly process that involves the following events:
   a. Platelet aggregation occurs in the central nervous system.
   b. There is a release of serotonin from the synaptic nerve endings.
   c. At the same time or following the release of serotonin, there is an increase and then a decrease in the levels of the blood-brain catecholamines norepinephrine and epinephrine. This is significantly different from previous ideas of spasm followed by rebound vasodilation that was purported to explain the vasoconstriction (aura), and vasodilatation (headache).

A9. **e.** Common triggers of migraine are as follows:
   a. Stress, worry, anxiety
   b. Menstruation
   c. Oral contraceptive pills
   d. Certain foods (aged cheese, chocolate)
   e. Alcohol
   f. Lack of sleep
   g. Glare, dazzle
   h. Weather or ambient temperature changes
   i. Physical exertion
   j. Fatigue
   k. Head trauma
Less common triggers of a migraine are as follows:
   a. High humidity
   b. Excessive sleep
   c. High altitude
   d. Excessive vitamin A
   e. Drugs: Nitroglycerin, reserpine, estrogens, hydralazine, ranitidine
   f. Pungent odors
   g. Fluorescent lighting

h. Allergic reactions
i. Cold foods
j. Refractory errors

A10. **a.** The drugs of first choice for the abortive treatment of acute severe to very severe migraine headache are the 5-HT$_1$ receptor agonists. Sumatriptan is the prototype. These drugs activate serotonin receptors. Oral, subcutaneous, and intranasal preparations are available. These are extremely effective in over 80% of cases.

In addition, intravenous DHE mesylate (1 mg) and ergotamine (rectal suppositories, sublingual tablets, and oral tablets) are also used to abort acute migraine headache in moderately severe cases of migraine.

Phenothiazines (such as chlorpromazine) and NSAIDs are useful as alternative agents in the treatment of migraine headaches and can be thought of as an alternative to the abortive agents just mentioned.

A11. **a.** Prophylactic pharmacotherapy for migraine headaches includes drugs from the following classes:
   a. β-Adrenergic blocking agents: Propranolol, nadolol, atenolol, timolol, metoprolol
   b. Tricyclic antidepressants: Amitriptyline, nortriptyline
   c. SSRIs: Fluoxetine, sertraline
   d. Calcium channel blockers: Verapamil, isradipine
   e. Serotonin antagonists: Methysergide
   f. Anticonvulsants: Valproic acid
   g. Antihistamine: Cyproheptadine

A12. **a.** This patient has chronic tension-type headache. Chronic tension-type headaches are often described as a steady, aching, "viselike" sensation that encircles the entire head. Chronic tension-type headaches are often accompanied by tight, tender muscles at the site of maximal pain, often in the posterior cervical, frontal, or temporal muscles. Tension headaches are recurrent and are often brought on by stress.

The pathogenesis of tension-type headaches is unclear. It may be related to the release of vasoactive substances that also explain migraine headaches. Often it is very difficult to separate the two syndromes.

A13. **f.** Chronic daily headaches (either tension-type or migraine-tension type) are usually related to causal factors that include the following: Stress and worry, depression, overwork, lack of sleep, incorrect posture, and marital and family dysfunction.

Treatment approaches for the relief of tension-type headaches should center on the following principles:
   a. Attempt to identify the causal factor(s).
   b. Attempt to modify or eliminate the stressor with behavior modification, biofeedback, relaxation therapy, yoga, exercise, and so on.

c. Consider the use of mild analgesics such as acetaminophen, NSAIDs, aspirin, tricyclic antidepressants, and SSRIs.
Codeine or other narcotic agents should be avoided.

A14. **f.** The total daily recommended dose of acetaminophen is 4000 mg/day. Even though this is a sporadic event, it would be wise to suggest a decrease to no more than 4 g/day, check her liver function now and (if she continues taking acetaminophen) continue checking it, and discuss the concept of analgesic rebound headaches with her.

A15. **d.** This patient has temporal arteritis (giant cell arteritis) until proven otherwise. When an elderly patient has a new-onset headache, temporal arteritis must be excluded. This patient has a unilateral headache with a tender temporal area, probably representing the inflamed temporal artery.

The most significant complication of temporal arteritis is sudden unilateral blindness caused by occlusion of the terminal branches of the ophthalmic artery. This is a completely preventable complication.

Temporal arteritis is often associated with polymyalgia rheumatica.

The ESR is a highly sensitive test in a patient you suspect of having temporal arteritis. The ESR is usually elevated above 50 mm/hr and may exceed 100 mm/hr.

The treatment of choice for a patient with temporal arteritis is high-dose prednisone. When temporal arteritis is diagnosed or even suspected, treatment should be started immediately with at least 50 mg of prednisone. If the diagnosis is confirmed, treatment should be continued for at least 4 weeks before any gradual reduction is instituted. If ocular complications have occurred, treatment should continue for 1 to 2 years.

A16. **e.** Because headache is such a common disorder and the excessive application of expensive and highly technical laboratory procedures to the diagnosis and management of benign headache is expensive and epidemiologically unsound, the following principles should apply to the investigation of headache:
   a. Patients with migraine headache with or without aura or tension-type headache rarely require more than a careful history and physical examination.
   b. Headaches of recent origin or progression deserve investigation. This is especially true of headaches that have a consistently focal distribution, headaches that follow trauma, or headaches that begin after age 40 years. CT or MRI scanning is recommended.

c. The EEG is almost never helpful in the diagnosis of primary headache.

d. Skull x-rays are useful only when abnormalities involving the base of the brain are suspected or immediately after head trauma.

e. Diagnostic lumbar puncture should be performed in any patient with a headache that is accompanied by fever or is explosive in nature. Lumbar puncture should, if possible, be deferred until after CT scanning in other forms of acute headache, especially if the patient has a stiff neck.

f. CT and MRI scans are the diagnostic modalities of choice in the evaluation of acute headache in which serious pathology is suspected.

A17. **b.** This is an extremely common scenario that is repeated thousands of times daily in Emergency Departments across North America. When these patients come through the Emergency Department doors, we all feel like "heading for the nearest exit." This patient is an excellent example of the mistakes made in treating this type of headache pattern, as listed here:

a. These patients should not be started on narcotic analgesics in the first place. Although there is a place in the rare patient for a one- or two-time dose of Demerol, that should be the limit.

b. When a patient with migraine headache tells you that "no abortive or prophylactic agent has ever worked," he/she is essentially telling you that this is not a migraine headache. We now realize the importance of the neurotransmitter serotonin in the pathogenesis of migraine headache. If none of the abortive prophylactic agents work, you can draw the reasonable conclusion that the major headache component is not dependent on serotonin. In this patient, there is no doubt that migraine headache was the beginning of the problem, but now rebound analgesic headache with migraine underlay is the most likely diagnosis and the treatment problem to be faced.

c. Status migrainous indicates a prolonged migraine attack usually lasting for more than 72 hours that does not resolve spontaneously.

A18. **e.** The treatment of this patient must include both an empathic physician who takes the time to explain what is happening to the patient and a physician who is prepared to do what needs to be done: Gradual reduction (suggested 10% a week) of the total narcotic dosage.

It would be very unwise to use large doses of non-narcotic analgesics in this patient. The most common cause of rebound analgesic headaches is, in fact, acetaminophen.

A19. **c.** This patient has a secondary headache (a headache resulting from a secondary disease or process). The description is a classic presentation of the headache of cerebral edema. In this case, the cerebral edema is caused by metastatic deposits related to the carcinoma of the lung that was previously resected and radiated. The classic symptoms in this case are fairly acute onset, constant headache, pressure-like sensation, and a progressively more severe headache every day.

A20. **d.** The treatment of choice for this patient is dexamethasone. The correct starting dose is 4 mg qid with ranitidine or omeprazole to protect the gastric mucosa and prevent peptic or stress ulceration.

A21. **c.** This patient has the classic description of a subarachnoid hemorrhage ("headache like I've never had before" and acute onset) and you should consider it subarachnoid hemorrhage until proven otherwise.

A22. **b.** This patient should have an immediate CT or MRI scan, and this should be followed by angiography or special MRI technique imaging to localize the blood vessel. The most common pathogenesis of subarachnoid hemorrhage is rupture of a berry aneurysm in the circle of Willis.

SOLUTION TO THE SHORT ANSWER MANAGEMENT PROBLEM

The reclassification of primary headache disorders (according to the International Headache Society) is as follows:

1. Migraine:
   a. Migraine without aura (common migraine)
   b. Migraine with aura (classic migraine)
   c. Complicated migraine (migraine with prominent neurologic symptoms)
   d. Basilar migraine
   e. Hemiplegic migraine
   f. Ophthalmoplegic migraine
2. Cluster headache:
   a. Episodic
   b. Chronic
3. Episodic tension-type headache
4. Chronic daily headache:
   a. Chronic tension-type headache
   b. Migraine-tension type headache complex (mixed or combined headache); usually evolved from migraine
   c. Analgesic/ergotamine rebound headache

Secondary headache is defined as a headache resulting from a disease or condition that is initially unrelated to the headache. The most common cause of secondary headache is probably related to side effects or adverse reactions produced by any number of pharmaceutical products.

SUMMARY OF THE DIAGNOSIS AND TREATMENT OF HEADACHE

This chapter has completely outlined the important points of the diagnosis and treatment of headache; the summary will take the form of a list of do's and don'ts in headache diagnosis and management.

1. Take a complete history and perform a complete physical (especially neurologic) examination.

2. Do not rely on CT or MRI scans to make the majority of your headache diagnoses.

3. Recognize that migraine headache in the same patient may have different presentations on different occasions.

4. Do not label a headache as tension headache unless the criteria for its diagnosis are met.

5. Attempt to discover the triggers or stresses that bring on both migraine-type and tension-type headaches.

6. Remember that the pathophysiology of migraine is related to serotonin depletion.

7. Recognize the contraindications to 5-HT$_1$ agonists:
   a. Ischemic heart disease/angina pectoris
   b. Previous myocardial infarction
   c. Uncontrolled hypertension
   d. Basilar artery migraine
   e. Hemiplegic migraine
   f. Patients taking monoamine inhibitors, SSRIs, or lithium

8. Avoid narcotics for the treatment of migraine headaches.

9. Recognize the underdiagnosis of rebound analgesia headache.

10. Beware of the patient with "migraine headache" for whom no abortive agent and no prophylactic agent works. The probability of that patient having migraine headache as the primary headache diagnosis is very low.

SUGGESTED READINGS

Fettes I: Menstrual migraine, *Postgrad Med* 101(5):67-77, 1997.

Mathew N: Headache. In Rakel R, ed: *Conn's current therapy*, Philadelphia, 1994, WB Saunders.

Newman LC et al: A pilot-study of oral sumatriptan as intermittent prophylaxis of menstruation-related migraine, *Neurology* 51(1): 307-309, 1998.

Welch KM: A 27-year-old woman with migraine headaches, *JAMA* 278(4):322-328, 1997.

PROBLEM · 25

SEIZURE DISORDERS

Seize the Moment.

Case 1 ■ A 65-Year-Old Male with a New-Onset Seizure

A 65-year-old male is brought to the Emergency Department after suffering a seizure while eating a meal in a restaurant. His wife states that he has never had anything like this before. Apparently, the patient developed convulsive jerking in his right arm and leg that lasted approximately 5 minutes. In addition, the patient lost consciousness for a short interval.

This patient's history includes smoking 80 packs of cigarettes per year and having chronic bronchitis.

The neurologic examination is completely normal. His blood pressure is 150/100 mm Hg. His pulse is 96 bpm and regular.

SELECT THE BEST ANSWER TO THE FOLLOWING QUESTIONS

Q1. Which of the following is the most correct statement regarding his seizure, history of smoking, and symptoms of bronchitis?
   a. there is probably no association between these conditions
   b. the nicotine in the cigarette smoke lowered his seizure threshold
   c. chronic hypoxemia increases the risk of seizure activity
   d. a complication of chronic cigarette smoking may first manifest as seizures
   e. chronic aspiration caused by bronchitis increases the risk of seizure activity

Q2. What is the type of seizure described in this patient?
   a. a simple partial seizure
   b. a complex partial seizure
   c. an absence seizure
   d. a tonic-clonic (grand mal) seizure
   e. a myoclonic seizure

Q3. What is the most common cause of a new-onset seizure in a patient of this age?
a. idiopathic
b. alcohol withdrawal
c. head trauma
d. brain tumor
e. an old stroke

Q4. Which of the following medications would not be a drug of first choice for the prevention of further seizures in this patient?
a. phenytoin
b. carbamazepine
c. phenobarbital
d. valproic acid
e. ethosuximide

Q5. Which of the following investigations is the most important study to be performed on this patient at this time?
a. a magnetic resonance imaging (MRI) scan of the brain
b. an electroencephalogram (EEG) study of the brain
c. angiography of the cerebral vessels
d. auditory- and brainstem-evoked potentials
e. a computed tomography (CT) scan of the chest

Case 2 ■ A 22-Year-Old Male Who Suddenly Lost Consciousness, Became Rigid, and Fell

A 22-year-old male is brought to the Emergency Department by his wife. While he was raking leaves in the backyard, he suddenly lost consciousness, became rigid, and fell to the ground. His respirations temporarily ceased. This lasted for approximately 45 seconds and was followed by a period of jerking of all four limbs lasting 2 to 3 minutes. The patient then became unconscious for 3 to 4 minutes.

On examination, the patient is drowsy. There is a large laceration on his tongue and a small laceration on his lip. The neurologic examination is otherwise normal. The vital signs are normal.

Q6. From what type of seizure is the patient in Case 2 suffering?
a. simple partial seizure
b. complex partial seizure
c. absence seizure
d. grand mal (tonic-clonic) seizure
e. myoclonic seizure

Q7. Which of the following medications would not be a drug of first choice for the prevention of further seizures in this patient?

a. phenytoin
b. carbamazepine
c. phenobarbital
d. primidone
e. ethosuximide

Case 3 ■ A 12-Year-Old Female Who Stares into Space

A mother comes to your office with her 12-year-old daughter. The mother states that for the past 6 months she and the girl's teacher have frequently noted the child staring into space. This lack of concentration usually lasts only 30 to 45 seconds. Sometimes there appears to be brief twitching of all limbs during this time.

The child's neurologic examination is normal.

Q8. What is the most likely cause of symptoms described in Case 3?
a. simple partial seizures
b. complex partial seizures
c. absence seizures
d. myoclonic seizures
e. none of the above

Q9. All of the following may be useful in the treatment of the patient in Case 3 except:
a. valproic acid
b. clonazepam
c. ethosuximide
d. phenytoin
e. all of the above are useful

Q10. Which of the following statements regarding beginning and stopping antiepileptic therapy is true?
a. antiepileptic therapy can safely be discontinued after a seizure-free interval of 1 year
b. antiepileptic medication should be started on every patient who has a seizure
c. antiepileptic medication should be started with a combination of two or more antiepileptic agents
d. the decision to stop antiepileptic medication should be guided by the results of the EEG
e. none of the above statements is true

Q11. Which of the following investigations is (are) useful in the initial evaluation of a patient with new-onset seizures?
a. EEG
b. MRI scan of the brain
c. serologic test for syphilis
d. carotid ultrasound
e. a, b, and c
f. all of the above

Q12. Which of the following statements regarding the diagnosis and treatment of status epilepticus is (are) true?
  a. poor compliance with the anticonvulsant drug regimen is the most common cause of tonic-clonic status epilepticus
  b. the mortality of status epilepticus may be as high as 20%
  c. the establishment of an airway is the first priority in the management of status epilepticus
  d. intravenous (IV) diazepam is the drug of first choice in the immediate management of status epilepticus
  e. all of the above statements are true

Q13. Which of the following is a (are) cause(s) of nonepileptic seizures?
  a. hypocalcemia
  b. hypomagnesemia
  c. pyridoxine deficiency
  d. thyrotoxic storm
  e. a, b, and c
  f. all of the above

Q14. Which of the following is most often confused with petit mal (absence) seizures in adults?
  a. benign rolandic epilepsy
  b. complex partial seizures
  c. myoclonic seizures
  d. simple partial seizures
  e. clonic seizures

Q15. Which of the following is the most common neurologic disorder?
  a. epilepsy
  b. multiple sclerosis
  c. stroke
  d. myasthenia gravis
  e. Bell's palsy

Q16. Which of the following primary brain tumors is most likely responsible for a new-onset seizure in a 68-year-old male?
  a. meningioma
  b. schwannoma
  c. ependymoma
  d. glioblastoma
  e. pituitary adenoma

SHORT ANSWER MANAGEMENT PROBLEM
Discuss the pathophysiology and treatment of febrile seizures in children.

ANSWERS

A1. **d.** There is a high probability of association between the patient's smoking and his seizures because in a patient older than age 40 years the most common cause of a new-onset seizure is a brain tumor (primary or secondary), and a history of chronic bronchitis and an 80-pack/year history of cigarette smoking suggests a significant probability of bronchogenic carcinoma. Consequently, seizure and cigarette smoking suggests a probability of primary bronchogenic cancer with secondary metastases to the brain.

A2. **a.** The seizure described in this patient is a simple seizure. The symptoms of simple seizure include focal motor symptoms and somatosensory symptoms that spread or "march" to other parts of the body. Other symptoms include special sensory symptoms that involve the visual, auditory, olfactory, or gustatory regions of the brain and autonomic symptoms or signs. Psychologic symptoms, often accompanied by an impaired level of consciousness, can also occur.

A3. **d.** As discussed in Answer 1, the most common cause of a new-onset seizure in patients in this age group is a brain tumor. As in this case a primary bronchogenic carcinoma with secondary brain metastases would be the most likely cause of a new-onset seizure in a 65-year-old heavy cigarette smoker with chronic obstructive pulmonary disease. The common causes of new-onset seizures by age are as follows:
  a. Less than 10 years:
    1) Idiopathic
    2) Congenital
    3) Birth injury
    4) Metabolic
  b. Age 10 to 40 years:
    1) Idiopathic
    2) Head trauma
    3) Preexisting focal brain disease
    4) Drug withdrawal
  c. Greater than age 40 years:
    1) Brain tumor
    2) Old stroke
    3) Trauma

A4. **e.** Partial seizures can be treated effectively with phenytoin, carbamazepine, phenobarbital, primidone, and valproic acid. Treatment with one drug is preferable to combination therapy.

Ethosuximide is not a good choice for the treatment of partial seizures. It is primarily indicated in petit mal (absence) seizures.

A5. **a.** The most important investigation in this patient at this time is an MRI scan of the brain, which will identify any cerebral or leptomeningeal mass that may be associated with the new-onset seizure. A CT scan would be a reasonable alternative. An EEG will identify the type of abnormal discharge and its location. It would, however, be a poor second choice.

A6. **d.** This patient has had a grand mal (tonic-clonic) seizure. Tonic-clonic seizures are often associated with a sudden loss of consciousness. The tonic phase is followed by a clonic phase characterized by generalized body musculature jerking. Following this is a stage of flaccid coma.

Associated manifestations include tongue or lip biting, urinary or fecal incontinence, and other injuries. An aura may precede a generalized seizure.

A7. **e.** As in partial (focal) seizures, the drugs of choice are phenytoin, carbamazepine, phenobarbital, primidone, and valproic acid. Ethosuximide is not an effective drug in the treatment of grand mal seizures.

A8. **c.** This patient has typical absence (petit mal) seizures. Petit mal seizures may present with impairment of consciousness, sometimes accompanied by mild clonic, tonic, atonic, or autonomic symptoms. These seizures, often brief in duration, interrupt the current activity and are characterized by a description of the patient "staring into space."

Petit mal seizures that begin in childhood are terminated by the beginning of the third decade of life. A bilaterally synchronous and symmetric 3-Hz "spike-and-wave" pattern is seen.

A9. **d.** Petit mal seizures can be effectively treated with ethosuximide, valproic acid, or clonazepam. Phenytoin is not an effective treatment for petit mal seizures.

A10. **d.** The criteria for deciding to treat or not to treat an initial seizure should include details of the seizure; adequate laboratory data, including measurement of glucose, electrolytes, alcohol, and other toxins; and the presence of EEG evidence of epileptic activity at least 2 weeks after the seizure. Careful reevaluation and monitoring are essential.

A consideration of discontinuation of medication can be made after a seizure-free period of 4 years. This decision should be confirmed by a lack of seizure activity on EEG.

A11. **e.** Laboratory investigations for a patient with an initial seizure should include a complete blood count (CBC), blood glucose determination, liver and renal function tests, and a serologic test for syphilis. Initial and periodic EEGs are mandatory. A CT or MRI scan should be performed in patients with focal neu-

rologic symptoms and/or signs, focal seizures, or EEG findings indicating a focal disturbance.

A chest x-ray film should be performed in all patients who are cigarette smokers; a primary lung neoplasm with secondary brain metastases producing cerebral edema and seizures is not uncommon. However, a plain x-ray film of the skull or a skull series is unlikely to produce any useful diagnostic information.

A12. **e.** Status epilepticus is a medical emergency, with a mortality of up to 20% and a high incidence of neurologic and mental sequelae in survivors.

Status epilepticus may be caused by poor compliance with medication, alcohol withdrawal, intracranial infection, neoplasm, a metabolic disorder, or a drug overdose. Prognosis depends on the length of time from the onset of the seizure activity to effective treatment.

The management of status epilepticus includes establishing an airway, giving 50% dextrose in case of hypoglycemia, giving IV diazepam, giving IV phenytoin, and treating resistant cases with IV phenobarbital.

A13. **f.** There are many causes of nonepileptic seizures. These are divided into the following categories:
a. Cardiogenic:
   1) Simple syncope
   2) Transient ischemic attacks
   3) Arrhythmias
   4) Sick sinus syndrome
b. Electrolyte imbalance:
   1) Hypocalcemia
   2) Hyponatremia and water intoxication
   3) Hypomagnesemia
c. Metabolic:
   1) Hypoglycemia
   2) Hyperglycemia
   3) Thyrotoxic storm
   4) Pyridoxine deficiency
d. Acute drug withdrawal:
   1) Alcohol
   2) Benzodiazepines
   3) Cocaine
   4) Barbiturates
   5) Meperidine
e. Drug intoxication:
   1) Cocaine
   2) Dextroamphetamine
   3) Theophylline
   4) Isoniazid
   5) Lithium
   6) Nitrous oxide anesthesia
   7) Acetylcholinesterase inhibitors

f. Metals:
   1) Mercury
   2) Lead
g. Infections:
   1) Gram-negative septicemia with shock
   2) Viral meningitis
   3) Bacterial meningitis (gram-negative or syphilitic)
h. Hyperthermia
i. Pseudoseizures (psychogenic)
j. Malignancies
k. Idiopathic (isolated unprovoked seizure)

A14. **b.** Absence (petit mal) seizures are often confused with complex partial seizures in adolescents and adults. An accurate diagnosis can often be made on the basis of history, the duration of the seizure, the presence of an aura and/or postictal confusion, the pattern of autonomic behavior, and the EEG.

In absence seizures, minor clonic activity (eye blinks or head nodding) is present in up to 45% of cases; the mean duration is seconds; and the EEG shows the typical bilateral symmetrical 3-cycle second spike and wave that may be easily provoked by hyperventilation. There is no aura or postictal confusion.

In contrast, complex partial seizures may be preceded by an aura, are followed by postictal confusion, last longer (1 to 3 minutes), and are associated with more complex automatisms and less frequent clonic components. The EEG tends to show focal slow or sharp and slow wave activity. The differentiation between these two types of seizures is important. Absence seizures tend to disappear in adulthood, but complex partial seizures do not. Furthermore, phenytoin (Dilantin) and carbamazepine (Tegretol) are effective in treating complex partial seizures but not absence attacks.

A15. **c.** The most common neurologic disorder is stroke. Epilepsy is the second most common disorder, with the prevalence ranging from 0.6% to 3.4% in the general population.

A16. **d.** The most common primary brain tumor in elderly patients is a glioma. Of the gliomas, the glioblastomas and the astrocytomas are by far the most common.

SOLUTION TO THE SHORT ANSWER MANAGEMENT QUESTION

Febrile seizures in children:
1. Age of risk: Age 6 months to 5 years
2. Risk factors for febrile convulsions:

a. Previous febrile convulsion: The risk of a subsequent febrile convulsion is 30% when the first seizure occurred between ages 1 and 3 years; 50% when it occurred first at other ages; and 50% after a second febrile seizure.
b. Family history of febrile convulsion (25%)
3. Prognosis: The prognosis for normal school progress and for seizure remission is excellent in children with febrile seizures.
4. Chances of progression of febrile seizures to epilepsy are very small: 98% of children with febrile seizures have no further seizures after age 5 years.
5. Factors that increase the chance of progression of febrile seizures to epilepsy:
   a. Presence of developmental delay
   b. Cerebral palsy
   c. Abnormal neurologic development
   d. History of epilepsy in a parent or sibling
   e. A seizure that has a focal onset, lasts more than 15 minutes, or recurs in the same febrile illness
6. Treatment: Prophylactic anticonvulsants
   a. Usually not indicated. If you do use prophylactic anticonvulsants, it will only be to treat the febrile seizure, not to prevent later epilepsy.
   b. Drug of choice when indicated: Rectal or oral diazepam 5 mg every 8 hours when the rectal temperature exceeds 38.5° C. The use of rectal diazepam at home to stop a febrile seizure not only increases the chance of preventing a prolonged febrile seizure but also gives the parent a sense of control over the situation.

SUMMARY OF THE DIAGNOSIS AND TREATMENT OF SEIZURES

1. Absolute rules concerning seizures:
   a. *Not all that seizes is epilepsy.*
   b. *Not all epilepsy seizes.*
   c. Many "seizures" are associated with other systemic disorders.

2. Major classification causes of nonepileptic seizures:
   a. Metastases to the brain
   b. Cardiogenic
   c. Electrolyte imbalance
   d. Metabolic causes
   e. Acute drug withdrawal
   f. Drug intoxication
   g. Heavy metal poisoning
   h. Infections

i. Hyperthermia
j. Pseudoseizures

3. Greatly simplified classification of epileptic seizures:
   a. Partial seizures:
      1) Simple partial seizures
      2) Complex partial seizures
   b. Generalized seizures:
      1) Petit mal (absence seizures)
      2) Tonic-clonic (grand mal) seizures
   c. Myoclonic seizures
   d. Tonic, clonic, or atonic seizures

4. Diagnosis and investigations:
   a. History (from a relative or bystander)
   b. Physical examination
   c. EEG
   d. CT and/or MRI scans
   e. Blood profile including CBC, blood glucose, liver function tests, renal function tests, human immunodeficiency virus serology (in high-risk groups), serum calcium level, and serologic test for syphilis

5. Treatment:
   a. Carefully evaluate whether or not the patient needs treatment after the first seizure.
   b. Drugs for generalized tonic-clonic (grand mal) seizures or partial seizures include the following:
      1) Phenytoin (drug of choice)
      2) Carbamazepine
      3) Phenobarbital
   c. Once antiepileptic drug therapy is initiated, it should be maintained for a time period measured in years, not months. Patients must be carefully considered for discontinuation of therapy
   d. Febrile seizures: Rectal suppository of diazepam 5 mg or oral diazepam every 8 hours is treatment of choice for prevention of subsequent seizures, if that has been carefully evaluated.
   e. Status epilepticus: Treatment is 50 mg dextrose, IV diazepam, IV phenytoin, and IV phenobarbital.

SUGGESTED READINGS

Farrell KF, Connolly MB: Epilepsy in infants and children. In Rakel R, ed: *Conn's current therapy*, Philadelphia, 1994, WB Saunders.

Uthman BM, Wilder BJ: Epilepsy in adolescents and adults. In Rakel R, ed: *Conn's current therapy*, Philadelphia, 1994, WB Saunders.

PROBLEM·26

STROKE AND STROKE-RELATED ILLNESS

"You Say My Husband Has an Overripe Berry in His Brain?"

Case 1 ■ A 67-Year-Old Male with a Sudden-Onset, Left-Sided Hemiplegia, Dysphagia, and a "Visual Problem"

A 67-year-old male is brought to the Emergency Department by ambulance after the gradual onset of the inability to move his right leg, followed by his right arm; speech impairment; and a "visual problem."

On examination, the patient has flaccid paralysis of the muscles of the right leg and the muscles (excluding the deltoid) of the right arm, a homonymous hemianopia, and dysphagia. In addition, he "does not recognize" that he is paralyzed, nor can he turn his eyes toward the right side. His deep tendon reflexes are hyperreflexic on the right side. His right great toe is upgoing.

It is now 6 hours since the symptoms began. It appears from talking to his wife that the symptoms are "still changing."

SELECT THE BEST ANSWER TO THE FOLLOWING QUESTIONS

Q1. What is the most likely diagnosis at this time?
   a. transient ischemic attack (TIA)
   b. completed stroke
   c. stroke-in-evolution
   d. subarachnoid hemorrhage
   e. complicated migraine

Q2. The location of symptoms at the site of the lesion correlates to which of the following?
   a. left middle cerebral artery
   b. right middle cerebral artery
   c. left anterior cerebral artery
   d. right anterior cerebral artery
   e. left posterior cerebral artery

Q3. What is the most likely pathophysiologic process involved at this time?
   a. a thrombotic stroke
   b. an embolic stroke
   c. a hemorrhagic stroke
   d. a lacunar stroke
   e. a subarachnoid hemorrhage

Q4. What is the most common pathophysiologic process in patients who have suffered a cerebrovascular accident (CVA)?
   a. a thrombotic stroke
   b. an embolic stroke

c. a hemorrhagic stroke
d. a lacunar stroke
e. a subarachnoid hemorrhage

Q5. In which of the following conditions would you most likely find an embolic phenomena as the pathophysiology of a CVA?
   a. hypertension
   b. atrial fibrillation
   c. ventricular fibrillation
   d. a young woman taking oral contraceptive pills
   e. b and d

Q6. What is the number one risk factor for CVAs?
   a. cigarette smoking
   b. hypertension
   c. hypercholesterolemia
   d. hypertriglyceridemia
   e. hypothyroidism

Q7. Lacunar strokes (lacunar infarcts) are most closely associated with which of the following?
   a. thrombosis
   b. embolization
   c. hypertension
   d. subarachnoid bleeding
   e. cerebral infarction

Case 2 ■ A 42-Year-Old Patient with Mental Status Impairment, Foot Drop, and Left-Sided Hemiplegia and Numbness

A 47-year-old patient develops the following symptoms and signs: impaired mental status including confusion, amnesia, perseveration, and personality changes; foot drop; apraxia on the affected side; left-sided hemiplegia; and left-sided numbness (both muscle power and sensation retained to some degree in left upper extremity).

Q8. This patient most likely has had a CVA affecting which of the following arteries?
   a. right middle cerebral artery
   b. posterior cerebral artery
   c. vertebral-basilar artery
   d. right anterior cerebral artery
   e. posterior/inferior cerebellar artery

Case 3 ■ A 77-Year-Old Female with Nystagmus, Homonymous Hemianopia, Facial Numbness, and Weakness

A 77-year-old female comes to the Emergency Department with the following signs and symptoms: dysar-thria and dysphagia, vertigo, nausea, syncope, memory loss and disorientation, and an ataxic gait.

On physical examination, the patient has nystagmus, homonymous hemianopia, numbness in the area of the twelfth cranial nerve, and facial weakness. You suspect a CVA.

Q9. Which of the following arteries is most likely to be involved?
   a. middle cerebral artery
   b. posterior cerebral artery
   c. vertebral-basilar artery
   d. anterior cerebral artery
   e. posterior/inferior cerebellar artery

Q10. There are many sources of potential emboli that may cause a CVA. The most common source of cerebral emboli is:
   a. the carotid arteries
   b. the aortic arch
   c. the heart
   d. the vertebral basilar arteries
   e. the middle cerebral artery

Q11. The role of computed tomography (CT) scanning within the first 24 hours of a stroke is:
   a. to exclude hemorrhages
   b. to exclude tumors
   c. to exclude abscesses
   d. to diagnose stroke
   e. a, b, and c

Q12. The use of anticoagulation is clearly effective in preventing recurrent cardioembolic strokes from atrial fibrillation, a recent myocardial infarction, valvular disease, or a patent foramen ovale. Contraindications to the use of anticoagulation would include:
   a. hemorrhage on a CT scan
   b. large cerebral infarctions
   c. evidence of bacterial endocarditis
   d. a and b above
   e. all of the above

Q13. A TIA is most closely associated with which of the following?
   a. amaurosis fugax
   b. subarachnoid hemorrhage
   c. lacunar hemorrhage
   d. intracranial aneurysm
   e. fusiform aneurysm

Q14. A ruptured berry aneurysm is usually located in which of the following?
   a. anterior cerebral artery distribution
   b. posterior cerebral artery distribution

c. circle of Willis
d. middle cerebral artery distribution
e. none of the above

Q15. A patient is suspected to have a cerebral infarction. If you had the opportunity to order only one investigation, which would you choose?
a. a regular angiogram of the cerebral circulation
b. a CT scan of the brain without contrast
c. a magnetic resonance imaging (MRI) angiogram of the brain
d. a digital subtraction angiogram of the brain
e. an immediate lumbar puncture

Q16. Which of the following is not a risk factor for the development of a CVA?
a. type 1 diabetes mellitus
b. type 2 diabetes mellitus
c. African-American race
d. cigarette smoking
e. diabetes insipidus

Q17. The incidence of stroke in the United States over the last 15 years has:
a. increased significantly
b. increased slightly
c. decreased significantly
d. decreased slightly
e. nobody really knows for sure

Case 4 ■ A 42-Year-Old White Male with a Curtain Coming Down Over His Eyes

A 42-year-old white male comes to your office with a complaint of decreased vision, which, with further questioning, he describes as "a curtain coming down over my eyes." The patient's past medical history includes hypertension and hyperlipidemia, and he recently admitted to extensive use of cocaine. He denies intravenous drug use, vertigo, diplopia, ataxia, or an abnormal heart rate.

Q18. If you had the choice of one test to help determine the cause of his symptoms, what would that be?
a. an ultrasound of the carotid arteries
b. a CT scan of the brain
c. an MRI scan of the brain
d. a fluorescein angiography of the fundi
e. a lumbar puncture

Q19. Which of the following statements regarding carotid endarterectomy (CEA) is true?

a. CEA is indicated in the presence of a completed stroke
b. CEA is indicated in the presence of a complete arterial occlusion
c. randomized, controlled trials have established the benefit of CEA over standard medical therapy for the treatment of carotid artery stenosis
d. CEA has been established as the treatment of choice in patients with a documented TIA and a tightly stenotic lesion exceeding 70%
e. nobody really knows for sure

Q20. In a patient with an asymptomatic carotid bruit who, on evaluation, reveals a high-grade stenosis, recommended treatment would include:
a. watchful waiting
b. anticoagulation therapy with aspirin or ticlopidine
c. CEA
d. CEA and aspirin
e. none of the above

Q21. In the diagnostic work-up of a patient with a TIA, a lumbar puncture should be used:
a. in all patients suspected of having a TIA
b. only when meningitis is suspected
c. in any patient considered to have a subarachnoid hemorrhage when a CT scan is not diagnostic
d. there are no clinical indications for a lumbar puncture in the work-up of a patient with a TIA or CVA

SHORT ANSWER MANAGEMENT PROBLEM
Define the following terms:
1. Transient ischemic attack
2. Stroke-in-evolution
3. Completed stroke

ANSWERS

A1. **c.** At this time the most likely diagnosis is stroke-in-evolution. The typical development of thrombotic stroke causes a clinical syndrome known as stroke-in-evolution. An intermittent or slow progression over hours to days is characteristic of stroke-in-evolution or slow hemorrhage.

A2. **a.** The symptoms that this patient is currently experiencing suggest a lesion of the left middle cerebral artery. The signs and symptoms of middle cerebral artery occlusion are as follows:
a. Dysphagia (left hemisphere involvement), dyslexia, dysgraphia

b. Contralateral hemiparesis or hemiplegia
c. Contralateral hemisensory disturbances
d. Rapid deterioration in consciousness from confusion to coma
e. Homonymous hemianopia
f. Denial of or lack of recognition of a paralyzed extremity
g. Eyes deviated to the side of the lesion, global aphasia if dominant hemisphere is involved

A3. **a.** The slow and continuing progression of the central nervous system symptoms is much more characteristic of a thrombotic stroke than of an embolic stroke.

A4. **a.** The pathophysiology of stroke, in order of frequency, is:
   a. Thrombotic stroke (most common)
   b. Embolic stroke
   c. Hemorrhagic stroke
   d. Lacunar stroke (lacunar infarct)
   e. Subarachnoid hemorrhage (least common)

A5. **b.** An embolic stroke involves fragments that break from a thrombus formed outside the brain in the heart, aorta, common carotid, or thorax. Emboli infrequently arise from the ascending aorta or the common carotid artery. The embolus usually involves small vessels and obstructs at a bifurcation or other point of narrowing, thus enabling ischemia to develop and extend. An embolus may completely occlude the lumen of the vessel, or it may remain in place or break into fragments and move up the vessel. The most common source of emboli is the heart.
   Conditions associated with the onset of an embolic stroke include the following:
   a. Atrial fibrillation
   b. Myocardial infarction
   c. Endocarditis
   d. Rheumatic heart disease
   e. Valvular prostheses
   f. Atrial septal defect
   g. Disorders of the aorta
   h. Disorders of the carotids
   i. Disorders of the vertebral-basilar system
   j. Other embolic phenomena: Air, fat, tumor
   k. Atrial myxoma

A6. **b.** CVAs or strokes remain the third leading cause of death in North America. The single most important risk factor for stroke is hypertension. The decrease in the incidence of stroke in North America is largely the result of the successful, aggressive, and ideal treatment of hypertension. The risk of stroke is three times higher in those with hypertension and is doubled in those with isolated systolic hypertension.
   Other factors important in the cause of stroke include the following:
   a. Age (the older the patient, the greater the risk)
   b. Other heart disease (valvular, conductive, infective, atherosclerotic)
   c. Cigarette smoking
   d. Diabetes mellitus (type 1 and type 2)
   e. Use of oral contraceptive pills when combined with smoking and older age
   f. Race: African-Americans are more prone than white Americans
   g. Family history of lipid disorders or cardiovascular diseases in general
   h. Gender (strokes are more common in females than in males)

A7. **c.** Lacunar strokes (lacunar infarcts) are smaller than 1 mm in size and involve the small perforating arteries predominately in the basal ganglia, pons, cerebellum, internal capsule, and, less commonly, the deep cerebral white matter. Lacunar infarcts are primarily associated with hypertension. Because of the subcortical location and small area of infarction, lacunar strokes may have pure motor and sensory deficits, ipsilateral ataxia, and dysarthria. They may appear on a CT scan as small hypodense areas. Prognosis and recovery are usually good.

A8. **d.** This patient most likely has a lesion in the area of the right anterior cerebral artery. Signs and symptoms of a CVA in the territory of the anterior cerebral artery include the following:
   a. Mental status impairments
      1) Confusion
      2) Amnesia
      3) Perseveration
      4) Personality changes: Flat affect, apathy
      5) Cognitive changes:
         a) Short attention span
         b) Slowness
      6) Deterioration of intellectual function
   b. Urinary continence (long duration)
   c. Contralateral hemiparesis or hemiplegia
   d. Sensory impairments (contralateral)
   e. Foot and leg deficits (more frequent than arm deficits), contralateral leg/foot paralysis
   f. Apraxia on affected side
   g. Expressive aphasia (for left hemisphere only)
   h. Deviation of the eyes and head toward the affected side
   i. Abulia (lack of initiative)
   j. Gait dysfunction

A9. **c.** This patient has had a CVA involving the vertebral-basilar system. The signs and symptoms of vertebral-basilar stroke are as follows:
  a. Dysarthria, dysphagia
  b. Vertigo, nausea, vomiting
  c. Disorientation
  d. Ataxic gait (ipsilateral cerebellar ataxia)
  e. Visual symptoms: Double vision, blurred vision
  f. Dysphagia
  g. Ocular signs: Nystagmus, conjugate gaze paralysis, ophthalmoplegia
  h. Akinetic mutism (locked-in syndrome when basilar artery occlusion occurs)
  i. Numbness of lips and face
  j. Facial weakness, alternating motor paresis
  k. Drop attacks, syncope

A10. **c.** The most common source of cerebral emboli is the heart.

A11. **e.** Strokes usually do not show up on a CT or MRI scan within the first 24 hours. Therefore the role of CT scanning is to rule out structural abnormalities such as hemorrhages, tumors, or abscesses.

A12. **d.** Bacterial endocarditis would not be considered a contraindication to anticoagulation therapy but would be considered a precaution with those bleeding tendencies and uncontrolled hypertension. Contraindications in this case would be a patient who has an extensive stroke, a hemorrhagic stroke, or severe thrombocytopenia.

A13. **a.** A TIA probably represents thrombotic particles causing an intermittent blockage of circulation or spasm. Amaurosis fugax, which is described by patients as "a curtain coming down in front of my eyes—a blackout," is really a TIA of the ophthalmic artery. This is associated primarily with the carotid circulation and may also be seen with contralateral weakness of the face, arm, or legs or as numbness.

A14. **c.** Intracranial aneurysms may result from arteriosclerosis, congenital abnormality, trauma, inflammation, and/or infection. Cocaine has recently been linked to aneurysm formation. The size may vary from 2 mm to 2 or 3 cm. Most aneurysms are located at bifurcations in or near the circle of Willis, particularly on the anterior or posterior communicating arteries. The aneurysm may be single, but in 20% of cases, more than one aneurysm is present. The peak incidence occurs between ages 35 and 60 years. Berry aneurysms are also known as saccular aneurysms and make up the majority of subarachnoid hemorrhages (51%).

A15. **b.** The diagnostic test of choice for a cerebral infarction is a CT scan of the head. A CT scan of the brain without contrast would allow exclusion of a cerebral hemorrhage. A CT scan is preferable to an MRI in the acute stages because it is quicker, and an MRI will not easily detect bleeding during the first 48 hours.

A16. **e.** The risk factors for CVAs include the following:
  a. Hypertension (single most important risk factor), including isolated systolic hypertension
  b. Hypercholesterolemia
  c. Hypertriglyceridemia (because it has been found to be an independent risk factor for vascular disease)
  d. African-American race (probably because of increased risk of hypertension)
  e. Obesity (also related to increased risk of hypertension)
  f. Sedentary lifestyle related to obesity, which is related to hypertension
  g. Cigarette smoking
  h. Women in their later reproductive years (age 37 to 45 years) who are heavy cigarette smokers and taking oral contraceptive pills
  i. Family history of CVAs
  j. Family history of hyperlipidemia
  k. Age over 65 years
  l. Types 1 and 2 diabetes mellitus
  m. Hypothyroidism (related to hyperlipidemia)
  Diabetes insipidus has nothing to do with CVA (with the possible exception of Sheenan's syndrome, and postpartum pituitary necrosis).

A17. **c.** Estimates vary widely. However, the incidence of stroke in the United States has declined dramatically in the last 15 years because of the relative success of the *Treatment of Hypertension* campaign. It should be noted, however, that the incidence increases almost twentyfold with age (from 100 per 100,000 people age 45 to 54 years to 1800 per 100,000 people at age 85 years).

A18. **a.** This patient has had a TIA. He has given a classic description of amaurosis fugax, and his cocaine use may have contributed to this. Cocaine probably caused an intense vasospasm; it is a powerful vasoconstrictor, much more powerful than either angiotensin II or thromboxane. This patient needs an ultrasound of his carotid arteries immediately.

A19. **d.** There has been a great deal of research about CEAs (when and when not to do). Studies have demonstrated that a CEA reduces the risk of subsequent stroke in patients who have had TIAs with a high-grade stenosis. One indication for performing a CEA is a documented TIA with a highly stenotic lesion, greater than 70%. If an ulcerated plaque is present with moderate stenosis, the risk of stroke increases, and patients benefit from CEA.

Further research is currently being conducted on the use of CEA for patients with carotid artery lesions between 30% and 70% and on patients with asymptomatic bruits with moderate stenotic lesions. These investigations may result in a recommendation to also do CEAs in such patients.

A20. **d.** Recent carotid artery studies report that treatment of asymptomatic patients having a high-grade carotid artery stenosis with CEA in combination with aspirin lowers the relative risk of stroke when compared to medical therapy alone.

A21. **c.** A lumbar puncture should be done in any patient considered to have a subarachnoid hemorrhage when a CT scan is not diagnostic. It should be performed in patients suspected to have infective endocarditis, meningitis, or inflammatory vasculitis, looking for the presence of cerebrospinal fluid leukocytosis.

SOLUTION TO THE SHORT ANSWER MANAGEMENT PROBLEM

Definitions:
1. *Transient ischemic attack:* A disturbance of the cerebrovascular system in which neurologic symptoms both appear and then disappear within 24 hours.
2. *Stroke-in-evolution:* The typical course of a thrombotic stroke. This is also known as a progressive stroke. It is best defined as an intermittent progression of a neurologic deficit over hours to days.
3. *Completed stroke:* A CVA that has reached its maximum destructiveness in producing neurologic deficits, although cerebral edema may not have reached its maximum.

SUMMARY OF THE DIAGNOSIS AND TREATMENT OF A CVA

1. Incidence: Very significant decrease over last 15 years as a result of hypertension control

2. Pathologic classification (in order of frequency):
   a. Thrombotic stroke
   b. Embolic stroke
   c. Hemorrhagic stroke
   d. Lacunar stroke
   e. Subarachnoid hemorrhage

3. Risk factors for CVA:
   a. Hypertension is the single most important risk factor.
   b. There is no such entity as mild hypertension any longer.
   c. See also Answer 16.

4. Classification of CVAs: See Short Answer Management Problem.
   It is important to evaluate and work up TIAs. Recent research concerning the benefits of CEA and aspirin therapy may prevent future TIAs or strokes.

5. Signs and symptoms: See details on arteries in Answers 2, 8, and 9.

6. Investigations and treatment:
   a. History
   b. Physical examination
   c. MRI angiogram or CT scan immediately
   d. If not hemorrhagic and not a completed stroke, consider heparin followed by warfarin. If it is already complete, do not follow this approach.
   e. Cerebral edema may become a major problem and corticosteroid therapy may be required.
   f. Unless contraindicated, all patients with TIAs, history of stroke, and risk factors for major stroke should be on aspirin prophylaxis.
   g. Rehabilitation: Aggressive, early, and forceful.

7. Concomitant conditions: Depression is the single most important coexisting or concomitant condition. Remember also that this applies to both the patient and the patient's caregiver.

8. The biopsychosocial model of illness: Few diseases are as devastating to a patient and a patient's family as stroke. Often the person who really gets lost in this whole ordeal is the spouse. Please remember the spouse.

9. Prevention:
   a. Treat hypertension aggressively
   b. Treat obesity and sedentary lifestyle aggressively
   c. Stop smoking
   d. Remember: An aspirin a day keeps the neurologist away.

SUGGESTED READINGS

Boss BJ et al: Alterations of neurologic function. In McCance KL, Huether SE, eds: *Pathophysiology: The biologic basis for disease in adults and children,* ed 2, St Louis, 1994, Mosby.

Ferri F et al: *Practical guide to the care of the geriatric patient,* St Louis, 1997, Mosby.

Tierney LM, McPhee SJ, Papadakis MA, eds: *Current medical diagnosis and treatment, 2000,* ed 39, Stamford, Conn, 1999, Appleton & Lange.

PROBLEM·27

ANEMIA

"I Hardly Have Enough Energy to Get Out of Bed."

Case 1 ■ A 35-Year-Old Female with Fatigue

A 35-year-old female comes to your clinic with a 4-month history of fatigue. Her history is unremarkable; she has had no major medical illnesses. She has noticed that during the past 12 months her menstrual periods have become heavier and longer; instead of lasting for only 4 days with bleeding that was "light to moderate," she now has a 7- to 9-day period with "very heavy flow." She is the mother of three healthy children.

On examination, the patient appears pale. Her lower eyelids are pale and so is her skin. Her blood pressure is 100/70 mm Hg. Physical examination, including a pelvic examination, is otherwise normal. Her blood smear reads as follows: Red blood cells (RBCs) are microcytic and appear to be hypochromic. Her platelet count is 175,000/mm^3. Her hemoglobin is 9.5 g/dl.

SELECT THE BEST ANSWER TO THE FOLLOWING QUESTIONS

Q1. What is the most likely cause of this patient's anemia?
a. iron deficiency anemia
b. hemolytic anemia
c. folic acid deficiency anemia
d. pernicious anemia
e. anemia of chronic disease

Q2. What is (are) the treatment(s) of choice to prevent this condition in this patient?
a. naproxen 375 mg bid (or a similar nonsteroidal antiinflammatory drug [NSAID]) during the last 2 weeks of the menstrual cycle
b. a low-dose oral contraceptive pill (OCP) given either continuously or in a cyclic manner
c. ferrous sulfate 300 mg tid to 300 mg qid

d. any of the above
e. none of the above

Q3. What is (are) the treatment(s) of choice to improve this patient's presenting symptoms?
a. naproxen 375 mg bid (or a similar NSAID) during the last 2 weeks of the menstrual cycle
b. a low-dose OCP given either continuously or in a cyclic manner
c. ferrous sulfate 300 mg tid to 300 mg qid
d. a or b
e. any of the above
f. none of the above

Case 2 ■ A Patient with Anemia and Severely Dysfunctional Uterine Bleeding with Unstable Vital Signs

Q4. What is the recommended first-line treatment?
a. intramuscular medroxyprogesterone acetate
b. intravenous (IV) conjugated estrogen
c. cryoprecipitate
d. fresh frozen plasma
e. high-dose OCPs given every hour

Q5. Which of the following disorders is a (are) possible secondary cause(s) of the disorder just described?
a. uterine fibroids
b. endometriosis
c. von Willebrand's disease
d. intrinsic factor deficiency
e. a, b, or c
f. any of the above

Q6. Which of the following investigations should be performed in this patient to rule out a secondary cause?
a. pelvic ultrasound with or without pelvic laparoscopy
b. coagulation profile
c. computed tomography (CT) scan of the abdomen and pelvis
d. a and b
e. all of the above
f. none of the above

Q7. What is the most sensitive test for the detection of the anemia described in Case 1?
a. serum iron
b. serum iron binding capacity
c. serum ferritin
d. serum transferrin
e. reticulocyte count

Case 3 ■ A Pregnant Woman at 22 Weeks' Gestation Who Has a 10.8-g/dl Hemoglobin Level

Q8. Which of the following statements regarding this patient's hemoglobin level is (are) true?
   a. this patient has, by definition, an iron deficiency anemia
   b. the reason for this hemoglobin level in this trimester is the relative expansion of the plasma volume relative to the RBC mass
   c. this patient should be treated with ferrous sulfate on a once or twice weekly basis
   d. all of the above
   e. none of the above

Case 4 ■ A 55-Year-Old Male Who's Been Feeling Fatigued for the Last 3 Months

A 55-year-old male comes to your office for a periodic health assessment. His only complaint is that he has been feeling quite fatigued during the last 3 months. He does not smoke and rarely drinks.

On physical examination, the patient appears pale. His blood pressure is 100/80 mm Hg. His pulse is 96 bpm and regular. No other abnormalities are found. A complete blood count reveals a hemoglobin level of 10.0 g/dl. His blood smear also shows a decreased mean corpuscular hemoglobin count and a decreased mean corpuscular volume (MCV).

Q9. Until proven otherwise, what is the most likely cause of his low hemoglobin level?
   a. lymphoma
   b. gastrointestinal malignancy
   c. lack of intrinsic factor
   d. dietary deficiency of folic acid
   e. dietary deficiency of iron

Case 5 ■ A 78-Year-Old Female Complaining of a "Lack of Energy"

A 78-year-old female comes to your office complaining of a "lack of energy" that began 8 months ago. On examination, the patient has marked pallor. Her hemoglobin level is 7.5 g/dl at this time. A peripheral blood smear reveals hypochromasia and microcytosis. Her hemoglobin was 13.0 g/dl 1 year ago.

Q10. What is the most likely cause of this patient's anemia?
   a. malnutrition
   b. pernicious anemia
   c. folic acid deficiency

d. gastrointestinal bleeding
e. hypothyroidism

Q11. The anemia of chronic disease is most often which of the following?
   a. hypochromic and normocytic
   b. hypochromic and microcytic
   c. normochromic and macrocytic
   d. normochromic and normocytic
   e. hyperchromic and macrocytic

Q12. What is the most common cause of anemia of chronic disease?
   a. chronic hepatic failure
   b. chronic renal failure
   c. congestive cardiac failure
   d. autoimmune disease
   e. chronic neurologic disease

Q13. Which of the following disorders is (are) associated with the anemia of chronic disease?
   a. rheumatoid arthritis
   b. non-Hodgkin's lymphoma
   c. chronic renal failure
   d. chronic hepatic failure
   e. all of the above

Q14. Which of the following is the most common type of anemia in the North American population?
   a. anemia of chronic disease
   b. iron deficiency anemia
   c. macrocytic anemia
   d. autoimmune hemolytic anemia
   e. iatrogenic anemia

Case 6 ■ A 75-Year-Old Female with Fatigue, Paresthesias, Weakness, and an Unsteady Gait

A 75-year-old female comes to your office with a 4-month history of fatigue, paresthesias, weakness, and an unsteady gait. These are new symptoms.

On examination, her skin is pale, as are her lower conjunctival lids. She has a number of interesting neurologic findings on physical examination, including patchy impairment of the sensations of touch and temperature, loss of both vibration and position sense, a positive Romberg sign, hyperreflexia, and bilateral upgoing Babinski signs. Her hemoglobin is 6.8 g/dl.

Q15. Which of the following statements regarding this patient's condition is (are) true?
   a. this patient has a hemolytic anemia
   b. a CT scan of the brain should be performed

c. hyposegmented neutrophils will be seen on the blood smear

d. the MCV value will exceed 100 mm^3

e. all of the above

Q16. If you could choose only one next investigation for this patient, what would it be?
a. reticulocyte count
b. serum folate
c. serum vitamin B$_{12}$ level
d. gastroscopy
e. bone marrow biopsy

Q17. The one next investigation confirms your suspicions. You now need to confirm the presence or absence of which of the following?
a. megakaryocytes in the bone marrow
b. hypersegmented neutrophils on the blood smear
c. intrinsic factor produced by the gastric parietal cells
d. extrinsic factor produced by the gastric secretin cells
e. folic acid synthesis precursors

Q18. During the first 2 weeks of therapy for the condition described in Case 6, which of the following is the most reasonable treatment regimen?
a. Oral (PO) folic acid 5 mg/day
b. PO vitamin B$_{12}$ 100 mg/day
c. subcutaneous vitamin B$_{12}$ 1000 mg/day
d. PO ferrous sulfate 300 mg/day; folic acid 5 mg/day; vitamin B$_{12}$ 100 mg/day
e. none of the above

Q19. The condition described in Case 6, when diagnosed by bone marrow biopsy, will most likely show which of the following?
a. neutropenia
b. thrombocytopenia
c. anemia
d. pancytopenia
e. leukopenia and anemia

Q20. Which of the following statements regarding folic acid deficiency is false?
a. folic acid deficiency demonstrates a macrocytic anemia
b. hypersegmented neutrophils are often seen on the peripheral blood smear
c. the most common cause of folic acid deficiency is an inadequate dietary intake of folic acid
d. folic acid deficiency is uncommon in patients who demonstrate alcohol abuse

e. reduced folate levels are usually seen in RBCs and in the serum

---

SHORT ANSWER MANAGEMENT PROBLEM
Distinguish between megaloblastosis and macrocytosis.

ANSWERS

A1. **a.** The patient in Case 1 has an iron deficiency anemia. This is the most common cause of anemia. In this patient the most likely cause of the anemia is excessive blood loss during her menstrual periods.

Pernicious anemia, folic acid deficiency anemia, hemolytic anemia, and anemia of chronic disease are not associated with the hypochromic, microcytic changes that characterize iron deficiency anemia.

A2. **b.** OCPs will reduce menstrual blood flow and is the drug of choice. An NSAID drug such as naproxen may have a profound effect on decreasing the menstrual blood flow in some patients; however, in many cases NSAIDs can increase menstrual flow.

A3. **c.** For the patient in Case 1 the appropriate symptomatic treatment to build up her iron stores is ferrous sulfate or ferrous gluconate. The initial dose of ferrous sulfate should be 300 mg tid. It may only be necessary to use ferrous sulfate for 1 to 2 months; at that time the patient can be taken off iron and remain on OCPs.

A4. **b.** The patient in Case 2 has severe menorrhagia with hemodynamic compromise or impending hemodynamic compromise, and the treatment of choice is IV conjugated estrogen, 25 mg repeated every 4 hours until the menorrhagia subsides.

A5. **e.** It is very important to rule out secondary causes of iron deficiency anemia caused by excessive menstrual bleeding, particularly if there has been a recent change from a normal flow as seen in Case 1. The most common secondary causes of iron deficiency anemia in menstruating women are either uterine fibroids or endometriosis. Von Willebrand's disease is certainly less common; it is, however, the most common inherited bleeding disorder and may often present as menorrhagia, metrorrhagia, or menometrorrhagia.

A6. **d.** Pelvic ultrasound, laparoscopy, and a coagulation profile should uncover the potential presence of uterine fibroids, endometriosis, or von Willebrand's disease, respectively. A CT scan of the abdomen and pelvis is not indicated.

A7. **c.** The most sensitive test for the diagnosis of iron deficiency anemia is the serum ferritin level. In iron deficiency anemia the serum ferritin level usually falls first. Thereafter, total iron-binding capacity increases and serum iron levels gradually decrease. The transferrin saturation will also decrease at this time. The reticulocyte count is not useful in assessing the degree of iron deficiency anemia.

A8. **b.** Extensive hematologic measurements have been made in healthy nonpregnant women, none of whom were either iron deficient or folate deficient. Anemia in nonpregnant women is defined as a hemoglobin concentration less than 12 g/dl. The hemoglobin concentration is lower in midpregnancy. In early pregnancy and again near term, the hemoglobin level of most healthy women with adequate iron stores is 11.0 g/dl. For these reasons, the Centers for Disease Control and Prevention has defined anemia as less than 11.0 g/dl in the first and third trimesters and less than 10.5 g/dl in the second trimester.

A9. **b.** Until proven otherwise, iron deficiency anemia in a middle-aged or elderly male is caused by gastrointestinal blood loss, the most sinister cause of which is a gastrointestinal malignancy. Carcinomas of the colon or rectum are the most important and most common malignancies found in this situation. This patient should have fecal occult blood testing followed by colonoscopy. Air-contrast barium enema may or may not be indicated for further elucidation. If all of the investigations are normal, the upper gastrointestinal tract should be investigated by gastroscopy.

Dietary iron deficiency or dietary folic acid deficiency is extremely unusual in a nonalcoholic male.

A lymphoma is more likely to produce a normochromic-normocytic blood smear rather than a hypochromic-microcytic picture.

Bleeding hemorrhoids may also produce iron deficiency anemia in middle-aged males.

Vitamin B_{12} deficiency resulting from lack of intrinsic factor would present as a macrocytic rather than a microcytic anemia.

A10. **d.** This patient's hypochromic-microcytic blood picture, coupled with a drop in hemoglobin from 13.0 to 7.5 g/dl in 1 year, is almost certainly caused by blood loss from a gastrointestinal malignancy or other bleeding source. The discussion in Answer 9 regarding the iron deficiency anemia in males also applies to postmenopausal females. The other common cause of iron deficiency in the anemia of elderly patients is malnutrition.

In contradistinction to hypochromic-microcytic anemia, the most common causes of megaloblastic anemia are vitamin B_{12} and folic acid deficiencies.

A11. **d.** The anemia of chronic disease is most often normochromic and normocytic.

A12. **b.**

A13. **e.** The anemia of chronic disease is most frequently associated with the following:
   a. Anemia of chronic inflammation:
      1) Infection
      2) Connective tissue disorders
      3) Malignancy (excluding malignancies where blood loss is a major factor, as in colon cancer)
   b. Anemia caused by chronic renal failure
   c. Anemia caused by endocrine failure
   d. Anemia of hepatic disease

Q14. **b.** In North America the most common category of anemia is iron deficiency anemia. In order of frequency, anemia prevalence is as follows:
   a. Iron deficiency anemia:
      1) Blood loss resulting from excessive menstrual flow
      2) Blood loss from the gastrointestinal tract
   b. Anemia of chronic disease, the most common causes being:
      1) Chronic renal failure
      2) Anemia caused by connective tissue disorders
   c. Macrocytic anemia:
      1) Pernicious anemia
      2) Folic acid deficiency anemia
   d. Hemolytic anemia:
      1) Autoimmune hemolytic anemias
      2) Nonautoimmune hemolytic anemias

A15. **d.** This patient has pernicious anemia. The signs and symptoms of pernicious anemia can be remembered well by the five Ps:
   a. Pancytopenia
   b. Peripheral neuropathy
   c. Posterior spinal column neuropathy
   d. Pyramidal tract signs
   e. Papillary (tongue) atrophy

The blood smear of a patient with pernicious anemia will show the following: megaloblastic anemia as demonstrated by MCV >100 mm^3, hypersegmented neutrophils, and oval macrocytes.

A16. **c.** Pernicious anemia is defined as a deficiency of vitamin B_{12} resulting from a lack of production of intrinsic factor by the gastric parietal cells (remember that vitamin B_{12} deficiency can also be produced by other causes such as a vegetarian diet).

A17. c. The deficiency of intrinsic factor is measured by the Schilling test. The Schilling test uses radiolabeled vitamin B_{12} and follows excretion with and without intrinsic factor.

A18. c. The acute treatment of pernicious anemia that is recommended is vitamin B_{12} 1000 mg/day subcutaneously for 1 week followed by 1000 mg/wk subcutaneously for 4 weeks and then followed by maintenance therapy of 1000 mg/mo. Since the root cause of the disease lies in an inability to absorb the vitamin, it cannot be administered orally.

A19. d.

A20. d. Folic acid deficiency is most commonly seen in alcoholics, patients with a malignancy, elderly patients, patients on a vegan diet, and pregnant patients. The most common cause of folic acid deficiency is inadequate intake.

Folic acid deficiency anemia, like vitamin B_{12} deficiency, is also a megaloblastic anemia. Patients with folic acid deficiency usually have normal vitamin B_{12} levels. Patients with folic acid deficiency anemia should be given 1 to 5 mg of folic acid per day. Remember that giving folic acid to a vitamin B_{12} patient will clear up the megaloblastic anemia but will have no effect on the neuropathy, which will continue to get worse.

SOLUTION TO THE SHORT ANSWER MANAGEMENT PROBLEM

The difference between macrocytosis and megaloblastosis is as follows:
1. Megaloblastosis: The macrocytes are oval.
2. Macrocytosis: The macrocytes are round.
3. Megaloblastic anemias are only one cause of macrocytosis.

The differential diagnosis of macrocytosis is as follows:
1. Megaloblastic anemias
2. Liver disease
3. Reticulocytosis
4. Myeloproliferative diseases (leukemia, myelofibrosis)
5. Multiple myeloma
6. Metastatic disease of bone marrow
7. Hypothyroidism
8. Aplastic anemia
9. Drugs (cytotoxic agents, alcohol)

10. Autoagglutination or cold agglutination disease

SUMMARY OF THE DIAGNOSIS AND TREATMENT OF ANEMIAS

1. Normal adult hemoglobin levels:
   a. Males: 14.0 to 18.0 g/dl
   b. Females: 12.0 to 16.0 g/dl

2. Classification of anemias on the basis of cause (production, destruction, loss)
   a. Production problems include the following:
      1) Hemoglobin synthesis disturbances as may be caused by iron deficiency, thalassemia, or chronic disease
      2) DNA synthesis disturbances, which lead to megaloblastic anemia
      3) Bone marrow infiltration in malignancies
      4) Stem cell disease, as in aplastic anemia or myeloproliferative disease
   b. Destruction problems include the following:
      1) Intrinsic hemolysis, as in spherocytosis, sickle cell anemia, or enzyme deficiencies
      2) Extrinsic hemolysis, as in infection, immune complexes, thrombocytopenic purpura, hemolytic/uremic syndrome, or mechanical valves
   c. Blood loss problems include:
      1) Excessive menstruation
      2) Bleeding in the gastrointestinal tract or genitourinary tract
      3) Trauma

3. Classification of anemias on the basis of cell size and appearance (microcytic, macrocytic, normocytic, hypochromic, normochromic)
   a. Microcytic anemias may result from the following:
      1) Iron deficiency, potentially caused by blood loss or nutritional deficiencies
      2) Thalassemias
      3) Chronic disease
   b. Macrocytic anemias are either:
      1) Megaloblastic, caused by folate or B_{12} deficiencies
      2) Nonmegaloblastic, such as that caused by chemotherapy

4. Iron deficiency anemia:
   a. Most common cause of anemia
   b. Most common cause in premenopausal women is excessive menstrual flow
   c. Iron deficiency anemia in males or in postmenopausal females should be considered to be from

gastrointestinal blood loss until proven otherwise; most common secondary cause is gastrointestinal malignancy

d. Iron deficiency anemia is hypochromic-microcytic; microcytosis comes first; hypochromasia is seen in advanced cases

e. Serum ferritin level is usually less than 12 mg/L and is the most sensitive test for iron deficiency

f. Most pregnant women with decreased hemoglobin are not truly anemic; they simply have a greater increase in plasma volume than in RBC mass; true anemia in pregnancy has been defined by the Centers for Disease Control and Prevention as follows:
   1) Hemoglobin in first and third trimesters is less than 11.0 g/dl
   2) Hemoglobin in second trimester is less than 10.5 g/dl

g. Investigations in women with excessive menstrual flow include pelvic ultrasound or laparoscopy (uterine fibroids, endometriosis) and coagulation disorders (von Willebrand's disease)

h. Treatment for iron deficiency anemia:
   1) Find the cause and correct if possible
   2) Ferrous sulfate 300 mg tid
   3) Menorrhagia: Prophylaxis is OCPs
   4) Severe menorrhagia with unstable vital signs: IV conjugated estrogen

5. Anemia of chronic disease:
   a. Anemia of chronic disease is normochromic-normocytic.
   b. Causes of anemia of chronic disease:
      1) Chronic renal failure (most common)
      2) Connective tissue disorders (autoimmune diseases)
      3) Malignancies (except gastrointestinal blood loss) such as multiple myeloma or lymphomas
      4) Inflammatory diseases
      5) Chronic hepatic disease
   c. Make the diagnosis (find the cause) and treat the cause.

6. Megaloblastic anemia resulting from a vitamin B_{12} deficiency:
   a. Pernicious anemia is the most common cause. The vitamin B_{12} deficiency results from a lack of intrinsic factor. Other causes of vitamin B_{12} deficiency are as follows:
      1) Total or subtotal gastrectomy
      2) A vegan diet
   b. Blood smear:
      1) MCV <100 mm^3

   2) Hypersegmented neutrophils
   3) Oval macrocytes
   c. Confirming tests:
      1) Serum vitamin B_{12} level
      2) Schilling test
   d. The five defining Ps:
      1) Pancytopenia
      2) Peripheral neuropathy
      3) Posterior spinal column neuropathy
      4) Papillary (tongue) atrophy
      5) Pyramidal tract signs
   e. Treatment:
      1) Vitamin B_{12} subcutaneously 1000 mg/day
      2) Vitamin B_{12} subcutaneously 1000 mg once/wk
      3) Vitamin B_{12} subcutaneously 1000 mg/mo
   f. Remember that a vitamin B_{12} deficiency may also induce a neuropathy

7. Megaloblastic anemia caused by a folic acid deficiency:
   a. Diagnosis: Blood smear with hypersegmented neutrophils and macro-ovalocytes
   b. Confirmation: Decreased serum folate or RBC folate levels
   c. Most common cause of folic acid deficiency is a dietary deficiency associated with alcoholism, vegan diet, and elderly patients on a "tea and toast" diet; also results from medications such as methotrexate and OCPs, pregnancy, and malignancy
   d. Folic acid supplementation (1 mg) is recommended for all pregnant women

8. Hemolytic anemias:
   a. Classification:
      1) Autoimmune hemolytic anemias
      2) Nonautoimmune hemolytic anemias
   b. Common causes:
      1) Most common cause of hemolytic anemia: Drugs (iatrogenic disease)
      2) Lymphoproliferative disorders: Chronic lymphocytic lymphoma, non-Hodgkin's lymphoma
      3) Connective tissue disorders: Systemic lupus erythematosus, rheumatoid arthritis
      4) Infections: Epstein-Barr virus, cytomegalovirus, *Mycoplasma pneumoniae,* human immunodeficiency virus (HIV)
      5) G6PDH deficiency
      6) Paroxysmal cold hemoglobinuria
   c. Diagnosis:
      1) Coombs test: Direct and indirect
      2) Reticulocyte count (elevated)
   d. Treatment:
      1) Corticosteroids

2) Splenectomy (in those who do not respond)
3) IV immunoglobulin

9. Miscellaneous disorders:
   a. Aplastic anemias
   b. Thalassemia
   c. Sickle-cell disease
   d. Hemophilia
   e. Platelet-associated bleeding disorders
   f. Disseminated intravascular coagulation

SUGGESTED READINGS

Little DR: Ambulatory management of common forms of anemia, *Am Fam Physician* 59(6):1598-1604, 1999.

Steinberg MH: Management of sickle cell disease, *N Engl J Med* 340(13):1021-1030, 1999.

Toh BH et al: Pernicious anemia, *N Engl J Med* 337(20):1441-1448, 1997.

PROBLEM·28

LYMPHOMAS AND MULTIPLE MYELOMAS

"Isn't Red Sternberg the Man Who Puts Out Oil Well Fires?"

Case 1 ■ A 16-Year-Old Male with a Mass in the Left Supraclavicular Area and Chest Pains

A 16-year-old male is brought to your office by his mother. He has noticed a significant swelling in the area of the left supraclavicular area that has been present for approximately 4 months. It has, according to the patient, not changed significantly in size over that time. He has had no fever, chills, nausea, vomiting, fatigue or malaise, weight loss, or other symptoms.

On examination, the abdomen is soft. No hepatomegaly or splenomegaly is present. No significant lymph node enlargement is present in the axillary chain, the cervical chain, or the inguinal chain.

A mass measuring 2.5 by 1.5 cm is felt to be attached to the muscular area above the left clavicle.

SELECT THE BEST ANSWER TO THE FOLLOWING QUESTIONS

Q1. What is the first step in the evaluation of this patient?
   a. a complete blood work-up
   b. an incisional biopsy
   c. an excisional biopsy
   d. a radical neck dissection
   e. none of the above

Q2. The evaluation produces a report that reads as follows: "Reed-Sternberg cells present." What is the most likely diagnosis?
   a. solitary lymph node enlargement
   b. acquired immunodeficiency syndrome (AIDS)
   c. metastatic carcinoma
   d. Hodgkin's disease
   e. non-Hodgkin's lymphoma

Q3. What is the next step in the investigation of this patient?
   a. staging of the disease
   b. radiation therapy
   c. combination chemotherapy
   d. bone scan
   e. computed tomography (CT) scan of the abdomen

Q4. In the staging of the disease from which this patient suffers, there are two distinct categories: A and B. To what do these two categories refer?
   a. the presence or absence of metastases
   b. the presence or absence of symptoms
   c. the presence or absence of bone marrow involvement
   d. the possibility or impossibility of cure
   e. the presence of absence or intraabdominal disease

Q5. Determining the stage of the disease includes all of the following except:
   a. CT scan of the abdomen
   b. CT scan of the brain
   c. lower lymphangiography
   d. bone marrow biopsy
   e. chest x-ray

Q6. The patient's disease is at stage IA. At this time, what would you do?
   a. do nothing; wait for further symptoms
   b. combination chemotherapy
   c. radiation therapy
   d. combination chemotherapy and localized radiotherapy
   e. radical surgery

Q7. With respect to the histologic pathology of this disease, which of the following patterns of disease is most common in North America?
   a. lymphocyte predominance type
   b. nodular sclerosis type
   c. mixed cellularity type
   d. lymphocyte depletion type
   e. none of the above

Case 2 ■ A 52-Year-Old Male with Swelling in His Neck and Elbows

A 52-year-old male comes to your office to reassure himself about "some swellings in my neck and elbows, as well as some chest pain." The other symptom is profound fatigue (for the last 3 months).

On examination, the patient has multiple enlarged cervical lymph nodes (as well as bilateral epitrochlear nodes). They measure anywhere from 1.0 to 2.0 cm in diameter. His liver edge is palpated approximately 3 cm below the left costal edge, and the tip of the spleen can be felt when he lies on his side.

Q8. If you could select only one test to perform on this patient, which of the following would you select?
   a. enzyme-linked immunosorbent assay (ELISA) human immunodeficiency virus (HIV) screening test
   b. immunoglobulin G-viral capsid antigen (IgG-VCA) antibody titer for cytomegalovirus
   c. IgG-VCA antibody titer for toxoplasmosis
   d. CT scan of the chest
   e. excisional lymph node biopsy

Q9. The test you ordered is performed. The result is which one of the following?
   a. diffuse small cleaved cell (diffuse poorly differentiated lymphocytic) histology
   b. nodular sclerosis histology: Reed-Sternberg cells present
   c. hilar mass seen on CT scan (measuring 6 cm to 20 cm)
   d. ELISA HIV test inconclusive
   e. IgG-VCA antibodies absent

Q10. Based on what you know at present, what is the most likely diagnosis?
   a. non-Hodgkin's lymphoma
   b. Hodgkin's disease
   c. systemic toxoplasmosis: systemic immune deficiency
   d. systemic cytomegalovirus: systemic immune deficiency
   e. AIDS

Q11. The treatment of choice based on all of your assumptions is which of the following?
   a. azidothymidine
   b. intensive chemotherapy and bone marrow transplantation
   c. α-interferon
   d. intensive chemotherapy only
   e. intensive therapy with ribavirin and acyclovir

Case 3 ■ A 75-Year-Old Male with "Bone Pain" in His "Breast Bone" and Head

A 75-year-old male comes with a chief complaint of "bone pain" in "my breast bone and my head, Doc." He tells you that he is sure he is OK but is here only because "the wife kept bugging me until I gave in."

The patient also appears somewhat pale and does tell you that he has been feeling tired lately and a bit "weak, depressed, and maybe confused."

He had a "touch of the flu" a few months ago. His wife tells you that this "touch of the flu" was actually bacterial pneumonia; the causative organism was *Streptococcus pneumoniae.* On examination, the patient has a tender sternum, tender occipital area of the skull, and pale conjunctiva.

Q12. With this information, if you could perform only one of the following initial tests, which one would you choose?
   a. electrolytes, blood urea nitrogen, creatinine
   b. complete blood count (CBC)
   c. erythrocyte sedimentation rate (ESR)
   d. serum calcium level
   e. platelet count

Q13. The laboratory test results are hemoglobin 8.5 g/dl: normochromic/normocytic anemia; ESR, 55 mm/hr; platelets, 15,000/mm^3; serum calcium level, 14 mg/dl; Na$^+$, 151 mEq/L; and serum creatinine, 53 mmol/L. Based on the information you now have for Case 3, what is the most likely diagnosis?
   a. metastatic carcinoma: metastasized to bone
   b. chronic lymphocytic leukemia
   c. multiple myeloma
   d. chronic renal failure: secondary to macroglobulinemia
   e. chronic myelogenous leukemia

Q14. Further investigations substantiate your findings. What is the treatment of choice at this time?
   a. bone marrow transplantation
   b. total body radiotherapy
   c. adjuvant combination chemotherapy: adriamycin, vincristine, bleomycin
   d. melphalan and prednisone
   e. none of the above

Q15. The patient's disease is caused by a proliferation of which of the following?
   a. myeloblasts
   b. lymphoblasts
   c. metastatic cancer cells
   d. plasma cells
   e. none of the above

Part A: Diseases

a. aplastic anemia
b. secondary polycythemia
c. hemolytic anemia
d. drug-induced thrombocytopenia
e. idiopathic thrombocytopenia purpura
f. sickle-cell disease
g. sickle-cell trait reaction
h. preleukemia
i. acute lymphocytic leukemia
j. disseminated intravascular coagulation
k. hemophilia
l. multiple myeloma
m. chronic lymphocytic leukemia

n. hemochromatosis
o. acute myelogenous
p. chronic myelogenous thrombocytopenia
q. cutaneous T-cell leukemia
r. neutrophilia
s. von Willebrand's disease
t. thalassemia
u. hairy cell leukemia
v. acute intermitten ptorphyria
w. polycythemia rubra vera
x. secondary leukemia
y. transfusion leukemia
z. myelofibrosis

Part B: Description

SAQ1. Clinical Case 1: Choice _____
1. Disease is associated with excessive proliferation of erythroid, granulocytic, and megakaryocytic precursors.
2. Splenomegaly is almost universal in this disease.
3. Disease has significantly elevated RBC mass.
4. Patient presents with plethora.
5. Disease characteristically has thrombocytosis.

SAQ2. Clinical Case 2: Choice _____
1. Disease produces a major disorder of the bone marrow.
2. Splenomegaly is present in all patients.
3. As the disease progresses, patients experience weight loss; skin and mucous membrane bleeding; and bone pain, jaundice, and lymphadenopathy.
4. Bone marrow tap is almost always unsuccessful: it is known as a "dry tap."
5. Bone marrow biopsy reveals fibrosis of marrow spaces and osteosclerosis.

SAQ3. Clinical Case 3: Choice _____
1. This disease has the presence of the Philadelphia chromosome.
2. When this disease is diagnosed, the total white blood cell (WBC) count often exceeds 200,000 cells/mm³.
3. This disease usually proceeds along the following course: (a) chronic phase of variable duration; (b) blastic transformation; with (c) some patients experiencing a distinct intermediate accelerated phase.
4. The most consistent physical finding is splenomegaly.
5. This is the most common serious hematologic disorder diagnosed in patients who survived the atomic bombs of Hiroshima and Nagasaki.

SAQ4. Clinical Case 4: Choice _____
1. This form of leukemia is the most common form in the United States.
2. The disease is usually seen in patients over age 50 years.
3. The abnormal cells morphologically resemble mature, small lymphocytes of the peripheral blood and accumulate in the bone marrow, blood, lymph nodes, and spleen in large numbers.

4. This disease has an "indolent nature."
5. Median survival exceeds 10 years, and many patients require no treatment.

SAQ5. Clinical Case 5: Choice _____
1. This disease has characteristic cells that exhibit cytoplasmic projections on their surfaces.
2. This disease results from an expansion of neoplastic type B lymphocytes.
3. This disease usually occurs in male patients over age 40 years.
4. Approximately 30% of patients with this disease have a vasculitis-like disorder.
5. The treatment of choice for this disease is very characteristic of the disease: Cladribine.

SAQ6. Clinical Case 6: Choice _____
1. This disease is a disease of children and young adults.
2. This disease is characterized by the clonal proliferation of immature hematopoietic cells.
3. The most common abnormal cells seen on bone marrow biopsy are immature lymphoblasts.
4. Infection is a nearly universal complication.
5. Approximately 50% of patients are either cured or characterized as being in long-term remission.

SAQ7. Clinical Case 7: Choice _____
1. The incidence of this disease increases with increasing age.
2. The most common abnormal cells seen on bone marrow biopsy are immature myeloblasts or immature promyelocytes.
3. Some patients with this disease develop the disease after either a preleukemia syndrome or a myelodysplastic syndrome.
4. Between 10% and 30% of patients with this disease survive 5 years; most of these patients are probably cured.
5. Bone marrow transplantation from either an identical twin or HLA-identical sibling is a very important part of treatment.

SAQ8. Clinical Case 8: Choice _____
1. This disease usually follows recovery from either a viral exanthem or a viral upper respiratory tract illness.
2. The acute form of this disease is caused by immune complexes containing viral antigens that bind to platelet receptors.
3. This disease produces a profound rapid decrease in the cell line in question.
4. Corticosteroids are the agents of choice in the treatment of this disease.
5. In severe cases of this disease, splenectomy may need to be performed.

SAQ9. Clinical Case 9: Choice _____
1. This is the most common inherited bleeding disorder.
2. The factor that is missing in this disease is responsible for platelet adhesion.
3. The factor that is missing in this disease also serves as a plasma carrier for factor VIII.
4. Women with this disorder may be initially diagnosed because of severe menorrhagia.
5. The treatment of choice for this disease is cryoprecipitate.

SAQ10. Clinical Case 10: Choice _____
1. This disease is most frequently associated with obstetric catastrophes.
2. Other major causes of this disease are major trauma, metastatic malignancies, and bacterial sepsis.
3. In this disease the combination of potent thrombogenic stimuli causes the deposition of small thrombi and small emboli throughout the microvasculature.
4. Most patients with this disease have extensive skin and mucous membrane bleeding and hemorrhage from multiple sites.
5. Patients with bleeding as a major symptom should receive fresh frozen plasma as therapy for the disorder.

ANSWERS

A1. c. This patient should have an excisional biopsy of the mass performed as soon as possible. Although a piece of tissue could be removed (an incisional biopsy), an excisional biopsy makes more sense.

A2. d. The anatomic pathology report of Reed-Sternberg cells present (these are large binucleate cells with a single distinct nucleoli) is pathognomonic of Hodgkin's disease. Hodgkin's disease is one of the most important success stories of medical oncology. It is a disease that used to be uniformly fatal; at this time, the vast majority of patients are cured.

One or two enlarged lymph nodes in a young person also indicates Hodgkin's disease until proven otherwise. Excisional biopsy should always be undertaken.

A3. a. After an anatomic diagnosis is made, the disease must be staged. Staging of Hodgkin's disease requires the following:
  a. Chest x-ray
  b. Bipedal lower extremity lymphangiography
  c. Liver scan
  d. Spleen scan
  e. CBC, platelet count, differential count
  f. Bone marrow aspiration and biopsy
  g. Serum liver enzyme levels, including alkaline phosphatase
  h. ESR
  i. CT scan of the abdomen
The Ann Arbor Staging Classification of Hodgkin's disease is as follows:
Stage I: Single lymph node (I) or single extralymphatic organ
Stage II: Two or more lymph nodes on the same side of the diaphragm
Stage III: Lymph nodes involved on both sides of the diaphragm or localized involvement of spleen or extralymphatic organ or both
Stage IV: Diffuse or disseminated disease or involvement of the liver or bone marrow

A4. b. The staging is further added to by the presence or absence of the following symptoms: fever, night sweats, and weight loss exceeding 10% in the last 6 months. The presence of any of the symptoms indicates that the stage of the disease should be labeled B. The absence of any of the symptoms indicates that the stage of the disease should be labeled A.

A5. b.

A6. c. The treatment of choice for stage IA and IIA disease is radiation therapy. This therapy is local, and extended field radiotherapy to contiguous node-bearing areas and adjacent regions has resulted in an 85% to 90% cure rate. Total nodal radiation therapy has been used in stages IB and IIB. Chemotherapy is added to radiation therapy when there is a large mediastinal mass, but research is ongoing to include chemotherapy for some patients treated with radiation and appears promising.

The current treatment recommendations for more localized disease (stages I, II, and III) are as follows:
  a. Radiation for IA and IIA disease
  b. Radiation and chemotherapy for stage III disease
    1) Adriamycin (Doxorubicin) (A)
    2) Bleomycin (B)
    3) Vinblastine (V)
    4) Dacarbazine (D) (six cycles of ABVD at 28-day intervals); positive response rates for stage III and IV disease are in the 80% range
  c. Involved region radiotherapy: This aggressive treatment regimen provides the best chance of cure.

A7. b. The histologic typing of Hodgkin's disease and the significance of some of the histologic types are as follows:
  a. Nodular sclerosis: Most common histologic type in North America and Western Europe
  b. Mixed cellularity: Second most common histologic type in North America
  c. Lymphocyte predominance:
    1) Abundance of Reed-Sternberg cells
    2) Associated with a favorable prognosis
  d. Lymphocyte depletion:
    1) Paucity of cellular elements
    2) Rarest histologic type
    3) Associated with advanced age, systemic symptoms, retroperitoneal nodes, and extra-anodal involvement
    4) Worst prognosis

A8. e.

A9. a.

A10. a. This patient has non-Hodgkin's lymphoma. The characteristics that suggest this diagnosis rather than Hodgkin's disease are the presence of lymph nodes draining Waldeyer's ring, the presence of epitrochlear lymph nodes, and the presence of chest pain, suggesting the involvement of lung tissue.

The lymph node histology involving non-Hodgkin's lymphoma will not be discussed in detail. However, the lymph node pathology of diffuse small cleaved cell (diffuse poorly differentiated lymphocytic) suggests a high-grade lymphoma with extensive involvement, including the liver, spleen, and bone marrow. Your physical examination confirms the possibility of the former two.

Staging is similar (although not identical) to the staging for Hodgkin's disease. Non-Hodgkin's lymphoma can be found in nodal sites, in viscera, or both. Extranodal disease is often solitary. Waldeyer's ring, upper gastrointestinal tract, testes, and bone are the most common extranodal sites. The staging of non-Hodgkin's lymphoma is divided into low grade, intermediate grade, and high grade. These are further divided into early stage and late stage.

A11. b. Treatment modalities are based on diagnosed staging and range from radiation for low-grade early stage to high-grade multiagent (cyclophosphamide, vincristine [CVP], and prednisone) chemotherapy, with possible autologous marrow transplantation for high-grade lesions.

A12. d. See Answer 13.

A13. c. The critical elements of this patient's history, physical, and laboratory data are as follows:
   a. Signs of bone pain (sternum and skull) and anemia
   b. Symptoms of weakness, depression, fatigue, and confusion
   c. Recent history of bacterial pneumonia; possible immune suppression
   d. Laboratory evidence of the following:
      1) Anemia, usually normocytic but rouleau formation is common
      2) Hypercalcemia
      3) Renal failure
      4) Thrombocytopenia
      5) Hyponatremia
      6) Elevated ESR

The combination of bone pain (location specific); hypercalcemia; normochromic or normocytic anemia; renal failure; weakness, depression, or confusion; and history of bacterial pneumonia points to the diagnosis of multiple myeloma.

The diagnosis will be substantiated by skull x-ray (showing punched-out lesions), serum electrophoresis with monoclonal peak, and demonstration of Bence-Jones protein in the urine.

Although you were asked to select only one laboratory test, you were given the results from all of the tests. In selecting, the one best test to perform among the tests listed is probably the serum calcium level.

Multiple myeloma is a disease of older patients, with the mean age being 68 years. It appears to be more common than average in farmers, petroleum workers, wood workers, and leather workers.

A14. d. The treatment of choice is a combination of melphalan and prednisone administered for 4 to 7 days every 4 to 6 weeks for 1 to 2 years. The disease is almost invariably fatal, but patients may live significantly long periods with virtually no symptoms once they are stabilized on therapy.

Recent chemotherapy with alkylating agents (vincristine, adriamycin, dexamethasone) is also being used, and the optimal chemotherapy regimen has not been determined. Autologous stem cell transplantation for patients younger than age 60 years is also being used. Additional treatment with radiation for bone pain and aggressive treatment for hypercalcemia is important.

A15. d. Pathologically, multiple myeloma is a plasma cell malignancy of proliferation.

SOLUTION TO THE SHORT ANSWER MANAGEMENT PROBLEM		
SAQ1. W	SAQ5. U	SAQ8. E
SAQ2. Z	SAQ6. I	SAQ9. S
SAQ3. P	SAQ7. O	SAQ10. J
SAQ4. M		

SUMMARY OF THE DIAGNOSIS AND MANAGEMENT OF LYMPHOMAS AND MULTIPLE MYELOMAS

1. Most common solid hematologic malignancies are the lymphomas:
   a. Disorders: Types and their prevalence:
      1) Non-Hodgkin's lymphoma: Most common (40,000 new cases per year in the United States)
      2) Hodgkin's lymphoma: Second most common (7500 new cases per year in the United States)
   b. Signs and symptoms:
      1) Most common sign or symptom is solitary or nonsolitary lymph node enlargement.
      2) The presence or absence of systemic symptoms not only is a staging phenomenon (A or B) but also is prognostic.
      3) Most common systemic symptoms include weight loss, night sweats, fevers, and pain.
   c. Differentiation of Hodgkin's from non-Hodgkin's:
      1) Systemic symptoms are more common in Hodgkin's lymphoma.
      2) Lymph node enlargement in the supraclavicular area is very common for Hodgkin's disease.

3) In non-Hodgkin's lymphoma the lymph nodes draining Waldeyer's ring and epitrochlear nodes are most commonly enlarged.
4) Non-Hodgkin's lymphoma often presents with mediastinal, abdominal, and extranodal symptomatology.
d. Prognosis:
1) Hodgkin's lymphoma has a better prognosis than non-Hodgkin's lymphoma, primarily because of less spread at the time of diagnosis.
2) Prognosis depends on accurate staging.
e. Treatment: Initially with chemotherapy for late stages, radiation for early stage disease IA-IIA

2. Multiple myeloma:
a. Prevalence: Multiple myeloma is mainly a disease of the elderly.
b. Pathology: Plasma cell malignancy/plasma cell proliferation
c. Signs and symptoms:
1) Bone pain (sternum, skull, ribs, and back)
2) Anemia: Normochromic/normocytic
3) Immune suppression (history of bacterial infections)
4) Renal failure
5) Hypercalcemia
6) Weakness, confusion, depression, fatigue
d. Diagnosis:
1) Serum protein electrophoresis
2) Bone marrow biopsy
3) Urine: Bence-Jones protein

3. Miscellaneous important hematologic conditions
a. Polycythemia rubra vera:
1) Plethora, sometimes cyanosis
2) Proliferation of all hematopoietic cell lines
3) Elevated hemoglobin, RBC mass, thrombocytosis
b. Myelofibrosis:
1) Weight loss
2) Bleeding from skin and mucous membranes
3) Bone marrow biopsy: Dry tap, normal bone marrow is replaced by fibrotic material
c. Chronic myelogenous leukemia:
1) Atomic bomb survivors
2) Philadelphia chromosome
3) WBC count at diagnosis often greater than 200,000/mm^3
4) Chronic phase followed by blastic phase
d. Chronic lymphocytic leukemia:
1) Most common leukemia in United States
2) Disease of older patients

3) Indolent nature; no treatment needed in many patients; median survival is 10 years
e. Hairy cell leukemia:
1) Cytoplasmic projections give disorder its name
2) Remarkably effective treatment with cladribine, usually presents with pancytopenia
f. Acute lymphocytic leukemia:
1) Disease of children
2) Immature lymphoblasts
3) Infections very common
4) 50% cure rate at present
g. Acute myeloblastic leukemia:
1) Most common acute leukemia of adults
2) Auer rods pathognomonic
3) Immature myeloblasts on smear
4) Infections very common
5) Bone marrow transplantation essential for survival (10% to 30%)
6) May follow myelodysplastic disorder or preleukemia
h. Idiopathic thrombocytopenic purpura:
1) Acute onset after viral exanthem or viral infection
2) Rapid drop in platelet count
3) Corticosteroids are treatment of choice; splenectomy in resistant cases
i. Von Willebrand's disease:
1) Most common inherited bleeding disorder
2) Results from a factor VIII deficiency
3) Often presents as severe menorrhagia in women
4) Factor VIII concentrates are treatment of choice
j. Disseminated intravascular coagulation:
1) Follows obstetric catastrophes, major trauma, metastatic malignancies, or bacterial sepsis
2) Microemboli or microthrombi in vasculature
3) Profuse bleeding from many sites
4) Treatment: Fresh frozen plasma for severe bleeding

SUGGESTED READINGS

Freedman AS, Nadler LM: Malignancies of lymphoid cells. In Fauci AS et al, eds: *Harrison's principles of internal medicine*, ed 14, New York, 1998, McGraw-Hill.

Spivak JL: Polycythemia vera and other myeloproliferative diseases. In Fauci AS et al, eds: *Harrison's principles of internal medicine*, ed 14, New York, 1998, McGraw-Hill.

Tierney LM, McPhee SJ, Papadakis MA, eds: *Current medical diagnosis and treatment, 2000*, ed 39, Stamford, Conn, 1999, Appleton & Lange.

Weitzler M, Bloomfield CD: Acute and chronic myeloid leukemias. In Fauci AS et al, eds: *Harrison's principles of internal medicine*, ed 14, New York, 1998, McGraw-Hill.

PROBLEM·29

RHEUMATOID ARTHRITIS

"I Hurt a Bit and Am Kind of Stiff When I Wake Up, but It's Not Serious, Is It?"

Case 1 ■ A 35-Year-Old Female with Malaise, Weight Loss, Vasomotor Disturbance, and Vague Periarticular Pain and Stiffness

A 35-year-old female comes to your office with a 6-month history of malaise, paresthesias in both hands, and vague pain in both hands and wrists. She has also felt extremely fatigued. She tells you that the pains in her joints are much worse in the morning. She is also beginning to notice pain and swelling in both knees.

The patient has a normal family history, with no significant diseases noted. The patient is taking no drugs and has no allergies.

On examination, there is a sensation of "bogginess" and slight swelling in both hands, in both wrists, and in the small bones of her hands. Both knees also feel somewhat "swollen and boggy." There are no other joint abnormalities, and the rest of the physical examination is normal.

SELECT THE BEST ANSWER TO THE FOLLOWING QUESTIONS

Q1. What is the most likely diagnosis in this patient?
a. nonarticular rheumatism
b. synovitis
c. gonococcal arthritis
d. rheumatoid arthritis
e. systemic lupus erythematosus

Q2. What is the most characteristic symptom of this disease?
a. early morning joint stiffness
b. progressive joint pain
c. predilection for the small joints
d. joint swelling
e. normal cartilage despite joint pain

Q3. What is the most characteristic sign of this disease?
a. joint swelling
b. bilateral (symmetrical) joint involvement
c. erythema surrounding the affected joints
d. joint bogginess
e. involvement of the glenohumeral joint in all cases

Q4. On what is the pathophysiology of this disease based?
a. bone destruction
b. bone spur formation
c. bone sclerosis
d. symmetrical joint involvement
e. synovial inflammation

Q5. In the course of the pathophysiology of this disease, which of the following is most characteristic of the disease?
a. synovial proliferation with cartilage erosion stimulated by cytokines
b. cartilage destruction stimulated by the proliferation of proteoglycans
c. cartilage destruction stimulated by the enzymatic action of proteoglycans
d. loss of the synovial membrane
e. none of the above; the pathophysiology of the disease is not known with any certainty

Q6. The disease described affects one particular part of the spine. What is the affected part, and what are the affected vertebrae?
a. cervical: C6-C7
b. cervical: C1-C2
c. thoracic: T7-T9
d. lumbar: L1-L3
e. lumbar: L4-L5

Q7. Which anemia usually accompanies this disease process?
a. microcytic: hypochromic
b. microcytic: normochromic
c. normocytic: normochromic
d. macrocytic: hyperchromic
e. normocytic: hypochromic

Q8. Which of the following is a (are) systemic complication(s) of the disease process?
a. vasculitis
b. pericarditis
c. pleural effusion
d. diffuse interstitial fibrosis of the lung
e. all of the above

Q9. Felty's syndrome is a complication of the described disorder. Which of the following is (are) part of Felty's syndrome?
a. splenomegaly
b. neutropenia
c. positive rheumatoid factor
d. a and b
e. all of the above

Q10. For the described disorder, which of the following is a (are) proven therapeutic agent(s)?
a. auranofin
b. hydroxychloroquine
c. methotrexate
d. D-penicillamine
e. all of the above

Q11. The patient develops a local flare-up in her right knee. Her left knee is affected to a small degree, but not nearly as severely as the right knee. Up to this time, remission had been induced and she was taking antiinflammatory agents to suppress inflammation. What is the treatment of choice for this local flare-up?
a. methotrexate
b. hydroxychloroquine
c. intraarticular corticosteroid injection
d. oral prednisone
e. auranofin

Q12. What is the drug of choice for the suppression of inflammation in a patient with this disease?
a. auranofin
b. methotrexate
c. oral prednisone
d. naproxen
e. D-penicillamine

Q13. Which of the following is not a classic radiologic feature of rheumatoid arthritis?
a. loss of juxtaarticular bone mass
b. narrowing of the joint space
c. bony erosions
d. subarticular sclerosis
e. all of the above are radiologic manifestations

SHORT ANSWER MANAGEMENT PROBLEM

Part A lists a number of different types of diseases in which arthritis is a major component. Part B lists characteristics of a number of different types of arthritis. Match the characteristics in Part B with the type of arthritis in Part A.

Part A: Type of Arthritis

SAQ1. ankylosing spondylitis
SAQ2. gonococcal arthritis
SAQ3. systemic lupus erythematosus
SAQ4. Lyme disease
SAQ5. rheumatic fever
SAQ6. gouty arthritis
SAQ7. juvenile rheumatoid arthritis
SAQ8. Reiter's disease
SAQ9. psoriatic arthritis
SAQ10. inflammatory bowel disease arthritis
SAQ11. calcium pyrophosphate arthritis
SAQ12. tuberculous arthritis

Part B: Characteristics

a. Positively birefringent under the polarizing microscope
b. Negatively birefringent under the polarizing microscope
c. Most common cause of infective arthritis in young adults
d. Conjunctivitis and urethritis are other features
e. Erythema chronicum migrans
f. Bamboo spine
g. Streptococcal pharyngitis usually occurs first
h. Arthritis may precede abdominal symptoms
i. Renal failure is major cause of death in this disease
j. Arthritis may appear before classic "silver-scaled" skin lesions
k. Major cause of arthritis in children
l. Lung disease is major manifestation of this disease in most patients

ANSWERS

A1. **d.** The most likely diagnosis is rheumatoid arthritis.

A2. **a.** The most characteristic symptom of rheumatoid arthritis is early morning stiffness. The total array of rheumatoid arthritic symptoms include the following:
a. Morning stiffness (characteristic symptom)
b. Pain on motion of joints
c. Tenderness in joints
d. Swelling (soft tissue inflammation of fluid, not bony overgrowth)
e. Symmetric joint involvement
f. Subcutaneous nodules
g. Positive agglutination (rheumatoid arthritis) factor
h. Characteristic histologic changes in the synovial membrane

A3. **b.** The most characteristic sign of rheumatoid arthritis is symmetrical joint involvement.

In most patients, rheumatoid arthritis starts out with a whimper and not a bang. The disease has an insidious start with nonspecific symptoms, such as fatigue and malaise, accompanied by arthralgias and low-grade fever. Later, polyarticular, symmetrical joint swelling begins (usually with the proximal interphalangeal, metacarpophalangeal, wrist, elbow, shoulder, knee, ankle, and metatarsophalangeal joints involved) but sparing the distal interphalangeal joints. Cervical spine involvement is common at the region C1-C2, but the remainder of the spine is usually spared.

A4. **e.**

A5. **a.** The pathophysiology of rheumatoid arthritis begins with synovial membrane swelling and synovial membrane proliferation. The synovium, which is normally only two cell layers thick, proliferates and erodes adjacent cartilage and adjacent bone. Cytokines, particularly interleukin-1 and tumor necrosis factor-α, that are secreted by macrophages produce the following:

a. Chondrocyte and osteoclast stimulation
b. Prostaglandin secretion and endothelial activation
c. CD4-positive T lymphocytes promote the inflammation early in the disease and are abundant in the synovium and the synovial fluid
d. Systemic effects such as fever and anemia are also effects of the macrophage/cytokine system

A6. **b.** Instability of the cervical spine is a life-threatening complication of rheumatoid arthritis. The instability results from a cervical ligament synovitis in the region of the first two cervical vertebrae. This complication occurs in 30% to 40% of patients who develop rheumatoid arthritis. Five percent of these patients eventually develop a myelopathy or cord injury as a result of this instability.

A7. **c.** The anemia that most often accompanies rheumatoid arthritis is characterized as mild, normochromic: normocytic. The characteristics at the cellular level of the anemia include the following: low to normal iron, low to normal iron-binding protein, and normal to low erythropoietin.

A8. **e.** Rheumatoid arthritis is a systemic disease. Some of the more important complications are as follows:

a. Vasculitis: From the very beginning of the synovial membrane thickening process, a microvascular vasculitis process is involved. This can progress to mesenteric vasculitis, polyarteritis nodosa, or other vascular syndromes.
b. Pericarditis: Fibrinous pericarditis is present in 40% of patients with rheumatoid arthritis at autopsy. Although infrequent, this pericarditis can occasionally be of the constricting type with life-threatening tamponade.
c. Pleural effusions: Rheumatic pleural effusions are extremely common.
d. Rheumatic nodules in the heart (affecting the conducting system): Rheumatic nodules may frequently lead to conducting disturbances, including heart block and bundle-branch blocks.
e. Rheumatic nodules in the lung can cavitate or become infected.
f. Diffuse interstitial fibrosis with a restrictive pattern on pulmonary function tests and with

a honeycomb pattern on chest x-ray may occur.

A9. **e.** Felty's syndrome usually occurs fairly late in the disease process. Felty's syndrome is manifested by splenomegaly, neutropenia, and a positive rheumatoid factor.

A10. **e.** All of the medications listed are disease-modifying antirheumatic drugs used in the treatment of rheumatoid arthritis.

A11. **c.** Because the flare-up is limited to one joint, it is reasonable to treat with a localized approach. An intraarticular corticosteroid injection may temporarily help control local synovitis.

A12. **d.** The drug(s) of choice for the suppression of inflammation in a patient with rheumatoid arthritis are the nonsteroidal antiinflammatory drugs (NSAIDs). Although aspirin is still theoretically the agent of first choice, patients are more likely to take 1 to 2 pills/day with NSAID therapy rather than the 10 to 12 required with aspirin therapy. Thus the answer to this question is naproxen. If an NSAID from a certain class does not work when given up to maximum dose, then try an agent from a second or different class. A cyclooxygenase-2 (COX-2) inhibitor may be preferable in long-term treatment because of decreased gastrointestinal side effects.

A13. **d.** In early rheumatoid arthritis, few radiologic findings are seen. Soft tissue changes in synovial fluid or capsular thickening may occasionally be seen on the radiograph but are more readily detected by physical examination. Loss of juxtaarticular bone mass (osteoporosis) is often detected near the finger joints and may be seen early in the disease. Narrowing of the joint space, due to thinning of the articular cartilage, is usually seen late in the disease. Bony erosions are seen best at the margins of the joint. Subarticular sclerosis is a feature of osteoarthritis, not rheumatoid arthritis.

SOLUTION TO THE SHORT ANSWER MANAGEMENT PROBLEM

SAQ1.	F	SAQ7.	K
SAQ2.	C	SAQ8.	D
SAQ3.	I	SAQ9.	J
SAQ4.	E	SAQ10.	H
SAQ5.	G	SAQ11.	A
SAQ6.	B	SAQ12.	L

SUMMARY OF THE DIAGNOSIS AND MANAGEMENT OF RHEUMATOID ARTHRITIS

1. Prevalence: Rheumatoid arthritis occurs in 1% of the population. Clinical risk for developing rheumatoid arthritis is highly associated with HLA DR4.

2. Signs and symptoms:
   a. Most common:
      1) Early morning stiffness is most common symptom.
      2) Symmetrical joint swelling is most common sign.
   b. Other signs and symptoms:
      1) Tenderness, swelling, and "bogginess" of joints
      2) Characteristic changes in the synovial membrane, including microvascular changes
      3) Positive rheumatoid factor
      4) Subcutaneous nodules
      5) Radiographic changes:
         a) Loss of juxtaarticular bone mass
         b) Joint space narrowing
         c) Bony erosions

3. Pathophysiology:
   a. Sequence and order of changes
      1) Macrophage activation
      2) Product(s) of activation is (are) production of cytokines: Interleukin and tumor necrosis factor
      3) Synovial membrane thickening, proliferation, and local "microvasculitis"
      4) Chondrocyte, osteoclast, CD4 positive T lymphocytes, endothelial proliferation
      5) Joint space narrowing
      6) Cytokines are also responsible for extra-articular symptoms such as fever and anemia

4. Systemic manifestations:
   a. Normochromic-normocytic anemia
   b. Fever
   c. Pericarditis
   d. Pleural effusion
   e. Rheumatoid nodules in lung
   f. Diffuse interstitial disease
   g. Felty's syndrome
   h. Rheumatoid nodules in heart causing heart block and bundle-branch block
   i. Systemic vasculitis

5. Treatment:
   a. Nonpharmacologic treatment:
      1) Systemic rest
      2) Articular rest—splints, braces, canes
      3) Physiotherapy, including heat, cold, joint range of motion, and exercise as tolerated
      4) Substitution of omega-3 for omega-6 fatty acids in the diet
   b. Disease-modifying agents: The early use of disease-modifying antirheumatic drugs for rheumatoid arthritis is beneficial.
      1) Gold compounds: Gold compounds are contraindicated in patients with hepatic or renal disease or blood dyscrasia.
      2) Hydroxychloroquine: Ophthalmologic screening is recommended before and routinely during the treatment with hydroxychloroquine.
      3) Sulfasalazine
      4) Penicillamine: CBC and urinalysis must be checked routinely while patient is on this medication.
      5) Azathioprine
      6) Methotrexate: Methotrexate is one of the most widely prescribed disease-modifying antirheumatic drugs for rheumatoid arthritis. It has a rapid onset of action (3 to 4 weeks), dependable clinical response, and is well-tolerated for long-term therapy. Side effects include reversible bone marrow suppression, hepatotoxicity, pulmonary hypersensitivity, and nephrotoxicity.
      7) Cyclosporine
      8) Leflunomide
      9) Minocycline
   c. Local remittent agents: First choice is injected corticosteroids
   d. Early disease or acute/chronic inflammation:
      1) First choice:
         a) NSAID: COX-2 inhibitors have decreased gastrointestinal toxicity
         b) Oxicams/indoleacetic acids (piroxicam/indomethacin)
      2) Alternative first choice: Aspirin
      3) Second choice: Nonacetylated salicylates
      4) Corticosteroids: Due to adverse effects with long-term use, corticosteriods should be used only after trials of other drugs. They are effective in suppressing inflammation rapidly.
      5) Surgery

SUGGESTED READINGS

Kandanoff RD: Rheumatoid arthritis. In Rakel R, ed: *Conn's current therapy,* Philadelphia, 1994, WB Saunders.

Kremer JM: Methotrexate and emerging therapies, *Rheum Dis Clin North Am* 24(3):651-658, 1998.

Sewell KL: Rheumatoid arthritis in older adults, *Clin Geriatr Med* 14(3):475-494, 1998.

OSTEOARTHRITIS

"Oh, How I Ache in the Evening."

Case 1 ■ An 80-Year-Old Female with Painful Finger Joints

An 80-year-old female complaining about a 6-month history of stiffness in her hands bilaterally is brought to your office by her daughter. The stiffness is worst in the evening and subsides thereafter. She has also noticed increasing (but not severe) pain in the lower back, both hips, and both knees.

On examination, the patient is obese. She has significant swelling of both the proximal interphalangeal (PIP) joints and the distal interphalangeal (DIP) joints. There is also deformity of both knees on examination. The rest of her physical examination is within normal limits.

SELECT THE BEST ANSWER TO THE FOLLOWING QUESTIONS

Q1. Which of the following statements regarding this patient's condition is true?
   a. the swelling present at the DIP joint may represent Bouchard's nodes
   b. the swelling present at the PIP joint may represent Heberden's nodes
   c. this patient will most likely demonstrate an elevated erythrocyte sedimentation rate (ESR) and a positive rheumatoid factor
   d. synovial fluid analysis will probably demonstrate a low viscosity and normal mucin clotting
   e. none of the above is true

Q2. Which of the following statements regarding the symptomatology of the condition described is false?
   a. pain is the chief symptom of osteoarthritis and is usually deep and aching in character
   b. stiffness of the involved joint is common but of relatively brief duration
   c. the pain of osteoarthritis is characteristically dull and aching
   d. the major physical finding in osteoarthritis is bony crepitus
   e. the presence of osteophytes is sufficient for the diagnosis of osteoarthritis

Q3. Which of the following statements concerning the condition described is false?

   a. this condition is the most common form of joint disease in the North American population
   b. 80% of the population have radiographic features of this condition in weight-bearing joints before age 65 years
   c. this condition has both primary and secondary forms
   d. narrowing of the joint space is unusual
   e. pathologically, the articular cartilage is first roughened and then finally worn away

Q4. A 65-year-old female with moderately severe osteoarthritis of her left hip comes to your office requesting an exercise prescription. She wishes to "get into shape." Which of the following would you recommend to this patient at this time?
   a. exercise is not good for osteoarthritis; rest is much more appropriate
   b. a graded exercise program consisting of brisk walking and gradually increasing the distance to 3 to 4 mi/day will probably not cause pain and will be good for her
   c. a passive isotonic exercise program is preferable to an active isometric exercise program
   d. any exercise program will probably hasten her need for total hip replacements
   e. swimming is the best exercise prescription you can give her; it promotes cardiovascular fitness and at the same time keeps pressure off the weight-bearing joints

Q5. Which of the following radiographic features is (are) usually seen with the condition just described?
   a. narrowing of the joint spaces
   b. bony sclerosis
   c. osteophyte formation
   d. subchondral cyst formation
   e. all of the above

Q6. Which of the following is a (are) useful treatment modality(ies) in the treatment of the condition just described?
   a. weight loss in obese patients
   b. canes, crutches, and walkers
   c. the application of heat to involved joints
   d. nonsteroidal antiinflammatory drugs (NSAIDs)
   e. all of the above

Q7. Which of the following statements concerning the incidence of the condition described above is (are) true?
   a. one third of adults age 25 to 75 years have radiographic evidence of osteoarthritis

b. cartilaginous fraying is common
c. mild synovitis may develop in response to crystals or cartilaginous debris
d. the most common sites for this disease are in the small joints of the hand, the foot, and the knees and/or hips
e. all of the above are true

Q8. What is (are) the major goal(s) of therapy in the disease just described?
a. minimize pain
b. prevent disability
c. delay progression
d. a and b only
e. all of the above

Q9. Which of the following statements regarding the use of NSAIDs in the condition described and as given to an elderly patient is true?
a. NSAIDs are generally very safe for the treatment of the condition described in elderly patients
b. NSAID toxicity in elderly patients is uncommon
c. NSAID toxicity in elderly patients is unlikely to be associated with renal insufficiency
d. the most common NSAID toxicity in elderly patients is gastrointestinal
e. none of the above is true

Q10. What is the drug of choice for the treatment of primary osteoarthritis?
a. acetaminophen
b. naproxen sodium
c. diclofenac
d. indomethacin
e. any of the above

SHORT ANSWER MANAGEMENT PROBLEM
Describe the nonpharmacologic and the pharmacologic management of the condition described.

ANSWERS

A1. **e.** This patient has obvious osteoarthritis. However, the location of Bouchard's nodes represents both overgrowth and significant osteoarthritic changes at the PIP joints (not the DIP joints), whereas Heberden's nodes represent bony overgrowth and significant osteoarthritic changes at the DIP (not the PIP) joints.

A significantly elevated ESR is seldom seen with osteoarthritis (except in the unusual cases in which there is a significant inflammatory component).

Synovial fluid analysis will most likely reveal a high (not low) viscosity and normal mucin clotting. The total leukocyte count in the synovial fluid will likely be less than 1000 cells/mm^3.

A2. **e.** The most common symptom in osteoarthritis is pain. The pain is described as dull, aching, aggravated by joint use, and relieved by joint rest. Joint stiffness in weight-bearing joints is common but usually is a very transient finding (especially in the morning). It also occurs after prolonged rest.

Osteoarthritis pain results from the movement of one joint surface against another with both joint surfaces exhibiting characteristic articular cartilage damage, including fraying and, ultimately, complete lack of cartilage. In addition, there are subchondral bone microfractures, irritation of the periosteal nerve endings, ligamentous stress, muscular strain, and soft tissue inflammation such as bursitis and tendinitis.

Bony crepitus is the most common physical finding in osteoarthritis. Osteophytes are a common radiologic finding, especially with advanced age. The diagnosis of osteoarthritis, however, is clinical, and the mere presence of osteophytes on an x-ray film is not sufficient for the diagnosis itself.

A3. **d.** Joint space narrowing is common. It is almost always associated with osteoarthritis. The pathologic process involved in osteoarthritis is as follows:
a. The primary defect in primary osteoarthritis and secondary osteoarthritis is loss of articular cartilage. In primary osteoarthritis this results from "normal" wear and tear. In secondary osteoarthritis the loss is caused by acute or chronic trauma, congenital deformities, metabolic disorders, septic and tubercular arthritis, and endocrine disorders such as acromegaly, obesity, or diabetes. The end result is that some 80% of the population have evidence of osteoarthritis in weight-bearing joints by the time they are age 65 years.
b. Cartilage changes progress as follows:
1) Glistening appearance is lost.
2) Surface areas of the articular cartilage flake off.
3) Deeper layers of the articular cartilage develop longitudinal fissures (fibrillation).
4) The cartilage becomes thin and eventually absent in some areas, leaving the underlying subchondral bone unprotected.
5) The unprotected subchondral bone becomes sclerotic (dense and hard).
6) Cysts develop within the subchondral bone and communicate with the longitudinal fissures in the cartilage.

7) Pressure builds up in the cysts until the cystic contents are forced into the synovial cavity, breaking through the articular cartilage on the way.

8) As the articular cartilage erodes, cartilage-coated osteophytes may grow outward from the underlying bone and alter the bony contours and joint anatomy. These spurlike bony projections enlarge until small pieces, called joint mice, break off into the synovial cavity.

9) The loss of articular cartilage probably takes place through the enzymatic breakdown of the cartilage matrix—the proteoglycans, glycosaminoglycans, and collagen are involved.

A4. **e.** Muscle spasm and muscle atrophy can be prevented in osteoarthritis by a graded exercise program. Active exercises are preferred to passive exercises; isometric exercises are preferred to isotonic exercises.

Because of minimal involvement of the weight-bearing joints, swimming can be recommended as an ideal exercise.

A graded exercise program that includes walking 3 to 4 mi/day will result in trauma to the joints and should be discouraged. It may very well hasten the need for total hip replacement.

A5. **e.** Radiographic changes in osteoarthritis include narrowing of the joint space caused by loss of articular cartilage, bony sclerosis resulting from thickening of subchondral bone, subchondral bone cysts, and osteophyte (bone spur) formation.

A6. **e.** The treatment of osteoarthritis includes non-pharmacologic measures and pharmacologic measures.

Nonpharmacologic measures include rest; the avoidance of overuse of the affected joint; walking aids such as canes, crutches, and walkers; weight loss; the application of heat; and other physiotherapy techniques.

Pharmacologic measures include simple analgesics such as acetaminophen, NSAIDs, and local steroid injections. Newer concepts in the treatment of osteoarthritis include chondroprotective agents, which conserve cartilage or stimulate cartilage repair within the osteoarthritic joint. These agents include tetracyclines, glycosaminoglycans, hyaluronan preparations, and gene therapy. Over-the-counter topical preparations, such as capsaicin cream are used for relief of pain. Other complementary approaches are under investigation.

Orthopedic surgery is used in severe cases. Joint replacement, especially of the knee and hip, is the treatment of choice when more conservative therapy has failed to control pain and maintain function.

A7. **e.** At least 33% of adults between ages 25 and 75 years have radiographic findings commonly seen in osteoarthritis. Some studies suggest that osteoarthritis begins as early as age 15 or 16 years.

The cartilaginous fraying associated with cartilage degeneration has been described. Associated with this may be a mild synovitis that develops in response to cartilaginous fragments (joint mice) in the joint space itself.

The most common sites for osteoarthritis to develop are the small joints of the hands, the small joints of the feet, the hips, the knees, and the vertebral column where the cartilaginous degeneration is of a somewhat different type (the intervertebral discs) but nevertheless is the same basic pathologic process.

A8. **e.** The goals for the patient with osteoarthritis are to minimize pain, prevent disability, and delay progression.

Some would argue that it is not possible to delay progression in osteoarthritis. However, this is false. Weight loss in an obese individual and decreased repetitive trauma or impact to a joint with osteoarthritis will delay progression.

A9. **d.** The most common type of toxicity associated with NSAIDs in elderly patients is gastrointestinal. This may take the form of an acute or chronic gastritis, a peptic ulcer, or a perforated duodenal ulcer. This may result in secondary anemia and other complications.

A10. **a.** NSAIDs (even though a mainstay of treatment for osteoarthritis) have very significant toxicity, especially when used in elderly patients with renal impairment or any other disease. Thus ordinary acetaminophen is safer and must be considered a drug of first choice.

If an NSAID is used for the treatment of osteoarthritis in elderly patients it is suggested that:
a. the dose be kept as low as possible
b. the drug be given with food and preferably with a cytoprotective agent such as misoprostol

Avoid NSAIDs with greater propensity to produce side effects (indomethacin, phenylbutazone, and the like).

Celecoxib and rofecoxib (cyclooxygenase-2 [COX-2] inhibitors) should have less risk for gastrointestinal complications and may become drugs of choice.

SOLUTION TO THE SHORT ANSWER MANAGEMENT PROBLEM

A. Nonpharmacologic treatment:
1. Weight loss
2. Exercise prescription: Strengthening, range of motion, and aerobic exercises including cycling, swimming, and cross-county trainers
3. Work modification (limit joint stress trauma)
4. Regular physiotherapy (heat, cold, ultrasound)
5. Transcutaneous electric nerve stimulation
6. Walking aids and braces

B. Pharmacologic treatment:
1. Acetaminophen: Drug of first choice
2. NSAIDs
3. Intraarticular steroid injection (improvement is usually only temporary)
4. Chondroprotective agents
5. Capsaicin cream

SUMMARY OF THE DIAGNOSIS AND TREATMENT OF OSTEOARTHRITIS

1. Diagnosis: A noninflammatory joint disease characterized by its lack of inflammatory signs and symptoms and by the loss of articular cartilage and degeneration in synovial joints.

2. Prevalence: Most common rheumatologic condition. Majority of people older than age 65 years have radiographic evidence of osteoarthritis.

3. Pathology: Proteolytic enzymes (proteoglycans, glycosaminoglycans) produce the characteristic changes in the articular cartilage just described.

4. Subtypes: Idiopathic and secondary. Secondary osteoarthritis is related to acute or chronic trauma, congenital abnormalities, and certain common conditions, including obesity and diabetes mellitus.

5. Treatment: Divided into nonpharmacologic and pharmacologic. The keys of nonpharmacologic treatment include weight loss; physiotherapy; stretching leading up to a mild aerobic, active, isometric exercise program (swimming is the single best exercise); work modification to limit weight bearing on affected joints; and use of aids such as canes and walkers.

The most important key of pharmacologic therapy is *primum non nocere*—first do no harm. Acetaminophen is the drug of choice because of its relative lack of toxicity in the elderly; if using NSAIDs, use cytoprotection or a COX-2 inhibitor. Limit intraarticular corticosteroid injections to large joints that fail to respond to other measures.

Consider surgery if all therapies fail or osteoarthritis is very severe.

SUGGESTED READINGS

Cardone DA, Tallia AF: Osteoarthritis. In Singleton J et al, eds: *Primary care*, Philadelphia, 1998, JB Lippincott.

Creamer P, Hochberg MC: Osteoarthritis, *Lancet* 350(9076):503, 1997.

Klippel JH et al, eds: *Primer on the rheumatic diseases: An official publication of the Arthritis Foundation*, ed 11, Marietta, Ga, 1998, Longstreet Press.

Kraus VB: Pathogenesis and treatment of osteoarthritis, *Med Clin North Am* 81:85-112, 1997.

Manek NJ, Lane NE: Osteoarthritis: Current concepts in diagnosis and management, *Am Fam Physician* 61(6):1795-1804, 2000.

Sack K: Osteoarthritis. In Rakel R, ed: *Conn's current therapy*, Philadelphia, 1994, WB Saunders.

PROBLEM·31

FIBROMYALGIA

"It's Awful; I Ache All Over."

Case 1 ■ A 35-Year-Old Female with Total Body Muscle Pain

A 35-year-old female comes to your office with a 1-year history of "aching and hurting all over." In addition, she complains of a chronic headache, difficulty sleeping, and generalized fatigue. When questioned carefully, she describes "muscle areas tender to touch." Although the pain is "worse in the back," there really is no place where "it doesn't exist." She also describes headaches, generalized abdomen pains, and some constipation.

On examination, the most striking finding is the presence of 13 discrete "trigger points" (tender muscle areas when palpated). These include the trapezius muscle, the sternomastoid, the masseter muscle, the levator scapulae, the muscles inserting into the area of the greater trochanter, the muscles inserting into the upper border of the patellae, and six areas on the back that together cover almost the entire back area.

The rest of the physical examination is normal. Her blood pressure is 120/70 mm Hg, and her cardiovascular, respiratory, and abdominal examinations are normal.

SELECT THE BEST ANSWER TO THE FOLLOWING QUESTIONS

Q1. What is the most likely diagnosis in this patient?
   a. polymyalgia rheumatica

b. masked depression
c. fibromyalgia
d. diffuse musculoskeletal pain, not yet diagnosed (NYD)
e. early rheumatoid arthritis

Q2. Which one of the following is not usually a site of tenderness in the disorder described?
a. the rectus abdominis muscle
b. the supraspinatus tendon
c. the lateral epicondyle of the humerus
d. the trapezius muscle
e. the middle gluteus muscle

Q3. The differential diagnosis of the condition described above includes which of the following?
a. chronic fatigue syndrome
b. hypothyroidism
c. masked depression
d. myofascial pain syndrome
e. all of the above

Q4. The diagnostic criteria of the disorder described include tenderness at how many of the 18 specific sites?
a. 5
b. 7
c. 9
d. 11
e. 13

Q5. What is the most characteristic symptom of the condition described?
a. pain in at least three or four body quadrants
b. "pain all over my body"
c. pain in specific bursae and tendons
d. pain in specific joints
e. pain in both arms, the posterior neck, and the upper back

Q6. What is the most important condition that must be considered in the differential diagnosis of the condition described?
a. generalized anxiety disorder
b. panic disorder
c. major depression
d. rheumatoid arthritis
e. osteoarthritis

Q7. What is the cause of this disorder?
a. an autoimmune process
b. a chronic inflammatory process
c. an acute inflammatory process
d. a slow or chronic virus infection
e. idiopathic

Q8. Which of the following statements regarding sleep disorders and the condition described is true?
a. there is no association between this condition and sleep disorders
b. patients with this disorder have an abnormal sleep pattern
c. patients with this disorder have difficult sleep induction, early morning wakening, and nightmares
d. patients with this disorder have profound insomnia
e. patients with this disorder usually have profound hypersomnia

Q9. Regarding therapy for this disorder, which of the following statements is (are) true?
a. use of nonsteroidal anti-inflammatory drugs (NSAIDs) have demonstrated a significant advantage over use of placebo
b. antidepressants are superior to placebo
c. muscle relaxants are superior to placebo
d. b and c
e. all of the above are true

Q10. Regarding the use of corticosteroids in the condition described, which of the following statements is true?
a. repetitive local injections with corticosteroids/lidocaine should be considered a first-line treatment option
b. oral prednisone has been shown to be effective
c. local injection of steroids/lidocaine should be reserved for resistant cases of this disorder
d. no benefit from oral steroids has been demonstrated
e. none of the above is true

SHORT ANSWER MANAGEMENT PROBLEM
Describe the criteria determined by the American Rheumatological Society as needed to establish a diagnosis of fibromyalgia.

ANSWERS

A1. **c.** This patient has fibromyalgia. Fibromyalgia is characterized by widespread musculoskeletal pain (defined as pain in the left and right side of the body, above and below the waist, plus axial pain) and the presence of 11 or more out of 18 specifically designated tender points or trigger points.

These musculoskeletal symptoms are often associated with total body pain, severe fatigue, nonrestorative sleep, postexertional increase in muscle pain, reduced functional ability, recurrent headaches, irritable bowel syndrome, atypical paresthesia, cold sensitivity (Raynaud's phenomenon), aerobic deconditioning, restless leg syndrome, sleep apnea, and nocturnal myoclonus.

Fibromyalgia is much more common in women than in men and is usually diagnosed between ages 20 and 50 years.

Rheumatoid arthritis is unlikely because of the lack of objective evidence of joint warmth, swelling, or deformity and the multiple soft tissue areas. Laboratory evaluation, however, is necessary to exclude this inflammatory condition.

Polymyalgia rheumatica occurs in an older age group and is discussed in Problem 117.

Diffuse musculoskeletal pain NYD is not a diagnosis.

A primary diagnosis of masked depression or a somatoform disorder should always be considered when vague somatic complaints are accompanied by sleep disturbance and fatigue. The multiple tender areas, however, are not usually seen in masked depression.

A2. **a.** Fibromyalgia is associated with tender points, or trigger points, at multiple characteristic locations, including the following:

a. The supraspinatus tendon
b. The costochondral junction
c. The lateral epicondyle of the humerus
d. The iliac crest
e. The greater trochanteric bursa of the femur
f. The medial fat pad of the knee
g. The suboccipital region of the head
h. The nuchal ligament
i. The trapezius muscle
j. The infraspinatus tendon
k. The rhomboid muscle
l. The erector spinae of the lumbar spine
m. The middle gluteus muscle
n. The piriformis muscle

An additional four, less anatomically descriptive areas are also included. The rectus abdominis muscle is not included.

The sensitivity of the trigger points can be assessed by measuring the exact amount of pressure applied over a certain anatomic site using a dolorimeter.

A3. **e.** Fibromyalgia certainly has some vague symptoms, and the trigger points are the most objective evidence of the disorder. Many health care professionals, however, still doubt its authenticity.

Hypothyroidism and chronic fatigue syndrome present with severe fatigue and share this major symptom with fibromyalgia.

Myofascial pain syndrome shares the symptom of trigger points with fibromyalgia and should be considered in the differential diagnosis.

A4. **d.** The number of trigger points identified by the American College of Rheumatology as being diagnostic of fibromyalgia is 11 or more.

A5. **b.** The most characteristic symptom of fibromyalgia is the symptom described by patients as "total body muscle pain." This is a symptom that from clinical experience appears to have reasonable sensitivity and specificity.

A6. **c.** The most important differential diagnosis of fibromyalgia is major depression or a somatoform disorder. Depression is a very common correlate with fibromyalgia, and it appears that many patients actually meet the criteria for both disorders. In addition, the tricyclic antidepressants (TCAs) are recommended for both conditions. In many cases the major depression that accompanies fibromyalgia is a masked depression, with many of the symptoms being somatic in origin.

A7. **e.** The cause of fibromyalgia is unknown. There is no significant evidence suggesting that the process is an autoimmune process, caused by a true acute or chronic inflammatory process (although this is a possibility), or the result of any type of viral infection.

A8. **b.** The many nonrheumatologic features of fibromyalgia include a pattern that is best described as a disorder of nonrestorative sleep (alpha nonrapid-eye-movement sleep anomaly). Although other sleep disorders, including sleep apnea in a small minority of patients, nocturnal myoclonus, and restless leg syndrome, are associated with fibromyalgia, a disorder of nonrestorative sleep (alpha-delta disorder) is the most common and the most diagnostic.

A9. **e.** There is certainly considerable controversy regarding which pharmacologic medications (if any) work and which do not. Results have been mixed, but it is fair to say that at least some studies have demonstrated favorable results for NSAIDs, tricyclics, fluoxetine, alprazolam, and cyclobenzaprine.

If the patient experiences sleep disturbances that are often associated with fibromyalgia, serotonin reuptake inhibitors (particularly fluoxetine) should only be used with caution for the treatment of this condition.

A10. **c.** It is currently recommended that local injections of corticosteroid/lidocaine combination be reserved for resistant trigger points because the risk-to-benefit ratio (especially for repeated injections) is questionable. Muscle atrophy, overlying skin atrophy, fibrosis, infection, abscess formation, and other complications may arise from repeated steroid injections.

SOLUTION TO THE SHORT ANSWER MANAGEMENT PROBLEM

The American College of Rheumatology diagnosis of fibromyalgia includes the following:

1. Widespread musculoskeletal pain in the left and right sides of the body, above and below the waist, plus axial pain; typically described by patient as "total body muscle pain" or "I hurt all over."
2. The presence of 11 or more out of a total of 18 specifically designated tender points or trigger points. The major clinical features of fibromyalgia include the following:
   a. Total body pain
   b. Multiple tender points on examination
   c. Severe fatigue
   d. Nonrestorative sleep (alpha nonrapid-eye-movement sleep anomaly)
   e. Postexertional increase in muscle pain
   f. Reduced functional ability
   g. Recurrent headaches
   h. Irritable bowel syndrome
   i. Atypical paresthesia
   j. Cold sensitivity (often Raynaud's phenomenon)
   k. Restless legs syndrome
   l. Aerobic deconditioning

SUMMARY OF THE DIAGNOSIS AND TREATMENT OF FIBROMYALGIA

1. Diagnosis: See the previous section.

2. Treatment:
   a. Nonpharmacologic:
      1) Physical therapy (heat, cold, ultrasound, TENS)
      2) Massage therapy
      3) Psychologic counseling
      4) Biofeedback
      5) Cardiovascular fitness training program
   b. Pharmacologic
      1) TCAs (low-dose): Amitriptyline, doxepin, nortriptyline, trazodone
      2) NSAIDs are of limited usefulness in fibromyalgia: Cyclobenzaprine, fluoxetine, alprazolam

Many of the positive effects of the medications tend to diminish over time.

SUGGESTED READINGS

Alarcon GS, Bradley LA: Advances in the treatment of fibromyalgia: Current status and future directions, *Am J Med Sci* 315(6):397-404, 1998.

Bennett R: Bursitis, tendinitis, myofascial pain and fibromyalgia. In Rakel R, ed: *Conn's current therapy*, Philadelphia, 1994, WB Saunders.

Bennet R: Fibromyalgia, chronic fatigue syndrome, and myofascial pain, *Curr Opin Rheumatol* 10(2):95-103, 1998.

Demitrack MA: Chronic fatigue syndrome and fibromyalgia, *Psychiatr Clin North Am* 21(3):671-692, 1998.

PROBLEM·32

CHRONIC FATIGUE SYNDROME

"Oh, How I Hate to Get Up in the Morning!"

Case 1 ■ A 25-Year-Old Female with Chronic Fatigue

A 25-year-old female comes to your office with a 9-month history of "unbearable fatigue." Before the fatigue began 9 months ago, she worked as a high school chemistry teacher. Since the fatigue began she has been unable to work at all. She tells you that "one day it just hit me—I literally could not get out of bed."

Her past history is unremarkable. She has a husband and two children who have been very supportive during her 9-month illness. She has no history of any significant illnesses, including no history of any psychiatric disease. There is no family history of psychiatric disease.

The other symptoms that the patient describes are difficulty concentrating, headache, sore throat, tender lymph nodes, muscle aches, joint aches, feverishness, difficulty sleeping, abdominal cramps, chest pain, and night sweats.

On physical examination, the patient has a low-grade fever (38.6° C), nonexudative pharyngitis, and palpable and tender anterior and posterior cervical and axillary lymph nodes.

SELECT THE BEST ANSWER TO THE FOLLOWING QUESTIONS

Q1. What is the most likely diagnosis in this patient?
   a. major depressive illness
   b. masked depression
   c. chronic fatigue syndrome
   d. fibromyalgia
   e. malingering

Q2. What is the cause of the condition presented here?
   a. unequivocally related to a viral infection
   b. associated with an imbalance of neurotransmitters in the brain

c. a factitious illness

d. associated with major psychiatric pathology in almost all cases

e. unknown

Q3. Which of the following statements regarding the condition described is false?

a. this condition is relatively new

b. this condition is also known as epidemic neuromyasthenia

c. this condition is also known as myalgic encephalomyelitis

d. this condition is also known as multiple chemical sensitivity syndrome

e. none of the above is false

Q4. Which of the following statements concerning the epidemiology of the condition described is (are) true?

a. patients with this condition are twice as likely to be women as to be men

b. patients with this condition are likely to be in the 25- to 45-year-old age bracket

c. clusters of outbreaks of this condition have occurred in many countries over the last 60 years

d. the primary symptom of this condition may be found in up to 20% of patients attending a general medical clinic

e. all of the above are true

Q5. Which of the following best describes the onset of the condition described in the majority of patients?

a. gradually increasing symptoms over a 3-month period

b. gradually increasing symptoms over a 6-month period

c. acute onset of symptoms in a previously healthy, well-functioning patient

d. chronic onset of symptoms over 1 to 2 years

e. the onset of symptoms is extremely variable; it is impossible to predict them with any degree of certainty

Q6. Which of the following is not a criterion in the diagnosis of the condition described?

a. sore throat

b. mild fever

c. prolonged generalized fatigue following previously tolerable levels of exercise

d. sleep disturbance

e. anxiety or panic attacks

Q7. Regarding the laboratory diagnosis of the condition, which of the following statements is true?

a. no laboratory test, however esoteric or exotic, can diagnose this condition or measure its severity

b. a well-defined laboratory test that is sensitive but not specific exists for diagnostic purposes

c. a well-defined laboratory test that is specific but not sensitive exists for diagnostic purposes

d. a well-defined laboratory test that is both sensitive and specific exists for diagnostic purposes

e. a number of laboratory tests in combination are used for definite confirmation of the condition

Q8. Which of the following has been shown to be the most effective therapy for the condition described?

a. use of a tricyclic antidepressant

b. use of a nonsteroidal antiinflammatory drug (NSAID)

c. a sensitive, empathetic physician who is willing to listen

d. cognitive psychotherapy

e. none of the above

Q9. The disorder described is associated with all of the following except:

a. hypothalamic dysfunction

b. conversion disorder

c. alpha-intrusion sleep disorder

d. chronic immune activation

e. myofascial pain

Q10. The disorder described is associated with which of the following symptoms?

a. sleep disruption

b. cognitive dysfunction

c. anxiety and/or depression

d. neurologic symptoms

e. all of the above

Q11. Some evidence suggests that symptoms of the disorder can be induced in healthy individuals through which of the following?

a. three nights of sleep deprivation

b. chronic pain resulting from a motor vehicle accident

c. leakage from silicon breast implants

d. *Mycoplasma pneumoniae* infections

e. all of the above

Q12. Empirical evidence suggests that the best drug to treat symptoms of the disorder is which of the following?

a. NSAIDs

b. antidepressants
c. clarithromycin
d. tryptophan
e. a and b

Q13. When using antidepressant medications to treat either the sleep disorder or the mood disorder associated with this condition, what should the dose be?
a. the usual dose given to treat depression
b. 1½ times the usual dose given to treat depression
c. ½ the usual dose given to treat depression
d. ¼ or less of the usual dose given to treat depression
e. twice the usual dose given to treat depression

Q14. What is the main therapeutic strategy used to reduce the symptoms of the disorder described?
a. correct the sleep disorder
b. provide psychotherapy for the conversion disorder
c. encourage the development of a support network
d. encourage the patient to return to work and full activity as soon as possible
e. none of the above

Q15. Most patients with the disorder:
a. fully recover with 2 years
b. partially recover with 2 years
c. never recover
d. are at risk for relapse following recovery
e. b and d

Q16. Risk factors for the development of the condition above include which of the following?
a. a family member with the condition
b. a recent motor vehicle accident
c. recurrent immune activation
d. a spouse with the disorder
e. all of the above

SHORT ANSWER MANAGEMENT PROBLEM
Describe the relationship between the described disorder and fibromyalgia.

ANSWERS

A1. **c.** This patient has the clinical manifestations that support a diagnosis of chronic fatigue syndrome. Clinically evaluated, unexplained chronic fatigue cases can be classified as chronic fatigue syndrome if the patient meets both of the following criteria:
a. Clinically evaluated, unexplained persistent or relapsing chronic fatigue that is of new or definite onset (i.e., not lifelong), is not the result of ongoing exertion, is not substantially alleviated by rest, and results in substantial reduction in previous levels of occupational, educational, social, or personal activities.
b. The concurrent occurrence of four or more of the following symptoms: Substantial impairment in short-term memory or concentration; sore throat; tender lymph nodes; muscle pain; multijoint pain without swelling or redness; headaches of a new type, pattern, or severity; unrefreshing sleep; and postexertional malaise lasting more than 24 hours. These symptoms must have persisted or recurred during 6 or more consecutive months of illness and must not have predated the fatigue.

The Centers for Disease Control and Prevention (CDC) in Atlanta has established a working definition of chronic fatigue syndrome in 1988, which was revised in 1993, namely: "*A thorough medical history, physical examination, mental status examination, and laboratory tests (diagram) must be conducted to identify underlying or contributing conditions that require treatment. Diagnosis or classification cannot be made without such an evaluation.*"*

A2. **e.** The cause of chronic fatigue syndrome is unknown. There are several common themes underlying attempts to understand the disorder. It is often postinfectious, is often accompanied by immunologic disturbances, and is commonly accompanied by depression. Viral agents that have been implicated as being associated with chronic fatigue syndrome include the lymphotropic herpesviruses, the retroviruses, and the enteroviruses.

A3. **a.** Chronic fatigue syndrome is not a new disease; it has been around for centuries. Certain individuals in the past have been labeled with a variety of diagnoses such as neurasthenia, effort syndrome, hyperventilation syndrome, chronic brucellosis, epidemic neuromyasthenia, myalgic encephalomyelitis, hypoglycemia, multiple chemical sensitivity syndrome, chronic candidiasis, chronic mononucleosis, chronic Epstein-Barr virus infection, and postviral fatigue syndrome.

A4. **e.** Patients with chronic fatigue syndrome are twice as likely to be women as men and are generally age 25 to 45 years.

*From Fukuda K et al: *Ann Intern Med* 121:953-959, 1994.

Cases are recognized in many developed countries. Most arise sporadically, but over 30 clusters of similar illnesses have been reported. The most famous of such outbreaks occurred in Los Angeles County Hospital in 1934; in Akureyri, Iceland, in 1948; in the Royal Free Hospital, London, in 1955; in Punta Gorda, Florida, in 1945; and in Incline Village, Nevada, in 1985.

The prevalence of chronic fatigue syndrome is difficult to estimate because this is entirely dependent on case definition. Chronic fatigue itself is a ubiquitous symptom, occurring in as many as 20% of patients attending a general medical clinic; the syndrome itself is much less common.

A5. **c.** The typical case of chronic fatigue syndrome arises suddenly in a previously active and healthy individual. An otherwise unremarkable flulike illness or some other acute stress is recalled with great clarity as the triggering event. Unbearable exhaustion is left in the wake of the incident. Other symptoms, such as headache, sore throat, tender lymph nodes, muscle and joint aches, and frequent feverishness lead to the belief that an infection persists. Then, over several weeks, the impact of reassurances offered during the initial evaluation fades as other features of the syndrome become evident, such as disturbed sleep, difficulty in concentration, and depression.

A6. **e.** Panic attacks and anxiety are not criteria in the CDC definition.

A7. **a.** No laboratory test, however exotic or esoteric, can make the diagnosis of chronic fatigue syndrome. Elaborate, expensive laboratory work-ups should be avoided; they only make an already complicated picture even more so. However, it is reasonable to perform testing in order to exclude other causes of fatigue.

A8. **c.** A sensitive, empathetic physician who is willing to listen is the most effective intervention that can be offered for chronic fatigue syndrome.

NSAIDs alleviate headache, diffuse pain, and feverishness. Nonsedating antidepressants improve mood and disordered sleep and thereby attenuate the fatigue to some degree.

The ingestion of caffeine and alcohol at night makes it harder to sleep, compounding fatigue, and should be avoided. Nothing, however, takes the place of an empathetic physician.

In terms of psychotherapy, the most effective therapy appears to be behavior-oriented therapy, not cognitive psychotherapy.

A9. **b.** Chronic fatigue syndrome is not a conversion disorder, nor is it a psychosomatic illness. Current re-search describes immune dysfunction in which T cells are chronically activated and hypothalamic dysfunction occurs, presumably because of cytokine penetration of the blood-brain barrier. Alpha-intrusion sleep disorder is probably also the result of cytokine penetration and may be worsened by myofascial pain, if present.

A10. **e.** Chronic fatigue syndrome may be classified as mild, moderate, or severe, depending on the number of symptoms present. Severe chronic fatigue syndrome may include not only fatigue, myofascial pain, and sleep disruption but also numerous neurologic complaints such as blurred vision, migrating paresthesias, and tinnitus. Mood disruption may be present; either depression or anxiety or both are often endogenous, reflecting neurochemical dysequilibrium. Cognitive dysfunction may be severe, with complaints of poor memory, poor concentration, and the inability to read.

A11. **e.** The symptoms of chronic fatigue syndrome can be induced in healthy individuals after only three nights of sleep disruption. This reduces stage 3, stage 4, or rapid-eye-movement (REM) sleep. Individuals who develop significant back pain after a motor vehicle accident (MVA) to the degree that it causes sleep disruption may also develop chronic fatigue syndrome. If immune activation is the initial trigger for the disease, it may be the result of many pathogens, although none of these has been identified.

A12. **e.** NSAIDs are often helpful in treating the symptoms of headache, diffuse pain, and feverishness. The nonsedating antidepressants may be useful in the treatment of depression, which is a predominant symptom in many patients.

A13. **d.** Empirical evidence suggests that patients with chronic fatigue syndrome lose their tolerance to many agents, including toxins such as secondhand cigarette smoke, certain fumes, alcohol, and medications. Antidepressants, such as amitriptyline, should be initially given to chronic fatigue patients in a dose approximately one fourth of the usual dose, although gradual tolerance may develop. When higher doses are used, physicians should carefully watch for symptoms of neurologic toxicity, which may, according to some, leave permanent deficits.

A14. **a.** The main therapeutic strategy in treating chronic fatigue syndrome should be to correct the sleep disorder. If the sleep disorder can be reduced and a period with more stage 3, stage 4, or REM sleep attained, the number of symptoms and their severity may be greatly reduced. This includes not only the symptoms of fatigue and pain but also the neurologic and mood/cognitive complaints. Patients required to return to work early when still symptomatic tend to suffer relapses and actually prolong their illness.

A15. **e.** Most patients with chronic fatigue syndrome partially recover within 2 years, often to the extent that they can return to work and resume most of the normal activities of their previous life. They are, however, at risk for relapse at any time (especially when they experience immune activation or sleep disruption).

A16. **e.** Risk factors for the development of chronic fatigue syndrome include a family member (especially a spouse) with the disorder, recurrent immune activation, and a recent MVA.

SOLUTION TO THE SHORT ANSWER MANAGEMENT PROBLEM

The relationship between chronic fatigue syndrome and fibromyalgia is fascinating. There certainly seems to be some connection between the two disorders. Some authorities believe that fibromyalgia and chronic fatigue syndrome are actually the same illness with different presentations. Clinicians see patients with more pain than fatigue, with more fatigue than pain, or with both fatigue and pain. Both fibromyalgia and chronic fatigue syndrome appear to share the alpha-intrusion sleep disorder.

SUMMARY OF THE DIAGNOSIS AND MANAGEMENT OF CHRONIC FATIGUE SYNDROME

1. Prevalence: Difficult to establish: The CDC estimated the prevalence to be 2 to 7 cases per 100,000 people (Straus). On the other hand, it is higher in specific subpopulations. For example, it has been estimated to be 5.1% (5100/100,000) among Gulf War veterans (Han et al).

   Chronic fatigue syndrome is not a new disease; it has been present for centuries. Most evidence for the disorder comes from outbreaks of the disorder, discussed earlier.

2. Etiology: The cause of chronic fatigue syndrome is unknown. Chronic fatigue syndrome, does, however, appear to be related to infectious agents (although none that has been investigated has been found to be linked to the disease) and immunologic

disturbances; T-cell activation may play a prominent role. Cytokines also appear to be involved. Alpha-intrusion sleep disorder appears to be related to cytokine involvement.

3. Signs and symptoms: The best diagnostic criteria at present have been set by the CDC. These criteria are listed in the Answer 1. It is important to diagnose and treat other syndromes, including major depressive disorder, which may present with complaints of chronic fatigue or that otherwise complicate the picture.

4. Course: Most patients partially recover within 2 years. All, however, are prone to relapse.

5. Treatment:
   a. Nonpharmacologic: An understanding physician who is prepared to spend time with the patient and listen and counsel in an empathetic fashion
   b. Pharmacologic: Empiric evidence suggests that the pharmacologic treatments of choice are L-tryptophan and clarithromycin. Please note that this is empiric evidence.

   Other pharmacologic agents that have been shown to be effective include NSAIDs and the tricyclic antidepressants. Select the dose carefully and begin at one fourth the usual dose.

SUGGESTED READINGS

Fukuda K et al: The chronic fatigue syndrome: A comprehensive approach to its definition and study, *Ann Intern Med* 121: 953-959, 1994.

Han KK et al: *Prevalence of chronic fatigue syndrome among U.S. Gulf War veterans.* Abstract3/4Biannual Research Conference, Cambridge, Mass, 1998, American Association for Chronic Fatigue Syndrome.

Straus S: Chronic fatigue syndrome. In Fauci AS et al, eds: *Harrison's principles of internal medicine,* ed 14, New York, 1998, McGraw-Hill.

PROBLEM·33

GOUT

"Ouch, My Big Toe!"

Case 1 ■ A 45-Year-Old Male with Excruciating Pain in His Left Foot

A 45-year-old obese male comes to the Emergency Department in the middle of the night screaming and holding his left foot. He tells you that he thinks he has an "acute blood vessel blockage" in his left toe. He wakes up the entire Emergency Department observation unit with his screams.

His history is significant for essential hypertension, for which he has been treated with a thiazide diuretic for the past 5 years. He categorically relates to you that he has never had the symptoms that he is experiencing now (and further adds that instead of all these questions he would prefer if you just got on with treatment).

On examination the patient's temperature is 38° C and his blood pressure is 170/110 mm Hg. He has an inflamed, tender, swollen left great toe. There is extensive swelling and erythema of the left foot, and his whole foot is tender. No other joints are swollen. No other abnormalities are found on physical examination.

SELECT THE BEST ANSWER
TO THE FOLLOWING QUESTIONS

Q1. What is the most likely diagnosis?
   a. acute cellulitis
   b. acute gouty arthritis
   c. acute rheumatoid arthritis
   d. acute septic arthritis
   e. acute vasculitis

Q2. Which of the following statements regarding this man's condition is false?
   a. the disease is more common in males than in females
   b. fever is unusual
   c. more than 50% of the initial attacks of this condition are confined to the first metatarsophalangeal joint
   d. peripheral leukocytosis can occur
   e. involvement is usually asymmetric

Q3. What is the definitive diagnostic test of choice for this patient's condition?
   a. a plasma level
   b. a random urine determination
   c. a 24-hour urine determination
   d. a synovial fluid analysis
   e. a Gram stain and culture and sensitivity

Q4. What is the most common metabolic abnormality found in the condition described in this patient?
   a. increased production of uric acid
   b. decreased renal excretion of uric acid
   c. increased production of uric acid metabolites
   d. decreased renal excretion of uric acid metabolites
   e. none of the above

Q5. What is the pharmacologic agent of choice for the initial management of this patient's condition?
   a. indomethacin
   b. colchicine
   c. acetaminophen
   d. aspirin
   e. phenylbutazone

Q6. Regarding the prophylaxis recommended for the prevention of future attacks of the condition described in the patient, which of the following would most accurately describe the current recommendation (as applied)?
   a. this patient probably should not be treated with a prophylactic agent
   b. this patient should be treated with a uricosuric agent as prophylaxis against future attacks of this condition
   c. this patient should be treated with a xanthine oxidase inhibitor as prophylaxis against future attacks of this condition
   d. this patient could be treated with either a uricosuric agent or a xanthine oxidase inhibitor as prophylaxis against future attacks of this condition
   e. none of the above

Q7. The determination of the agent of choice for the prophylaxis of the condition described is made by which of the following?
   a. a serum blood level
   b. a joint fluid aspiration
   c. a 24-hour urine determination of uric acid
   d. a joint x-ray
   e. none of the above

Q8. Which of the following drugs increase(s) the excretion of uric acid?
   a. sulfinpyrazone
   b. probenecid
   c. allopurinol
   d. a and b only
   e. all of the above

Q9. In patients started on prophylactic therapy, which of the following statements regarding the use of prophylactic agents is (are) true?
   a. the patient who is begun on a prophylactic agent should also be started on colchicine
   b. colchicine should be added and maintained for 3 to 6 months
   c. indomethacin can replace colchicine in this instance
   d. none of the above statements is true
   e. all of the above statements are true

Q10. Which of the following drugs would be most likely to provide significant relief in the case of an acute attack of the condition described?
a. oral prednisone
b. oral dexamethasone (Decadron)
c. intravenous (IV) hydrocortisone (Solu-Cortef)
d. IV methylprednisolone (Solu-Medrol)
e. intraarticular methylprednisolone acetate

Q11. Which of the following classes of drugs is most likely to precipitate the condition described?
a. thiazide diuretics
b. calcium channel blockers
c. angiotensin-converting enzyme (ACE) inhibitors
d. β-blockers
e. α-blockers

Case 2 ■ A 55-Year-Old Male with Joint Pain

A 55-year-old male patient comes to your office complaining about joint pain. He states that he has had pain in both ankles for the past 4 months, which has been getting progressively worse. He also states that, on occasion, he also has pain in his wrists. Although his blood pressure is now within normal limits (138/75 mm Hg), he states that for the last 5 years he has been treated with 50 mg of hydrochlorothiazide per day for hypertension.

As part of a routine work-up you find that he has a serum uric acid level of 12.4 mg/dl.

Q12. Which of the following statements is (are) true?
a. the uric acid blood level is elevated
b. the uric acid blood level is depressed
c. the uric acid blood level is within the normal range
d. if the uric acid blood level is abnormal, treatment should be considered to prevent the condition described even if there are no symptoms
e. a and d are true

SHORT ANSWER MANAGEMENT PROBLEM
Discuss the indications for the use of prophylactic agents in hyperuricemic states.

ANSWERS

A1. **b.** This patient has acute gouty arthritis. This is a very typical presentation for gout. With acute gout, the patient usually develops an acute pain in a joint of the lower extremity, with the most common joint being the metatarsophalangeal joint of the big toe. The pain of acute gout often wakes the patient from sleep, and the patient ends up in the Emergency Department with a pain that is described as crushing or excruciating.

The joint rapidly becomes erythematous, swollen, warm, and extremely tender. The skin surrounding the joint is usually tense and shiny. The swelling in acute gout often extends well beyond the joint itself and may involve the entire foot (or other part of the extremity). This swelling, resulting from periarticular edema, makes the differentiation from septic arthritis particularly difficult. Often the patient is unable to bear weight on the affected foot.

A2. **b.** Fever may occur in patients with gout, especially in patients with polyarticular disease. The temperature may reach 39.5° C (103° to 104° F).

The metatarsophalangeal joint is the location of the acute gouty attack in over 50% of patients experiencing their first attack. Obviously the big toe is not the initial site for a significant minority of patients. Most first attacks are asymmetric. If untreated, involvement of other joints of the foot may occur simultaneously or follow rapidly. Acute gout may also involve the bursae or the tendon sheaths.

Leukocytosis may also be seen. Tophi are occasionally seen with the first attack. Usually, however, there is a time interval (often 10 years or more) between the initial attack and the appearance of the complication of a gouty tophus.

Gout is more common in men than in women. In women it most often occurs after menopause.

A3. **d.** The ultimate diagnosis of gout is made by demonstrating negatively birefringent, needle-shaped crystals under a polarizing microscope. This examination should be attempted in all patients suspected of having gout. Although an elevated serum uric acid concentration is usually seen with acute gout, it is neither as sensitive nor as specific a test as the demonstration of uric acid crystals in synovial fluid under the microscope.

The diagnosis of septic arthritis can be ruled out by appropriate Gram stains and cultures of the same specimen of synovial fluid as obtained for examination with the polarizing microscope.

A4. **b.** The most common metabolic abnormality associated with gout is decreased renal excretion of uric acid. This may be a primary or a secondary event. Secondary causes such as chronic renal disease, acute ethanol ingestion, and diuretic (especially thiazide diuretic) therapy are associated with the development of elevated serum uric acid levels and subsequent gout.

The most common cause of overproduction of uric acid is a myeloproliferative or lymphoproliferative disorder. In addition, when a patient is undergoing cancer chemotherapy there is a very significant liberation of uric acid from dying cells. The greater the responsiveness of the tumor to chemotherapy or radiotherapy, the quicker is the tumor breakdown and the more extensive the breakdown of uric acid.

A5. **a.** Until recently, colchicine was the drug of choice for the treatment of acute gout. This agent, however, has many gastrointestinal side effects that limit its usefulness, especially with the frequency and dose needed in acute gout (hourly).

NSAIDs such as indomethacin 50 mg tid are now the drugs of choice in most settings. The NSAIDs should ideally be given for a 1- to 2-week period until treatment aimed at decreasing the uric acid pool is begun.

Aspirin taken in small doses can actually aggravate the problem. Acetaminophen has no antiinflammatory activity and is not indicated in the acute treatment of gout. Phenylbutazone is an excellent antiinflammatory agent but has been associated with bone marrow suppression and aplastic anemia. Systemic corticosteroid therapy can be used to treat patients with acute gout who have not responded to other therapies and patients in whom other therapies are contraindicated. Intraarticular injections of a corticosteroid are usually very effective in patients with acute monarticular gout.

A6. **a.** From the history, you gather that this is the first attack of acute gout in this patient. The current recommendation suggests that it is not advisable to begin prophylactic therapy until the patient has had at least two attacks, or perhaps three. This recommendation is made for the following two reasons:
a. If there is a precipitating secondary cause (as in this patient with the treatment of hypertension using a thiazide diuretic), it may very well be able to be eliminated.
b. Because a second attack may not occur for years (if at all), the risk-to-benefit ratio for prophylactic medication is not favorable.

A7. **c.** The choice of a prophylactic agent (if one is going to be used) is made by determining the 24-hour secretion of uric acid.

A8. **d.** If the patient excretes significantly more uric acid than 750 mg/24 hours, he is producing too much uric acid, and the production should be slowed by treatment with a drug that inhibits production. The rate-determining step in the synthetic pathway depends on the enzyme xanthine oxidase. Allopurinol, the usual drug given, is an inhibitor of xanthine oxidase. If the patient excretes less than 750 mg/24 hours of uric acid, then the metabolic problem rests with the failure to excrete the uric acid once it is produced. In this case, drugs that increase the excretion rate, known as uricosuric agents, should be used. The two most common drugs in this class are probenecid and sulfinpyrazone.

A9. **e.** As previously discussed, the prophylactic agents for the prevention of gouty arthritis fall into two classes: The xanthine oxidase inhibitors (which inhibit the formation of uric acid) and the uricosuric agents (which increase the excretion of uric acid).

When prophylaxis against recurrent attacks is begun, either colchicine or an NSAID such as indomethacin should be added to the choice of the prophylactic agent for 3 to 6 months. The colchicine or indomethacin can then be discontinued, and the patient can remain on the uricosuric agent or the xanthine oxidase inhibitor indefinitely.

If the uricosuric agent is the preferred treatment because of the 24-hour urine uric acid determination, the following rules should be followed:
a. Uricosuric agents should be used only in patients with normal renal function.
b. Uricosuric agents should be used only in patients who have no history of renal stone formation.
c. Uricosuric agents should be used only in patients who do not overproduce uric acid.

Allopurinol is indicated in patients with urate overproduction, history of renal stones, and renal impairment.

A10. **e.** A local injection of a corticosteroid such as methylprednisolone acetate into an inflamed gouty joint reliably produces resolution of the acute gouty condition. This treatment appears to be most beneficial in patients with acute gouty monarthritis of a large joint (which may receive injections reliably) and in patients with resistant attacks in whom coexistent infection has been excluded.

A11. **a.** Diuretics in general, and thiazide diuretics in particular, elevate the serum uric acid level. Although the vast majority of patients who are receiving thiazide diuretics do not develop gout, those who do tend to be on relatively high doses of thiazide (anything greater than 25 mg) and have other coexistent reasons for the development of gout (such as acute ethanol intake).

It has been conclusively shown that increasing the dosage of a thiazide diuretic above 25 mg/day will not improve hypertension control; instead it will simply increase the probability of significantly elevated uric acid levels.

The six metabolic side effects of thiazide diuretics are as follows: hyperuricemia, hyperglycemia, hyperlipidemia, hypokalemia, hyponatremia, and hypomagnesemia.

A12. **a.** The condition being discussed in this question is asymptomatic hyperuricemia. The symptoms described do not suggest gout and are unlikely to be related to the uric acid level. The question that arises from this condition is, "Should the hyperuricemia be treated?" The answer is no.

Asymptomatic hyperuricemia results most commonly from a pharmacologic agent; that pharmacologic agent is most commonly a thiazide diuretic. Even though a thiazide diuretic (especially in high dose) can produce a very significant increase in the serum uric acid level, well over 95% of patients with asymptomatic hyperuricemia remain asymptomatic. Thus the treatment of asymptomatic hyperuricemia is not recommended.

SOLUTION TO THE SHORT ANSWER MANAGEMENT PROBLEM

The prophylactic agents used in the prevention of recurrence of acute gout have been discussed in detail. In brief review, prophylactic agents should be used only if the patient has had more than one attack of gout, a gouty tophus develops, there is x-ray evidence of joint destruction from the gouty arthritis, or there is a history of urolithiasis.

SUMMARY OF THE DIAGNOSIS AND TREATMENT OF ACUTE GOUT

1. Diagnosis: Firmly established by examination of joint aspirate under a polarizing microscope (negatively birefringent uric acid crystals)

2. Symptoms: Acute onset of pain in a joint of the lower extremity, most commonly the first metatarsophalangeal joint. Along with the pain there are associated tenderness, erythema, and swelling of the surrounding tissues.

3. Differential diagnosis: The most important differential diagnosis in acute gout is septic arthritis.

4. Pathophysiology: Acute gout is most often associated with a decreased renal excretion of uric acid (rather than an overproduction of uric acid).

5. Treatment:
   a. Acute attack: Indomethacin; colchicine is an alternative agent
   b. Prophylactic treatment:
      1) Not given after only one attack
      2) Choose either a uricosuric agent or a xanthine oxidase inhibitor. Choice is based on the results of the 24-hour urine uric acid determination plus other factors previously discussed.
      3) If prophylaxis is given, then use either indomethacin or colchicine in low dose in addition to your prophylactic agent for 3 to 6 months.
      4) Do not treat asymptomatic hyperuricemia.

SUGGESTED READING
Yood R: Hyperuricemia and gout. In Rakel R, ed: *Conn's current therapy*, Philadelphia, 1994, WB Saunders.

PROBLEM·34

GLOMERULONEPHRITIS

"The Blood in My Urine Came from My Sore Throat?"

Case 1 ■ A 29-Year-Old Female with Fatigue, Anorexia, and Bloody Urine

A 29-year-old female comes to your office with symptoms of extreme fatigue, no appetite, and bloody urine. She developed a very sore throat 3 weeks ago, but did not have it examined or treated. Her 6-year-old daughter had a similar sore throat 1 week before her. Her doctor (over the phone) said, "You probably have a viral infection from your daughter. Don't worry about it."

Three days ago she began to have bloody urine and swelling of her hands and feet, and she felt terrible. Her past health had been excellent. There is no family history of significant illness. She has no allergies.

On examination, she has significant edema of both lower extremities. Her blood pressure is 170/105 mm Hg. Her blood pressure was last checked 1 year ago; at that time it was normal.

SELECT THE BEST ANSWER TO THE FOLLOWING QUESTIONS

Q1. What is the most likely diagnosis in this patient at this time?
   a. hemorrhagic pyelonephritis
   b. IgA nephropathy (Berger's disease)
   c. poststreptococcal glomerulonephritis
   d. hemorrhagic cystitis
   e. membranous glomerulonephritis

Q2. Which of the following is pathognomonic of the disorder described in Case 1?
a. macroscopic hematuria
b. microscopic hematuria
c. eosinophils in the urine
d. red blood cell casts
e. protein 1.0 g/24 hours

Q3. Approximately 4 weeks after the mother develops her symptoms, her daughter comes down with an illness characterized by swelling of a number of joints with erythema and pain, bumps on both of her elbows, significant fatigue, fever, and a skin rash covering her body. On examination, the daughter has a grade III/VI pansystolic murmur. Her blood pressure is 100/70 mm Hg. What is the most likely diagnosis in her daughter's case?
a. juvenile rheumatoid arthritis
b. Still's disease
c. postviral arthritis syndrome
d. rheumatic fever
e. autoimmune complex disease

Q4. Which of the following statements regarding the prevention of the problems experienced by the patient and her daughter is true, assuming both are treated with 10 days of penicillin?
a. the mother's condition was preventable by penicillin; the daughter's condition was not
b. the mother's condition was not preventable by penicillin; the daughter's condition was
c. both the mother's and the daughter's conditions were preventable by treatment with penicillin
d. neither the mother's condition nor the daughter's condition could have been prevented by treatment with penicillin
e. prevention is variable with both conditions: penicillin may prevent both conditions, but it may not prevent either

Q5. What is the treatment of choice for the condition described in the mother?
a. penicillin
b. gentamicin
c. prednisone
d. a and b
e. none of the above

Q6. Which of the following statements concerning prognosis of the condition described in the mother is (are) true?
a. most patients with this disorder eventually develop end-stage renal failure
b. the prognosis in the mother depends on how aggressively the antecedent streptococcal infection is treated
c. most patients with the acute disease recover completely within 1 to 2 years
d. 5% to 20% of patients with this acute disease end up with progressive renal disease
e. c and d

Q7. Which of the following is a (are) complication(s) of the disease process described in the mother?
a. hypertensive encephalopathy
b. congestive cardiac failure
c. acute renal failure
d. a and b
e. all of the above

Q8. Which of the following subtypes of the disease presented in the mother is associated with group A β-hemolytic streptococcus?
a. minimal change
b. focal segmental sclerosis
c. membranous
d. diffuse proliferative
e. crescentic

Q9. Which of the following subtypes of the disease presented in the mother is most closely associated with nephrotic syndrome?
a. minimal change
b. focal segmental sclerosis
c. membranous
d. diffuse proliferative
e. crescentic

Q10. What is the most common cause of chronic renal failure?
a. glomerulonephritis (acute to chronic)
b. chronic pyelonephritis
c. diabetes mellitus
d. hypertensive renal disease
e. congenital anomalies

Q11. What is the least common cause of chronic renal failure among the following causes?
a. glomerulonephritis (acute to chronic)
b. chronic pyelonephritis
c. hypertensive renal disease
d. diabetes mellitus
e. congenital anomalies

Q12. Which of the following antihypertensive agents is contraindicated in patients with chronic renal disease?
a. hydrochlorothiazide-triamterene
b. furosemide

c. prazosin
d. nifedipine
e. α-methyldopa

Q13. What is the major cause of death in patients with chronic renal failure?
   a. uremia
   b. malignant hypertension
   c. hyperkalemia-induced arrhythmias
   d. myocardial infarction
   e. subarachnoid hemorrhage

Q14. What is the anemia usually associated with chronic renal failure?
   a. hypochromic
   b. macrocytic
   c. normochromic: normocytic
   d. microcytic
   e. hypochromic: microcytic

Q15. Which of the following may be indicated in the treatment of a patient with chronic renal failure?
   a. limitation of dietary protein
   b. sodium supplementation
   c. calcium supplementation
   d. a and b
   e. all of the above

Q16. Which of the following is (are) associated with nephrotic syndrome?
   a. proteinuria, 3.5 g/day
   b. edema
   c. hypoalbuminemia
   d. hypercholesterolemia
   e. all of the above

Q17. Which of the following statements regarding nephrotic syndrome is false?
   a. most patients with nephrotic syndrome progress to chronic renal failure
   b. some cases of nephrotic syndrome are drug induced
   c. Hodgkin's disease may lead to nephrotic syndrome
   d. preeclamptic toxemia may lead to nephrotic syndrome
   e. none of the above statements is false

Q18. Which of the following statements regarding diabetes mellitus and chronic renal failure is true?
   a. diabetes mellitus is an uncommon cause of chronic renal failure
   b. diabetes mellitus type 1 is a more common cause of chronic renal failure than diabetes mellitus type 2

c. diabetes mellitus type 2 is a more common cause of chronic renal failure than diabetes mellitus type 1
   d. diabetes mellitus type 2 does not lead to chronic renal failure
   e. diabetes mellitus type 1 does not lead to chronic renal failure

Q19. The treatment of nephrotic syndrome includes which of the following?
   a. corticosteroids
   b. loop diuretics
   c. thiazide diuretics
   d. protein restriction
   e. all of the above

Q20. What percentage of patients with any of the primary glomerulonephropathies present with a nephrotic syndromelike picture?
   a. 10%
   b. 20%
   c. 40%
   d. 50%
   e. 75%

Q21. Comparing the recommended treatment of poststreptococcal glomerulonephritis (PSGN) with the recommended treatment on non-poststreptococcal glomerulonephritis (NPSGN), which of the following statements is most accurate?
   a. the treatment protocols are the same
   b. corticosteroid treatment is indicated for both PSGN and NPSGN
   c. corticosteroid treatment is generally not indicated in for PSGN but is for NPSGN
   d. corticosteroid treatment is generally indicated for PSGN but not for NPSGN
   e. the prognosis of neither PSGN nor NPSGN depends on the presence or absence of treatment

SHORT ANSWER MANAGEMENT PROBLEM
Discuss the importance of the use of nonsteroidal antiinflammatory drugs (NSAIDs) as a cause of renal dysfunction in elderly patients.

ANSWERS

A1. **c.** This patient has poststreptococcal glomerulonephritis. Poststreptococcal glomerulonephritis is the most common cause of acute glomerulonephritis. The syndrome may begin as early as 2 weeks after the initial streptococcal infection. In patients with mild disease, there may be no signs of symptoms. In more severe disease, the symptoms of malaise, headache, mild fever, flank pain, edema, hypertension, and pulmonary edema may occur. Oliguria is common. The urine is often described as bloody, coffee colored, or smoky.

A2. **d.** The red blood cell casts are found in the urine of patients with acute glomerulonephritis and are pathognomonic for this condition. Other notable abnormalities include an elevated erythrocyte sedimentation rate (ESR) and an elevated antistreptolysin O (ASO) titer.

A3. **d.** In this case, the daughter of the patient has developed rheumatic fever. The Jones criteria for the diagnosis of rheumatic fever include the following:

Major Criteria	Minor Criteria
(1) Carditis	(1) Arthralgias
(2) Polyarthritis	(2) Fever
(3) Chorea	(3) Elevated ESR
(4) Erythema marginatum	(4) Elevated C-reactive protein
(5) Subcutaneous nodules	(5) Prolonged PR interval on ECG

Two major criteria or one major criterion and two minor criteria are virtually diagnostic of rheumatic fever.

It is important to realize that in some parts of the United States, the incidence of rheumatic fever is rising, not falling. This has been a relatively recent phenomenon and is a cause for concern in terms of the treatment (or lack of treatment) of streptococcal pharyngitis.

A4. **b.** Poststreptococcal glomerulonephritis is not preventable by penicillin; rheumatic fever, on the other hand, is preventable. In both conditions, the cause of complications is group A β-hemolytic streptococcus. Once the clinical or laboratory diagnosis of streptococcal pharyngitis is made, therapy with penicillin should be instituted and continued for a period of 10 days.

A5. **e.** The primary treatment of acute glomerulonephritis associated with streptococcal infection is symptomatic. Although penicillin will eradicate the carrier state of group A β-hemolytic streptococci, it will not influence the course of the glomerulonephritis.

Symptomatic treatment should include bed rest and protein restriction (if the blood urea nitrogen [BUN] or

creatinine level is elevated). Fluid overload should be treated with loop diuretics such as furosemide or ethacrynic acid. If acute renal insufficiency develops and volume overload is unresponsive to diuretics, hemodialysis should be considered.

A6. **e.** Most patients with acute glomerulonephritis recover completely within 1 to 2 years. On the other hand, 5% to 20% of patients will end up with progressive renal damage. As indicated above, the treatment of the antecedent streptococcal infection has no bearing on the prognosis.

A7. **e.** Complications of acute poststreptococcal glomerulonephritis include hypertensive encephalopathy, congestive cardiac failure, acute renal failure, chronic renal failure (5% to 20%), and nephrotic syndrome.

A8. **d.** Poststreptococcal glomerulonephritis usually presents as a diffuse proliferative glomerulonephritis.

A9. **a.** Nephrotic syndrome usually presents as minimal change glomerulonephritis.

A10. **c.** The most common cause of chronic renal failure is diabetes mellitus, not glomerulonephritis. Forty percent of patients with type 1 diabetes mellitus eventually develop diabetic nephropathy chronic renal failure. Twenty percent of patients with type 2 diabetes mellitus develop diabetic nephropathy and subsequent chronic renal failure.

A11. **b.** Chronic pyelonephritis is the least likely cause of chronic renal failure of those listed. Chronic pyelonephritis rarely leads to chronic renal failure in the absence of obstruction.

A12. **a.** Potassium-sparing diuretics such as the triamterene component of a mixed thiazide—potassium-sparing diuretic combination can cause hyperkalemia. All of the other agents, including hydrochlorothiazide (alone), furosemide, prazosin, nifedipine, and α-methyldopa are safe to use in chronic renal failure. The dosage of all of these agents, however, should be reduced when renal failure supervenes.

In addition to the potassium-sparing diuretics, the ACE inhibitors and angiotensin receptor blockers can also significantly raise the serum potassium level. Thus they must never be used in patients with chronic renal failure who are receiving any kind of potassium-sparing diuretic or other potassium supplement for any reason. Second, they are at least relatively contraindicated when patients develop the degree of renal insufficiency necessary to produce chronic renal failure.

A13. **d.** The major causes of death in patients with chronic renal failure are myocardial infarction and cardiovascular accidents (CVAs), secondary to atherosclerosis and arteriolosclerosis. Uremia itself can be controlled by dialysis or renal transplantation. Hypertension is usually controllable by individualized antihypertensive therapy. Arrhythmias, although they do occur in these patients, are not the major cause of death. Subarachnoid hemorrhage, as a subset of a CVA, does occur but is less common as a cause of death than myocardial infarction.

A14. **c.** The anemia of chronic renal failure is usually normochromic:normocytic. Hematocrit often starts to decrease when the serum creatinine level reaches 200 to 300 μmol/L (2 to 3 mg/dl) or when the glomerular filtration rate has decreased to about 20 to 30 ml/min.

The etiology of the normochromic:normocytic anemia is probably a decreased synthesis of erythropoietin by the kidney.

A15. **e.** Treatment of chronic renal failure may include any of the following:
  a. Limitation of dietary protein
  b. Careful control of water balance: Fluid intake should be sufficient to maintain adequate urine volume, but no attempt should be made to force diuresis. If edema is present, a cautious trial of furosemide or ethacrynic acid is indicated, with careful monitoring of serum electrolyte levels.
  c. Electrolyte supplementation/restriction: Sodium supplements may be required to restore sodium losses. Potassium intake may have to be restricted or supplemented. In severe hyperkalemia, acute measures to remove potassium may be required.
  d. Mineral supplementation/restriction: In the presence of bone disease (renal osteodystrophy), treatment with phosphate binders and supplemental calcium may be necessary.

A16. **e.** Nephrotic syndrome, as previously mentioned, is most closely associated with minimal change glomerulonephritis.

Nephrotic syndrome is characterized by albuminuria (3.5 g/day), hypoalbuminemia, hyperlipidemia, edema, hypertension, and renal insufficiency.

A17. **a.** Most cases of nephrotic syndrome do not in fact lead to chronic renal failure. It depends entirely on the etiology. The causes of nephrotic syndrome are as follows:
  a. Primary glomerular diseases (all subtypes)

  b. Secondary to infections (including poststreptococcal glomerulonephritis)
  c. Drugs (such as penicillamine and gold)
  d. Neoplasia (as in Hodgkin's disease)
  e. Multi-system disease (systemic lupus erythematosus [SLE], Goodpasture's syndrome)
  f. Endocrine diseases (diabetes mellitus)
  g. Miscellaneous (preeclamptic toxemia)

A18. **c.** As stated before, diabetes mellitus is the most common cause of chronic renal failure. Although the prevalence is less common in type 2 (20%) as opposed to type 1 (40%) diabetes, the prevalence of type 2 diabetes is actually 10 times the prevalence of type 1 diabetes. The logical conclusion from this consideration is that type 2 diabetes mellitus is a more common cause of chronic renal failure than type 1 diabetes mellitus.

A19. **e.** Nephrotic syndrome is treated with nonpharmacologic symptomatic therapies such as protein restriction and excessive fluid restriction, pharmacologic symptomatic therapies such as thiazide and loop diuretics, and antiinflammatory/immunosuppressive therapies (prednisone and cytotoxic drugs).

It has been demonstrated that antiinflammatory drugs such as prednisone enhance the potential for the disorder to attain remission. The usual protocol includes high-dose corticosteroid therapy followed by a gradual reduction to the point where alternate-day therapy with prednisone is introduced.

A20. **b.** The natural history proposed for nephrotic syndrome suggests that approximately 20% of patients who have a primary glomerulonephropathy of some kind will develop nephrotic syndrome.

A21. **c.** The most important difference in therapy between PSGN and NPSGN is corticosteroid therapy (useful in NPSGN but not in PSGN). In NPSGN, corticosteroids can be used both in the primary presentation and in recurrences.

SOLUTION TO THE SHORT ANSWER MANAGEMENT PROBLEM

NSAIDs are a major concern because of their ability to induce nephrotoxicity, especially in elderly patients. Nephrotoxicity as a potential problem when beginning or maintaining elderly patients on NSAIDs is frequently either not thought of or ignored. The NSAID sulindac has been suggested as a possible exception to this problem, as it may be the one NSAID that will not cause nephrotoxicity. However, extreme caution is still required. NSAID use is the most common cause of renal insufficiency in the elderly. When considering prescribing an NSAID to an elderly patient, it is wise to follow clinical practice guidelines that resemble the following Clinical Practice Guidelines:

1. Establish a definitive diagnosis.
2. Ask yourself this question: Is this an inflammatory condition? If yes, an NSAID is reasonable (as in rheumatoid arthritis). If no (as in osteoarthritis), is there an alternative medication that will provide relief with minimal adverse effects, such as acetaminophen plain or acetaminophen with a small amount of codeine (8 mg)?
3. If you decide to start an elderly patient on an NSAID, perform baseline renal function tests, including a 24-hour urine for creatinine clearance and protein.
4. Consider choosing an NSAID with a favorable efficacy/renal toxicity profile (such as sulindac).
5. Begin with the lowest dose.
6. Consider gastric protection to avoid gastric problems, such as gastritis, peptic ulcer, and reflux esophagitis. If you decide to use an H2 blocker, consider one demonstrated to have a favorable efficacy/side effect profile in the elderly (such as ranitidine).
7. Recheck the patient's renal function in 3 months.
8. Continue to monitor the efficacy/side effect profile at all times and always ask yourself this question: Are you doing more good than harm?
9. Never combine an NSAID and a potassium-sparing diuretic, or an NSAID and an ACE inhibitor, in an elderly patient. This can and will produce rapid and potentially fatal hyperkalemia.

Remember, first do no harm.

SUMMARY OF THE DIAGNOSIS AND TREATMENT OF RENAL DISEASES

1. Glomerulonephritis:
   a. Classification (simplified):
      1) Poststreptococcal glomerulonephritis (PSGN)
      2) Nonpoststreptococcal glomerulonephritis (NPSGN) (many subtypes)
   b. Symptoms and signs:
      1) Malaise
      2) Headache
      3) Anorexia
      4) Low-grade fever
      5) Edema
      6) Hypertension
      7) Gross hematuria with red blood cell casts
      8) Proteinuria
      9) Impaired renal function

   Remember: *Not all that appears to be congestive heart failure actually is.* For example, uremic pericarditis is often diagnosed as congestive heart failure and mistreated with diuretic therapy. Increased jugular venous pressure does not always equal congestive heart failure. (See also Problem 4.)
   c. Treatment:
      1) PSGN that is symptomatic: Protein restriction, fluid restriction, thiazide and loop diuretics
      2) NPSGN that is symptomatic: As described for PSGN plus corticosteroids; initially high dose with gradual tapering; alternate-day therapy suggested as ideal

2. Nephrotic syndrome:
   a. Etiology and prevalence:
      1) Many and diverse causes
      2) 20% of primary glomerulonephropathies develop into nephrotic syndrome
   b. Signs and symptoms:
      1) Edema
      2) Hypoalbuminemia
      3) Hyperalbuminuria (greater than 3.5 g/day)
      4) Hypertension
      5) Hyperlipidemia
      6) Renal insufficiency
   c. Treatment: Symptomatic:
      1) Protein restriction
      2) Fluid restriction
      3) Thiazide and loop diuretics
      4) Prednisone
      5) Cytotoxic agents

3. Chronic renal failure:
   a. Cause: Most common cause is diabetes mellitus; most common type of diabetes mellitus is type 2
   b. Symptoms, signs, and laboratory findings:
      1) Weakness
      2) Fatigability
      3) Headaches
      4) Anorexia
      5) Nausea and vomiting
      6) Pruritus
      7) Polyuria
      8) Nocturia
      9) Hypertension
      10) Congestive heart failure
      11) Pericarditis
      12) Anemia
      13) Azotemia
      14) Acidosis

15) Elevated serum potassium levels
16) Decreased serum potassium levels
17) Decreased serum protein levels
   c. Treatment:
      1) Protein restriction
      2) Careful fluid balance
      3) Potassium restriction or supplementation
      4) Calcium supplementation
      5) Phosphate removal
      6) Hypertension control
      7) Hemodialysis or peritoneal dialysis
      8) Renal transplantation

SUGGESTED READINGS

Cattran DC: Primary glomerular diseases. In Rakel R, ed: *Conn's current therapy*, Philadelphia, 1994, WB Saunders.

Jennette JC, Falk RJ: Diagnosis and management of glomerular diseases, *Med Clin North Am* 23:477, 1997.

Palmer BF: Chronic renal failure. In Rakel R, ed: *Conn's current therapy*, Philadelphia, 1994, WB Saunders.

Walker R: General management of end stage renal disease, *Br J Med* 315:1429, 1997.

PROBLEM·35

URINARY TRACT INFECTIONS AND PYELONEPHRITIS

"Let's Avoid Dialysis If We Can."

Case 1 ■ ■ A 27-Year-Old Female with Spina Bifida and Bilateral Costovertebral Angle Pain

A 27-year-old female comes to the Emergency Department with a 4-day history of fever, chills, and bilateral costovertebral angle (CVA) pain. She has an indwelling urinary catheter and describes to you "at least 12 of these episodes before this current one." She has been seeing the same family physician since birth and has been diagnosed as having "nervous bladder and kidney syndrome." He has prescribed some over-the-counter (OTC) "kidney pills" in the past for these symptoms. She tells you that they "never really worked," and she has often found herself bed-bound with symptoms for several weeks before the fever broke.

You, the Emergency Department doctor on shift, are somewhat skeptical about the nervous bladder and kidney syndrome.

On examination, the patient is flushed. Her temperature is 40° C. She has intermittent shaking rigors. She has CVA tenderness bilaterally. Her abdomen is somewhat tender to palpation. There is blood in the catheter collection bag.

SELECT THE BEST ANSWER TO THE FOLLOWING QUESTIONS

Q1. What is the most likely diagnosis in this patient?
   a. nervous bladder and kidney syndrome
   b. acute hemorrhagic cystitis
   c. acute urethritis
   d. acute pyelonephritis
   e. the newly named spina bifida bladder spasm syndrome (SBBSS)

Q2. What would be the most likely organism in this patient?
   a. a gram-positive coccus
   b. a gram-positive rod
   c. an anaerobic organism
   d. a fungal organism
   e. a gram-negative organism

Q3. Which of the following bacteria would not likely be considered as a highly probable cause of this problem?
   a. *Pseudomonas aeruginosa*
   b. *Klebsiella pneumoniae*
   c. *Enterobacter*
   d. group A β-hemolytic streptococcus
   e. *Proteus*

Q4. After obtaining a urinalysis and a urine specimen for culture and sensitivity, you should now treat the patient with which of the following?
   a. the OTC kidney pills
   b. ciprofloxacin 500 mg tid PO (outpatient)
   c. Septra DS two tabs bid PO (outpatient)
   d. intravenous (IV) antibiotics in the hospital
   e. no medications are indicated at this time

Q5. What is (are) the antibiotic(s) of first choice for this patient?
   a. IV ceftriaxone (Rocephin) or cefotaxime (Claforan)
   b. IV trimethoprim-sulfamethoxazole (TMP-SMX)
   c. IV ciprofloxacin
   d. IV ampicillin and gentamicin
   e. any of the above

Q6. The investigations that should be performed on this patient at this time include which of the following?
   a. serum blood urea nitrogen (BUN)/creatinine
   b. renal ultrasound
   c. blood cultures
   d. complete blood count (CBC) with differential
   e. all of the above

Q7. The renal ultrasound shows small, shrunken kidneys, with no enlargement of the ureters and no stones. What is the most likely diagnosis in this patient?
a. chronic pyelonephritis
b. uterovesical reflux
c. hydronephrosis
d. vesicular diverticula
e. none of the above

Q8. Which of the following statements regarding chronic prophylaxis in this patient is true?
a. chronic prophylaxis is not indicated
b. chronic prophylaxis is unlikely to be of any benefit
c. chronic prophylaxis may make a significant difference in the preservation of this patient's renal function
d. chronic prophylaxis will be difficult because of resistant organisms
e. none of the above is true

Case 2 ■ A 34-Year-Old Female with Hematuria, Dysuria, Increased Urinary Frequency, and Nocturia

A 34-year-old female comes with a 3-day history of hematuria, dysuria, increased urinary frequency, and nocturia. She has had no fever, no chills, and no back pain.

On examination, she does not look ill. Her temperature is 37.5° C. Her abdomen is nontender. There is no CVA tenderness.

Q9. What is the most likely diagnosis?
a. Berger's disease (IgA nephropathy)
b. acute hemorrhagic cystitis
c. acute hemorrhagic urethritis
d. acute glomerulonephritis
e. acute cystitis with concomitant coagulation disorder

Q10. What is the treatment of choice for the patient described in Case 2?
a. a 10-day course of ampicillin and probenecid
b. a 7-day course of ampicillin and probenecid
c. a 3-day course of TMP-SMX
d. a 1-day course of TMP-SMX
e. a single dose of ampicillin 3.5 g and probenecid 1 g

Q11. You have now decided on your therapeutic plan for the patient described in Case 2. At what time would you implement this plan?
a. right away: forget about the cultures—you likely have a big enough "gun" to kill everything in sight anyway
b. right away: start therapy immediately after taking the urine specimen for culture and sensitivity
c. tomorrow: send the urine culture stat and order the pathologist to call you with the result personally
d. tomorrow: send the urine culture and ask the pathology department for a report as soon as possible without aggravating the pathologist
e. whenever: send the urine culture and when you get it back call the patient; if the symptoms have not cleared up, consider starting the antibiotic

Q12. What is the most likely organism involved in the infection that has developed in the patient described in Case 2?
a. *Pseudomonas aeruginosa*
b. *Providencia*
c. *Escherichia coli*
d. *Klebsiella*
e. *Enterococcus*

Q13. The quinolone antibiotics (such as ciprofloxacin and levofloxacin) are a very significant advance in antimicrobial treatment. They also work by a unique mechanism. The mechanism(s) of action is (are):
a. bactericidal mode of action
b. inhibits DNA gyrase
c. blocks protein synthesis
d. inhibits cell wall synthesis
e. a and b

SHORT ANSWER MANAGEMENT PROBLEM
Discuss a classification of urinary tract infections in adult males and adult females.

ANSWERS

A1. **d.** This patient has acute pyelonephritis. First, she has very significant predisposing factors for urinary tract infections, including an indwelling urinary catheter and a neurologic condition that increases the probability of same. Second, she seems to have had some less than optimal medical diagnoses. Third, she almost certainly has had recurrent episodes of pyelonephritis. This raises the possibilities of chronic pyelonephritis, reflux kidney damage, and resistant organisms. Fourth, the symptoms fit. Fever, chills, and CVA pain in a patient with a neurologic predisposing condition and an indwelling catheter equals acute pyelonephritis.

A2. **e.** First, this patient is classified as having a complicated urinary tract infection, which occurs when any of the following are present in the patient: Obstruction (stones), indwelling urinary catheter, high postvoid residual urine volume, anatomic or functional genitourinary abnormalities, renal impairment, and renal transplantation.

Although the most common organism is a gram-negative organism, it is frequently an organism that would not occur in patients without urinary tract disease. Examples include *Proteus, Providencia, Serratia, Pseudomonas, and Klebsiella.* Overall, *Escherichia coli* (one of many serotypes and one likely to be resistant to multiple antibiotics) is probably still the most common organism.

A3. **d.** The only organism listed that is an unlikely candidate is group A β-hemolytic streptococcus.

A4. **d.** This patient has not had any of the following at any time in the past:
 a. A proper assessment
 b. An accurate diagnosis
 c. Proper treatment
At this time, she should be hospitalized, treated with IV fluids and IV antibiotics, and have a complete assessment of both urinary tract function and urinary tract damage. In addition, ways of preventing future infections should be considered.

A5. **e.** Any of these regimens could be used for the treatment of acute pyelonephritis. Quinolones (such as ciprofloxacin or levofloxacin) are indicated for the treatment of complicated urinary tract infections and will cover most if not all gram-negative organisms, including *Proteus* and *Pseudomonas.* It would also be reasonable to use gentamicin, a combination of ampicillin and gentamicin, or a third-generation cephalosporin.

A6. **e.** At this time, a complete work-up should be done, including the following (as a minimum):
 a. Blood:
  1) CBC with differential
  2) Serum BUN/creatinine
  3) Electrolytes
  4) Blood cultures
 b. Urine:
  1) Complete urinalysis
  2) Urine for culture and sensitivity
  3) Urine for white blood cell and red blood cell casts
 c. Diagnostic imaging:
  1) Renal and abdominal ultrasound
  2) Intravenous pyelogram (IVP)

A7. **a.** This patient's abnormal ultrasound shows small, shrunken kidneys secondary to repeated urinary tract infections that have gone untreated. It is important from this time onward to measure renal function regularly and do everything possible to preserve this patient's renal function.

A8. **c.** First, repeated urine cultures must be done to determine the dominant organisms growing. Next, the susceptibility and resistance of these organisms must be determined to guide prophylactic therapy. It is difficult to say at this time what that therapy should be; it all depends on the results, but it certainly needs to be done.

A9. **b.** This patient has acute hemorrhagic cystitis, which is simply a variant of acute cystitis. It is no more difficult to treat and does not have any more complications than other forms of acute cystitis.

A10. **c.** Patients with uncomplicated urinary tract infections respond well to a 3-day treatment regimen. This abbreviated course of management is a good compromise between a 1-day course of therapy and the conventional 7- to 14-day regimens. The relapse rate with the 3-day regimen is comparable to longer courses of therapy. An abbreviated therapy is also more cost-effective and is associated with fewer adverse drug effects than the more prolonged courses of therapy.

TMP-SMX is certainly a drug of first choice for uncomplicated urinary tract infections at the present time. The other drug of first choice would be a quinolone such as norfloxacin, ciprofloxacin, or levofloxacin.

A11. **b.** You should not wait to begin therapy. Start immediately after you obtain the urine specimen for culture. Ask for the result as soon as possible, but do not aggravate the pathologist.

A12. **c.** This is a case of uncomplicated urinary tract infection. Hemorrhagic cystitis cannot really be considered a complication. With an uncomplicated infection, you are likely going to be dealing with an uncomplicated organism. Therefore *Escherichia coli* is the most likely organism involved in the infection.

There are many serotypes of *E. coli* that can produce urinary tract infection; some serotypes are more likely to produce hemorrhagic cystitis; others are more likely to produce nonhemorrhagic cystitis.

A13. **e.** The quinolone antibiotics are a significant advance in antimicrobial therapy. They use a totally unique mechanism of action. These antibiotics are extremely effective against many gram-positive and especially gram-negative organisms. The quinolone antibiotics work essentially at a molecular genetic level.

The quinolone antibiotics are bactericidal in action. Action is achieved mainly by inhibition of the DNA gyrase. This is an essential component of the bacterial DNA replication system. The inhibition of the α-subunit of the DNA gyrase blocks the resealing of the nicks on the DNA strands induced by this α-subunit, leading to the degradation of the DNA by exonucleases.

SOLUTION TO THE SHORT ANSWER MANAGEMENT PROBLEM

A. Females:
  1. Uncomplicated lower tract infections:
     a. Acute cystitis
     b. Acute hemorrhagic cystitis
  2. Complicated upper tract infections:
     a. Acute pyelitis
     b. Acute pyelonephritis
  3. Conditions likely to increase the risk of acquiring a complicated urinary tract infection:
     a. Diabetes mellitus
     b. Stone disease
     c. Chronic indwelling catheterization
     d. Immunosuppression
     e. Pregnancy
     f. Neuropathic bladder
     g. Congenital anomalies (reflux)
     h. Urethral stenosis
     i. Urinary tract obstruction
  4. Sexually transmitted urinary tract infections: Acute urethritis
     a. *Chlamydia trachomatis*
     b. *Mycoplasma hominis*
     c. *Ureaplasma urealyticum*
     d. *Neisseria gonorrhea*
B. Males:
  1. Uncomplicated urinary tract infection: Very rare in the absence of obstruction except for acute prostatitis
  2. Complicated urinary tract infections:
     a. Acute cystitis: Must be investigated with renal ultrasound
     b. Acute pyelitis
     c. Acute pyelonephritis
     d. Chronic prostatitis

The most common complicating factor in males is obstruction caused by benign prostatic hypertrophy/hyperplasia. However, all males with a urinary tract infection not caused by a sexually transmitted disease need to be investigated. The minimal investigation is a renal ultrasound.

3. Sexually transmitted diseases:
  a. Acute urethritis:
     1) *Chlamydia trachomatis* (nongonococcal urethritis [NGU])
     2) *Mycoplasma hominis* (NGU)
     3) *Ureaplasma urealyticum* (NGU)
     4) *Neisseria gonorrhea* (gonococcal urethritis)
  b. Acute epididymo-orchitis: *Chlamydia trachomatis*

SUMMARY OF THE DIAGNOSIS AND TREATMENT OF URINARY TRACT INFECTION

1. Classification: See the short answer management problem.

2. Signs and symptoms:
   a. Lower tract: Dysuria, frequency, nocturia, hematuria, terminal dribbling, discharge (sexually transmitted diseases)
   b. Upper tract: Same as lower tract plus fever, chills, CVA pain/tenderness

3. Laboratory:
   a. Urinalysis, testing for culture and sensitivity (lower tract)
   b. CBC, blood cultures, 24-hour urine for creatinine clearance and protein, renal ultrasound, IVP

4. Complications:
   a. Evaluate each patient in terms of risk factors.
   b. Avoid indwelling catheterization whenever possible.

5. Treatment:
   a. Lower tract (females):
      1) Three-day course of TMP-SMX
      2) Pyridium for analgesia
   b. Upper tract:
      1) Quinolone (such as ciprofloxacin or levofloxacin)
      2) Ampicillin and gentamicin
      3) Third-generation cephalosporin with or without gentamicin
   c. Inpatient versus outpatient: Acute pyelonephritis: hospitalize those with complications or complicating diseases; otherwise outpatient IV port therapy daily or high-dose oral therapy
   d. Prophylaxis: Consider for high-risk patients: first choice, quinolones or macrodantin
   e. STDs:
      1) Gonorrhea: Rocephin IM (250 mg) and azithromycin (1 g single dose) or doxycycline for 7 days

2) NGU: Azithromycin (1 g single dose) or doxycycline for 7 days

SUGGESTED READING
Arsdalen K: The urogenital tract. In Rakel R, ed: *Conn's current therapy*, Philadelphia, 1994, WB Saunders.

PROBLEM·36

ACNE

"Hit That Zit!"

Case 1 ■ A 15-Year-Old Distressed Adolescent with "The Zits"

A 15-year-old female comes to your office with a complaint of the "zits." She has been attempting to treat these with frequent washings and avoidance of cosmetics and other facial products. She is very distressed and breaks down crying. She is afraid that "no boys will ever be interested in me with such an ugly face." Her past history is unremarkable. She is taking no medications at present. She has no allergies. Her family history is unremarkable.

On physical examination the patient has multiple maculopapular-pustular lesions with comedones on her face and back. No other abnormalities are found on examination.

SELECT THE BEST ANSWER TO THE FOLLOWING QUESTIONS

Q1. What is the diagnosis in this patient?
    a. acne vulgaris
    b. ecthyma
    c. acne fulminans
    d. rosacea
    e. *Propionibacterium* acne class II

Q2. What is the treatment of first choice in this patient at this time?
    a. topical tretinoin
    b. intralesional corticosteroids
    c. topical benzoyl peroxide
    d. topical erythromycin
    e. oil-based antiacne moisturizers

Q3. The patient returns. There has been an improvement of about 20% in the skin lesions since her first visit. She has gradually increased the strength of the preparation you gave her. What would you do at this time?

    a. discontinue the first agent and treat her with topical benzoyl peroxide
    b. discontinue the first agent and treat her with topical tretinoin
    c. continue the first agent and add topical tretinoin
    d. discontinue the first agent and treat her with topical erythromycin
    e. continue the first agent and add topical erythromycin

Q4. The patient returns again in another 4 weeks. She has now sustained an improvement of about 35% in the lesions since her first visit and continues to execute your instructions faithfully. However, she is still not satisfied, and neither are you. What would you do at this time?
    a. discontinue the first and second agents and substitute a systemic antibiotic
    b. continue the first and second agents and add a systemic antibiotic
    c. continue the first and second agents and add topical clindamycin or erythromycin
    d. continue the first and second agents and add oral 13-cis-retinoic acid
    e. continue the first and second agents, and add a new "oil-free" product that through your local pharmaceutical detail man you have learned "kills acne bugs dead"

Q5. The patient, as instructed, returns again in 1 month. She has now sustained an improvement of about 50% but is still not satisfied. What would you do at this time?
    a. throw up your hands in disgust and say "I give up"
    b. refer her to the first dermatologist who comes to mind
    c. tell her to "hang in there" for a little longer
    d. stop all the medication you have started her on and try something else
    e. continue all three agents you have started her on and add a systemic antibiotic

Q6. An 18-year-old male comes with moderately severe nodular-pustular acne on his face and back. What would be your agent of first choice in this case?
    a. topical benzoyl peroxide
    b. topical tretinoin
    c. systemic tetracycline
    d. penicillin
    e. 13-cis-retinoic acid

Q7. The patient described in Question 6 returns in 6 weeks with only moderate improvement. What would you now prescribe?
   a. systemic tetracycline
   b. systemic erythromycin
   c. cyproterone acetate
   d. 13-cis-retinoic acid
   e. none of the above

Q8. Closed comedones are associated with the condition described. What is a closed comedone also known as?
   a. a whitehead
   b. a blackhead
   c. a pustule
   d. a maculopapule
   e. a carbuncle

Q9. Open comedones are associated with the condition described. What is an open comedone also known as?
   a. a whitehead
   b. a blackhead
   c. a pustule
   d. a maculopapule
   e. a carbuncle

Q10. Which of the following statements concerning the association of certain foods with certain diseases and health care outcomes is true?
   a. chocolate can exacerbate acne vulgaris
   b. shellfish can exacerbate acne vulgaris
   c. nuts can exacerbate acne vulgaris
   d. shellfish and nuts, although not associated with acne, are associated with certain other important public health outcomes
   e. none of the above

Q11. Which of the following bacteria is (are) associated with the condition described above?
   a. *Staphylococcus aureus*
   b. *Streptococcus viridans*
   c. *Propionibacterium acnes*
   d. all of the above
   e. none of the above

Q12. Which of the following is (are) essential for a good skin-care program specifically designed for patients with the described disorder?
   a. oil-free products
   b. gentle, nonabrasive cleansing
   c. manual manipulation of skin lesions
   d. a and b
   e. all of the above

Q13. On further questioning you learn that the patient described in Case 1 has just stopped the oral contraceptive pill (OCP) last month. Which of the following statements regarding the possible use of oral/topical antibiotics in the patient above is (are) true?
   a. if the patient goes back on the pill, oral tetracycline is the systemic agent of choice for her acne
   b. if the patient goes back on the pill, oral tetracycline (for acne) is unlikely to have any effect on the OCP's efficacy
   c. if the patient goes back on the pill, because of the potential interaction with certain antibiotics, a very low-dose OCP should be used
   d. all of the above
   e. none of the above

Q14. What is (are) the absolute contraindication(s) to the use of oral isotretinoin for the treatment of acne vulgaris?
   a. children under age 14 years
   b. women of childbearing potential who are not adequately protected against pregnancy
   c. allergy to topical tretinoin
   d. all of the above
   e. none of the above

Q15. Which of the following is (are) true concerning rosacea?
   a. rosacea occurs in middle-aged individuals
   b. rosacea consists of papules and pustules on the face
   c. rosacea produces a background erythema and telangiectasias on the face
   d. all of the above
   e. none of the above

Q16. What is the first-line treatment of rosacea?
   a. topical benzoyl peroxide
   b. topical tretinoin
   c. topical erythromycin or clindamycin
   d. topical metronidazole
   e. none of the above

Q17. What is the second-line treatment of rosacea?
   a. topical metronidazole
   b. oral metronidazole
   c. oral tetracycline
   d. oral 13-cis-retinoic acid
   e. oral erythromycin

Q18. Which of the following conditions is sometimes associated with rosacea?
   a. rhinophyma

b. cellulitis
c. multiple carbuncle formation
d. cavernous sinus thrombosis
e. anaerobic septicemia

SHORT ANSWER MANAGEMENT PROBLEM
Describe the pathophysiology of acne vulgaris.

ANSWERS

A1. **a.** This patient has acne vulgaris. Acne vulgaris affects most teenagers and continues to affect many patients into their twenties and their thirties.

A2. **c.**

A3. **c.**

A4. **c.**

A5. **e.**

A6. **c.**

A7. **d.** The treatment of choice for acne can take many forms, but a recommended approach is outlined below. In this approach, only one drug is added at a time; this allows you to evaluate clearly the efficacy of that agent. This approach may need to be amended if the patient has a nodular-pustular acne in the beginning (as in Questions 6 and 7); see below.
   a. Treatment protocol for mild to moderate acne:
      1) Begin with topical benzoyl peroxide 2.5%. Increase to 5% and 10% rapidly. This product is preferably given in gel form because it is less drying. Benzoyl peroxide is best given in the morning.
      2) Add topical tretinoin or adapalene. These are applied at bedtime. Remember to tell your patient to expect redness and irritation of the face, especially in the initial period. Urge the patient not to discontinue the product because of this side effect.
      3) Add topical erythromycin or topical clindamycin. This should be used in combination with 1 and 2. If there are significant lesions on the back that are difficult to get at for the patient (even at the beginning of treatment) you may need to prescribe a systemic antibiotic from the beginning.
      4) Add systemic tetracycline to the topical benzoyl peroxide and topical tretinoin. Continue the topical antibiotic.

b. Moderate to severe nodular pustular acne:
   1) The choices for systemic antibiotic therapy include tetracycline, minocycline, doxycycline, erythromycin, clindamycin, and trimethoprim-sulfamethoxazole.
   2) In severe cystic acne an oral retinoid, 13-cis-retinoic acid, may be necessary.

A8. **a.**

A9. **b.** Acne vulgaris is the result of the obstruction of sebaceous follicles by sebum and desquamated epithelial cells. An anaerobic organism, *Propionibacterium acnes,* will proliferate, which leads to inflammation. Clinically these pathophysiologic events lead to noninflammatory open and closed comedones and, in more severe cases, inflammatory papules, pustules, and nodules. Most patients have a mixture of both noninflammatory and inflammatory lesions.

A10. **d.** There is no indication that the intake of certain foods is associated with acne. This includes chocolate, nuts, and shellfish. Shellfish and nuts have important public health consequences related to food allergies and anaphylaxis. Many Americans die each year as a result of anaphylaxis and subsequent angioneurotic edema, and shock.

A11. **c.** Acne vulgaris is associated with the bacterium *Propionibacterium acnes.*

A12. **d.** A good skin-care program contains the following: Gentle, nonabrasive cleansing; the use of oil-free products; and leaving the skin lesions alone.

A13. **e.** Broad-spectrum antibiotics may reduce the effectiveness of oral contraceptives. Certain oral contraceptives may be used in the treatment of moderate acne vulgaris in females age 15 years or older who desire contraception, have achieved menarche, and are unresponsive to topical antiacne medications.

A14. **b.** The single most important absolute contraindication to the use of 13-cis-retinoic acid (Accutane) is women in the reproductive years. Accutane is teratogenic and should never be used in this age group. Children under age 14 years and individuals with allergic reactions (not the redness that is characteristic of topical isotretinoin) should also not be given Accutane.

A15. **d.** Rosacea is an acneiform condition that affects middle-aged patients. It is characterized by papules and pustules occurring on a background of erythema and telangiectasia of facial skin. The main area affected is the middle third of the face, from the forehead to the chin. With rosacea, comedones are typically absent. There is, however, a tendency for the facial skin of patients affected by rosacea to become thickened and to produce enlarged sebaceous glands. When this happens in the area of the nose, the condition is known as rhinophyma. Rosacea is more common in women, but affected men seem more prone to develop a severe case of rhinophyma.

A16. **d.** The first-line treatment for rosacea is a topical antibiotic. The antibiotic of choice is metronidazole (MetroGel) applied twice daily. Topical tretinoin and topical benzoyl peroxide preparations aggravate the erythema and are usually not helpful. Topical corticosteroids also aggravate the condition.

A17. **c.** The second-line treatment for rosacea is a systemic antibiotic. Tetracycline is the drug of choice. After the first month, the dosage can often be lowered and then ultimately discontinued. Recurrences are common, however, and repeated courses of antibiotics are often needed. Systemic antibiotics are also useful in treating the associated keratitis and blepharitis that are occasionally associated with rosacea.

Systemic therapy with erythromycin, minocycline, doxycycline, or metronidazole is effective if tetracycline is ineffective.

Rosacea that fails to respond to the treatment alternatives just outlined may respond to oral isotretinoin.

A18. **a.** The rhinophyma has been thought to be associated with alcohol abuse and alcoholism: the "W.C. Field's syndrome." It is unclear how strong this connection is. There certainly are many exceptions, but it may warrant consideration when evaluating a patient (especially a middle-aged male to elderly male) with rhinophyma.

SOLUTION TO THE SHORT ANSWER MANAGEMENT PROBLEM

The pathophysiology of acne vulgaris involves the following six steps:
1. The androgen stimulation of sebum production
2. Keratinous obstruction of the sebaceous follicle outlet
3. Accumulation of keratin and sebum with the formation of open and closed comedones (blackheads and whiteheads)
4. Bacterial colonization of the trapped sebum with *Propionibacterium acnes*
5. Inflammatory reaction to the colonization of the trapped sebum

6. Production of inflammatory papules, pustules, nodules, and cysts

SUMMARY OF THE DIAGNOSIS AND TREATMENT OF ACNE VULGARIS AND ROSACEA

1. Acne vulgaris:
   a. Prevalence: 75% of teenagers and young adults (up to and including patients in their twenties and thirties)
   b. Pathophysiology: See the short answer management problem.
   c. Causative organism: *Propionibacterium acnes*
   d. Classification of acne vulgaris:
      1) Obstructive acne:
         a) Closed comedones (whiteheads)
         b) Open comedones (blackheads)
      2) Inflammatory acne: Formation of lesions generally proceeds in the following order:
         a) Papules/pustules
         b) Nodules
         c) Cysts
         d) Scars
   e. Treatment measures:
      1) Nonpharmacologic:
         a) Gentle face washing
         b) Avoidance of manipulation of acne lesions
         c) Using water-based cosmetics only
         d) Using oil-free moisturizers only
      2) Pharmacologic: The treatment of acne vulgaris can be seen as a series of discrete steps:
         a) Step 1: Begin with benzoyl peroxide gel
         b) Step 2: Add topical tretinoin or adapalene
            Consider using step 1 in the morning and step 2 in the evening.
         c) Step 3: Add topical antibiotic (erythromycin, clindamycin)
            Consider using step 3 along with a combination of steps 1 and 2.
         d) Step 4: Systemic antibiotics such as tetracycline, minocycline, doxycycline, erythromycin, clindamycin, or trimethoprim-sulfamethoxazole
            Consider using combination of steps 1, 2, 3, and 4.
         e) Step 5: For severe nodular-cystic acne only, use oral isotretinoin (associated with serious, dose-related side effects)
   f. Common myths believed by patients:
      1) Acne is caused by failure to wash away dirt and oil with sufficient zeal. Not true; acne can be made worse by washing too vigorously and causing irritation. Gentle washing with normal soap is sufficient.

2) Too much junk food causes acne. Not true; no connection between diet and acne has ever been established.

3) "Unhealthy" sex habits, including masturbation, same sex play, or even simple indulgence can cause acne. Not true; sex with the wrong person can cause rashes but it will not be acne.

4) Stress can cause acne. Not true; however, stress can increase a nervous tendency to pick, squeeze, and/or rub pimples and make them worse.

5) Acne is a normal adolescent problem of no consequence that should be allowed to run its course. Not true; the physical and psychologic consequences of acne can be cataclysmic. Prompt treatment can prevent severe outbreaks and avoid physical and emotional scarring.

6) Acne vulgaris always clears up after adolescence. Not true; over 10% of individuals continue to have this form of acne well into adulthood.

2. Rosacea:
   a. Definition: Acneiform eruption that affects middle-aged patients. Characterized by papules and pustules occurring on a background of erythema and telangiectasia of facial skin.
   b. Complications: Thick skin forms on face (especially on nose). This condition is called rhinophyma.
   c. Treatment:
      1) Step 1: Topical metronidazole
      2) Step 2: Systemic therapy using tetracycline, erythromycin, minocycline, doxycycline, metronidazole, or isotretinoin.

SUGGESTED READINGS

American Academy of Dermatology, 1999; http//: www.aad.org.
Lookingbill DP: Acne vulgaris and rosacea. In Rakel R, ed: *Conn's current therapy*, Philadelphia, 1994, WB Saunders.

PROBLEM·37

INFERTILITY

"Doctor, I'll Just Die if I Don't Have a Baby Now!"

Case 1 ■ A Couple That Has Been Unsuccessful in Conceiving after 18 Months of Trying

A 28-year-old female and her 27-year-old husband have been trying to conceive for the past 18 months. They are extremely anxious, and during the interview the wife begins to cry.

You go through a short history on both members of the couple today in preparation for a more thorough investigation. You discover that the wife has a history of pelvic inflammatory disease (PID; one episode at age 18 years). The husband is healthy and has had no major medical problems.

SELECT THE BEST ANSWER TO THE FOLLOWING QUESTIONS

Q1. What is the next most appropriate step in the evaluation of this couple?
   a. tell the couple that the infertility is the result of previous PID and refer them to an adoption agency
   b. refer them to a gynecologist to break the news of the infertility
   c. begin the wife on clomiphene citrate
   d. refer the couple to a psychiatrist
   e. none of the above

Q2. Primary infertility is defined as inability to conceive despite unprotected intercourse for how many months?
   a. 6 months
   b. 12 months
   c. 18 months
   d. 24 months
   e. none of the above

Q3. Secondary infertility is defined as the inability to conceive despite unprotected intercourse, following a previous conception, for how many months?
   a. 6 months
   b. 12 months
   c. 18 months
   d. 24 months
   e. none of the above

Q4. In attempting to obtain a history from both husband and wife that will lead you to a diagnosis of infertility, which of the following is the most important question?
   a. the current medications that both partners (but especially the husband) are taking
   b. the frequency of intercourse
   c. the position(s) when intercourse takes place
   d. the amount of time that the female spends trying to maximize the tilt of the vagina after intercourse
   e. the age of the husband

Q5. What is the prevalence of primary infertility in American couples?
   a. <1%
   b. 4% to 6%
   c. 10% to 15%
   d. 20% to 25%
   e. 30% to 35%

Q6. In the United States, the male is principally responsible for what percentage of infertility in couples attempting to conceive?
   a. 10%
   b. 20%
   c. 30%
   d. 40%
   e. 50%

Q7. In the United States, the female is principally responsible for what percentage of infertility in couples attempting to conceive?
   a. 10%
   b. 20%
   c. 30%
   d. 40%
   e. 50%

Q8. Which of the following statements regarding the occurrence of ovulation is true?
   a. the female partner should keep a basal body temperature chart for at least 6 months before ovulation can be precisely determined
   b. a woman who has a menstrual period every 6 months may still be ovulating on a monthly basis
   c. a woman who has regular menstrual cycles associated with premenstrual symptoms is almost certainly ovulating
   d. the only accurate method of determining ovulation is by endometrial biopsy
   e. if a woman has been anovulatory for a period of greater than 1 year, it is unlikely that she will ever ovulate again

Q9. Which of the following statements regarding the physiology of infertility is false?
   a. the hypothalamic-pituitary-ovarian axis must be functional in order to stimulate normal folliculogenesis
   b. an adequate increase in progesterone production must be present to stimulate the luteinizing hormone (LH) surge
   c. intercourse must take place at mid-cycle, placing sperm into the upper vagina
   d. adequate numbers of sperm must arrive in the distal oviduct to fertilize the egg
   e. none of the above

Q10. Which of the following statements concerning the investigation of infertility is false?
   a. both male and female partners should be investigated simultaneously
   b. ovulation can be confirmed by recording of the basal body temperature
   c. the adequacy of the luteal phase is assessed by midluteal progesterone levels
   d. anything less than 90% normal sperm morphology is cause for infertility
   e. none of the above statements is false

Q11. The World Health Organization (WHO) has issued parameters for the assessment of a normal sperm analysis. Which of the following is not part of the WHO's criteria for a normal sperm analysis?
   a. total count greater than 20 million sperm/ml
   b. sperm demonstrate greater than 50% motility
   c. sperm demonstrate greater than 50% normal morphology
   d. total semen volume is greater than 2.0 ml
   e. all of the above are part of WHO's definition

Q12. What is the most common identified female factor responsible for infertility?
   a. ovulatory/luteal phase dysfunction
   b. cervical mucus abnormality
   c. tubal adhesions and scarring
   d. endometriosis
   e. autoantibodies to sperm

Q13. What is the most common identified male factor responsible for infertility?
   a. previous mumps infection
   b. primary testicular failure
   c. idiopathic low motility
   d. testicular varicocele
   e. previous history of epididymitis

Q14. Which of the following is (are) true regarding varicoceles?
   a. varicoceles are caused by incompetent valves in the testicular vein
   b. 90% of varicoceles occur on the left side
   c. treatment consists of operative ligation of the spermatic vein
   d. a and c
   e. all of the above are true

Q15. Which of the following statements most correctly describes the manner in which a family physician should conduct an infertility investigation?
   a. the partners should be assessed one at a time;

if no cause is found in the wife, the husband should then be checked

b. the family physician should assess one factor at time; the infertility investigation should be completed within approximately 9 months

c. the family physician should recommend an immediate referral to a gynecologist for the woman; if no infertility factor is found, the physician should refer the husband to a urologist for a fertility work-up

d. the family physician should assess both husband and wife at the same time; preliminary investigations should be completed within 2 months

e. none of the above is true

Q16. What is the drug of choice for induction of ovulation?
a. clomiphene citrate
b. danazol
c. bromocriptine
d. gonadotropins
e. none of the above

SHORT ANSWER MANAGEMENT PROBLEM
Because of the significant impact of acute PID on future fertility, discuss how you would approach a young girl who asked you for a prescription for the oral contraceptive pill.

ANSWERS

A1. **e.** The most appropriate first step is to perform a complete history and physical examination on both partners.

A2. **b.** Primary infertility is defined as the inability of a couple to achieve a pregnancy after at least 12 months of unprotected intercourse, with adequate frequency of intercourse a necessary prerequisite. Within 1 year, 90% of "normal" couples should achieve a pregnancy.

A3. **b.** Secondary infertility is defined as the inability to achieve conception despite unprotected intercourse for 12 months following a previous conception. If conception does not occur within that time, a complete evaluation of both partners is indicated. In the female, a complete history including the menstrual history, previous surgery, and previous pelvic infections should be documented. The physical examination of the woman should evaluate any signs of endocrine disorder, and a complete pelvic examination (including rectovaginal) should be performed. In the male, a

history of mumps, current medications, and a history of epididymitis or other male genitourinary infection is important. The physical examination should include testicular size, location of the urethral meatus, and the presence or absence of a varicocele. The prostate should be examined.

A4. **b.** There are many factors affecting reproductive performance. The most important of these factors include the following:

a. The age of the female partner: At age 40 years, women have a 50% decreased fertility rate and three-fold increase risk of spontaneous abortion compared with younger women.

b. The age of the male partner: Until age 65 years, a man's age does not affect sperm or ability to fertilize eggs.

c. Coital frequency: Although frequency of intercourse is positively correlated with pregnancy rates, infrequent coitus is an uncommon cause of infertility.

d. Timing of intercourse: Intercourse before ovulation is key to maximizing the chance of pregnancy.

e. Coital technique

f. The use of lubricants: Some lubricants have spermicidal properties.

g. The use of douching after intercourse

h. A history of multiple sexual partners (in either partner, but especially in the female)

i. A history of sexually transmitted diseases: This is mediated through tubal adhesions.

j. The history of previous pregnancies

k. A history of sickle-cell disease

l. Nutrition (especially in the female): Female body weight 15% below normal may reduce fertility.

m. Exposure to toxic agents

n. A history of smoking and/or alcohol use in either partner

o. Medication use in either partner

p. A history of surgery involving reproductive structures in either partner

q. Exposure to radiation

r. Excessive physical exertion and heat

Of the choices offered in the question, the most important factor listed is the frequency of intercourse. Often a couple who comes in for assessment of infertility is found to have a problem with the frequency of intercourse (in that they are having intercourse only one or two times per month). This will greatly increase the time required to achieve a successful pregnancy.

A5. **c.** The prevalence of infertility in American couples is approximately 10% to 15%. This represents the number of couples who are not able to conceive within 12 months if they are using no contraception and attempting to achieve a pregnancy. It must be recognized that this merely represents an aggregate summary statistic and usually is of little value when counseling an individual or couple regarding the chance of conception. The factors listed in Answer 4 all influence this infertility prevalence.

A6. **d.**

A7. **d.** In the United States the male and the female are each responsible for 40% of infertility. In 20% the cause is unknown or problems exist with both partners.

A8. **c.** If a woman has regular menstrual cycles associated with cyclic premenstrual sensations or symptoms (molimina), she is almost certainly ovulating. A woman who is menstruating regularly does not have to keep taking her basal body temperature for 6 months; to do so is both unnecessary and anxiety provoking. On the other hand, a woman who has a menstrual period only every 6 months is almost certainly not ovulating.

Ovulation is most easily assessed by a history of regular cyclical menses; endometrial biopsy is rarely necessary. Many women who are anovulatory for long periods of time can have ovulation induced with clomiphene; therefore a 1-year history of anovulation is not at all hopeless.

A9. **b.** A successful pregnancy is dependent on the following male and female factors:
   a. The hypothalamic-pituitary-ovarian axis must be functional in order to stimulate normal folliculogenesis and recruitment of the dominant follicle.
   b. An adequate increase in estrogen production must be present to stimulate the LH surge, which leads to ovulation.
   c. The fimbria must be able to sweep the egg into a patent, functional oviduct.
   d. The testes must be able to produce mature, functional spermatozoa.
   e. Intercourse must take place at midcycle, placing sperm into the upper vagina.
   f. Cervical mucus quality must facilitate sperm entry and storage.
   g. Adequate numbers of sperm must arrive in the distal oviduct to fertilize the egg.
   h. Transport of the conceptus toward the uterine cavity must be facilitated by a patent, functional oviduct.
   i. The endometrium must have been prepared by adequate levels of progesterone to allow implantation by the blastocyst, but not to stimulate the LH surge.

A10. **d.** Both male and female partners should initially be investigated simultaneously using inexpensive and noninvasive testing.
   a. In the male: A semen analysis should be performed. Ejaculation should be avoided for 2 to 7 days. The semen specimen should be obtained by masturbation and examined within 30 to 60 minutes of specimen collection. Parameters evaluated include for semen volume (2 to 5 ml), sperm concentration (>20 million sperm/ml), sperm morphology (>30% normal forms), and sperm motility (>50% motile). At least 75% of fertile men will have at least one abnormal characteristic; 25% will have two abnormalities. It is more important to consider the number of abnormal parameters than an abnormality in a single parameter. An abnormal semen analysis should be repeated on two or three occasions at least a month apart.
   b. In the female:
      1) Ovulation can usually be assessed by history. If cycles are regular by history, obtain a mid-luteal progesterone level (>10 mg/ml) for indirect evidence of ovulation as well as to document normal luteal function. A basal body temperature (BBT) chart may also provide indirect evidence of ovulation. Following ovulation the BBT will show an increase of 0.5° to 1.0° F. A 2- or 3-month period of charting should be adequate. If cycles are irregular or absent, begin ovulation induction even though occasional ovulatory cycles may occur.
      2) Ovarian reserve is assessed if the female partner is over age 35 years by obtaining a follicle-stimulating hormone (FSH) level on the third day of the cycle. An elevated level (>12 mIU/ml) indicates impending ovarian failure.
      3) Tubal disease risk is assessed by obtaining a chlamydia IgG antibody level. If it is negative, the risk of tubal disease is less than 5%.
      4) An ovarian endometrioma is ruled out by a pelvic sonogram.
      5) The postcoital test was used in the past to assess how favorable the cervical mucus was to sperm. With the advent of intrauterine insemination (IUI), this test is no longer used, since IUI completely bypasses the cervical mucus.
      6) Tubal patency is assessed by hysterosalpingography (HSG) in the first week after menses. Diagnostic laparoscopy is indicated only

if the HSG shows any tubal disease or if the sonogram shows an endometrioma.

A11. **d.** The WHO's definition of a normal sperm analysis is as follows:
  a. Sperm concentration: >20 million/ml (15 to 20 million/ml is suboptimal but still capable of producing a pregnancy)
  b. Percentage of sperm that demonstrate forward motility: >50% of total number
  c. Percentage of sperm that exhibit what is considered to be a "normal morphology": >50%

The WHO does not comment on semen volume in its "normal" parameters.

A12. **c.** The most commonly identified female cause of infertility is associated with tubal factors (40%), particularly tubal adhesions and scarring from previous PID. Other factors are ovulatory problems (10% to 15%), and cervical factors (10%).

A13. **d.** The most commonly identified male factor associated with infertility is a testicular varicocele. Second on the list is primary testicular failure, followed by epididymitis as the third most common factor.

A14. **e.** Varicocele is the most common identifiable cause of male infertility. Varicocele results from incompetent valves in the testicular vein, permitting the transmission of hydrostatic venous pressure; distention and tortuosity of the pampiniform plexus result. Varicoceles are present on the left side in 90% of cases, presumably because of venous drainage of the left testes to the left renal vein, causing increased retrograde venous pressure.

Surgical treatment of varicoceles should take place only if the varicocele appears to be a cause of infertility or the varicocele is symptomatic (a dragging scrotal sensation is a problem).

A15. **d.** Infertility investigations should be conducted quickly, and both husband and wife should be evaluated at the same time. The emotional impact of infertility can be very traumatic to a young couple. The longer the time taken to complete the investigations, the greater is the emotional trauma. The family physician can perform baseline complete histories and baseline physical examinations on both members of the couple, semen analysis on the husband (repeated), basal body temperature charting on the female, and midluteal serum progesterone determination on the female partner. These investigations can be completed in a short time. If no cause is found (and this would suggest a tubal or peritoneal factor), referral to a gynecologist should be made as quickly as possible.

A16. **a.** If the female partner is not ovulating or has irregular cycles, ovulation induction using medical therapy can be successful in more than 90% of patients. Clomiphene citrate is the usual initial agent used. It is a synthetic, weak estrogen that competes with endogenous estrogen for estrogen-binding sites in the hypothalamus. As it blocks the endogenous estrogen negative feedback, it leads to enhanced gonadotropic hormone (GnRH) release. A low dose (50 mg) is administered for 5 days in the early follicular phase, increasing until there is evidence of ovulation. Ovulation is successful in 70% of women, with a pregnancy rate of 50%. Twin pregnancy rates are 8% with clomiphene.

SOLUTION TO THE SHORT ANSWER MANAGEMENT PROBLEM

The advice you would give your young patient should include the following:
  1. Because of the risk of sexually transmitted diseases (STDs, including acquired immunodeficiency syndrome [AIDS]) and subsequent PID, you would recommend the use of a barrier method of contraception (such as condoms) along with the oral contraceptive pill (OCP).
  2. You should make the patient aware that although the OCP may protect against one type of PID (gonococcal PID), it does not protect against, and may even promote, chlamydial PID.
  3. Reinforce the importance of limiting sexual partners (to one) if possible.
  4. Reinforce the importance of telling your young patient that she should not have sex if her partner refuses to wear a condom.
  5. Ask her to return regularly for counseling and support.

SUMMARY OF THE DIAGNOSIS AND MANAGEMENT OF INFERTILITY

1. Definition: Failure to achieve a pregnancy after at least 12 months of unprotected intercourse

2. Prevalence: The prevalence of infertility in the American population is 10% to 15%.

3. Most common causes:
  a. Female:
    1) Tubal adhesions and scarring from PID
    2) Anovulatory cycles
    3) Other abnormalities in tubes and uterus
    4) Amenorrhea as a result of anorexia nervosa or continuing vigorous exercise (long-term)
    5) Hyperprolactinemia

b. Male:
   1) Varicocele
   2) Primary testicular failure
   3) Previous epididymitis or mumps orchitis

4. Investigations:
   a. Complete histories (both partners)
   b. Complete physical examinations (both partners)
   c. Semen analysis (repeated twice): Male factor
   d. Basal body temperature monitoring and/or assessment of regular menstrual cycles: Ovulatory factor
   e. Midluteal progesterone: Luteal phase factor

5. Referrals:
   a. Referral to a gynecologist for assessment of tubal and peritoneal factors
   b. Referral to a urologist if a varicocele is detected

6. Treatment options:
   a. Male infertility: Artificial donor insemination (ADI): particular attention must be paid to ensuring that the donor is free from STDs (especially AIDS). The current recommendation is for the sperm to be stored for 6 months and, if the donor is still HIV negative, to inseminate at that time.
   b. Female infertility:
      1) Cervical mucus problems: Cervical mucus problems impairing conception may be treated with insemination or uterine instillation of a small amount of specially prepared sperm.
      2) Ovarian disorders: Ovulation disorders can be treated with drugs to induce ovulation. Clomiphene citrate suppresses estrogen's ovulation-suppressive effect. In women whose ovulation is suppressed by hyperprolactinemia (high blood levels of the pituitary hormone prolactin), ovulation may be induced with prolactin-suppressing drugs such as bromocriptine.
      3) Uterine/tubal abnormalities: Specific corrective surgical procedures (for PID adhesions and scarring and for endometriosis); gamete intrafallopian tube transfer (GIFT); in vitro fertilization
   c. Adoption: Adoption may be the only vehicle left to some couples. To maximize the ability to cope, it is recommended that this subject be raised early rather than later.

SUGGESTED READINGS

Hatcher RA: *Contraceptive technology*, ed 17, New York, 1998, Ardent Media.
Mishell DR et al: *Comprehensive gynecology*, St Louis, 1997, Mosby.
Speroff L et al: *Clinical gynecologic endocrinology and infertility*, Baltimore, 1994, Williams & Wilkins.

PROBLEM·38

SLEEP DISORDERS

"Sweet Sleep, Where Are You?"

Case 1 ■ A 48-Year-Old Male with a 6-Month History of Snoring, Nocturnal Breath Cessations, and Excessive Daytime Sleepiness

A 48-year-old male comes to your office with his wife. His wife complains to you that "he is constantly snoring" and she has put up with all she can. This has been going on for a number of years, but it has been getting worse lately. His wife also tells you that "sometimes he even stops breathing during the night."

When you ask the patient directly, he says, "Well, I may snore a bit, but I think my wife is exaggerating." You somehow doubt the latter statement.

On examination, the patient weighs 310 pounds. His blood pressure is 200/105 mm Hg (measured with a large cuff). There is a grade III/VI systolic murmur present along the left sternal edge. You believe that there is elevated jugular venous pressure when he lies at a 45-degree angle.

SELECT THE BEST ANSWER TO THE FOLLOWING QUESTIONS

Q1. What is the most likely diagnosis in this patient?
   a. narcolepsy
   b. obstructive sleep apnea syndrome
   c. generalized poor physical condition
   d. central sleep apnea syndrome
   e. adult-onset adenoid hypertrophy

Q2. To what is the pathophysiology of this condition related?
   a. collapse of the pharyngeal walls repetitively during sleep
   b. failure of upper airway dilator muscle activity
   c. sleep-related upper airway obstruction and cessation in ventilation (apneas)
   d. a and c
   e. all of the above

Q3. This condition is accompanied by which of the following?
   a. hypoxemia
   b. hypercarbia

c. metabolic acidosis
d. respiratory acidosis
e. a, b, and d
f. all of the above

Q4. What is (are) the major symptom(s) of this disorder?
a. loud snoring
b. daytime hypersomnolence
c. disturbed nonrefreshing sleep
d. weight gain
e. a, b, and c
f. all of the above

Q5. What is (are) the clinical feature(s) associated with the condition described?
a. systemic hypertension
b. inhibited sexual desire
c. depression
d. a and b
e. all of the above

Q6. What is (are) the factor(s) that predisposes to this condition?
a. alcohol intake
b. benzodiazepines
c. hyperthyroidism
d. a and b
e. all of the above

Q7. What is the treatment of first choice for this disorder?
a. uvulopalatopharyngoplasty (UPP) surgery
b. tracheostomy
c. continuous positive airway pressure (CPAP)
d. nortriptyline
e. alprazolam

Q8. Which of the following drugs is contraindicated in the treatment of the disturbed, nonrefreshing sleep that is associated with the condition described?
a. fluoxetine
b. sertraline
c. alprazolam
d. phenelzine
e. paroxetine

Case 2 ■ A 35-Year-Old Male with Weak Muscles after Laughing

A 35-year-old male comes to your office with a chief complaint of "weak muscles," especially after laughing. On further questioning you discover that the pa-

tient has excessive daytime sleepiness and "weird imaginings" just before going to sleep at night. The patient appears anxious and tense.

Q9. What is your tentative diagnosis?
a. narcolepsy
b. hysterical conversion reaction
c. psychosomatic symptoms secondary to chronic anxiety
d. hypochondriasis
e. obstructive sleep apnea

Q10. Which of the following is not a symptom of the disorder described in Case 2?
a. catalepsy
b. hypnagogic hallucinations
c. sleep paralysis
d. restless and disturbed sleep
e. persistent daytime sleepiness

Q11. The daytime symptoms of the disorder described are treated well with which of the following medications?
a. methylphenidate
b. dextroamphetamine
c. mazindol
d. a and b only
e. all of the above

Q12. The nighttime symptoms of the disorder described in Case 2 are best treated by which of the following?
a. alprazolam
b. nortriptyline
c. protriptyline
d. b or c
e. all of the above

Q13. The diagnosis for the problem described in Case 2 is best established by which of the following?
a. nocturnal polysomnogram (NPSG)
b. multiple sleep latency test (MSLT)
c. either a or b
d. a and b together
e. neither a nor b

Q14. What percentage of adult Americans experience significant sleep difficulties in any given year?
a. 5%
b. 10%
c. 15%
d. 25%
e. 50%

Q15. Insomniacs often compensate for lost sleep by delaying their morning awakening time or by napping, which actually may have the effect of further fragmenting their nocturnal sleep. What is this disorder known as?
a. mixed-up insomniac syndrome
b. insufficient sleep syndrome
c. inadequate sleep hygiene
d. adjustment sleep disorder
e. psychophysiologic insomnia

Q16. Insomniacs who voluntarily curtail their time in bed, usually in response to social and/or occupational demands, are best diagnosed with which of the following?
a. workaholic sleep loss syndrome
b. inadequate sleep hygiene
c. insufficient sleep syndrome
d. adjustment sleep disorder
e. psychophysiologic insomnia

Q17. Insomniacs who develop anticipatory anxiety over the prospect of another night of sleeplessness followed by another day of fatigue in response to a previously resolved stressor are known to have which of the following?
a. adjustment sleep disorder
b. psychophysiologic insomnia
c. inadequate sleep hygiene
d. insufficient sleep syndrome
e. generalized anxiety disorder insomnia

Q18. A 73-year-old male is admitted to the hospital for a transurethral resection of the prostate (TURP) procedure. The procedure is postponed because of some abnormal test results. The patient tells you that he has had extreme difficulty in sleeping since coming into the hospital. What is the most likely diagnosis in this patient?
a. adjustment sleep disorder
b. psychophysiologic insomnia
c. inadequate sleep hygiene
d. insufficient sleep syndrome
e. sudden-onset central sleep apnea

Q19. What is the major difference between idiopathic hypersomnolence and narcolepsy?
a. daytime somnolence
b. frequent daytime naps
c. awakening unrefreshed versus awakening refreshed from these frequent daytime naps
d. significant differences in treatment
e. none of the above

Q20. What is the difference between periodic limb movement disorder (nocturnal myoclonus) and restless legs syndrome?
a. kicking of the lower extremities in nocturnal myoclonus versus sensory loss in restless legs syndrome
b. patient awareness with nocturnal myoclonus versus patient unawareness with restless legs syndrome
c. kicking of the lower extremities in restless legs syndrome versus sensory loss in nocturnal myoclonus
d. patient awareness with restless legs syndrome versus patient unawareness in nocturnal myoclonus
e. none of the above

SHORT ANSWER MANAGEMENT PROBLEM
Discuss the principles of use for hypnotic agents in the management of sleep disorders.

ANSWERS

A1. **b.** This patient has obstructive sleep apnea. The major symptoms of obstructive sleep apnea syndrome are as follows:
a. Loud snoring
b. Reports of prolonged pauses in respiration during sleep
c. Daytime hypersomnolence
d. Disturbed nonrefreshing sleep
e. Weight gain

A2. **e.** The pathophysiology of obstructive sleep apnea syndrome (OSA) includes the following:
a. The pharyngeal walls collapse repetitively during sleep, causing intermittent sleep-related upper airway obstruction and cessation in ventilation (apneas).
b. The cessation of ventilation is related to a concomitant loss of inspiratory effort.
c. Upper airway closure in OSA results from a failure of the genioglossus and other upper airway dilator muscles. Apnea results.

A3. **e.** OSA produces the following acid-base balance situation:
a. Apnea causes hypercarbia, hypoxemia, and a resulting respiratory acidosis.
b. Only if there is another preexisting condition associated with OSA will metabolic acidosis be produced.

A4. **f.** See Answer 1.

A5. **e.** Associated clinical features of OSA include systemic hypertension; inhibited sexual desire; impotence; ejaculatory impairment; depression; deficits in attention, motor efficiency, and graphomotor ability; deterioration in interpersonal relationships; marital discord; and occupational impairment.

A6. **d.** Factors that predispose to OSA include sedating pharmacologic agents such as alcohol and benzodiazepines (all are contraindicated in OSA); nasal obstruction; large uvula; low-lying soft palate; retrognathia, micrognathia, and other craniofacial abnormalities; pharyngeal masses such as tumors or cysts; macroglossia; tonsillar hypertrophy; vocal cord paralysis; obesity; hypothyroidism; and acromegaly.

A7. **c.** Although CPAP is the best choice of these listed, always consider weight reduction in obese individuals.

A8. **c.** The most established management options, in order of most preferred option first, are the following:
    a. CPAP
    b. UPP
    c. Tracheostomy
Additional measures are as follows:
    a. Weight loss should be encouraged.
    b. Antidepressants that are stimulating, such as protriptyline, fluoxetine, sertraline, and paroxetine, are best suited to manage coexistent depression. Chronic anxiety, which may complicate the OSA picture, should not be managed with benzodiazepines. Instead, the nonbenzodiazepine buspirone, which does not appear to aggravate OSA, should be used, along with behavioral treatments. Thus alprazolam is contraindicated.

A9. **a.** This patient has narcolepsy.

A10. **a.** The major symptoms of narcolepsy are as follows:
    a. Persistent daytime sleepiness
    b. Cataplexy (not catalepsy)
    c. Hypnagogic or hypnopompic hallucinations
    d. Sleep paralysis
    e. Restless and disturbed sleep
Definitions:
    a. Cataplexy: An abrupt paralysis or paresis of skeletal muscles that usually follows emotional experiences such as anger, surprise, laughter, or physical exercise.
    b. Hypnagogic (or hypnopompic) hallucinations: Hallucinations that are vivid and often frightening dreams occurring after falling asleep (or on awakening).
    c. Sleep paralysis: A global paralysis of voluntary muscles that usually occurs shortly after falling asleep and lasts a few seconds or minutes.
Cataplexy, hypnagogic hallucinations, and sleep paralysis are thought to be manifestations of an underlying aberration in the control of the timing of rapid-eye-movement (REM) sleep that in turn results in "attacks" of REM sleep during wakefulness.

A11. **e.** Medications commonly used to control excessive daytime sleepiness include pemoline 18.75 to 112.5 mg/day, methylphenidate 5 to 60 mg/day, and dextroamphetamine 5 to 60 mg/day. In refractory cases, mazindol 3 to 6 mg/day, a tricyclic compound with anorexic properties, may be used. Tolerance may be minimized by prescribing the lowest effective dose and asking patients to take regular drug holidays on days when their need for alertness is lowest.

A12. **d.** The REM-related symptoms of cataplexy (hypnagogic hallucinations and sleep paralysis) can be controlled with REM-suppressant medications such as the tricyclic antidepressants protriptyline 5 to 30 mg/day, imipramine 50 to 200 mg/day, or nortriptyline 50 to 100 mg/day. Many narcoleptics also require emotional support.

A13. **d.** Other than the obvious behavioral manifestations of excessive daytime sleepiness (yawning, drooping eyelids, psychomotor retardation), physical examination is typically unrevealing in narcolepsy. If the diagnosis is suspected, it must be confirmed by NPSG and MSLT.

A14. **d.** Approximately 25% of all American adults express sleep-related complaints over the course of a 1-year period.

A15. **c.** Many individuals unknowingly engage in habitual behaviors that harm sleep, that is, they have poor or inadequate "sleep hygiene." Insomniacs, for example, often compensate for lost sleep by delaying their morning awakening time or by napping. These behaviors actually have the effect of further fragmenting nocturnal sleep. Instead, insomniacs should be advised to adhere to a regular awakening time regardless of the amount of sleep that they have gotten and to avoid naps.

A16. **c.** Individuals who voluntarily curtail their time in bed, usually in response to social and occupational demands, have what is best termed insufficient sleep syndrome. Although sleep reduction may be as little as 1 hour per night, over long periods of time such a pattern may lead to daytime hypersomnolence and result in impairment.

A17. **b.** Patients who develop anticipatory anxiety over the prospect of another night of sleeplessness followed by another day of fatigue have what is known as psychophysiologic insomnia. Anxiety typically increases as bedtime approaches and reaches maximum intensity after retiring. Sufferers often spend hours in bed awake, focused on and brooding over their sleeplessness, which in turn aggravates their insomnia even further. Persistent psychophysiologic insomnia often complicates other insomnia disorders.

A18. **a.** This patient has adjustment sleep disorder. This common disorder is caused by acute emotional stressors such as job loss or hospitalization. The result is insomnia, typically difficulty in falling asleep, mediated by tension and anxiety. Symptoms usually remit shortly after abatement of the stressors. Treatment is warranted if daytime sleepiness and fatigue interfere with functioning or if the disorder lasts for more than a few weeks.

A19. **c.** Idiopathic hypersomnolence is a lifelong and incurable disorder that has a variable age of onset. The most prominent symptom of this disorder is unrelenting daytime somnolence. Patients spend lengthy periods of time sleeping at night only to awaken feeling more sleepy. They take frequent and lengthy daytime naps. However, unlike patients with narcolepsy, they awaken from these naps feeling unrefreshed.

A20. **d.** Periodic limb movement disorder (nocturnal myoclonus) is characterized by the repetitive (usually every 20 to 40 seconds) twitching or kicking of the lower extremities during sleep. Patients usually have the complaint of unrelenting insomnia, most often characterized by repeated awakenings after sleep onset.

Restless legs syndrome is a creeping, crawling sensation in the lower extremities manifested by irresistible leg kicks that affect patients on reclining before falling asleep. Unlike periodic limb movement disorder, however, the patient is very aware of this phenomenon and resorts to moving the affected extremity by stretching, kicking, or walking to relieve symptoms. Many patients are depressed, irritable, and angry. Psychosocial impairment such as job loss and relationship difficulties are quite common.

SOLUTION TO THE SHORT ANSWER MANAGEMENT PROBLEM

The use of hypnotic agents in sleep disorders is a subject of great controversy (mainly because of their very wide and sometimes very inappropriate use). There are many factors that influence the decision of whether to prescribe a hypnotic agent and which hypnotic agent to prescribe.

The disadvantages of prescribing a hypnotic agent include the following:
1. There is a propensity for daytime somnolence with the use of an agent that has either a medium half-life or a long half-life.
2. A second factor is the propensity for the development of drug tolerance. Larger and larger quantities of the drug are needed to produce the same effect.
3. Hypnotics may produce symptoms of autonomic hyperactivity and irritability the following day. This is a particular problem with those hypnotics that have a very short half-life. Next-day tremor and nervousness are good examples of this phenomenon.
4. In the vast majority of cases, although hypnotics are specifically indicated for only short periods of time, they are used for longer and longer periods of time. The result is that after approximately 3 weeks, the hypnotic agents begin working in the opposite manner to which they were intended: instead of helping sleep, they actually hinder sleep.

SUMMARY OF THE DIAGNOSIS AND TREATMENT OF SLEEP DISORDERS

1. Prevalence: The overall prevalence of sleep disorders and sleep difficulties in the American population is estimated to be approximately 25% in any given year. This includes, of course, all forms of sleep disturbance, both long- and short-term.

2. Sleep phases and laboratory investigation:
   a. Human sleep: Human sleep is made up of basically two types of sleep patterns: non-REM sleep and REM sleep. Non-REM sleep has four stages and accounts for approximately 75% of total sleep. REM sleep occupies approximately 25% of total sleep.
   b. Sleep investigations: All sleep investigations should be performed in a proper, accredited sleep laboratory. The two basic tests indicated in sleep disorders are the NPSG and the MSLT.

3. Specific sleep disorders:
   a. OSA: Consists of loud snoring; prolonged pauses in breathing during sleep; daytime hypersomnolence; disturbed, nonrefreshing sleep; and weight gain.
      1) Pathophysiologic abnormalities produce apnea.
      2) Associated conditions include obesity, systemic hypertension, sexual dysfunction, depression, and anxiety.
      3) Treatment of choice: CPAP. Second and third management choices include UPP surgery and tracheostomy.
         a) Weight loss should be encouraged; alcohol should be discouraged; benzodiazepines should be prohibited; and systemic hypertension should be treated.
         b) Depression should be treated with a nonsedating antidepressant (SSRIs or protriptyline).
   b. Central sleep apnea (CSA): A rare syndrome characterized by cessation of ventilation related to a concomitant loss of inspiratory effort.
   c. Narcolepsy:
      1) Symptoms: Cataplexy, hypnagogic or hypnopompic hallucinations, and sleep paralysis.
      2) Associated conditions: Persistent daytime sleepiness and restless and disturbed sleep.
      3) Treatment: Medications used to combat excessive sleepiness include pemoline, methylphenidate, and dextroamphetamine. Mazindol is used in resistant cases. The REM-related symptoms of cataplexy and hypnagogic hallucinations are best treated with a stimulating tricyclic antidepressant such as nortriptyline or protriptyline.
   d. Idiopathic hypersomnolence: A lifelong and incurable disorder that has, as its most prominent feature, unrelenting daytime somnolence. Patients spend lengthy periods of time sleeping at night only to awaken feeling more sleepy. Unlike the narcoleptic, they awaken from their frequent daytime naps feeling unrefreshed.
   e. Periodic limb movement disorder (nocturnal myoclonus): A disorder characterized by repetitive (usually every 20 to 40 seconds) twitching or kicking of the lower extremities during sleep. Patients usually complain of unrelenting insomnia, most often characterized by repeated awakenings after sleep onset. Baclofen, clonazepam, and carbidopa-levodopa may relieve these symptoms.
   f. Restless legs syndrome: The hallmark of this disorder is a "creeping sensation" in the lower extremities and irresistible leg kicks that affect patients on reclining before falling asleep. Unlike periodic limb movement disorder, the patients are very well aware of these symptoms and resort to moving the affected extremity by stretching, kicking, or walking to relieve the symptoms.

4. Hypnotic agents: In most primary care practices, the distinct disadvantages just described outweigh any possible benefit, especially on a long-term basis.

SUGGESTED READINGS

American Psychiatric Association: *Diagnostic and statistical manual,* ed 4, Washington, DC, 1994, American Psychiatric Association Press.

Doghramji K: The evaluation and management of sleep disorders. In Stoudemire A, ed: *Clinical psychiatry for medical students,* ed 2, Philadelphia, 1994, Lippincott.

Tierney LM, McPhee SJ, Papadakis MA, eds: *Current medical diagnosis and treatment, 2000,* ed 39, Stamford, Conn, 1999, Appleton & Lange.

PROBLEM · 39

PAIN MANAGEMENT

"The Only Thing That Helps Is Demerol. How About Another Prescription?"

Case 1 ■ A 21-Year-Old Male with Chronic Back Pain

A 21-year-old male comes to your office with a chief complaint of chronic back pain. He states that he fell off a ladder 3 years ago and broke his back. Since that time he has been unable to work and has been able to function only when taking a combination of pentazocine (Talwin) and meperidine (Demerol). He walks slowly and carefully and states that he is unable to flex or extend his lumbar spine because of pain. He points to the lower lumbar area as the point of maximum pain. He states that he doesn't like to take drugs but he has to; taking drugs is the only way he can continue to function.

SELECT THE BEST ANSWER TO THE FOLLOWING QUESTIONS

Q1. What is the most likely diagnosis in this patient?
   a. congenital vertebral deformity with secondary lumbar fractures
   b. old lumbar fractures with chronic paravertebral muscle spasm
   c. chronic lumbar pain syndrome
   d. narcotic drug abuse
   e. somatoform pain disorder

Q2. Your suspicions are confirmed. What should your next step be?
a. order a CT scan of the lumbar spine
b. order an MRI scan of the lumbar spine
c. refer the patient for an orthopedic consultation
d. refer the patient for a neurosurgical consultation
e. none of the above

Q3. After the initiation of the most appropriate investigative procedure (or other intervention or non-intervention), what would you do then?
a. prescribe Demerol and Talwin for 1 month and see the patient for review at that time
b. prescribe Talwin but not Demerol in an effort to cut down on the amount of narcotic analgesic used
c. prescribe Tylenol with Codeine instead of Talwin and Demerol in an effort to decrease the addiction potential of the drug used
d. begin to prescribe Demerol or Talwin for short periods of time (1 week) in an effort to monitor drug intake carefully
e. none of the above

Q4. Which of the following statements regarding drug abuse and drug dependence is true?
a. drug dependence is defined as the inappropriate use of a drug in terms of either the medical indications or its dose
b. drug abuse refers to physical or psychologic dependence on drugs
c. prescription drug abuse includes legal drugs that find their way into the illicit drug market
d. drug abuse may or may not lead to drug dependence
e. none of the above statements is true

Q5. Which of the following prescription drugs are unlikely to be abused?
a. narcotic analgesics
b. sedative-hypnotics
c. benzodiazepines
d. amphetamine-like substances
e. anticonvulsants

Q6. Which of the following benzodiazepines is less likely to be associated with rebound anxiety?
a. triazolam
b. lorazepam
c. alprazolam
d. flurazepam
e. all of the above may cause rebound anxiety

Q7. Which of the following groups of physicians are likely to be responsible for drug diversion?
a. impaired physicians
b. dishonest physicians
c. duped physicians
d. dated physicians
e. all of the above may be responsible for drug diversion

Q8. Which of the following drugs may be helpful in the treatment of chronic low back pain?
a. amitriptyline
b. methocarbamol
c. acetaminophen
d. naproxen
e. all of the above

Q9. Which of the following statements regarding chronic low back pain treated with narcotic analgesics is true?
a. narcotic analgesics are absolutely contraindicated in all cases of chronic low back pain
b. narcotic analgesics are likely to add to the patient's problems rather than helping them
c. narcotic analgesics are rarely used in the management of chronic low back pain
d. narcotic analgesics are likely to have a significant positive impact on the patient's low back pain
e. none of the above

Q10. Which of the following conditions is the most frequent diagnosis in which narcotic analgesics are used for a chronic nonmalignant pain problem?
a. migraine headaches
b. rheumatoid arthritis
c. chronic pelvic pain
d. abdominal pain
e. ischemic vascular disease

SHORT ANSWER MANAGEMENT PROBLEM
Describe a set of conditions under which the use of narcotic analgesics for the management of chronic nonmalignant pain may be considered appropriate.

ANSWERS

A1. **d.** The most likely diagnosis in this patient is narcotic drug abuse. If he himself is not a narcotic abuser, he may very well be a prescription drug trafficker.

The most common office presentations of opioid abusers are complaints of chronic pain, often related to previous trauma. Chronic back pain or other orthopedic pain related to an old injury and chronic headache are the two most common complaints.

A valuable clue to narcotic abuse in this patient is his statement that his pain is relieved only by taking a combination of pentazocine and meperidine. A patient who names his analgesics of choice is almost certainly either a narcotic drug addict or a drug trafficker.

A2. e. The ordering of a CT scan, an MRI scan, or the referral to a consultant orthopedic surgeon or neurosurgeon would not be valuable in this patient. In most cases, even if the appointment was made, the patient would not keep it. There is a significant probability that no such injury occurred, and the whole episode is fictitious. On the other hand, it is possible that the injury occurred and that the patient has become dependent on and/or addicted to narcotic analgesics.

The appropriate "investigation" in this case would be to attempt to elicit a more complete history regarding the patient's injury, including initial emergency treatment and other physicians consulted, and to discuss with the patient your serious concerns regarding his use of narcotic analgesics.

His response to your concerns will, in all likelihood, further elucidate the diagnosis. The chronic pain patient may be too frightened of recurrence or too dependent on narcotic analgesics to consider alternative forms of pain management; the prescription drug trafficker will either increase pressure or become angry or even violent; and the patient who is going through withdrawal may admit to this at this point.

A3. e. If the patient is a true narcotic drug addict, the most reasonable course of action is to attempt to convince him to enter an inpatient drug rehabilitation program. In programs of this type, methadone is often available for the slow tapering of the narcotic dosage.

All of the other options are inappropriate. If the patient is a narcotic addict, you have simply continued to supply his habit. If he is a drug trafficker, you have just supplied him with drugs to peddle to other narcotic addicts.

A4. d. Drug abuse is defined as inappropriate use of a drug in terms of either its medical indications or its dose. Drug dependence refers to physical or psychologic dependence on drugs. Drug abuse may or may not lead to drug dependence.

Prescription drug abuse refers to the abuse of drugs that are obtained by physician prescription. It does not include legal drugs that find their way into the illicit drug market.

A5. e. The four main classes of psychoactive drugs that tend to be chronically abused include the narcotic analgesics, the sedative-hypnotics, the benzodiazepines, and the amphetamine-like substances.

Some of the commonly abused prescription drugs include the following: Dilaudid, Fiorinal, morphine, Percocet/Percodan, Valium, and a combination of Talwin and Ritalin.

The anticonvulsant medications (such as carbamazepine and valproic acid) are unlikely to be associated with abuse.

A6. d. Rebound anxiety after discontinuation of a sedative-hypnotic can produce severe symptoms. The syndrome, however, is transient and lasts for a relatively short time.

The risk of rebound anxiety is directly related to the elimination half-life after short-term use. Short-acting agents such as triazolam, lorazepam, and bromazepam carry a greater risk than a longer-acting agent such as flurazepam.

A7. e. Doctors responsible for drug diversion and the continuation of prescription drug abuse can be divided into the four Ds: the "disabled or impaired physicians" who prescribe medications for themselves; the "dishonest doctors" who consciously misprescribe for profit; the "duped doctors" who easily give in to patient demands for drugs; and the "dated doctors" who lack medical knowledge regarding the effects of their prescriptions.

A8. e. Patients with chronic low back pain should be treated with anything but narcotic analgesics. Direct analgesics such as acetaminophen, aspirin, and nonsteroidal antiinflammatory agents (NSAIDs) such as naproxen can be very helpful. Skeletal muscle relaxants such as methocarbamol may reduce skeletal muscle spasm around the injured or chronic pain area. Adjuvant analgesics such as desipramine (a tricyclic antidepressant) are very useful in chronic back syndromes, especially neuropathic chronic pain syndromes.

A9. b. Narcotic analgesics are likely to add to the patient's problems rather than help or diminish them. Essentially, what started out as one problem (the chronic low back pain) has become two problems (the chronic low back pain plus narcotic dependence and/or addiction).

Although not absolutely contraindicated in the management of low back pain, they should not be used unless all of the following conditions have been fulfilled:

a. You are absolutely sure that the patient has a "real" chronic pain syndrome that is anatomically and physiologically based (this is quite rare).

b. You have tried all aspects and types of nonpharmacologic therapy and all other types of pharmacologic management before resorting to narcotic analgesics.

c. A colleague or specialist in pain management has been consulted.

A complete list of conditions is covered in the summary at the end of this problem.

Narcotic analgesics do not create a positive impact on your patient's life and your patient's pain. Usually you start the patient on a low dose and the dose gradually increases. The patient returns and the pain is no better or only minimally better. Therefore you prescribe an increased dose of the narcotic, and the cycle begins to repeat itself again and again.

In the general population of patients with chronic pain syndromes, narcotic analgesics are used much more often than they should be. Once the cycle is established, it is very difficult to break.

A10. **a.** The most frequent nonmalignant pain diagnosis leading to the prescription of narcotic analgesics is migraine headache. Patients with chronic migraine headache frequently come to the Emergency Department of hospitals seeking injections of meperidine and dramamine. The patient tells you that "this is the only combination that works." The probability that this patient has a nonmalignant pain syndrome without some degree of narcotic dependence or narcotic addiction is very low.

SOLUTION TO THE SHORT ANSWER MANAGEMENT PROBLEM

The answer includes a summary of rules that may be helpful in managing patients with chronic nonmalignant pain. These represent the guidelines established by the College of Physicians and Surgeons, Province of Alberta. Guidelines vary from state to state and from province to province. Please consult your state licensing authority before adhering to these guidelines.*

GUIDELINES FOR THE MANAGEMENT OF CHRONIC NONMALIGNANT PAIN

1. Take a complete pain history and do a complete physical examination.
2. Assess the patient for the possibility of coexistent depression, sleep disorder, personality disorder,

---

*The College of Physicians and Surgeons of Alberta, Canada: *Guidelines for the management of chronic non-malignant pain*, Edmonton, Canada, 1993.

poorly developed coping skills, and level of social function.
3. Obtain all relevant documentation concerning prior investigations and consultations.
4. Consider ways in which the patient can be empowered to assume responsibility for the problem.
5. Long-term treatment with analgesic medication should be administered only if analgesics result in relief of pain, functional improvement, or both.
6. Opioids are not first-line drugs in the management of chronic nonmalignant pain but are occasionally helpful. One must carefully weigh the potential problems associated with such medications against possible benefit when considering prescribing them.
7. A multidisciplinary team approach to pain management is essential.

GUIDELINES FOR OPIOID USE IN CHRONIC NONMALIGNANT PAIN

1. Diagnosis of the underlying medical condition causing the pain problem must be established.
2. A history of recent or remote substance abuse is a relatively strong contraindication to the use of any opioid; the available evidence suggests that chronic opioid therapy in such patients should be considered only under extraordinary circumstances.
3. An adequate trial of nonopioid analgesics and adjuvant analgesics should have been carried out without success.
4. Only one physician should prescribe opioids.
5. To start a patient on an opioid, the principles of the World Health Organization's "analgesic ladder" should be employed. Patients should first be started on opioids in combination with NSAIDs or acetaminophen. Only after a good trial on a weak opioid should a strong opioid be considered.
6. Treatment of pain with opioids is actually a treatment trial and, like all therapeutic trials, may be effective or ineffective. Effective therapy may be defined as identification of a dose associated with meaningful partial analgesia and no adverse effects severe enough to compromise comfort or function.
7. If a fixed preparation of a weak opioid and nonopioid analgesic is not satisfactory, then oral morphine may be tried on the patient.
8. Parenteral dosing of opioids to treat chronic nonmalignant pain should be strongly discouraged and daily IM injections avoided.
9. There should be an agreement between the patient and the prescribing physician that clearly delineates that there can be no unsanctioned dose esca-

lation, no selling of the opioids, no seeking of opioids from another physician, and no hoarding of opioids.

10. The patient should be seen and assessed at least every 9 weeks and more frequently if there is a history of previous substance abuse. At each visit the clinician should evaluate the patient for several distinct aspects of therapy, including the following:
    a. Analgesic efficacy
    b. Adverse pharmacologic events
    c. Function (physical and psychologic)
    d. The occurrence of apparent drug-abuse-related behaviors

Documentation is very important with this therapy, and physicians should keep careful records that include reference to the various aspects of therapy.

11. Flares of pain can be treated with small extra doses of opioid by mouth; each monthly prescription should include a few extra doses for this purpose.

The goal of chronic opioid therapy is not the elimination of pain (which may be impossible) but rather the control of pain to a tolerable level; there is clear emphasis on level of function of the patient in his/her social, work, and personal life.

SUGGESTED READINGS

American Psychiatric Association: *Diagnostic and statistical manual*, ed 4, Washington, DC, 1994, American Psychiatric Association Press.

The College of Physicians and Surgeons of Alberta, Canada: *Guidelines for the management of chronic non-malignant pain*, Edmonton, Canada, 1993.

National Cancer Institute: *Guidelines for pain management*, 1999; *http://www.nci.nih.gov.*

Weiss K, Greenfield P: Prescription drug abuse, *Psychiatr Clin North Am* 9(3):475-490, 1986.

PROBLEM·40

ETHICS

"Beware! There May Be a Surreptitious Price to Pay!"

Case 1 ■ A Pharmaceutical Company That Is Paying for a "Weekend Getaway" for All of the Family Practice Residents

A pharmaceutical company has just produced another "marvelous" scientific advance (in their own words) in the treatment of peptic ulcer disease. The local representative advises you, the chief family medicine resident, of their desire to send all 24 of your residents on an "all-expenses-paid weekend" to attend a CME event on peptic ulcer disease. There will, of course, be

time for certain "organized and expense-paid recreational activities" following the 1½ hours of lecture each day on a 3-day weekend. Included in the offer are the following:

1. Air transportation for you and a significant other to a "getaway retreat" on the Eastern seaboard
2. All hotel accommodations for you and your significant other
3. All meals for you and your significant other
4. Conference registration
5. All recreational activities, including golf at a six-star golf course, white-water rafting, snorkeling, horseback riding, and even a "shopping spree" for the shoppers in the crowd. As the chief resident you are responsible for making the final decision on whether or not this should take place.

SELECT THE BEST ANSWER TO THE FOLLOWING QUESTIONS

Q1. You consider the event to be:
   a. unequivocally ethical and would personally support it
   b. ethical enough that it deserves your support
   c. of a questionable ethical nature that you may or may not support depending on the nature of additional information received concerning it
   d. of sufficient ethical doubt to cause you to seriously consider not supporting it
   e. unequivocally unethical and will not support it in any way

Q2. You, a practicing family physician, are invited to attend an "evening under the stars" featuring a 3-hour river cruise and a gourmet meal for you and your "significant other." Of course, a short (1-minute) scientific presentation on the merits of the sponsoring company's drug will be the true highlight of the evening. You consider the event to be:
   a. unequivocally ethical and would personally support it
   b. ethical enough that it deserves your support
   c. of a questionable ethical nature that you may or may not support depending on the nature of additional information received concerning it
   d. of sufficient ethical doubt to cause you to seriously consider not supporting it
   e. unequivocally unethical and will not support it in any way

Q3. You, the principal investigator for a phase IV (post-marketing) trial, are invited to organize and attend an international 1-day symposium on the preliminary results of the "research." The symposium is being held in a luxury hotel on the French Riviera. Your 10 co-investigators are also invited. You consider the event to be:

a. unequivocally ethical and would personally support it
b. ethical enough that it deserves your support
c. of a questionable ethical nature that you may or may not support depending on the nature of additional information received concerning it
d. of sufficient ethical doubt to cause you to seriously consider not supporting it
e. unequivocally unethical and will not support it in any way

Q4. You, the director of CME for a major hospital, are offered the use of an "audience response system" donated to your department (an audience response system allows the responses of a CME audience to be measured one-to-another and compared to the correct response). The cost of the system is $10,000. The company representatives insist that "there are no strings attached." You consider the offer to be:

a. unequivocally ethical and would personally support it
b. ethical enough that it deserves your support
c. of a questionable ethical nature that you may or may not support depending on the nature of additional information received concerning it
d. of sufficient ethical doubt to cause you to seriously consider not supporting it
e. unequivocally unethical and will not support it in any way

Q5. The representative of a large company specializing in the development of new antihypertensive agents offers to sponsor a "dinner meeting" for 100 physicians. At this dinner meeting a well-known expert (remember the definition of an expert: Someone from out of town with a tray full of slides) will present his views on the "new drug treatments for hypertension." The dinner meeting will be held at a world-class French restaurant and will feature "exquisite French cuisine prepared by a chef flown in from Paris for the specific purpose of preparing the meal." You consider the event to be:

a. unequivocally ethical and would personally support it
b. ethical enough that it deserves your support
c. of a questionable ethical nature that you may or may not support depending on the

nature of additional information received concerning it
d. of sufficient ethical doubt to cause you to seriously consider not supporting it
e. unequivocally unethical and will not support it in any way

Q6. A well-known pharmaceutical company offers to donate $1,000,000 for a "resident scholarship" to attend a major scientific meeting. The funds will be made available to the residency program director and the selection made by the department of family medicine itself. You consider the event to be:

a. unequivocally ethical and would personally support it
b. ethical enough that it deserves your support
c. of a questionable ethical nature that you may or may not support depending on the nature of additional information received concerning it
d. of sufficient ethical doubt to cause you to seriously consider not supporting it
e. unequivocally unethical and will not support it in any way

Q7. A pharmaceutical company representative makes an appointment to see you, the chief resident in the department of family medicine, to discuss the sponsoring of "noon rounds" for the next 4 weeks. He apparently has "drug videos" that he wishes to familiarize your resident colleagues with. He, of course, will provide all the necessary refreshments and food for the entire group. You consider the event to be:

a. unequivocally ethical and would personally support it
b. ethical enough that it deserves your support
c. of a questionable ethical nature that you may or may not support depending on the nature of additional information received concerning it
d. of sufficient ethical doubt to cause you to seriously consider not supporting it
e. unequivocally unethical and will not support it in any way

Q8. Fifty pharmaceutical companies agree to "buy booths" at a major national scientific meeting. You are the chairperson of the scientific meeting and are asked to make the final decision in this case. You consider the event to be:

a. unequivocally ethical and would personally support it
b. ethical enough that it deserves your support

c. of a questionable ethical nature that you may or may not support depending on the nature of additional information received concerning it

d. of sufficient ethical doubt to cause you to seriously consider not supporting it

e. unequivocally unethical and will not support it in any way

Q9. The same situation as described in Question 8 occurs in this case. The only difference, however, is that each pharmaceutical company is attempting to outdo the other with "tokens of appreciation." These vary from simple pens and pencils to entire sets of golf clubs. You consider the event to be:

a. unequivocally ethical and would personally support it

b. ethical enough that it deserves your support

c. of a questionable ethical nature that you may or may not support depending on the nature of additional information received concerning it

d. of sufficient ethical doubt to cause you to seriously consider not supporting it

e. unequivocally unethical and will not support it in any way

Q10. A pharmaceutical company asks you, a family physician with expertise in cancer pain management, to speak at a "dinner meeting." The dinner meeting is being held at a "middle-class" restaurant. You will be paid $2000 for your services. You consider the event to be:

a. unequivocally ethical and would personally support it

b. ethical enough that it deserves your support

c. of a questionable ethical nature that you may or may not support depending on the nature of additional information received concerning it

d. of sufficient ethical doubt to cause you to seriously consider not supporting it

e. unequivocally unethical and will not support it in any way

ANSWERS

A1. **d.** The following "acid tests" produced by the American College of Physicians should help you to come to a reasonable conclusion on all of the ethical problems presented. The two acid tests that can be used in every case are as follows:

a. Would this event withstand both public and professional scrutiny?

b. Would you want these arrangements to be generally known?

In this case, the payment for airfare, accommodation, meals, recreational events, and apparently everything else is completely contrary to the guidelines established by the American Academy of Family Physicians. In addition, it is extremely doubtful that these arrangements would withstand either public or professional scrutiny, nor would many feel comfortable with their publication in the local newspaper the next day.

Suppose, for example, the event is being sponsored by company X marketing drug Y. You are a heart patient taking company X's drug. Furthermore, assume that the drug is very expensive and you are on a fixed income. On reading about this in your local paper, your response would likely be less than positive.

A2. **e.** You may think that this is a complete exaggeration and that no one would seriously consider only a 1-minute presentation. This, in fact, is a true scenario that attracted 75 physicians and their spouses.

A3. **d.** There are enough serious questions that arise from this description to place the event in the d category.

On the ethical side, you, the principal investigator, and your 10 co-investigators are being invited to a meeting to discuss "research" results.

On the very questionable side are the following:

a. This is a post-marketing study and cannot in any meaningful way be classified as research. These studies are most often uncontrolled and simply require the "researcher" to fill in a simple form, for which a computer system (which, of course, the "researcher" gets to keep) is provided.

b. As another acid test, it has been suggested that you must determine the primary attraction to the event. Is it the scientific meeting itself or the social venue? In this case, the social venue would probably win out.

Q4. **a.** In this case, the fiduciary relationship of patient and physician is not compromised. In fact, it could be argued that because the audience response system increases the interactive nature of any CME event, the "probability of learning" among the participants will increase. This should result in improved patient care.

A5. **e.** This case reeks of possible "influence peddling" and "peer selling"; what you might as well refer to as a "hit man" for the company presents views on why this company's product is superior to anything else produced by humanity to date.

Only if the following conditions were satisfied would an affair of this nature be acceptable to both public and professional scrutiny:

a. The speaker presented an independent, unbiased assessment of hypertensive drug treatment. This must include not only an analysis of new products but a comparison (both efficacy and cost) with older products.

b. The affair was held at a somewhat less elaborate restaurant with a somewhat less elaborate menu.

A6. **a.** This is, it appears, a highly ethical proposal that presents few if any problems. The major consideration in this case is the control of the funds and the selection of the resident by the department of family medicine itself.

A7. **d.** Although "noon rounds" should and usually do have significant educational value, you must be very cautious about the nature of the drug videos. If they portray a reasonable summary of the disease condition and its treatment in a balanced perspective (with the company's product mentioned by generic name only and mentioned as one of the treatment options), then it may be a reasonable request. If the drug videos are, as in most cases, strictly promotional in nature, then on the basis of the importance of maintaining a completely ethical relationship with the pharmaceutical industry, you would probably have to refuse the request.

A8. **a.** The fact of the matter is that we, as physicians, must work in close cooperation with the pharmaceutical industry. Continuing medical education would suffer greatly and in many cases be completely eliminated without the support of industry. The buying of booths for a major meeting or the buying of advertising space at national and regional medical publications is common practice and considered to be completely ethical by most concerned.

A9. **d.** There is considerable debate on this subject. The major contention by those who consider this practice to be unethical is that the pharmaceutical companies are, by their actions, attempting to "buy" the physicians. It appears to many, however, to be a matter of degree. In my opinion, a pen is unlikely to buy a physician; a complete set of golf clubs is a different story.

A10. **d.** The ethical difficulty with this problem is not the topic, the speaker, or the restaurant; rather, it is the amount of money that both the public and your professional colleagues would consider to be reasonable

for a 1-hour presentation. You could even argue that because cancer pain is an area in which family physicians can use considerable education, this activity should be encouraged. Dr. Swanson donated the $2000 to the Residency Trust Fund when faced with this very issue.

SUMMARY OF ETHICAL CONSIDERATIONS FOR PHYSICIANS AND THE PHARMACEUTICAL INDUSTRY

1. *Primum non nocere*—"First do no harm" (including no harm in inflating drug costs by your acceptance of pharmaceutical offerings that are clearly unethical).

2. The acid tests for dealing with industry:
   a. Would you want these arrangements generally known?
   b. Would this withstand public and professional scrutiny?

3. Physicians and the pharmaceutical industry must work together. That working together, however, must be on terms that never compromise the fiduciary relationship between patient and physician or pass the cost for these events onto those who can least afford it.

4. Residents beware: As the prescribers of tomorrow, you are the number one target of the pharmaceutical industry.

5. Consider the primary purpose of the event in question: Is it the event itself or the social venue?

6. Remember to call research and marketing what they are. Be cautious of the real purpose of your involvement in post-marketing research—in most cases it is marketing and not research.

7. Beware of experts from afar: They may be "snake-oil salesmen" in disguise.

SUGGESTED READINGS

American Academy of Family Physicians approves statement on the ethics of proprietary relationship with industry, *Am Fam Physician* 44(6):2233-2239, 1991.

E-Addendum 11: *Clarification of gifts to physicians from industry,* Council on Ethical and Judicial Affairs *(E- 8.061),* 1999; *Policy Finder @http://www.ama-assn.org.*

Newton W et al: There is no such thing as a free lunch. Developing policies on pharmaceutical industry support, *J Fam Practice* 34(1):32-34, 1992.

C·H·A·P·T·E·R 2

Obstetrics

FAMILY-CENTERED MATERNITY CARE

"Doctor, Will You Help Me Make This a Family Affair?"

Case 1 ■ A 26-Year-Old Primigravida Who Wishes to Discuss a Birth Plan

A 26-year-old woman comes to your office at 14 weeks' gestation for her initial prenatal visit. You have been referred to her by friends who are your patients. She would like you to assume her prenatal care and deliver her child.

Her uterus feels 14 weeks by size and her blood pressure is 100/70 mm Hg. All other aspects of the initial complete physical examination are normal.

SELECT THE BEST ANSWER TO THE FOLLOWING QUESTIONS

Q1. The patient asks you about birth plans during her initial visit and inquires as to your attitudes toward pregnant couples who wish to participate in decision-making regarding the conduct of labor and delivery. How would you respond?
   a. birth plans are not a good idea; usually something goes wrong and the couple is disappointed
   b. birth plans are not a good idea; they frequently lead to unresolved guilt in the couple
   c. birth plans should be avoided; perinatal morbidity and mortality is usually increased
   d. birth plans are an excellent idea; everything always goes according to plan
   e. birth plans are a good idea; they involve the couple in the planning for their baby's delivery and can be a very important part of the prenatal, postnatal, and postpartum care

Q2. On the next prenatal visit, the couple wishes to discuss your feelings concerning a number of issues. The first issue is electronic fetal monitoring. The couple is aware that, in some hospitals and with some physicians, continuous electronic fetal monitoring (EFM) in labor is standard procedure.

Which of the following statements regarding continuous routine EFM is true?
   a. the perinatal mortality rate in laboring patients who undergo continuous EFM is lower than in those who do not
   b. the perinatal morbidity rate in laboring patients who undergo EFM is lower than in those who do not
   c. the incidence of cesarean section in laboring patients undergoing EFM is not statistically different from those who do not
   d. there is no significant difference in perinatal outcomes between those patients who undergo EFM and those who do not
   e. the incidence of admission to the intensive care nursery is greater in those patients whose fetuses do not undergo EFM

Q3. The couple then asks you about routinely ordering ultrasound in pregnancy. Which of the following statements regarding the use of routine ultrasound in pregnancy is false?
   a. routine prenatal ultrasound has been shown by U.S. studies to be justified from a cost-benefit standpoint
   b. repetitive studies by independent researchers have not found any consistently adverse effects of obstetric ultrasound on perinatal outcome
   c. first-trimester ultrasound gestational age assessment should be performed on patients scheduled for elective repeat cesarean section
   d. vaginal bleeding in pregnancy should be assessed by ultrasound examination
   e. a size-date discrepancy in fundal height of 3 cm or more is an indication for obstetrical ultrasound

Q4. The couple inquires about the routine administration of intravenous (IV) fluids during labor. Concerning this issue, which of the following statements is false?
   a. the use of routine IV fluids does not limit ambulation in the first stage of labor

b. if epidural analgesia is to be administered, an IV line must be in place

c. if the first stage of labor is prolonged, an IV line should be in place to prevent dehydration

d. if a patient has a history of a severe postpartum hemorrhage, an IV line should be established

e. none of the above statements is false

Q5. When you mention the words "epidural analgesia," the couple becomes quite agitated. They state quite emphatically that they do not wish, under any circumstances, to have an epidural anesthetic. What should your response to this request be?

a. "you really have to leave it up to me to decide that"

b. "epidural analgesia is one of many noncompulsory methods to relieve labor pain"

c. "you better track down another doctor"

d. "epidurals have no complications; you should really reconsider your position"

e. none of the above

Q6. Which of the following statements regarding epidural analgesia is (are) true?

a. maternal hypertension is a common side effect of epidural analgesia

b. high spinal anesthesia is one of the most serious complications of epidural analgesia

c. unintentional dural puncture occurs in 10% of attempted epidural analgesia

d. prolongation of all stages of labor by epidural analgesia has been established

e. fetal bradycardia is consistently seen with epidural analgesia

Q7. The couple has registered in Lamaze classes. Lamaze can best be described as which of the following?

a. a method emphasizing the psychoprophylaxis of labor

b. a method describing how to keep away from physicians at all costs

c. a method concentrating on the difficulties physicians cause in obstetrics

d. a method emphasizing the importance of "toughing things out"

e. all of the above

Q8. The couple's final question concerns "routine episiotomy." They have been told that the medical profession is "cut-happy" and that the vast majority of episiotomies are unnecessary. Which of the following statements regarding routine episiotomy is true?

a. episiotomy pain may be more severe and last longer than the pain from perineal lacerations

b. episiotomy repairs heal more rapidly than do vaginal and perineal tears

c. dyspareunia is more common after vaginal lacerations and perineal tear than after episiotomy

d. episiotomy reduces the rate of subsequent pelvic relaxation problems

e. episiotomy reduces the rate of third- and fourth-degree perineal lacerations

Q9. Which of the following is (are) an indication for the performance of an episiotomy?

a. nonreassuring fetal heart rate in the second stage of labor

b. significant maternal cardiac disease

c. operative delivery using obstetric forceps

d. delivery of the fetus with shoulder dystocia

e. all of the above

Q10. Which of the following statements regarding the presence or absence of a supportive person (or coach) in labor is (are) true?

a. the presence of a support person or coach decreases the need for analgesia in labor

b. the presence of a support person or coach decreases the need for operative interventions such as forceps or vacuum extraction

c. the presence of a support person or coach decreases the cesarean section rate

d. all of the above are true

e. none of the above is true

SHORT ANSWER MANAGEMENT PROBLEM
A 28-year-old primigravida presents at 16 weeks' gestation for her first prenatal visit. She is accompanied by her husband. As you begin to discuss your routine with respect to prenatal care, the couple presents you with a "list of demands." These demands include the right to decide whether an IV will be inserted, when the fetal heart can be auscultated, when the physician can "interfere" with the natural birth process, and how the infant is to be resuscitated. Describe how you would deal with this problem.

ANSWERS

A1. **e.** Birth plans are an integral component of what has become known as family-centered maternity care. Family-centered maternity care allows pregnant couples the opportunity of going through labor and delivery in an informal setting, preferably with minimal medical intervention. Family-centered maternity care involves the husband or significant other as a coach in labor and allows for immediate bonding of infant to both parents.

Breast-feeding is encouraged, and rooming-in is available. A trusting doctor-patient relationship is essential to family-centered maternity care. If the couple is confident in their doctor, they feel secure that any intervention that is considered will obviously be discussed with them. If the couple is involved in the decision-making process throughout labor and delivery, any unresolved guilt related to the birth process will be avoided.

A2. **d.** Well-controlled studies have shown that intermittent auscultation of the fetal heart rate is equivalent to EFM in assessing fetal condition when performed at specific intervals with a 1:1 nurse-to-patient ratio. EFM is associated with a small but significant increase in the incidence of delivery by cesarean section due to presumed "fetal distress." Perinatal outcomes as assessed by intrapartum stillbirths, low Apgar scores, need for assisted ventilation of the newborn, admission to neonatal intensive care unit, and the onset of neonatal seizures are similar with both intermittent auscultation and EFM.

A3. **a.** Although obstetric ultrasound studies are performed routinely in many European countries, in the United States the routine use of ultrasonography cannot be supported from a cost-benefit standpoint. However, a 1984 consensus development conference convened by the National Institute of Child Health and Human Development proposed 27 indications for ultrasonography in pregnancy. These indications include estimation of gestational age for patients scheduled for elective cesarean delivery, identification of the cause of vaginal bleeding in pregnancy, and evaluation of significant uterine size-clinical dates discrepancy. Ultrasound exposure at intensities usually produced by diagnostic ultrasound instruments has not been found to cause any harmful biologic effects on fetuses. Infants exposed in utero have shown no significant differences in birth weight or length, childhood growth, cognitive function, acoustic or visual ability, or rates of neurologic deficits. The use of diagnostic obstetric ultrasound on an as-needed basis has been supported by the American College of Obstetricians and Gynecologists.

A4. **a.** An IV line can limit ambulation in the first stage of labor. Although it is customary in many hospitals to start IV infusions early in labor, there is seldom any real need to do so in women with uncomplicated pregnancies at least until analgesia is admin-

istered. Listed below are situations in which IV hydration is indicated:
   a. for prehydration when epidural analgesia is about to be administered
   b. to prevent dehydration and acidosis in the presence of a prolonged first stage of labor
   c. to administer oxytocin prophylactically to prevent postpartum hemorrhage

A5. **b.** Epidural analgesia should be viewed as an option and only as an option. It is highly effective at significantly reducing or completely eliminating pain in the second stage of labor. There is some evidence that severe pain in labor may cause maternal vasoconstriction and subsequent decreased oxygen flow to the fetus; however, this has not been established. As with any invasive procedure, use of epidural analgesia may be associated with severe but rare complications.

A6. **b.** One of the most serious immediate complications of epidural analgesia is a high or total spinal. Signs and symptoms include numbness and weakness of upper extremities, dyspnea, inability to speak, and finally apnea and loss of consciousness. Maternal hypotension, not hypertension, is common and can be minimized by prophylactic intravascular volume expansion with 500 to 1000 ml of non-glucose-containing isotonic crystalloid solution. Unintentional dural puncture, resulting in a spinal headache, occurs in less than 2% of cases. Randomized controlled trials have shown conflicting results regarding the effect of epidurals on progress of labor. Fetal bradycardia may be occasionally seen with epidural analgesia, but it is usually easily treated by IV fluid administration and conservative management.

A7. **a.** Patients who utilize the Lamaze technique have been schooled in the psychoprophylaxis of labor. Some people regard Lamaze as "anti-physician," "anti-all-intervention," and "anti-everything else." This is somewhat unfair. The Lamaze technique, if properly utilized, can help a select group of patients achieve the goals they have identified for their labor and delivery experience.

A8. **a.** Episiotomy pain may be more severe and long-lasting than the pain of vaginal and perineal lacerations. Healing time for vaginal and perineal lacerations is generally shorter than the healing time for an episiotomy. Dyspareunia is more common after episiotomy than after vaginal and perineal tears, resulting in a prolongation of time before return to normal sexual activity.

Routine episiotomy neither increases nor decreases the incidence of subsequent pelvic relaxation. All randomized prospective studies have shown the rate of third- and fourth-degree perineal lacerations are increased rather than reduced by routine episiotomy.

A9. **e.** Indications for episiotomy include nonreassuring fetal heart rate findings in the second stage of labor, significant maternal cardiac disease, prophylactic forceps, shoulder dystocia, and infants in the breech presentation when vaginal delivery is anticipated.

Contraindications to episiotomy include inflammatory bowel disease, lymphogranuloma venereum, or severe perineal scarring or malformation. Complications of episiotomy include excessive blood loss and increased rates of lacerations into the anal sphincter and anal mucosa as well as infections.

Episiotomy rates can be reduced by following these indications and contraindications and by not performing an episiotomy routinely. Vaginal and perineal tears may be avoided by perineal massage and stretching exercises before delivery. Communication with the patient during perineal stretching will help reduce the degree and number of tears during childbirth. Also, controlling professional urgency for rapid delivery provides extra time for the fetal head to stretch the perineum, resulting in an increased possibility for an intact perineum.

Episiotomy does shorten the second stage of labor, but that in and of itself is not a reason for its performance.

A10. **a.** The presence of a support person or coach decreases the need for subsequent analgesia in labor. This does not, however, apply to subsequent operative interventions including forceps delivery, vacuum extraction, or cesarean section.

SOLUTION TO THE SHORT ANSWER MANAGEMENT PROBLEM

This particular scenario, which is not uncommon, can be described in one way only: bad news. It is reasonable to attempt to talk to this couple in an effort to try and discover why they feel the way they do about the medical profession. Have they had a bad experience? Do they have any trust in you, to whom they have come seeking prenatal care? These issues in this case can be summarized as follows:
1. Is the couple prepared to accept your decisions regarding when medical intervention is necessary provided you consult and explain your position to them?
2. Is the couple prepared to allow you, as the physician, to perform your duly responsible medical functions in this case?

3. Is the couple willing to trust you, providing that you earn their trust?

If the answers to all three questions can be eventually negotiated to yes, it would be appropriate to proceed with the care of this patient's pregnancy. If, however, the answer to one or more of the questions is no, the best and safest course of action would be to inform the patient and her husband that in all good conscience you cannot look after their pregnancy. You, as a physician, have that ethical right except in the event of an emergency. In many cases it would be better for all concerned if the physician were to suggest that another care provider be sought. You must, however, continue to look after the patient until the time that a care provider is identified.

The patient should be sent a registered letter to that effect and a copy sent to the College of Physicians and Surgeons in the state or province in which you practice.

SUMMARY OF SOME OF THE ISSUES CONCERNED WITH NATURAL CHILDBIRTH

1. Birth plans: If prudently developed and open to negotiation and change, they may be of benefit in a couple's pregnancy. They have the potential to foster good doctor-patient communication.

2. Continuous EFM is no more effective than intermittent auscultation in lowering perinatal morbidity and mortality in low-risk pregnancies.

3. Current recommendations are that obstetrical ultrasound should only be used for specific indications even though no adverse perinatal outcomes have been demonstrated in repetitive studies.

4. Intravenous therapy: Specific indications include long labor with ketones, use of epidural analgesia, and history of severe postpartum hemorrhage; it is not routinely needed in low-risk pregnancies.

5. Anesthesia: Epidural is the analgesic of choice and should be available should women choose it. Prepared childbirth classes may enhance the number of women seeking unmedicated childbirth.

6. Episiotomy: An episiotomy does not heal more quickly; is more painful, has greater incidence of dyspareunia, increases the risk of third-degree and fourth-degree lacerations, and does not change the incidence of later pelvic relaxation. Although it does shorten the second stage of labor, that shortening in and of itself offers no definitive benefit to either mother or baby.

SUGGESTED READINGS

American Institute of Ultrasound in Medicine: *Bioeffects and safety of diagnostic ultrasound*, Rockville, Md, 1993, AIUM.

Banta D, Thacker S: The risks and benefits of episiotomy: A review, *Birth* 9:25-30, 1982.

Cunningham FG et al: *Williams' obstetrics*, ed 20, Norwalk, Conn, 1997, Appleton & Lange.

Hoult IJ et al: Lumbar epidural analgesia in labor: Relation to fetal malposition and instrument delivery, *Br Med J* 1:14-16, 1977.

Leveno K et al: A prospective comparison of selective and universal fetal monitoring in 34,995 pregnancies, *N Engl J Med* 315:10-16, 1986.

Lyons EA et al: In utero exposure to diagnostic ultrasound: A 6-year follow-up, *Radiology*, 166:687-690, 1988.

MacDonald D et al: The Dublin randomized controlled trial of intrapartum fetal heart rate monitoring, *Am J Obstet Gynecol* 152:524-539, 1985.

PROBLEM·42

PREGNANCY CAN BE UNCOMFORTABLE

"Read My Lips, Doctor. I'm Never Going to Let This Happen Again."

Case 1 ■ A 23-Year-Old Primigravida with Many Physical Complaints

A 23-year-old primigravida comes to your office for her second prenatal visit. You first saw her 4 weeks ago at 7 weeks' gestation. At that time you performed a complete history, a complete physical examination, and all necessary blood work. Today you note she has gained 3 pounds in the last 4 weeks. She has been nauseated every day, with one episode of emesis a day.

On examination, her blood pressure is 110/70 mm Hg and her general and pelvic examination is unremarkable.

SELECT THE BEST ANSWER TO THE FOLLOWING QUESTIONS

Q1. Nausea and/or vomiting in pregnancy affects approximately 80% of women at some time during pregnancy. Current theory suggests that these symptoms are due to increased levels of which of the following hormones?
   a. estrogen
   b. progesterone
   c. human chorionic gonadotropin
   d. human placental lactogen
   e. androstenedione

Q2. Which of the following should not be part of your initial advice or treatment for this patient?

   a. reassurance that this is a self-limiting condition
   b. eating small, frequent meals
   c. discontinuation of oral iron therapy
   d. avoid contact with cooking odors
   e. prescription of an antinausea medication

Q3. What is the drug of choice for severe hyperemesis gravidarum in pregnancy?
   a. prochlorperazine
   b. promethazine
   c. chlorpromazine
   d. metoclopramide
   e. ondansetron

Case 2 ■ A 29-Year-Old Multigravida with an Unrelenting Backache

A 29-year-old multigravida (gravida 5, para 4) comes to your office at 36 weeks' gestation with the following complaint: "I've had the worst backache in my life for the last 10 days. I've put heat on it, I've put cold on it, and I've tried rest. Nothing helps, Doctor."

On examination, the patient has no costovertebral angle (CVA) tenderness. There is moderate paralumbar tenderness. She has had no urinary tract symptoms that would suggest urinary tract infection (UTI). Flexion, extension, lateral rotation, and lateral bending all enhance the pain. She tells you that she does not recall any injury. However, the onset of the backache appeared to correspond with the baby dropping into her pelvis. She has not had any problems with her back in other pregnancies.

The patient describes the pain as dull, constant, and centered in the L2-L5 area, with no radiation to either the right leg or the left leg. It is aggravated by walking, moving, and bending. It is relieved somewhat by rest.

Q4. Which of the following is (are) the most likely reason for her back pain?
   a. motion of the symphysis pubis
   b. motion of the lumbosacral joints
   c. general relaxation of the pelvic ligaments
   d. any of the above
   e. b or c

Q5. What is (are) the management of choice for this patient's condition?
   a. nonpharmacologic therapy: massage, physiotherapy
   b. acetaminophen
   c. acetaminophen and codeine
   d. any of the above
   e. a and/or b only

Case 3 ■ A Pregnant 37-Year-Old Professional Woman with Varicose Veins

A 37-year-old woman (gravida 2, para 1) comes to your office at 16 weeks' gestation with severe vulvar and lower extremity varicosities. They are bilateral and extend from her feet to her thighs. The varicosities began approximately 4 weeks ago and have been gradually increasing in severity. She is a physician and works full-time in her practice. The varicosities are unsightly and cause severe pain, especially as the day goes on. The worst varicosities are her vulvar varicosities.

Q6. What would you recommend at this time for the patient in Case 3?
   a. discontinue work duties until after pregnancy
   b. inject sclerosing agents into the most severe veins
   c. elevate her legs and wear support hose
   d. a and c
   e. all of the above

Q7. Which is the most common complication of varicosities in pregnancy?
   a. deep venous thrombosis
   b. pulmonary embolism
   c. superficial thrombophlebitis
   d. ovarian vein thrombosis
   e. septic pelvic thrombophlebitis

Case 4 ■ A 25-Year-Old Primigravida with Severe Rectal Pain

A 25-year-old primigravida at 36 weeks' gestation comes to your office with severe rectal discomfort of 3 weeks' duration. On examination, you notice several hemorrhoids that are 1 cm in diameter.

Q8. Which of the following statements about hemorrhoids in pregnancy is false?
   a. hemorrhoids are varicosities of the rectal veins
   b. constipation in pregnancy aggravates the formation of hemorrhoids
   c. obstruction of venous return by the enlarged uterus worsens hemorrhoids
   d. bleeding from rectal veins may result in folate-deficiency anemia
   e. thrombosis of a rectal vein can cause significant pain

Case 5 ■ A 28-Year-Old Multigravida with Gastroesophageal Reflux Disease

A 28-year-old multigravida comes to your office at 30 weeks' gestation with heartburn. The symptoms are severe enough that the patient is in pain for the majority of the day.

On examination, the abdomen is soft. The patient's blood pressure is 110/70 mm Hg. There is no evidence of other conditions that may have precipitated this.

Q9. Which of the following statements regarding heartburn in pregnancy is false?
   a. relaxation of the lower esophageal sphincter allows reflux of stomach contents into the esophagus
   b. upward displacement and compression of the stomach by the uterus worsens symptoms
   c. usually symptoms are mild and can be relieved by small, frequent meals
   d. aluminum and magnesium hydroxide are first-line antacid choices
   e. sodium bicarbonate is an antacid that is free of side effects

Q10. Bizarre cravings develop during pregnancy, sometimes to the point that foods or substances considered hardly edible or nonedible are consumed in great quantities. This condition is known as and is associated with which of the following?
   a. pica associated with macrocytic anemia
   b. pica associated with iron-deficiency anemia
   c. amylophagia associated with iron-deficiency anemia
   d. geophagia associated with macrocytic anemia
   e. pica associated with none of the above

Case 6 ■ A Pregnant Woman with Swollen Legs

A patient at 32 weeks' gestation with increased swelling in both lower extremities comes to your office. The previous week she went to another physician with bilateral lower extremity swelling from the knees down. She was prescribed both a thiazide diuretic and a loop diuretic. Now she has come to see you.

Q11. What should you do at this time?
   a. tell her to continue the thiazide diuretic but stop the loop diuretic
   b. tell her to continue the thiazide diuretic and the loop diuretic and add a potassium-sparing diuretic

c. tell her to continue the thiazide diuretic and the loop diuretic, and add an extended release potassium capsule

d. tell her to stop both the thiazide diuretic and the loop diuretic

e. tell her to wait a few minutes, warm up the big office computer, and try to obtain the information from a data bank

Case 7 ■ A 29-Year-Old Primigravida with Copious Vaginal Discharge

A 29-year-old primigravida comes to your office complaining of increased vaginal discharge. She is 33 weeks pregnant.

On speculum examination, you confirm a copious clear vaginal discharge. There is no significant odor, a wet prep is normal, and culture results are negative. No pooling of fluid is seen in the posterior fornix.

Q12. Which of the following statements regarding increased vaginal discharge during pregnancy is (are) true?
a. in most cases, the discharge is physiologic
b. physiologic discharge arises from estrogen-mediated increased cervical mucus
c. monilia may be identified in up to 25% of pregnant women
d. monilia should be treated in both symptomatic women and asymptomatic women
e. a, b, and c are true

Case 8 ■ A Constipated 29-Year-Old Multigravida

A 29-year-old multigravida at 22 weeks' gestation comes to your office with a chief complaint of constipation. She states that she is having only one bowel movement every 5 or so days.

Q13. With regard to this complaint, which of the following statements is (are) true?
a. constipation is uncommon in pregnancy
b. constipation is more common in early pregnancy than in late pregnancy
c. constipation does not need to be treated in pregnancy
d. all of the above are true
e. none of the above is true

Q14. Which of the following has (have) been implicated in the pathogenesis of constipation in pregnancy?
a. reduced gut motility
b. mechanical obstruction by the uterus

c. increased water resorption
d. increased estrogen levels
e. a, b, and c

Q15. The treatment(s) of choice for constipation in pregnancy include which of the following?
a. discontinuing iron supplements
b. increasing the amount of fiber in her diet
c. increasing her physical activity
d. addition of a bulk-forming agent
e. all of the above

SHORT ANSWER MANAGEMENT PROBLEM
List three complaints of pregnant women other than the ones already listed and their causes.

ANSWERS

A1. **c.** Nausea and vomiting in pregnancy are common complaints, especially during the first trimester. Nausea, vomiting, or other gastrointestinal symptoms may occur in up to 80% of pregnant women. The hormonal basis for the nausea and vomiting of pregnancy is not entirely clear. Severe hyperemesis is much more frequent with molar pregnancies with high levels of human chorionic gonadotropin (HCG). Empiric data supporting this includes the finding that as the level of HCG declines at the end of the first trimester, the nausea and vomiting usually subside.

A2. **e.** Nausea in pregnancy should be treated with conservative management whenever possible. Medications should be prescribed only if conservative approaches fail. Small, frequent meals, the avoidance of foods with a high-fat content, an intake of dry foods, and reassurance may be all that is necessary. If iron therapy has been started, it should be discontinued. Avoidance of contact with situations that may induce nausea (such as cooking odors) is also recommended.

If persistent vomiting leads to weight loss, ketonuria, or electrolyte imbalance, hospitalization is necessary. With persistent severe symptoms, it is imperative a workup be undertaken to rule out other serious conditions such as: molar pregnancy, hyperthyroidism, pancreatitis, cholecystitis, appendicitis, hepatitis, and peptic ulcer disease.

A3. **d.** If conservative therapy fails, antinauseants are indicated. The category B drug that can be used in severe hyperemesis gravidarum is metoclopramide, which increases gastrointestinal motility. The category C drugs include promethazine, prochlorperazine, and chlorpromazine. These drugs are used in moderately severe hyperemesis gravidarum.

Categories B and C refer to the risk of using the drug in pregnancy. With drugs that are either category B or category C, the benefit often outweighs the risk.

Ondansetron is a new serotonin antagonist that is being used for severe nausea, particularly the nausea induced by cancer chemotherapy. No experience with pregnant patients is available yet.

A4. **d.** Backache occurs to some extent in most pregnant women in minor degrees following excessive strain or fatigue and excessive bending, lifting, or walking. A mild backache usually requires little more than elimination of the strain. In some pregnant women, as in this patient, motion of the symphysis pubis and lumbosacral joints, as well as general relaxation of pelvic ligaments, may be demonstrated. The most important disease to rule out is UTI (especially ascending).

A5. **e.** Treatment of this condition involves education regarding back pain in pregnancy, rest for much of the remaining pregnancy as possible, massage and physiotherapy, and acetaminophen. Codeine should be avoided; it has habituation potential when used chronically and can aggravate constipation as well.

A6. **d.** Varicosities, generally resulting from congenital predisposition, are exaggerated by prolonged standing and advanced maternal age in pregnancy. They arise in up to 40% of pregnant women. Femoral venous pressure increases by twofold to threefold in pregnancy. The symptoms produced by varicosities vary from cosmetic blemishes on the lower extremities and mild pain to quite severe pain, tenderness, discomfort, and prominence. The suggested treatment is daily, frequent periods of rest and elevation of the lower extremities.

A7. **c.** The most common complication of superficial varicosities is superficial thrombophlebitis. This should be treated with cold packs and rest. Superficial thrombophlebitis is not related to deep venous thrombosis, ovarian vein thrombosis, septic pelvic thrombophlebitis, or pulmonary embolism.

A8. **d.** Hemorrhoids are varicosities of the rectal veins that are most often related to increased pressure on the rectal veins caused by obstruction of venous return by the large uterus, and by the tendency to be constipated in pregnancy.

Pain and swelling can usually be relieved by topically applied anesthetics, warm soaks, and agents that soften the stool. Thrombosis of a rectal vein can cause considerable pain, and when this happens (usually re-

lated to an external rectal vein), the clot should be evacuated. Bleeding from the rectal veins can occasionally result in the loss of sufficient blood to cause an iron-deficiency (not folate-deficiency) anemia. The loss of only 15 ml of blood results in the loss of 6 to 7 mg of iron, an amount that is equal to the daily requirements during later pregnancy.

A9. **e.** Heartburn, an extremely common complaint in pregnancy, is caused by the reflux of gastric contents into the lower esophagus. The increased frequency of regurgitation during pregnancy most likely results from the upward displacement and compression of the stomach by the uterus combined with decreased gastrointestinal motility. In most pregnant women the symptoms are mild and are relieved by a regimen of small, frequent meals and avoidance of bending over.

Antacid preparations may provide considerable relief, and most are completely safe. Aluminum hydroxide, magnesium hydroxide, and magnesium trisilicate, alone or in combination, should be used in preference to sodium bicarbonate. The pregnant woman who tends to retain sodium can become edematous as the result of ingestion of excessive amounts of sodium bicarbonate.

A10. **b.** Occasionally during pregnancy bizarre cravings for strange foods develop. These cravings may be for materials hardly considered edible. Some of those substances have included laundry starch, baking powder, baking soda, clay, baked dirt, powered bricks, and frost scraped from the refrigerator.

Ingestion of starch (amylophagia) or clay (geophagia) or related items is practiced more often by socioeconomically less-privileged pregnant women. The desire for dry lump starch, chopped ice, or even refrigerator frost has been considered by some to be triggered by severe iron deficiency. Although women with severe iron deficiency sometimes crave these items, and although craving is usually ameliorated after correction of the iron deficiency, not all pregnant women with pica are iron deficient.

A11. **d.** Lower extremity edema, a common complication of late pregnancy, occurs because the pelvic veins and inferior vena cava are occluded as a result of the pressure from the enlarging uterus. Treatment consists of avoiding prolonged standing, elevating the lower extremities, and wearing support hose. Thiazide diuretics reduce intravascular volume as do loop diuretics. Both classes are contraindicated in pregnancy. In this patient, you should:
   a. Discontinue the thiazide
   b. Discontinue the loop diuretic

c. Suggest elevation of extremities for 1 hour three times a day

d. Suggest that she stay off her feet as much as possible

Warming up the big computer is never a bad idea. This would be a good second choice.

A12. **e.** The most common vaginal discharge in pregnancy is a physiologic discharge. The discharge is caused by increased formation of mucus by the cervical glands under the influence of estrogen. However, it is important to rule out ruptured membranes and leaking amniotic fluid. This is accomplished by performing a speculum examination looking for pooling of fluid in the posterior fornix and identifying whether or not the fluid present turns nitrazine paper blue and if ferning is seen on microscopic examination when the fluid is allowed to air dry on a glass slide.

Monilia may be identified in the vagina in up to 25% of women in late pregnancy. If the patient is symptomatic, she should be treated. If she is not symptomatic, treatment is not needed. The drugs of choice for the treatment of symptomatic monilia in pregnancy are either clotrimazole or miconazole.

A13. **e.**

A14. **e.** The cause of constipation in pregnancy is multifactorial. Potential causes include hormonally mediated smooth muscle relaxation and mechanical pressure from the enlarging uterus.

A15. **e.** Increasing the intake of fluids, increasing the intake of fiber, and increasing the amount of exercise (especially walking) should be encouraged. If these measures are not effective, then a bulk-forming agent such as psyllium or methylcellulose may be added. Laxatives should be used with caution because of the habituation potential.

SOLUTION TO THE SHORT ANSWER MANAGEMENT PROBLEM

Three additional common complaints of pregnancy are:

a. Ptyalism: profuse salivation
1) Cause: stimulation of the salivary glands by the ingestion of starch
2) Treatment: the cause should be looked for and eradicated if possible

b. Fatigue: in early pregnancy; most pregnant women complain of fatigue and desire excessive periods of sleep

c. Headache: in early pregnancy; a frequent complaint

1) Cause:
a) In the vast majority of cases, no cause can be demonstrated.
b) A few cases may result from sinusitis or ocular strain caused by refractive errors.
c) Pregnancy-induced hypertension is a potential cause in later pregnancy; at this stage any woman who presents with a headache should be assessed for pre-eclampsia.
2) Treatment: largely symptomatic; by midpregnancy most of these headaches decrease in severity or disappear.

SUMMARY OF THE DIAGNOSIS AND TREATMENT OF COMMON COMPLAINTS IN PREGNANCY

1. Nausea and vomiting:
   a. Pathophysiology: increased levels of circulating HCG
   b. Treatments:
      1) Reassurance
      2) Small, frequent meals and dry food
      3) Discontinuation of iron therapy (if patient is on supplemental iron)
      4) Antinauseants if moderately severe:
         a) Promethazine
         b) Chlorpromazine
         c) Prochlorperazine
         d) If severe, metoclopramide

2. Constipation:
   a. Pathophysiology: reduced gastrointestinal motility, mechanical obstruction of the uterus, increased water resorption
   b. Treatments:
      1) Discontinuation of iron therapy (if patient is on iron)
      2) Increasing amount of fiber in the diet
      3) Increasing the amount of total fluid intake
      4) Increasing the amount of physical activity

3. Back pain:
   a. Pathophysiology: motion of the symphysis pubis and lumbosacral ligaments, relaxation of the pelvic ligaments and the round ligament of the uterus
   b. Treatment: symptomatic: heat, ice, acetaminophen, avoidance of activities that aggravate the problem

4. Hemorrhoids:
   a. Pathophysiology: increased pressure in the rectal vein system secondary to increased intravascular volume

b. Treatment:
1) Recumbent position
2) TUCKS-witch hazel pads
3) Hemorrhoidal cream and hydrocortisone cream
4) Excision of external thrombosed hemorrhoid

5. Varicosities:
a. Pathophysiology: congenital predisposition in weakness of vein valves, increased pressure secondary to increased intravascular volume
b. Treatment: rest, elevation, compression stockings
c. Complication: superficial thrombophlebitis most common

6. Heartburn:
a. Pathophysiology: displacement of uterus upward, exerting pressure on the diaphragm; and decreased pressure in lower esophageal sphincter
b. Treatment: antacids: magnesium hydroxide and aluminum hydroxide

7. Lower extremity edema:
a. Pathophysiology: increased intravascular volume (increased by 50%), gravity
b. Treatment:
1) avoid diuretics, which will further reduce the intravascular volume
2) rest, recumbency

8. Increased vaginal discharge:
a. Pathophysiology: almost always normal; due to increased hormone levels, especially estrogen
b. Treatment:
1) Rule out ruptured membranes and vaginitis or cervicitis
2) Reassurance

SUGGESTED READING

Cunningham FG et al: *Williams obstetrics,* ed 20, Norwalk, Conn, 1997, Appleton & Lange.

PROBLEM·43

ROUTINE PRENATAL CARE

"Shouldn't You See Me More Often, Doctor?"

Case 1 ■ A 24-Year-Old Primigravida at 8 Weeks' Gestation

A 24-year-old primigravida presents at 8 weeks' gestation for her first prenatal visit. She has asked you to be her family doctor and to look after her during the entire pregnancy. You agree to provide her pregnancy care. During your first visit you explain your general philosophy regarding prenatal care and perinatal care.

SELECT THE BEST ANSWER TO THE FOLLOWING QUESTIONS

Q1. The Department of Health and Human Services Expert Panel on Prenatal Care has recommended which of the following regarding routine prenatal care?
a. that the number of routine office visits be significantly reduced for women at low risk
b. that focus should be on the total health and well being of the family including medical, psychologic, social, and environmental barriers affecting health
c. that provision of systematic health care start long before pregnancy because it was proven to be beneficial to the physical and emotional well being of the prospective mother and child
d. all of the above are true
e. b and c only are true

Q2. The Expert Panel on Prenatal Care has recommended that office visits be limited to visits for specific purposes during the first how many months of pregnancy?
a. 2 months
b. 3 months
c. 4 months
d. 5 months
e. 6 months

Q3. A 26-year-old primigravida conceived on September 9, 1998. According to Nägele's rule, what is the patient's estimated date of delivery (assume a 28-day cycle)?
a. June 2, 1999
b. June 16, 1999
c. July 2, 1999
d. July 9, 1999
e. June 23, 1999

Q4. The American College of Obstetricians and Gynecologists has recommended intervals for routine and indicated tests in the prenatal period. Which of the intervals shown below is (are) recommended?
a. initial visit: as early as possible
b. obstetric ultrasound: 18 weeks gestation
c. screening for gestational diabetes: 26 to 28 weeks' gestation

d. hepatitis B virus screen: as early as possible (first visit)

e. all of the above

Q5. What is the recommended entire weight gain recommended by the National Academy of Sciences for a pregnant woman who is 65 inches tall with a prepregnancy weight of 225 pounds?
a. 5 to 15 pounds
b. 10 to 20 pounds
c. 15 to 25 pounds
d. 25 to 35 pounds
e. 28 to 40 pounds

Q6. The number of calories recommended for women in pregnancy is approximately how many greater than for nonpregnant women?
a. 200
b. 300
c. 500
d. 750
e. 900

Q7. Which of the following statements would be regarded as reasonable nutritional advice standards in pregnancy?
a. supplementation with 30 to 60 mg of iron daily after the first 4 months
b. supplementation with folic acid 1 mg daily throughout pregnancy
c. a regular diet with salt added to taste
d. seek weight gain based on prepregnancy weight
e. all of the above

Q8. Which of the following statements regarding smoking in pregnancy is (are) true?
a. the risk of spontaneous abortion is significantly increased
b. perinatal mortality rates are significantly increased
c. abruptio placenta rates are significantly increased
d. birth weights are significantly decreased
e. all of the above are true

Q9. Which of the following statements regarding alcohol consumption in pregnancy and fetal alcohol syndrome is (are) true?
a. limit alcohol intake to one or two glasses of wine
b. abstain completely from alcohol during pregnancy
c. fetal alcohol syndrome is decreasing in the United States

d. a and c
e. b and c

Q10. Which of the following Caldwell-Moloy pelvic shape classification is (are) both the most common and the most functional for delivery?
a. gynecoid pelvis
b. android pelvis
c. anthropoid pelvis
d. platypelloid pelvis
e. a and c are equally common and equally functional

Q11. Which of the following clinical examination measurements is the most critical in determining the ability of the fetus to pass through the pelvis in labor?
a. obstetrical conjugate
b. diagonal conjugate
c. pelvic inlet
d. midpelvis
e. pelvic outlet

Q12. When is the fetal head said to be engaged?
a. when the frontal diameter has passed through the pelvic inlet
b. when the occipital diameter has passed through the pelvic inlet
c. when the biparietal diameter has passed through the pelvic inlet
d. when the biparietal diameter has passed through the midpelvis
e. when the occipital diameter has passed through the midpelvis

Q13. The stage and phases of labor describe the various parts of the parturition process. Which of the following describes when effacement of the cervix primarily occurs?
a. Stage 1, latent phase
b. Stage 1, active phase
c. Stage 2
d. Stage 3

Q14. The active phase in a nullipara, according to the graphic labor curve of Friedman, should produce cervical dilatation of how many centimeters per hour?
a. 0.5 cm
b. 1.0 cm
c. 1.2 cm
d. 1.5 cm
e. 2.0 cm

Q15. The third stage of labor begins when the baby is delivered. What is the most frequent mistake made by physicians in this phase?
- a. allowing the third stage to progress at a very slow pace
- b. allowing the third stage to progress on its own
- c. attempting to pull or tug at the umbilical cord
- d. attempting to stop the "gush of blood" that normally accompanies the third stage of labor
- e. massaging the uterus and injecting oxytocin into the uterus

Q16. Which of the following statements regarding amniotomy is true?
- a. amniotomy does not change the length of labor
- b. amniotomy decreases the cesarean section rate
- c. amniotomy improves newborn Apgar scores
- d. amniotomy may result in prolapse of the umbilical cord
- e. none of the above

Q17. Which of the following has (have) been demonstrated to be of benefit in decreasing the risk of postpartum hemorrhage following the delivery of the placenta?
- a. massage of the fundus of the uterus
- b. injection of intravenous (IV) or intramuscular (IM) oxytocin
- c. injection of IV or IM ergonovine maleate
- d. traction on the umbilical cord
- e. a, b, and c
- f. all of the above

Q18. What are the average durations of the first stage of labor in a nullipara and the first stage of labor in a multipara?
- a. 10 hours (nullipara), 7 hours (multipara)
- b. 8 hours (nullipara), 5 hours (multipara)
- c. 12 hours (nullipara), 6 hours (multipara)
- d. 14 hours (nullipara), 8 hours (multipara)
- e. 9 hours (nullipara), 6 hours (multipara)

Q19. What are the average durations of the second stage of labor in a nullipara and the second stage of labor in a multipara?
- a. 1 hour 40 minutes (nullipara), 55 minutes (multipara)
- b. 1 hour 20 minutes (nullipara), 45 minutes (multipara)
- c. 50 minutes (nullipara), 20 minutes (multipara)
- d. 40 minutes (nullipara), 10 minutes (multipara)
- e. 1 hour 30 minutes (nullipara), 1 hour (multipara)

Q20. Which of the following options is (are) correct regarding intrapartum antibiotic prophylaxis of group B beta *Streptococcus* (GBBS) sepsis?
- a. antibiotics are not effective in decreasing GBBS sepsis
- b. antibiotics are administered only to women with risk factors
- c. antibiotics are administered only to women with positive late pregnancy GBBS vaginal cultures
- d. antibiotics can completely prevent GBBS sepsis
- e. b and c

SHORT ANSWER MANAGEMENT PROBLEM
Matching Problem: Part A lists 10 drugs that may be useful in pregnancy. Part B lists 10 indications for treatment with those drugs. Match the numbered drug with the proper lettered condition in each case.

Part A
1. Aspirin
2. Zidovudine
3. Ergonovine
4. Aldomet
5. Magnesium sulfate
6. Hydralazine
7. Penicillin
8. Ritodrine
9. Hydrochlorothiazide
10. Captopril

Part B
a. Severe hypertension in pregnancy
b. Prophylaxis against group B streptococcus
c. Drug of choice: preeclampsia and eclampsia
d. Possibly useful in the prevention of preeclampsia
e. Postpartum agent to enhance uterine contractions
f. Can prevent human immunodeficiency virus (HIV) infection in the infant of an infected mother
g. Teratogenic drug
h. No possible use in normal pregnancy
i. Treatment of choice in chronic hypertension
j. Treatment for preterm labor

ANSWERS

A1. **d.**

A2. **e.** The Department of Health and Human Services Expert Panel on Prenatal Care has suggested that women at low risk can reduce the number of prenatal visits significantly. This recommendation (office visits limited to those visits necessary for indicated procedures and intervals) is for the first 6 months of pregnancy. This is a significant change from standard practice, but there is no difference in demonstrated quality of care between low-risk women who had regular "monthly" office visits and women who had prenatal visits at the time of recommended intervals for indicated tests and procedures.

Detailed recommendations have also been made regarding preconception care beginning within a year of a planned pregnancy. There should be an emphasis on prenatal care that provides an opportunity to focus on the total health and well being of the family, including medical, psychologic, social, and environmental barriers affecting health. Systematic health care beginning long before pregnancy proves beneficial to the prospective mother and infant.

The American College of Obstetricians and Gynecologists suggests that the pregnant patient not only see her physician at the first indication that she is pregnant, but also take special care during the year before she plans to get pregnant to ensure the healthiest possible outcome. Exercise, a healthy diet, and other healthy lifestyles should be encouraged many months before attempting to conceive.

A3. **a.** Nägele's rule identifies the estimated date of delivery for women that have a 28-day menstrual cycle. The mean duration of pregnancy calculated from the first day of the last normal menstrual period (LNMP) for a large number of healthy women has been identified as to be very close to 280 days, or 40 weeks. Nägele's rule estimates the expected date of delivery by adding 7 days to the date of the first day of the LNMP and counting back 3 months. If a woman's menstrual periods are 35 days apart, add 14 days rather than 7 days. If her periods are 21 days apart, add 0 days rather than 7 days.

A4. **e.** On the first prenatal visit, the following investigations should be performed: hemoglobin and hematocrit; urinalysis; blood group, Rh type, antibody screen, rubella antibody titer, syphilis screen, hepatitis B virus screen, and cervical cytology. HIV testing should be recommended for all pregnant women.

Obstetric ultrasound may be performed for dating of the pregnancy (accurate dating) at 18 weeks' gestation. Also at that time a maternal serum alphafetoprotein (screening for neural tube defects) or triple marker screen (screening for both neural tube defects and trisomy 18/trisomy 21) should be offered.

At 26 to 28 weeks' gestation the patient should have the following procedures performed: routine screen for diabetes mellitus, repeat hemoglobin or hematocrit, and repeat antibody test for unsensitized Rh-negative patients. At that time also, prophylactic administration of Rho(d) immunoglobulin can be administered to patients who are Rh negative.

At 32 to 36 weeks' gestation, testing for sexually transmitted diseases and repeat hemoglobin or hematocrit may be performed, if indicated.

A5. **c.** The average total pregnancy weight gain for normal healthy women eating without restrictions is 27.5 pounds (12.5 kg). However, the National Academy of Science summarized the published studies on weight gain during pregnancy and found that the amount of ideal weight gain varied inversely with the prepregnancy weight of the woman. Their pregnancy weight gain recommendations, based on percentage of ideal body weight (IBW), are as follows: underweight women (<90% of IBW) should gain 28 to 40 pounds (12.5 to 18 kg); normal weight women (90% to 135% of IBW) should gain 25 to 35 pounds (11.5 to 16 kg); overweight women (>135% of IBW) should gain 15 to 25 pounds (7 to 11.5 kg). Of the recommended weight gain, approximately 9 kg comprise the normal physiologic events and features of pregnancy. These include the fetus, placenta, amniotic fluid, uterine hypertrophy, increase in maternal blood volume, breast enlargement, and dependent maternal edema as the consequence of mechanical factors. The remaining 1 to 3 kg is mostly fat.

Pregnant women should be encouraged to gain an adequate amount of weight. However, wide ranges of maternal weight gains are compatible with good clinical outcomes.

A6. **b.** The recommended National Research Council Recommended Daily Dietary Allowances for women before, during pregnancy, and during lactation are as follows:

	Nonpregnant	Pregnant	Lactating
Kilocalories	2200	2500	2600
Protein (g)	55	60	65

A7. **e.** In general, the pregnant woman should eat what she wants to eat in amounts she desires and with salt added to taste. Care should be taken to make sure there is enough food to eat, especially in the case of the socioeconomically deprived woman.

As stated before, the pregnant woman's ideal pregnancy weight gain will be determined by her prepregnancy weight.

Periodically explore the food intake by dietary recall to uncover the ingestion of any bizarre foods. In this way, the occasional nutritionally absurd diet (pica) will be discovered.

Give tablets of simple iron salts to pregnant women that provide between 30 and 60 mg of iron per day.

Supplement the pregnant patient's diet with 1 mg of folic acid per day.

Recheck the hematocrit or hemoglobin concentration at 28 to 32 weeks' gestation to detect any significant decrease.

A8. **e.** Pregnancy outcomes are adversely affected by maternal cigarette smoking: spontaneous abortion rates are doubled; perinatal mortality rates are significantly increased; abruptio placenta is almost twice as common in smokers, and mean birth weights of smokers are almost 200 g less than nonsmokers. This decrease in birth weight is a combined result of preterm deliveries and growth restriction of term babies. It is estimated that 4600 infants die annually in the United States because of maternal smoking. Other conditions linked with maternal smoking include placenta previa, premature rupture of the membranes, chorioamnionitis, placental calcifications, and placental hypoxia.

The pathophysiology of maternal smoking includes the following:
a. Carbon monoxide and its functional inactivation of fetal and maternal hemoglobin
b. Vasoconstrictor action of nicotine, causing reduced placental perfusion
c. Reduced appetite, and, in turn, reduced caloric intake
d. Decreased maternal plasma volume

A9. **b.** The safest policy for maternal alcohol use is no use. No safe level of alcohol intake in pregnancy has been identified. Even a few drinks at a critical time in organogenesis can be teratogenic. The incidence of fetal alcohol syndrome in the United States is increasing, not decreasing. Fetal alcohol syndrome is the most common preventable cause of mental retardation.

A10. **a.** The Caldwell-Moloy classification of four pelvis types is an attempt to predict how much difficulty there is going to be in the actual delivery of the infant before delivery. The type that is both most common and most suited for delivery is the gynecoid pelvis.

The android pelvis has convergent sidewalls, ischial spines that are prominent, and a subpubic arch that is narrow.

The anthropoid pelvis is a pelvis in which the ischial spines are narrow. This type of pelvis is much more common in black women; the android pelvis is more common in white women.

The platypelloid pelvis has a flattened gynecoid shape. It is quite rare; only 3% of women have this type of pelvis.

A11. **b.** The diagonal conjugate is the most important overall pelvic dimension. It is the distance from the sacral promontory to the lower margin of the symphysis pubis. It is the measurement that directly determines the dimensions of the pelvic inlet. The obstetric conjugate is determined by subtracting 1.5 to 2.0 cm from the diagonal conjugate. If the diagonal conjugate is greater than 11.5 cm, it is reasonable to assume that the pelvic inlet is of adequate size.

A12. **c.** The fetal head is said to be engaged when the biparietal diameter of the fetal head has passed through the pelvic inlet. Although engagement of the fetal head is usually regarded as a phenomenon of labor, in nulliparas it commonly occurs during the last few weeks of pregnancy.

A13. **a.** The stages and phases of labor can be described as follows:
a. Stage 1, latent phase: It has its onset with the onset of regular uterine contractions. It ends with acceleration of the cervical dilatation slope (usually at 3 cm or more dilatation). The purpose of the latent phase is for coordination of contractions as well as cervical softening and effacement. It normally lasts less than 14 hours in a multipara or less than 20 hours in a primipara.
b. Stage 1, active phase: It has its onset with acceleration of the cervical dilatation slope. It ends with complete cervical dilatation at 10 cm. The purpose is threefold: active dilatation of the cervix, beginning the descent of the presenting fetal part, and beginning of the cardinal movements of labor. It normally lasts less than 4 hours in a multipara or less than 5 hours in a primipara.
c. Stage 2: It has its onset with complete cervical dilatation. It ends with delivery of the neonate. The purpose is to complete the descent of the presenting fetal part through the pelvis and completion of the cardinal movements of labor. It normally lasts less than 30 minutes in a multipara or less than 60 minutes in a primipara.
d. Stage 3: It has its onset with delivery of the neonate. It ends with delivery of the placenta. The purpose is to shear off the anchoring villi and to deliver the placenta. It normally lasts less than 30 minutes.

A14. **c.** The graphic labor curve of Friedman is a visual representation of cervical dilatation versus time. In a primigravida the average dilatation during the first stage of labor is 1.2 cm/hr; in multiparas the average cervical dilatation is 1.5 cm/hr.

A15. **c.** The most frequent mistake that is made in the third stage of labor is putting undue and unnecessary tension on the umbilical cord. This can cause premature separation of the placenta from the uterus and breaking or tearing of the umbilical cord. Rarely it may cause an inversion of the uterus, a life-threatening problem that is associated with severe postpartum hemorrhage.

A16. **d.** Amniotomy describes the artificial rupture of the membranes to either induce or augment labor contractions. Other common indications for amniotomy include placement of internal electronic fetal monitoring devices when external devices do not produce a satisfactory tracing and placement of intrauterine pressure catheters for assessment of uterine contraction quality when labor progress in inadequate. The data from multiple studies show that the mean length of labor is shortened up to hours but the cesarean rates and perinatal outcomes are unchanged. Before performing amniotomy it is important to ensure that the fetal head is well applied to the cervix. Otherwise prolapse of the umbilical cord may occur jeopardizing fetal oxygenation and requiring a crash cesarean delivery.

A17. **e.** The third stage of labor is best managed by massaging the uterine fundus as soon as the placenta is delivered. An intravenous or intramuscular injection of either oxytocin or ergonovine maleate will contract the uterus. Traction on the umbilical cord will not speed up the contraction of the uterus, which is the primary mechanism for separating the placenta from its implantation site.

A18. **b.**

A19. **c.**

	Nullipara	Multipara
Average length		
Stage 1	8 hours	5 hours
Stage 2	50 minutes	20 minutes

A20. **c.** GBBS is a part of normal human bacterial flora with reservoirs of colonization in otherwise healthy individuals. Vaginal colonization can be as high as 35%. GBBS sepsis attacks two infants per 1000 births with a 50% mortality rate. Highest risk is found in GBBS carriers with preterm delivery, rupture of membranes greater than 12 hours, onset of labor or rupture of membranes at less than 37 weeks' gestation, or intrapartum fever. With so serious an impact on newborns, prophylactic antibiotics, often using ampicillin, have successfully been used to decrease the GBBS attack rate. Concerns have been raised, however, that widespread intrapartum prophylaxis will lead to emergence of resistant pathogens. In 1996 the Centers for Disease Control and Prevention issued the

following recommendations for the active prevention of GBBS: that antibiotic prophylaxis should be used with penicillin, that prophylaxis should be provided based on either positive late prenatal culture or a strategy based solely on clinical risk factors, and that all women with a previous GBBS-infected infant be prophylactically treated.

SOLUTION TO THE SHORT ANSWER MANAGEMENT PROBLEM

1. D	5. C	8. J
2. F	6. A	9. H
3. E	7. B	10. G
4. I		

SUMMARY OF CERTAIN ANTEPARTUM AND PERIPARTUM EVENTS

1. Routine checkups in pregnancy: Not indicated nearly as frequently as commonly practiced, especially in the first trimester

2. Recommended initial screening (as soon as possible after diagnosis):
   a. Complete blood count (CBC)
   b. Blood group and atypical antibody screen
   c. Rh status
   d. Rubella antibody status
   e. Syphilis
   f. HIV (high risk)
   g. Hepatitis B virus

3. Recommended initial 18-week screening:
   a. Obstetrical ultrasound screening for fetal anomaly screening
   b. Maternal serum alpha-fetoprotein
   c. Triple marker screen

4. Recommended initial 28-week screening:
   a. Gestational diabetes screening: 1-hour, 50-g glucose tolerance test; if results are 140 mg%, perform a 3-hour, 100-g glucose tolerance test
   b. Repeat atypical screen for Rh-negative women and administer Rh immunoglobulin, if indicated
   c. Repeat CBC

5. Recommended initial 36-week screening: Optional GBBS vaginal culture

6. Prenatal surveillance (every prenatal visit):
   a. Fetal:
      1) Fetal heart rate
      2) Fundal height, actual and amount of change

3) Presenting part and station (late in pregnancy)
4) Fetal activity
b. Maternal:
1) Blood pressure: actual and extent of change
2) Weight: actual and amount of change
3) Symptoms, including epigastric pain, headache, and altered vision

7. Other prenatal factors:
a. Nägele's rule: First day LNMP + 7 days − 3 months = Estimated date of delivery
b. Weight gain: ideal amount is based on maternal prepregnancy weight
c. Calories: 300 additional calories in pregnancy; 400 additional calories in lactation
d. Supplementation: iron 30 to 60 mg after 4 months; folic acid 1 mg/day
e. Smoking: stop; 4600 perinatal deaths per year in United States due to smoking
f. Alcohol: none

8. Perinatal summary:
a. Graphic labor curve of Friedman: active stage of labor (Stage 2) is 1.2 cm/hr for nullipara and 1.5 cm/hr for multipara
b. Stage 2 of labor: 60 minutes for nullipara; 30 minutes for multipara
c. Stage 3 of labor: 30 minutes. Use oxytocin, ergonovine, or Hemabate to enhance uterine contractility after the placenta is expelled.
d. Engagement: when the biparietal diameter passes the pelvic inlet
e. Conjugates and pelvis:
1) Diagonal conjugate is the measurement from the sacral promontory to the symphysis pubis. It is the most important pelvic dimension. If >11.5 cm, the pelvic inlet is adequate.
2) Most favorable pelvic shape: gynecoid (occurs in 50% of women)

SUGGESTED READINGS

American College of Obstetricians and Gynecologists Technical Bulletin: *Smoking and Women's Health*, Number 240, Sept, 1997.
American College of Obstetricians and Gynecologists Technical Bulletin: *Substance abuse and pregnancy*, Number 195, July, 1994.
Centers for Disease Control and Prevention: Prevention of perinatal group B *Streptococcal* disease: A public health perspective, *MMWR* 45(RR-7):1-24, 1996.
Cunningham FG et al: *Williams obstetrics*, ed 20, Norwalk, Conn, 1997, Appleton & Lange.
Rosen MG et al: Caring for our future: A report by the expert panel on the content of prenatal care, *Obstet Gynecol* 77:782, 1991.

PROBLEM · 44

MANAGEMENT OF THE FIRST AND SECOND STAGES OF LABOR

There Is a Time to Sow, a Time to Reap, and a Time to Deliver.

Case 1 ■ A 28-Year-Old Primigravida in Labor

A 28-year-old primigravida at term is admitted to the delivery suite with contractions 5 minutes apart. Her cervix is found to be 3 cm dilated and 90% effaced. When examined 5 hours later she has progressed to 4 cm dilated and is 100% effaced. The station of the head is zero (0). Her contractions are mild to moderate and have become more irregular during the past 3 hours. She has been ambulating, but this has not changed the strength or the frequency of her contractions. Her membranes are intact and bulging. The baseline fetal heart rate (FHR) is 150 bpm. The monitor tracing shows frequent heart rate accelerations.

SELECT THE BEST ANSWER TO THE FOLLOWING QUESTIONS

Q1. What is the most appropriate course of action at this time?
a. perform an amniotomy
b. begin oxytocin stimulation for hypotonic labor
c. call the anesthesiologist to administer epidural analgesia
d. reassure the patient that her contractions will eventually pick up
e. none of the above

Q2. The appropriate action is taken. After 4 more hours, her contractions are still mild to moderate and irregular in frequency. The cervix is now 5 cm dilated. The electronic fetal monitor strip is reactive. What would be the most appropriate course of action at this time?
a. perform an amniotomy
b. begin oxytocin stimulation for hypotonic labor
c. call the anesthesiologist to administer epidural analgesia and prepare the patient for cesarean section
d. tell the patient and the nursing staff to relax; everything takes time
e. none of the above

Q3. With the appropriate intervention the patient progresses to full cervical dilatation. After pushing for 2 hours, the patient is exhausted. The fetal scalp is visible at the introitus. The position of the head is occiput anterior. The FHR tracing is reac-

tive with a baseline rate of 150 bpm. Her contractions are strong, lasting 50 seconds, and are 2 to 3 minutes apart. What would you do at this time?
a. increase the oxytocin
b. explain to the patient that she'll just have to try a little harder
c. attempt delivery with outlet forceps
d. attempt delivery with a vacuum extractor
e. either c or d

Q4. Which of the following statements concerning the use of the vacuum extractor and/or outlet forceps in the second stage of labor is true?
a. the perinatal morbidity of infants delivered with outlet forceps is higher than if a vacuum extractor is used
b. the perinatal morbidity of infants delivered with a vacuum extractor is higher than if outlet forceps are used
c. intracranial compression with the vacuum extractor is higher than that with outlet forceps
d. Apgar scores of infants delivered by the vacuum extractor are higher than those of infants delivered by outlet forceps
e. the perinatal morbidity and Apgar scores of infants delivered by outlet forceps and vacuum extractor are similar

Q5. Which of the following is (are) essential for a forceps delivery to be classified as outlet forceps?
a. the scalp is or has been visible at the introitus
b. the skull has reached the pelvic floor
c. the sagittal suture is in the anteroposterior diameter of the pelvis
d. the orientation of the fetal head must be unequivocally identified
e. all of the above

Q6. Which of the following is (are) maternal indications for forceps delivery?
a. maternal exhaustion
b. need to avoid voluntary expulsive efforts
c. lack of maternal cooperation in pushing
d. excessive maternal analgesia
e. all of the above

Q7. Which of the following FHR patterns suggests a need for a forceps delivery if all other criteria have been met?
a. fetal heart tones with a persistent baseline rate of >150 bpm
b. repetitive late decelerations dropping 20 bpm lasting 20 seconds
c. repetitive early decelerations dropping 20 bpm lasting 20 seconds

d. repetitive variable decelerations dropping 20 bpm lasting 20 seconds
e. repetitive accelerations of 20 bpm lasting 20 seconds

Q8. Which of the following conditions must be met before a forceps delivery is attempted?
a. the cervix must be fully dilated
b. the membranes must be ruptured
c. the head must be engaged
d. the bladder must be empty
e. all of the above

Q9. Which of the following statements regarding induction of labor by stripping the membranes is (are) true?
a. stripping of the membranes has been firmly established as a safe and efficient method to induce labor
b. stripping of the membranes has not been associated with infection
c. stripping of the membranes has not been associated with subsequent vaginal bleeding
d. stripping of the membranes appears to induce labor through a prostaglandin stimulation/mediation
e. all of the above are true

Q10. Which of the following is (are) risks of administering oxytocin for the induction of labor?
a. uterine rupture
b. fetal hypoxia
c. uterine hypertonia
d. all of the above
e. none of the above

SHORT ANSWER MANAGEMENT PROBLEM
Discuss the major issues when considering the use of oxytocin for the induction of labor.

ANSWERS

A1. **a.** This patient has hypotonic labor. When a patient in the active phase of labor (cervical dilatation ≥4 cm dilation) develops hypotonic or dysfunctional uterine contractions and if the fetal head is engaged, it is appropriate to perform an amniotomy. This may augment and shorten labor. The mechanism of augmentation of contractions is thought to be release of prostaglandins from the fetal membranes when they are artificially ruptured. The patient should be kept in the Fowler's position after amniotomy to facilitate drainage of the amniotic fluid. Amniotomy should be performed under sterile conditions only if the fetal head is engaged and is well applied to the cervix. There is no indication for epidural analgesia at this time.

A2. **b.** In this patient, amniotomy has not enhanced uterine contraction regularity, intensity, and frequency. Oxytocin stimulation for hypotonic labor should now be considered. The following guidelines should be adhered to:

a. The patient must be in the active phase of labor with cervical dilatation of at least 3 cm.
b. The fetal head is engaged or descends through the pelvic inlet with fundal pressure.
c. The fetus should be in a cephalic presentation.
d. There should be no polyhydramnios.
e. The patient's parity should be less than 6.
f. The patient should not have a previous uterine scar.
g. The fetal status should be reassuring.
h. Oxytocin infusion is immediately turned off if hyperstimulation of the uterus occurs. When infusion is restarted, it should be at half the previous dose.
i. There should be continuous electronic monitoring of the fetal heart and uterine activity.

A3. **e.** The mother is exhausted. Her contractions are strong and 2 to 3 minutes apart and are therefore not hypotonic. It would be inappropriate to increase the rate of oxytocin infusion. The head is on the perineum. Therefore delivery of the infant by either an outlet forceps or a vacuum extractor would be appropriate. When a mother has been pushing for 2 hours and is exhausted, it is inappropriate to advise her to "try" harder.

A4. **e.** The perinatal morbidity rates and Apgar scores on infants delivered by outlet forceps and by a vacuum extractor are similar. The vacuum extractor is used more commonly in Europe and Canada than in the United States. The soft silastic vacuum extractor has the advantage over older metal models of being able to be applied immediately to the fetal head. The pressure should be decreased between contractions. There is lower intracranial compression with the vacuum extractor, but there is no significant difference in perinatal morbidity or Apgar scores between infants delivered by the vacuum extractor and infants delivered by outlet forceps.

In the hands of experienced operators, both instruments are effective and safe. Proper cup placement is the most important determinant of success in vacuum extraction. The center of the cup should be over the sagittal suture and about 3 cm in front of the posterior fontanelle. Such placement prevents iatrogenic deflexion and asynclitism of the fetal head.

A5. **e.** Forceps deliveries are classified as follows (with all criteria being present):

a. Outlet forceps: This refers to the application of forceps when the scalp is visible at the introitus without the need to separate the labia, the fetal skull has reached the pelvic floor, the sagittal suture is in the anteroposterior diameter of the pelvis, and rotation does not exceed 45 degrees.
b. Low forceps: This refers to the application of forceps when the skull has reached a station of at least +2 but is not on the pelvic floor; and when the sagittal suture is in the anteroposterior or oblique diameter of the pelvis.
c. Midforceps: This refers to the application of forceps when the head is engaged but has not reached a station of +2.
d. High forceps: This refers to the application of forceps at any time before engagement of the head. There are no indications for high forceps deliveries in present-day obstetric practice.

A6. **e.** Maternal indications for outlet forceps include maternal exhaustion, need to avoid voluntary expulsive effort (e.g., certain cardiac or cerebrovascular disease), lack of maternal cooperation in pushing or excessive analgesia impairing voluntary expulsive efforts.

A7. **b.** The major fetal indication for termination of the second stage of labor is a *nonreassuring fetal heart rate pattern*. This phrase has replaced the old term, *fetal distress*, because of the imprecision and inaccuracy of the latter. Nonreassuring patterns may be manifested by persistent and repetitive findings of the following: baseline FHRs of <100 or >160 bpm, late deceleration patterns of any degree, and severe variable decelerations. Severe variable decelerations can be described using the "Rule of 60's": the decelerations last longer than 60 seconds, drop to lower than 60 bpm, or drop 60 beats below the baseline.

Accelerations are always reassuring. Early decelerations (head compressions) are benign and are not an indication for the termination of the second stage of labor. Variable decelerations (cord compressions) of a mild or moderate degree are not indications for intervention, but late decelerations, even 20 bpm, are nonreassuring and suggest a need for forceps delivery.

A8. **e.** The use of forceps is permissible only when all of the following conditions are present, regardless of the urgency of delivery:

a. The cervix must be fully dilated.
b. The membranes must be ruptured.
c. The head must be engaged, preferably at station +2 or below.

d. The head must present in either vertex or face presentation with chin anterior.
e. Cephalopelvic disproportion must have been ruled out.
f. The bladder must be empty.

A9. **d.** Induction of labor by stripping the membranes is a relatively common practice, although few reports documenting its efficacy and safety have been published. The potential for infection and bleeding from a previously undiagnosed placenta previa or from a low-lying placenta, as well as accidental rupture of the membranes, should be considered. Only one randomized study involving 180 pregnancies has demonstrated that membrane stripping is safe and associated with a decreased incidence of postterm gestation. If it is effective, the mechanism of action is likely to be mediated by the stimulation of prostaglandins located in the membrane itself.

A10. **d.** Oxytocin is a powerful drug and has been associated with uterine rupture, hypertonic uterine contractions, and fetal hypoxia resulting from uterine hypertonia. Oxytocin must be administered on a risk-benefit basis. The risks have been previously discussed. The benefits include decreased risk of maternal exhaustion, decreased risk of intrapartum infection, and decreased risk of traumatic operative delivery. As well, failure to treat uterine dysfunction may expose the fetus to an appreciably higher risk of death.

SOLUTION TO THE SHORT ANSWER MANAGEMENT PROBLEM

Almost a quarter of all labors are induced or augmented using oxytocin. The following protocol should be observed:
a. Close observation
b. Continuous FHR monitoring
c. Continuous uterine activity monitoring
d. Parity less than 6
e. Reassuring FHR and pattern
f. Thick meconium absent

Numerous protocols exist for oxytocin augmentation of labor with respect to the initial dose, incremental dose increases, and intervals between dose increases. There are advantages and disadvantages to both high- and low-dose regimens. Either dosing schema is acceptable, providing the guidelines discussed above are adhered to before and during oxytocin administration. Low-dose regimens begin at 0.5 to 1 mU/min, increasing the dose 1 mU/min every 30 to 40 minutes up to a maximum dose of 20 mU/min. High-dose regimens start at 6 mU/min, advancing by 3 mU/

min every 20 to 40 minutes up to a maximum dose of 42 mU/min. If hyperstimulation occurs, the oxytocin infusion is immediately turned off. When infusion is restarted, it should be at half the previous dose.

SUMMARY OF ACTIVE MANAGEMENT OF THE FIRST AND SECOND STAGES OF LABOR

1. Hypotonic labor:
   a. Establish that the patient is in true labor.
   b. If true labor is established and is not progressing, consider amniotomy.
   c. If amniotomy is performed or membranes have ruptured spontaneously and labor is not progressing, consider oxytocin augmentation adhering to protocol.
   d. Consider stripping of the membranes.

2. Operative vaginal delivery:
   a. Forceps and vacuum are equally effective and safe if properly used.
   b. Follow maternal and fetal indications for operative delivery.
   c. If considering operative vaginal delivery for fetal distress or other emergency situations, weigh carefully the risks and benefits of both vaginal and abdominal delivery before making a decision.

SUGGESTED READINGS

American College of Obstetricians and Gynecologists Technical Bulletin: *Dystocia and the augmentation of labor,* Number 218, December, 1995.
Cunningham FG et al: *Williams obstetrics,* ed 20, Norwalk, Conn, 1997, Appleton & Lange.

PROBLEM · 4 5

HYPERTENSION IN PREGNANCY

"Will the Lid Blow Off?"

Case 1 ■ A 35-Year-Old Primigravida with Hypertension

A 35-year-old primigravida comes to your office at 16 weeks' gestation. She is a new patient. She is excited about her new pregnancy and asks you to be her primary care physician who will deliver her baby. Her husband accompanies her to the visit and appears to be highly supportive of the pregnancy.

Her medical history is unremarkable. She denies a history of hypertension although she has not had her blood pressure measured for 5 years. On physical examination, her blood pressure after 5 minutes of rest is

160/100 mm Hg. A repeat measurement 1 week later is 154/98 mm Hg. Funduscopy is normal, and no other abnormalities are determined.

SELECT THE BEST ANSWER
TO THE FOLLOWING QUESTIONS

Q1. What is the most likely diagnosis in this patient?
   a. preeclampsia
   b. chronic hypertension
   c. chronic hypertension with superimposed pre-eclampsia
   d. transient hypertension
   e. labile hypertension

The patient is followed on a weekly basis. Her blood pressure remains at or around 155/98 until 26 weeks' gestation, when it is noted to have increased to 170/106 mm Hg. She also is found to have 2+ proteinuria. The 24-hour urine protein level is 300 mg/day.

Q2. At this time what is the most likely diagnosis?
   a. preeclampsia
   b. chronic hypertension with superimposed eclampsia
   c. chronic hypertension with superimposed pre-eclampsia
   d. transient hypertension
   e. hemolysis, elevated liver enzymes, and low platelet count syndrome

Q3. Now what is the treatment of choice?
   a. increased rest at home; increase the frequency of office visits to twice weekly
   b. admit the patient to the hospital for bed rest and further evaluation
   c. admit the patient to the hospital; begin pharmacologic therapy
   d. institute pharmacologic therapy as an outpatient; see the patient in the office twice weekly
   e. admit the patient to the hospital for bed rest and pharmacologic therapy

The patient's blood pressure responded to the treatment initiated at 26 weeks' gestation by dropping to a level of 140/90 mm Hg and stayed at that level. Now, at 34 weeks' gestation, her proteinuria has increased to 6 g/day. A biophysical profile is performed. The non-stress test is reactive. Fetal breathing movements, gross body movements, and extremity tone are present. However, the amniotic fluid index is 4 cm, with the largest single pocket of only 1.5 cm.

Q4. What is the next step in management?
   a. begin pharmacologic therapy with a thiazide diuretic
   b. begin pharmacologic therapy with a beta-blocker
   c. begin pharmacologic therapy with a calcium channel blocker
   d. begin pharmacologic therapy with a direct vasodilator
   e. none of the above

Case 2 ■ A Hypertensive 25-Year-Old Primigravida Who Is Taking a Thiazide Diuretic

A 25-year-old primigravida is a known hypertensive who is presently on a thiazide diuretic. On examination at 8 weeks' gestation her blood pressure is 120/85 mm Hg.

Q5. What should you do at this time?
   a. discontinue the thiazide diuretic and substitute atenolol
   b. discontinue the thiazide diuretic and substitute methyldopa
   c. discontinue the thiazide diuretic and substitute nothing
   d. continue the thiazide diuretic and see the patient every 2 weeks
   e. none of the above

Q6. The patient described in Case 2 has her blood pressure well controlled until 18 weeks' gestation. At that time her blood pressure rises to 160/102 mm Hg. What should you do at this time?
   a. reinstitute the thiazide diuretic
   b. start the patient on an angiotensin-converting enzyme (ACE) inhibitor
   c. start the patient on a calcium channel blocker
   d. start the patient on alpha methyldopa
   e. start the patient on a β-adrenergic blocker

Q7. What is the pharmacologic agent of choice for the treatment of chronic hypertension in pregnancy?
   a. atenolol
   b. propranolol
   c. alpha methyldopa
   d. nifedipine
   e. captopril

Q8. Which of the following antihypertensive drug classes are contraindicated for use in pregnancy?
   a. thiazide diuretics
   b. ACE inhibitors
   c. calcium channel blockers
   d. a and b only
   e. all of the above

Q9. What is the drug of choice for the management and control of the seizures associated with eclampsia?
    a. intravenous (IV) phenytoin
    b. IV diazepam
    c. IV methyldopa
    d. IV clonidine
    e. IV MgSO$_4$

Q10. Regarding the use of aspirin to prevent preeclampsia in normotensive women, which of the following statements is true?
    a. aspirin has been conclusively shown to provide a reduction in maternal morbidity
    b. aspirin has been conclusively shown to provide a reduction in maternal mortality
    c. aspirin has been conclusively shown to provide an improved fetal outcome
    d. aspirin has been conclusively shown to lower morbidity in preeclampsia
    e. none of the above

Q11. What is the cause of preeclampsia currently thought to be?
    a. a deficiency of endothelin-1
    b. a deficiency of endothelium-derived relaxing factor (EDRF)
    c. a change in the ratio of prostacyclin to thromboxane
    d. an increase in free radical formation
    e. none of the above

Q12. The pathophysiology of preeclampsia is primarily due to which of the following?
    a. vascular endothelial cell proliferation
    b. diffuse vascular vasospasm
    c. glomerular cell hypertrophy
    d. placental vessel hyperplasia
    e. carotid body hypoplasia

SHORT ANSWER MANAGEMENT PROBLEM
Discuss the risk factors for pregnancy-induced hypertension.

ANSWERS

A1. **b.** This patient most likely has chronic hypertension. Chronic hypertension is defined as a blood pressure >140 mm Hg systolic or > 90 mm Hg diastolic either predating pregnancy or occurring before the 20 weeks' gestation.

Pregnancy-induced hypertension, or preeclampsia, is defined as a sustained rise in arterial blood pressure after 20 weeks' gestation to a level ≥140 mm Hg systolic or ≥90 mm Hg diastolic. Alternatively, pregnancy-induced hypertension can be defined by a 30- or 15-mm Hg increase in systolic pressure, respectively. In the latter case, transient hypertension lacks a proteinuria, but a proteinuria of ≥300 mg/24 hr denotes sustained hypertension or preeclampsia. Weight gain and edema are frequently present; they are not necessary, however, to make the diagnosis of preeclampsia.

Eclampsia and the presence of generalized or grand mal seizures are the major complication of preeclampsia.

A patient who has chronic hypertension with superimposed preeclampsia is defined as a patient who, having preexisting hypertension, has a further increase in blood pressure or worsening of proteinuria after 20 weeks' gestation.

A2. **c.** At this time, the patient has chronic hypertension with superimposed preeclampsia. This condition is associated with significant fetal morbidity and mortality, and the fetus should, therefore, be monitored extremely closely for the duration of the pregnancy.

A3. **b.** This patient has developed chronic hypertension with superimposed preeclampsia. She should be admitted to the hospital for bed rest and for further investigation and evaluation. Bed rest and reduced activity are essential.

The patient should be placed in the left lateral position, which will hopefully result in:
    a. Lower blood pressure readings
    b. Mobilization of extravascular fluid
    c. Decreased endogenous excretion of catecholamines
    d. Increased renal perfusion and diuresis
    e. Improvement in uterine blood flow

Further investigation and evaluation should include the evaluation of renal function (including 24-hour urine for total protein and creatinine clearance) and coagulation parameters (including platelets, prothrombin time, partial thromboplastin time, fibrinogen, and fibrin degradation products), liver function tests, and uric acid levels.

Pharmacologic therapy should not be instituted unless the blood pressure remains significantly elevated (diastolic pressure >100 mm Hg) in spite of bed rest.

Rest at home and institution of outpatient pharmacologic therapy would not be appropriate at this time.

A4. **e.** The treatment of choice for this patient at this time is delivery. The low amniotic fluid indicates this fetus is in jeopardy. This patient, with a 24-hour urine protein exceeding 5 g/day, now has chronic hypertension with superimposed severe preeclampsia. The patient should receive a 5-g IV bolus dose of magnesium sulfate followed by 2 g/hr infusion and induction of labor initiated if fetal status is stable.

Although in this scenario the patient's blood pressure is not in the severe category, if the blood pressure should reach a mean arterial pressure (MAP) ≥130 mm Hg or a diastolic pressure ≥110 mm Hg, IV hypertensives should be instituted to avoid or limit end-organ damage, particularly cerebral hemorrhage. The diastolic blood pressure should be brought down to between 90 and 100 mm Hg. Reducing blood pressure lower than this could jeopardize placental perfusion. IV boluses of hydralazine or labetalol are indicated. Sodium nitroprusside is reserved for resistant cases in which blood pressure does not respond.

A5. **c.** Patients who become pregnant while on antihypertensives and who are well controlled should have their medications discontinued. Therapy should be reinstituted if the MAP increases to ≥117 mm Hg or the diastolic pressure rises to ≥100 mm Hg. There is no evidence that treating diastolic blood pressure below 100 mm Hg improves either maternal or fetal outcome.

A6. **d.**

A7. **c.**

A8. **b.** The best option of the drugs listed is alpha methyldopa. It has been investigated with randomized, prospective studies and found to improve both maternal and fetal outcomes. Although a beta-blocker could be used, a potential concern is association with intrauterine growth restriction (IUGR). Thiazide diuretics should not be initiated in pregnancy because they tend to decrease intravascular volume initially. However, women who conceive while on chronic diuretic therapy may safely continue these agents. Thiazides have been associated with neonatal thrombocytopenia. ACE inhibitors are contraindicated because of their association with fetal hypocalvaria, renal failure, oligohydramnios, and fetal and neonatal death. Women who conceive while using such agents should be advised to discontinue them immediately. Calcium channel blockers, although not contraindicated in pregnancy, have a relatively short track record compared with drugs such as alpha methyldopa and are not recommended as drugs of first or second choice.

A9. **e.** The drug of choice for the control of seizures associated with eclampsia is magnesium sulfate. A commonly used regime is as follows:
   a. Control of convulsions with magnesium sulfate.

An IV loading dose of 5 g is administered followed by a 2-g/hr IV infusion.
   b. Intermittent IV injections of hydralazine to lower blood pressure to between 90 and 100 mm Hg.
   c. Avoidance of diuretics and hyperosmotic agents
   d. Limitation of IV fluid administration unless fluid loss is excessive
   e. Delivery by the most appropriate route based on obstetric indications. If the patient's cervix is favorable, induction of labor can be attempted after stabilization of the patient if fetal well being is ensured.

A10. **e.** Initial studies, designed to prevent preeclampsia in normotensive primigravidas by use of aspirin, showed a decrease in preeclampsia but an increase in abruptio placenta. Subsequent larger prospective studies question whether preeclampsia rates can even be decreased. Studies on women at increased risk for preeclampsia suggest administration of low-dose aspirin (60 to 80 mg) may be an appropriate option. However, use of aspirin is not recommended for preeclampsia prophylaxis in unselected, normotensive multiparas or nulliparous patients.

A11. **c.**

A12. **b.** The pathophysiology at the cellular level and the pathologic process that begins preeclampsia are still unknown. There are many possible factors that may play a role. These include endothelins (which are potent vasoconstrictors), EDRF, and the ratio of two particular prostaglandins that have opposite actions (the vasodilating prostacyclin and the vasoconstricting thromboxane).

In terms of the actual pathophysiology, there is little doubt that the major contributing factor that gives rise to all of the complications of preeclampsia and eclampsia is an intense vasospasm or vasoconstriction.

SOLUTION TO THE SHORT ANSWER MANAGEMENT PROBLEM

The established risk factors for preeclampsia include:
   a. Nulliparity
   b. Small vessel disease (e.g., systemic lupus erythematosus, long-standing type 1 diabetes mellitus)
   c. Chronic hypertension
   d. Hydatidiform mole
   e. Preexisting renal disease
   f. Multiple gestation
   g. Young nulliparous teenagers
   h. "Elderly" pregnant women

SUMMARY OF THE DIAGNOSIS AND TREATMENT OF HYPERTENSION IN PREGNANCY

1. Diagnosis and classification:
   a. Pregnancy-induced hypertension:
      1) Hypertension without proteinuria or edema (also known as *transient hypertension*)
      2) Preeclampsia
         a) Mild
         b) Severe
      3) Eclampsia
   b. Chronic hypertension:
      1) Without superimposed preeclampsia
      2) With superimposed preeclampsia
      3) With superimposed eclampsia
   c. Transient hypertension

2. Definition of hypertensive disorders:
   a. Preeclampsia: either systolic blood pressure ≥140 mm Hg or diastolic blood pressure of ≥90 mm Hg or an increase in systolic blood pressure of 30 mm Hg or in diastolic blood pressure of 15 mm Hg after the 20 weeks' gestation
   b. Chronic hypertension: a systolic blood pressure ≥140 mm Hg systolic or a diastolic blood pressure of ≥90 mm Hg either predating pregnancy or occurring before 20 weeks' gestation or that persists postpartum
   c. Chronic hypertension with superimposed preeclampsia: a further increase in blood pressure or a worsening of proteinuria after 20 weeks' gestation in a patient with established hypertension
   d. Pregnancy-induced hypertension without proteinuria or pathologic edema: this used to be called *transient, or late, hypertension.*

3. Treatment of hypertensive disorders in pregnancy:
   a. Patients with chronic hypertension on medication who become pregnant should discontinue all antihypertensive agents in early pregnancy if the blood pressure is normal. The reason for this is that perinatal outcome and the incidence of chronic hypertension with superimposed preeclampsia are not altered by drug treatment.
   b. Reinstitute therapy if the MAP is ≥117 mm Hg or if the diastolic pressure is ≥100 mm Hg during the second trimester or if the MAP is ≥127 mm Hg or the diastolic pressure is ≥110 mm Hg during the third trimester.
   c. Drugs of choice in the treatment of hypertension in pregnancy:
      1) Chronic hypertension:
         a) First choice: alpha methyldopa
         b) Second choices: atenolol, labetalol

   2) Pregnancy-induced hypertension with preeclampsia:
      a) Mild: no drug treatment
      b) Severe: intravenous antihypertensives (first choice: IV labetalol to keep diastolic pressure <100 mm Hg to avoid end-organ damage, particularly cerebral hemorrhage). Deliver the fetus once the fetal lung maturity is established, in the presence of IUGR or fetal distress, or if there is further deterioration in the maternal condition.

4. Pathophysiology of pregnancy-induced hypertension with preeclampsia or eclampsia: Unknown, but probably involves endothelins, EDRF, and altered ratio of vasodilating prostacyclin to vasoconstricting thromboxane. Vasospasm is the major pathophysiologic process responsible.

SUGGESTED READINGS

American College of Obstetricians and Gynecologists Technical Bulletin: *Hypertension in pregnancy,* Number 219, January, 1996.

Cunningham FG et al: *Williams obstetrics,* ed 20, Norwalk, Conn, 1997, Appleton & Lange.

Idama TO, Lindow SW: Magnesium sulfate: A review of clinical pharmacology applied to obstetrics, *Br J Obstet Gynecol* 105:260-268, 1998.

Whitlin AG, Sibai BM: Magnesium sulfate therapy in preeclampsia and eclampsia, *Obstet Gynecol* 92:883-889, 1998.

PROBLEM · 46

DIAGNOSIS AND MANAGEMENT OF INTRAUTERINE GROWTH RESTRICTION

Is It Too Small or Too Immature?

Case 1 ■ A 36-Year-Old Multigravida with a Uterus Too Small for Dates

A 36-year-old female (gravida 4, para 2, aborted 1) is seeing you for the first time at 34 weeks' gestation. She recently moved to your area and was receiving prenatal care with another physician before her move. She brought a copy of her previous prenatal records with her.

She has noticed decreased fetal movements for the past 2 days. She states pregnancy has been complicated by chronic hypertension, and her previous prenatal visit blood pressure readings have been in the vicinity of 150/90 mm Hg.

On examination, her blood pressure is 155/95 mm Hg and she has 3+ pitting edema. Her fundal height is 29 cm. The fetus' presentation is cephalic and the fetal heart rate is 125 bpm.

SELECT THE BEST ANSWER
TO THE FOLLOWING QUESTIONS

Q1. Which of the following would be of most help at this point in time in arriving at a working diagnosis with this pregnancy?
a. take a repeat blood pressure after 5 minutes of left lateral rest
b. confirm gestational age from a first-trimester sonogram report
c. perform a nonstress test (NST)
d. perform a contraction stress test (CST)
e. check a spot urine sample for degree of proteinuria

Q2. Assume that a first-trimester sonogram was performed that did confirm her current gestational age to be 34 weeks. What is the most appropriate next step in management?
a. perform an amniocentesis for fetal lung maturity studies
b. hospitalize the patient on the maternity unit for observation
c. perform an obstetric sonogram for fetal measurements
d. perform an immediate cesarean section for fetal indications
e. send the patient home for bed rest

Q3. The sonogram shows the composite of fetal measurements is 30 weeks' gestation. Which of the following statements regarding the decreased fetal growth do you know is true for sure?
a. the fetus is small for gestational age (SGA)
b. the fetus has suffered brain damage
c. the fetus has a congenital infection
d. the fetus is constitutionally small
e. the fetus has abnormal chromosomes

Q4. The fetal measurements by sonogram showed head measurements appropriate for 33 weeks' gestation but abdominal circumference at 27 weeks' gestation. Which of the following causes for SGA would be most consistent with these findings?
a. maternal smoking
b. congenital rubella infection
c. maternal lead exposure
d. monosomy X (Turner's syndrome)
e. maternal chronic hypertension

Q5. What is the leading cause of perinatal death in intrauterine growth restriction (IUGR) infants?
a. intrauterine asphyxia
b. preeclampsia in the mother
c. diabetes in the mother

d. meconium aspiration
e. none of the above

Q6. What is the single most preventable cause of IUGR in pregnancy?
a. maternal hyperglycemia
b. maternal malnutrition
c. maternal cigarette smoking
d. maternal hypertension
e. maternal illicit drug abuse

Q7. What is the most common maternal disease causing IUGR?
a. maternal hypertension
b. maternal anemia
c. maternal renal disease
d. maternal inflammatory bowel disease
e. maternal valvular heart disease

Q8. What is the single screening clinical modality for a possible IUGR fetus?
a. inadequate maternal weight gain
b. inadequate fundal height growth
c. maternal hypertension
d. maternal fetal risk status
e. none of the above

Q9. IUGR is associated with which of the following neonatal conditions?
a. hypothermia
b. hypoglycemia
c. hypothyroidism
d. a and b
e. all of the above

Q10. Which of the following statements concerning fetal alcohol syndrome is (are) false?
a. fetal alcohol syndrome will lead to symmetrical IUGR
b. fetal alcohol syndrome is not seen when maternal intake is limited to 1 to 2 drinks a day
c. the prevalence of fetal alcohol syndrome is extremely high in many parts of the United States
d. all of the above are false
e. none of the above is false

Q11. Which of the following statements regarding cigarette smoking in pregnancy is false?
a. impairment of fetal growth is directly related to the number of cigarettes smoked
b. smoking is associated with preterm birth, placenta previa, and placenta abruptio
c. presenting the fetal hazards of cigarette smoking to a pregnant woman almost always causes her to quit

d. cigarette smoking produces symmetric IUGR
e. none of the above is false

Q12. Which of the following maternal drugs poses the greatest danger in terms of fetal growth restriction and other fetal and newborn problems?
a. phenytoin
b. digoxin
c. prednisone
d. selective serotonin reuptake inhibitors
e. acetaminophen

Q13. Which of the following antepartum fetal testing methods offers the most specific evaluation of fetal jeopardy?
a. fetal movement charts
b. biophysical profile (BPP) testing
c. CST
d. NST
e. none of the above

Q14. Which of the following parameters define(s) a reactive NST?
a. the absence of late decelerations
b. the absence of variable decelerations
c. the absence of early decelerations
d. all of the above
e. none of the above

Q15. Which of the following parameters define(s) a positive CST?
a. the presence of late decelerations
b. the presence of variable decelerations
c. the presence of early decelerations
d. all of the above
e. none of the above

Q16. Which of the following is (are) components of BPP testing?
a. gross fetal movements
b. fetal breathing movements
c. fetal tone
d. amniotic fluid volume and amniotic fluid pockets
e. all of the above

Q17. Of the components of the BPP, which is the best predictor of fetal outcome with IUGR?
a. gross fetal movements
b. fetal breathing movements
c. fetal tone
d. reactive NST
e. amniotic fluid volume

Q18. The presence of decelerations on an electronic fetal monitor strip during labor is variably important depending on the type of deceleration in relation to its occurrence relative to the uterine contraction. Each type of deceleration conveys a certain interpretation or a certain meaning. Which of the following pairs of deceleration type and deceleration meaning is (are) correct?
a. early deceleration = head compression
b. variable deceleration = cord compression
c. late deceleration = fetal distress
d. all of the above are correct
e. none of the above is correct

SHORT ANSWER MANAGEMENT PROBLEM

The terminology related to decreased growth of the fetus in utero is confusing. There are two basic nomenclatures: the SGA nomenclature and the asymmetric/symmetric IUGR nomenclature. Define these two nomenclatures and select the one considered most appropriate.

ANSWERS

A1. **b.** In this case the discrepancy in assumed gestational age and fundal height is greater than 3 cm. After 20 weeks' gestation the fundal height in centimeters and the gestational age in weeks should approximate each other. This appears to be a case of fundal height less than dates. To make that assumption, however, it is important that the dates be accurate. A first-trimester ultrasound measurement of the fetal crown-rump length is accurate to within ±5 days. If the patient's records reveal an early sonogram, the results would be most helpful in identifying if this uterus is truly small for dates. Repeating the blood pressure would be helpful in confirming the hypertension, but since her blood pressure is not significantly higher than it was previously, this would not give us a diagnosis. Performing an NST or a CST would assess fetal well being but would not assess if the fundus is truly too small for dates. Assessing proteinuria would assess maternal well being but would not confirm suspicions of being small for dates.

A2. **c.** The early sonogram provides a benchmark from which the adequacy of fetal growth can be assessed. A sonogram at this time will allow you to assess if appropriate fetal growth has taken place since then. A fundus smaller than dates can be due to examiner measurement error, particularly if the patient is obese. However, if the fundus is truly too small for dates, possible causes could be decreased amniotic fluid (oligohydramnios) or decreased fetal size. The acronym IUGR, formerly stood for "intrauterine growth *retardation*" but now has been replaced with "intrauterine growth *restriction*." The change in terminology came about because these small fetuses are not retarded.

A3. **a.** Fetuses in the less than tenth percentile are considered to be SGA. SGA infants are associated with higher rates of mortality and morbidity for their gestational ages but do better than infants with the same weight delivered at earlier gestational ages. SGA infants can be divided into two groups: those with a decreased growth potential and those with a normal potential for growth but who are prevented from reaching it because of decreased nutrition and oxygen transmission across the placenta. Although it is possible for the small fetus to have brain damage, to suffer from a congenital infection, to be constitutionally small, or to have abnormal chromosomes, the only fact we know for sure is that it is SGA.

A4. **e.** Disproportionately small SGA fetuses (wasting of the torso while preserving the brain) are described as having *asymmetric* IUGR, whereas proportionately small SGA fetuses (the torso and brain are both small) are described as having *symmetric* IUGR. The fetus described in Question 4 falls into the former category. Asymmetric IUGR has been associated with fetuses who have normal growth potential that is decreased by maternal factors such as maternal hypertension, chronic renal disease, small vessel disease, or severe malnutrition. Symmetric IUGR has been associated with fetuses that have decreased growth potential due to abnormal chromosomes, intrauterine infections, teratogens, anatomic anomalies, and toxins.

A5. **a.** The leading cause of perinatal death in IUGR is intrauterine asphyxia. Diminished placental function due to factors such as cigarette smoking, diminished perfusion, placental infarction, and intrauterine infection is the most common causative factor in IUGR. The IUGR fetus is at risk for in utero complications including hypoxia and metabolic acidosis, which may occur at any time but are particularly likely to occur during labor.

A6. **c.** Cigarette smoking is the single most common preventable cause of IUGR in North America today. Cigarette smoking is more common among women of childbearing age than is alcoholism or illicit drug abuse. Birth weight is reduced by an average of 200 g in infants of smoking mothers. The amount of reduction is related to the number of cigarettes smoked per day. Infants of smoking mothers are also shorter in

length, and there is a greater risk of perinatal death or compromise in labor.

A7. **a.** Hypertension is the single most common maternal disease causing IUGR in pregnancy. Hypertension results in decreased blood flow through the spiral arteries of the placenta, resulting in decreased delivery of oxygen and nutrients to the placenta and to the fetus. Hypertension may also be associated with placental infarction. Other maternal diseases associated with IUGR include maternal anemia, severe maternal malnutrition, maternal renal disease, maternal malabsorption, multiple pregnancy, extrauterine pregnancy, and maternal valvular disease. The common factor in each of these diseases is interference with uptake or delivery of nutrients or oxygen to the fetus.

A8. **a.** Maternal weight gain, maternal blood pressure, maternal risk status, and especially a history of a previous IUGR fetus are all very important with respect to fetal IUGR. The most important screening clinical modality is a series of carefully performed fundal height measurements throughout gestation. A tape, calibrated in centimeters, is applied over the abdominal curvature from the top of the symphysis to the top of the uterine fundus. Between 18 and 30 weeks the measurement should be within 2 to 3 cm from the gestational age in weeks.

A9. **d.** IUGR fetuses must be observed carefully during the first few hours of life. A blood sugar level should be drawn immediately and the infant should be wrapped up in layers of blankets or placed under a warming light. These maneuvers are necessary because IUGR babies are very prone to both hypoglycemia and hypothermia. Hypothyroidism is not increased in IUGR neonates.

A10. **b.** Fetal alcohol syndrome has a high prevalence in some areas of the United States. Prevalence rates in some populations are up to 50% of all children born. Fetal alcohol syndrome leads to symmetric IUGR. Contrary to public opinion, no amount of alcohol is a safe amount of alcohol for a pregnant woman. The prevalence of fetal alcohol syndrome in pregnant women who have an average of 1 to 2 drinks a day may be as high as 10%.

A11. **c.** Cigarette smoking and its dangers increase proportionally with the number of cigarettes smoked. Cigarette smoking produces symmetric IUGR. Cigarette smoking is also associated with many other abnormal conditions in pregnancy including placenta abruptio, placenta previa, and preterm labor. It is difficult to get pregnant women to quit smoking, although success rates are greater than among nonpregnant women. If a woman does stop smoking in pregnancy, she is very likely to start again following the end of pregnancy. The most common response, when pregnant women are told of the risks to their babies, is, "It won't happen to me."

A12. **a.** Certain anticonvulsants, especially phenytoin and trimethadione, may produce specific and characteristic syndromes that include symmetric IUGR as well as fetal anomalies. The other medication options in this question are not associated with fetal growth problems.

A13. **b.** The purpose of antepartum fetal assessment is to identify potential fetal compromise early enough to allow successful intervention and to avoid morbidity and mortality. The specificity of any test modality is its ability to exclude normal results. Not all antepartum fetal testing have the same specificity. The most specific fetal test is the BPP with 70% specificity. When the BPP is low, 70% of the time the fetus is truly compromised. The other options have the following specificities: CST = 50%, NST = 20%, and fetal movement charting = 20%.

A14. **e.** An NST is based on the assumption that fetal heart rate (FHR) accelerations are associated with fetal movements after 30 weeks' gestation and indicate a normally functioning uteroplacental unit. An NST is evaluated on the presence or absence of FHR accelerations. An FHR acceleration peaks at least 15 bpm above the baseline and lasts at least 15 seconds from baseline to baseline. An NST is considered *reactive* (or reassuring) if there are at least two accelerations within a 20-minute period, with or without fetal movements discernible by the mother. An NST is considered *nonreactive* if there are insufficient FHR accelerations after observing for a 40-minute period. Lack of FHR accelerations can occur with any of the following: gestational age <30 weeks, fetal sleep cycles, fetal central nervous system anomaly, fetal sedation by maternal medications, or fetal hypoxia (in a minority of cases). If the NST is nonreactive without explanation, a vibroacoustic stimulation should be administered. A healthy fetus will move its extremities and accelerate its heart rate in response to sound and vibratory stimulation directed through the maternal abdominal and uterine walls.

A criterion for NST evaluation is independent of uterine decelerations.

A15. **a.** A CST is based on the assumption that uterine contractions diminish the flow of oxygenated intervillous blood to the fetus. A fetus with adequate metabolic reserve can cope satisfactorily with transient oxygen deprivation (i.e., FHR remains at stable baseline through contractions, whereas a compromised fetus will show late decelerations [FHR decelerations persisting after a contraction]). A CST is evaluated on the presence or absence of repetitive late decelerations. If they are present with three consecutive contractions in 10 minutes, the CST is positive. This is not reassuring. If late decelerations are absent, the CST is negative, which is reassuring regarding fetal status.

A16. **e.** The BPP has five components: the NST, fetal breathing movements, fetal gross body movements, fetal tone, and amniotic fluid volume. Each of these five parameters is assigned a maximum value of two points. Thus a perfect BPP is 10/10. BPP scores of 8/10 or 10/10 are reassuring of fetal well being. These fetuses are at low risk for chronic fetal hypoxia or asphyxia. Scores of 4/10 or 6/10 are concerning. These fetuses should be delivered if they are near term, otherwise the BPP should be repeated within 24 hours. Scores of 0/10 or 2/10 are ominous. These fetuses should be delivered expeditiously regardless of gestational age.

A17. **e.** The best predictor of fetal outcome with IUGR is the sonographic evaluation of amniotic fluid volume. The finding of a single vertical pocket of amniotic fluid measuring 3 cm or more is reassuring. If the vertical fluid pocket is less than 3 cm, the perinatal mortality rises significantly.

A18. **d.** The definition and significance of FHR decelerations during labor are as follows:
  a. Early decelerations:
    1) Deceleration type: early in relation to the onset of the accompanying uterine contraction. They are mirror images of the contractions and are mediated by vagal stimulation.
    2) Response to: head compression by the force of uterine contractions.
    3) Significance: are not clinically significant.
  b. Variable decelerations:
    1) Deceleration type: variable in relation to the onset of the accompanying uterine contraction. They are characterized by a sudden decrease in heart rate with a sudden return to baseline.
    2) Response to: umbilical cord compression by fetal movement or uterine contractions.
    3) Significance: mild to moderate variable decelerations are not clinically significant. Severe variable decelerations (prolonged, repetitive, and deep) are not reassuring. Severe variable decelerations meet the "rule of 60s": last

longer than 60 seconds, drop to lower than 60 beats per minute, or drop 60 beats per minute below the baseline.

c. Late decelerations:

1) Deceleration type: late in relation to the onset of the accompanying uterine contraction. They are characterized by gradual decreases in fetal heart with a gradual return after the end of the contraction.

2) Response to: uteroplacental insufficiency.

3) Significance: they are never reassuring, especially if they are associated with decreased variability or tachycardia. They tend to be less dramatic on the recording paper and can actually be missed if the recording paper is not turned to a vertical position to read the strip. If persistent, late decelerations necessitate immediate intervention to correct the fetal hypoxia or asphyxia.

SOLUTION TO THE SHORT ANSWER MANAGEMENT PROBLEM

a. The SGA nomenclature

1) Definition: An SGA fetus or neonate is defined as one below the tenth percentile of the mean for a given population.

2) Problems with this definition:

a) Definition of the tenth percentile depends on many factors. Many reference tables use standards derived from a Denver, Colorado population. Since Denver is at an elevation of 5000 feet, babies born in that city tend to be smaller than babies born at sea level. The birth weight considered to be in the tenth percentile at 5000 feet is less than the birth weight considered to be in the tenth percentile at sea level.

b) Although all growth-restricted infants are SGA, not all SGA infants are growth restricted. Of SGA infants, 10% are small due to constitutional factors in the mother. These latter factors include maternal ethnic group, maternal parity, maternal weight, and maternal height.

b. The asymmetric IUGR fetus versus the symmetric IUGR fetus

1) Definition: the definition of asymmetric versus symmetric defines the relationship between the size of the fetal head versus the size of the rest of the fetal body.

2) Explanation of the definition:

a) Asymmetric IUGR refers to fetuses with normal growth potential that are pre-

vented from being actualized. Different anatomic sites respond differently to diminishing placental function. Head size is determined by brain size. As placental function diminishes, the fetal brain tends to be spared by preferential shunting of oxygen and nutrients through the foramen ovale and ductus arteriosus, allowing normal head growth. Because placental insufficiency may result in diminished glucose transfer and hepatic storage, fetal abdominal circumference (which reflects liver size) would be reduced. Muscle mass is also reduced, as are subcutaneous tissue fat stores. Asymmetric fetal IUGR is attributed to placental insufficiency due to a variety of hypertensive complications of pregnancy as well as advanced diabetes mellitus with small vessel disease.

b) Symmetric IUGR refers to fetuses with decreased growth potential due to a variety of causes that impacted on the fetus early in pregnancy (e.g., abnormal chromosomes, intrauterine infections, teratogens, anatomic anomalies, and toxins). These causative factors tend to affect all organs equally, including the brain and the liver. Thus fetal body measurements are all decreased.

c. The terminology of choice: previously, the terminology of choice was *SGA*. Current terminology uses asymmetric or symmetric IUGR because they tend to reflect underling pathophysiology. However, there is considerable evidence that fetal growth patterns are more complex and attempts to prenatally classify the cause of IUGR in fetuses is not as clear and precise as previously thought. Although all fetuses with IUGR are also SGA fetuses, not all SGA fetuses are IUGR fetuses.

SUMMARY OF THE DIAGNOSIS AND MANAGEMENT OF INTRAUTERINE GROWTH RESTRICTION

1. Definitions:

a. See the Short Answer Management Problem. Current terminology uses two IUGR subtypes:

1) Symmetric

2) Asymmetric

2. Prevalence: The true prevalence of IUGR among all pregnant women is estimated at approximately 5%. Not all SGA fetuses are restricted in their growth potential.

3. Differentiation: The importance of differentiating the various types of IUGR is that it allows you to propose a management plan that is based on the pathologic condition involved. It is especially important, based on the old terminology, to separate normal from abnormal. Using the old terminology, a fetus whose mother was of a particular ethnic group, of a certain parity, of a certain weight, or of a certain height would be considered SGA and the baby probably labeled as IUGR when in fact this was not the case.

4. Risk status: True IUGR babies are at extremely high risk for perinatal morbidity and mortality.

5. Important connections:
   a. Asymmetric IUGR: most commonly associated with either some form of maternal hypertensive process or collagen vascular process or maternal diabetes mellitus with small vessel disease.
   b. Symmetric IUGR: most commonly associated with the following:
      1) Chromosomal abnormalities
      2) Cigarette smoking
      3) Fetal alcohol syndrome
      4) Intrauterine infections

6. Clinical clues and investigations:
   a. Physical examination and clinical correlates:
      1) Fundal height is less than expected by dates
      2) Failure to achieve adequate maternal weight gain
   b. Investigations:
      1) Establish whether gestational age is accurate
      2) Confirm IUGR by obstetric sonogram fetal measurements
      3) Identify if IUGR is asymmetric or symmetric
      4) If risk factors for IUGR are present, deal with them at each prenatal visit (e.g., smoking, drinking alcohol)
      5) A sonographic search for fetal anatomic or chromosomal anomalies should be performed
      6) Initiate fetal surveillance with a 3-cm amniotic fluid pocket being the best predictor of fetal well being

7. Antepartum management:
   a. If IUGR is diagnosed before 34 weeks' gestation and amniotic fluid volume and antepartum fetal surveillance is normal, observation is recommended. Assess fetal growth by sonography every 2 to 3 weeks. As long as there is continued growth and fetal evaluation remains normal, conservative management is appropriate. In most cases neither a precise cause nor a specific therapy is apparent. There is no specific treatment that has been shown to improve perinatal outcome. With evidence of fetal jeopardy on antepartum surveillance, delivery should be initiated promptly.
   b. If IUGR is diagnosed near term, prompt delivery is likely to afford the best outcome for the fetus. If the diagnosis is uncertain, expectant management with regular fetal surveillance should be followed until fetal lung maturity can be assured.

8. Intrapartum management: A trial of vaginal delivery is appropriate in many cases. However, it is important to recognize that if the IUGR is caused by placental insufficiency, the fetus may be unable to tolerate labor. If amniotic fluid is decreased, umbilical cord compression is more often identified. This can be alleviated with amnioinfusion. Emergency cesarean delivery is more frequently necessary.

9. Postpartum management: Complications in neonates include hypoglycemia (caused by decreased liver glycogen reserves), hypothermia (caused by decreased subcutaneous tissue), and polycythemia (caused by relative intrauterine hypoxia). If the fetus is hypoxic at birth, meconium aspiration is more likely. Specialized neonatal care may well be needed for these IUGR babies.

SUGGESTED READINGS

American College of Obstetricians and Gynecologists Technical Bulletin: *Antepartum fetal surveillance,* Number 188, January, 1994.
Cunningham FG et al: *Williams obstetrics,* ed 20, Norwalk, Conn, 1997, Appleton & Lange.

PROBLEM · 47

POSTTERM PREGNANCY

"Is It Late, Doctor?"

Case 1 ■ A 24-Year-Old New Patient Who Allegedly Has Gone Past Her Due Date

A 24-year-old woman (gravida 2, para 1) comes to you as a new patient recommended by a friend. She has recently moved to your community with her 2-year-old daughter. She regrets that she lost her prenatal records when packing, but she claims to be 43 weeks pregnant by dates. When you ask her who her previous doctor was she tells you that she only went to her doctor three or four times because she didn't have time and that she forgot the doctor's name.

She has not been keeping a fetal kick chart, but she says the baby has been moving. She has not had an obstetric ultrasound. On examination, her fundal height is 36 cm. Her cervix is soft, 25% effaced, and 1 cm dilated. The fetus' presentation is cephalic and the fetus weighs 6 to 7 pounds. The fetal heart rate is 142 bpm and regular.

SELECT THE BEST ANSWER TO THE FOLLOWING QUESTIONS

Q1. At this time, what would you do?
   a. tell her to come back in a week while you think about things
   b. perform a biophysical profile and sonogram for fetal weight
   c. schedule her for induction of labor at the maternity unit
   d. schedule her for cesarean section just to be on the safe side
   e. do nothing now; make an appointment to see her in 1 week

Q2. A pregnancy is defined as being postterm if it exceeds how many days of gestation?
   a. 280 days
   b. 287 days
   c. 294 days
   d. 273 days
   e. 301 days

Q3. What is the approximate prevalence of postterm pregnancy based on the last menstrual period (LMP)?
   a. 25%
   b. 15%
   c. 10%
   d. 5%
   e. 3%

Q4. What is the approximate true prevalence of postterm pregnancy based on the date of conception?
   a. 25%
   b. 15%
   c. 10%
   d. 5%
   e. 3%

Q5. Which of the following parameters is the most sensitive test for the prediction of fetal asphyxia and resultant perinatal mortality in postterm pregnancy?
   a. a weekly nonstress test (NST)
   b. a biweekly NST

   c. lack of a 3-cm vertical pocket of amniotic fluid on ultrasound
   d. lack of a 1-cm vertical pocket of amniotic fluid on ultrasound
   e. a contraction stress test (CST)

Q6. What is the most common cause of a diagnosis of postdated pregnancy?
   a. lack of an obstetric ultrasound in pregnancy
   b. inaccurate dating using the LMP
   c. the postmaturity syndrome
   d. intrauterine growth restriction
   e. none of the above

Q7. Which of the following statements regarding postterm pregnancy is (are) true?
   a. the perinatal mortality rate is increased in patients who have, in fact, gone past 42 completed weeks' gestation
   b. the incidence of meconium staining and meconium aspiration is increased in patients who have gone beyond 42 completed weeks' gestation
   c. the true postterm fetus may continue to gain weight in utero and present a problem at birth because of fetal size
   d. the intrauterine environment in a true postterm pregnancy may predispose to the development of a dysmature or dystrophic infant
   e. all of the above are true

Q8. To what does the term *postmature* refer?
   a. all infants delivered by mothers diagnosed as postterm
   b. all infants verified by objective criteria to be greater than 42 weeks' gestation
   c. infants displaying specific characteristics delivered after 42 weeks' gestation
   d. it is no longer a useful description
   e. none of the above

Q9. A colleague of yours describes his approach to postterm gestation: "I deliver all my patients at 42 weeks." Without inquiring about his perinatal morbidity and mortality statistics, which of the following is (are) reason(s) not to follow his example?
   a. it is difficult to predict which fetuses will develop significant problems
   b. induction of labor is not always successful in leading to vaginal delivery
   c. delivery by cesarean section increases the risk of serious maternal morbidity

d. the majority of fetuses who are truly more than 42 weeks fare well

e. all of the above are true

Q10. At this time, which of the following is (are) true regarding those women who have been established to be truly postterm (greater than 42 weeks' gestation)?

a. there are two approaches to managing these pregnancies: one is conservative and the other is aggressive

b. there appears to be no difference in perinatal outcome between aggressive management and conservative management if conservative management includes an appropriate protocol for fetal surveillance

c. aggressive management appears to result in lower perinatal morbidity and mortality than conservative management

d. a and b

e. a and c

SHORT ANSWER MANAGEMENT PROBLEM

You are a family physician doing obstetrics in your local hospital. You have been asked to develop a clinical practice guideline (CPG) for the management of postterm pregnancy. Prepare this CPG based on your knowledge of the subject.

ANSWERS

A1. **b.** This patient presents a dilemma because the data you need to accurately identify her gestational age are not available. Although she appears to be in the third trimester of pregnancy by fundal height, her dates are suspect because she appears to be a poor historian. The most appropriate action at this time is to confirm fetal well being by means of a biophysical profile, and at the same time to obtain an estimate of fetal weight. The ultrasound examination cannot be expected to provide a due date at this point in her pregnancy. The normal variation in fetal size is so great in the third trimester that ultrasound estimates will vary by as much as 3 weeks plus or minus. Scheduling induction or cesarean delivery is premature at this point. Doing nothing is inappropriate. Ideally assessment of gestational age is confirmed early in pregnancy using the following parameters:

a. Menstrual history: The LMP tends to be reliable if the patient is sure of her dates, if the pregnancy was planned, if the menstrual cycle was regular, if the menstrual cycle was usual for the patient, and if there is no recent history of oral contraceptive use, abortion, pregnancy,

or lactation (all of which are associated with anovulation).

b. Clinical parameters include pregnancy landmarks that are identified as early as they appear: uterine size estimated by an early pelvic examination (before 12 weeks' gestation), fetal heart tones detected by Doppler stethoscope (before 12 weeks gestation), fundal size estimated by abdominal palpation at the symphysis pubis (at 12 weeks' gestation) and the umbilicus (at 20 weeks' gestation); maternal report of feeling fetal movement (quickening) at 16 to 18 weeks in a multigravida and 18 to 20 weeks in a primigravida, fetal heart tones heard with a fetoscope (at 18 to 20 weeks' gestation).

c. Ultrasound parameters include crown-rump length (between 8 and 12 weeks' gestation [accurate to within 5 days]) and fetal biparietal diameter (between 12 and 18 weeks' gestation [accurate to within 7 days]).

A2. **c.**

A3. **c.**

A4. **e.** A pregnancy is defined as being postterm if it persists beyond 294 days (or 42 weeks' gestation) from the first day of the LMP, assuming ovulation occurred on day 14 of the menstrual cycle. More precisely however, postterm pregnancy should be defined as one that persists beyond 280 days from conception. Since only 15% of women's menstrual cycles are exactly 28 days long, many women ovulate more than 14 days after their LMP. Thus even though their pregnancies go beyond 294 days from the LMP, they have not gone beyond the 280 days from conception and are not truly postterm.

The pseudoprevalence of postterm pregnancy (the prevalence of the label of postterm pregnancy being applied or documented in the chart based on LMP) is approximately 10%. However, the true prevalence of postterm pregnancy is approximately 3%.

A5. **c.** The most sensitive test for the prediction of fetal asphyxia and resultant perinatal mortality in postterm pregnancy is decreased amniotic fluid on ultrasound. The largest study to date, the Canadian Postterm Pregnancy Trial, found that using the lack of a 3-cm pocket as a test for the basis for intervention was associated with a lower perinatal mortality rate than using either an NST or a CST. Thus the performance of a biophysical profile on a biweekly basis, with the demonstration of a 3-cm amniotic fluid pocket, is a reassuring sign that suggests that the fetal status is reassuring.

A6. **b.** Postdated pregnancy is most commonly diagnosed because of incorrect or inaccurate dates based on the first day of the LMP. Although not performing an obstetric ultrasound during pregnancy will increase the probability of that diagnosis being made, it is not the true cause.

A7. **e.** The perinatal mortality rate and the incidence of meconium staining and meconium aspiration are increased when the gestational age is 42 weeks or beyond. In true postterm pregnancy, placental function is unchanged and the fetus may continue to gain weight in utero resulting in a macrosomic fetus. This occurs in 70% of cases. In other cases the placenta may undergo aging, infarction, and calcification. In these pregnancies the intrauterine environment may predispose for loss of fetal weight, loss of subcutaneous fat and muscle, and a dystrophic or dysmature appearance. This occurs in 30% of cases.

A8. **c.** The term *postmature* as applied to neonates refers to a specific subset of infants delivered of mothers who are truly postterm and who display the following characteristics:
   a. Underweight due to loss of subcutaneous fat
   b. Long and thin in girth
   c. Skin with patchy areas of desquamation
   d. Skin sometimes covered with meconium
   e. Wrinkled hands and feet on the ventral surfaces
   f. Long nails stained with meconium

A9. **e.**

A10. **d.** The following five reasons serve to discourage a policy of delivering all fetuses whose gestational age is merely suspected to be at least 42 weeks' gestation:
   a. Gestational age is not always known precisely, thus the fetus may actually be less mature than believed.
   b. It is difficult to identify with precision those fetuses likely to develop significant morbidity if left *in utero*.
   c. The majority of these fetuses fare rather well.
   d. Induction of labor is not always successful.
   e. Delivery by cesarean section appreciably increases the risk of serious maternal morbidity not only in this pregnancy but also to a degree in subsequent ones.

When a pregnancy is definitely confirmed to be 42 or more weeks in length, two management approaches appear to be equally appropriate. A randomized investigation by Hannah et al. compared elective induction with antepartum surveillance (NST, amniotic fluid volume, and fetal movement counting). Women were randomized to either induction of labor at 42

weeks' gestation or serial antenatal fetal testing. The findings showed that induction of labor at 42 weeks' gestation resulted in a lower rate of cesarean section (21%) than in the antenatal surveillance group (25%), with equivalent infant outcomes in the two study groups.

SOLUTION TO THE SHORT ANSWER MANAGEMENT PROBLEM

The following are the steps that should be in the guidelines you have prepared for the management of postterm pregnancy.
   a. Review the entire prenatal history. Establish whether or not the LMP was a normal one and calculated an estimated date of conception (EDC) based on dates.
   b. Review the early pregnancy landmarks that are documented on the prenatal chart.
   c. Review any obstetric ultrasounds performed during the pregnancy and calculate an EDC. If more than one ultrasound was performed, use the date established by the ultrasound earliest in the pregnancy.
   d. Compare the EDC by dates and compare it to the EDC from the early pregnancy landmark and the ultrasound data.
   e. Determine your best estimate of the EDC from all the information available.
   f. Begin antenatal monitoring at 41 weeks' gestation by best estimate EDC: charting fetal movement daily, performing NSTs twice weekly, and looking for at least one 3-cm pocket of amniotic fluid volume twice weekly.
   g. Perform a pelvic examination at 42 weeks' gestation and evaluate cervical effacement and cervical dilatation. Begin induction of labor if the cervix is ripe. If not, then ripening of the cervix with a prostaglandin gel is indicated before formal induction with oxytocin.
   h. Obtain a consultation from an obstetrician at this time (if one has not already been done).
   i. If induction is unsuccessful or if fetal well being cannot be assured during induction, proceed to cesarean section.

SUMMARY OF THE DIAGNOSIS AND MANAGEMENT OF POSTTERM PREGNANCY

A good summary of this chapter is provided by the clinical practice guideline given in the Solution to the Short Answer Management Problem.

SUGGESTED READINGS

American College of Gynecologists and Obstetricians Practice Patterns: *Management of postterm pregnancy,* Number 6, October, 1997.

Cunningham FG et al: *Williams obstetrics,* ed 20, Norwalk, Conn, 1997, Appleton & Lange.

Hannah ME et al: Canadian multicenter post-term pregnancy trial group: Induction of labor as compared with serial antenatal monitoring in post-term pregnancy, *New Engl J Med* 326:1587, 1992.

PROBLEM·48

SPONTANEOUS ABORTION

"Will We Make It to Term?"

Case 1 ■ A 25-Year-Old with Vaginal Bleeding at 11 Weeks' Gestation

A 25-year-old female (gravida 2, para 0) comes to your office at 11 weeks' gestation with vaginal bleeding and mild lower abdominal cramping. She is crying and upset. Her previous pregnancy ended in a miscarriage at 9 weeks' gestation.

On examination, a bright red flow is seen coming from the cervical os. Her cervix is closed. The uterus by palpation is 8 to 9 weeks' gestation. Her blood pressure is 120/70 mm Hg and her pulse rate is 96. No other abnormalities are found.

**SELECT THE BEST ANSWER
TO THE FOLLOWING QUESTIONS**

Q1. What is the most likely diagnosis of this patient's condition at this time?
 a. threatened abortion
 b. inevitable abortion
 c. incomplete abortion
 d. recurrent spontaneous abortion
 e. complete abortion

Q2. The vaginal blood flow in this patient increases slightly while in your office. She is now soaking through approximately one pad every 2 hours. What would you do at this time?
 a. observe carefully at home; order outpatient investigations
 b. admit the patient to the hospital and obtain an obstetric sonogram to assess pregnancy viability
 c. observe the patient at home; tell her not to worry about anything
 d. admit the patient to the hospital for observation only; no testing is indicated at this time
 e. it doesn't really matter

Q3. Taking into account your management, the patient goes on to abort the fetus 3 days later. Her bleeding is minimal and her vital signs are stable. On examination, it appears that most of the placental tissue is present. A sonogram shows an empty uterus with a normal endometrial stripe. What would you now recommend?
 a. no further treatment
 b. ergonovine maleate to contract the uterus
 c. prophylactic antibiotics to prevent infection
 d. dilatation and curettage
 e. serial beta human chorionic gonadotropin (bHCG) titers

Q4. What is the spontaneous abortion rate in North American women?
 a. 10%
 b. 20%
 c. 25%
 d. 50%
 e. 75%

Q5. Spontaneous abortion is defined as which of the following?
 a. pregnancy loss at any gestational age
 b. pregnancy loss before 20 weeks' gestation
 c. delivery of a fetus-neonate under 250 g
 d. delivery of a fetus-neonate under 500 g
 e. none of the above

Q6. What is the most commonly recognized precipitating factor in spontaneous abortion?
 a. chromosomal abnormality
 b. advanced maternal age
 c. preexisting chronic maternal disease
 d. alcohol intake
 e. cigarette smoking

Q7. What is the most commonly recognized chromosomal anomaly associated with first-trimester spontaneous abortion?
 a. autosomal trisomy
 b. monosomy
 c. tetraploidy
 d. autosomal monosomy
 e. sex chromosome polysomy

Q8. Which of the following maternal conditions is (are) associated with an increased incidence of abortion?
 a. hypothyroidism
 b. controlled diabetes mellitus
 c. uncontrolled diabetes mellitus
 d. all of the above
 e. none of the above

Q9. Which of the following statements regarding cigarette smoking and spontaneous abortion is (are) true?
   a. smoking has been associated with an increased risk of euploidic abortion
   b. in women who smoke more than 14 cigarettes per day, the risk of spontaneous abortion is twice that of women who do not smoke
   c. smoking increases the risk of abortion by a factor of 1.2 for each 10 cigarettes smoked per day
   d. all of the above are true
   e. none of the above is true

Q10. Which of the following statements regarding the risk of spontaneous abortion and alcohol intake is (are) true?
   a. the risk of spontaneous euploidic abortion is increased even when alcohol is consumed "in moderation" during pregnancy
   b. the spontaneous abortion rate is doubled in women who drink twice weekly
   c. the spontaneous abortion rate is tripled in women who consume alcohol daily
   d. all of the above are true
   e. none of the above is true

Q11. Which of the following antibodies is most clearly associated with spontaneous abortion?
   a. anticardiolipin antibody
   b. antithyroid antibody
   c. antinuclear antibody
   d. rheumatoid factor
   e. antismooth muscle antibody

SHORT ANSWER MANAGEMENT PROBLEM
Describe the currently recommended classification of spontaneous abortion.

ANSWERS

A1. **a.** The diagnosis is threatened abortion. Threatened abortion is defined as minimal vaginal bleeding, with or without mild cramping, in the first 20 weeks of pregnancy. The interval cervical os is closed. Sonographically the gestational sac appears normal and a viable embryo or fetus is noted with cardiac motion. The incidence of threatened abortion in pregnancy is 20% to 25%; of that number, half go on to abort the fetus. Threatened abortion is associated with a higher risk of preterm labor, low birth weight, and perinatal mortality. There is, however, no increased risk of fetal malformations.

Inevitable abortion is defined as profuse vaginal bleeding and, during the first half of pregnancy, is accompanied by cervical dilatation and rupture of the gestational sac. No passage of tissue has yet occurred.

Incomplete abortion is defined when the criteria for inevitable abortion are met, and some, but not all placental tissue has been passed. A sonogram can be helpful in identifying if products of conception remain in the uterine cavity.

Completed abortion is defined when bleeding, dilatation of the cervix, and complete passage of products of conception have occurred during the first half of pregnancy. This diagnosis is best confirmed with a sonogram

Recurrent spontaneous abortion refers to three or more consecutive abortions.

A2. **b.** In any patient with more than slight bleeding, hospitalization is wise. With the associated cramping in this patient there is a high probability that she will go on to abort. Investigations in the hospital should include a bHCG level and an obstetric ultrasound to assess pregnancy viability and to determine intrauterine contents.

A3. **e.** The patient appears to have undergone a completed abortion. Performing a dilatation and curettage is unnecessary if the products of conception have already been removed from the uterus. The sonogram is strongly suggestive that this is the case. However, if serial weekly bHCG levels fall to zero, it can safely be assumed that all viable trophoblastic villi are out of the uterus.

Ergonovine maleate and prophylactic antibiotics are most useful when excessive bleeding occurs in the postpartum period and is not thought to be caused by retained products of conception.

A4. **b.** The spontaneous abortion rate in North American women is approximately 15% to 20%.

A5. **b.** Spontaneous abortion is defined as the termination of pregnancy before 20 weeks' gestation based on the last menstrual period.

A6. **a.** The most commonly recognized precipitating factor in spontaneous abortion is chromosomal anomaly. Up to 50% of clinically recognized pregnancy losses are have cytogenetic abnormalities. When chorionic villus sampling is performed on the placental tissue of first-trimester embryonic demises, up to 75% will be chromosomally abnormal.

A7. **a.** The most commonly recognized chromosomal abnormality associated with first-trimester spontaneous abortion is autosomal trisomy. It can be the result of an isolated nondisjunction, maternal or paternal balanced translocation, or balanced chromosomal inversion.

A8. **c.** Uncontrolled diabetes mellitus has been associated with an increased incidence of spontaneous abortion. Well-controlled diabetes, however, is not. There is also no association between hypothyroidism and spontaneous abortion.

A9. **d.** Cigarette smoking is associated with an increased risk of euploidic abortion. For women who smoke more than 14 cigarettes per day, the risk of spontaneous abortion is approximately twice that of nonsmokers. This is independent of either maternal age and alcohol ingestion. The risk of spontaneous abortion increases in a linear fashion by a factor of 1.2 for each 10 cigarettes smoked per day.

A10. **d.** The incidence of spontaneous euploidic abortion is increased even when alcohol is consumed even "in moderation." Recent studies have indicated that the abortion rate is doubled in women who consume alcohol twice weekly and is tripled in women who consume alcohol daily when compared to nondrinkers. Increased euploidic abortion is strong evidence that both tobacco and alcohol are toxic to embryos.

A11. **a.** Autoimmune mechanisms are those in which a cellular or humoral response is directed against a specific site within the host. Connective-tissue disorders such as systemic lupus erythematosus are associated with increased abortion and fetal death.

Antiphospholipid antibodies, including the lupus anticoagulant and anticardiolipin antibodies, are examples of autoimmune disease states that are associated with recurrent abortion. Treatment includes low-dose aspirin, subcutaneous heparin injections, or oral steroids.

SOLUTION TO THE SHORT ANSWER MANAGEMENT PROBLEM

The classification of spontaneous abortion is as follows:
   a. Threatened abortion: any bloody vaginal discharge or vaginal bleeding that occurs before 20 weeks' gestation (based on gestational age, not on embryologic age).
   b. Inevitable abortion: rupture of the membranes in the presence of cervical dilatation during the first 20 weeks' gestation.
   c. Missed abortion: retention of nonviable products of conception in utero for up to 4 weeks.

   d. Recurrent spontaneous abortion: previously known as habitual abortion. Defined by various criteria of number and sequence. The most generally accepted definition refers to three or more consecutive spontaneous abortions.

SUMMARY OF THE DIAGNOSIS AND MANAGEMENT OF SPONTANEOUS ABORTION

1. Classification: See the Short Answer Management Problem in this problem.

2. Investigation of threatened abortion:
   a. Serial bHCG levels
   b. Ultrasound (if inconclusive, repeat in 1 to 2 weeks)

3. Management of threatened abortion:
   a. There is no evidence that bed rest changes the pregnancy outcome in the first trimester
   b. There is no evidence that administering any pharmacologic agent changes the outcome
   c. Conservative management if bleeding slows down or stops (document live fetus by ultrasound)
   d. Dilatation and curettage if heavy bleeding continues or ultrasound reveals a nonviable pregnancy live fetus

SUGGESTED READING
Cunningham FG et al: *Williams obstetrics*, ed 20, Norwalk, Conn, 1997, Appleton & Lange.

PROBLEM · 49

POSTPARTUM BLUES, DEPRESSION, AND PSYCHOSES

"A Bundle of Joy: So Why Is Mom So Sad?"

Case 1 ■ A 26-Year-Old Primigravida Who Is Tearful and Depressed 4 Days Postpartum

A 26-year-old primigravida delivers a healthy male infant at 40 weeks' gestation. She is doing fairly well until the fourth day postpartum. At that time she develops insomnia, fatigue, and feelings of sadness and depression.

The patient has a history of bipolar disorder, but she has not had an episode of either hypomania or depression for the last 5 years.

Despite your concern regarding her history of bipolar disorder, she begins to improve on the eighth day postpartum and returns to her normal mental state at 2 weeks postpartum. When you see her in the office in 6 weeks she is well.

SELECT THE BEST ANSWER TO THE FOLLOWING QUESTIONS

Q1. What is the most likely diagnosis in this patient?
a. postpartum depression
b. postpartum blues
c. a mild depression, definitely associated with her previous disease
d. postpartum anxiety
e. postpartum psychosis

Q2. What is the best initial choice of treatment for the patient presented in Case 1?
a. a tricyclic antidepressant
b. lithium carbonate
c. a monoamine oxidase inhibitor (MAOI)
d. a selective serotonin reuptake inhibitor (SSRI)
e. supportive psychotherapy alone

Q3. Considering this patient's history of bipolar disorder, which of the following statements is true?
a. the probability of a recurrence is no greater after pregnancy than in the nonpregnant state
b. the probability of a recurrence is actually decreased in the postpartum state
c. the probability of a recurrence is increased in the postpartum state
d. none of the above
e. nobody knows for sure

Case 2 ■ A 28-Year-Old Primigravida Who Is Guilt Driven, Tearful, and Depressed

A 28-year-old primigravida delivers a healthy female infant at 39 weeks' gestation. She is well until the fourth postpartum day, when she develops tearfulness, despondency, guilt, anorexia, depression, insomnia, and feelings of inadequacy in coping with her infant. These feelings continue and she is in marked distress when seen for her 3-week check up.

Q4. What is the most likely diagnosis in this patient?
a. postpartum depression
b. postpartum blues
c. adjustment disorder with depressed mood
d. early bipolar disorder
e. none of the above

Q5. What is (are) the treatment(s) of choice for the patient described in Case 2?
a. a tricyclic antidepressant
b. a MAO inhibitor
c. an SSRI
d. supportive psychotherapy
e. c and d

Case 3 ■ A 29-Year-Old Primigravida Who Is in Orbit

A 29-year-old primigravida is found on the fourth postpartum day loudly singing hymns at 4 AM in the hospital corridor. During the next 24 hours she causes significant turmoil on the maternity ward. She is found rushing into other patients' rooms announcing that she is about to start classes in "bioenergetics" and urges them to participate. She refuses meals and denies any need to sleep because she is "in touch with the source of superior power." She is hyperactive and talkative and invites her obstetrician to make love to her.

Q6. Which of the following statements is (are) true concerning this patient?
a. this patient has a postpartum psychosis
b. this patient probably has schizophrenia
c. this patient most likely has postpartum depression
d. a and c
e. b and c

Q7. What is (are) the greatest risk(s) at this time for this patient?
a. suicide
b. infanticide
c. homicide
d. degeneration into a more or less permanent paranoid state
e. a and b

Q8. Which of the following is the initial treatment of choice for this patient?
a. intensive observation alone
b. lithium carbonate
c. antipsychotic medication
d. an SSRI
e. diazepam

Q9. Which of the following statements regarding the effects of maternal depression in older children is (are) true?
a. behavioral problems are more common in children whose mothers have had a postpartum depression

b. significant emotional problems may occur in children whose mothers have an episode of depression in the first postpartum year
c. there is a significant correlation between reading difficulties in children and depression in their mothers
d. all of the above are true
e. none of the above is true

Q10. What is the single most important risk factor for the development of a postpartum depression?
a. a history of depression
b. a history of bipolar disorder
c. a greater-than-average postpartum drop in the serum progesterone level
d. a recent stressful life event
e. the mother's experience as a child in her family of origin

SHORT ANSWER MANAGEMENT PROBLEM
The relationship between the patient and her physician makes a significant difference when considering the probability that postpartum depression will develop, the early and successful recognition of mood disturbances in the postpartum period, and the successful treatment of same. This will decrease the length and severity of those mood disturbances. Provide specific suggestions to accomplish this goal.

ANSWERS

A1. **b.** This patient has postpartum blues, the common name for mild depressive symptoms that occur during this period. Postpartum blues occur in about 50% to 80% of puerperal women. The syndrome is transitory, resolving spontaneously within a few days to 2 weeks. Postpartum blues usually starts with a brief period of weeping on the third or fourth day after delivery and peaks between the fifth and tenth day after delivery. Symptoms include anxiety, headaches, poor concentration, and confusion.

The cause of postpartum blues is unknown, but a hormonal basis is suspected. Of the hormones involved, the most likely candidate is progesterone, and the most likely alteration is progesterone deficiency.

A2. **e.** The treatment of choice for postpartum blues includes supportive psychotherapy; family (especially spousal) support, understanding, and reassurance; and patient education (reassuring the patient that this is completely normal). In the patient described, it is especially important to reinforce that there is no connection between the postpartum blues now experienced

and her previous bipolar illness; resolution of "the blues" will occur within 2 weeks, but monitoring her condition is necessary to ensure both maternal and fetal health.

A3. **c.** In a patient with a history of bipolar disorder there is actually an increased chance of reoccurrence in the postpartum period.

Of the 50% to 80% of women who develop postpartum blues, only 10% will go on to have a true *postpartum depression,* the common term for a major depressive disorder with postpartum onset.

A4. **a.** This patient has a true postpartum depression because she has a major depressive episode. Postpartum depression, as discussed previously, occurs in approximately 10% of women. In postpartum depression, in contradistinction to postpartum blues, the patient is disabled for a period of time greater than 2 weeks. The major symptoms are a depressed mood, a real concern about the ability to cope with the new infant, and increased guilt. Other symptoms include tearfulness, despondency, worrying about not loving the baby enough, worrying about doing something "irrational" to the baby, anxiety regarding feeding the baby, fear about the baby's sleep, fear about older siblings' jealousy, hypochondriac symptoms, irritability, impaired concentration, poor memory, and extreme fatigue.

Multiple risk factors for postpartum depression have been suggested and include:
a. Hormonal deficiency: progesterone
b. Family history of depression
c. The conduct and stress of the labor itself
d. History of inadequate nurturing in childhood
e. Lack of an intimate confiding relationship with her partner
f. Inadequate commitment of the father to the whole process of pregnancy, labor, and delivery
g. Concurrent presence of stressful life events including family crises, bereavement, change in housing, financial problems, and caring for her other children.

A5. **e.** The treatment of choice for postpartum depression is a combination of supportive psychotherapy and antidepressants. SSRIs are usually the antidepressant medications of first choice since they are safer and have fewer potentially serious side effects than do tricyclic antidepressants or MAOIs. Breast feeding should be avoided since antidepressants and their metabolites may be present in breast milk. Addressing these risk factors will probably decrease the duration and the severity of the postpartum depression. The best strategy appears to involve the health care professionals (doctor, public health nurse, psychiatric nurse), the patient's immediate family (especially a supportive husband), supportive friends and relatives, and group psychotherapy (where postpartum women with this condition compare their experiences).

A6. **a.** This patient has a postpartum psychosis. Postpartum psychoses occur in 1 to 2 per 1000 postpartum women. The presentation may be dominated by bizarre, persecutory, or grandiose delusions or thought disorganization. Manic symptoms may also be present.

Postpartum psychosis may occur as an exacerbation of preexisting bipolar disorder, major depressive disorder, or schizophrenia. When such history is absent, the diagnosis is often brief psychotic disorder with postpartum onset.

This patient is having a hypomanic episode. She is likely to have had a personal or family history of mood disorder.

A7. **e.** A patient with postpartum psychosis is at risk for suicide and infanticide. In one study, 5% of patients committed suicide and 4% of patients committed infanticide.

A8. **c.** Acute treatment for this patient consists of administering an antipsychotic drug to control psychosis and agitation. A high potency antipsychotic medication such as risperidone or haloperidol might be good first choices. At the same time, the patient should be closely observed by hospital staff.

Depending on the presence of an underlying psychiatric disorder or of persistent mood symptoms, antidepressant or mood-stabilizing medication may be initiated after acute control of the psychotic behavior. Additionally, supportive individual and family psychotherapy should be given. Once the psychotic episode is resolved, long-term therapy should be started. After discharge it is prudent to arrange regular visits by a mental health worker to measure general day-to-day coping skills immediately postpartum and for an extended time.

A9. **d.** Enduring postpartum depression may have subtle effects on the older children of the mother. Behavioral and emotional problems and learning difficulties may develop as a result of postpartum or chronic maternal depression.

A10. **d.** Of all the factors discussed previously, the single most important risk factor for the development of postpartum depression is a recent stressful life event.

SOLUTION TO THE SHORT ANSWER MANAGEMENT PROBLEM

Specific suggestions to alter the course of postpartum mood disturbances in your patients should include:

a. Encouraging the attendance of the husband or significant other at prenatal visits
b. Questioning the couple about prenatal education received concerning mood changes in pregnancy, during labor, and after pregnancy
c. Providing patient education materials on specific mood disturbances
d. Emphasizing the importance of the husband or significant other in all aspects of the pregnancy, labor and delivery, puerperium, and care of the new family member
e. Discussing with both members of the couple the social and emotional joys and challenges of childbirth
f. Describing all tests, all examination procedures, the reason(s) for all routine questions, and any deviation from normal protocol that may occur during pregnancy
g. Discussing all of the uncomfortable physiologically based problems of pregnancy (edema, heartburn, ligament relaxation, hemorrhoids, and so on) that might be expected
h. Providing clear instructions to the couple regarding when to call you and when to go to the hospital and reassuring the couple that you "would rather receive a call than not receive a call"
i. Making at least one visit to the patient during early labor
j. Explaining every possible intervention during labor and the reason(s) for same (such as artificial rupture of the membranes, internal fetal monitoring, and augmentation of labor)
k. Encouraging the patient at every opportunity during labor and delivery
l. Assessing the patient immediately postpartum and monitoring her condition carefully. Pay particular attention to a patient history of bipolar disorder or major depressive disorder, a family history of depression or any other significant psychiatric disease, and a patient who is going through or recently has gone through a major life stressor.

SUMMARY OF POSTPARTUM DEPRESSION DIAGNOSIS AND TREATMENT

1. Postpartum blues:
   a. Incidence: 50% to 80%
   b. Evolution: begins on or about the third day postpartum and resolves by 2 weeks

c. Treatment: reassurance, supportive psychotherapy; involvement of spouse or significant other is critical

2. Postpartum depression:
   a. Incidence: 10%
   b. Evolution: begins on the third to fifth day postpartum and lasts longer than 2 weeks
   c. Treatment: psychotherapy and pharmacologic antidepressant therapy

3. Postpartum psychosis:
   a. Incidence: 0.1% to 0.2%
   b. Treatment:
      1) Acute: antipsychotic medication, close observation to prevent self-harm and harm to the infant
      2) Long-term:
         a) Mood stabilizer if underlying bipolar disorder, manic phase is present; mood stabilizer and antidepressant if bipolar disorder, depressive phase is present.
         b) Antidepressant if underlying major depressive disorder is present
         c) Psychotherapy: supportive group or individual. Involvement of spouse or significant other is critical.

4. Prevention of postpartum psychopathology:
   a. Education in the prenatal period: this education must include significant attention to the psychological consequences of pregnancy, labor and delivery, and the impact of the neonate on the family.
   b. Explanation of all procedures and interventions to allow the patient as much control as possible during labor.
   c. Significant involvement of the husband or significant other in the process is critical.

SUGGESTED READINGS

American Psychiatric Association: *Diagnostic and statistical manual of mental disorders,* ed 4, Washington, DC, 1994, American Psychiatric Association Press.

Holden J: Postnatal depression: Its nature, effects, and identification using the Edinburgh Postnatal Depression Scale, *Birth* 18(4):211-221, 1991.

Kaplan HI, Sadock BJ, eds: *Kaplan and Sadock's synopsis of psychiatry: Behavioral sciences/clinical psychiatry,* ed 8, Baltimore, 1998, Williams & Wilkins.

Robinson G, Stewart D: Postpartum psychiatric disorders, *Can Med Assoc J* 134(1):31-36, 1986.

Shaner R: *Psychiatry,* Baltimore, 1997, Williams & Wilkins.

C·H·A·P·T·E·R 3

Women's Health

PROBLEM·50

OSTEOPOROSIS

"Am I Shrinking?"

Case 1 ■ A 61-Year-Old Female with Severe Back Pain

A 61-year-old female comes to your office for assessment of severe back pain, which she has had for the past 2 years and has been getting progressively worse. The pain is described in the following manner: (1) *location:* midthoracic area (on the spine itself); (2) *quality:* basically a dull pain with sharp, shooting exacerbations; (3) *severity:* baseline severity 7/10; incremental increase to 9/10; incremental decrease to 6/10; (4) *chronology:* Pain began 2 years ago when she slipped, fell, and injured her back on a newly waxed floor in her home. Since that time, the pain has been getting progressively worse; (5) *constant/intermittent:* dull pain relatively constant, sharp pain comes and goes; (6) *aggravating factors:* movement of any kind; lateral rotation of the spine; (7) *alleviating factors:* rest and acetaminophen; (8) *pain history:* no previous significant chronic pain syndromes until this pain began 2 years ago; (9) treatments employed: (a) nonpharmacologic (physical therapy has helped) and (b) pharmacologic (acetaminophen 500 mg tid); (10) *physical examination:* pain elicited on pressing on T7 and T8; (11) *quality of life:* Before the pain began (10/10), the patient was active in her garden and participated in social activities. At this time, however, she is severely limited (3/10).

On examination, the patient has obvious kyphosis. As mentioned, she is tender at both T7 and T8 on the midpoint of the vertebrae. The patient has a body mass index of 19. No other abnormalities are found on physical examination.

SELECT THE BEST ANSWER
TO THE FOLLOWING QUESTIONS

Q1. The patient's pain as described is most likely due to which of the following:

a. degenerative arthritis
b. vertebral compression fractures secondary to osteoporosis
c. osteoarthritis
d. an intervertebral disc that has been dislocated
e. spinal stenosis

Q2. What is the most likely pathologic condition of the patient described?
a. primary osteoporosis
b. secondary osteoporosis
c. osteoarthritis type 1
d. osteoarthritis type 2
e. nerve root impingement secondary to spinal stenosis

Q3. How is osteoporosis defined?
a. an increased turnover of calcium in newly formed bone
b. a failure to deposit inorganic mineral in newly formed organic bone matrix
c. a lack of calcium in newly formed bone
d. bone mineral density of 2.5 standard deviations below the mean for normal healthy adults aged 30 to 40 years
e. a decrease in both bone mass and matrix in trabecular and cortical bone

Q4. How is osteomalacia defined?
a. an increased calcium turnover
b. a failure to deposit inorganic mineral in newly formed organic bone matrix
c. a lack of calcium in newly formed bone
d. a decrease in bone mass in the absence of a mineralization defect
e. a decrease in both bone mass and matrix in trabecular and cortical bone

Q5. Which of the following is not an established risk factor for osteoporosis?
a. postmenopausal status
b. sedentary lifestyle
c. cigarette smoking

d. obesity

e. alcohol intake

Q6. What is the most common presenting condition of osteoporosis?
   a. wrist fracture (Colles' fracture)
   b. vertebral compression fracture
   c. fracture of the neck of the femur
   d. fracture of the head of the femur
   e. fracture of the proximal tibia

Q7. What is the most common site for type 1 osteoporotic fractures?
   a. the distal radius
   b. the thoracic vertebra
   c. the lumbar vertebra
   d. the head of the femur
   e. the neck of the femur

Q8. What is the most common site for type 2 osteoporotic fractures?
   a. the neck of the femur
   b. the head of the femur
   c. the thoracic vertebrae
   d. the lumbar vertebrae
   e. the pelvis

Q9. Which of the following sites of osteoporosis is most commonly associated with morbidity and mortality?
   a. the head of the femur
   b. the neck of the femur
   c. the thoracic vertebrae
   d. the lumbar vertebrae
   e. the distal radius

Q10. What is the treatment of first choice for the prevention of primary osteoporosis?
   a. conjugated estrogen 0.625 mg/day and medroxyprogesterone acetate 10 mg/day on days 1 to 13 of the calendar month
   b. conjugated estrogen 1.25 mg/day and medroxyprogesterone acetate 10 mg/day on days 1 to 13 of the calendar month
   c. calcium carbonate 1000 to 1500 mg/day
   d. conjugated estrogen 1.25 mg/day
   e. etidronate (Didronel) 16 mg/day

Q11. Which of the following statements regarding the use of calcium carbonate in the treatment of osteoporosis is true?
   a. calcium carbonate (1000 to 1500 mg/day) should begin at menopause
   b. calcium carbonate (1000 to 1500 mg/day) should begin within 2 years of the onset of menopause
   c. calcium carbonate (1000 to 1500 mg/day) should begin between 35 and 40 years of age
   d. calcium carbonate has not been shown to be beneficial in the prevention or treatment of osteoporosis
   e. calcium carbonate is contraindicated in the management of osteoporosis

Q12. Which of the following is (are) recommended for treatment of established osteoporosis?
   a. calcitonin
   b. calcium carbonate
   c. estrogen
   d. diphosphonate etidronate
   e. all of the above

Q13. In the diagnosis of osteoporosis, abnormal laboratory values include:
   a. hypocalcemia
   b. decreased 25-hydroxy vitamin D
   c. hypophosphatemia
   d. all of the above
   e. none of the above

Q14. The test of choice in the diagnosis of osteoporosis is:
   a. single-photon absorptiometry
   b. double-photon absorptiometry
   c. dual-energy x-ray absorptiometry (DEXA)
   d. quantitative computed tomography (CT) scan
   e. plain x-ray of the thoracic spine

Q15. The World Health Organization's (WHO) definition for osteopenia includes:
   a. a bone mineral density between 0 and 1.0 standard deviation below the mean for normal healthy adults aged 30 to 40 years
   b. a bone mineral density between 1.0 and 2.5 standard deviations below the mean for normal healthy adults aged 30 to 40 years
   c. a bone mineral density greater than 2.5 standard deviations below the mean for normal healthy adults aged 30 to 40 years
   d. a bone mineral density between 1.0 and 2.5 standard deviations above the mean for normal healthy adults aged 30 to 40 years
   e. none of the above

Q16. Conditions that warrant prescription of bone mass measurements include:
   a. perimenopausal or estrogen-deficient females who are considering long-term therapy

b. patients with osteopenia or vertebral fractures revealed on x-ray
c. monitoring efficacy of long-term treatment of osteoporosis
d. patients on long-term glucocorticoid therapy
e. a, b, and c
f. all of the above

Q17. The treatment of osteoporosis includes all of the following except:
a. calcium supplementation
b. vitamin D supplementation
c. vitamin E supplementation
d. exercise
e. estrogen replacement therapy for postmenopausal females

Q18. Which of the following patients should not be given a routine DEXA test:
a. a 65-year-old postmenopausal woman who has been on estrogen replacement therapy
b. a 75-year-old male
c. a 65-year-old male who, for some 10 years, has been taking Lasix for hypertension and an aluminum-based antacid for digestive upset
d. a 60-year-old African-American woman who has not been on estrogen replacement therapy
e. all of the above should be screened for potential osteoporosis

SHORT ANSWER MANAGEMENT PROBLEM
Discuss the relationship between the treatment of osteoporosis and the prevention of cardiovascular disease in postmenopausal women.

ANSWERS

A1. **b.** This patient has one or more vertebral compression fractures at midthoracic sites. This is a common cause of back pain in this age group, especially among women, and especially among women who also have kyphosis, another manifestation of osteoporosis. The pain associated with vertebral compression fractures can be severe and should be treated accordingly.

The 11-point pain history described was purposefully put into the question. This can serve as a valuable tool in the evaluation of patients with any pain syndrome.

A2. **a.** Osteoporosis can be divided into two subtypes:
a. Primary osteoporosis: An age-related loss of bone in both women and men but most commonly in estrogen-deficient postmenopausal women
b. Secondary osteoporosis: Osteoporosis that develops secondary to an underlying condition such as osteomalacia, multiple myeloma, diabetes, hyperthyroidism, nutritional deficiencies, and immobility, and to medications such as glucocorticoids, excessive thyroid supplementation, heparin, phenytoin, phenobarbital, and methotrexate when combined with steroids

A3. **d.** WHO defines osteoporosis as a bone mineral density that is 2.5 standard deviations below the mean for healthy adults aged 30 to 40 years.

A4. **b.** Osteomalacia is defined as a failure to deposit inorganic mineral in newly formed organic bone matrix, leading to a decreased bone density from diminished mineralization.

A5. **d.** The established risk factors for osteoporosis include the following:
a. female sex
b. postmenopausal status and early menopause
c. low body weight
d. sedentary lifestyle and lack of exercise
e. cigarette smoking or excessive alcohol intake
f. Caucasian or Asian race
g. low calcium intake throughout life
h. family history of osteoporosis in first-degree relatives
i. Drugs such as loop diuretics, phenytoin, and carbamazepine and other antiseizure drugs such as heparin, warfarin, excess thyroid hormone, lithium, isoniazid, glucocorticoids, cyclosporine A, methotrexate, and antiacids containing aluminum

Obesity, one of the choices listed, appears to be protective against osteoporosis.

A6. **b.** Vertebral compression fracture is the most common presenting condition of osteoporosis. Wrist fracture (Colles' fracture) is the second most common presenting condition.

A7. **b.** Type 1 osteoporosis (not to be confused with primary osteoporosis) occurs primarily in postmenopausal females and results in a decrease in trabecular bone. The most common site for type 1 osteoporosis fracture is the thoracic vertebra (usually around T7 to T9).

A8. **a.** Type 2 osteoporosis occurs in both sexes, generally becoming evident by the seventh decade of life and resulting in a decrease in both trabecular and cortical bone mass. The most common fracture site resulting from type 2 osteoporosis is the neck of the femur.

A9. **b.** In addition to being the most common site for type 2 osteoporosis, fracture of the neck of the femur is also the most common cause of osteoporosis-related morbidity and mortality.

A10. **a.** The recommended treatment for the prevention of osteoporosis in women is conjugated estrogens 0.625 mg/day continually and medroxyprogesterone acetate 10 mg from days 1 to 13 of the calendar month. Other modalities include calcium supplementation, vitamin D supplementation, and weight-bearing exercise. (See Answer 12 for a description of potential therapeutic modalities.)

A11. **c.** It is recommended to initiate supplementation with calcium carbonate to age 35 to 40 years to reduce the risk of osteoporosis in later life. Recent research suggests that calcium supplementation should even be started earlier to more effectively increase bone mass before menopause.

Despite claims made for various calcium products on the market, there is no convincing evidence that more expensive supplements are absorbed appreciably better in patients with normal gastric function. Once in the acidic environment of the stomach, the calcium salt will ionize and no longer be associated with whatever anion it was ingested with.

A12. **e.** The following summarizes treatments available for the management of established osteoporosis:

   a. Estrogen 0.625 mg/day throughout the month; Progesterone 10 mg on days 1 to 13 of the calendar month. Estrogen therapy is the primary tool available for prevention and management of postmenopausal osteoporosis.
   b. Raloxifene (Evista) is a relatively newly developed analogue of estrogen that acts on bone and, like estrogen, decreases serum lipid levels. However, it appears to be an estrogen antagonist in uterine and breast tissue. Although studies have shown raloxifene to decrease the rate of bone loss relative to placebos, trials relating to its effect on fractures have not yet been completed.
   c. Calcium carbonate 1500 mg/day (NOTE: begin calcium carbonate as preventative therapy). For maximum efficiency, 1500 mg should be ingested in increments throughout the day. For patients who normally do not ingest significant amounts of calcium with their meals, a convenient suggestion is for them to take a third of their daily dose with each meal.
   d. Vitamin D 400 IU/day. Increase to 600 to 800 IU/day in the elderly. Since vitamin D is required for efficient absorption of calcium, adequate intake must be assured throughout life.
   e. Alendronate (Fosamax), 10 mg, is approved by the Food and Drug Administration for the treatment and prevention of osteoporosis. It should be taken in the morning with 8 ounces of water on an empty stomach, and the patient should be sitting or standing for at least 30 minutes, preferably for an hour, to prevent esophagitis. Because the bisphosphonates tend to form insoluble complexes with a host of substances no food or drink other than water should be ingested during this time.

   Etidronate, another bisphosphonate, is less effective but less expensive and often better tolerated than alendronate. It is given cyclically in a dose of 400 mg/day for 4 weeks every 3 months.

   Risedronate (Actonel) recently has been evaluated by the Vertebral Efficacy with Risedronate Therapy (VERT) study group and found to be effective and well tolerated in the treatment of women with oseoporosis. The primary advantage may prove to be even greater tolerance because it can be administered orally in lower dosages than the other antiresorptive bisphosphonates.

   Pamidronate is a parenteral bisphosphonate that can be used as an intravenous infusion in osteoporotic patients who cannot tolerate oral bisphosphonates.
   f. Weight-bearing exercise. Any activity that loads bone will help keep them strong and should be recommended throughout life for men and women as a preventative modality. Obviously, activities will have to be limited as a therapeutic option in fragile individuals, but, as a general rule, walking at least 6 mi/wk is ideal. Although only mildly weight bearing, Chinese tai chi can also improve balance and prevent injury from falls. Swimming is not a weight-bearing exercise, but aqueous weight-bearing exercises can be designed to meet special needs.
   g. Calcitonin (Calcimar, Miacalcin), 50 to 100 IU/day subcutaneously or, more recently, by nasal spray (200 IU/day). It is primarily recommended for individuals who will not take estrogen (usually women who fear an increased risk of breast cancer) but might also include men.

Sodium fluoride has not been found to be effective in the treatment of established osteoporosis.

It should be noted that not all of these medications need to be taken at the same time because they may have antiresorptive properties and act similarly. Also, if yearly DEXA measurements show continued bone loss in a patient with osteopenia, it generally would be wise to start therapeutic treatment before frank osteoporosis develops.

A13. **e.** Serum calcium, phosphate, and parathyroid hormone levels are normal in patients with primary osteoporosis. The values listed are all consistent with osteomalacia. Although alkaline phosphatase activity is usually normal in osteoporosis, it may be slightly elevated if there has been a fracture.

A14. **c.** The diagnostic test of choice is the DEXA scan. It can measure bone mineral density at both the spine and hip and only has a small amount of radiation exposure.

A15. **b.** WHO defines osteopenia as a bone mineral density 1.0 to 2.5 standard deviations below the mean for normal healthy adults aged 30 to 40 years. Osteoporosis is more then 2.5 standard deviations below the mean.

A16. **e.**

A17. **c.** Common treatment modalities for the treatment of osteoporosis include the following:
  a. calcium supplementation of 1000 to 1500 mg/day (1500 mg/day for the elderly).
  b. Vitamin D 400 IU/day (600 to 800 IU/day for the elderly)
  c. Weight-bearing exercise: Helps maintain bone density and includes walking, jogging, and weight training
  d. Estrogen replacement therapy
  e. Bisphosphonates
  f. Calcitonin

It should be noted the Selective Estrogen Receptor Modulators such as raloxifene can also be used in postmenopausal females in place of estrogen for the prevention of osteoporosis. It is sometimes used because it does not cause hyperplasia of the endometrium or breasts. It has no effect on coronary plaque of hot flushes and can increase the risk of thromboembolism.

A18. **e.** Although petite Caucasian and Asian postmenopausal women who have not been on estrogen therapy have the greatest risk for developing osteoporosis, it also is true that women on estrogen replacement therapy, African-American women and males are not immune. In fact about 20% of the 28 million Americans with osteoporosis are males and some 3 million more are at risk. That National Osteoporosis foundation reports that a man older than 50 is more likely to suffer an osteoporosis-induced fracture than he is to develop prostate cancer. Aluminum-based ant-

acids and loop diuretics such as Lasix are just two of the many medications that increase the risk of osteoporosis in males as well as females. (For a more comprehensive list of drugs that increase the risk of osteoporosis see Answer 5.)

SOLUTION TO THE SHORT ANSWER MANAGEMENT PROBLEM

The relationship between the treatment of osteoporosis in postmenopausal women and the prevention of cardiovascular disease is estrogen. Estrogen (usually given in the form of Premarin 0.625 mg/day or alternatively as an Estraderm patch 50 mg twice a week) has been found to be protective against the development of all forms of atherosclerotic vascular disease in postmenopausal women. Estrogen decreases the risk of cardiovascular disease significantly in the postmenopausal period (some studies indicating a 33% risk reduction). Having stated this, however, there still is not enough evidence to recommend that all woman in the postmenopausal period be treated with estrogen replacement; rather, it should be on the basis of a risk factor analysis.

SUMMARY OF THE DIAGNOSIS AND TREATMENT OF OSTEOPOROSIS

1. Definition: Decrease in bone mass in absence of mineralization defect. Differentiate osteoporosis from osteomalacia, the latter being a group of diseases characterized by failure to deposit the inorganic mineral into newly formed bone.

2. Classification and pathologic condition:
  a. Type 1: Common in postmenopausal women, primarily affecting trabecular bone in vertebrae as well as the distal forearm.
  b. Type 2: Common in individuals of both sexes, particularly after the seventh decade, and involves the loss of cortical and trabecular bone affecting the femoral neck, proximal humerus, proximal tibia, and pelvis as well as the vertebrae and distal forearm.

3. Treatment: Estrogen or progesterone, calcitonin, calcium carbonate, bisphosphonate (alendronate and others in Answer 12), vitamin D, and weight-bearing exercise.

SUGGESTED READINGS
Barzel U: Osteoporosis. In Rakel R, ed: *Conn's current therapy*, Philadelphia, 1994, WB Saunders.
Eastell R: Treatment of postmenopausal osteoporosis, *N Engl J Med* 338(11):736-746, 1998.

Tierney LM, McPhee SJ, Papadakis MA, eds: *Current medical diagnosis and treatment, 2000,* Stamford, Conn, 1999, Appleton & Lange.

Harris ST et al: Effects of risedronate treatment on vertebral and nonvertebral fractures in women with postmenopausal osteoporosis: A randomized controlled trial. Vertebral Efficacy with Risedronate Therapy (VERT) study group, *JAMA* 282(14):1344-1352, 1999.

Orwoll ES: Osteoporosis in men, *N Dimen Osteoporosis* 1(5):2-8, 1999.

PROBLEM · 5 1

VULVOVAGINITIS

"I'm On Fire Below!"

Case 1 ■ A 21-Year-Old Female with a Curdy-White Vaginal Discharge

A 21-year-old woman comes to your office complaining of perineal itching and vaginal discharge. On inspection of the external genitalia you note vulvar erythema and curdy, white discharge. On speculum examination you note the discharge is thick and adherent to the vaginal walls. The vaginal pH is 4.0, and there is no amine odor.

SELECT THE BEST ANSWER TO THE FOLLOWING QUESTIONS

Q1. What is the most likely diagnosis in this patient?
   a. physiologic discharge
   b. bacterial vaginosis (BV)
   c. candidiasis
   d. trichomoniasis
   e. none of the above

Q2. What is the treatment of choice in this patient?
   a. metronidazole vaginal cream
   b. oral (PO) ampicillin
   c. miconazole vaginal cream
   d. PO nystatin tablets
   e. none of the above

Q3. The patient does not respond to the treatment you prescribed. At this time, what should you do?
   a. repeat the treatment offered first
   b. repeat the treatment offered first and double the dose
   c. prescribe PO fluconazole in a single dose
   d. reculture the patient
   e. reconsider the diagnosis

Q4. Which of the following is (are) established risk factors for recurrent candidal vulvovaginitis?

   a. diabetes mellitus
   b. long-term antibiotic therapy
   c. human immunodeficiency virus (HIV) infection
   d. all of the above
   e. none of the above

Case 2 ■ A 25-Year-Old Female with a Gray-Green Malodorous Vaginal Discharge

A 25-year-old female comes to your office complaining of itching and a profuse malodorous vaginal discharge. On inspection of the external genitalia you find vulvar edema and erythema. Speculum examination reveals profuse, gray-green, malodorous discharge that is adherent to the vaginal walls. The pH is 6.0. Microscopic examination of the discharge in a saline preparation shows 15 white blood cells per high-power field (WBC/s/HPF) and many motile flagellated organisms.

Q5. What is the most likely diagnosis in this patient?
   a. candidiasis
   b. trichomoniasis
   c. BV
   d. physiologic discharge
   e. nonspecific vaginitis

Q6. What is the treatment of choice for the patient described in Case 2?
   a. intravaginal miconazole
   b. intravaginal clotrimazole
   c. PO metronidazole 250 mg tid
   d. PO ampicillin 500 mg tid
   e. PO 2-g stat dose of metronidazole

Case 3 ■ A 29-Year-Old Female with a Gray Malodorous Vaginal Discharge

A 29-year-old female comes to your office with a 2-week history of profuse, malodorous discharge. On examination, the discharge is present at the introitus. It is gray. It is homogeneous and has a low viscosity. It is adherent to the vaginal walls. The pH is 6.5. An amine odor is present. On microscopic examination, "clue cells" are present but WBCs are absent.

Q7. What is the most likely diagnosis in this patient?
   a. BV
   b. trichomoniasis
   c. candidiasis
   d. HIV
   e. none of the above

Q8. What is the treatment of choice for the condition described in case 3?
    a. intravaginal miconazole (one tablet) for 7 days
    b. intravaginal clotrimazole (one tablet) for 7 days
    c. PO 2-g stat dose of metronidazole
    d. PO metronidazole 250 mg tid for 7 days
    e. PO erythromycin 500 mg tid

Q9. What is the most common class of organism associated with the condition most likely responsible for the symptoms described in Case 3?
    a. gram-positive aerobic cocci
    b. gram-negative aerobic rods
    c. gram-negative aerobic cocci
    d. anaerobic bacteria
    e. gram-positive rods
    f. a fungus or yeast
    g. a protozoa

Q10. The "whiff test" or "amine odor" test is of use in diagnosing which of the following vaginal infections?
    a. trichomoniasis
    b. BV
    c. candidiasis
    d. physiologic discharge
    e. all of the above

Q11. What is the most common form of vaginitis?
    a. vulvovaginal candidiasis
    b. trichomoniasis
    c. BV
    d. chlamydial vaginitis
    e. none of the above

SHORT ANSWER MANAGEMENT PROBLEM

Describe the differentiation of a vaginal discharge based on pH, WBCs, amine odor test, consistency, color, and presence of clue cells.

ANSWERS

A1. **c.** This patient has candidiasis. *Candida albicans* is a commensal organism in most women. When *Lactobacilli* and specific fungal inhibitory factors are suppressed, an infection can result.

Pruritus is the most common symptom in vaginal candidiasis. Discharge may be normal or increased and is usually described as white and curdy, like cottage cheese. Irritation and soreness may be present. Vulvar burning may be noted, which can be exacerbated with micturition or sexual intercourse. Erythema of the vulva is common.

Predisposing factors for vaginal candidiasis include the premenstrual phase of the menstrual cycle, antibiotic use, and coitus. There is no direct relationship between vaginal candidiasis and oral contraceptive pills.

Physical examination often reveals vulvar erythema and edema. The discharge is often adherent to the vaginal walls. The vaginal pH is usually normal (<4.5). Amine odor is absent, and WBCs are not prominent. Mycelia or spores may be seen on microscopic examination of potassium hydroxide (KOH) preparations of vaginal discharge.

A2. **c.** The treatment of choice in this patient is an imidazole cream or suppository. Many regimens using imidazoles or clotrimazole have shown high cure rates. The treatment regimens vary from 1 to 7 days. Because of the presence of both internal and external symptoms, the use of a preparation containing both vaginal miconazole ovules (one per night for three nights) and external miconazole cream (to be applied to the vulvar area once or twice a day) can be recommended. Loose-fitting clothing and cotton underwear will decrease colonization rates.

In recurrent candidiasis, 1% gentian violet or oral nystatin or ketoconazole can be used.

Treatment of the male partner is usually unnecessary unless he has symptoms of yeast balanus or he is uncircumcised. Under these conditions, a reservoir of yeast in the man may serve as a source of reinfection of the woman.

A3. **c.** A single 150-mg dose of PO fluconazole is at least as effective as intravaginal treatment for vulvovaginal candidiasis. Compliance is high with single-dose therapy. This is the only oral agent approved by the U.S. Food and Drug Administration for this use. Ketoconazole 200-mg PO tablet bid for 5 days has been effective in treating resistant and recurrent candidal infections. The effectiveness of these oral agents is believed to be due to the elimination of the rectal reservoir of yeast. Both these agents can cause significant liver toxicity, so they should be used with caution in patients with altered liver function tests. However, fluconazole appears to present a much lower risk of liver toxicity.

A4. **d.** Risk factors for vaginal candidiasis include:
    a. Physical disruption of the integument
    b. Pregnancy
    c. Antibiotic therapy
    d. Diabetes mellitus
    e. Immunologic deficiencies (including HIV infection)
    f. Tight-fitting clothing
    g. Sexual behavior (including oral-genital and anal sex)

The oral contraceptive pill does not seem to increase the incidence of symptomatic candidiasis, although it may increase the frequency of the carrier state.

A5. **b.** This patient has trichomoniasis. The symptoms of trichomoniasis include a malodorous, copious, grayish-green vaginal discharge that adheres to the vaginal walls. Vulvar erythema, pruritus, and edema may be present. Erythema of the vaginal mucosa is common. The pH is usually greater than 5.0. Motile trichomonads and numerous WBCs are often seen on microscopic examination of saline preparations of vaginal discharge.

A6. **e.** The treatment of choice for trichomoniasis is metronidazole. The recommended treatment protocol is a single 2-g PO dose. Patients who fail to respond to a single PO dose of 2 g should be given extended therapy consisting of a dose of 500 mg of metronidazole for 7 days.

Because trichomoniasis is a sexually transmitted disease, simultaneous treatment of the male partner(s) is essential. Reinfection is a major cause of recurrence.

A7. **a.** This patient has BV. BV is the most common cause of vaginal discharge. BV has been known as nonspecific vaginitis, *Gardnerella* vaginitis, *Haemophilus* vaginitis, *Corynebacterium* vaginitis, mixed bacterial vaginitis, and anaerobic vaginitis. BV is caused by an alteration of the normal vaginal flora.

The dominant species, *Lactobacillus acidophilus,* normally suppresses the growth of the gram-negative and gram-positive facultative and obligate anaerobes and maintains normal pH through the production of lactic acid. Lactobacilli also produce hydrogen peroxide, which is toxic to the anaerobes. When the dominance of *Lactobacilli* is upset and other bacterial species overgrow, the result is BV, which frequently is asymptomatic. Symptomatic patients usually see their physicians, complaining of a fishy odor along with vaginal discharge. The discharge is present at the introitus, is gray in color, and is homogenous. It has a low viscosity and is adherent to the vaginal walls. The pH is >5.0, and an amine odor is present on exposure to KOH. Clue cells (vaginal epithelial cells with an obscured border resulting from adherence of anaerobic bacteria to the cell border) are often seen. WBCs are absent.

A8. **d.** The treatment of choice for BV is PO metronidazole 250 mg tid or 500 mg bid for 7 days. Recently, a single 2-g dose has been demonstrated to be adequate. Treating the patient's sexual partner does not alter the recurrence rate. Alternatively, 0.75% met-

ronidazole vaginal cream for 7 days can be used. The patient should be counseled that all alcohol products should be avoided with any metronidazole regimen because profuse nausea and vomiting (disulfiram reaction) may occur. A second antianaerobic agent that can be used is clindamycin. This can be taken either orally (300 mg for 7 days) or intravaginally (2% clindamycin cream for 7 days).

A9. **d.** The anaerobic bacteria are most commonly associated with BV. The anaerobic bacteria such as peptostreptococci interact with other bacteria including *Corynebacterium, Haemophilus,* and other species to produce the characteristic findings.

A10. **b.** The whiff test, or amine odor test, is of use in the diagnosis of a BV. It reflects the production of amines by the anaerobic bacteria themselves.

A11. **c.** The most common cause of abnormal vaginal discharge is BV. BV accounts for 35% to 50% of all cases of vaginal discharge. Candidiasis accounts for 20% to 40%, and trichomoniasis for 10% to 20%.

SOLUTION TO THE SHORT ANSWER MANAGEMENT PROBLEM

Vaginal discharge may be differentiated on the basis of several characteristics. These include pH, the presence or absence of WBCs, the amine odor test, the presence or absence of clue cells, consistency, and color. The differentiation is as follows:

 a. Normal (physiologic) vaginal discharge:
   1) Clear or white discharge
   2) Nonhomogenous
   3) Scant to moderate
   4) pH <4.5
   5) Amine odor negative
   6) Clue cells absent
   7) Trichomonads absent
   8) Mycelia absent
   9) The presence of normal epithelial cells and lactobacilli
 b. BV:
   1) Malodorous discharge
   2) White or gray; homogeneous
   3) Moderate in amount
   4) pH >4.5
   5) Amine test positive
   6) Clue cells present
   7) Trichomonads absent
   8) Mycelia absent
   9) Predominance of coccobacilli
   10) Few to no leukocytes

c. Vulvovaginal candidiasis:
   1) Pruritus
   2) Thick, white discharge
   3) Homogeneous
   4) Thick clumps of curdy material
   5) Vulvar, introital, and vaginal edema and erythema
   6) pH <4.5
   7) Amine test absent
   8) Clue cells absent
   9) Trichomonads absent
   10) Mycelia present
   11) Normal flora on microscopy
d. Trichomoniasis:
   1) Pruritus
   2) Fishy odor
   3) Gray or yellow-green
   4) Thin
   5) Homogeneous ± vulvar and vaginal erythema
   6) pH >4.5
   7) Amine test absent
   8) Clue cells absent
   9) Trichomonads present
   10) Mycelia absent
   11) Many polymorphonuclear leukocytes, large amounts of cellular debris

SUMMARY OF THE DIAGNOSIS AND TREATMENT OF VULVOVAGINITIS

1. Diagnosis: See the differentiation given in the Solution to the Short Answer Management Problem in this problem.

2. Treatment:
   a. Normal vaginal discharge: no treatment necessary
   b. BV: PO metronidazole 250 mg tid or 500 mg tid for 7 days; PO clindamycin 300 mg bid for 7 days; 0.75% metronidazole vaginal cream for 7 days; 2% clindamycin vaginal cream for 7 days.
   c. Trichomoniasis: single stat PO dose of metronidazole (2 g for both the patient and the sexual partner)
   d. Candidiasis: imidazole cream or suppository; clotrimazole cream or suppository; single 150-mg PO dose of fluconazole

SUGGESTED READINGS

American College of Obstetricians and Gynecologists: Vaginitis, *Tech Bull* No. 226, 1996.
Brooks L: Vulvovaginitis. In: Rakel R, ed: *Conn's current therapy,* Philadelphia, 1997, WB Saunders.
Oral fluconazole for vaginal candidiasis, *Med Lett* 36(631):1-2, 1994.

PROBLEM · 52

EVALUATION AND MANAGEMENT OF CERVICAL ABNORMALITIES

"Papa Smear: Who Is That?"

Case 1 ■ A 26-Year-Old Female with an Abnormal Pap Smear

A 26-year-old woman comes to your office for her periodic health assessment. She is married, has two children, and has had no major medical illnesses. She has been a regular patient of yours for many years. She is a cigarette smoker with a 10-pack/yr history. She has used combination oral contraceptive pills as a means of contraception for 9 months. She has a lifetime history of 10 sexual partners, but does not recall ever having contracted a sexually transmitted disease (STD).

Her blood pressure is 100/70 mm Hg, and her pulse is 72 and regular. Her pelvic examination is unremarkable including external genitalia, vagina, cervix, uterus and adnexa. Her Papanicolaou (Pap) smear comes back 3 days later and is reported as grade 1 cervical intraepithelial neoplasia (CIN-1), or low-grade squamous intraepithelial lesion (LGSIL).

SELECT THE BEST ANSWER TO THE FOLLOWING QUESTIONS

Q1. At this time, assuming that this patient is reliable in follow-up, what should you do?
   a. repeat the Pap smear in 1 year
   b. repeat the Pap smear in 4 to 6 months
   c. repeat the Pap smear in 1 to 3 months
   d. refer the patient for colposcopy
   e. refer the patient for a bone biopsy

Case 2 ■ A 28-Year-Old Female with a *Trichomonas vaginalis* Infection

A 28-year-old female comes to your office for a routine periodic health assessment. A Pap smear is performed and the result comes back CIN-1/LGSIL with *Trichomonas vaginalis* present.

Q2. What would you do at this time?
   a. treat the infection and repeat the Pap smear at the next recommended screening interval
   b. treat the infection and repeat the Pap smear in 6 weeks
   c. treat the infection in the patient and in her partner and repeat the Pap smear at the next recommended screening interval

d. treat the infection in the patient and in her partner and repeat the Pap smear in 6 weeks
e. refer the patient for colposcopy

Q3. Which of the following statements regarding carcinoma of the cervix or analysis of the Pap smear is false?
a. carcinoma of the cervix can be regarded as an STD
b. case-finding for carcinoma of the cervix can stop at age 65, providing the patient has been adequately screened before and has had no new sexual partners after that time
c. an Ayres spatula is a sufficient tool for obtaining a specimen of the endocervix for Pap smear analysis
d. carcinoma of the cervix is a disease with a long lead time
e. none of the above statements is false

Q4. Carcinoma of the cervix is usually associated with which of the following viruses?
a. Herpes simplex virus (HSV) type 1
b. HSV type 2
c. human papillomavirus (HPV)
d. human parvovirus
e. adenovirus

Q5. Which of the following is not a documented direct risk factor for carcinoma of the cervix?
a. a partner who has had multiple sexual partners
b. an early age of first intercourse
c. intercourse with more than three partners
d. a clinical history of condyloma acuminata
e. a HSV type 2 infection

Q6. You are beginning the transformation of your practice into an evidence-based practice in which the recommendations of the U.S. Preventive Services Task Force on the Periodic Health Examination are followed. One of the most important recommendations made by that task force is regular screening of all women for cervical cancer.

If this were to occur and every female patient in your practice under the age of 65 years was screened with the Pap smear at the intervals recommended for cervical cancer, what percentage of cervical cancers could be prevented (actual effectiveness, not theoretical effectiveness)?
a. 100%
b. 92%
c. 80%
d. 64%
e. 51%

Q7. The current recommendation for screening by Pap smear for carcinoma of the cervix includes which of the following classification structures or provisions?
a. all women who are or who have been sexually active should have regular Pap smears
b. all women who have reached the age of 18 years should have regular Pap smears
c. after three normal Pap smears, the interval time between Pap smears can be lengthened in low-risk patients
d. Pap smear screening intervals are recommended on the basis of classification of women into three risk categories that include most women
e. all of the above are included in the current recommendation

Q8. Which of the following is the greatest concern when considering Pap smear interval screening?
a. the false positive rate of the Pap smear
b. the false negative rate of the Pap smear
c. the positive predictive value of the Pap smear
d. the method of performing the Pap smear
e. the decreased ability to interpret Pap smear slides because of air drying

Q9. A Pap smear report on a patient of yours who you examined 1 week ago comes back from the laboratory. The report reads, "unsatisfactory for evaluation." At this time, what should you do?
a. phone the cytopathologist and tell him to get with it; you haven't time for his mistakes
b. repeat the Pap smear immediately
c. repeat the Pap smear; but no sooner than 6 weeks from the previous smear
d. repeat the Pap smear in 4 to 6 months if the patient is low risk
e. repeat the Pap smear only if it seems reasonable

Q10. What is the most cost-effective and least invasive mode of treating SILs of the cervix?
a. laser therapy
b. 5-fluorouracil
c. cryotherapy
d. electric cauterization
e. any of the above

Q11. Cervical neoplasia is related to which of the following anatomic sites?
a. the squamous epithelium
b. the columnar epithelium
c. the squamocolumnar junction

d. the exterior of the cervical os

e. the interior of the cervical os

SHORT ANSWER MANAGEMENT PROBLEM
Discuss the new Bethesda classification system for Pap smear reporting. Compare it to the cervical intraepithelial classification system and correlate these results with cytopathologic findings on the Pap smear.

ANSWERS

A1. **b.** The class system of smear reporting has been significantly revised, and that aspect will be discussed in another question. With this change, the management of CIN-1/LGSIL has become more conservative and more controversial. Only 15% to 20% of CIN-1/LGSIL lesions will progress to a higher grade lesion. In light of this relatively slow temporal progression of CIN-1 lesions, expectant management of women with low-grade CIN on a single Pap smear is acceptable, assuming that they are good follow-up candidates. In this situation, Pap smears may be repeated every 4 to 6 months for three intervals. If any subsequent Pap smear report over the next 12 to 18 months shows premalignant change, the woman must be referred for colposcopic evaluation. Conversely, if all Pap smears are reported as normal during this period of increased surveillance, the woman may return to a routine screening pattern afterward. Women who are not good follow-up risks should be advised to receive colposcopic evaluation of a single low-grade CIN Pap smear reading.

A2. **c.** The recommended procedure in this case is to treat the *Trichomonas vaginalis* infection if it has not been treated in both the patient and her partner. As in the first case, the recommendations for follow-up have changed. Because the Pap smear is very specific for detecting *Trichomonas,* there is no need to perform "hanging drop" preparations or any other test to confirm Trichomoniasis. Repeat the Pap smear at the next routine screening interval and repeat every 4 to 6 months for three intervals, unless the narrative report mentions obscuring inflammation and indicates the need to repeat the Pap smear after treatment has been completed.

A3. **c.** Sampling the exocervix is performed using an Ayres or similar spatula. The spatula is inadequate for sampling the endocervical canal (EC). The EC should be sampled with a brush sampling device if the woman is not pregnant; a cotton-tip applicator is used during pregnancy.

Carcinoma of the cervix is an STD. Risk factors include early onset of intercourse, three or more sexual partners, a male sexual partner who has had other partners, a clinical history of condyloma acuminata, and cigarette smoking.

Postmenopausal women may cease to have Pap smears after the age of 65 years provided they have no new sexual partners after that time. The other stipulation to this is that adequate screening has occurred previously.

Carcinoma of the cervix is a disease with a long lead time. Lead time is the period of time between the detection of a medical condition by screening and the time when it ordinarily becomes symptomatic. Diseases with long lead times usually lend themselves to effective screening programs.

The steps in obtaining an adequate Pap smear include:

a. Collect cells before the bimanual examination.

b. Avoid contaminating the sample with lubricant.

c. Obtain the Pap smear specimen before sampling for gonococcus and chlamydia.

d. View the entire portion when obtaining the Pap smear.

e. Remove excessive vaginal discharge with a large cotton-tipped applicator.

f. Obtain the exocervical smear first, then the endocervical specimen by gently rotating the brush to avoid bleeding.

g. A single slide can be used combining both specimens together.

h. Apply the collected material uniformly to the glass slide fixing the specimen rapidly to avoid air drying artifact. Endocervical cells can become air dried in a matter of seconds.

A4. **c.** Carcinoma of the cervix is usually associated with the HPV. The type of the HPV involved is important in determining the malignant potential of the virus. HPV types 6 and 11 frequently are isolated from cervical condylomata and low-grade lesions and are believed to be of low-risk low-malignant potential. In contrast, HPV types 16, 18, 31, 33, and 35 are considered to be high-risk HPV types. Although they may be found in low-grade lesions, they are more commonly present in high-grade lesions in cervical squamous cell carcinoma and adenocarcinoma.

A5. **e.** HSV type 2 is not considered an identifiable risk factor for carcinoma of the cervix. Indirectly, of course, as an STD, an episode of HSV type 2 tends to go hand in hand with the epidemiologic risk factors just listed. HPV alone is insufficient to initiate the development and proliferation of a premalignant lesion. Thus another factor, commonly referred to as a cofactor or a facilitating factor, is necessary to act in concert with HPV to initiate these premalignant changes. As an example, cigarette smoking has been identified as an extremely important cofactor—so important as to double a smoker's risk of cervical cancer in comparison with nonsmokers.

In addition, epidemiologic data are consistent with the biologic mechanism just cited. The primary epidemiologic risk factors that have been estimated include the following:

a. Early onset of intercourse: this is defined as intercourse before the age of 20 years. Metaplasia is most active during adolescence, making a young woman much more vulnerable to cervical cellular changes.

b. Three or more sexual partners: this refers to three or more sexual partners in one lifetime. The equation is simple: the greater the number of sexual partners, the greater the risk of acquiring a high-risk type of HPV.

c. Male sexual partner who has had other partners: this is especially true if a previous partner had cervical cancer.

d. Clinical history of condyloma acuminata

A6. **b.** A reproductive health care visit represents an ideal opportunity to offer cancer screening tests. The Pap smear, more than many other screening tests, has proven its cost-effectiveness over the years. If your office is equipped with an ideal information management system and you were able to recall all of your female patients under the age of 65 at appropriate screening intervals, it is estimated that 92% of cervical cancers could be prevented. The other 8% would escape detection because of improper technique, imperfections in cytologic technology, and the biologic behavior of the malignant lesions.

A7. **e.** All women who are or who have been sexually active or who have reached 18 years of age should have an annual Pap test and pelvic examination. After a woman has three or more consecutive normal annual cervical cytologic reports, the Pap test may be performed less frequently at the discretion of the physician.

Pap smear screening intervals are determined by the risk status of the individual patient. The risk status is divided into three levels or categories of risk.

a. Extremely low-risk patients:
1) Virginal patients
2) Those patients with more than five benign Pap smears and a hysterectomy for benign disease
3) Those patients with more than 10 benign Pap smears, including one at age 60 or older, and who are presently over the age of 65 years
Recommendation: Pap smear is unnecessary

b. Low-risk patients:
1) Those patients with the onset of sexual activity before 20 years of age
2) Those patients with less than three sexual partners in a lifetime
3) Those patients who use barrier contraceptive methods
4) Those patients who are nonsmokers
5) Those patients with a previously normal Pap smear
Recommendation: Pap smears yearly for 3 years, then every 2 to 3 years

c. High-risk patients:
1) Onset of sexual activity at older than 20 years of age
2) Three or more sexual partners in a lifetime
3) Those patients with a history of HPV or STDs
4) Those patients with a previously abnormal Pap smear
5) Patients who are cigarette smokers
Recommendation: Pap smear yearly

A8. **b.** A central concern in determining the appropriate screening intervals for Pap smears is the risk of a false-negative Pap smear. A false-negative Pap smear will occur when a smear has been interpreted as normal when, in fact, it is not normal. The longer the sampling interval, the greater the risk that a false-negative Pap smear will result in a delay in lesion detection.

The currently quoted rate of false-negative Pap smear results is approximately 20%. The currently quoted specificity for the Pap smear is 70%. If two Pap smears are performed in a short time interval, the rate of false-negative smears drops to 4%. If three smears are performed in a relatively short time interval, the false negative rate falls to 0.8%.

A9. **c.** A Pap smear that comes back labeled "unsatisfactory for evaluation" may be a result of inadequate sampling, air drying, excessive red or white blood cells, and other factors that make interpretation difficult or impossible. The recommended procedure in this case is as follows:

a. Repeat the Pap smear, preferably when the woman is at midcycle and has not had intercourse or used vaginal products for at least 24 hours.

b. Repeat the Pap smear in a time frame no less than 6 weeks after the previous smear.

The reason for this latter part of the recommendation is that repetitive sampling over short periods may actually increase the risk of false-negative results because of decreased exfoliation of abnormal cells and a greater likelihood of reparative changes.

A10. **c.** The most cost-effective and least invasive mode of treating SILs of the cervix is cryotherapy using nitrous oxide or carbon dioxide as a refrigerant. The lesions must be completely covered by the probe and must not extend into the EC. A double-freeze technique is used to extend the thermal injury 4 to 5 mm beyond the edge of the probe.

A recent therapeutic modality is the loop electrode excision procedure (LEEP). A thin wire loop electrode is used to excise the entire cervical transformation zone under local infiltration anesthesia. This technique provides a tissue specimen suitable for histologic evaluation and may be used as both a diagnostic and treatment procedure.

A11. **c.** At puberty, when estrogen levels rise and *Lactobacillus* species consequently colonize the vagina, the vaginal pH drops into an acidic range. This environment changes the exposed fragile columnar epithelial cells around the cervical os, leading to their replacement by squamous epithelium, a process referred to as *squamous metaplasia*. As this process proceeds over decades, the advancing edge of the squamous epithelium, also known as the *squamocolumnar junction (SCJ)*, migrates centrally toward the cervical os and ultimately into the EC. Squamous metaplasia is most rapid during adolescence and accelerates further during pregnancy. Cervical neoplasia tends to occur between the original and the new SCJ.

SOLUTION TO THE SHORT ANSWER MANAGEMENT PROBLEM

Bethesda System	CIN Classification	Pap Smear Findings
1. Low-grade SIL	HPV changes	Atypia, koilocytotic, warty condylomatous
	CIN I	Mild dysplasia
2. High-grade SIL	CIN II	Moderate dysplasia
	CIN III	Severe dysplasia, carcinoma-in-situ

SIL, Squamous intraepithelial lesion; *HPV*, human papillomavirus; *CIN*, cervical intraepithelial neoplasia.

SUMMARY OF CERVICAL ABNORMALITIES

1. Cost-effectiveness of the Pap smear: The Pap smear has proven to be one of the most cost-effective preventative medicine tools for the primary care physician.

2. Goal of screening and case finding: The goal is to ensure that every female patient between the ages of 18 and 65 years of age is screened at appropriate intervals.

3. Specificity of Pap smear: 70%. If two Pap smears are done 1 year apart, the specificity for picking up cervical cancer increases to 96%.

4. Interval of screening: According to risk—extremely low risk, low risk, and high risk. See Answer 7.

5. U.S. Preventive Task Force screening recommendation for low-risk women: Three normal Pap smears 1 year apart followed by screening every 2 to 3 years up to the age of 65

6. New Bethesda reporting system for Pap smears: The old system includes HPV change; CIN-I, CIN-II, and CIN-III; the new system is based on SIL.
   a. Low-grade SIL (corresponds to HPV change and CIN-I) and cellular changes including atypia and mild dysplasia
   b. High-grade SIL (corresponds to CIN-II and CIN-III) and cellular changes including moderate dysplasia, severe dysplasia, and carcinoma-in-situ (i.e., squamous cell carcinoma).

7. Cause of cervical cancer: HPV types 16, 18, 31, 33, and 35 acting along with cofactors, which include cigarette smoking and risk factors for cervical cancer, namely early first intercourse, three or more partners in a lifetime, partner who has had multiple sexual partners, and a clinical history of condyloma acuminata.

8. Abnormal descriptive diagnoses on Pap smear reporting:
   a. Infection:
      1) Fungus consistent with *Candida* species
      2) *Trichomonas vaginalis*
      3) Predominance of coccobacilli consistent with shift in vaginal flora
      4) Bacteria morphologically consistent with *Actinomyces* species associated with an intrauterine device (IUD)
   b. Reactive and reparative:
      1) Reactive cellular changes associated with inflammation
      2) Atrophy with inflammation
      3) IUD
   c. Squamous cell abnormalities:
      1) Atypical squamous cell of undetermined significance
      2) LGSIL
      3) High-grade SIL

4) Atypical glandular cells of undetermined significance
5) Squamous cell carcinoma, endocervical adenocarcinoma

9. Treatment of SILs:
   a. Cryotherapy is the treatment of choice for most lesions. LEEP is a new modality that provides a histologic specimen.
   b. Laser therapy or conization may be needed.

SUGGESTED READINGS

American College of Obstetricians and Gynecologists: Cervical cytology: Evaluation and management of abnormalities, *Tech Bull* No. 183, 1993.
Mishell DR et al: *Comprehensive gynecology,* St Louis, 1997, Mosby.

PROBLEM · 53

PREMENSTRUAL SYNDROME

Flowing Along with the Moon

Case 1 ■ A 35-Year-Old Female with Premenstrual Syndrome

A 35-year-old woman comes to your office with a 6-month history of fatigue, breast tenderness, abdominal bloating, fluid retention, anxiety, irritability, depression, difficulty concentrating, and insomnia. These symptoms occur on a regular basis during the 8 days before the onset of her menstruation.

There is no significant lack of interest in life, no guilt, no hopelessness, no appetite disturbance, no psychomotor retardation or psychomotor agitation, and no other symptoms.

Her physical examination is normal. Her blood pressure is 110/75 mm Hg. Her pelvic examination is normal. There is no cervical-motion tenderness. The uterus is normal in size and mobility.

SELECT THE BEST ANSWER TO THE FOLLOWING QUESTIONS

Q1. What is the most likely diagnosis in this patient?
   a. generalized anxiety disorder
   b. masked depression
   c. major depressive illness
   d. premenstrual syndrome (PMS)
   e. hypochondriasis

Q2. What is the prevalence of the disorder described among American women in the reproductive years?

a. 1%
b. 10%
c. 25%
d. 50%
e. 75%

Q3. The most important element in establishing the diagnosis in a patient such as this is a good history. What is the most important information in the history?
   a. the severity of the symptoms
   b. the number of symptoms
   c. the timing of the symptoms relative to the menstrual cycle
   d. the presence and severity of the depression or anxiety
   e. all of the above are of equal importance

Q4. The symptoms described in Case 1 are most common in what phase of the menstrual cycle?
   a. premenstrual for 1 to 14 days
   b. during menstruation
   c. after menstruation for 1 to 14 days
   d. premenstrual for 15 to 18 days
   e. after menstruation for 15 to 18 days

Q5. The cause of the condition described is unknown. However, of the choices listed below, which one has been shown in placebo-controlled trials to be involved in the signs and symptoms of the syndrome?
   a. an estrogen-deficiency syndrome
   b. a progesterone-deficiency syndrome
   c. a progesterone-excess syndrome
   d. an estrogen-excess syndrome
   e. a serotonin deficiency

Q6. What is the condition most commonly confused with this condition?
   a. generalized anxiety disorder
   b. panic disorder
   c. major depression
   d. schizo-affective disorder
   e. none of the above

Q7. What is the treatment of choice for patients manifesting mild symptoms of this disorder?
   a. intensive psychotherapy
   b. single-agent pharmacotherapy
   c. multiagent pharmacotherapy
   d. intensive psychotherapy and multiagent pharmacotherapy
   e. none of the above

Q8. Which of the following over-the-counter (OTC) medications may be helpful in the treatment of the condition described?
   a. ibuprofen
   b. vitamin E
   c. vitamin C
   d. vitamin B$_6$
   e. all of the above

Q9. Regarding the use of hormone therapy in the disorder described, which of the following has (have) been shown to be effective?
   a. medroxyprogesterone acetate
   b. oral contraceptive pills
   c. natural progesterone suppositories
   d. a and b only
   e. all of the above

Q10. Regarding the use of pharmacologic therapy in the treatment of the disorder described, which of the following has (have) been shown to reduce the severity of symptoms?
   a. paroxetine
   b. buspirone
   c. fluoxetine
   d. alprazolam
   e. all of the above

SHORT ANSWER MANAGEMENT PROBLEM
Discuss the prevalence, the definition, and the importance of premenstrual symptoms, PMS, and late luteal phase dysphoric disorder (premenstrual dysphoric disorder). Clearly distinguish between them. Also, discuss the statement, "Premenstrual syndrome is a psychiatric disorder."

ANSWERS

A1. **d.** This patient has PMS. PMS is a syndrome of unknown etiology causing a recurrent profile of symptoms that are annoying for many women but can be debilitating for a small minority (especially in the decade before menopause).

Symptoms include psychologic symptoms and physical symptoms. Because of the multitude of symptoms, the diagnosis is often missed. The cyclic manifestation of these symptoms in rhythm with the menstrual cycle is pathognomonic for PMS.

For the diagnosis of PMS to be established, the following criteria have to be met:
   a. Symptoms are significant and are repetitive with each menstrual cycle and begin at or after ovulation.
   b. Symptoms resolve near menses.

   c. The patient is symptom free from the cessation of menses until the time of ovulation (at least 7 symptom-free days are present in each cycle).
Symptoms of PMS may include:
   a. Physical: abdominal bloating, edema, weight gain, constipation, hot flashes, breast pain, headache, acne, rhinitis, palpitation, muscle aches, joint aches, and cramping.
   b. Psychologic: anxiety, depression, irritability, mood swings, increased appetite, lethargy, fatigue, forgetfulness, sleep disorders, phobias, and crying.

A2. **b.** Although premenstrual symptoms occur in up to 90% of women, severe symptoms that interfere with work or social activities occur in, at most, 10% of women in the reproductive years.

A3. **c.** The timing of the symptoms to the rest of the menstrual cycle is the most important factor in establishing a diagnosis of PMS. The relationship of symptoms to the rest of the menstrual cycle is best established by a calendar that is kept for at least three consecutive menstrual cycles. Included in the calendar should be the first day of the cycle, a daily rating of the menstrual flow (slight, moderate, heavy, or heavy with clots), and the symptoms experienced (rated on a scale of 1 to 3).

A4. **a.** The symptoms described occur in the premenstrual period. The symptoms last anywhere from 1 to 14 days.

A5. **e.** The cause of PMS is unknown. Various hypotheses involving the female sex steroids have been proposed. However, prospective studies have shown that estrogen and progesterone levels throughout the menstrual cycle appear to be similar in women with PMS and asymptomatic women. Other unproven hypotheses include personality traits, psychosocial stress, elevated prolactin levels, hypoglycemia, and vitamin deficiencies.

Recent evidence provides strong support for the hypothesis that severe premenstrual dysphoric symptoms are the result of disturbances in central neurotransmitter regulation involving opioids and serotonin.

A6. **c.** The condition most closely associated with PMS is major depression. It is imperative that the physician rule out depression (including masked depression) before making a definitive diagnosis of PMS. Although PMS symptoms are cyclical with each menstrual cycle, the symptoms of depression are persistent throughout repetitive cycles.

A7. **e.** Because the underlying cause of PMS remains uncertain, most treatments for PMS are aimed at alleviating symptoms. This can be done primarily with a combination of lifestyle changes, with particular emphasis in exercise. There is evidence that women who exercise have milder PMS symptoms. Elimination of caffeine and chocolate has been recommended for women particularly bothered by mastalgia.

A8. **a.** Prostaglandin inhibitors such as mefenamic acid (Ponstel) and naproxen sodium (Anaprox), as well as OTC nonsteroidal antiinflammatory drugs (NSAIDs) such as ibuprofen, are effective therapies for dysmenorrhea and have also been shown in some studies to decrease the symptoms of PMS, including depression and irritability. However, vitamins E, C and B₆ have not been shown to have any therapeutic advantage in the treatment of PMS.

A9. **b.** Progesterone vaginal suppositories, widely used in the past, are no more effective than placebo. They can potentially induce menstrual cycle irregularities and should be avoided. Synthetic progestins such as medroxyprogesterone acetate (Provera), may create mild PMS symptoms rather than alleviating them. Some studies, however, suggest that combination oral contraceptive pills may reduce PMS symptoms. A nonhormonal potassium-sparing diuretic (spironolactone) has been shown to be beneficial in treating some of the physical symptoms of PMS. Physical symptoms, refractory to spironolactone, may be helped by hydrochlorothiazide.

A10. **e.** All of the choices have been helpful. In women with a main symptom of depression, selective serotonin reuptake inhibitors have been shown to be effective. Examples include fluoxetine and paroxetine. Because of a lengthy buildup of this drug to a therapeutic range, it should be used continuously.

In women in whom the main symptom is anxiety, the two medications that have been shown to be effective are alprazolam (Xanax) and buspirone (BuSpar).

SOLUTION TO THE SHORT ANSWER MANAGEMENT PROBLEM

a. Prevalence:
1) Premenstrual symptoms: 80% of all women in their reproductive years have premenstrual symptoms.
2) PMS: 10% to 20% of all women in their reproductive years have PMS.
3) Late luteal phase dysphoric disorder and premenstrual dysphoric disorder: 2% to 3% of women in the reproductive years have late luteal phase dysphoric disorder (premenstrual dysphoric disorder).

b. Definition:
1) Premenstrual symptoms: the presence of one or more of the many symptoms that have been discussed
2) PMS: the presence of a relatively large number of symptoms at the right time and with at least one symptom-free week following menstruation
3) Late luteal phase dysphoric disorder (DSM-III-R) and premenstrual dysphoric disorder (DSM-IV) are two different names for the same disorder. The critical difference between late luteal phase dysphoric disorder (premenstrual dysphoric disorder) and PMS is that the symptoms are of sufficient severity and duration to interfere with social or occupational functioning, academic work, or productivity in whatever way that is defined. Only 2% to 3% of women have the symptoms and the disorder to such a degree that it interferes with social functioning, occupational functioning, academic functioning, or productivity.

The statement, "Premenstrual syndrome is a psychiatric disorder" is false.

SUMMARY OF THE DIAGNOSIS AND MANAGEMENT OF PREMENSTRUAL SYNDROME

1. Diagnosis: Multiple physical and psychologic symptoms occurring in the premenstrual period (see the list in Answer 1).

2. Cause: Unknown.

3. History: History is most important. It must be confirmed by charting symptoms for at least 2 months.

4. Treatment:
   a. Nonpharmacologic:
   1) Low-fat, high-complex carbohydrate diet
   2) Aerobic exercise
   3) Avoid caffeine
   4) Avoid alcohol
   5) Relaxation techniques
   b. Pharmacologic:
   1) Hormonal: Oral contraceptive pill or Danazol
   2) Nonhormonal: NSAIDs such as mefenamic acid (Ponstel), naproxen sodium (Anaprox), fluoxetine (Prozac), alprazolam (Xanax), and buspirone (BuSpar)
   c. Diuretic therapy: Spironolactone or hydrochlorothiazide.

SUGGESTED READINGS

American College of Obstetricians and Gynecologists Committee Opinion: *Premenstrual syndrome*, No. 155, 1995.

Chihal HJ: Premenstrual syndrome. In Rakel R, ed: *Conn's current therapy*, Philadelphia, 1994, WB Saunders.

Mishell DR et al: *Comprehensive gynecology*, St Louis, 1997, Mosby.

PROBLEM·54

POSTMENOPAUSAL SYMPTOMS AND THEIR SEQUELAE

"Turn on the Air Conditioner."

Case 1 ■ A 48-Year-Old Female with Hot Flashes

A 48-year-old woman (gravida 3, para 3) has had increasingly irregular menses. Her last period was 12 months ago. She had been experiencing sudden on-set of profuse, embarrassing diaphoresis and sensation of heat occurring both during the day and at night. She finds her emotional state increasingly labile. She also is experiencing sleep disturbances and anxiety. Her pelvic examination reveals atrophic external genitalia, a small anteverted uterus, and no adnexal masses with unremarkable rectovaginal examination.

SELECT THE BEST ANSWER TO THE FOLLOWING QUESTIONS

Q1. What is the most likely diagnosis in this patient?
   a. pheochromocytoma
   b. hyperthyroidism
   c. menopause
   d. generalized anxiety disorder
   e. panic attacks

Q2. What is the treatment of choice for this patient?
   a. thyroid replacement
   b. estrogen with progestin
   c. antidepressants
   d. estrogen alone
   e. progestogen alone

Q3. What is the recommended dosage for postmeno-pausal hormone replacement in women with an intact uterus?
   a. 0.625 mg/day conjugated estrogen
   b. 0.625 mg/day conjugated estrogen and 10 mg medroxyprogesterone acetate (MPA) for days 1 to 13 of the calendar month
   c. 0.625 mg/day conjugated estrogen and 2.5 mg/day MPA continuously
   d. 10 mg/day MPA
   e. 150 mg/month Depo-Provera

Q4. Calcium intake is related to the prevention and treatment of postmenopausal osteoporosis. Which of the following statements regarding calcium in-take is true?
   a. estrogen decreases calcium absorption
   b. dietary calcium without estrogen can com-pletely prevent postmenopausal bone loss
   c. calcium intake during adolescence is unrelated to postmenopausal bone density
   d. obtaining calcium from dietary sources is preferable to obtaining it from calcium sup-plements
   e. sufficient vitamin E intake is necessary to en-sure dietary calcium is absorbed

Q5. Which of the following statements regarding es-trogen and heart disease is true?
   a. estrogen significantly decreases the risk of coronary artery disease in women
   b. estrogen has no effect on coronary artery dis-ease rates in women
   c. estrogen increases the risk of coronary artery disease in women
   d. no firm relationship between estrogen use and coronary artery disease risk in women has been established
   e. the effect of estrogen on coronary artery dis-ease risk in women is unknown

Q6. Hormone replacement therapy is begun on a pa-tient who presents with vasomotor menopausal symptoms. For this condition it is recommended that hormone therapy be given for how long?
   a. until the symptoms abate
   b. 1 to 2 years
   c. 3 to 5 years
   d. 10 years
   e. the ideal length of time for replacement is un-known at this time

Q7. The effect of estrogen replacement therapy on plasma lipids shows which of the following?
   a. estrogen increases serum low-density lipopro-tein (LDL)
   b. estrogen increases serum high-density li-poprotein (HDL)
   c. estrogen decreases serum LDL
   d. estrogen decreases serum HDL
   e. estrogen increases serum HDL and decreases serum LDL

Q8. Which of the following is (are) risk factors for postmenopausal osteoporosis?
   a. cigarette smoking
   b. lean body mass

c. sedentary lifestyle
d. Caucasian race
e. all of the above

Q9. Which of the following statements concerning osteoporosis is true?
  a. symptoms are noted as soon as bone density falls below a given threshold
  b. bone fractures appear most commonly in the femoral neck
  c. both estrogen and progestin replacement therapy preserve bone mass
  d. the protective effect of estrogen on bone mass is permanent, even if estrogen is discontinued
  e. aerobic exercise of any kind prevents the bone loss that occurs postmenopausally

Q10. Oral progestational agents have which of the following effects on plasma lipids?
  a. raise HDL and LDL
  b. lower HDL and LDL
  c. raise HDL and lower LDL
  d. lower HDL and raise LDL
  e. raise very low-density lipoprotein (VLDL) and lower LDL and HDL

SHORT ANSWER MANAGEMENT PROBLEM
List four contraindications to the use of postmenopausal estrogens.

ANSWERS

A1. **c.** The most likely diagnosis in this patient is menopause. The diagnosis is based on the appropriate age of a female patient for menopause, symptoms of classic "hot flashes" coming on daily and frequently, and the association of these symptoms with the cessation of menses. Menopause is a retrospective diagnosis based on 12 or more months of amenorrhea occurring at a mean age of 51 years. Perimenopause is the diagnosis when the same symptoms occur but when amenorrhea has been less than 12 months.

Hyperthyroidism would be a greater possibility in the absence of some of the other symptoms.

Hot flashes may accompany generalized anxiety disorder and panic disorder. These disorders, however, have many other symptoms as well.

A2. **b.** In this case, pheochromocytoma should receive only brief consideration. The preferred treatment regime for hot flashes or other menopausal symptoms

is a combination of estrogen and progestin. The progestin protects the endometrium from unopposed estrogen-induced endometrial hyperplasia and possibly endometrial carcinoma.

A3. **c.** The most common regimen of hormone replacement therapy in the United States for women with an intact uterus is 0.625 mg/day conjugated estrogen and 2.5 mg/day MPA continuously. The cyclic administration results in progestin withdrawal bleeding, which many postmenopausal women consider a nuisance. The continuous administration results in the majority of women becoming amenorrheic within a few months. The Postmenopausal Estrogen/Progestin Interventions (PEPI) trial (see Suggested Readings) showed that the protective effect of progestin on the endometrium was similar whether the MPA was given for 5 or 10 mg for 14 days each month or it was given continuously with a dose of 2.5 or 5 mg. Progestin therapy is of no benefit to women without a uterus because its sole purpose is to prevent endometrial hyperplasia.

A4. **d.** Both retrospective and prospective studies have shown that estrogen increases calcium absorption. Increasing dietary calcium without estrogen can decrease but not completely prevent postmenopausal bone loss. Ingesting the recommended daily intake of dietary calcium (1200 to 1500 mg/day) during the adolescent years results in greater adult bone mass than occurs if insufficient calcium is ingested. Calcium supplementation is only of benefit for those women who have an inadequate daily ingestion (less than 500 mg/day). It is preferable to main adequate calcium intake from foods containing this mineral rather than by supplemental calcium sources. All individuals need sufficient amounts of vitamin D, not vitamin E, to ensure that dietary calcium is absorbed.

A5. **a.** One of the positive side effects of estrogen replacement therapy in postmenopausal women is protection from coronary artery disease. Cardiovascular disease (CVD) is the leading cause of death among women in industrialized countries, resulting in greater than 50% of deaths in postmenopausal women. Estrogens have a significant protective effect against atherosclerosis in postmenopausal women. For example, the rate of cardiovascular mortality in premenopausal women is approximately 20% of age-matched men; following menopause, however, the risk among postmenopausal women catches up to age-matched men unless the women are on estrogen replacement therapy.

The relative risk of CVD among postmenopausal estrogen users compared to nonusers has been compared in several studies. All have shown reduced risk in estrogen users, although the decrease of risk reduction has been quite variable. Women with risk factors for CVD appear to benefit the most from estrogen.

A6. **e.** Evidence suggests that estrogen protection against osteoporosis (even if the patient is not a high-risk candidate) may be sufficient reason to consider estrogen supplementation for an indefinite period once started for treatment of hot flashes. At this point it is unclear for how long hormone replacement optimally should be provided. The most prudent approach is to individualize decision-making with each patient, taking into consideration her individual risk factors for osteoporosis, CVD, and breast cancer.

A7. **e.** Exogenous estrogens have a favorable effect on the lipid profile: they raise HDL by 16% to 18%, and they lower atherogenic LDL by 15% to 19%. Both these changes significantly reduce cardiac risk.

A8. **e.** A significant risk of estrogen deficiency in postmenopausal women is osteoporosis. The risk factors for osteoporosis include:
  1) Female gender
  2) Postmenopausal status
  3) Caucasian or Asian race
  4) Positive family history
  5) Early spontaneous or surgical menopause
  6) Sedentary lifestyle
  7) Cigarette smoking
  8) High caffeine intake
  9) High alcohol intake
  10) High protein intake
  11) Lean body mass

A9. **c.** Osteoporosis is a major complication of postmenopausal estrogen deficiency. It is an asymptomatic disorder, and its presence usually goes undetected until a fracture occurs many years after bone density falls below the fracture threshold. At least 25% of the bone needs to be lost before osteoporosis is diagnosed by routine x-ray examination. Dual-energy x-ray absorptiometry is the preferred technique to measure bone density. Postmenopausal bone loss occurs more rapidly in trabecular than cortical bone with compression fractures of the vertebrae being the most common site. Fractures of the distal radius and the femoral neck are next in frequency. Estrogen replacement therapy and progestin therapy contribute to preservation of bone mass. The greatest benefit of estrogen replacement therapy occurs when it is initiated within 5 years of menopause. The protective effect of estrogen on bone mass is not permanent. Within 3 months of discontinuing estrogen the rate of bone loss rapidly in-

creases. Weight-bearing aerobic exercise will retard but not prevent postmenopausal bone loss.

A10. **d.** In contradistinction to estrogens, progestational agents tend to have the opposite effect on plasma lipids. Progestational agents raise LDL and lower HDL. However, in the PEPI trial discussed previously, the beneficial changes in lipid metabolism observed with estrogen alone were only slightly reduced with the addition of a synthetic progestin and not changed when micronized progesterone was given sequentially.

Moreover, the major mechanism whereby estrogen reduces CVD is by a direct action on the arterial wall, not through changes in serum lipids. The mechanism of beneficial effect of estrogen on the endothelium may be by increasing the synthesis and release of nitric oxide, reduction of serum angiotensin-converting enzyme activity, as well as increasing vascular anti-oxidant activity. All of these mechanisms result in a cardiovascular protection effect in normal women as well as those with existing heart disease. These effects do not appear to be reduced by the addition of progestins.

SOLUTION TO THE SHORT ANSWER MANAGEMENT PROBLEM

Four contraindications to the use of postmenopausal estrogen replacement therapy are:
  a. Known or suspected endometrial or breast cancer
  b. Genital bleeding of uncertain origin
  c. Active liver disease
  d. Active thromboembolic disease or a history of estrogen-related thromboembolic disease

SUMMARY OF THE DIAGNOSIS AND TREATMENT OF POSTMENOPAUSAL SYMPTOMS AND THEIR SEQUELAE

1. Classification of symptoms:
   a. Vasomotor symptoms: Hot flushes/hot flashes develop in 75% of postmenopausal women.
   b. Urogenital symptoms: Dyspareunia, vaginal itching, vaginal dryness, burning, and urgency and frequency of urination.

2. Investigations: All patients being considered for hormonal replacement therapy should have a complete history and physical with special attention given to blood pressure measurement, breast and pelvic examination, and Pap smear. Mammography should be performed initially to avoid estrogen ad-

ministration in a patient with preexisting subclinical breast cancer; it should be repeated yearly after age 50.

3. Treatment:
   a. Hormone replacement therapy: Women without a uterus should take continuous estrogen only. Women with an intact uterus should take estrogen and progestins to prevent endometrial hyperplasia from unopposed estrogen. Most commonly used estrogens are oral (PO) 0.625 mg conjugated estrogen or estrone sulfate or 1 mg of micronized estrogen. An alternative is transdermal estradiol with a daily dose of 0.05 mg. The theoretic advantage of the transdermal route is the avoidance of the first-pass liver metabolism. The vaginal route for estrogen administration is suboptimal because absorption is variable among women. Most commonly used progestin is oral MPA.

   Administration regimen may be continuous estrogen and progestin, which avoids withdrawal bleed in most women, or continuous estrogen with progestin 10 to 14 days/mo.

   The length of time that estrogen should be given is unknown. The best current advice is to take the estrogen indefinitely. Osteoporosis is a major cause of morbidity and mortality in elderly women and should be considered serious enough to use a prophylactic regime (as previously discussed), especially in high-risk women.

   b. Progesterone: Progestins relieve hot flashes in 70% of women who have a contraindication to estrogen. The usual dose of MPA is 10 mg/day PO or 50 to 150 mg of Depo-MPA intramuscularly every 3 months.

   c. Alpha-adrenergic agonist (Clonidine): An alternative for the treatment of hot flashes (effective in 30% to 40% of cases) is Clonidine, a centrally acting alpha-adrenergic agonist. Clonidine, usually administered in an initial dose of 0.1 mg bid, has significant side effects (primarily orthostatic hypotension and typical anticholinergic effects).

   d. Megestrol acetate: A recent report suggests that megestrol acetate may prevent and relieve hot flashes and hot flushes. This drug, an androgenic agent given in a dosage of 20 mg/day, is well tolerated by most menopausal women.

4. Controversy: Should all postmenopausal women be treated with exogenous estrogen in the postmenopausal period to prevent osteoporosis? Probably not. Base your decision on risk factors.

SUGGESTED READINGS

Loprinzi C et al: Megestrol acetate for the prevention of hot flashes, *N Engl J Med* 331(6):347-352, 1994.

Mishell DR et al: *Comprehensive gynecology*, St Louis, 1997, Mosby.

Walsh BW, Schiff I: Menopause. In Rakel R, ed: *Conn's current therapy*, Philadelphia, 1994, WB Saunders.

The Writing Group for the PEPI Trial: Effects of hormone replacement therapy on endometrial histology in postmenopausal women, *JAMA* 275(5):370-375, 1996.

PROBLEM · 55

DYSMENORRHEA

"Why Do I Get This Terrible Stomachache Every Month?"

Case 1 ■ A 14-Year-Old Female with Lower Midabdominal, Colicky Pain with Her Menstrual Cycle

A 14-year-old female comes to your office with a 6-month history of lower midabdominal pain. The pain is colicky in nature, radiates through to the back and upper thighs, begins within a few hours of the onset of menstruation, and lasts from 2 to 4 days. Menarche (initially irregular but now regular) began 18 months ago. Her menstrual periods became regular 6 months ago. The patient is not sexually active.

On physical examination, the patient appears unremarkable with normal secondary sexual development. Abdominal examination results are normal. Rectal examination reveals a normal sized, mobile uterus. No other abnormalities are detected.

SELECT THE BEST ANSWER TO THE FOLLOWING QUESTIONS

Q1. What is the most likely diagnosis in this patient?
   a. primary dysmenorrhea
   b. pelvic inflammatory disease (PID)
   c. secondary dysmenorrhea
   d. endometriosis
   e. psychogenic abdominal pain

Q2. Which of the following has (have) been shown to be consistently associated with the pain produced by the condition described?
   a. elevation of myometrial resting tone
   b. elevation of contractile myometrial pressure
   c. increased frequency of uterine contractions
   d. dysrhythmia of uterine contractions
   e. all of the above

Q3. The disorder described appears to be mediated by which of the following?
   a. increased levels of prostaglandin synthetase

b. decreased levels of prostaglandin synthetase
c. increased levels of cyclic adenosine mono-phosphate (cAMP)
d. decreased levels of cAMP
e. none of the above

Q4. The pathophysiology of the disorder described involves which of the following?
a. vasodilatation of the uterine arteries
b. vasoconstriction of the uterine arteries
c. venous vasodilatation of the uterine veins
d. venous vasodilatation of the pelvic veins
e. none of the above

Q5. The disorder described usually begins at what age?
a. 15 to 25
b. 20 to 30
c. 30 to 40
d. 40 to 45
e. within 2 years of the onset of menstruation

Q6. Which of the following is not directly associated with secondary dysmenorrhea?
a. ectopic pregnancy
b. endometriosis
c. adenomyosis
d. chronic PID
e. placement of an intrauterine device (IUD)

Q7. What is the prevalence of secondary dysmenorrhea among American women of childbearing age?
a. 5% to 10%
b. 15% to 25%
c. 30% to 40%
d. 50% to 75%
e. >90%

Q8. Which of the following drugs has (have) been demonstrated to be efficacious in the treatment of secondary dysmenorrhea?
a. ibuprofen
b. naproxen
c. acetylsalicylic acid
d. a and b
e. all of the above

Q9. A patient with the condition described is being treated with a fenamate (Ponstel [mefenamic acid]). She has received some benefit from this treatment, which was initiated 3 months ago, but it has only lowered the pain from a level of 7/10 to a level of 4/10. At this time, what would you do?
a. continue the fenamate
b. discontinue the fenamate and begin oxycodone

c. switch to oral contraceptive pills (OCPs)
d. switch to danazol
e. switch to a nonsteroidal antiinflammatory drug (NSAID) of a different class

Case 2 ■ A 24-Year-Old Female with Lower Midabdominal, Colicky Pain with Her Menstrual Cycle

A 24-year-old nulligravida woman comes to your office with an 18-month history of cyclic pelvic pain related to her regular and predictable menses. On further questioning you find she has been engaging in regular intercourse without contraception since she got married 2 years ago but has been unable to conceive. Upon pelvic examination, you find a normal-sized, immobile, retroverted uterus with nodularity and tenderness on palpation of the uterosacral ligaments. She denies ever being diagnosed with any sexually transmitted disease (STD).

Q10. Which of the following is the most likely diagnosis for the patient in Case 2?
a. PID
b. endometriosis
c. leiomyomata uteri
d. adenomyosis
e. sarcoidosis

Q11. Which of the following diagnostic modalities would be the one of choice to establish a diagnosis in this condition?
a. hysteroscopy
b. sonography
c. laparoscopy
d. hysterosalpingogram (HSG)
e. magnetic resonance imaging (MRI) scan

Q12. Which of the following medical therapies would be appropriate in treating this condition?
a. danazol
b. gonadotropin-releasing hormone (GnRH) agonist
c. OCPs
d. progestins
e. all of the above

SHORT ANSWER MANAGEMENT PROBLEM
Discuss the two most commonly recommended treatments for the primary form of the condition described in Case 1 and how you would decide on your treatment of choice.

ANSWERS

A1. a. This young woman has primary dysmenorrhea. Primary dysmenorrhea is the most common gynecologic complaint experienced by young women. Of menstruating women, 50% to 75% experience this symptom; in 10% of menstruating women it is severe.

Primary dysmenorrhea usually begins within 6 to 12 months of menarche. The pain is in the lower abdomen and is often colicky. The pain associated with each cycle usually begins within a few hours of the beginning of the onset of menstrual flow. The pathophysiology is initiated by progesterone withdrawal, which releases prostaglandins that cause excessive myometrial contractions leading to decreased uterine blood flow and uterine ischemia. (As would be expected, anovulatory cycles without progesterone withdrawal are usually not associated with primary dysmenorrhea.) Symptoms associated with primary dysmenorrhea include nausea, vomiting, diarrhea, headache, breast tenderness, and fatigue.

Secondary dysmenorrhea is dysmenorrhea caused by an underlying pelvic pathologic condition. PID and endometriosis are two primary causes of secondary dysmenorrhea.

Psychogenic factors, although previously thought to be a cause of primary dysmenorrhea, are unlikely to be related to the disorder.

A2. e. Primary dysmenorrhea is associated with the following:
a. An elevation of myometrial resting tone to above 10 mm Hg
b. An elevation of contractile myometrial pressure to above 120 mm Hg
c. An increased frequency of uterine contractions
d. Dysrhythmia of uterine contractions
These physiologic changes result in increased production of vasoconstrictive prostaglandins causing uterine hypoxia.

A3. a.

A4. b. Primary dysmenorrhea is pathologically mediated by an increase in the level of the enzyme prostaglandin synthetase. Elevated levels of the enzyme produce vasoconstricting prostaglandins that are responsible for uterine hypoxia, or uterine angina, which produces the pain of dysmenorrhea. The vasoconstriction itself takes place in the branches of the uterine artery.

A5. e. One of the most important distinguishing characteristics of primary dysmenorrhea is the age of onset. Primary dysmenorrhea almost always begins within 2 years of the onset of menstruation. The tran-

sition from the anovulatory and irregular cycles immediately following puberty to the regular ovulatory cycles of the adult years takes place within the first 2 years after menarche. Primary dysmenorrhea is related to ovulatory cycles with progesterone withdrawal triggering endometrial spiral arteriolar spasm leading to prostaglandin release and uterine ischemia. If dysmenorrhea begins at a later time, secondary dysmenorrhea is much more likely.

A6. e. Ectopic pregnancy is not directly associated with secondary dysmenorrhea. It is, however, indirectly related because of the secondary dysmenorrhea/PID link.

Secondary dysmenorrhea is defined as dysmenorrhea caused by a concurrent organic pelvic pathologic process; it can be caused by any one of the following:
a. Endometriosis
b. Leiomyomas
c. Adenomyosis
d. Endometrial polyps
e. Cervical stenosis
f. PID
g. The presence of an IUD

A7. d. Of American women of childbearing age, 50% to 75% experience dysmenorrhea. Many of these women (>90%) will also have experienced primary dysmenorrhea. As just discussed, however, there are numerous secondary causes. These secondary causes usually produce symptoms at a significantly later age.

A8. e. NSAIDs are a mainstay of treatment for primary dysmenorrhea. This includes acetylsalicylic acid (aspirin). NSAIDs exert their effect by inhibiting the production of prostaglandins through inhibition of the enzyme prostaglandin synthetase.

A9. e. NSAIDs are the drugs of choice for the treatment of primary dysmenorrhea. A reasonable length of time for a trial of one agent is 3 months. If, after that time, there has not been a significant change in the pain and discomfort, an agent of another class should be tried.

Following are the classes of NSAIDs and examples of each:

Group	Agent
Benzoic acid derivatives	Aspirin
Butyrophenone	Phenylbutazone
Indole acetic acid derivative	Indomethacin
Fenamates	Mefenamic acid (Ponstel)
Propionic acid derivatives	Ibuprofen (Motrin)
	Naproxen (Naproxen)
	Naproxen sodium (Anaprox)
Piroxicam	Feldene

In general, the groups of choice include the fenamates and the propionic acid derivatives. In the patient described, a reasonable choice would be to switch the patient to a propionic acid derivative such as naproxen sodium (Anaprox) for a 3-month period. If that is ineffective, a switch to OCPs would be the next logical alternative. NSAIDs should not be given to patients who have nasal polyps, angioedema, and bronchospasm related to aspirin or other NSAIDs.

A10. **b.** The presentation is that of secondary dysmenorrhea, which can be defined as painful menses developing after onset of ovulatory cycles with the finding of a specific pelvic pathologic condition. It can be caused by endometriosis, leiomyomas, adenomyosis, endometrial polyps, cervical stenosis, PID, or an IUD.

The first four options in Question 10 (i.e., PID, endometriosis, leiomyomata uteri, or adenomyosis) can all result in secondary dysmenorrhea. The normal sized uterus tends to eliminate leiomyomata and adenomyosis as the probable diagnosis. PID and endometriosis could both cause a retroverted uterus, infertility, and painful menses. The negative history for STDs tends to eliminate PID, leaving endometriosis as the most likely diagnosis. Sarcoidosis is not associated with secondary dysmenorrhea.

Endometriosis is a benign condition in which endometrial glands and stroma are found outside the uterine cavity. It is estimated to occur in 15% of women and is the most common gynecologic diagnosis responsible for hospitalization of women in the United States in their reproductive years. The degree of symptomatology may be unrelated to the gross extent of the disease. It is often associated with dyspareunia (painful intercourse), dyschezia (painful defecation), and infertility. However, 30% of patients with endometriosis are asymptomatic.

A11. **c.** The diagnosis of endometriosis can be strongly suspected on the basis of a careful history and physical examination. However, confirmation of the diagnosis requires direct surgical visualization of lesions, which is usually performed by laparoscopy. Hysteroscopy and HSG are not helpful diagnostically because they assess only the internal uterine anatomy, not the external pelvic cavity and peritoneal surfaces. Ultrasound and MRI may give useful information in differentiating solid from cystic lesions, but they cannot be used for primary screening.

A12. **e.** The primary goal of hormonal treatment of endometriosis is induction of amenorrhea, which will hopefully result in atrophy of the ectopic endometrial tissue. Appropriate patients are those with symptomatic disease who desire fertility. Approaches that can be used include pseudomenopause and pseudopregnancy. Induction of pseudomenopause utilizes either danazol, which produces a hypoestrogenic and hyperandrogenic response, or GnRH agonists, which suppress gonadotropin secretion with a secondary decrease in ovarian estrogen production. Induction of pseudopregnancy utilizes continuous use of OCPs or continuous use of progestins (oral or injectable), which results in endometrial gland and stromal atrophy. Thus all the options listed in Question 12 are appropriate medical therapies for endometriosis.

SOLUTION TO THE SHORT ANSWER MANAGEMENT PROBLEM

The two recommended treatments for primary dysmenorrhea are the NSAIDs (discussed previously) and OCPs. Both of these treatments are highly effective in reducing the pain and symptoms associated with the condition. The manner in which you decide first and second choice depends on the additional need for contraceptive protection. If she is sexually active, then the OCP would be your first choice. If, on the other hand, she is not sexually active and does not intend to become sexually active, an NSAID may be preferable.

SUMMARY OF THE DIAGNOSIS AND TREATMENT OF DYSMENORRHEA

1. Diagnosis:
   a. Primary dysmenorrhea: Begins within 2 years of the onset of menarche. Presents with colicky, midabdominal pain, spasmodic in nature, starting with or a few hours after the onset of the menstrual flow and usually lasting for 2 to 4 days.
   b. Secondary dysmenorrhea: Usually begins later (in relation to menarche) and is often associated with irregular cycles and anovulatory bleeding. Causes include endometriosis, adenomyosis, endometrial polyps, myomas, cervical stenosis, PID, and use of an IUD.

2. Treatment:
   a. Primary dysmenorrhea:
      1) NSAIDs (in patients not needing contraceptive protection): Most commonly used classes are fenamates and propionic acid derivatives. If a drug from one class is not effective after three cycles, try a drug from the other class. If this is not successful, proceed to the OCP.
      2) OCP is the treatment of choice in those young women requiring contraceptive protection.

b. Secondary dysmenorrhea: Establish and treat the cause.

SUGGESTED READINGS
American College of Obstetrics and Gynecology: Chronic pelvic pain, *Tech Bull* No. 223, 1996.
Barmat L, Schinfeld J: Dysmenorrhea. In Rakel R, ed: *Conn's current therapy,* Philadelphia, 1994, WB Saunders.
Mishell DR et al: *Comprehensive gynecology,* St Louis, 1997, Mosby.

PROBLEM · 56

DYSFUNCTIONAL UTERINE BLEEDING

"Doctor, I'm Using a Gross of Sanitary Napkins Each Month."

Case 1 ■ A 35-Year-Old Female with Heavy Menstrual Periods

A 35-year-old woman (gravida 4, para 3, aborted 1) comes to your office complaining of irregular and heavy menstrual periods for the past year. She underwent a laparoscopic bilateral tubal sterilization after her last pregnancy 4 years ago.

On physical examination, her blood pressure is 120/80 mm Hg. She is appropriate weight for height. Examination of the head and neck, cardiovascular system, respiratory system, abdomen, musculoskeletal system, and neurologic systems are normal. Pelvic examination reveals normal external genitalia; mobile, nontender cervix, and a normal-sized uterus. Her ovaries are appropriately sized with no other adnexal masses.

SELECT THE BEST ANSWER TO THE FOLLOWING QUESTIONS

Q1. What would you do at this time?
   a. reassure the patient that the periods will eventually settle down
   b. prescribe estrogen replacement therapy with progesterone to take care of the problem
   c. provide a monthly injection of intramuscular (IM) Depo-Provera to take care of the problem
   d. prescribe a sedative; the basic problem is rattled nerves caused by heavy flow
   e. none of the above

Q2. Which of the following should be considered in the differential diagnosis of this patient's problem?
   a. uterine polyp
   b. submucous fibroid

   c. adenomatous hyperplasia
   d. adenomyosis
   e. all of the above

Q3. What is the most likely diagnosis in this patient?
   a. menopause
   b. "nervous uterus"
   c. dysmenorrhea complicated by bleeding
   d. dysfunctional uterine bleeding (DUB)
   e. none of the above

Q4. What is the most likely underlying cause of this patient's abnormal bleeding?
   a. anovulation
   b. multiple ovulation
   c. a coagulation defect
   d. uterine pathology
   e. none of the above

Q5. What is the average volume of blood loss during normal menstruation?
   a. 10 cc
   b. 30 cc
   c. 50 cc
   d. 80 cc
   e. 100 cc

Q6. What is the most common physiologic correlate of DUB?
   a. estrogen withdrawal
   b. estrogen breakthrough
   c. progesterone withdrawal
   d. progesterone breakthrough
   e. none of the above

Q7. What is the definition of DUB?
   a. menstrual bleeding, either excessive in duration or amount or unpatterned with no anatomic cause
   b. painful, irregular bleeding secondary to systemic disease; no cause demonstrated
   c. abnormal vaginal bleeding of endometrial origin
   d. uterine bleeding at the extremes of life
   e. none of the above

Q8. Which of the following systemic diseases is (are) associated with abnormal vaginal bleeding?
   a. hypothyroidism
   b. hyperthyroidism
   c. cirrhosis
   d. renal failure
   e. all of the above

Q9. Which of the following laboratory investigations may be indicated in the evaluation of abnormal uterine bleeding?
   a. serum or urine pregnancy test
   b. serum T4 and thyroid-stimulating hormone (TSH)
   c. basal body temperature charting
   d. pelvic ultrasound
   e. all of the above

Q10. Anovulatory DUB accounts for approximately what percentage of total DUB?
   a. 10%
   b. 25%
   c. 50%
   d. 75%
   e. 90%

Q11. The hormonal treatment(s) of choice for anovulatory DUB may include which of the following?
   a. ethinyl estradiol
   b. medroxyprogesterone acetate
   c. progesterone
   d. combination oral contraceptive pills (OCPs)
   e. all of the above

Case 2 ■ A 24-Year-Old Female with Heavy Uterine Bleeding

A 24-year-old obese female with a history of irregular menstrual periods presents to the Emergency Department with a 10-day history of heavy uterine bleeding. She is soaking through 20 pads per day. Her hemoglobin, when last measured 6 months ago, was 14 g/dl. Today it is 9.0 g/dl. You suspect significant blood loss caused by chronic anovulation.

Q12. What is the treatment of choice at this time in this patient?
   a. IM medroxyprogesterone acetate
   b. IV Premarin
   c. IV danazol
   d. factor VIII cryoprecipitate
   e. a high-dose OCP

SHORT ANSWER MANAGEMENT PROBLEM
Describe the origin of oligomenorrhea and amenorrhea in women athletes who exercise strenuously.

ANSWERS

A1. **e.** All of the choices offered are inappropriate. The first and most important question you have to ask

regarding any patient in the reproductive years with abnormal bleeding is "Could this patient be pregnant?" Accordingly, the next step in management is to order a urine or serum beta-human chorionic gonadotropin pregnancy test. Once pregnancy has been ruled out, you can proceed for a further workup. If there is a secondary cause, the cause should be identified and corrected if possible. DUB refers to uterine bleeding (either unpredictable or excessive in amount or duration) for which no specific genital tract lesion or systemic cause is found.

A2. **e.** This question asks you to identify the secondary causes of heavy menstrual periods, or menorrhagia. If the periods are heavy only, the appropriate term is *menorrhagia.* If the periods are irregular only, then the appropriate term is *metrorrhagia.* If the periods are both heavy and irregular, then the appropriate term is *menometrorrhagia.*

The secondary causes that should be considered in this case include the following:
   a. Uterine fibroids
   b. Submucous fibroids
   c. Endometriosis
   d. Adenomyosis
   e. Chronic pelvic inflammatory disease
   f. Endometrial polyps
   g. Coagulation defects
   h. Massive obesity
   i. Ovarian abnormalities
   j. Severe hypothyroidism
   k. Adenomatous hyperplasia
   l. Endometrial carcinoma

A3. **d.** The most likely diagnosis in this patient is DUB.

A4. **a.** The most common cause of DUB is anovulatory bleeding. When the uterine lining is sequentially proliferated by estrogen then ripened with progesterone, the endometrium is structurally stable. Sloughing of the endometrium does not occur unless progesterone withdrawal takes place. When progesterone is withdrawn, the tissue breakdown is orderly and progressive. Bleeding is limited in both amount and duration by spiral arteriolar vasoconstriction. Menstrual shedding is simultaneous in all endometrial segments of the uterus. This is why ovulatory cycles are regular and predictable from month to month.

When the uterine lining is proliferated by estrogen alone without progesterone to stabilize it, the endometrium continues to thicken. When the endometrial proliferation reaches a given thickness, it starts to shed, but this bleeding is not accompanied by spiral arteriolar vasoconstriction. Therefore it is not limited in either amount or duration; it can occur at any time. Endometrial shedding occurs at random times from random sites within the uterus. This is why anovulatory bleeding is irregular and unpredictable.

Ovulatory uterine bleeding may be associated with oligomenorrhea, menorrhagia, or menometrorrhagia.

DUB usually occurs at the extremes of the reproductive years—during puberty and before menopause. It is less common in the reproductive years, although ovulatory DUB does occur during this time. Ovulatory DUB may be associated with midcycle spotting, premenstrual spotting, or postmenstrual spotting. Ovulatory DUB accounts for less than 10% of all DUB.

A5. **b.** The usual duration of menstrual flow is 4 to 6 days and the average blood loss during that time is 30 cc. The duration of flow appears to be related to estrogen stimulation. Nonsteroidal antiinflammatory drugs (NSAIDs) appear to be effective in decreasing the endometrial bleeding with ovulatory DUB but not with anovulatory DUB. The mechanism of reduction of menstrual blood loss in ovulatory DUB is related to a differential effect on various prostaglandin moieties. Prostacyclin is a vasodilator, so it tends to increase bleeding. Thromboxane is a vasoconstrictor, so it tends to decrease bleeding. All NSAIDs are cyclooxygenase inhibitors and thus block the formation of both prostacyclin and thromboxane. NSAIDs possibly suppress prostacyclin to a greater degree than thromboxane.

A6. **b.** The most common physiologic correlate of anovulatory DUB is estrogen breakthrough. Anovulation results in a unopposed endometrial estrogen stimulation; this eventually results in a buildup of the endometrial lining beyond the capacity of the stroma to support.

A7. **a.** This answer gives more detail regarding definition of DUB.

DUB can be defined as vaginal bleeding of endometrial origin that may be excessive (greater than 80 ml), prolonged (greater than 7 days), or unpatterned in which no specific genital tract lesion or systemic cause is found.

A8. **e.** DUB can be associated with hypothyroidism, hyperthyroidism, cirrhosis, renal failure, diabetes mellitus, hyperprolactinemia, polycystic ovarian syndrome, premature menopause, blood dyscrasia, emotional and physical stress, and nutritional disorders including morbid obesity and anorexia nervosa.

In the evaluation of abnormal uterine bleeding, it is often helpful to group causes according to age:
  a. Menarche to age 20: Greater than 95% of abnormal uterine bleeding is dysfunctional and an-

ovulatory. A careful history and physical examination is usually all that is required in the evaluation. OCPs and NSAIDs are of particular therapeutic benefit.
  b. Ages 20 to 40: Anovulation is uncommon in this age group as a cause of DUB. A careful history and physical examination should precede any investigations. A hysteroscopy, endometrial sampling, and laparoscopy may, however, eventually be indicated in the evaluation.
  c. Age greater than 40: Anovulation is a major cause of abnormal uterine bleeding in this age group. Uterine fibroids, cervical polyps, and endometrial carcinoma, must, however, be excluded. Endometrial sampling is recommended.

A9. **e.** Because of the numerous causes of abnormalities in uterine bleeding already discussed, serum T4, serum TSH, basal body temperature monitoring, serum pregnancy test, and pelvic ultrasound are all tests that may be indicated depending on the circumstances including history, physical examination, and age.

A10. **e.** Anovulatory DUB accounts for greater than 90% of all DUB; ovulatory DUB accounts for the remaining 10%.

A11. **e.** Once an accurate diagnosis of anovulation (or progesterone deficiency) has been established, the primary goal is to normalize the bleeding pattern by adding back to the patient the progesterone or progestin deficiency. All of the options in the question provide that critical ingredient.

If ovulation is not desired but contraception is, then a combination OCP will accomplish these goals. A possible advantage of the OCPs is their tendency to produce a lighter withdrawal flow. The pills are started on day 5 of the first cycle and then given for 21 continuous days, with an interruption of 7 days between each course of medication. Withdrawal flow should be anticipated during the days when no medication is taken. An alternative approach consists of the cyclic administration of 10 days of oral ethinyl estradiol, 10 days of oral medroxyprogesterone acetate or single IM progesterone-in-oil injection at 4-week intervals.

For patients in whom hormonal therapy has failed and who have completed childbearing, options include endometrial ablation by thermal injury using a hysteroscopic laser or roller ball as well as an endometrial balloon. Hysterectomy should be considered (1) only for patients who have had multiple curettage and (2) when thorough diagnostic evaluation has failed to reveal a specific or correctable pathologic condition.

A12. **b.** The treatment of choice for this type of heavy DUB is IV estrogen (Premarin 25 mg IV q4h for 3 to 4 doses). In this patient the endometrial lining that is remaining (the basal layer) will be less responsive to progestin therapy. The high-dose estrogen rapidly proliferates the thinned basal endometrium stopping the bleeding. The estrogen administration must be followed by 10 days of a progestin to allow a normal progestin withdrawal flow to occur. As an alternative to IV Premarin, the OCP can be given four times per day for 5 to 7 days. This, however, would likely be associated with significant nausea.

SOLUTION TO THE SHORT ANSWER MANAGEMENT PROBLEM

Women who exercise excessively or frequently have not only oligomenorrhea but also amenorrhea that may have been going on for many months or even years. The origin of this oligomenorrhea or amenorrhea in nearly all cases is anovulation of hypothalamic-pituitary origin. Because of the potential danger of unopposed endometrial estrogen buildup without shedding, it is reasonable to try a uterine bleed with hormonal therapy (estrogen or progesterone depending on the circumstances of the individual case).

SUMMARY OF THE DIAGNOSIS AND TREATMENT OF DYSFUNCTIONAL UTERINE BLEEDING

1. Definition: Abnormal uterine bleeding that cannot be attributed to any specific genital tract lesion or systemic disease

2. Classification of DUB:
   a. Anovulatory: Prevalence is 90%
      1) Oligomenorrhea
      2) Menorrhagia
      3) Menometrorrhagia
   b. Ovulatory: Prevalence is 10%
      1) Midcycle spotting
      2) Premenstrual spotting

3. Considerations regarding patient age: In patients older than 20 years, a pathologic condition of the pelvis must be excluded before making the diagnosis of DUB. Also consider the other causes that may be associated with DUB.

4. Treatment:
   a. Anovulatory DUB:
      1) OCPs
      2) Cyclic progestins: Ethinyl estradiol, medroxyprogesterone acetate, progesterone-in-oil.

      3) Endometrial ablation if none of these is effective
   b. Ovulatory DUB:
      1) Midcycle spotting: Ethinyl estradiol or OCPs
      2) Premenstrual spotting: Cyclic progestins
      3) Postmenopausal spotting: NSAIDs or OCPs
   c. Acute hemorrhage caused by DUB: Premarin IV, or OCPs 4 times/day for 5 to 7 days followed by OCPs or oral Provera

SUGGESTED READINGS

American College of Obstetricians and Gynecologists: Dysfunctional uterine bleeding, *Tech Bull* No. 134, 1989.

Friedman C: Dysfunctional uterine bleeding. In Rakel R, ed: *Conn's current therapy*, Philadelphia, 1994, WB Saunders.

PROBLEM·57

ECTOPIC PREGNANCY

"I Missed My Period, but I Have Pain and I Am Still Spotting."

Case 1 ■ A 28-Year-Old Female with Pelvic Pain and Vaginal Bleeding

A 28-year-old woman comes to your office with a 2-week history of pelvic pain and scant vaginal bleeding. There has been no vaginal discharge. She is married, has no children, and has been trying to become pregnant for the past 18 months. Her menstrual periods have always been regular, but she is now 3 weeks past the date at which she would have expected her last period.

Her uterus feels slightly enlarged and boggy. There is a small amount of "dark brownish-red" blood in the vaginal pool. Her left adnexa are somewhat tender. Her right adnexa are normal.

SELECT THE BEST ANSWER TO THE FOLLOWING QUESTIONS

Q1. At this time, what is the most important diagnosis to exclude?
   a. ruptured corpus luteum cyst
   b. acute pelvic inflammatory disease (PID)
   c. ectopic pregnancy
   d. threatened abortion
   e. incomplete abortion

Q2. In taking a complete history from this patient, which of the following questions would be of particular importance?
   a. history of fever within the last 24 hours

b. history of dysmenorrhea
c. history of menorrhagia
d. history of last menstrual period
e. history of previous miscarriages

Q3. What is the most important single laboratory/imaging test to be performed at this time in this patient?
   a. serum or urine beta-human chorionic gonadotropin (HCG) test
   b. hysterosalpingogram
   c. culdocentesis
   d. pelvic ultrasound
   e. laparoscopy

Q4. Regarding the epidemiology of the condition described, which of the following statements is (are) true?
   a. there has been marked increase in the incidence of this condition in the United States over the past 20 years
   b. there has been marked increase in the prevalence of this condition among women in the childbearing years in the United States over the past 20 years
   c. the absolute number of cases of this condition in the United States has increased out of proportion to population growth over the last 20 years
   d. all of the above statements are true
   e. none of the above statements is true

Q5. Regarding the risks of morbidity and mortality associated with this condition in the United States, which of the following statements is (are) true?
   a. this condition remains the third most common cause of maternal death in the United States
   b. the mortality rate could be decreased by at least one third with earlier diagnosis and management
   c. most maternal deaths from this condition occur as a result of intraabdominal hemorrhage
   d. all of the above are true
   e. none of the above is true

Q6. Anatomically speaking, the condition described is most commonly associated with which of the following structures?
   a. the ampulla of the fallopian tube
   b. the isthmus of the fallopian tube
   c. the interstitial portion of the fallopian tube
   d. the interstitial portion of the ovary
   e. the endometrial lining

Q7. The condition described often goes undiagnosed in a young woman for some time. Which of the following symptoms or signs is the earliest indication of this problem?
   a. tachycardia
   b. acute severe abdominal pain
   c. a vasovagal attack or a feeling of dizziness and lightheadedness, especially on assuming the upright position
   d. severe vaginal hemorrhage
   e. severe swelling and bloating of the abdomen

Q8. The diagnosis you suspected in the patient described in Case 1 is confirmed. Which of the following is (are) common signs or symptoms in this condition?
   a. abdominal pain
   b. irregular vaginal bleeding
   c. abdominal tenderness
   d. amenorrhea
   e. all of the above

Q9. What is (are) the major complication(s) of the condition described?
   a. intraabdominal hemorrhage
   b. hypovolemia and shock
   c. fetal death
   d. a and b
   e. all of the above

Q10. Which of the following is (are) documented risk factors for the condition described?
   a. endosalpingitis
   b. paratubal adhesions
   c. tubal ligation
   d. prolonged infertility
   e. all of the above

Q11. Which of the following organisms is (are) most closely associated with the condition described?
   a. *Bacteroides fragilis*
   b. *Klebsiella pneumoniae*
   c. *Escherichia coli*
   d. group A beta-hemolytic streptococcus
   e. all of the above

Q12. What is the medical treatment of choice for the condition described?
   a. intravenous estrogen
   b. oral (PO) estrogen
   c. PO progesterone
   d. intramuscular (IM) medroxyprogesterone acetate
   e. IM methotrexate

ANSWERS

A1. **c.** The most important diagnosis to exclude at this time in this patient is ectopic pregnancy. In a patient who is in the childbearing age group, any of the three As (amenorrhea, abdominal pain, and abnormal vaginal bleeding) should suggest the possibility of an ectopic pregnancy.

The differential diagnosis of ectopic pregnancy includes the following problems: spontaneous abortion, molar pregnancy, ruptured corpus luteum, acute PID, adnexal torsion, degenerating leiomyoma, PID, acute appendicitis, pyelonephritis, diverticulitis, regional ileitis, and ulcerative colitis.

A2. **d.** The most important question to ask at this time is for the patient to define for you the history of her last menstrual period. The patient, in fact, tells you that she missed her last menstrual period. Many women with an ectopic pregnancy will tell you that their menstrual period occurred at the regular time but that the flow volume was significantly less than normal. This, in anatomic pathologic terms, corresponds to the shedding of the uterine decidual tissue secondary to necrosis of the trophoblastic tissue.

A3. **a.** Based on this patient's history and physical examination, the probability of an ectopic pregnancy is very high. Therefore a qualitative serum or urine beta-HCG is the most important investigation to perform at this time. If the qualitative HCG is negative, ectopic pregnancy is ruled out. If the qualitative HCG is positive, it is vital to establish whether the pregnancy is intrauterine or extrauterine. This is accomplished by a combination of quantitative serum HCG and pelvic sonography.

The discriminatory threshold is the critical serum quantitative HCG titer above which a normal gestational sac should be seen in the uterus by sonography. The discriminatory threshold is 1500 mIU/ml when using transvaginal sonography or 6500 mIU/ml with abdominal sonography. Failure to find a gestational sac in the uterus when either of these thresholds is reached is presumptive evidence of an ectopic pregnancy.

If the serum HCG titer does not exceed the threshold and no intrauterine gestational sac is seen, it is impossible to differentiate a normal pregnancy from an ectopic pregnancy. Since the serum HCG titer should double in 48 hours, repeat the HCG titer and sonography every 2 days until the threshold is reached or an intrauterine pregnancy has been confirmed.

A4. **d.** There has been a marked increase in incidence, prevalence, and absolute number and rate of ectopic pregnancies in the United States over the past 2 decades. The actual number has increased out of proportion to the growth in the population; in fact, it has increased fivefold between 1970 and 1989. There is a marked increase in the rate of ectopic pregnancies with increasing age. Most ectopic pregnancies occur in multigravida women, with only 10% to 15% occurring in nulligravida women. Rates of ectopic pregnancies are up to 30% higher in nonwhite women.

A5. **d.** Ectopic pregnancy is the most common cause of maternal death in the first half of pregnancy. It is the most common single cause of all maternal deaths among black women. Overall, the risk of death from ectopic pregnancy is 10 times greater than the risk of childbearing and more than 50 times greater than the risk of legal abortion. The major cause of death from ectopic pregnancy is blood loss (88%), with infection (3%) and anesthesia complications (2%) much less common. Patient delay in consulting a physician after development of symptoms accounts for a third of the deaths, whereas treatment delay resulting from misdiagnosis contributes to half of the deaths. More than 50% of women died of hemorrhage without emergency surgery.

Although the diagnosis of ectopic pregnancy has increased over the past 20 years, the maternal mortality rate has decreased. The dramatic decrease in death rate from ectopic pregnancy is a result of improved diagnosis and treatment.

A6. **a.** The most frequent site of extrauterine implantation is the ampulla of the fallopian tube (78%) where most fertilizations occur. The isthmus of the fallopian tube is the next most common site of implantation (12%). Cornual pregnancies are uncommon, representing only 2% to 3% of the total. Abdominal, ovarian, and cervical pregnancies are rare.

A7. **c.** The signs and symptoms of this condition are discussed at length in a subsequent question. However, it is important to recognize the earlier signs and the earlier symptoms that will allow the diagnosis to be made before significant damage occurs or a major complication arises.

An early response to moderate intraabdominal hemorrhage may range from no change in pulse, blood pressure, or syncope to a slight rise in blood pressure, or a vasovagal response with bradycardia and hypotension. This can be manifested by any significant change in blood pressure that occurs upon assuming the upright position from a supine position. Thus either a vasovagal attack or significant difference in standing and supine blood pressures may indicate hypovolemia secondary to as-yet undetected bleeding into the abdominal cavity from an ectopic pregnancy that is rupturing.

A8. **e.** There are no absolutely pathognomonic signs or symptoms of an early ectopic pregnancy. The most common symptoms noted are the three As (abdominal pain, abnormal vaginal bleeding, and amenorrhea). Between 96% and 100% of patients with ectopic gestation complain of pain, even before rupture. No specific type of pain is diagnostic. With tubal rupture, the pain becomes more severe.

Amenorrhea or a history of abnormal menses is reported in 75% to 95% of patients with ectopic pregnancy. A careful history with respect to the character and timing of the last two or three menstrual cycles (amount of flow and number of days of flow) is important. Initially patients will often state that they have not missed a period; however, when questioned carefully, they may describe the period as being different (lighter than usual or irregular in timing). This bleeding may, in fact, represent bleeding from an endometrial slough. Profuse bleeding is uncommon.

Common symptoms of early pregnancy such as nausea and breast tenderness are present in only 10% to 25% of patients with ectopic pregnancies. Symptoms of dizziness and fainting (vasovagal symptoms as mentioned previously) are present in 20% to 35% of patients. A few patients will state that they, in fact, passed tissue (a decidual cast). Most patients are afebrile.

Abdominal tenderness is present in most patients (80% to 95%). Rebound tenderness may or may not be present. A mass is palpable in 50% of patients with ectopic pregnancy. If there is uterine enlargement, it is not to the degree that would be expected for the duration of amenorrhea.

A9. **d.** The major complications of ectopic pregnancy are intraabdominal hemorrhage, hypovolemia, and shock secondary to rupture. Rupture of the ectopic pregnancy is responsible for almost all maternal morbidity and mortality.

Fetal death cannot be classified as a major complication because of its inevitability in ectopic pregnancy.

A10. **e.** The following is a list of suggested risk factors.
  a. Previous salpingitis, especially endosalpingitis (8 times increased risk)

  b. Previous ectopic pregnancy (50% increased risk)
  c. Paratubal adhesions caused by postabortal, puerperal infection; appendicitis; endometriosis
  d. Tubal ligation (in the last 2 years)
  e. Tubal surgery
  f. Infertility
  g. Cigarette smoking

A11. **a.** *B. fragilis* and *Peptostreptococcus* are the anaerobic organisms that, in combination with *Neisseria gonorrhea* or *Chlamydia trachomatis,* are usually responsible for acute PID. Acute PID results in tubal adhesions, tubal scarring, and occlusion that subsequently increase the risk of ectopic pregnancy.

A12. **e.** The medical management of choice for ectopic pregnancy is IM methotrexate. Methotrexate is a folic acid antagonist that destroys rapidly growing tissue including chorionic villi. It does have the potential for serious toxicity. A single dose is successful in resolving 90% of ectopic pregnancies. Declining serum HCG titers indicate success. Failure of titers to decrease at least 15% by day 4 to 7 posttreatment indicates the need for an additional dose or surgery. The cumulative success rate is 95% with subsequent evidence of tubal patency in 80% and fertility in almost 70%. These rates are similar to those reported with treatment of unruptured tubal pregnancy by salpingostomy. Methotrexate is optimal for small, unruptured ectopic pregnancies and should be considered only if the following conditions apply:
  a. Early gestation (preferably <8 weeks)
  b. Patient desires future fertility
  c. Nonlaparoscopic diagnosis
  d. Patient is hemodynamically stable without signs of hemoperitoneum
  e. Patient has normal hemoglobin, liver function, and renal function
  f. Patient is able to return for follow-up care

SOLUTION TO THE SHORT ANSWER MANAGEMENT PROBLEM

The significant increase in incidence, prevalence, and the absolute number of ectopic pregnancies in the United States during the last 20 years, and the number of ectopic pregnancies out of proportion to the growth of the population appears to be the result of an increased risk and increased rate of sexually transmitted disease (STD), particularly acute PID and chronic PID. These STD increases are primarily caused by infection with two organisms: *N. gonorrhea* and *C. trachomatis.* Secondary bacterial invaders can be involved, including *B. fragilis* and *Peptostreptococcus.*

SUMMARY OF THE DIAGNOSIS AND TREATMENT OF ECTOPIC PREGNANCY

1. Prevalence rates per 1000 pregnancies (live births, legal abortions, and ectopic pregnancies): 1970, 4.5/1000 pregnancies; 1989, 16.0/1000 pregnancies. Increasing prevalence appears to be due to increasing prevalence of STDs, especially acute PID.

2. Pathogenesis: Major risk factors include previous ectopic pregnancy, acute or chronic PID with tubal scarring and tubal adhesions, and cigarette smoking.

3. Signs and symptoms:
   a. The three As: Abdominal pain, amenorrhea, abnormal vaginal bleeding indicate an ectopic pregnancy until proven otherwise.
   b. Vasovagal attacks and orthostatic hypotension are strong indicators of tubal rupture.

4. Major complications: Tubal rupture is indicated by intraabdominal hemorrhage or hypovolemia and shock.

5. Investigations if missed or abnormal menstrual period:
   a. Qualitative urine or serum beta-HCG; if positive, obtain quantitative serum HCG
   b. Transvaginal ultrasound looking for intrauterine gestational sac

6. Treatment:
   a. Medical management: Methotrexate should be used only in patients who are hemodynamically stable with a normal hemoglobin, normal liver function tests, and normal renal function.
   b. Surgical management: Laparotomy with:
      1) Salpingectomy
      2) Tubal sterilization
      3) Fallopian tube conservative surgery:
         a) Salpingostomy
         b) Segmental resection and anastomosis
         c) Fibril evacuation

SUGGESTED READINGS

American College of Obstetricians and Gynecologists Practice Bulletin: *Medical management of tubal pregnancy,* No. 3, 1998.
Cunningham FG et al, eds: *Williams obstetrics,* ed 19, Norwalk, Conn, 1993, Appleton & Lange.
Mishell DR et al: *Comprehensive gynecology,* St Louis, 1997, Mosby.

PROBLEM·58

MANAGEMENT OF CONTRACEPTION

"Doctor, I'll Just Die if I Have a Baby Now!"

Case 1 ■ A 23-Year-Old Hypertensive Female Requesting a Prescription for Oral Contraceptive Pills

A 23-year-old nulligravida comes to your office requesting oral contraceptive pills (OCPs). She states she has never had any major medical problems. She denies a history of liver disease, sexually transmitted diseases (STDs), migraine headaches, or estrogen-dependent neoplasia.

On examination, her blood pressure is 160/100 mm Hg (large cuff). Her weight is 220 pounds, and she is 5 feet, 5 inches tall. Other than obesity, her general examination is normal. Her pelvic examination is unremarkable. You perform a Papanicolaou (Pap) smear.

SELECT THE BEST ANSWER TO THE FOLLOWING QUESTIONS

Q1. What would you do at this time?
   a. prescribe OCPs and be done with it
   b. prescribe an amphetamine for weight reduction and see her in 1 month
   c. tell her to forget it; you are not interested in giving her the pill
   d. tell her that she is really far too overweight to take the pill
   e. none of the above

Q2. What would your next step be?
   a. obtain a more detailed history today and retake her blood pressure
   b. refer her to one of your partners who specializes in this area
   c. refer her to a rapid weight-loss center
   d. just give her the pill; the whole thing is not worth the trouble
   e. none of the above

Q3. You see the same patient the next week and her blood pressure is 150/105 mm Hg after 5 minutes of rest. What would you do at this time?
   a. give her OCPs
   b. give her a thiazide diuretic
   c. give her a stern lecture on the dangers of smoking
   d. start her on an 800-calorie diet
   e. none of the above

Q4. The patient returns in another week. Her blood pressure is 140/100 mm Hg. No other changes are

found (in either history or physical examination). At this time, what would you do?
a. start her on OCPs
b. ask her to consult your partner, who specializes in weight management
c. tell her to stop smoking
d. put in an intrauterine device (IUD)
e. none of the above

Q5. Which of the following is (are) side effects of OCPs?
a. headaches
b. nausea and vomiting
c. cervical ectopia
d. hepatocellular adenomas
e. all of the above

Q6. Which of the following cancers has (have) OCPs definitely been associated with (either increasing or decreasing the risk)?
a. ovarian carcinoma
b. breast carcinoma
c. cervical carcinoma
d. all of the above
e. none of the above

Q7. Which of the following statements regarding the relationship between OCPs and STDs is true?
a. OCPs protects against gonococcal infections
b. OCPs protect against chlamydial infections
c. OCPs protect against both gonococcal and chlamydial infections
d. OCPs protect against gonococcal infections but may enhance chlamydial infections
e. OCPs protect against chlamydial infections but may enhance gonococcal infections

---

Case 2 ■ A 21-Year-Old Female with Multiple Sexual Partners

A 21-year-old female comes to your office for OCPs. She is healthy, has had no major medical problems, and is a nonsmoker, a nondrinker, and an exercise enthusiast. She is not obese.

On examination, her blood pressure is 110/70 mm Hg. Her pulse is 72 and regular. General examination and pelvic examination are normal. Her Pap smears have been normal. She states she has multiple sexual partners.

Q8. What would you do at this time?
a. prescribe OCPs without further counseling
b. prescribe OCPs but advise her to limit sexual partners

c. prescribe OCPs but stress only condoms will protect against STDs
d. tell her to use condoms only since they will both protect against STDs and prevent pregnancy
e. none of the above

Case 3 ■ A 16-Year-Old Female Who Fears Pregnancy 4 Hours after Sexual Intercourse

A 16-year-old female comes to the Emergency Department at 4 AM. She had sexual intercourse at 12 AM and is absolutely frantic because she was not using any contraception. She asks for emergency contraception.

Q9. Which of the following are effective strategies for postcoital contraception?
a. 5 mg ethinyl estradiol for 5 days
b. 30 mg conjugated estrogens for 5 days
c. any estrogen-progestin OCP, four tablets immediately then repeated in 12 hours
d. 500 mg danazol immediately then repeated in 12 hours
e. all of the above

Q10. Of the following OCPs, which would be your first choice for a patient (all other things being equal)?
a. Loestrin 1/20 (20 mg ethinyl estradiol and norethindrone)
b. Low Ovral (30 mg ethinyl estradiol and levonorgestrel)
c. Ovral (50 mg ethinyl estradiol and levonorgestrel)
d. any of the above
e. none of the above

Case 4 ■ A 17-Year-Old Female Who Is Being Pressured by Her Boyfriend to Have Sexual Intercourse

A 17-year-old female comes to your office for a consultation. Her 18-year-old boyfriend has been pressuring her to have sex, but she is confused. On the one hand, she is scared that if she says no that the word will get around the school that she is a square. On the other hand, if she says yes, she believes that she will be violating herself.

Q11. Based on this information, what would be your next step in management?
a. refer her to a counselor who will help her deal with her ambivalence
b. assume a nondirective counseling approach reflecting her question back to her

c. tell her it is OK to say yes; just be careful
d. tell her it is OK to say no, especially in the age of STDs
e. refer her to her spiritual counselor

Q12. Which of the following statements regarding condoms is (are) true?
a. condoms prevent both unintended pregnancy and STDs
b. condoms are the most effective method for preventing human immunodeficiency virus (HIV) infection
c. condoms are the only reliable, readily reversible male method of contraception
d. condoms rarely break during vaginal intercourse
e. a, b, and c
f. all of the above

Q13. Which of the following statements regarding vaginal spermicides is (are) true?
a. vaginal spermicides must be used with the diaphragm, cervical cap, and the cervical sponge
b. vaginal spermicides reduce the risk of transmission of *Neisseria gonorrhea*
c. vaginal spermicides reduce the risk of transmission of *Chlamydia trachomatis*
d. vaginal spermicides reduce the risk of transmission of HIV infection
e. a and c
f. a, b, and c
g. all of the above

Q14. Which of the following are noncontraceptive health benefits of OCPs?
a. decreased risk of benign breast changes
b. decreased rate of ectopic pregnancy
c. decreased incidence of iron-deficiency anemia
d. decreased incidence of endometrial carcinoma
e. all of the above

Q15. Which of the following statements concerning the use of the diaphragm, cervical cap, and cervical sponge is (are) true? It has been definitely established that:
a. they are simple and noninvasive
b. they reduce the risk of transmission of gonorrhea
c. they reduce the risk of transmission of chlamydia
d. they reduce the risk of transmission of HIV
e. a, b, and c
f. all of the above

Q16. Which of the following statements concerning the use of OCPs during lactation is (are) true?
a. the very low-dose, combined OCPs can be used in lactation
b. the estrogen in the low-dose combined OCPs may decrease breast milk production
c. a small amount of estrogen in the low-dose combined OCPs does enter the breast milk
d. all of the above are true
e. none of the above is true

Q17. The long-acting intramuscular hormonal contraceptive approved by the Food and Drug Administration in the United States is which of the following?
a. Danazol
b. Bromocriptine
c. Depo-Provera
d. Depo-Premarin
e. Norplant

Q18. The major indication for the use of the minipill is a woman:
a. who only wishes to expose her body to one hormone
b. who wants to take the lowest possible dose of contraceptive
c. who has no intention of staying on the pill for a long time
d. who has relative or absolute contraindications to the estrogen component of the combined OCP
e. in whom the combination OCPs failed

Case 5 ■ A 22-Year-Old Para 2, Gravida 2 Female Who Does Not Want to Get Pregnant Again

A 22-year-old woman (para 2, gravida 2) has a history of thrombophlebitis during her last pregnancy. She is sure that she does not want to go through another pregnancy for at least 4 years (and perhaps ever).

Q19. Which of the following contraceptives should she be placed on?
a. Depo-Provera
b. Norplant
c. a combined OCP
d. the minipill
e. a or b

Q20. Which of the following medications may interact with the combined OCPs to decrease its efficacy?
a. phenytoin
b. rifampin

c. diazepam
d. amitriptyline
e. all of the above

SHORT ANSWER MANAGEMENT PROBLEM
Part A: List the contraindications to the insertion of an IUD.
Part B: Discuss the advantages and disadvantages of permanent female sterilization.
Part C: Discuss the advantages and disadvantages of permanent male sterilization.

ANSWERS

A1. **e.** At this point, you need to obtain more specific and detailed information on the following problems you have identified:
a. Morbid obesity
b. Elevated blood pressure reading
c. Nicotine addiction
d. No stated reason for OCP use at this time
e. No discussion about STDs

A2. **a.** It is important to obtain a more complete history before she leaves the office today and to focus on some of these major questions:
a. Is she sexually active at this time?
b. If yes, how many current sexual partners does she have?
c. How many lifetime sexual partners has she had?
d. Is she planning to use condoms as well as OCPs?
e. Has she ever tried to stop smoking?
f. Does she want to quit smoking?
g. Has she ever tried to lose weight?
h. Does she want to lose weight?
At the same time, you can recheck her blood pressure under the following conditions:
a. Left arm, supine after 5 minutes of rest
b. Large blood pressure cuff (or leg cuff)

A3. **e.** This patient still cannot be labeled as hypertensive; she has only two readings that are elevated and that are separated by 1 week.

It is reasonable to begin discussing a smoking cessation regimen, modifying food intake, or initiating an exercise program. It would not be appropriate to take on all three at the same time. In addition, the patient needs to have one more blood pressure readings taken at least 1 week from now.

A4. **e.** This patient has one relative contraindication to OCPs (heavy smoking), but she also has risk factors for thrombophlebitis, pulmonary emboli, and other cardiovascular diseases (heavy smoking, obesity, and hypertension).

Considering the risk/benefit ratio in this patient, a contraceptive method other than OCPs might be preferable.

A5. **e.** Clinicians can enhance their patients' contraceptive success by fully discussing side effects with them before initiating OCPs, then managing these side effects as they occur. The following is a partial list of possible side effects:
a. Unwanted menstrual cycle changes: Intermenstrual, or breakthrough, spotting and bleeding occur in 25% of OCP users during the first 3 months of use but decrease over time. This can result from insufficient estrogen, excess progestin, or both.
b. Nausea and vomiting: Nausea may occur in the first cycle or so of OCP use but seldom continues. This is an estrogen-induced effect.
c. Headaches: These are occasionally reported by OCP users. Tensions headaches are not related to OCP use. The effect of OCPs on migraine headaches is variable. Women experiencing classic migraines should use another form of contraception.
d. Hypertension: Mild elevation of blood pressure may occur but is usually reversible. This tends to be an estrogen-induced effect.
e. STDs: See Answer 7.
f. Thrombophlebitis, pulmonary emboli, and stroke: These life-threatening conditions are increased in: heavy smokers, obese women over age 40, women who are hypertensive, and women who are diabetics. Since the risk rises in direct relationship to increasing estrogen doses, the lowest doses of estrogens should be prescribed. A history of OCP use does not increase the risk of cardiovascular disease.
g. Glucose intolerance: This is related to the dose, potency, and chemical structure of the progestin component. The mechanism appears to induce insulin resistance.
h. Gallbladder disease: The formation of gallstones does not appear to be increased by OCP use, but the growth of existing gallstones may be augmented.
i. Lipid profile: Estrogens and progestins have opposite effects on the lipid profile. The estrogen component of OCPs causes an increase in high-density lipoprotein (HDL) cholesterol, a decrease in low-density lipoprotein (LDL) cholesterol, and an increase in total cholesterol and triglycerides. The progestin component causes a decrease in HDL cholesterol, an increase in LDL

cholesterol, and a decrease in total cholesterol and triglycerides. Older OCP formulations with high progestin doses, had adverse effects on the lipid profile. With current low-dose formulations the estrogen and progestins offset each other so LDL, HDL, and total cholesterol levels are unchanged. However, triglycerides are raised.

j. Hepatocellular adenomas: Although benign hepatocellular adenomas can be produced by the estrogen component of OCPs, they have become rare since the advent of low-dose OCPs. There is no relationship between OCPs and liver cancer.

A6. **a.** There is no convincing evidence that OCPs lead to an increase in any type of cancer, including cervical and breast cancer. Conflicting findings of epidemiologic studies regarding OCPs and cervical cancer may be attributed to several potential biases, for which these studies have not been consistently controlled. A history of cervical intraepithelial neoplasia does not contraindicate the use of hormonal contraception.

Numerous metaanalyses have looked at the relationship between OCPs and breast cancer. There is no demonstrable increase of breast cancer in current users or in past users.

There is, however, convincing evidence that OCPs lead to a decrease in the incidence of ovarian carcinoma (by decreasing the number of ovulatory disruptions of the ovarian capsule) and endometrial carcinoma (by increasing the duration of endometrial exposure to progestins).

A7. **d.** OCPs protect against gonococcal infections but may actually enhance chlamydial infections. Chlamydial cervicitis is 2 to 3 times more common in women taking OCPs. OCPs are associated with cervical ectropion, a broadening of the area on the ectocervix covered by the mucus-secreting columnar cell that normally lines the cervical canal. It is theorized that the area of ectropion of OCP users may be more vulnerable to *C. trachomatis* infection. Although the prevalence of lower genital tract chlamydial infection (cervicitis) is increased, the risk of upper genital tract chlamydial infection (acute pelvic inflammatory disease [PID]) is decreased by two thirds.

A8. **c.** This is a very common scenario and one that is frequently mismanaged. What ends up happening in a lot of cases is that the patient is simply given a prescription for OCPs and allowed to leave the office without the benefit of either contraceptive counseling or STD counseling. Although you may argue that telling the patient to use condoms only would be a better choice, it would not. This patient has specifically re-

quested OCPs, and it is reasonable to give OCPs to her once you have done the following:
   a. Counseled her regarding the possible side effects of OCPs
   b. Counseled her regarding the risks and benefits of OCPs
   c. Counseled her about safe sexual practices
   d. Counseled her about the importance of always using condoms along with OCPs to protect against STDs in her present situation (multiple sexual partners).

A9. **e.** A wide variety of agents are successful postcoital treatments for preventing pregnancy. The most effective method is high-dose estrogen (ethinyl estradiol or conjugated estrogen) for 5 days with a failure rate of 1%. The most widely used is four tablets of combination OCPs taken in two doses 12 hours apart with a failure rate of 2%. Nausea and vomiting occur in such high rates with the estrogenic medications that prophylactic antiemetics should be prescribed. The antiestrogen, danazol, in two doses 12 hours apart, has a failure rate of 2% but causes less nausea and vomiting. Placement of a copper IUD has a failure rate of less than 1%, but cost considerations as well as concerns regarding infection have limited this use. Mifepristone, administered as a single 600-mg dose, is as effective as OCPs. With all these methods, intervention should occur within 72 hours of the sexual exposure.

A10. **a.** The OCP with the lowest estrogen content would be the OCP of choice from those listed. There are so many OCPs on the market that it is a good idea for a physician to become accustomed to using two or three of them and using them well. There are biphasic pills and triphasic pills; there are progestin-only pills and there are pills that vary in both the content of estrogen and progesterone and the particular progesterone.

As general rules in prescribing OCPs you should ask yourself the following questions: Can this individual be prescribed an OCP with estrogen? If yes, then consider the following factors in your decision:
   a. The number of micrograms of ethinyl estradiol
   b. The availability of that particular OCP
   c. Ease of remaining on the schedule imposed by that particular OCP
   d. Price of pills to the clinic
   e. Price of pills to the patient
   f. Prior experience of this woman or the clinician caring for this woman with a special pill
If estrogens are contraindicated, then consider the following:
   a. Progestin-only preparation: the mini-pill, Depo-Provera, or Norplant
   b. IUD

c. Condoms
d. Diaphragm, cervical cap
e. Foam
f. Cervical sponge

A11. **d.** Initiation of sexual activity is a very personal decision and should not take place as a result of coercion. One sign of an unhealthy relationship is when one partner seeks to exploit or manipulate the other partner. This case is an example of such a relationship. The young woman can benefit from your giving her permission to say "No" to a sexual relationship she is not ready for.

A12. **f.** The following are facts concerning condoms:
a. Unlike nonbarrier contraceptives, condoms, if used consistently and correctly, prevent both unintended pregnancy and sexually transmitted infection.
b. When used consistently and correctly, condoms are the most effective method for preventing HIV infection.
c. Condoms can be used with other contraceptives when STDs are a concern. Other more effective contraceptives such as sterilization, OCPs, Norplant implants, Depo-Provera, and IUDs do not prevent HIV infection or other STDs.
d. Except for coitus interruptus, condoms are the only readily reversible method of birth control for men.
e. Condoms rarely break during vaginal intercourse. Further, not every broken condom results in pregnancy or infection.
f. The provision of condoms in large numbers at a low or no cost and the promotion of positive images of condoms need to become major public health priorities.

A13. **f.** Vaginal spermicides have the following important qualities:
a. Vaginal spermicides are simple, free of systemic side effects, available without a prescription, and can be used intermittently, with little planning needed.
b. Vaginal spermicides are an integral component of vaginal barrier methods, including the cervical diaphragm, the cervical sponge, and the cervical cap.
c. Vaginal spermicides reduce the transmission of important STDs including *N. gonorrhea* and *C. trachomatis.*
d. Vaginal spermicides have been shown to inactivate HIV *in vitro,* but data are unclear *in vivo.* They should not be relied upon to prevent HIV. Condoms are more reliable for prevention of HIV transmission.

A14. **e.** OCPs are effective in reducing the risk of the following:
a. Carcinoma of the endometrium (discussed earlier)
b. Carcinoma of the ovary (discussed earlier)
c. Benign fibrocystic breast changes
d. Iron-deficiency anemia (due to a significant decrease in blood loss during menstruation)
e. Reduced incidence of gonorrhea
f. Reduced incidence of ectopic pregnancy

A15. **e.** The following are true of diaphragms, caps, and sponges (DCS):
a. They are simple to use and noninvasive.
b. Women who use a DCS method have reduced rates of gonorrhea, chlamydia, ectopic pregnancy, and the serious sequelae of PID.
c. Regarding the impact of DCS methods on HIV risk of transmission, abstinence is the safest choice, and using latex condoms can reduce the risk.
d. Unlike male condoms or spermicide, a woman can use a vaginal barrier without the direct cooperation of her partner. Correct use does not require an interruption in lovemaking.
e. Consistent and correct use is essential for success with vaginal barrier methods; most failures occur because the method is not used.

A16. **d.** Although safety is not a problem, it is not recommended that lactating women use low-dose combination OCPs because milk production can be suppressed because of the estrogen component. This is primarily a concern in the initiation of breastfeeding. There is no concern regarding infant safety, since only a small amount of ethinyl estradiol is passed through the breast milk to the baby. However, it may decrease breast milk production.

A17. **c.** The long-acting progestin approved for intramuscular use is depot-medroxyprogesterone acetate (DMPA) [Depo-Provera]. A deep intramuscular injection of 150 mg of DMPA will reliably prevent pregnancy for at least 14 weeks, giving a 2-week grace period for women receiving injections every 3 months. The failure rate is one of the lowest of all contraceptive methods at 0.3/100 woman-years, similar to surgical sterilization and subcutaneous implants. Although use of DMPA does not permanently suppress fertility, return of fertility may be delayed up to 18 months. Depo-Provera acts by a number of mechanisms: its primary action is to inhibit ovulation, but it also changes cervical mucus so it is hostile to sperm passage and induces endometrial atrophy. No fetal anomalies have been confirmed if pregnancy occurs while on DMPA. It has been associated with hematologic improvement in women with sickle cell disease and reduced seizure frequency in women with seizure disorders. Persistent irregular bleeding is the main reason for discontinuance of DMPA. A reversible reduction in bone density has been reported in DMPA users.

A18. **d.** The major indication for the Progestin-only pill (e.g., Norethindrone or Norge-sterol) is for patients who have either an absolute or a relative contraindication to the estrogen component of the combined OCP. Most of the health benefits of progestin-only pills are similar to the combined OCPs. The mini-pill has the advantage of being immediately reversible. The mechanism of action of the mini-pill is primarily on producing a hostile cervical mucus and less by suppression of ovulation. Because the effect of the progestin on the cervical mucus does not last much more than 24 hours, the mini-pill must be taken as close to possible the same time each day.

A19. **e.** The risk of thrombosis appears to be related to the estrogen component. Thus this patient should avoid the combination OCPs, and rather select a progestin-only method. Since the patient has indicated she wants to defer pregnancy for a prolonged period, the two choices that make the most sense are Norplant (a long-acting subcutaneous implant contraceptive that prevents pregnancy for up to 5 years) and Depo-Provera. Although the mini-pill could be used, the need to remember the pill each day may be a drawback.

A20. **e.** Medications that are known to interact with OCPs with a potential to decrease their efficacy can be divided into the following categories:
   a. The anticonvulsants: phenobarbital, carbamazepine, primidone, phenytoin, and ethosuximide.
   b. Lipid agents: some lipid-lowering drugs (especially Clofibrate)
   c. The antibiotics: rifampin, isoniazid, penicillin, ampicillin, metronidazole, tetracycline, neomycin, chloramphenicol, sulfonamides, and nitrofurantoin
   d. Sedatives, hypnotics, tricyclic antidepressants, and antipsychotics

SOLUTION TO THE SHORT ANSWER MANAGEMENT PROBLEM

Part A: Contraindications to the insertion of an IUD are as follows:
   a. Absolute contraindications:
      1) Confirmed or suspected pregnancy
      2) Known or suspected pelvic malignancy
      3) Undiagnosed vaginal bleeding
      4) Known or suspected pelvic infection, acute or chronic, including STDs and genital actinomycosis
      5) Reported behaviors placing an individual at high risk for STDs
      6) Hyperbilirubinemia secondary to Wilson disease (only true for copper IUDs)
   b. Relative contraindications:
      1) Uterine size or shape incompatible with effective IUD use
      2) Medical conditions (e.g., corticosteroid therapy, valvular heart disease, and any incidence of immune suppression) increasing the risk of infection
      3) Nulligravidity
      4) Abnormal Pap smear (until managed)
      5) History of ectopic pregnancy

Part B: The advantages and disadvantages of female sterilization are as follows:
   a. Advantages:
      1) Permanent
      2) Highly effective
      3) Inexpensive in the long run
      4) Decreased risk of ovarian cancer and acute PID
      5) Partner compliance not required
      6) No interruption in lovemaking
   b. Disadvantages and cautions:
      1) Reversibility difficult and expensive
      2) Requires surgeon, operating room (aseptic conditions), trained assistants, medications, surgical equipment
      3) Expensive at the time performed
      4) Morbidity and mortality high when considered for 1 year
      5) Regret can occur if: age less than 30, medically indicated procedure, recent emotional trauma (e.g., divorce, death, or sickness), coercion from spouse or family
      6) If sterilization fails, ectopic pregnancy is a risk
      7) No protection from STDs, including HIV

Part C: The advantages and disadvantages of male sterilization are as follows:
   a. Advantages:
      1) Permanent
      2) Highly effective
      3) Inexpensive in the long run
      4) Safe
      5) Quickly performed as an outpatient procedure
   b. Disadvantages:
      1) Reversibility difficult and expensive (requires a surgeon, aseptic conditions, medications, and technical assistance)

2) Expensive at the time performed
3) Regret in 5% to 10% of patients
4) No protection against STDs, including HIV
c. Comments:
  1) Sperm antibodies develop in 50% to 66% of all men who undergo a vasectomy; no consistent relationship found between sperm antibodies and atherosclerotic vascular disease
  2) No consistent relationship found between vasectomy and prostate cancer

SUMMARY OF THE MANAGEMENT OF CONTRACEPTION

1. First things first:
   a. History and physical examination
   b. When a patient presents with requests for contraception, the physician must consider not only the prevention of pregnancy, but also the protection against STDs.

2. OCPs:
   a. For OCP users: Use OCP and a barrier method.
   b. Consider relative and absolute contraindications; also consider whether or not the risks outweigh the benefits.
   c. Use the lowest estrogen dose possible when using OCPs.
   d. Considerations that should be taken seriously:
      1) Smoking
      2) Obesity
      3) Hypertension
   e. Learn to use two or three OCPs well
   f. A low-dose combination OCP may be used in lactation but may decrease milk production.
   g. The combination OCP is protective against ovarian cancer and endometrial cancer.
   h. The combination OCP is protective against benign breast changes. It has no effect on the incidence of breast cancer.

3. Barrier methods:
   a. Condoms (male and female)
   b. Cervical cap
   c. Contraceptive diaphragm
   d. Vaginal sponge

4. Abstinence: This is a reasonable and acceptable option, particularly in younger patients.

5. IUD:
   a. Efficacy: High
   b. 98% of IUD users say they are happy with this method, and 60% of women with IUDs are repeat users.

c. The Cu T380 A (ParaGuard) offers 10 years of very effective protection, with only about 2% of women becoming pregnant within the first year of use.

6. Progesterone-containing contraceptives: Main indication is a contraindication to the estrogen component of combined OCPs.
   a. The minipill
   b. Depo-Provera
   c. Norplant

7. Permanent sterilization:
   a. Female sterilization
   b. Male sterilization

SUGGESTED READINGS

Hatcher R et al: *Contraceptive technology,* ed 17, New York, 1998, Ardent Media.
Mishell DR et al: *Comprehensive gynecology,* St Louis, 1997, Mosby.

PROBLEM · 5 9

SEXUALLY TRANSMITTED DISEASE

"We Had a Great Time, Honey, but That's Your Problem Now."

Case 1 ■ A 24-Year-Old Female with Abdominal Pain, Pelvic Pain, and Adnexal Tenderness

A 24-year-old female comes to the Emergency Room with a 2-day history of lower abdominal pain, pelvic pain, fever, chills, and malaise. Associated with these symptoms, the patient has also felt nauseated for the last 48 hours and has vomited twice.

On physical examination, there is bilateral adnexal tenderness, bilateral lower abdominal tenderness, and tenderness on cervical motion.

The patient has a temperature of 40° C. Her last menstrual period was 5 weeks ago, but she has had a small amount of spotting during the last few days. She had one previous episode of these symptoms 15 months ago.

SELECT THE BEST ANSWER TO THE FOLLOWING QUESTIONS

Q1. What is the most likely diagnosis in this patient?
   a. acute appendicitis
   b. chronic salpingitis
   c. acute salpingitis
   d. ectopic pregnancy
   e. endometritis

Q2. Which of the following statements regarding the relationship between oral contraceptive pills (OCPs) and the disease described is true?
   a. OCPs protect against all forms of this condition
   b. OCPs protect against one form of this condition but not another
   c. OCPs protect against none of the forms of this condition
   d. OCPs have nothing to do with this condition
   e. nobody really knows for sure

Q3. Which of the following organisms is not associated with this condition?
   a. *Neisseria gonorrhea*
   b. *Chlamydia trachomatis*
   c. *Mycoplasma hominis*
   d. peptostreptococcus
   e. beta-hemolytic streptococcus

Q4. Which of the following is not a risk factor for this condition?
   a. age <25 years
   b. multiple sexual partners
   c. a barrier contraceptive method
   d. a history of previous episodes of the same condition
   e. time of the last menstrual period

Q5. What is the most appropriate intervention and treatment of this patient?
   a. hospitalize the patient and begin treatment
   b. begin treatment as an outpatient, but recheck the patient's condition within 24 hours
   c. begin treatment as an outpatient and make an appointment for her to see a gynecologist
   d. begin treatment as an outpatient but recheck her if the condition worsens
   e. nobody really knows for sure

Q6. If hospital management was chosen for this patient, which of the following treatment options would be the most appropriate first-line treatment?
   a. intravenous (IV) ampicillin and gentamycin
   b. IV cefoxitin and doxycycline
   c. IV ampicillin and tobramycin
   d. IV ciprofloxacin
   e. IV ampicillin

Q7. If outpatient management was chosen for this patient, which of the following treatment regimens would be the most appropriate first-line treatment?
   a. oral (PO) cefoxitin, probenecid, and doxycycline

   b. intramuscular (IM) ceftriaxone, PO probenecid, and PO doxycycline
   c. IM aqueous procaine penicillin G, PO probenecid, and PO doxycycline
   d. any of the above
   e. none of the above

Q8. What is the current United States Public Health Service recommendation for the treatment of uncomplicated genital, rectal, or pharyngeal gonococcal infection?
   a. PO ampicillin and PO probenecid
   b. PO ciprofloxacin
   c. IM ceftriaxone followed by PO doxycycline
   d. PO cefixime followed by PO doxycycline
   e. c or d

Case 2 ■ A 24-Year-Old Male with a Mucoid Urethral Discharge

A 24-year-old male comes to your office with a mucoid urethral discharge. This was preceded by a 2-day history of urgency and frequency. He has no other symptoms.

Q9. What is the most likely diagnosis in this patient?
   a. gonorrhea
   b. acute prostatitis
   c. epididymitis
   d. nongonococcal urethritis (NGU)
   e. bacterial cystitis

Q10. What is the most likely organism causing the condition described in Case 2?
   a. *C. trachomatis*
   b. *Ureaplasma urealyticum*
   c. *Trichomonas vaginalis*
   d. *N. gonorrhea*
   e. nobody really knows for sure

Q11. What is the treatment of first choice for the probable condition described in Case 2?
   a. PO ciprofloxacin
   b. PO doxycycline
   c. PO erythromycin
   d. PO ampicillin and PO probenecid
   e. none of the above

Q12. Which of the following statements regarding *N. gonorrhea* infections is (are) false?
   a. the spectrum of illness caused by *N. gonorrhea* ranges from uncomplicated urethritis to septicemia

b. a Gram stain of a tissue or secretion sample with *N. gonorrhea* infection will show gram-positive intracellular diplococci
c. many *N. gonorrhea* strains have become resistant to penicillin
d. many *N. gonorrhea* strains have become resistant to tetracycline
e. all of the above statements are false

Q13. Many patients presenting with gonococcal genital infections have concomitant infections with *C. trachomatis.* To what percentage of patients does this statement apply?
a. 10%
b. 20%
c. 45%
d. 30%
e. 25%

Q14. Which of the following is (are) a common symptom(s) of *N. gonorrhea* in males?
a. dysuria
b. increased frequency
c. greater urgency
d. a and b
e. all of the above

Q15. Which of the following is (are) a complication(s) of disseminated gonococcal infection (DGI)?
a. arthritis
b. tenosynovitis
c. bacteremia
d. b and c only
e. all of the above

Case 3 ■ A 24-Year-Old Male with a Mucoid Urethral Discharge and a History of Greater Urgency and Frequency

A 24-year-old male comes to your office with a mucoid urethral discharge. This was preceded by a 2-day history of greater urgency and frequency. He has had no other symptoms. He has no previous history of sexually transmitted diseases (STDs).

Q16. What is the most likely diagnosis in this patient?
a. *C. trachomatis* urethritis
b. *N. gonorrhea* urethritis
c. nonspecific urethritis
d. *Escherichia coli* urethritis
e. none of the above

Case 4 ■ A 24-Year-Old Female with Dysuria and Painful Genital Lesions

A 24-year-old female comes to your office with a 2-day history of dysuria accompanied by painful genital lesions that have coalesced to form ulcers. The patient also describes systemic symptoms including fever, malaise, myalgias, and headache. There is no previous history of this condition.

Q17. Which of the following statements concerning the patient described in Case 4 is false?
a. the most likely diagnosis is herpes simplex type 2
b. this patient is unlikely to experience a recurrence of these symptoms at a later date
c. the duration of viral shedding may be reduced by treatment with acyclovir
d. the time to heal these lesions may be reduced by treatment with acyclovir
e. severe or frequent recurrences can be treated by the administration of acyclovir prophylactically

---

Case 5 ■ A 25-Year-Old Female with Vulvar "Growths"

A 25-year-old female comes to your office with a 2-week history of "growths" in the vulvar region. On examination, you find multiple verrucous lesions on the labia majora and the labia minora.

Q18. What is the most likely diagnosis in this patient?
a. condyloma lata
b. condyloma acuminatum
c. herpes simplex type 1
d. herpes simplex type 2
e. none of the above

Q19. What is the treatment of choice for the patient described in Case 5?
a. podophyllin in benzoin
b. trichloracetic acid
c. carbon dioxide laser
d. 5-fluorouracil cream
e. acyclovir

Q20. Which of the following statements regarding syphilis is true?
a. *Treponema pallidum,* the causative organism, is becoming resistant to penicillin
b. Syphilis has become an uncommon STD
c. Treatment of syphilis with ceftriaxone and doxycycline is ineffective

d. The Jarisch-Herxheimer reaction is a very common reaction in patients with syphilis who are effectively treated with antibiotics

e. none of the above statements is true

Q21. What is the treatment of choice for primary or secondary syphilis?

a. IM benzathine penicillin G

b. PO ciprofloxacin

c. IM ceftriaxone

d. PO trimethoprim-sulfamethoxazole (TMP-SMX)

e. PO tetracycline

Case 6 ■ A 17-Year-Old Male with a Mucoid Urethral Discharge

A 17-year-old male comes to your office with a mucoid urethral discharge for 3 days. He claims to only have had one sexual encounter in his life with a very sweet young girl that he met 2 weeks ago at a school dance. His symptoms include associated dysuria and increased frequency and urgency. You decide to treat him with oral thymidine monophosphate-sulfamethoxazole.

He returns in 3 days with a tender scrotum, with scrotal skin that is red, warm, and tense, and with partial obstruction of the rugal folds. The upper part of the scrotal structure appears to be acutely tender.

Q22. What is the most likely diagnosis at this time?

a. *C. trachomatis* urethritis with complicating orchitis

b. *C. trachomatis* urethritis with complicating epididymitis

c. *E. coli* epididymitis

d. *E. coli* orchitis

e. *M. hominis* urethritis with complicating epididymitis

Q23. What is the treatment of choice for the patient just described?

a. PO doxycycline

b. PO thymidine monophosphate

c. PO ampicillin and probenecid

d. IM benzathine penicillin G

e. IM ceftriaxone

SHORT ANSWER MANAGEMENT PROBLEM
List the risk factors and the complications of acute pelvic inflammatory disease (PID) in women.

ANSWERS

A1. **c.** This patient meets the clinical diagnostic criteria for acute salpingitis which are: (1) abdominal direct tenderness (with or without rebound tenderness), tenderness with motion of cervix and uterus, and adnexal tenderness and (2) elevated temperature, elevated white blood cell count or erythrocyte sedimentation rate (ESR), positive culdocentesis, an inflammatory mass on pelvic examination or sonography, or a positive Gram stain or smear.

The differential diagnosis of acute PID includes disorders of any of the three organ systems within the pelvis: (1) reproductive tract (adnexal torsion, ectopic pregnancy, bleeding corpus luteum, and endometriosis), (2) gastrointestinal tract (appendicitis, diverticulitis, regional ileitis, and ulcerative colitis), and (3) urinary tract (cystourethritis and pyelonephritis).

The patient described in Case 1, however, is more likely to have acute salpingitis than any other diagnosis. Although the patient has had one previous episode of these symptoms, a diagnosis of chronic salpingitis cannot be made without laparoscopy. An infection confined to the endometrium (endometritis) is unlikely in this patient. The adnexal tenderness is much more comparable with acute salpingitis. Endometritis usually occurs postpartum (retained products of conception) or after a procedure such as a suction dilatation and curettage for therapeutic abortion.

A2. **b.** OCPs protect against gonococcal PID. The incidence of genital tract infection with *C. trachomatis* infection in the lower reproductive tract may actually be increased when taking OCPs. However, upper reproductive tract disease, such as acute salpingitis, does not appear to be increased by the use of OCPs.

The protective effect against gonococcus may be associated with a decreased average amount of menstrual blood flow, with menstrual blood acting as a culture medium; a decreased permeability of cervical mucus to the infective organism; a decreased cervical dilatation at mid-cycle and menstruation; and a decrease in the strength of uterine contractions.

A3. **e.** The most common organisms associated with acute PID are *N. gonorrhea* and *C. trachomatis*. *M. hominis* is rarely involved. Many episodes of PID are polymicrobial and involve anaerobic organisms such as *Bacteroides fragilis* and peptostreptococcus, in addition to the two most common organisms, *N. gonorrhea* and *C. trachomatis*. Beta-hemolytic streptococcus (the streptococcus associated with bacterial pharyngitis) is not associated with acute PID.

A4. **c.** Barrier contraceptive methods (such as a condom or diaphragm) are protective against, rather than contributory to, acute PID. Risk factors for acute PID include age (<25 years), multiple sexual partners, nonbarrier contraceptive methods (especially the intrauterine device [IUD]), time of the last menstrual period (the closer the time of onset to the last menstrual period, the greater the risk), a history of a previous episode of documented PID, and symptoms of urethritis in a sexual partner.

A5. **a.** Early treatment of acute PID decreases the probability of tubal scarring and subsequent infertility. The incidence of infertility is 15% after one episode of untreated or inadequately treated PID. Most cases of PID can be treated on an outpatient basis. However, the Centers for Disease Control and Prevention recommends aggressive management, including hospitalization and inpatient treatment for the following criteria:
 a. All nulliparous women
 b. Presence of tuboovarian complex or abscess
 c. All adolescents (compliance with therapy unpredictable)
 d. Concurrent HIV infection
 e. Uncertain diagnosis
 f. Gastrointestinal symptoms
 g. Peritonitis in upper quadrants
 h. Presence of an IUD
 i. History of operative or diagnostic procedures
 j. Inadequate response to outpatient therapy

A6. **b.** The recommended regimen for inpatient management of PID is one of the two following regimens:
 a. Cefoxitin (Mefoxin), 2.0 g IV q6h or cefotetan (Cefotan), 2 g IV q12h and doxycycline, 100 mg q12h PO or IV. This regimen is given for at least 48 hours after the patient improves clinically. After discharge from the hospital, continuation of doxycycline, 100 mg PO bid for a total of 10 to 14 days.
 b. Clindamycin (Cleocin), 900 mg IV q8h, and gentamicin (Garamycin) loading dose IV or IM (2 mg/kg) followed by a maintenance dose (1.5 mg/kg) q8h. This regimen is given for at least 48 hours after the patient improves clinically. After discharge from the hospital, continuation of doxycycline, 100 mg PO bid for 10 to 14 days.

A7. **b.** The recommended treatment regime for patients treated on an outpatient basis includes the following:
 a. IM ceftriaxone 250 mg
 b. PO probenecid
 c. PO doxycycline
The probenecid can be given as a one-time dose (250 g); the doxycycline should continue for 14 days (100 mg PO bid).

A8. **e.** The preferred treatment of uncomplicated adult gonococcal urethritis, adult gonococcal cervicitis, and adult gonococcal proctitis is:
 a. Ceftriaxone 250 mg IM or Cefixime 400 mg PO once
 b. Doxycycline 100 mg PO bid for 7 days

A9. **d.** The most likely diagnosis in this patient is NGU.

A10. **a.** The most likely organism causing this condition is *C. trachomatis.*
 Symptoms in men include dysuria, frequency, and mucoid to purulent urethral discharge. Some men have asymptomatic infections. Female sexual partners of men with *C. trachomatis* NGU are likely to have a mucopurulent discharge. Next in order of frequent causative agents to *C. trachomatis* for NGU is *Ureaplasma urealyticum.*
 Men with typical clinical symptoms are presumed to have NGU when their urethral (gram-stained) smear shows WBCs with no gram-negative diplococci or their rapid antigen-detection test is positive. In addition, cultures for *N. gonorrhea* should confirm the absence of this organism.

A11. **b.** The recommended regimen for treating uncomplicated urethral *C. trachomatis* infections is doxycycline, 100 mg PO bid for 7 days. A good substitute is tetracycline 500 mg PO qid for 7 days. In addition, it is imperative that all recent sexual contacts be treated.
 Alternative regimens include erythromycin base 250 mg PO qid for 7 days or erythromycin ethylsuccinate 400 mg PO qid for 7 days. If erythromycin is not tolerated, sulfisoxazole 500 mg PO qid for 10 days may be effective.
 A recent controlled trial of a single dose of azithromycin for the treatment of chlamydial urethritis has been shown to be as effective as a 7-day course of doxycycline.

A12. **b.** *N. gonorrhea* has become, in many parts of the world, resistant to both penicillin and tetracycline. Thus, even in areas where there is a relatively low incidence of antibiotic-resistant gonorrhea, the treatment of choice has become ceftriaxone 250 mg IM or cefixime 400 mg PO once.
 The spectrum of disease created by *N. gonorrhea* ranges from a mild urethritis to septicemia with many systemic complications, including septicemia and arthritis.
 The Gram stain of a WBC containing *N. gonorrhea* shows gram-negative intracellular diplococci, not gram-positive intracellular diplococci.

A13. **c.** As many as 45% of patients with gonococcal genital infection have concomitant infection with *C. trachomatis.* Because current diagnostic tests for chlamydial infection do not permit a timely or reliable diagnosis, patients should be treated presumptively for that organism as well as for gonococcus. Sexual partners of infected patients should be evaluated, have cultures taken, and be treated presumptively for gonococcal and chlamydial infection, regardless of their symptom status.

A14. **e.** *N. gonorrhea* in males may produce dysuria, frequency, and urgency.

A15. **e.** Gonococcal arthritis-dermatitis syndrome is the most common clinical manifestation of DGI and consists of tenosynovitis, arthritis, and a pustular or papular rash. Meningitis and endocarditis may complicate bacteremic gonococcal infection. Gonococcal infection at other sites in adults includes gonococcal conjunctivitis and gonococcal epididymitis.

A16. **a.** This patient most likely has *C. trachomatis* urethritis. It is the most common cause of NGU. Symptoms in men include dysuria, frequency, and mucoid to purulent urethral discharge. Some men have asymptomatic infections. Female partners of men with *C. trachomatis* are likely to have chlamydial mucopurulent cervicitis. The second most common etiologic agent in NGU is *U. urealyticum.*

Men with typical clinical symptoms are presumed to have NGU when their urethral (Gram-stained) smear shows WBCs with no gram-negative diplococci or when their rapid antigen-detection test is positive. Furthermore, cultures for *N. gonorrhea* should confirm the absence of this organism.

A17. **b.** This patient has a primary genital herpes infection. The most common symptom of genital herpes infection is a cluster of painful genital lesions. With primary infection, the multiple vesicles that are initially present coalesce to form intensely painful ulcers. Most lesions are found on the vulva and vaginal mucosa. Other symptoms include fever, malaise, myalgias, and headache. Dysuria and vaginal discharge are also common. Recurrences are common; the severity of the primary disease symptoms bears no relationship to the chance of acquiring recurrent disease. The diagnosis of genital herpes should always be confirmed by culture.

The treatment of choice for primary herpes simplex genital viral infection is acyclovir. Acyclovir has been shown to shorten the duration of viral shedding and to shorten the time of lesion healing. The recommended dose is 200 mg PO 5 times a day for 10 days. Famciclovir and valacyclovir are antiviral agents also used with the benefit of requiring fewer doses per day.

Patients with severe or frequent recurrences can be treated with acyclovir prophylactically. General supportive measures including povidone-iodine will often provide relief. Bacterial superinfection can be treated with a topical antibiotic such as fusidic acid ointment or cream.

A18. **b.** This patient has condyloma acuminatum. This is caused by the human papillomavirus (HPV). Condyloma lesions may appear on the introitus, the labia majora, the labia minora, the perineal area, and the urethra. Patients with condyloma are four times more likely to develop cervical carcinoma *in situ* and subsequent invasive cervical cancer. These women should have yearly Papanicolaou smears. If any cytologic abnormalities are found, colposcopically directed biopsies should be performed.

Patients with condyloma acuminatum should also be carefully screened for other STDs.

An association has been demonstrated between condyloma acuminatum and laryngeal papillomas in the newborn, but this is extremely rare.

A19. **c.** The treatment that has been reported to have the highest cure rate in patients with condyloma acuminatum is the carbon dioxide laser. Cure rates with this form of therapy approach 90%. The primary goal of treating visible HPV is removal of symptomatic warts. Current treatments probably do not significantly affect the natural history of HPV infections or prevent the development of cervical carcinoma. Other treatment options include topical therapy (podofilox, podophyllin, trichloroacetic acid, 5-fluorouracil, and imiquimod), destructive procedures (cryotherapy, electrodesiccation, and surgical excision), and immunotherapy (with interferon).

A20. **d.** *T. pallidum,* the causative organism of syphilis, is not becoming resistant to penicillin. This is an exception to the increasing prevalence of usual antibiotic resistant organisms. However, syphilis is not going away; there were, in fact, alarming increases in incidence rates for new cases of syphilis in the late 1980s. Although the rate has recently declined somewhat, syphilis has, in a very real sense, grown along with acquired immunodeficiency syndrome.

The Jarisch-Herxheimer reaction is a common reaction that occurs within several hours of initiating therapy in patients with syphilis. It occurs in all women with primary syphilis and half of women with secondary syphilis. It consists of constitutional symptoms (headache, fever, and myalgia), mild hypotension, and worsening of specific syphilis manifestations. This phenomenon should be treated with salicylates (acetaminophen in pregnant women) or, in severe cases, with prednisone.

A localized Jarisch-Herxheimer reaction also may manifest as transient worsening of neurologic, otic, or ophthalmologic symptoms soon after therapy and should be treated with prednisone. Patients should be warned of the possibility of the Jarisch-Herxheimer reaction before therapy begins and instructed with regard to self-medication and the need for contacting the physician.

A21. **a.** Although benzathine penicillin G remains the drug of choice for the treatment of syphilis, a combination of doxycycline and ceftriaxone is also effective.

A22. **b.** Despite his relative sexual innocence, this patient almost certainly has a primary NGU caused by *C. trachomatis* with a complicating epididymitis.

The symptoms of acute epididymitis include scrotal skin that is red, warm, and tense, with partial or total obliteration of the rugal folds. The epididymis is tender to the touch, indurated, and enlarged.

A23. **a.** If a patient presents with what appears to be an acute epididymitis or an acute orchitis and the inflammation or swelling does not improve on antibiotic therapy, a neoplasm should be suspected and an ultrasound of the testicle performed.

The most common bacterial cause of acute epididymitis is *E. coli*. The most common pathogens in general are *C. trachomatis* and *M. hominis.*

SOLUTION TO THE SHORT ANSWER MANAGEMENT PROBLEM

a. Risk factors for PID:
   1) Age (women between the ages of 18 and 25)
   2) Multiple sexual partners
   3) Initial sexual encounter at an early age
   4) Nonwhite women have a greater risk than whites
   5) Instrumentation of the endometrial cavity (that is, insertion of an IUD)
   6) Nonbarrier contraceptive methods
   7) Relationship of infection to last normal menstrual period (LNMP) (the closer the time of organism infection to the LNMP, the greater the risk)
   8) History of previous PID
   9) Symptoms of urethritis in a sexual partner

b. Complications of acute PID:
   1) Progression of the infection to tuboovarian abscess and subsequent peritonitis
   2) Bacteremia from diffuse pelvic involvement
   3) Resultant tubal scarring, which leads to the following:
      a) Chronic pelvic adhesions
      b) Chronic pelvic pain syndrome
      c) Ectopic pregnancy
      d) Subsequent infertility

SUMMARY OF THE DIAGNOSIS AND TREATMENT OF SEXUALLY TRANSMITTED DISEASES

1. PID:
   a. Signs and symptoms of acute salpingitis:
      1) Lower abdominal pain
      2) Lower abdominal tenderness
      3) Cervical motion tenderness
      4) Adnexal tenderness accompanied by at least one of the following:
         a) elevated temperature
         b) elevated WBC
         c) elevated ESR
         d) positive culdocentesis
         e) an inflammatory mass on pelvic examination or ultrasound
         f) a positive Gram stain or smear.
   b. Differential diagnosis:
      1) Acute appendicitis
      2) Endometritis
      3) Corpus luteum bleeding
      4) Benign ovarian tumor
      5) Chronic salpingitis
   c. Laboratory evaluation and procedures:
      1) complete blood count
      2) ESR
      3) ultrasound
      4) beta-HCG
      5) laparoscopy
   d. Pathophysiology:
      1) Microbiology: Polymicrobial infection most likely; an anaerobic organism is almost always involved. Major anaerobic organisms include *B. fragilis* and peptostreptococcus.
      2) Pathophysiology involves inflammation of the fallopian tubes (acute salpingitis) with extension in either direction into uterus or into ovaries. An extension into the ovaries may lead to the formation of a tuboovarian abscess.
   e. Treatment of PID:
      1) Inpatient treatment:
         a) IV cefoxitin and IV doxycycline

b) IV clindamycin and IV gentamicin followed by PO doxycycline
   2) Outpatient treatment: IM cefoxitin or ceftriaxone, PO probenecid, and either PO doxycycline or PO tetracycline
f. Risk factors for PID: See the Solution to the Short Answer Management Problem
g. Complications of PID: See the Solution to the Short Answer Management Problem
h. Key issue in PID: To hospitalize or not to hospitalize. See Answer 5.

2. Gonococcal urethritis:
   a. Organism: *N. gonorrhea*
   b. Symptoms: Dysuria, frequency, discharge (initially serous or milky that changes to a yellow, creamy discharge with significant urethral pain); may be asymptomatic in women
   c. Treatment: IM ceftriaxone (one dose) and either PO doxycycline or PO cefixime (one dose) or PO cefixime and PO doxycycline

3. NGU:
   a. Organism: *C. trachomatis or U. urealyticum*
   b. Symptoms: Dysuria, frequency, mucoid to purulent urethral discharge; may be asymptomatic in men as well as in women, although more common in women
   c. Laboratory diagnosis: Urethral, cervical, rectal, and pharyngeal swab to demonstrate coexisting gram-negative intracellular diplococci
   d. Treatment: PO doxycycline or PO tetracycline

4. Epididymitis:
   a. Organisms:
      1) Most common cause: *C. trachomatis*
      2) Most common bacterial cause: *E. coli*
      3) Other organism that may be involved: *U. urealyticum, Mycoplasma*
   b. Symptoms: Painful and red scrotum, and tenderness in epididymis and scrotum
   c. Differential diagnosis: Testicular tumor, and testicular torsion

d. Treatment: PO doxycycline, nonsteroidal antiinflammatory drug (Indocin), scrotal elevation, and ice packs

5. Syphilis:
   a. Organism: *T. pallidum*
   b. Sign: Painless ulcer in genital region (primary syphilis)
   c. Laboratory diagnosis: Darkfield examination for *T. pallidum*
   d. Treatment: IM benzathine penicillin

6. Herpes genitalis:
   a. Organism: Herpes simplex type 2
   b. Symptoms and signs: Painful ulcers in genital area and associated swelling and lymphadenopathy
   c. Laboratory diagnosis: Viral culture
   d. Treatment: Acyclovir, famciclovir and valacyclovir
   e. Recurrences: Recurrences are common

7. Condyloma acuminatum:
   a. Organism: HPV
   b. Sign and symptoms: Cauliflower-like lesion in genital area
   c. Treatment: Cryosurgery
   Remember, STDs go together; where one is discovered, others may also be found. The major public health initiatives involve prevention (education) and contact tracing.

SUGGESTED READINGS
Althausen A: Epididymitis. In Rakel R, ed: *Conn's current therapy,* Philadelphia, 1994, WB Saunders.
American College of Obstetrics and Gynecology: Chronic Pelvic Pain, *Tech Bull* No. 223, 1996.
Hatcher RA et al, eds: *Contraceptive technology,* ed 17, New York, 1998, Ardent Media.
Mata J: Nongonococcal urethritis. In Rakel R, ed: *Conn's current therapy,* Philadelphia, 1994, WB Saunders.
Mishell DR et al: *Comprehensive gynecology,* St Louis, 1997, Mosby.

C·H·A·P·T·E·R 4

Psychiatry, Behavioral Science, and Communication

PROBLEM·60

DEPRESSIVE DISORDERS

When the Blues Become Black

Case 1 ■ A 34-Year-Old Female Who Is Tearful and Sad

A 34-year-old female comes to your office in a state of depression. She tells you that she has been "way down" for the past several months and has not felt much like doing anything. For the past 4 months she has been on long-term disability leave. For some 18 months before that, she had been working approximately 75 hr/wk, dealing with daily difficulties and conflicts as a business executive. She found work to be increasingly stressful, ultimately compelling her to take a leave of absence.

She expresses her current situation by saying, "I have no joy left in life; I don't enjoy doing anything, nor do I have any interest in any of my previous activities." Her other symptoms include sleeping approximately 14 hr/day, almost continual feelings of guilt and hopelessness, a state of having almost no energy "all of the time," decreased ability to concentrate, no appetite—resulting in a 24-pound weight loss, and being unable to "move around" or get anything done.

She is married and has three children. Her marriage is described as "excellent" and her husband is very supportive. She does admit, however, to a significant decrease in sexual interest and activity. Her past health has been excellent, except for a "nervous breakdown' when she was 22 years old. Both her mother and father were alcoholics, but she only drinks on occasion, is on no drugs, and has no allergies. Her physical examination is completely normal in all systems.

SELECT THE BEST ANSWER TO THE FOLLOWING QUESTIONS

Q1. What is the most likely diagnosis in this patient?
   a. adjustment disorder with depressed mood
   b. generalized anxiety disorder
   c. major depressive disorder (MDD)
   d. mood disorder caused by a general medical condition
   e. dysthymic disorder

Q2. Which of the following types of psychotherapy is generally considered most effective in the illness previously described?
   a. psychoanalytic psychotherapy
   b. behavioral psychotherapy
   c. psychodynamic psychotherapy
   d. cognitive psychotherapy
   e. supportive psychotherapy

Q3. The goals of the psychotherapy for this condition include which of the following?
   a. providing a therapeutic rationale or explanation for the patient's symptoms
   b. providing ongoing education regarding the illness, prognosis, and treatment
   c. guiding the patient with respect to interpersonal relationships, work, and major life adjustments
   d. helping to bolster the patient's morale
   e. all of the above

Q4. What is the pharmacologic agent of choice in the disorder described?
   a. a selective serotonin reuptake inhibitor (SSRI)
   b. a tricyclic antidepressant (TCA)
   c. a nonselective monoamine oxidase inhibitor (MAOI)
   d. a selective MAOI
   e. lithium carbonate

Case 2 ■ A 41-Year-Old Male Who Is Chronically Depressed

A 41-year-old male comes to your office with a 3-year history of a "depressed mood." He states that he feels "depressed most of the time," although there are periods when he feels better than others. He feels chronically tired, has some difficulty concentrating at work, and has found it difficult to remain productive and efficient as chief executive officer of a major company. He has had no other symptoms. His health is otherwise good. He is on no medications.

Q5. This 41-year-old male most likely suffers from which of the following?
   a. adjustment disorder
   b. dysthymic disorder
   c. MDD
   d. mood disorder caused by a general medical condition
   e. none of the above

Q6. What is the treatment of choice for the patient in Case 2?
   a. a TCA
   b. an SSRI
   c. cognitive psychotherapy
   d. a and c
   e. b and c

Case 3 ■ A 35-Year-Old Female Who Is Distressed at Work

A 35-year-old female comes to your office with a 3-month history of feeling "depressed." She feels "extremely distressed" at work and tells you that she is "burned out." You discover that she moved into a managerial position at work 4 months ago and is having a great deal of difficulty (interpersonal conflict) with two of her employees.

The patient has no history of psychiatric illness. She has no other symptoms. She is on no medications.

Q7. What is the most likely diagnosis in this patient?
   a. adjustment disorder with depressed mood
   b. dysthymic disorder
   c. MDD
   d. mood disorder caused by a general medical condition
   e. burnout

Q8. What is the treatment of choice for the patient described in Case 3?
   a. a TCA
   b. an SSRI
   c. supportive psychotherapy
   d. a and c
   e. b and c

Case 4 ■ A Hard-Driving 45-Year-Old Male Who Is "Burned Out"

A 45-year-old male who is a "hard-driving" executive comes to your office with a 4-month history of feelings

of sadness, irritability, loss of appetite, inability to concentrate, and a significantly decreased ability to function in his role as the manager of a division of a major corporation. He tells you that he is "completely burned out."

When you question him, he tells you that "he has been using anything and everything possible to try to relax." He has missed a number of days of work recently because he "hasn't felt up to it." He also complains of increasing stomach pains and headaches over the last 2 months.

Q9. From the history given, what is the most likely diagnosis in this patient?
   a. MDD
   b. dysthymic disorder
   c. mood disorder caused by a general medical condition
   d. substance-induced mood disorder
   e. adjustment disorder with depressed mood

Q10. What is the treatment of choice for the patient described in Case 4?
   a. an SSRI
   b. a TCA
   c. an MAOI
   d. lithium carbonate
   e. none of the above

Case 5 ■ A 61-Year-Old Retired Male Who Is Depressed

A 61-year-old male, a patient whom who you have known for 20 years, comes to your office with a 4-month history of depression. He has no previous history of psychiatric illness, nor is there any evidence of psychiatric illness in his family. He has also been feeling extremely fatigued, has lost his appetite, has lost 20 pounds, and has begun to experience "stomach pains" diagnosed by an Emergency Room doctor as "irritable bowel syndrome." He retired from his position as an administrative assistant with the Internal Revenue Service 6 months ago, and his symptoms began 2 months after that event.

On examination, the patient fits the criteria for MDD. However, he also has other findings that concern you. He is having many more episodes of the "irritable bowel syndrome" pain than he previously did. He is also experiencing more "constipation" There is a definite difference in the periumbilical region on percussion (tympany changes to dullness over a 6-cm area).

Q11. On the basis of the information given, which of the following conditions is the most likely possibility in this patient?

a. MDD
b. substance-induced mood disorder
c. adjustment disorder with depressed mood
d. mood disorder caused by a general medical condition
e. dysthymia disorder

Q12. What is the primary treatment for the patient described in Case 5?
a. an SSRI
b. a TCA
c. an MAOB inhibitor
d. lithium carbonate
e. none of the above

Q13. What is the most likely diagnosis based on the signs and symptoms reported in Case 5?
a. carcinoma of the stomach
b. carcinoma of the pancreas
c. early delirium
d. early Alzheimer's disease
e. dysthymic disorder

Q14. As physicians, we need to inform our patients that depression is a disease like any other; it often affects body chemistry, just as diseases such as hypothyroidism, hyperthyroidism, and diabetes mellitus do. Which of the following hypotheses support(s) this argument?
a. Loss of the normal feedback mechanism inhibiting adrenocorticotropic hormone
b. The lack of normal suppression of blood cortisol following the administration of dexamethasone
c. The generalized decrease in noradrenergic function in depressed patients
d. a and b
e. all of the above

Q15. Which of the following neurotransmitters appears to be the most important mediator of depressive illness in humans?
a. norepinephrine
b. acetylcholine
c. dopamine
d. serotonin
e. tryptophan

Q16. A complete psychiatric history is most important in evaluating depressed patients. In taking a history from a patient with depression, which of the following questions is the most important question to ask?
a. inquiry into the family history of psychiatric disorders
b. inquiry into the personal history of previous episodes of depression
c. inquiry into suicidal ideation
d. inquiry into the presence or absence of hallucinations
e. inquiry into the presence or absence of delusion

SHORT ANSWER MANAGEMENT PROBLEM
Discuss a strategy for the pharmacological management of MDD.

ANSWERS

A1. **c.** The diagnosis in this patient is MDD. This is based on the presence for at least 2 weeks of a distinct change in mood (sadness or lack of pleasure) accompanied by changes in appetite and activities including decreased energy, psychomotor agitation or retardation, decreased appetite for food or sex, weight loss, changes in sleep-wake cycles, and depressive rumination or thoughts of suicide. Adjustment disorder with depressed mood is not diagnosed when symptoms are severe enough to be considered MDD.

Generalized anxiety disorder is characterized by excessive worry and nervousness about many problems. Mood disorders caused by general medical conditions are initiated and maintained by physiologic problems.

Dysthymic disorder is characterized by a depressed mood that persists for over 2 years without the other features of MDD. The criteria for MDD according to the *Diagnostic and Statistical Manual of Mental Disorders, fourth edition* (DSM-IV) are as follows:

a. Five or more of the following symptoms present during the same 2-week period and representing a change from previous functioning. At least one of those two symptoms must be either 1) or 2) from the following list:
1) Depressed mood most of the day, nearly every day, as indicated by either subjective report (such as feeling sad or empty) or observation made by others (e.g., appears tearful).
2) Markedly diminished interest or pleasure in all or almost all activities most of the day, nearly every day (as indicated by either subjective account or observation made by others).
3) Significant weight loss when not dieting or weight gain (e.g., a change of more than 5% of body weight in a month) or a decrease or increase in appetite nearly every day.
4) Insomnia or hypersomnia nearly every day.
5) Psychomotor agitation or retardation nearly every day (observable by others and not

merely subjective feelings of restlessness or being slowed down).

6) Fatigue or loss of energy nearly every day.

7) Feelings of worthlessness or excessive or inappropriate guilt (which may be delusional) nearly every day (not merely self-reproach or guilt about being sick).

8) Diminished ability to think or concentrate or indecisiveness nearly every day (either by subjective account or observed by others).

9) Recurrent thoughts of death (not just fear of dying), recurrent suicidal ideation without a specific plan, a suicide attempt, or a specific plan for committing suicide.

b. The symptoms do not meet the criteria for a mixed episode (manic depression).

c. The symptoms cause clinically significant distress or impairment in social, occupational, or other important areas of functioning.

d. The symptoms are not caused by the direct physiologic effects (such as drug abuse or a medication) or a general medical condition (hypothyroidism).

e. The symptoms are not accounted for by bereavement (after the loss of a loved one); the symptoms persist for longer than 2 months or are characterized by a marked functional impairment, morbid preoccupation with worthlessness, suicidal ideation, psychotic symptoms, or psychomotor retardation.

A mnemonic for MDD is SIG-EM-CAPS (A diagnosis is made if a patient has five out of the nine symptoms, which must include Energy/fatigue or Mood).

a. S = **S**leep (hypersomnia or insomnia)

b. I = **I**nterest (lack of interest in life in general)

c. G = **G**uilt or hopelessness

d. E = **E**nergy/fatigue

e. M = **M**ood (depressed, sadness)

f. C = **C**oncentration (lack of)

g. A = **A**ppetite (increased or decreased; weight loss or weight gain)

h. P = **P**sychomotor (retardation or agitation)

i. S = **S**uicidal ideation

The other choices in this question are discussed in various other problems in this chapter.

A2. d. Most studies suggest that cognitive psychotherapy is the type of psychotherapy most effective in treatment of depression. Cognitive therapy changes the way that patients interpret events and encourages a greater sense of optimism and empowerment. This method of brief psychotherapy was developed over the last two decades by Aaron T. Beck. It is primarily used for the treatment of mild to moderate depression and for patients with low self-esteem. It is similar to behavioral therapy in that it aims at the direct removal of symptoms rather than the resolution of underlying conflicts such as is attempted in psychodynamic psychotherapies. Cognitive therapists view the patient's conscious thoughts as central to production. Both the content of thoughts and thought processes are seen as disordered in people with such symptoms. Therapy is directed at identifying and altering these cognitive distortions.

A3. e. There are a wide range of psychotherapeutic interventions that may be useful in the treatment of mood disorders, particularly depressive mood disorders. The establishment of a relationship is often crucial in the treatment of the depressed patient. Elements of an effective psychotherapeutic relationship include the following:

a. Providing a therapeutic rationale or explanation for the patient's symptoms

b. Providing ongoing education and feedback about the patient's illness, prognosis, and treatment

c. Guiding the patient with respect to interpersonal relationships, work, and major life adjustments

d. Helping to bolster the patient's morale

e. Setting realistic goals

f. Being available in time of crisis

These important aspects of treatment, sometimes referred to as supportive psychotherapy, are components of most other therapies, including psychodynamic, behavioral, and cognitive psychotherapies.

A4. a. The pharmacologic treatment of choice in most patients with MDD is currently a member of the class of drugs known as SSRIs. The agents in this class include fluoxetine (Prozac), sertraline (Zoloft), paroxetine (Paxil), fluvoxamine (Luvox), and citalopram (Celexa). These agents have significantly fewer side effects than the TCAs. The major side effects include gastrointestinal distress, tremor, insomnia, somnolence, decreased libido and inhibited orgasm, and dry mouth.

The SSRIs have replaced the TCAs as the drugs of first choice for MDD in adults. The SSRIs act exactly as they are named—they block the reuptake of serotonin in the brain. Other antidepressants currently used when SSRIs are ineffective or contraindicated include trazodone (Desyrel), nefazodone (Serzone), bupropion (Wellbutrin), venlafaxine (Effexor), and mirtazapine (Remeron).

TCAs are less commonly used because they are more severely toxic. Major anticholinergic side effects exhibited by TCAs include dry mouth, urinary retention, constipation, and blurred vision. Other serious significant side effects include orthostatic hypotension (an alpha-blockade side effect), cardiac conduction abnormalities (an increased risk for patients with second-degree and third-degree heart block or right or left bundle branch block due to a quinidine-like action) and excessive sedation due to an antihistamine-like action.

Antidepressants all have comparable efficacy overall, but individual patients may respond to some antidepressants but not others. It is impossible to predict with certainty which antidepressant will be effective for a particular patient, so trial of two or more antidepressants is sometimes necessary. A patient should be switched to a different antidepressant if he or she does not respond after 4 weeks or if side effects are intolerable.

Selection of particular antidepressants should be based on the individual patient's clinical presentation. If the patient's symptoms include fatigue, hypersomnia, and lethargy, a minimally sedating antidepressant such as fluoxetine, venlafaxine, desipramine, or nortriptyline should be used. If, on the other hand, the patient's symptoms include anxiety, insomnia, and irritability, a more sedating antidepressant such as nefazodone, mirtazapine, or trazodone would be more appropriate. If sexual side effects occur with use of an SSRI, bupropion, an antidepressant with minimal sexual side effects (decreased libido), is often substituted.

Antidepressants exert multiple effects on central and autonomic nervous system pathways, at least partially by presynaptic blockade of norepinephrine or serotonin reuptake. The mechanism of antidepressant action is not clearly understood.

MAOIs such as phenelzine or tranylcypromine may be effective in cases of treatment-resistant MDD. MAOIs are effective antidepressants whose mode of action is to block irreversibly postsynaptic inactivation of epinephrine, norepinephrine, dopamine, and serotonin.

MAOIs do not exhibit the anticholinergic side effects seen with tricyclics. The most common side effects of these drugs are dizziness, orthostatic hypotension, sexual dysfunction, insomnia, and daytime sleepiness. The greatest risk with MAOIs is the occurrence of hypertensive crises, which may be induced by the consumption of large amounts of certain foods (i.e., aged cheese, red wine) or drugs containing sympathetic stimulant activity.

If several antidepressant medications are ineffective in treating individuals with MDD, augmentation of response by adding lithium or thyroxine may be attempted.

Pharmacologic treatment of MDD is effective in approximately 70% to 75% of cases. Electroconvulsive therapy (ECT) is often useful for individuals who do not respond to antidepressants, have contraindications to antidepressants, or are in immediate danger of committing suicide. Unlike antidepressants, which often take 4 to 6 weeks to have a full effect, ECT is effective almost immediately.

A5. **b.** This patient has a dysthymic disorder. Dysthymic disorder is defined as a depressive syndrome in which the patient is bothered all or most of the time by depressive symptoms. These symptoms are not of sufficient severity to warrant a diagnosis of major depressive episode.

Adjustment disorder is generally more time limited and related to a specific stressor.

Mood disorders caused by general medical conditions have specific physiologic causes.

A6. **e.** Because of the long history, this patient should probably be treated with a combination of psychotherapy and pharmacotherapy.

The pharmacologic class of choice at this time is the SSRIs such as fluoxetine (Prozac) 20 to 40 mg/day, sertraline (Zoloft) 50 to 200 mg/day, or paroxetine (Paxil) 20 to 50 mg/day.

Psychotherapy (either supportive psychotherapy or cognitive psychotherapy as described earlier) is an important component of the treatment of this condition.

A7. **a.** This patient has an adjustment disorder with depressed mood, which is defined as a reaction to some identifiable psychosocial stressor(s) that occurs within 3 months of the onset of the depressed mood. The major characteristic of the disorder is an impairment in occupational or social functioning. The severity of the depression is not sufficient to warrant a diagnosis of MDD. Treatment of individuals with adjustment disorder includes counseling about stress management and brief psychotherapy.

Dysthymic disorder is characterized by 2 or more years of chronically depressed mood. Mood disorder caused by a general medical condition is caused by a known pathophysiologic process.

Substance-induced mood disorder is directly caused by a particular substance, commonly alcohol or psychostimulants. Substance-induced mood disorder should be considered in individuals with depressive symptoms, especially those who may be under psychologic stress and using inappropriate coping mechanisms such the use of alcohol or drugs.

A8. **c.** The treatment of choice for adjustment disorder is brief psychotherapy consisting of counseling and stress management. If possible, the stressor should be removed. If not possible, relaxation therapy, biofeedback, and exercise are useful for improving the ability to cope with stress. The physician should discuss specific coping strategies with specific goals and objectives negotiated with the patient.

A9. **d.** This patient most likely has a substance-induced mood disorder. The "tip-offs" to this diagnosis in this patient are as follows:

    a. Symptoms and signs of depression

    b. A self-described "burnout syndrome"

    c. The missing of a number of days of work recently

    d. The clue of "I am using anything and everything to try to relax."

The sequence of events that likely took place in this patient is as follows. The drive to keep going faster and faster "to stay on the treadmill" eventually led to a depressive disorder and occupational burnout. This was followed by inappropriate "coping mechanisms" including the use of alcohol or drugs to keep going. Eventually he reached a point where he was unable to function because of depression, "burnout syndrome," and the number of days missed at work. Therefore his work suffered.

A10. **e.** The steps that should be pursued in this patient's case are as follows:

    a. Ask the patient about alcohol intake (specific amounts, specific times, and total intake).

    b. Administer an alcohol abuse questionnaire if possible.

    c. Interview the patient's wife.

    d. If possible speak to the patient's colleagues, being cognizant of the patient's right to confidentiality.

    e. Confirm or refute the hypothesis of depressive disorder caused by substance-induced mood disorder.

    f. If confirmed, begin assertive intervention.

    g. Assertive intervention should include an intensive recovery program. This should include a detoxification program if necessary. In-patient rehabilitation treatment, including individual, group, and family psychotherapy, is sometimes necessary. Referral to a 12-step program such as Alcoholics Anonymous is extremely useful for both rehabilitation and relapse prevention.

A11. **d.** This patient most likely has a mood disorder caused by a general medical condition. The single most likely diagnosis is carcinoma of the pancreas. This is especially suspicious based on the change in the percussion note from tympany to dullness and the associated symptoms including weight loss and stomach pains.

The major differential diagnosis in this patient would be adjustment disorder with depressed mood associated with his retirement. The physical signs, however, point away from this.

A12. **e.** The "primary treatment" in this case is to confirm "mood disorder" secondary to general medical condition. An antidepressant agent, particularly an SSRI with few side effects, would not be inappropriate in this patient at this time. This is, however, a secondary treatment.

A13. **b.** See Answer 11.

A14. **e.**

A15. **d.** One of the most difficult challenges physicians face is helping our patients understand that many cases of depression represent illnesses that have biologic components. Physiologic abnormalities are sometimes associated with depressive disorders. In the case of a MDD, we are aware of the following physiologic abnormalities.

    a. There is a "neurotransmitter imbalance" that appears to be caused by a relative deficiency of the neurotransmitter serotonin. The new SSRIs add confirming evidence to this hypothesis.

    b. We know that patients with MDD have hyperactivity of the hypothalamic-pituitary-adrenal axis. This results in elevated plasma cortisol levels and nonsuppression of cortisol following a dexamethasone suppression test.

    c. There is blunting of the normally expected increase in plasma growth hormone induced by alpha-2-adrenergic receptor agonists.

    d. There is blunting of serotonin-mediated increases in plasma prolactin.

A16. **c.** The single most important question to ask in a patient who presents with signs and symptoms of depression is whether or not they have contemplated suicide. The questioning and the rationale should proceed as follows:

    a. Have you ever considered that "life really isn't worth it" and that "you should end it all?"

    b. If you have, have you thought of the means by which you would do it?

    c. Have you considered a specific plan for ending your life?

    d. Do you feel that your situation is hopeless?

The overall mortality from suicide in individuals with MDD is 15%. Symptoms that place a depressed patient at higher risk for suicide are a practical and lethal plan, with feelings of hopelessness. Patients must be directly asked about such symptoms, and steps must be taken to protect those at high risk. Such steps include close observation, immediate availability of the therapist, or hospitalization.

SOLUTION TO THE SHORT ANSWER MANAGEMENT PROBLEM

A strategy for the pharmacologic management of MDD is as follows:
a. Identify and treat causes unrelated to MDD (such as hypothyroidism or substance abuse).
b. Use single-agent pharmacotherapy as the first step. (Unless contraindicated, the use of an SSRI is now the drug of first choice). This class includes:
   1) Sertraline (Zoloft)
   2) Paroxetine (Paxil)
   3) Fluoxetine (Prozac)
c. Alternative drug selection: If there is no satisfactory response after 4 weeks or if the patient cannot tolerate the first drug, switch to a different drug. The new drug should be one that minimizes the troublesome side effects or comes from a different chemical class, other than MAOIs.
d. If trials of two or three antidepressants are ineffective, augment the best-tolerated antidepressant with lithium carbonate.
e. If the best-tolerated antidepressant with lithium carbonate is ineffective, consider substituting an MAOI.
f. ECT should be used if several antidepressant trials have been ineffective, if there are contraindications to the use of antidepressants, or if there is a high risk of immediate suicide.

SUMMARY OF THE DIAGNOSIS AND MANAGEMENT OF MAJOR DEPRESSIVE DISORDER

1. Prevalence:
   a. MDD:
      1) Lifetime prevalence: 3.5% to 5.8% of the population
      2) Gender difference: Higher in women than in men
   b. Dysthymia:
      1) Lifetime prevalence: 2.1% to 4.7%
      2) Gender difference: Higher in women than in men
   c. Prevalence for depression in medical settings, which select for patients with emotional distress or physical illness has been reported to be as high as 15%.

2. Differential diagnosis of MDD: DSM-IV criteria: American Psychiatric Association, 1994
   a. MDD
   b. Dysthymia
   c. Depression caused by a general medical condition
   d. Adjustment disorder with depressed mood
   e. Substance-induced mood disorder
   f. Manic episodes with irritable mood
   g. Mixed episodes (depression, hypomania)

3. MDD versus dysthymia:
   a. MDD: In addition to depressed mood, there are significant changes in appetite and activities, such as sleep disturbance, weight loss, severe fatigue or lack of energy, and suicidal rumination.
   b. Dysthymia: Perhaps best described as "a chronic ongoing depressed mood" that lasts years rather than weeks or months.

4. Subclassifications of MDD: Once a diagnosis of depression has been made, the clinician should further characterize the syndrome if possible into the following categories:
   a. Unipolar versus bipolar:
      1) MDD, unipolar
      2) Affective disorder, bipolar
   b. Melancholic versus nonmelancholic: 40% to 60% of all hospitalizations are for melancholic depression. Symptoms include anhedonia, excessive or inappropriate guilt, early morning waking, anorexia, psychomotor disturbance, and diurnal variation in mood. The depressed melancholic patient may appear frantic, fearful, agitated, or withdrawn.
   c. Psychotic versus nonpsychotic: Psychotic depressions are not rare. Studies suggest that approximately 10% to 25% of patients hospitalized for major depression have a psychotic depression.
   d. Atypical depression: Atypical depression denotes symptoms that include hypersomnia instead of insomnia, hyperphagia (sometimes as a carbohydrate craving) rather than anorexia, and reactivity (mood changes with environmental circumstances), as well as a long-standing pattern of interpersonal rejection sensitivity. It is much more common in women. Patients with atypical depression are frequently reported to have an anxious or irritable mood rather than dysphoria.
   e. Masked depression: Masked depression is similar to atypical depression. Instead of overt depression, the depression is expressed as many psychosomatic signs and symptoms.

5. Treatment:
   a. Follow the guidelines provided in the Short Answer Management Problem.
   b. Consider the SSRIs as the drugs of first choice unless specific medical contraindications to their use are present.
   c. Treat for at least 4 weeks before you consider the therapy you are using to be a therapeutic failure.
   d. Remember that MDD is a recurrent disease: At 1 year following the start of therapy, 33% will be free of the disease, 33% will have had a relapse, and 33% will still be depressed.
   e. Remember that MDD should be treated with a combination of pharmacotherapy and psychotherapy (psychotherapy to be discussed in Problem 72).

6. Three-phase approach to the treatment of depression:
   a. Acute treatment phase, phase 1: Time = 6 to 12 weeks
      Goal: The goal of this phase of therapy is the remission of symptoms of depression.
   b. Continuation treatment, phase 2: Time = 4 to 9 months
      Goal: The goal of this phase of therapy is to prevent a relapse of the depressive symptoms.
   c. Maintenance treatment, phase 3: Time = 1 to an indeterminate number of years
      Goal: The goal of this phase of therapy is to treat patients who have had three or more episodes of depression. Prevention of recurrence is the treatment end point.

There is broad consensus among consultants that the continuation treatment phase is the most critical in determining a successful clinical outcome. The panel recommends that through the continuation treatment phase that medication is indicated at full dose. The danger that needs to be avoided is not to stop or decrease medication too soon.

Too often medication is tapered or discontinued shortly after symptoms have been brought under control; this greatly increases the patient's risk of relapse. There is no justification for lowering the effective dose of an antidepressant drug during maintenance treatment.* During this phase you should see the patient once a week for the first 6 to 8 weeks, depending on the individual. Once the patient is stable, you should see the patient every other week for 4 weeks; following that, the patient should be seen once a month. If the patient is on one of the TCAs and there is a partial

---

*From American Psychiatric Association: *Diagnostic and statistical manual of mental disorders,* ed 4, Washington, DC, 1994, American Psychiatric Association Press.

or inadequate response, plasma concentrations of the drug should be obtained.

Once the patient is asymptomatic for at least 6 months following a depressive episode, recovery from the episode is declared.

The termination of therapy must be accompanied by patient education. The key concern is the likelihood of a recurrent episode. If this is the patient's first bout of depression that needed to be treated, the recurrence rate is approximately 50%. If there have been previous episodes of depression or a family history of depression, the probability of a recurrence is increased significantly. The patient must be made aware of the symptoms that indicate when another episode is likely. You need to remember that if therapy is initiated early in the disease course, it is more likely to be effective faster. You need to tell the patient that subsequent attacks can be treated effectively.

SUGGESTED READINGS

American Psychiatric Association: *Diagnostic and statistical manual of mental disorders,* ed 4, Washington, DC, 1994, American Psychiatric Association Press.

Bell I, Gelenberg A: Mood disorders. In Rakel R, ed: *Conn's current therapy,* Philadelphia, 1994, WB Saunders.

Risby E, Risch SC, Stoudemire A: Mood disorders. In Stoudemire A, ed: *Clinical psychiatry for medical students,* ed 2, Philadelphia, 1990, JB Lippincott.

Steer RA et al: Dimensions of the Beck depression inventory-II in clinically depressed outpatients, *J Clin Psychol* 55(1):117-128, 1999.

PROBLEM · 61

BIPOLAR DISORDER

"I Can Do Anything You Can Do, Better."

Case 1 ■ A 42-Year-Old Computer Science Professor Who Has Just Been Anointed By God as the New Head of the Computer Age

A 42-year-old computer science professor is brought to the Emergency Room by his wife, who complains that for the last 4 weeks her husband has become increasingly irritable, angry, and suspicious. She states: "His personality has completely changed"; "He has not slept for 6 nights and has been found by the local police using his laptop under a lamppost to work on his computer programs."

He has become preoccupied with the belief that God has anointed him as the "new leader of the computer age." Fearing that his ideas will be stolen by INTERPOL, the CIA, the State Police, and the "Red Coated Mounties" from Canada, he has constructed an elaborate mathematical code that allows only him and his appointed prophets to understand the programs. He quite proudly states that "Albert Einstein wouldn't have a chance at this; it's even too clever for him!"

His wife further volunteers that the patient has been depressed on and off throughout his life and has been on "all kinds of junk" for the depression, none of which helped at any time. However, she claims the patient has never had a substance abuse problem of any kind. She describes her husband's family as "a whole bunch of nuts." She continues to tell you that his mother calls him at 3 AM each morning (just as he is getting his equipment and extension cords set up outside, rooting through the garage, knocking everything over, and waking up the entire neighborhood). He has devised the "world's longest telephone cord" (he takes the calls from his mother in the middle of the street). His father has been admitted to a psychiatric hospital on a number of occasions, sometimes for alcoholism and sometimes for "weird behavior." He has been treated with shock treatments. One of his sisters is a drug addict; another sister is a "friend of the earth" and lives in a commune.

During the interview the patient volunteered little information, is extremely agitated, and paces the floor. He makes a number of sexual advances toward the nurse who is observing him.

SELECT THE BEST ANSWER TO THE FOLLOWING QUESTIONS

Q1. Based on the history given, what condition best describes the behavior exhibited in this patient?
 a. acute hypomania
 b. acute mania
 c. acute anxiety
 d. dementia
 e. delirium

Q2. Based on the patient's personal history, the condition applied in Question 1, and the family history described, this is most likely a part of a condition known as which of the following?
 a. bipolar disorder
 b. alcohol intoxication
 c. major depressive disorder (MDD)
 d. schizoid personality disorder
 e. schizophrenia

Q3. In the *Diagnostic Statistical Manual of Mental Disorders, fourth edition* (DSM-IV) this condition is further subclassified into which of the following?
 a. schizophrenia: catatonic type
 b. schizophrenia: paranoid type

 c. bipolar I disorder
 d. bipolar II disorder
 e. atypical insanity

Q4. At this time, what would you do?
 a. prescribe diazepam and tell his wife that you will review the situation
 b. prescribe lithium carbonate on an outpatient basis and see the patient in 3 months
 c. prescribe fluphenazine on an outpatient basis and see the patient in 1 week
 d. prescribe a tricyclic antidepressant (TCA) on an outpatient basis and see the patient in 1 week
 e. none of the above

Q5. Your mother has just been told that she has the illness that has just been described. You begin to wonder about the inheritability of such a disorder. What is your relative risk of developing the disorder described compared with someone without a first-degree relative with the disease?
 a. half as much
 b. equal to
 c. 24 times as much
 d. twice as much
 e. 3.5 times as much

Q6. Which of the following statements regarding lithium carbonate in the treatment of the disorder described is (are) true?
 a. lithium carbonate is a drug of choice in the treatment of this disorder
 b. lithium prevents relapses of depressive episodes in this disorder
 c. lithium is not metabolized and therefore problems related to active metabolites or inactive metabolites do not exist
 d. the average daily dose of lithium required to treat bipolar disorder is 900 mg
 e. all of the above

Q7. Patients with this disorder who are refractory to lithium carbonate should be treated with which of the following?
 a. carbamazepine
 b. L-tryptophan
 c. divalproex
 d. a and c only
 e. all of the above

Q8. Which of the following neurotransmitters is (are) most clearly implicated in the cause of the acute manic or acute hypomanic episodes in bipolar disorder?

a. norepinephrine
b. dopamine
c. serotonin
d. a and b
e. all of the above

Q9. Which of the following best conceptualizes the definition of cyclothymic disorder?
   a. cyclothymic disorder is best described as a less severe form of bipolar disorder
   b. cyclothymic and dysthymic disorders are virtually identical
   c. cyclothymic disorder is a more severe, more chronic form of bipolar disorder
   d. cyclothymic disorder, by definition, has none of the elements of positive family history that characterize bipolar disorder
   e. none of the above is true

Q10. Which is the pharmacologic treatment of choice for cyclothymic disorder?
   a. a serotonin reuptake inhibitor
   b. a TCA
   c. an monoamine oxidase inhibitor
   d. divalproex
   e. lithium carbonate

SHORT ANSWER MANAGEMENT PROBLEM

Describe the basic diagnostic features of bipolar disorder: manic episode and hypomanic episode.

ANSWERS

A1. **b.** The most likely diagnosis in this patient at this time is acute mania. Mania is defined as a distinct period of abnormally and persistently elevated, expansive, or irritable mood. It may include inflated self-esteem or grandiosity, decreased need for sleep, loquaciousness, flight of ideas, distractibility, increase in goal-directed activity, activities such as unrestrained buying sprees, sexual indiscretions, and foolish business investments. These symptoms cause a marked impairment in occupational functioning.

The basic difference between mania and hypomania is that in mania there are often psychotic symptoms and a more severe impairment in normal functioning (social, occupational, etc.). In addition, the mood disturbance is more severe.

With no history of substance abuse problems, memory impairment or general medical conditions, delirium and dementia are less likely. A diagnosis of acute anxiety would not account for many of the presenting symptoms.

Schizophrenia is less likely because of the good premorbid functioning and the family history of mood disorder. Schizoaffective disorder is unlikely because the patient's delusions are associated in time with his affective symptoms only.

A2. **a.** This episode of acute mania is part of a bipolar disorder. To make the diagnosis of bipolar disorder you need at least one episode of mania or hypomania. This patient has a history that is very suggestive of major depression, and this provides further evidence for a diagnosis of bipolar disorder.

His mother may have bipolar disorder, indicated by her 3 AM phone calls. Also, his father obviously had an MDD treated with electroconvulsive therapy.

A3. **c.** DSM-IV subdivides bipolar disorder into two types: bipolar I and bipolar II. Bipolar I disorder identifies a patient who has had at least one true manic episode. A history of depression or hypomania may also be present in the patient with bipolar I disorder, but neither of these conditions is essential for the diagnosis. Patients with bipolar II disorder have a history of hypomania and major depressive episodes but no history of mania.

A4. **e.** The treatment of choice at this time is admission to a hospital and treatment with an antipsychotic agent such as risperidone or haloperidol until the psychotic symptoms subside. He should be placed on lithium carbonate at the same time. Lithium carbonate is the drug of choice for the treatment of bipolar disorder. The usual dosage is 900 to 1200 mg (with blood level monitoring).

Lithium carbonate is effective treatment for acute mania and prevents relapses of both manic and depressive episodes in bipolar disorder. In the treatment of acute mania, it may be 10 to 14 days before the full therapeutic effect of lithium is felt. Lithium is not metabolized and therefore does not accumulate active metabolic products.

Patients with bipolar disorder who do not respond to lithium carbonate should be treated with either one of two anticonvulsants medications: carbamazepine or divalproex acid. These agents are as effective as lithium carbonate in the treatment of bipolar disorder. They may also be used in situations in which lithium is contraindicated because of a general medical condition or a potential for noncompliance with monitoring. About 30% of patients with bipolar disorder will not respond to lithium and will have to be treated with other agents.

Outpatient therapy is often impossible in patients with acute mania. Diazepam or a TCA is not the recommended agent for the treatment of acute mania.

A5. **c.** The genetic evidence is very strong for bipolar disorder. First-degree relatives of patients with bipolar illness are reported to be at least 24 times more likely to develop bipolar illness than relatives of control subjects. The incidence of bipolar illness and MDD is much higher in first-degree relatives of patients with bipolar illness than in the general population. On the other hand, first-degree relatives of patients with MDD have an increase in the incidence of unipolar depression only.

A6. **e.**

A7. **d.**

A8. **d.** The most relevant pharmacologic data relating to theories of acute mania and acute hypomania is the consistent finding that direct or indirect norepinephrine and dopamine agonists (those drugs that stimulate the noradrenergic and dopaminergic receptors or increase concentrations of these neurotransmitters in the brain) can precipitate mania or hypomania in patients with underlying bipolar illness. Stimulants such as amphetamines and cocaine can induce maniclike syndromes in patients who do not appear to have an underlying vulnerability to develop a bipolar disorder. This suggests an association of mania or hypomania with hyper-adrenergic or hyperdopaminergic states.

A9. **a.** Cyclothymic disorder is best conceptualized as a relatively less severe form of bipolar illness. The data indicate that approximately 30% of individuals with cyclothymia have a positive family history for bipolar illness. By definition, cyclothymic disorder is a chronic mood disturbance of at least 2 years' duration and involving numerous hypomanic and mild depressive episodes that do not meet the diagnostic criteria for mania or major depression with no periods of euthymia greater than 2 months.

A10. **e.** As with bipolar disorder, the treatment of choice is lithium carbonate.

SOLUTION TO THE SHORT ANSWER MANAGEMENT PROBLEM

a. Key features of bipolar disorder: Manic episode:
1) A distinct period of abnormally and persistently elevated, expansive, or irritable mood lasting at least 1 week and of sufficient severity to cause marked impairment in social or occupational functioning

2) During this period, at least three of the following symptoms are also present:
   a) Grandiosity
   b) Decreased need for sleep
   c) Hyperverbal or pressured speech
   d) Flight of ideas or racing thoughts
   e) Distractibility
   f) Increase in goal-directed activity or psychomotor agitation
   g) Excessive involvement in pleasurable activities that have a high potential for painful consequences
3) There is no evidence of a physical or substance-induced cause or the presence of another major mental disorder to account for the patient's symptoms.
b. Key features of hypomanic episodes:
1) A distinct mood of sustained elevated, expansive, or irritable mood lasting for at least 4 days that is clearly different from the individual's nondepressed mood yet does not cause marked impairment in social or occupational functioning such as in acute mania.
2) During the mood disturbance at least three of the following symptoms are also present to a significant degree:
   a) Inflated self-esteem or grandiosity
   b) Decreased need for sleep
   c) More talkative than usual
   d) Flight of ideas or racing thoughts
   e) Distractibility
   f) Increase in goal-directed activity or psychomotor agitation
   g) Excessive involvement in pleasurable activities that have a high potential for painful consequences
3) The episode is not physical or substance-induced.

SUMMARY OF THE DIAGNOSIS AND TREATMENT OF BIPOLAR DISORDER

1. Prevalence:
   a. The prevalence of bipolar disorders varies from 0.7% to 1.6% (lifetime).
   b. The prevalence is greater in women than in men.
   c. In general medical settings (settings that select for patients with emotional distress and physical illness), the prevalence rate is probably between 5% and 10% (lifetime).

2. Classification of bipolar disorders:
   a. Bipolar disorder I: A patient with bipolar disorder who has had at least one episode of true mania

b. Bipolar disorder II: A patient with bipolar disorder who has not had at least one episode of true mania

c. Cyclothymic disorder: A less severe form of bipolar disorder

3. Heritability of bipolar disorder:
   a. First-degree relatives of patients with bipolar affective disorder are at least 24 times more likely to develop bipolar illness than relatives of control subjects.
   b. The incidence of both bipolar illness and MDD is much higher in first-degree relatives of patients with bipolar illness than in the general population.

4. Diagnostic criteria:
   a. See diagnostic criteria for acute mania and acute hypomania in the Short Answer Management Problem.
   b. The other mood component of bipolar disorder is, of course, depression, which is discussed in Problem 60.

5. Cyclothymic disorder:
   a. Cyclothymic disorder is defined as a less severe form of bipolar disorder. By definition, it is a chronic mood disturbance of at least 2 years' duration and involves numerous hypomanic and mild depressive episodes. These episodes do not meet the diagnostic criteria for bipolar disorder or MDD.
   b. In cyclothymic disorder there are no periods of euthymia greater than 2 months' duration.

6. Treatment:
   a. Acute treatment:
      1) Hospitalization for acute mania with psychosis
      2) High potency antipsychotic agents (risperidone, haloperidol) when psychosis is present
      3) Benzodiazepines (lorazepam, clonazepam) may be useful for severe agitation during mania
   b. Maintenance and prevention of relapse:
      1) Lithium carbonate is the agent of first choice (usual dosage is 900 to 1200 mg/day).
      2) Carbamazepine and divalproex are useful when lithium is ineffective or contraindicated.
      3) Other anticonvulsants such as lamotrigine and gabapentin may be used when the previously mentioned agents are ineffective when used alone or in combination.

SUGGESTED READINGS

American Psychiatric Association: *Diagnostic and statistical manual of mental disorders*, ed 4, Washington, DC, 1994, American Psychiatric Association Press.

Kaplan HI, Sadock BJ, eds: *Kaplan and Sadock's synopsis of psychiatry: Behavioral sciences/clinical psychiatry*, ed 8, Baltimore, 1998, Williams & Wilkins.

Risby E, VanSant S, Stoudemire A: Mood disorders. In Stoudemire A, ed: *Clinical psychiatry for medical students*, ed 3, Philadelphia, 1998, JB Lippincott.

Shaner R: *Psychiatry*, Baltimore, 1997, Williams & Wilkins.

PROBLEM · 62

SCHIZOPHRENIA

"You Had Better Do What I Say; I Get My Orders from Lucifer, Himself."

Case 1 ■ A 22-Year-Old Male Brought to the Emergency Room by the Paramedics

A 22-year-old male is brought to the Emergency Room (ER) by the paramedics accompanied by his parents. He had begun to cut himself with a sharp knife at home and his father had called 911. The father tells you that this was the last straw. He tells you that his son has been acting very strangely for the past 15 months.

The patient himself stares straight ahead and refuses to answer any questions. He does, however, ask the nurse if she wants to kneel and kiss his hand. When she declines, the patient replies by saying, "You are the first woman who has refused the invitation to kiss the god of the Milky Way's hand." He points to the door entrance and remarks to the nurse, "You know, I could have you killed by my space soldiers; all it would take is one zap with the green ray gun from one of them."

The patient's father tells you that his son has essentially locked himself in his room for the past year. He eats all his meals there. He has some carpentry skills, and he built a large "dinner decontamination center" by knocking out three of the major upstairs walls. This occurred while his father and mother were on vacation. When they do see him, he seems very sad and depressed, and his voice can sometimes barely be heard.

The patient had a job at a fast-food restaurant but was fired 9 months ago when he started to "inject all the hamburgers with a decontamination substance," which turned out to be a thick mixture of pulverized leeches. It was at that point that he locked himself in his room for good. He has had no other medical conditions in the past 7 years. Before that he had suffered from episodes of major depression. He dropped out of school halfway through grade 8. His other significant history includes enuresis, encopresis, and separation anxiety as a child. His father is confident that his son is on no drugs, prescription or otherwise.

When you ask about family history of psychiatric disorders, alcoholism, or drug use, the father replies that "some quack of a psychiatrist labeled me as an alcoholic, which of course I am not." When you ask the patient's father what he drinks, he replies, whiskey. You deliberately overestimate the amount: "Sir, would you drink two bottles per day?" He replies, "No, of course not; one 26-ounce would be tops."

The patient states that he was appointed as the god of the Milky Way 14 months ago when the spaceship first landed in the back yard after having been searching for him for 400 years.

The mental status examination on this patient is difficult to complete because the patient is uncooperative with testing and is mute for prolonged periods. The patient's blood pressure is normal, as is the rest of the physical examination.

SELECT THE BEST ANSWER TO THE FOLLOWING QUESTIONS

Q1. What is the most likely diagnosis in this patient at this time?
a. schizoaffective disorder
b. schizophrenia
c. schizophreniform disorder
d. bipolar disorder
e. delusional disorder

Q2. Of the following features, which one is most suggestive of the diagnosis?
a. disorganized speech
b. delusions
c. hallucinations
d. the presence of both positive and negative symptoms
e. disorganized or catatonic behavior

Q3. How is the term *delusion* defined?
a. a false belief that is fixed and not explainable based on the cultural background of the individual
b. a disorder of the form of thought
c. a convincing feeling that one is being persecuted
d. a convincing feeling that one is being controlled by a supernatural force
e. the experiencing of stimuli in any of the senses in the absence of external stimulation

Q4. The differential diagnosis of this disorder described includes which of the following?
a. bipolar disorder
b. schizoaffective disorder
c. delusional disorder
d. brief psychotic disorder
e. all of the above

Q5. How is the term *psychosis* best defined?
a. behavior marked by a break from reality
b. behavior marked by a fixed false belief not in keeping with current life situation or circumstance
c. behavior not in keeping with the current environment in which the individual finds himself or herself
d. behavior marked by the sight of objects that are not present
e. behavior marked by the hearing of sounds that are not present

Case 2 ■ A 19-Year-Old Hallucinating Male Brought to the Emergency Department by His Parents

A patient comes to the ER with almost identical symptoms to the patient described in Case 1. However, the time from the beginning of the illness (the onset of the first symptom) to the termination of all symptoms is only 4 months.

Q6. What is the most likely diagnosis in this patient?
a. schizophrenia
b. schizoaffective disorder
c. schizophreniform disorder
d. bipolar disorder
e. brief psychotic disorder

Case 3 ■ A Patient with Acute Psychiatric Symptoms but with More Prominent Depression Symptoms

A patient develops acute psychiatric symptoms much like those described in Case 1 but in whom the symptoms of depression or mania are more prominent than the psychotic symptoms.

Q7. This patient would most likely have developed which of the following conditions?
a. schizophrenia
b. schizoaffective disorder
c. schizophreniform disorder
d. bipolar disorder
e. brief psychotic disorder

Q8. Disturbances in which of the following pairs of neurotransmitter systems are most clearly implicated in the pathogenesis of the condition described in Case 1?
   a. serotonin/dopamine
   b. serotonin/norepinephrine
   c. serotonin/gamma-aminobutyric acid (GABA)
   d. acetylcholine/dopamine
   e. acetylcholine/GABA

Q9. Which of the following is the drug of first choice for the patient presented in Case 1?
   a. risperidone
   b. clozapine
   c. haloperidol
   d. lithium carbonate
   e. fluoxetine

Q10. Which of the statements regarding the condition described in Case 1 is (are) most accurate?
   a. there is a documented genetic component in the cause of the condition described in Case 1
   b. environmental factors affect the expression of the condition
   c. lateral ventricular enlargement is common in this condition
   d. increased width of the third ventricle is common in this condition
   e. all of the above statements are true

SHORT ANSWER MANAGEMENT PROBLEM
Describe the differential diagnosis of psychosis.

ANSWERS

A1. **b.** The most likely diagnosis in this patient is schizophrenia. The following features characterize schizophrenia:
   a. Psychotic symptoms, at least two, present for at least 1 month.
      1) Hallucinations
      2) Delusions
      3) Disorganized speech (incoherence, evidence of a thought disorder)
      4) Disorganized or catatonic behavior
   b. Negative symptoms (flattening of affect, lack of motivation)
   c. Impairment in social or occupational functioning
   d. Duration of the illness for at least 6 months
   e. Symptoms are not primarily a result of a mood disorder or schizoaffective disorder
   f. Symptoms are not caused by a medical, neurologic, or substance-induced disorder.

A2. **d.** The most suggestive symptom of schizophrenia is the presence of both positive and negative symptoms.

Positive symptoms include the psychotic symptoms just described. The dramatic symptoms of hallucinations and delusions are the most reliably recognized symptoms of the illness.

Negative symptoms include the flattening of affect (emotional blunting), apathy, and the lack of motivation. Negative symptoms are sometimes called deficit symptoms.

A3. **a.** A delusion is defined as a fixed false belief that cannot be explained on the basis of the cultural background of the individual.

A4. **e.** The differential diagnosis of schizophrenia includes the following:
   a. Delusional disorder: A delusional disorder is a condition in which the patient has a delusion lasting for at least 1 month in the absence of prominent hallucinations or bizarre behavior.
   b. Brief psychotic disorder: A brief psychotic disorder is a disorder characterized by a relatively sudden onset of psychosis that lasts for a few hours to a month with a return to normal premorbid functioning at that time.
   c. Schizoaffective disorder: A schizoaffective disorder is a psychotic disorder that is differentiated from schizophrenia by either depressive symptoms or manic symptoms that are prominent and consistent features of a patient's long-term psychotic illness (see Answer 7). In contrast, a schizophreniform disorder is a disorder displaying the signs and symptoms of schizophrenia but lasting less than 6 months (see Answer 6).
   d. Bipolar disorder is distinguished from schizophrenia by a history of discrete mood episodes (mania and depression). Psychosis is only present during the mood episodes. During periods of euthymia, no psychosis is present.
   e. Psychotic disorder caused by a general medical condition
   f. A substance-induced psychotic disorder: Substances commonly associated with this condition include amphetamines, cocaine, various "designer drugs" (e.g., methylenedioxymethamphetamine), and some hallucinogens.

A5. **a.** *Psychosis* is a generic descriptive term applied to behavior marked by a break or loss of contact with reality. This often presents as disorganization of mental processes, emotional aberrations, difficulty in interpersonal relationships, and a decrease in functional capacity. In a patient with psychosis, mundane daily responsibilities may become burdensome or impossible to manage.

A6. **c.** A patient with schizophrenia-like symptoms that last for a period shorter than 6 months is classified as having schizophreniform disorder. Patients with schizophreniform disorder can be classified into those with or without good prognostic features. Good prognostic features include an acute onset, good premorbid functioning, and the absence of a flat affect. Patients without good prognostic features are more likely to have a condition that persists longer than 6 months. When symptoms persist past this point, the diagnosis is changed to schizophrenia.

A7. **b.** This patient has a schizoaffective disorder. A schizoaffective disorder is usually diagnosed when depressive or manic symptoms are a prominent and consistent feature of a patient's long-term psychotic illness. The diagnosis can be substantiated if the longitudinal course is consistent with schizophrenia and if residual schizophrenic-like symptoms persist when the patient is not depressed or manic. If, on the other hand, the psychotic symptoms are present only when the patient is depressed or manic and the patient has a relatively good interim functioning between episodes, the patient should be considered to have a primary mood disorder (either a major depressive disorder with psychotic features) or a bipolar disorder.

A8. **a.** The neurochemical basis of schizophrenia is not yet understood. However, medications that blockade some dopamine receptors (D2 and D4) and some serotonin receptors (5-HT2) ameliorate symptoms of the illness. The drugs that stimulate dopamine receptors (such as amphetamines) can produce schizophrenic-like symptoms. Drugs that stimulate serotonin receptors (such as lysergic acid) cause hallucinations.

A9. **a.** Risperidone and other newer antipsychotic medications, including olanzapine and quetiapine, present advantages over older agents and should be used as drugs of first choice. These medications have minimal or absent extrapyramidal movement side effects and may also be more effective for treatment of negative symptoms of schizophrenia. In addition to blockading dopamine receptors, newer antipsychotic medications blockade serotonin (5-HT2) receptors. Like newer antipsychotic medications, clozapine blockades both dopamine and serotonin receptors, has no movement side effects, and may be effective for negative symptoms of schizophrenia. However, it has a 5% incidence of seizures and a 1% incidence of agranulocytosis. Therefore it is not used as a first-line medication.

A10. **e.** There is considerable evidence that schizophrenia is an illness that runs in some families, although the majority of patients do not have a first-degree relative with schizophrenia. The morbid risk of a first-degree relative of a schizophrenic individual developing schizophrenia is approximately 10%.

There are also unknown environmental factors that influence the expression of schizophrenia.

There is a discordance rate of 10% to 30% for schizophrenia in identical twins. Furthermore, there is a seasonal variation in the birth dates of individuals with schizophrenia. Slightly more individuals with schizophrenia are born in the winter months.

Computed tomography and magnetic resonance imaging studies have demonstrated that in some schizophrenic patients there is enlargement of the lateral ventricles, increased width of the third ventricle, and sulcal enlargement suggestive of cortical atrophy.

SOLUTION TO THE SHORT ANSWER MANAGEMENT PROBLEM

A differential diagnosis of psychosis is as follows:
  a. Schizophrenia
  b. Schizophreniform disorder
  c. Schizoaffective disorder
  d. Bipolar disorder (manic phase)
  e. Delusional disorder
  f. Brief psychotic disorder
  g. Psychotic disorder caused by a general medical condition
  h. Substance-induced psychotic disorder

SUMMARY OF THE DIAGNOSIS AND TREATMENT OF SCHIZOPHRENIA

1. Prevalence: The lifetime prevalence of schizophrenia is 1% to 2%.

2. Characteristics of psychotic symptoms:
   a. Psychotic symptoms are nonspecific and occur in a variety of medical, psychiatric, neurologic, and substance-induced disorders.
   b. First-onset psychosis after the age of 45 generally suggests a neurologic disorder, a medical condition, a substance-induced disorder, or a psychotic depression. The onset of schizophrenia after the age of 45 is rare.

3. Main diagnostic clues to the diagnosis of schizophrenia are positive symptoms and negative symptoms:
   a. Positive symptoms include hallucinations, delusions, and bizarre behavior.

b. Negative symptoms include emotional blunting, apathy, or avulsion.

4. Differential diagnosis of schizophrenia and clues to each one:
   a. Delusion disorder: A disorder in which a delusion lasts at least 1 month. No other positive symptoms or negative symptoms of schizophrenia are present.
   b. Brief psychotic disorder: A disorder that is characterized by a relatively sudden onset of psychosis that lasts for a few hours to a month with a return to premorbid functioning thereafter. No other positive or negative symptoms are present.
   c. Bipolar I disorder: A disorder in which the psychotic symptoms are present only when the patient is depressed or manic; the patient has relatively good interim functioning between episodes.
   d. Major depressive disorder with psychotic features: A disorder in which the psychotic symptoms are present only when the patient is depressed; the patient has relatively good interim functioning between episodes.
   e. Schizophreniform disorder: Both the positive and the negative symptoms of schizophrenia are present, but the patient either recovers without residual symptoms within a 6-month period or has symptoms for less than 6 months.
   f. Schizoaffective disorder: If a patient has symptoms of depression or mania with psychosis and the depressive or manic symptoms are a prominent and consistent feature of the patient's long-term psychotic illness, schizoaffective disorder is the most likely diagnosis.
   g. Psychotic disorder caused by a general medical condition: A disorder that may produce psychotic symptoms include cerebral neoplasms, cerebrovascular disease, epilepsy, thyroid disorders, parathyroid disorders, hypoxia, hypoglycemia, hepatic disorders, renal disorders, and autoimmune disorders.
   h. Substance-induced psychotic disorder: This most commonly occurs with the amphetamines.

5. Symptoms and signs of schizophrenia:
   a. Psychotic symptoms are present for at least 1 month including two of the following:
      1) Delusions
      2) Disorganized speech (incoherence, evidence of a thought disorder)
      3) Disorganized or catatonic behavior
   b. Negative symptoms are present (affective flattening, lack of motivation).

c. Impairment in social or occupational functioning
d. Duration of the illness for at least 6 months.
e. Symptoms are not caused by a mood disorder or schizoaffective disorder.
f. Symptoms are not caused by a medical, neurologic, or substance-induced disorder.

6. Subtypes of schizophrenia:
   a. Catatonic: Dominated by motoric abnormalities such as rigidity and posturing
   b. Disorganized: Marked by flat affect and disorganized speech and behavior
   c. Paranoid: Paranoid symptoms in the absence of catatonic and disorganized features
   d. Undifferentiated: None of the above symptoms predominate
   e. Residual: Only negative symptoms or attenuated symptoms remain after an active phase

7. Causation:
   a. Schizophrenia is believed to have a pathogenesis that consists of an interaction between genetic influences and environmental variables.
   b. There are gross morphologic and cytoarchitectural abnormalities in the brains of some individuals with schizophrenia, but there are no pathognomonic findings. An increased prevalence of perceptual-motor and cognitive abnormalities is described in many studies.

8. Treatment:
   a. Active phase:
      1) Hospitalization for severely disorganized or dangerous behavior
      2) Antipsychotic medications, with newer antipsychotic medications being the drugs of first choice.
      3) Reassurance and support for both patient and family members
   b. Chronic phase:
      1) Continued antipsychotic medication at the lowest effective dose often prevents relapse for long periods.
      2) Psychosocial treatment: Underlying goals are treatment of symptoms, reduction of stress, mobilization of social supports, assistance with deficits in daily living skills caused by the illness, and gradual rehabilitation to the most autonomous level of functioning possible for the individual patient.

SUGGESTED READINGS

American Psychiatric Association: *Diagnostic and statistical manual of mental disorders,* ed 4, Washington, DC, 1994, American Psychiatric Association Press.

Kaplan HI, Sadock BJ, eds: *Kaplan and Sadock's synopsis of psychiatry: Behavioral sciences/clinical psychiatry*, ed 8, Baltimore, 1998, Williams & Wilkins.

Ninan P et al: Schizophrenia and other psychotic disorders. In Stoudemire A, ed: *Clinical psychiatry for medical students*, ed 3, Philadelphia, 1998, JB Lippincott.

Shaner R: *Psychiatry*, Baltimore, 1997, Williams & Wilkins.

PROBLEM·63

ALCOHOL DEPENDENCE AND ALCOHOL ABUSE

"Doc, I'll Never Be an Alcoholic; I Have a Hollow Leg."

Case 1 ■ A 45-Year-Old Male with an Enlarged Liver

A 45-year-old executive comes to your office for his periodic health assessment. He tells you that he has been feeling "tired, and just not myself lately." He also tells you that he has been so tired that he "has had to stay home from work for many days at a time." He is beginning to question his ability to function effectively as the chief executive officer of a transportation company. When you inquire about other symptoms, he tells you that he has also suffered from "profound headaches" and that his sex life with his wife is "the pits." On direct questioning he tells you that the headaches "have been a problem for the past 6 months" and his "lack of interest in sex" for about the same amount of time.

He has had no serious medical, surgical, or psychiatric illnesses to date. He tells you that he is taking no over-the-counter or prescription drugs.

The patient describes himself as a "social drinker," and his use of alcohol as "strictly to relax." He then states, "I certainly hope you do not think I am an alcoholic, Doctor!" Moreover, there is no evidence of acute intoxication at this time.

He does state, on more persistent questioning, "Well, maybe I am using more alcohol than I did a few years ago," "Oh sometimes, I might get a few shakes the next day if I have had too many drinks," and "Well, I have spent some time trying to hide it around the house, Doctor." His last statement, however, is "But Doctor, I am not an alcoholic, you know."

His father died of complications of "yellow jaundice" at age 61. His mother died of complications of "heart failure" at age 69. He has three brothers and two sisters; all are well.

On physical examination, his blood pressure is 160/104 mm Hg. His pulse is 96 and regular. Examination of the head and neck, respiratory system, and musculoskeletal system are normal. Examination of the cardiovascular system reveals a point of maximum impulse (PMI) in the fifth intercostal space on the anterior axillary line. He subsequently describes recent episodes of "waking up at night short of breath" as well as "shortness of breath on exertion." Examination of the gastrointestinal system reveals no tenderness or rebound tenderness. The liver edge is palpated approximately 8 cm below the right costal margin. Examination of the neurologic system reveals intermittent carpal spasms of both extremities. He cannot perform serial 7s and has difficulty with recall of information on the mental status examination.

SELECT THE BEST ANSWER TO THE FOLLOWING QUESTIONS

Q1. With the history given, what is the best description of the most likely diagnosis in this patient?
   a. somatization disorder
   b. adjustment disorder with depressed and anxious mood
   c. major depressive disorder
   d. alcohol dependence
   e. alcohol abuse

Q2. Which of the following signs or symptoms further substantiate your diagnosis in this patient?
   a. the location of the PMI
   b. the patient's elevated blood pressure
   c. the abdominal signs on physical examination
   d. none of the above
   e. all of the above

Q3. What were the total direct and indirect social costs in the United States in 1995 resulting from the disorder diagnosed in Question 1?
   a. $50,000,000
   b. $100,000,000
   c. $1,000,000,000
   d. $150,000,000,000
   e. impossible to calculate

Q4. What is the most likely cause of the patient's liver edge palpated at 8 cm below the right costal margin?
   a. tricornute liver (congenital malformation)
   b. alcoholic hepatitis
   c. alcoholic (Laënnec's) cirrhosis
   d. "the deep diaphragm pushing the liver down" syndrome
   e. hepatorenal syndrome

Q5. There is a high correlation between the disorder diagnosed in Question 1 and which of the following syndromes?
   a. generalized anxiety disorder
   b. major depressive disorder

c. schizophrenia

d. opioid abuse

e. all of the above

f. b and d only

Q6. The patient's inability to perform serial 7s and information recall is most likely caused by which of the following?

a. benign senile forgetfulness syndrome

b. alcoholic dementia

c. alcoholic amnestic syndrome

d. all of the above are equally likely

e. b and c

Q7. Which of the following neurotransmitters has been most clearly implicated in the disease process established by the diagnosis made in Question 1?

a. dopamine

b. angiotensin

c. serotonin

d. aldosterone

e. acetylcholine

Q8. Regarding risk factors for the condition diagnosed in Question 1, which of the following statements most accurately reflects risk factor status and identification?

a. there are no risk factors for this disease; it just happens

b. there is no single factor that accounts for increased relative and absolute risk in first-degree relatives of patients with this disorder

c. genetic, familial, environmental, occupational, socioeconomic, cultural, personality, life stress, psychiatric comorbidity, biologic, social learning, and behavioral conditioning are all risk factors or risk environments for this disorder

d. there is a clear risk factor stratification for this disorder

e. b and c

Q9. What are the concordance rates for this disorder among identical twins and fraternal twins, respectively?

a. 35% and 70%

b. 3% and 3%

c. 70% and 35%

d. 50% and 50%

e. 25% and 75%

Q10. How is *alcohol dependence syndrome* best defined?

a. a state in which a syndrome of drug-specific withdrawal signs and symptoms follows reduction or cessation of drug use

b. a state in which the physiologic or behavioral effects of a constant dose of a psychoactive substance decreases over time

c. a physiologic state that follows cessation or reduction in the amount of drug used

d. a and b

e. all of the above

Q11. How is *alcohol withdrawal syndrome* best defined?

a. a state in which a syndrome of drug-specific withdrawal signs and symptoms follows the reduction or cessation of drug use

b. a state in which the physiologic or behavioral effects of a constant dose of a psychoactive substance decreases over time

c. a pathologic state that follows cessation or reduction in the amount of drug used

d. a and b

e. all of the above

Q12. How is *alcohol abuse syndrome* best defined?

a. a maladaptive state leading to clinically significant impairment

b. a maladaptive state leading to clinically significant distress

c. a maladaptive state leading to laboratory significant impairment

d. either a or c

e. either a or b

Q13. Considering the patient described, which of the following diagnostic imaging procedures is (are) definitely indicated?

a. chest x-ray

b. cardiac echocardiogram

c. computed tomography (CT) scan of the head

d. a and c only

e. all of the above

Q14. Which of the following explanations is the most likely explanation for the tremors observed on physical examination?

a. delirium tremens (early)

b. alcohol withdrawal syndrome

c. thiamine deficiency

d. alcoholic encephalopathy (early)

e. Korsakoff's psychosis

Q15. 26-year-old male comes to your office for a periodic health examination before he gets married. When you question him about his lifestyle and ask him about his alcohol intake, he replies that he is a "social drinker." Once that is established what should you do?

a. congratulate him on avoiding problems with alcohol

b. accept "social drinking" at face value and move onto the next question

c. ask him whether he ever has a drink while alone

d. ask him to very specifically define social drinking

e. first establish what he drinks; following that, overestimate the daily consumption and then come down from there

---

Case 2 ■ A Patient with Short-Term Memory Deficits

A patient whom you suspect of alcohol dependence demonstrates significant short-term memory deficits. He then tries to cover up those deficits by, in your opinion, making up answers to questions.

Q16. Which of the following is the most likely diagnosis?
a. Wernicke's encephalopathy
b. alcohol-induced persisting amnestic disorder (Korsakoff's psychosis)
c. alcohol-induced psychotic disorder with delusions
d. alcohol-induced psychotic disorder with hallucinosis
e. alcohol-induced persisting dementia

Q17. The feature described as "making up answers to questions" is known as which of the following?
a. confabulation
b. alcoholic lying
c. alcoholic delirium
d. alcoholic paranoia
e. memory loss encephalopathy

Q18. What is the cause of the disorder described in Case 2?
a. riboflavin deficiency
b. thiamine deficiency
c. zinc deficiency
d. cerebral atrophy caused by alcohol abuse
e. cerebellar atrophy caused by alcohol abuse

Q19. The word *alcoholism* means different things to different people. Of the following, which is the best definition of alcoholism?
a. alcohol abuse and alcohol dependency
b. alcohol abuse but not alcohol dependency
c. alcohol abuse or alcohol dependency
d. alcohol abuse and/or alcohol dependency
e. none of the above represent an adequate definition of alcoholism

Q20. What is the percentage of the American population who use at least some alcohol (or have used some alcohol)?
a. 50%
b. 60%
c. 70%
d. 90%
e. 94%

SHORT ANSWER MANAGEMENT PROBLEM

Part A: Provide a screening test for alcohol abuse that can be easily administered in the office setting.

Part B: List five objectives for short-term treatment of the patient and the patient's family in a case of alcohol dependence.

ANSWERS

A1. **d.** This patient has alcohol dependence, which is defined as at least three of the following occurring over a 12-month period:
a. Tolerance: the need for increased amounts of a substance to achieve intoxication or another desired effect or markedly diminished effect with use of the same amount of the substance.
b. Characteristic withdrawal symptoms or the use of alcohol (or a closely related substitute) to relieve or avoid withdrawal
c. Substance often taken in larger amounts over a longer period than the person intended
d. Persistent desire or one or more unsuccessful attempts to cut down or quit drinking
e. A great deal of time spent in getting the alcohol, drinking it, or recovering from its effects
f. Important social, occupational, or recreational activities are given up or reduced because of the alcohol
g. Continued alcohol use despite the knowledge of having a persistent or recurrent social, psychologic, or physical problem that is caused by, or exacerbated by, use of alcohol.

A2. **e.** The physical signs and symptoms actually substantiate the diagnosis of alcohol dependence, not alcohol abuse. Alcohol dependence is defined as a maladaptive pattern of alcohol use with adverse clinical consequences. These physical symptoms include the following:
a. The PMI: the location of the PMI in the fifth intercostal space suggests cardiomegaly. This could be on the basis of either alcoholic cardiomyopathy or hypertension (most likely also related to alcohol intake).

b. The obvious hepatomegaly suggests either alcoholic hepatitis or cirrhosis of the liver.

c. The fine tremor suggests early alcoholic encephalopathy. This is substantiated by the cognitive dysfunction (lack of ability to perform serial 7s).

d. The patient's hypertension suggests alcohol as a potential cause.

A3. **d.** The direct and indirect social costs of alcohol-related disorders in the United States in 1995 were estimated at $150 billion. Of this, approximately 15% are health care costs and 60% is lost productivity.

A4. **c.** The most likely cause of the hepatomegaly is alcoholic (Laënnec's) cirrhosis. Although in many patients this could represent alcoholic hepatitis, the presence of other central nervous system symptoms and signs suggests alcoholic cirrhosis.

A5. **e.** The National Institute of Mental Health Epidemiologic Catchment Area Program found a very high correlation rate between alcoholism and the following:
  a. Suicide
  b. Homicide
  c. Accidents
  d. Anxiety disorders
  e. Major depressive disorder
  f. Schizophrenia
  g. Narcotic drug abuse
  h. Cocaine abuse

A6. **e.** Chronic alcohol use is associated with the cognitive and memory deficits of alcoholic dementia (alcohol persisting dementia) and the more restrictive memory deficits of alcohol amnestic disorder. Patients with alcohol-related amnestic syndrome have the most difficulty with short-term memory (remembering recent events). However, deficits may be noted in long-term memory as well.

A7. **c.** Ethyl alcohol (ethanol) has been demonstrated to have significant effects on several brain neurotransmitter systems. Acute exposure to alcohol appears to inhibit excitatory N-methyl-D-aspartate (NMDA) receptors, whereas chronic alcohol exposure causes a sensitization of NMDA receptors. Alcohol also affects the activity of the beta-adrenergic receptors and the adenosine neurotransmitter receptors linked to adenylate cyclase. Alcohol causes the release of serotonin from neurons, and chronic use may lead to depletion of brain serotonin. Alcohol has been shown to modify the binding of gamma-aminobutyric acid (GABA) to its receptors and augments the electrophysiologic and behavioral effects of GABA in animals.

A8. **e.** Factors that determine an individual's susceptibility to a substance use disorder are not well understood. Studies of populations at risk for developing substance abuse have identified many factors that foster the development and continuance of substance use, including genetic, familial, environmental, occupational, socioeconomic, cultural, personality, life stress, psychiatric comorbidity, biologic, social learning, and behavioral conditioning.

A9. **c.** The concordance rate for alcoholism among identical twin pairs is twice that of fraternal twin pairs. The rates are 70% and 35%, respectively.

A10. **d.** See Answer 1.

A11. **a.** Alcohol withdrawal syndrome is a substance-specific syndrome that develops following cessation of or reduced intake of alcohol.

A12. **a.** Alcohol abuse describes patterns of alcohol use that do not meet the criteria for alcohol dependence. Alcohol abuse is defined as a maladaptive pattern of substance use that causes clinically significant impairment. This may include impairments in social, family, or occupational functioning; the presence of psychologic or physical problems; or the use of alcohol while or before driving a motor vehicle. Alcohol abuse commonly progresses to alcohol dependence.

A13. **e.** The imaging studies indicated in this patient include a chest x-ray, a CT or magnetic resonance imaging scan of the head, and an echocardiogram. An echocardiogram should be done to define the thickness of the left ventricular wall to determine whether or not left ventricular hypertrophy is, in fact, present, as is indicated by the position of the PMI. A chest x-ray can be justified on the basis of probable cardiac enlargement, that is, to measure the cardiac/thoracic ratio. A CT scan is justified to rule out causes of cognitive disturbances that may be related to alcohol abuse, including intracranial bleeding. It may also detect causes of cognitive disturbances unrelated to alcohol.

A14. **d.** The movement disorder that is demonstrated on physical examination suggests the early stages of liver failure and alcoholic encephalopathy. It may develop into asterixes (an arrhythmic flapping tremor of the fully extended hand), sometimes referred to as *liver flap.*

A15. **e.** *Social drinking* is a term with little meaning. It is important to more precisely determine drinking patterns.

The first step is to determine whether or not a patient drinks. The second step is to determine how much alcohol a patient drinks. Because of the tendency of individuals who drink alcohol excessively to minimize their problems, one way of obtaining an accurate assessment of alcohol intake is to greatly overestimate what you believe to be the worst case scenario and then come down. For example, you might say, "Well, if it's beer you drink, do you drink one case (24 cans) per day?"

It may surprise you how often the response comes back: "Oh no, Doctor, it wouldn't be any more than half that much."

A common instrument for screening for alcoholism in the primary care office setting is the CAGE questionnaire. The CAGE questionnaire includes four questions:
   a. Have you ever felt the need to **C**ut down on your drinking?
   b. Have you ever felt **A**nnoyed by criticisms of your drinking?
   c. Have you ever had **G**uilty feelings about drinking?
   d. Have you ever taken a morning **E**ye-opener?

With the CAGE questionnaire, any more than one positive answer may suggest alcohol abuse.

Another reliable screening tool for heavy alcohol use is the Michigan Alcohol Screening Test (MAST). This 25-item scale identifies abnormal drinking through its social and behavioral consequences with a sensitivity of 90% to 98%. The Brief MAST, a shortened 10-item test, has been shown to have similar efficacy.

A16. **b.** This patient has alcohol-induced persisting amnestic disorder, called *Korsakoff's psychosis.* Patients with alcohol-related amnestic disorder have the most difficulty with short-term memory (remembering recent events), although deficits in long-term memory may be noted as well.

A17. **a.** Patients often try to conceal or compensate for their memory loss by confabulation (making up answers or talking around questions that require them to use their memory).

A18. **b.** The cause of this particular disorder is a chronic deficiency in the vitamin thiamine. For that reason, whenever a patient is in a confused state that may be related to alcohol abuse, intravenous thiamine should be administered.

A19. **e.** Alcoholism is defined as a repetitive but inconsistent and sometimes unpredictable loss of control of drinking that produces symptoms of serious dysfunction or disability.

A20. **d.** It is estimated that 90% of the American population uses at least some alcohol.

SOLUTION TO THE SHORT ANSWER MANAGEMENT PROBLEM

Part A: A good primary care screening test for alcoholism is the CAGE questionnaire. The CAGE questionnaire has been described in Answer 15. Alternatives are the MAST (25 items) and the Brief MAST (10 items).

Part B: Five objectives for the short-term treatment of alcohol dependence in the patient and the patient's family include the following:
   a. Relieving subjective symptoms of distress and discomfort caused by intoxication or withdrawal
   b. Preventing or treating serious complications of intoxication, withdrawal, or dependence
   c. Establishing sobriety
   d. Preparing for and referral to long-term treatment or rehabilitation
   e. Engaging the family in the treatment process

SUMMARY OF THE DIAGNOSIS AND TREATMENT OF ALCOHOL DEPENDENCE AND ALCOHOL ABUSE

1. Prevalence: An estimated 5% to 7% of Americans have alcoholism in any given year and 13% will have it sometime during their lifetime.

2. Economic costs: The direct economic costs of alcoholism in the United States are staggering. In 1995 total economic losses from lost productivity in the United States were $90 billion. This does not include indirect economic costs and noneconomic costs and losses.

3. Definitions:
   a. Alcoholism: A repetitive but inconsistent and sometimes unpredictable loss of control of drinking that produces symptoms of serious dysfunction or disability.
   b. Alcohol dependence: A maladaptive pattern of alcohol use that includes three of the following:
      1) Tolerance
      2) Withdrawal
      3) Increasing amounts of consumption
      4) Desire or attempts to cut down or quit
      5) Substantial time spent in "hiding the habit"
      6) Important social, occupational, or recreational dysfunction
      7) Continued use of alcohol despite knowledge of having a persistent or recurrent social, psychologic, or physical problem

c. Alcohol abuse: A residual category that describes patterns of alcohol use that do not meet the criteria for alcohol dependence

d. Alcohol intoxication: Reversible, alcohol-specific physiologic and behavioral changes caused by recent exposure to alcohol

e. Alcohol withdrawal: An alcohol-specific syndrome that develops following cessation of or reduced intake in the amount of alcohol.

f. Alcohol-persisting disorder: An alcohol-specific syndrome that persists long after acute intoxication or withdrawal abates (such as memory impairments or dementia)

4. Systemic disease association: The following disease states are directly linked to the toxic effects of alcohol:
   a. Alcoholic cardiomyopathy
   b. Systemic hypertension
   c. Alcoholic hepatitis
   d. Laënnec's (alcoholic) cirrhosis
   e. Esophageal varices, gastritis, ascites, edema
   f. Peripheral neuropathy
   g. Alcoholic encephalopathy

5. Neurologic syndromes:
   a. Alcoholic dementia
   b. Alcoholic amnestic disorder
   c. Korsakoff's psychosis
   d. Wernicke's encephalopathy
   e. Alcoholic hallucinosis
   f. Alcoholic paranoia
   g. Alcohol delirium

6. Screening:
   a. The CAGE questionnaire
   b. The MAST questionnaire
   c. The Brief MAST questionnaire

7. Laboratory testing: There are no diagnostic tests that are specific for alcohol dependence, but mean corpuscular volume, liver transaminases (SGOT, SGPT), and gamma-glutamyl transferase are the three most common tests. The accuracy of a diagnosis of alcoholism increases when all three tests are used together.

8. Treatment:
   a. General considerations: See the Short Answer Management Problem.
   b. Long-term treatment must have the following characteristics to maximize its potential:
      1) Active involvement with comprehensive rehabilitation and recovery program
      2) Relapse prevention program with peer support components and possibly pharmacologic components, including disulfiram or naltrexone.
      3) Inclusion of family and significant others in recovery process
   c. Goals of long-term treatment:
      1) Maintain sobriety
      2) Make significant changes in lifestyle, work, and friendships
      3) Treat underlying psychiatric illness (dual diagnosis)
      4) Ongoing involvement in Alcoholics Anonymous or similar groups for relapse prevention

SUGGESTED READINGS

American Psychiatric Association:. *Diagnostic and statistical manual of mental disorders,* ed 4, Washington, DC, 1994, American Psychiatric Association Press.

Kaplan HI, Sadock BJ, eds: *Kaplan and Sadock's synopsis of psychiatry: Behavioral sciences/clinical psychiatry,* ed 8, Baltimore, 1998, Williams & Wilkins.

Shaner R: *Psychiatry,* Baltimore, 1997, Williams & Wilkins.

Swift R: Alcoholism and substance abuse. In Stoudemire A, ed: *Clinical psychiatry for medical students,* ed 3, Philadelphia, 1998, JB Lippincott.

PROBLEM·64

DRUG ABUSE

One Minute, Euphoric; the Next, Down in the Dumps

Case 1 ■ A 32-Year-Old Administrator with "Rapidly Swinging Moods"

A 32-year-old man is brought into the Emergency Room (ER) by his wife one evening. She tells you that "something is desperately wrong with my husband." She states he used to be kind, even-keeled, and fun to be with, but during the last year, she says, he has "changed drastically."

He now exhibits behavior that can best be described as "very erratic." He will go from periods of extreme depression to short intervals of "being on top of the world," "extremely elated," with "extremely fast speech and restlessness." After a few hours, he goes back into a state of depression. His wife brought him into the ER tonight because he was in a period of elation and euphoria.

She also tells you that her husband has not been performing well at work lately and that "some of his colleagues have noticed some strange behavior." In addition, his wife tells you that "money seems to be disappearing from our bank account at a rate far faster than I can explain."

On examination, the patient is obviously euphoric and elated. When you ask him why he agreed to come tonight, he tells you that he feels so good, he would do anything to please his wife. His speech appears extremely pressured.

On physical examination, his blood pressure is 190/110 mm Hg. His pulse is 128 and regular. His pupils are widely dilated, and he is sweating profusely.

SELECT THE BEST ANSWER TO THE FOLLOWING QUESTIONS

Q1. With this history and physical examination, what is the most likely diagnosis?
  a. bipolar I disorder, rapid cycling
  b. bipolar II disorder, rapid cycling
  c. amphetamine intoxication
  d. cocaine intoxication
  e. schizophrenia: catatonic subtype

Q2. At this time, what would be the most appropriate course of action?
  a. arrange for a routine psychiatric consultation on an elective basis
  b. arrange for a social worker to see the patient and his wife now
  c. arrange for an immediate psychiatric consultation
  d. call the appropriate consultant and relate the history, your findings and diagnosis, and appropriate acute intervention
  e. prescribe diazepam and follow up as an outpatient in 1 week

Q3. The term *dual diagnosis* in psychiatry refers to which of the following?
  a. any two closely related psychiatric disorders in the same patient
  b. any two relatively unrelated psychiatric disorders in the same patient
  c. the manic and depressive episodes of bipolar disorder
  d. the existence of both a psychiatric disorder and a substance abuse disorder in the same patient
  e. the existence of both a chronic medical disorder and a psychiatric disorder in the same patient

Q4. What is the most effective interview strategy to motivate this patient to engage in treatment?
  a. to focus on the precise details of the euphoria and the elation the patient is experiencing
  b. to focus on the precise details of the longer periods of the depression the patient is experiencing
  c. to focus on the precise details of the negative consequences that have resulted from the patient's symptoms
  d. to focus on the relationship between the patient's symptoms and the possible use or abuse of alcohol
  e. focusing on the relationship between the patient's symptoms and the relationship with his wife

Q5. Of the following substances listed, which has undergone the most dramatic epidemic increase in the last decade in the United States?
  a. anabolic steroids
  b. crack cocaine
  c. hallucinogens
  d. cannabis
  e. alcohol

Q6. Following informed consent, which of the following laboratory tests will yield the most significant information concerning the confirmation of the diagnosis made in this patient?
  a. serum cotinine level
  b. urine benzoylecgonine level
  c. urine opioid and serum opioid metabolite levels
  d. serum gamma glutamyl transferase
  e. serum barbiturate level

Q7. Which of the following is (are) a complication(s) of the disorder diagnosed in the patient described?
  a. sudden cardiac death
  b. cerebral hemorrhage
  c. respiratory arrest
  d. convulsions
  e. all of the above

Q8. Which of the following statements regarding opioid abuse in the United States is (are) true?
  a. The prevalence of human immunodeficiency virus (HIV) infection among intravenous (IV) drug abusers in the United States continues to increase
  b. Opioid overdose should be suspected in any patient who is in a coma and has respiratory depression
  c. Nausea, vomiting, cramps, and diarrhea are symptoms of opioid withdrawal
  d. b and c
  e. all of the above are true

Q9. Which of the following substances is responsible for the most mortality in our society?
  a. nicotine

b. alcohol
c. cocaine
d. heroin
e. cannabis

Q10. Which of the following drugs most effectively ameliorates the symptoms of heroin withdrawal?
a. naloxone
b. naltrexone
c. clonidine
d. disulfiram
e. methadone

Q11. Which of the following is a specific benzodiazepine antagonist?
a. flumazenil
b. naltrexone
c. clonidine
d. methadone
e. sertraline

Q12. Which of the following drugs is most effective for alcohol and benzodiazepine detoxification?
a. flumazenil
b. naltrexone
c. carbamazepine
d. lorazepam
e. clonidine

SHORT ANSWER MANAGEMENT PROBLEM

Describe the general principles of interviewing a patient you suspect of having a substance-abuse problem but who denies the problem.

ANSWERS

A1. **d.** This patient most likely has cocaine intoxication. Cocaine intoxication is characterized by elation, euphoria, excitement, pressured speech, restlessness, stereotyped movements, and bruxism. Sympathetic stimulation occurs, including tachycardia, hypertension, mydriasis, and sweating. Paranoia, suspiciousness, and psychosis may occur with prolonged use. Overdose produces hyperpyrexia, hyperreflexia, seizures, coma, and respiratory arrest. Amphetamine produces similar symptoms, but rapid changes in mood from elation to depression are less common because of its longer half-life. It is also much less expensive than cocaine and less likely to rapidly deplete someone's savings.

A2. **d.** The treatment of choice is detoxification and drug rehabilitation. The therapy should include individual psychotherapy and group (family) psychotherapy.

A3. **d.** The term *dual diagnosis* is most often used in psychiatry to denote the occurrence of substance abuse and another psychiatric illness. It is also used to refer to the co-occurrence of a developmental disorder (e.g., mental retardation) and another psychiatric illness.

A4. **c.** The most effective strategy for engaging individuals in substance abuse treatment is to focus on the negative consequences resulting from drug abuse. This will produce the greatest likelihood of convincing the patient that he or she has a problem. Substance abuse treatment is rarely successful when patients do not believe that their problem is serious.

A5. **b.** Of the drugs listed, the one having undergone the most substantial increase in use over the last decade is crack cocaine. In younger populations, the use of inhalants, especially gasoline, has also greatly increased.

A6. **b.** The metabolite of cocaine that can be detected in the urine is benzoylecgonine. It should be tested for as soon as possible.

A7. **e.** The complications of cocaine intoxication include the following:
a. Sudden cardiac arrhythmias
b. Convulsions
c. Respiratory arrest
d. Cerebral hemorrhage
e. Sudden cardiac death

A8. **e.** Despite declines in some other populations such as educated gay males, the prevalence of HIV infection among IV drug abusers continues to increase. Opioid overdose should be suspected in any patient who presents to the ER with coma, convulsions, and respiratory depression. Therefore naloxone, an opioid antagonist, is often indicated even before confirmation of opioid toxicosis. Nausea, vomiting, cramps, and diarrhea are common signs and symptoms of opioid withdrawal. Other signs and symptoms include generalized pain, dysphoria, lacrimation, yawning, rhinorrhea, and piloerection.

A9. **a.** Nicotine addiction and tobacco use are legally sanctioned, although restrictions on exposure of others to secondhand smoke have increased. Tobacco accounts for over 350,000 premature deaths per year in the United States, far more than any other recreational substance.

A10. **e.** Methadone most effectively treats the symptoms of heroin withdrawal and is often used acutely for this purpose. As a component of detoxification treatment, methadone is then gradually reduced to minimize withdrawal symptoms. The alpha$_2$-adrenergic agonist clonidine hydrochloride may also be used to suppress some of the signs and symptoms of opioid withdrawal. Clonidine acts at presynaptic noradrenergic nerve endings in the locus ceruleus of the brain and blocks the adrenergic discharge produced by opioid withdrawal. In most studies clonidine has been shown to suppress approximately 75% of opioid withdrawal signs and symptoms, especially autonomic hyperactivity and gastrointestinal symptoms. Withdrawal symptoms that are not significantly ameliorated by clonidine include drug craving, insomnia, arthralgias, and myalgias.

A11. **a.** Flumazenil (Romazicon) is a benzodiazepine antagonist that binds competitively and reversibly to the GABA-benzodiazepine receptor complex and inhibits the effects of the benzodiazepines. The drug is approved for the treatment of benzodiazepine overdose or the reversal of benzodiazepine sedation.

A12. **d.** Tapering doses of lorazepam or other benzodiazepines are the most effective treatment for most serious alcohol and benzodiazepine withdrawals. Carbamazepine has been demonstrated to be an effective treatment for alcohol and benzodiazepine withdrawal and has less potential than benzodiazepines for causing drug dependence. However, the adverse effects of carbamazepine, including blood dyscrasias and hepatitis, make it less useful than benzodiazepines for this indication. Animal studies suggest that periodic administration of flumazenil during the chronic administration of benzodiazepines may attenuate the subsequent withdrawal syndrome, but this is not a practical clinical treatment.

SOLUTION TO THE SHORT ANSWER MANAGEMENT PROBLEM

The general principles of interviewing a potentially drug-abusing patient who initially denies drug abuse (and that includes most patients) includes the following:
   a. Attempt to obtain a detailed history of any substance use (start with nicotine and alcohol).
   b. Inquire about physical and behavioral problems.
   c. Provide empathy and concern to encourage trust on the part of the patient.
   d. Avoid judgmental attitudes and pejorative statements.

   e. The most effective interview strategy is to focus on whether or not the patient has experienced negative consequences due to his or her use of psychoactive substances, has poor control of use, or has been criticized by others concerning his or her pattern of behavior or use of the substance.
   f. Confront the patient if you have absolute evidence.
   g. Include input from family members and significant others whenever possible.

SUMMARY OF THE DIAGNOSIS AND TREATMENT OF DRUG ABUSE

Many ramifications that concern drug abuse are also outlined in Problem 63, concerning alcoholism. Others are as follows:

1. Gateway drugs: Individuals with substance use disorders often first started to abuse alcohol and marijuana and then progressed to cocaine, opioids, or other dangerous drugs.

2. Recreational substance that causes most morbidity and mortality worldwide: Nicotine, via cigarette smoking

3. Stimulant abuse: Crack cocaine abuse is still common in the United States, and amphetamine abuse is quickly escalating.

4. Opioid abuse: IV heroin users are now the second largest group of patients with acquired immunodeficiency syndrome in the United States.

5. Specific drugs:
   a. Cocaine: Cocaine increases the sympathetic stimulation of the central nervous system (CNS) and produces initial euphoria as a high. Cocaine (crack) is potent and significantly less expensive than many other drugs.
   b. Caffeine: Caffeine and related methylxanthines are ubiquitous drugs in our society. These drugs produce sympathetic stimulation, diuresis, bronchodilatation, and CNS stimulation.
   c. Cannabis: Marijuana, although illegal, has been used at one time or another by 64.8% of adult Americans. Cannabis intoxication is characterized by tachycardia, muscle relaxation, euphoria, and a sense of well being. Tachycardia, time sense alteration, and emotional lability are common.
   d. Anabolic steroids: Some data suggest that 6.5% of adolescent American boys and 1.9% of adoles-

cent American girls have used anabolic steroids. The medical complications of these drugs include myocardial infarction, stroke, and hepatic disease. Psychiatric symptoms associated with anabolic steroid use include severe depression, psychotic (paranoid) symptoms, aggressive behavior, homicidal impulses, euphoria, irritability, anxiety, racing thoughts, and hyperactivity. (All of these symptoms decline or are eliminated upon discontinuation of the drug.)

e. Hallucinogens: The hallucinogens include lysergic acid diethylamide, mescaline, psilocybin, dimethyltryptamine, hallucinogenic amphetamines, and methylenedioxyamphetamine. The mechanism of action of these substances includes stimulation of CNS dopamine or serotonin.

f. Inhalants: Inhalants are volatile compounds that are inhaled for their intoxicating effects. Substances in this class include organic solvents (e.g., gasoline, toluene, and ethyl ether). Inhalants are ubiquitous and readily available in most households. These are drugs of choice for many disadvantaged youths in both urban and rural environments.

g. Nicotine: More than 50 million Americans smoke cigarettes daily, and another 10 million use other forms of tobacco. Nicotine addiction and tobacco use are generally legally sanctioned for adults. Tobacco accounts for over 350,000 premature deaths per year, primarily as a result of cardiovascular disease and cancer.

h. Opioids: Opioid dependence remains a significant sociologic and medical problem in the United States. There are an estimated 500,000 opioid addicts. Opioid addicts are frequent users of medical and surgical services due to multiple medical sequelae of IV drug use and associated lifestyle.

6. Treatment:
a. The general characteristics of drug abuse treatment have already been outlined; however, the most important principles include the following:
1) Detoxification and elimination of withdrawal symptoms
2) Initial admittance of a problem and alignment of social support systems (the family)
3) Long-term intensive individual and group therapy
4) Inclusion of the family members in therapy
b. Special treatments:
1) Methadone: For opioid withdrawal
2) Naltrexone (a long-acting orally active opioid antagonist): When taken regularly, entirely

blocks m-opioid receptors, thus blocking the opioid euphoric, analgesic, and sedative properties
3) Clonidine: Blocks many symptoms of opioid withdrawal
4) Flumazenil (Romazicon) is the first benzodiazepine antagonist to be approved by the Food and Drug Administration.
5) Carbamazepine (Tegretol) has been shown to be effective for ethanol and sedative detoxification.

SUGGESTED READINGS

American Psychiatric Association: *Diagnostic and statistical manual of mental disorders,* ed 4, Washington, DC, 1994, American Psychiatric Association Press.
Kaplan HI, Sadock BJ, eds: *Kaplan and Sadock's synopsis of psychiatry: Behavioral sciences/clinical psychiatry,* ed 8, Baltimore, 1998, Williams & Wilkins.
Shaner R: *Psychiatry,* Baltimore, 1997, Williams & Wilkins.
Swift R: Alcoholism and substance abuse. In Stoudemire A, ed: *Clinical psychiatry for medical students,* ed 3, Philadelphia, 1998, JB Lippincott.

PROBLEM·65

EATING DISORDERS

"I Watch My Diet and Run 5 Miles Every Day, but I'm Still So Fat That I Can't Stand Looking in the Mirror."

Case 1 ■ A 19-Year-Old Female with Rapid Weight Loss and an Intense Fear of Gaining Weight

A 19-year-old female comes to your office with a 30-pound weight loss during the last 6 months. She states that she has an intense fear of gaining weight. She also admits to amenorrhea of 4 months duration. When questioned about her perception of her weight, she states, "I still feel fat."

She denies episodes of binge eating and purging. She also denies the use of laxatives or diuretics.

On examination, the patient is approximately 25% below expected body weight. There is evidence of significant muscle wasting. Her blood pressure is 90/70 mm Hg, and her heart rate is 52 and regular. There appears to be a significant fine hair growth over her entire body.

SELECT THE BEST ANSWER TO THE FOLLOWING QUESTIONS

Q1. What is the most likely diagnosis in this patient?
a. borderline personality disorder
b. bulimia nervosa

c. anorexia nervosa
d. generalized anxiety disorder
e. masked depression

Q2. Diagnosis of this disorder requires the maintenance of body weight at what percentage below
ideal body weight?
a. 5%
b. 10%
c. 15%
d. 20%
e. 25%

Q3. What percentage of individuals with the disorder described has an accompanying major depressive disorder (MDD) or a coexisting anxiety
disorder?
a. 10%
b. 20%
c. 30%
d. 50%
e. 75%

Q4. What is the lifetime prevalence of obsessive
compulsive disorder (OCD) in patients with this
disorder?
a. 5%
b. 15%
c. 25%
d. 50%
e. 75%

Q5. Which complication has the greatest potential for
immediate lethality?
a. muscle wasting
b. generalized fatigue and weakness
c. hypokalemia
d. bradycardia
e. hypotension

Q6. Which of the following is (are) true regarding *The
Diagnostic and Statistical Manual of Mental Disorders, fourth edition* (DSM-IV) classification of eating disorders?
a. there are two types of anorexia nervosa specified in DSM-IV: the restricting type and the
binge-eating/purging type
b. there are two types of bulimia nervosa specified in DSM-IV: the purging type and the nonpurging type
c. anorexia nervosa and bulimia nervosa may be
comorbidly diagnosed in a given patient
d. a and b
e. all of the above are true

Case 2 ■ A 26-Year-Old Binge-Eating Female Who Vomits to Prevent Weight Gain

A 26-year-old patient comes to your office with recurrent episodes of binge eating (approximately 4 times a
week) after which she vomits to prevent weight gain.
She says that "she has no control" over these episodes
and becomes depressed because of being unable to
control herself. These episodes have been occurring for
the past 2 years. She also admits to using self-induced
vomiting, laxatives, and diuretics to lose weight.

On examination, the patient's blood pressure is
110/70 mm Hg and her pulse is 72 and regular. Examination also shows that the cardiovascular system, the
respiratory system, the abdomen, the musculoskeletal
system, and the neurologic systems are all normal.

Q7. What is the most likely diagnosis in this patient?
a. borderline personality disorder
b. anorexia nervosa
c. bulimia nervosa
d. masked depression
e. generalized anxiety disorder

Q8. Examination of which of the following is most
likely to be abnormal in patients with the disorder described in Case 2?
a. the mouth
b. the cervical and axillary lymph nodes
c. the right upper quadrant of the abdomen
d. the sensory component of the neurologic
system
e. the motor component of the neurologic
system

Q9. Regarding the prevalence of the disorders described in the previous two cases, which of the
following statements is true?
a. the prevalence of the disorder described in
Case 1 is increasing, whereas the prevalence of
the disorder described in Case 2 is decreasing
b. the prevalence of the disorder described in
Case 1 is decreasing, whereas the prevalence of the disorder described in Case 2 is
increasing
c. the prevalence of both disorders is increasing
d. the prevalence of both disorders is decreasing
e. the prevalence of both disorders has remained
unchanged over the past decade

Q10. The patient described in Case 1 should be
treated in which manner?
a. as an outpatient: treatment focused on pharmacotherapy, psychotherapy, and behavior
modification

b. as an inpatient: treatment focused on pharmacotherapy, psychotherapy, and behavior modification

c. as an inpatient: treatment focused on psychotherapy and behavior modification

d. as an outpatient: treatment focused on psychotherapy and behavior modification

e. as an outpatient: treatment focused on pharmacotherapy

Q11. Which of the following drugs has (have) been shown to be of benefit in the treatment of the disorder described in Case 2?

a. monoamine oxidase inhibitors
b. tricyclic antidepressants
c. selective serotonin reuptake inhibitors (SSRIs)
d. b and c
e. all of the above

Q12. Which of the following psychotherapies is (are) generally considered most effective for the treatment of the disorder described in Case 2?

a. supportive psychotherapy
b. psychodynamic psychotherapy
c. psychoanalytic psychotherapy
d. cognitive-behavioral psychotherapy
e. a, b, and d

SHORT ANSWER MANAGEMENT PROBLEM

List the psychiatric disorders and associated conditions that have been shown to be related to the conditions described in this chapter.

ANSWERS

A1. **c.** This patient has anorexia nervosa

A2. **c.** Anorexia nervosa is characterized by the following:

a. A patient who refuses to maintain her minimal normal body weight for age and height leading to maintenance of body weight 15% below that which is expected or a patient who fails to gain weight as expected during growth, leading to body weight 15% below that which is expected.

b. Even though underweight, she has an intense fear of gaining weight or becoming fat.

c. The patient experiences her body weight, size, or shape in a disturbed fashion, such as claiming to feel fat even when she is clearly underweight.

d. In female patients, at least three menstrual periods that should otherwise have been expected to occur have not occurred.

A3. **e.** Up to 75% of anorexia nervosa patients have a coexisting MDD or anxiety disorder, and up to 25% of anorexia nervosa patients develop an obsessive compulsive disorder in their lifetimes.

A4. **c.**

A5. **c.** The medical complications of anorexia nervosa include muscle wasting, fatigue, depression of cardiovascular function leading to bradycardia and hypotension, and depression of body temperature mechanisms leading to hypothermia. The abnormality with the greatest immediate potential lethality, however, is hypokalemia, with resultant cardiac dysrhythmias and possibly sudden death.

A6. **d.** There are two types of anorexia nervosa and two types of bulimia nervosa. The two types of anorexia nervosa are the restricting type and the binge-eating/purging type. Restricting-type patients avoid weight gain primarily through limiting food intake and do not usually engage in binge eating, self-induced vomiting, or misuse of diuretics or laxatives. The binge-eating/purging type of patients regularly engages in binge eating and purging (self-induced vomiting or misuse of laxatives or diuretics).

The two types of bulimia nervosa are the purging type and the nonpurging type. Abnormalities of eating behavior, including binge eating and purging, occur in both anorexia nervosa and bulimia nervosa. A diagnosis of bulimia nervosa is not made if the diagnostic criteria for anorexia nervosa are present.

A7. **c.** This patient has bulimia nervosa. Bulimia nervosa is characterized by the following:

a. The patient engages in repeated episodes of binge eating large amounts of food in brief periods.

b. The patient regularly engages in severe compensatory behaviors to prevent weight gain, such as self-induced vomiting, misuse of laxatives or diuretics, diet pills, fasting, very strict diets, and/or very vigorous exercise.

c. The patient engages in at least two binge eating and purging/severe compensatory behaviors per week for a minimum of 3 months

d. The patient is relentlessly overconcerned regarding weight and body shape.

As is the case for anorexia nervosa, two subtypes of bulimia nervosa are recognized: the purging type of patient, who regularly engages in self-induced vomiting or misuse of laxatives or diuretics and the nonpurging type of patient, who usually does not self-induce vomiting or misuse laxatives or diuretics to lose weight. Instead, the nonpurging type of patient engages in other severe compensatory behaviors such as fasting or excessive exercise.

A8. **a.** A frequently observed abnormality in bulimia nervosa is an abnormality in the examination of the head and neck (specifically the mouth). Examination of the mouth reveals the evidence of dental caries and periodontal disease that occur because of the effects of repeated vomiting.

A9. **c.** Studies suggest that among adolescent and young adult women in high school and college settings, the prevalence of clinically significant eating disorders is approximately 4% and, for more broadly defined syndromes, may be as high as 8%. The prevalence of these disorders seems to have increased over the past several decades. The prevalence of eating disorders may be influenced by societal attitudes regarding beauty and fashion.

A10. **c.** A 30-pound weight loss in 6 months suggests that this patient is at immediate risk for life-threatening complications. Most clinicians in this circumstance would suggest inpatient therapy with a focus on reestablishing a reasonable weight through calorie supplementation, behavioral modification, and possibly other forms of psychotherapy. SSRI antidepressant medication may be indicated for comorbid depression that commonly accompanies anorexia nervosa.

A11. **c.** SSRI agents such as fluoxetine or sertraline have been shown to be successful in reducing binge eating and purging episodes, whether or not there is comorbid depression.

A12. **d.** Cognitive-behavioral psychotherapy appears most effective for treatment of bulimia nervosa. This includes several stages, each consisting of several weeks or biweekly individual or group sessions. The first stage emphasizes the establishment of control over eating; this utilizes behavioral techniques such as self-monitoring. The second stage focuses on attempts to restructure the patient's unrealistic cognitions about eating and body image and instill more effective modes of problem solving. The third stage emphasizes maintaining the gains and preventing relapse, and often provides 6 months to a year of weekly sessions to provide close follow-up during times when relapse is common. Self-help groups, especially Overeaters Anonymous, may also be useful for individuals with bulimia nervosa.

SOLUTION TO THE SHORT ANSWER MANAGEMENT PROBLEM

The psychiatric disorders that are related to the eating disorders described include the following:
a. MDD
b. An anxiety disorder (75% of patients with an eating disorder have either MDD or an anxiety disorder at the same time)
c. Chemical dependency and substance abuse
d. Personality disorders

SUMMARY OF THE DIAGNOSIS AND TREATMENT OF EATING DISORDERS

1. Prevalence:
   a. The prevalence of eating disorders is 4%.
   b. The prevalence of abnormal eating behaviors may be as high as 8%.
   c. The prevalence of these disorders has increased significantly over the past several decades.

2. Symptoms: The symptoms of both anorexia nervosa and bulimia nervosa have been described previously. The major diagnostic clues are as follows:
   a. Anorexia nervosa:
      1) Failure to maintain normal weight (less than 85% of ideal weight)
      2) An intense fear of gaining weight
      3) A distorted body image (feeling fat in spite of being grossly underweight)
      4) Amenorrhea
   b. Bulimia nervosa:
      1) Repeated episodes of rapid binge eating
      2) Severe compensatory behaviors to lose weight
      3) Unrelenting over concern with weight and body image

3. Relationships between the two disorders:
   a. Both disorders involve abnormal eating behaviors and concern with body image.
   b. Of individuals with anorexia nervosa, 50% have binge-eating and purging behavior
   c. A diagnosis of bulimia nervosa is not made if the criteria for diagnosis of anorexia nervosa are present.

4. Complications:
   a. Anorexia nervosa: The physical complications of starvation:
      1) Depletion of fat
      2) Muscle wasting (including cardiac muscle in severe wasting)

3) Bradycardia

4) Cardiac arrhythmias (sudden death may follow)

5) Leukopenia, hypercortisolemia, osteoporosis

6) Cachexia

7) Lanugo (fine body hair)

b. Bulimia nervosa:

1) Dental caries and dental disease from vomiting

2) Metabolic abnormalities (hypokalemia secondary to vomiting)

3) Melanotic stool from laxative abuse

5. Treatment:

a. Anorexia nervosa:

1) Hospitalization to reestablish weight and correct metabolic abnormalities

2) Behavior modification, cognitive-behavioral psychotherapy, and family therapy

3) SSRI antidepressants for coexisting depression

b. Bulimia nervosa:

1) Cognitive-behavior psychotherapy

2) SSRIs used to treat the binge-eating component

SUGGESTED READINGS

American Psychiatric Association: *Diagnostic and statistical manual of mental disorders,* ed 4, Washington, DC, 1994, American Psychiatric Association Press.

Kaplan HI, Sadock BJ: Eating disorders. In Kaplan HI, Sadock BJ, eds: *Kaplan and Sadock's synopsis of psychiatry: Behavioral sciences/clinical psychiatry,* ed 8, Baltimore, 1998, Williams & Wilkins.

Shaner R: *Psychiatry,* Baltimore, 1997, Williams & Wilkins.

Yager U: Eating disorders. In Stoudemire A, ed: *Clinical psychiatry for medical students,* ed 3, Philadelphia, 1998, JB Lippincott.

PROBLEM · 6 6

GENERALIZED ANXIETY DISORDER

"My Mom Won't Let Me Play Outside. She Is Afraid I Will Get Run Over by a Truck."

Case 1 ■ A 36-Year-Old Female with Shortness of Breath and Palpitations

A 36-year-old female comes to your office with an 8-month history of shortness of breath, palpitations, dizziness, trouble swallowing, restlessness, fatigue, and anxiety regarding her job and the health of her two children. She tells you that she constantly worries about what could happen to her children when they are playing with other children in their homes (where she cannot be constantly supervising their play activities). She also worries about them dying in a car crash. She tells you, "Well, I'm very concerned about them not only being in an automobile accident but also about the possibility of the seat belts coming loose."

When you directly question her about some of these worries she readily admits to you that "I know I'm worrying too much, Doctor, but I just can't help it."

She also admits to muscle tension, easy fatigability, difficulty concentrating, having trouble falling and staying asleep, and irritability.

At this point in the interview she becomes very tense and tells you, "You know, Doctor, this is really getting out of control; it's getting so bad that it is interfering with my everyday life." On physical examination, the patient's thyroid gland is slightly larger than normal but still within normal limits. Her blood pressure is 160/60 mm Hg, and her pulse is 108 and regular. Examination of the abdomen is completely normal. All other systems are completely normal.

SELECT THE BEST ANSWER TO THE FOLLOWING QUESTIONS

Q1. What is the most likely diagnosis in this patient?

a. panic disorder

b. major depressive disorder

c. generalized anxiety disorder (GAD)

d. hypothyroidism

e. hypochondriasis

Q2. Of patients with the disorder described, what percentage has at least one other similar disorder at some time in their life?

a. 10%

b. 30%

c. 50%

d. 80%

e. no data available

Q3. What is the most common error made in the diagnosis of the disorder described?

a. misdiagnosing this disorder when it is actually related to any one of several other general medical or mental conditions

b. misdiagnosing this disorder as depression

c. misdiagnosing this disorder as hyperthyroidism

d. misdiagnosing this disorder as pheochromocytoma

e. misdiagnosing this disorder as a multiple endocrine neoplasia syndrome

Q4. Which of the following symptoms is generally not characteristic of the disorder described?
a. awakening with apprehension and unrealistic concern regarding future misfortune
b. worry out of proportion to the likelihood or impact of feared events
c. a 6-month or longer course of anxiety and associated symptoms
d. association of the anxiety described with depression
e. anxiety exclusively focused on health concerns

Q5. Which of the following statements regarding the disorder described above is (are) true?
a. this disorder may develop between attacks in panic disorder
b. the symptoms of this disorder are often present in episodes of depression
c. medical conditions that produce the major symptom associated with this disorder must be excluded
d. the disorder is accompanied by symptoms of motor tension, autonomic hyperactivity, vigilance, and scanning
e. all of the above are true

Q6. What is the psychotherapy or therapy of choice in this disorder?
a. behavioral psychotherapy
b. hypnosis
c. cognitive therapy
d. psychoanalytic psychotherapy
e. supportive psychotherapy

Q7. What is the pharmacologic agent of choice in this disorder?
a. alprazolam
b. buspirone
c. amitriptyline
d. fluoxetine
e. imipramine

Q8. Which of the following pharmacologic agents is not recommended in the treatment of this disorder?
a. diazepam (Valium)
b. chlordiazepoxide (Librium)
c. clorazepate (Tranxene)
d. clozapine (Clozaril)
e. clonazepam (Klonopin)

Q9. This disorder is more common in which of the following?
a. young to middle-aged females
b. ethnic minorities
c. those currently not married
d. those of lower socioeconomic class
e. all of the above

Q10. Which of the following statements is (are) true regarding this disorder?
a. this disorder displays autosomal-dominant genetic transmission
b. the major symptom of this disorder may be a conditioned response to a stimulus that the individual has come to associate with danger
c. there is little relationship between the onset of this disorder and the cumulative effects of stressful life events
d. b and c
e. all of the above

SHORT ANSWER MANAGEMENT PROBLEM
Part A: List three substances that may precipitate the major symptom associated with this condition.
Part B: List two contraindications to using benzodiazepines to treat this disorder.

ANSWERS

A1. **c.** This patient has GAD, which is defined as unrealistic or excessive worry about several life events or activities for a period of at least 6 months during which the person has been bothered more days than not by these concerns. In addition, the following six symptoms are present: muscle tension, restlessness or feeling keyed up or on edge, easy fatigability, difficulty concentrating or a sensation of the "mind going blank" because of anxiety, trouble falling or staying asleep, and irritability. Finally, the anxiety, worry, or physical symptoms significantly interfere with the person's normal routine or usual activities or cause marked distress.

A2. **d.** Of patients with GAD, at least 80% of patients have had at least one other anxiety disorder in their lifetime.

A3. **a.** The most common diagnostic error made is misdiagnosing GAD when another disorder is the actual cause of the anxiety. This leads to inappropriate and ineffective treatment decisions. The symptom of anxiety is prominent in a number of conditions, including the following:
a. Depressive disorders
b. Psychotic disorders
c. Substance abuse disorders
d. Somatoform disorders

e. Other medical conditions (especially those associated with dyspnea)

f. Medication side effects (sympathomimetic agents)

A4. **e.** GAD is characterized by awakening with apprehension and concern regarding future misfortune, worry out of proportion to the likelihood or impact of feared events, a duration of 6 months or more of anxiety or associated symptoms, and an association with depressed moods.

GAD is usually not associated exclusively with health concerns. When health concerns become the focus of worry, a diagnosis of hypochondriasis or another somatoform disorder becomes more likely.

A5. **e.** Generalized persistent anxiety may develop between attacks in panic disorder. GAD symptoms are often present during episodes of depression. As with panic disorder, medical conditions that may produce anxiety symptoms such as hyperthyroidism or caffeine intoxication must be excluded.

GAD is characterized by chronic anxiety about life circumstances accompanied by symptoms of motor tension, autonomic hyperactivity, vigilance, and scanning.

A6. **a.** Behavioral treatment of GAD is often effective, and includes relaxation exercises, systematic desensitization, and biofeedback. Cognitive therapy, especially when combined with systematic desensitization in imagination or relaxation, may improve GAD symptoms; however, cognitive therapy alone is not usually as effective.

A7. **b.** Buspirone, a nonbenzodiazepine anxiolytic, is a pharmacologic treatment of choice for GAD. The mechanism of action is not established, but pharmacologic activity includes a decrease in serotonin and an increase in dopamine and norepinephrine activity. Buspirone does not produce drowsiness or impair driving skill and lacks abuse potential. Long-acting benzodiazepines such as diazepam (Valium) and chlordiazepoxide (Librium) are also commonly used to treat GAD. Short-acting benzodiazepines, especially alprazolam, are generally avoided for treatment of GAD because of their increased incidence of withdrawal symptoms and drug dependency.

A8. **d.** Benzodiazepines, including diazepam (Valium), flurazepam (Dalmane), chlordiazepoxide (Librium), clorazepate (Tranxene), and clonazepam (Klonopin), are employed in the treatment of GAD. Clozapine is an antipsychotic agent that has shown superior efficacy over other antipsychotic medications in the treatment of refractory schizophrenic patients. It has no role in the treatment of GAD.

A9. **e.** GAD is slightly more common in young to middle-aged females, ethnic minorities, those not currently married, and those of lower socioeconomic class status.

A10. **b.** There is no convincing evidence of a specific form of genetic transmission of GAD. Behavioral theories consider anxiety, like panic disorder, a conditioned response to a stimulus that the individual has come to associate with danger. There is also some suggestion that the onset of GAD may be related to the cumulative effects of several stressful life events.

SOLUTION TO THE SHORT ANSWER MANAGEMENT PROBLEM

Part A: Five substances that can produce significant anxiety include the following:
   a. Caffeine
   b. Cocaine
   c. Amphetamines (methylphenidate, dextroamphetamine)
   d. Lysergic acid diethylamide, mescaline, psilocybin, dimethyltryptamine
   e. Alcohol

Part B: A history of substance abuse, especially alcohol and other anxiolytics, sedatives, and hypnotics, is a relative contraindication for treatment with benzodiazepines. Buspirone is not contraindicated with a history of alcohol or drug abuse.

SUMMARY OF THE DIAGNOSIS AND TREATMENT OF GAD

1. Epidemiology: A 1-month prevalence rate of 2.5% for GAD using research diagnostic has been demonstrated.

2. Differential diagnosis:
   a. Panic disorder
   b. Somatoform disorder
   c. Hypochondriasis
   d. Psychoactive substance use
   e. Depression (with secondary anxiety)
   f. Hyperthyroidism
   g. Caffeinism

3. Symptoms:
   a. GAD is characterized by chronic excessive anxiety concerning life circumstances accompanied

by symptoms of motor tension, autonomic hyperactivity, vigilance, and scanning.
b. The symptoms of anxiety, worry, or physical symptoms significantly interfere with the person's normal routine of usual activities and cause marked distress.

4. Treatment:
a. Nonpharmacologic treatments:
   1) Relaxation techniques (muscle relaxation, guided imagery)
   2) Systematic desensitization
   3) Cognitive therapy
b. Pharmacologic treatments:
   1) Long-acting benzodiazepines (e.g., diazepam)
   2) Buspirone, a nonbenzodiazepine anxiolytic
   3) Antidepressant medication when major depressive disorder is also present

SUGGESTED READINGS

American Psychiatric Association: *Diagnostic and statistical manual of mental disorders*, ed 4, Washington, DC, 1994, American Psychiatric Association Press.
Kaplan HI, Sadock BJ: Anxiety disorders. In Kaplan HI, Sadock BJ, eds: *Kaplan and Sadock's synopsis of psychiatry: Behavioral sciences/clinical psychiatry*, ed 8, Baltimore, 1998, Williams & Wilkins.
Nagy L et al: Anxiety disorders. In Stoudemire A, ed: *Clinical psychiatry for medical students*, ed 3, Philadelphia, 1998, JB Lippincott.
Shaner R: *Psychiatry*, Baltimore, 1997, Williams & Wilkins.

PROBLEM·67

FACTITIOUS DISORDER

"I Most Certainly Need Another Operation. You Must Be Incompetent!"

Case 1 ■ A 26-Year-Old Female with an "Abdomen Full of Scars"

A 26-year-old female comes to the Emergency Room (ER) with a 6-month history of "severe abdominal pain" that is relieved only by meperidine (Demerol). The patient self-reports "many, many operations" on her stomach, gallbladder, common bile duct, pancreas, large bowel, small bowel, spleen, and others that she can't remember.

She tells you when you introduce yourself that "she has heard all about you" and is certainly glad that "you are here to solve her problems." She further tells you that she "was on the brink" until she called the Emergency Department and found out that you were the ER doctor in charge of care today.

When you try to obtain a more complete history regarding all of her abdominal problems, she tells you that she has been in 57 different hospitals in the last 37 months. She goes back to her original statement about her delight with you being on duty today.

On examination, the patient's blood pressure is 120/79 mm Hg. Her pulse is 72 and regular. Examination of the head and neck reveals "multiple scars" on her face from "gland surgery." Her abdomen has 9 scars in different locations. When you press gently on her abdomen she screams very loudly. It is 3 AM and anyone in the 36-room ER who did happen to be asleep is no longer in that state.

SELECT THE BEST ANSWER TO THE FOLLOWING QUESTIONS

Q1. On the basis of the history and physical examination, what is the most likely diagnosis in this patient?
a. borderline personality disorder
b. antisocial personality disorder
c. somatization disorder
d. factitious disorder with predominant physical signs and symptoms (Munchausen syndrome)
e. malingering

Q2. Which of the following descriptions best fits patients with this disorder?
a. "scarface personality"
b. "gridiron abdomen"
c. "lost love syndrome"
d. "deceptive fever syndrome"
e. "multiple personality disorder"

Q3. In which of the following demographic groups does this disorder occur more commonly?
a. males
b. females
c. health care workers
d. b and c
e. a and c

Q4. The prevalence of factitious disorders among patients admitted to general hospitals (primary and secondary care) in the United States is approximately which of the following?
a. 0.05% of all admissions
b. 0.1% of all admissions
c. 0.5% of all admissions
d. 1.0% of all admissions
e. 5.0% of all admissions

Q5. Which of the following criteria is (are) important in establishing the diagnosis?

a. intentional production or feigning of physical symptoms
b. intentional production or feigning of psychological symptoms
c. motivation to assume the sick role
d. a and b only
e. all of the above

Q6. Which of the following signs or symptoms is most predictive of this disorder?
a. signs and symptoms of a major depressive disorder or a brief depressive disorder
b. an obvious, recognizable goal in producing the signs and symptoms
c. pathologic lying, lack of close relationships with others, hostile and manipulative manner, and associated substance and criminal behavior
d. multiple admissions to different hospitals, multiple referrals to different physicians, and multiple surgical procedures
e. the involuntary production of multiple symptoms as opposed to the voluntary production of multiple symptoms

Q7. When physical symptoms predominate in this disorder, what eponym is sometimes used?
a. Briquet's syndrome
b. Ganser syndrome
c. Munchausen syndrome
d. doctor abuse syndrome
e. none of the above

Q8. A patient who comes to the local ER with these signs and symptoms may produce which of the following behaviors?
a. self-injection of insulin when not a diabetic
b. self-bloodletting and putting of same into urine to imitate hematuria
c. allowing the thermometer used to take temperature to be immersed in hot water
d. when producing a urine sample contaminating it with feces
e. all of the above

Q9. Which of the following disorders is (are) part of the differential diagnosis of the condition described?
a. somatoform disorder
b. antisocial personality disorder
c. malingering
d. Ganser syndrome
e. all of the above

Q10. Which of the following disorders is most likely to have occurred previously in a patient who has the disorder described?
a. major depressive disorder
b. generalized anxiety disorder
c. childhood abuse or deprivation
d. childhood depression
e. infantile autism

Q11. Which of the following traits is (are) often present in patients who have this disorder?
a. decreased self-worth and self-esteem
b. poor identity formation
c. masochistic personality traits
d. all of the above
e. a and b only

Q12. What is the most effective treatment for this disorder?
a. early diagnosis and careful documentation
b. extensive psychoanalysis-type with a focus on early childhood trauma
c. cognitive psychotherapy
d. behavior-oriented psychotherapy
e. repeated confrontation about the bizarre nature of the symptoms

SHORT ANSWER MANAGEMENT PROBLEM
Discuss the manner in which the condition described begins.

ANSWERS

A1. **d.** This patient has a factitious disorder of the predominantly physical subtype. This is known as Munchausen syndrome.

A core feature of patients with this disorder is their intentional production of physical symptoms, often resulting in hospital admission. To support their history, the patients may feign symptoms suggestive of a disorder involving any organ system. They are often surprisingly familiar with complex medical diagnoses and may give realistic histories that deceive even experienced physicians.

The presentations that these patients manifest are myriad and include hematoma, hemoptysis, abdominal pain, fever, hypoglycemia, lupuslike syndrome, nausea, vomiting, dizziness, and seizures. As well, the urine of these patients is sometimes intentionally contaminated with blood or feces, anticoagulants are taken to simulate bleeding disorders, and insulin is used to produce hypoglycemia. (These are just a few of the symptoms produced in this disorder and the lengths gone to produce disease.)

One of the most common acts in factitious disorder patients is heating a thermometer. In this case, a patient who does not appear to be ill presents with a temperature of 104° F. This is often produced by hot water or a hot lamp.

A2. **b.** The patients may acquire what is classically referred to as a "gridiron abdomen" from multiple surgical procedures. Complaints of pain, especially that simulating renal colic, are common. The classic description of this patient includes someone who comes in seeking meperidine (Demerol). In one of the typical scenarios, once the patient is in hospital he or she will continue to be demanding and difficult. As each test is returned and the result is negative, the patient may actually accuse the doctor of incompetence, threaten litigation, and become abusive. Some patients may discharge themselves abruptly, especially when and if they begin to suspect that the staff is catching on or when the staff begins to confront the patient. From there the patient moves on to another hospital in the same or another city and the cycle begins again.

Some of the risk factors for this behavior and this disorder include the following:
a. Specific predisposing factors and actual physical disorders during childhood leading to extensive medical treatment
b. Anger against the medical profession or health care workers
c. Employment as a medical professional or medical paraprofessional
d. Any type of important relationship with a physician in the past

A3. **e.** Factitious disorder is more common in the following:
a. Males
b. Health care workers
c. Health care professionals
d. Individuals with a history of abuse in their family

A4. **e.** The prevalence of factitious disorders in admissions to primary and secondary general hospitals in the United States is thought to be about 5%. This figure may reflect an under diagnosis of factitious disorder. Clinicians may not yet consistently recognize psychologic conditions that influence interactions with health care resources.

A5. **e.** *The Diagnostic and Statistical Manual of Mental Disorders, fourth edition* (DSM-IV) has established the following diagnostic criteria for factitious disorder:
a. The patient intentionally produces or feigns physical or psychologic signs or symptoms.

b. The motivation for the patient is to assume the "sick role."
c. External incentives for the behavior (such as economic gain, avoiding legal responsibility, or improving physical well being) are absent or secondary.

The subtypes of factitious disorder are as follows:
a. Factitious disorder with predominantly psychologic signs and symptoms (if psychologic signs and symptoms predominate in the clinical presentation)
b. Factitious disorder with predominantly physical signs and symptoms (if physical signs and symptoms predominate in the clinical presentation)
c. Factitious disorder with combined psychologic and physical signs (the classification when combined psychologic and physical signs and symptoms are present, but neither predominate)

A6. **d.** The most characteristic findings in factitious disorder are multiple doctors, multiple referrals, multiple hospitals, and multiple surgical procedures. Although the items in option **c** may also occur, these are often seen in antisocial personality disorder. The symptoms produced by factitious disorder patients are voluntary, not involuntary.

A7. **c.** Factitious disorder with predominantly physical signs and symptoms has been called *Munchausen syndrome*. This syndrome is named after an 18th-century German baron named Baron von Munchausen who told exaggerated stories. Other names for the condition are hospital addiction, polysurgery addiction, and professional patient syndrome.

A8. **e.** A patient who comes to the local ER with signs or symptoms of a factitious disorder may well self-inject insulin when not a diabetic, produce by bloodletting enough blood to simulate macroscopic or microscopic hematuria when mixed with urine, heat a thermometer either with hot water or under a lamp to produce a grossly elevated temperature reading, or mix feces with urine to simulate the possible diagnosis of an abdominal or pelvic fistula.

All of these behaviors are designed by the patient to generate among his or her physicians and other health care workers an appearance of serious organic illnesses.

A9. **e.** Any disorder in which the physical signs and symptoms are prominent should be considered in the differential diagnosis of factitious disorder. The possibility of many organic diseases that may mimic factitious disorder or are part of the total disease picture must be considered. The major differential diagnosis lies between factitious disorder and the following:

a. Somatoform disorders: The somatoform disorders consist of the following:

1) Somatization disorder: A factitious disorder is differentiated from somatization disorder (Briquet's syndrome) by the voluntary production of factitious symptoms, the extreme course of multiple hospitalizations, and the patient's seeming willingness to undergo an extraordinary number of mutilating procedures.

2) Conversion disorder: A factitious disorder is differentiated from conversion disorder by the following: conversion patients are not usually conversant with medical terminology and hospital routines, and conversion patients have symptoms that bear a direct temporal relation or symbolic reference to specific emotional conflicts. Conversion patients do not volitionally produce their symptoms.

3) Hypochondriasis: A factitious disorder is differentiated from hypochondriasis in that hypochondriacal patients do not usually voluntarily initiate the production of symptoms, and hypochondriacal patients typically have a later age of onset.

b. Personality disorders:

1) Antisocial personality disorder has been discussed.

2) Histrionic personality disorder is associated with a "dramatic flair"; this, however, is not found in all patients with factitious disorder.

3) Borderline personality disorders and schizotypal personality disorders also need to be considered as comorbid diagnoses in patients with factitious disorder.

c. Malingering disorders: Factitious disorders must be distinguished from malingering disorders. Malingerers have an obvious recognizable, external incentive for producing the signs and symptoms that they exhibit (for example, they do not want to return to work). Reasons for not wanting to return to work include financial remuneration or compensation (by far the most common), evading the police, avoiding having to go back to a job that they detest, or simply wanting shelter for the night.

d. Substance abuse: If a patient who has a documented factitious disorder also has a substance abuse problem, it is very important that both conditions be evaluated, diagnosed, assessed, and treated.

e. Ganser syndrome: Ganser syndrome refers to a behavior often exhibited during medical exami-

nation by inmates in correctional facilities. It is characterized by the subject's using an approximate answer. For example, patients with the disorder may respond to a simple question with astonishingly incorrect answers. For example, an inmate is asked the color of a blue sweater; he says, "red."

A10. **c.** Individuals with factitious disorder often have histories of abuse and/or deprivation during childhood. Some clinicians believe that this has etiologic significance. In such an environment the patient learns to expect rejection and abuse and may learn to use the facsimile of genuine illness to create a closer bond with caregivers. Later in life, the patient repeats these interactions with health care personnel, desperately seeking their attention and angrily expecting rejection.

A11. **d.** Factitious disorder is associated with the following:

a. Decreased self-worth and self-esteem
b. Inadequate identity formation
c. Masochistic personality traits
d. Learned helplessness as a child if abuse was present
e. Tendency to seek approval from anyone and everyone

A12. **a.** Treatment is best focused on management rather than on cure. Unfortunately, there is little evidence for long-term effectiveness of specific forms of psychotherapy for this disorder.

The single most important factor in successful management of this condition is a physician's early recognition of the disorder with a goal of averting iatrogenic complications. As with other covert conditions such as spousal abuse, it is important to consider factitious disorder as a potential diagnosis; you will not make this diagnosis unless you think about it as a possible diagnosis.

SOLUTION TO THE SHORT ANSWER MANAGEMENT PROBLEM

Factitious disorders usually begin in early adult life. They occasionally begin in childhood or in adolescence. Characteristically, the following series of events begins the chain reaction of seeing doctors, referral to more doctors, admission to hospitals, voluntary discharge from the hospital if the situation becomes uncomfortable, and quickly checking into a new hospital.

a. The onset of the disorder or of discrete episodes of treatment seeking may follow a real illness, a loss (and subsequent adjustment reaction), or an abandonment (and subsequent adjustment reaction).

b. Usually the patient or a close relative of the patient had a hospitalization in childhood or early adolescence for a genuine physical illness. Thereafter a long pattern of successive hospitalizations unfolds, beginning insidiously, and progressing in a spiral that is difficult to stop.

SUMMARY OF THE DIAGNOSIS AND MANAGEMENT OF FACTITIOUS DISORDERS

1. Prevalence: Approximately 5% of admissions to primary and secondary care hospitals

2. Etiology: Etiology is associated with child abuse or child deprivation in the family of origin. In addition, there is often a history of genuine physical illness in the patient or a close relative or caregiver during childhood.

3. The cycle begins: The cycle begins in early adult life usually following discrete episodes of treatment following a real illness. Thereafter a long pattern of successive hospitalizations unfolds, beginning insidiously.

4. Demographic characteristics: Factitious disorder is more common in males, hospital workers, and health care workers.

5. DSM-IV criteria for factitious disorder:
   a. The patient intentionally produces or feigns physical or psychologic signs or symptoms.
   b. The motivation for the behavior is to assume the sick role.
   c. External activities for the behavior such as economic gain, avoiding legal responsibility, or improving physical well-being (as in malingering disorders) are absent.
   DSM-IV subtypes:
   1) Predominantly psychologic signs and symptoms
   2) Predominantly physical signs and symptoms (Munchausen syndrome)
   3) Combined psychologic and physical signs and symptoms

6. Differential diagnosis of factitious disorder:
   a. Somatoform disorders:
   1) Somatization disorder
   2) Conversion disorder
   3) Hypochondriasis

   b. Personality disorders:
   1) Antisocial personality disorder
   2) Borderline personality disorder
   3) Histrionic personality disorder
   c. Malingering: Most important distinguishing feature of factitious disorder from malingering is that in malingering there is an obvious, recognizable, environmental goal in producing signs and symptoms.
   d. Substance abuse syndrome
   e. Ganser syndrome: Usually confined to prison populations. Patients intentionally give the wrong answers to questions.

7. Course and prognosis:
   a. Begins in early adult life.
   b. Usual history is one of severe, incapacitating emotional trauma or untoward reactions.
   c. Overall prognosis for establishing a normal life is poor.

8. Treatment: Most important factor in any kind of successful management is to get to the patient and make the diagnosis before the abdomen looks like a football field. If you do not think of the diagnosis, then you will not make the diagnosis!

SUGGESTED READINGS

American Psychiatric Association: *Diagnostic and statistical manual of mental disorders*, ed 4, Washington, DC, 1994, American Psychiatric Association Press.

Kaplan HI, Sadock BJ: Factitious disorders. In Kaplan HI, Sadock BJ, eds: *Kaplan and Sadock's synopsis of psychiatry: Behavioral sciences/clinical psychiatry*, ed 8, Baltimore, 1998, Williams & Wilkins.

Shaner R: *Psychiatry*, Baltimore, 1997, Williams & Wilkins.

PROBLEM · 68

SOMATOFORM DISORDERS

"Dr. X Told Me It Is Just My Imagination, but I Really Do Hurt Bad."

Case 1 ■ A 27-Year-Old Female with 22 Different Symptoms

A 27-year-old female comes to your office for an initial consultation. She has heard from her best friend that "you are the most competent physician in the city." The symptoms described include chest pain, palpitations, "beating thyroid gland," nausea, periodic vomiting, abdominal pain, diarrhea, dizziness, gait disturbance, double vision, blurred vision, "seizures" (she falls down in the middle of crowds of people), pain on urination, back pain, abdominal pain, neck pain, headaches, vaginal paraesthesia, intolerance to fatty foods, intolerance to high-fiber foods, heartburn, and "constant gas." She tells you in a very dramatic and authoritative manner, "I just can't take it any more, Doctor, and I guess that is why I have come to you; I hear you are so good!"

Although you intend to pursue more of a history, you take an educated guess as to the diagnosis.

SELECT THE BEST ANSWER TO THE FOLLOWING QUESTIONS

Q1. What is your best educated guess as to the diagnosis in this patient?
a. somatization disorder
b. conversion disorder
c. somatoform disorder
d. hypochondriasis
e. masked depression

Q2. At this time, what would you do?
a. step out of the room and ask your secretary to page you in 5 minutes
b. tell the patient that you believe she is exaggerating her symptoms
c. prescribe a benzodiazepine (alprazolam)
d. make another appointment with the patient to delve into the patient's personal history and family history
e. tell the patient that her problems are most likely emotionally based and refer her to a psychotherapist

Q3. What is the pharmacologic treatment of choice for the disorder described?
a. a benzodiazepine
b. divalproex
c. a selective serotonin reuptake inhibitor (SSRI)
d. an monoamine oxidase inhibitor (MAOI)
e. none of the above

Case 2 ■ A 23-Year-Old Female Complaining of Having a "Peculiarly Prominent Jaw"

A 23-year-old female comes to your office with a chief complaint of having "a peculiarly prominent jaw." She tells you that she has seen a number of plastic surgeons about this problem, but "every one has refused to do anything."

On examination, her jaw appears to you to be completely normal. There is no protrusion that you can see, and it appears to you that she not only has a completely normal jaw but also a completely normal face.

Her mental status examination and her Beck Depression Inventory suggest some degree of underlying depression. The rest of her physical examination is completely normal.

Q4. What is the most likely diagnosis in this patient?
a. dysthymia
b. major depressive disorder (MDD) with somatic concerns
c. somatization disorder
d. body dysmorphic disorder
e. hypochondriasis

Q5. Therapies that have reportedly produced successful results in this disorder include which of the following?
a. pimozide
b. SSRIs
c. tricyclic antidepressants (TCAs)
d. individual or group psychotherapies
e. all of the above

Case 3 ■ A Mother of Five with a Constant Headache

A 29-year-old mother of five comes to your office with a "constant headache." Upon meeting her, you note that she uses crutches to walk. She states that this is because of her neck, abdominal, pelvic, and rib pain. She goes on to say that she has been diagnosed as having fibromyalgia. After performing a complete history, physical examination, and laboratory and radiologic workup, you make a diagnosis of tension headache. She then tells you that she has seen a number of other physicians about the same problem and that they have come to the same conclusion (which she believes is totally incorrect). You ask her to return for a further discussion about this problem next week, shake hands, and are about to leave. However, she continues to discuss the details of her pain and the difficulties that the pain causes her.

You tell her that you will continue discussion of these problems with her when you see her next week. You again attempt to leave the office.

Q6. What is the most likely diagnosis in this patient?
a. fibromyalgia
b. somatoform pain disorder
c. pain disorder associated with psychologic factors
d. somatization disorder
e. none of the above

Q7. What is the preferred treatment for this patient?
a. weekly (daily, if needed) visits with you

b. group psychotherapy
c. individual cognitive psychotherapy
d. individual behavior modification therapy
e. treatment in a multidisciplinary pain clinic

Case 4 ■ A 27-Year-Old Woman Complaining of Suddenly Becoming Blind

A 27-year-old patient comes to the Emergency Room (ER) with a complaint of "having suddenly gone blind." Apparently, she was walking down the street on her way to work and, suddenly, she could not see. The visual impairment that she describes is bilateral, complete (no vision), and associated with "numbness and tingling" in both lower extremities.

Her husband accompanies her to the ER and gruffly tells you, "Whatever it is, Doc, I want you to fix it and fix it fast."

The physical examination of the patient suggests a significant difference between the subjective symptoms and the objective complaints. Specifically, both the knee jerks and the ankle jerks are present and brisk; there is, however, no motor power in either lower extremity.

Q8. Based on the information provided, what is the most likely diagnosis?
   a. somatization disorder
   b. conversion disorder
   c. bilateral: ophthalmic artery occlusion and spinal artery occlusion
   d. histrionic personality disorder
   e. none of the above

Q9. What is the most appropriate step at this time?
   a. call an ophthalmologist immediately (stat)
   b. call a neurologist stat
   c. call a psychiatrist stat
   d. call a social worker stat
   e. reassure the patient and inquire about stressors

Case 5 ■ A 41-Year-Old Male Requesting a Cancer Checkup

A 41-year-old male comes to you for his first visit, requesting a "complete cancer checkup." This patient, you come to understand, has had eight complete cancer checkups already this year. He has had four of the eight done at "executive check-up centers." He is the chief executive officer of a large company and thus has the opportunity to take advantage of some "health perks." He provides a list of the tests he wishes to have done, including a complete history, a complete physi-

cal examination, a complete laboratory profile (this includes 157 different tests), a colonoscopy, a gastroscopy, a skeletal survey, x-rays of all body parts, a "head-to-toe" computed tomography scan, and a "head-to-toe" magnetic resonance imaging scan.

You learn that this patient is afraid that he has cancer, especially afraid that he has cancer of the colon. A relative had a colon cancer resected 2 years ago and advised him to get checked as often as possible.

You are amazed that he actually has time to function as the CEO of his company. The truth is, however, that he doesn't. He admits that this fear is greatly interfering with his work and social life.

Q10. What is the most likely diagnosis in this patient?
   a. somatization disorder
   b. hypochondriasis
   c. factitious disorder
   d. obsessive compulsive disorder (OCD)
   e. MDD

Q11. What is the treatment of choice for the patient described?
   a. weekly reassurance that he does not have cancer after performing all the tests he has requested
   b. weekly assurance that he does not have cancer without performing all the tests he has requested
   c. weekly assurance that he does not have cancer after refusing to perform all the tests he has requested
   d. collaboration between yourself (the primary care physician) and a psychiatrist, the goal of which is the development of a plan for regularly assessing this patient's ongoing psychosocial history and its manifestations, educating the patient, and providing appropriate supportive, behavioral, or cognitive psychotherapy
   e. all of d and lithium carbonate prophylactically and an SSRI agent

Q12. The term *somatothymia*:
   a. denotes the inability to describe or be aware of emotional feelings
   b. denotes a specific neuroendocrine syndrome
   c. communicates the inability to express physical distress in psychologic language
   d. denotes the use of somatically based words to describe emotional feelings
   e. denotes the inability to express psychologic distress in psychologic-based verbal language

ANSWERS

A1. **a.** This patient has somatization disorder. Somatization disorder is characterized by the following symptoms:

   a. Multiple physical complaints of long-standing occurrence

   b. These have usually resulted in significant medical diagnostic testing, medical intervention, and other iatrogenic problems.

   c. The symptoms have resulted in significant occupational or social malfunction.

   d. The symptoms that have occurred include symptoms that are not fully explained by a known medical condition or by clinical findings.

   e. The symptoms include pain symptoms in at least four different sites, including headache or related pain, abdominal pain, back pain, joint pain, extremity pain, chest pain, rectal pain, dyspareunia.

   f. The symptoms include two or more gastrointestinal (GI) symptoms including nausea, diarrhea, bloating, vomiting, and food intolerance.

   g. The symptoms include one or more sexual symptoms including erectile or ejaculatory dysfunction, irregular or excessive bleeding, or decreased libido or indifference.

   h. The symptoms include one or more pseudoneurologic symptoms including a conversion symptom or a dissociative symptom.

A2. **d.** In this patient another visit is reasonable to try to establish some reasonable baseline history and physical examination. Assessment and treatment of somatization disorder include the following principles:

   a. The presentation must be considered in terms of the psychosocial nature of the symptoms, both current and past.

   b. The diagnostic procedures and therapeutic interventions must be based on objective, rather than subjective, findings.

   c. The physician must form a good "therapeutic alliance" with the patient.

   d. The patient's social support system must be both extensively reviewed and utilized to maximum potential.

   e. A regular appointment schedule with the physician must be established for the patient.

   f. The dialogue that occurs between the doctor and the patient must address symptoms and signs from a both a somatic and psychologic viewpoint, focusing in part on the emotional implications of the debilitating complaints.

   g. The need for referral should be recognized early, especially in chronic cases where many physicians have been involved over time and concurrently.

   h. The physician should be cognizant of the likelihood of comorbid psychiatric disorders, especially mood disorders.

   i. The significance of personality features, substance abuse, and self-destructive behavior must be determined and addressed.

   j. The therapeutic alliance between the physician and the patient must be refocused to address the problem from the perspective of management rather than cure.

A3. **e.**

A4. **d.** This patient has body dysmorphic disorder, a condition characterized by the following:

   a. A preoccupation with an imagined or grossly exaggerated body defect.

   b. Clinically apparent distress associated with social, occupational, or functional impairment.

   c. Anorexia nervosa, psychotic disorders, OCD, or any other psychiatric disorders cannot account for the preoccupation and the impairment.

The differential diagnosis of body dysmorphic disorder includes the following:

   a. Anxiety disorder

   b. MDD

   c. Hypochondriasis

   d. Other somatoform disorders

   e. Factitious disorders

   f. Malingering

Associated features of body dysmorphic disorder include "doctor shopping," medication problems, conflicting opinions from multiple physicians, and iatrogenic disease.

A5. **e.** General principles discussed for somatization disorders discussed in the previous question apply to management of body dysmorphic disorder; however, the somatic preoccupations are often persistent. Individual or group psychotherapy is sometimes useful. SSRIs may be useful for some patients. Pimozide, TCAs, and MAOIs have also been used.

A6. **c.** The diagnosis for the patient in Case 3 is pain disorder associated with psychologic factors. The criteria for this diagnosis are as follows:

   a. Pain is the prominent clinical presentation and is of sufficient severity to require assessment.

b. The pain results in social, occupational, or functional impairment or clinically significant distress.

c. Psychologic factors precipitate, exacerbate, or maintain the pain or contribute to the severity of the pain.

d. The pain is not a component of somatization disorder or other psychiatric disorders including sexual dysfunction.

In many situations, however, the patient may have a bona fide physical illness (such as lumbar disk disease), but psychologic factors appear to predominate. If the medical disorder appears to be present and is making a significant contribution to the patient's pain complaints, the patient may be diagnosed with pain disorder associated with both psychologic factors and a general medical condition.

As many as 40% of patients with chronic pain have pain that is primarily psychogenic in origin. Pain that is associated with prominent psychologic features is diagnosed in women twice as frequently as in men. Evidence exists to suggest a familial pattern, with first-degree biologic relatives being at higher risk for developing the disorder. A known familial pattern that includes a history of anxiety, depression, or alcohol dependence occurs at greater frequency than would be expected in the general population. Comorbid MDD is extremely common. Substance abuse, especially analgesics and anxiolytics and other sedatives and hypnotics, is also extremely common.

The differential diagnosis of pain disorder must take into consideration other psychiatric disorders such as a psychologic factors affecting a general medical condition, somatization disorder, hypochondriasis, depressive disorders, generalized anxiety disorder, factitious disorder, and malingering.

Full appreciation of the etiologic factors involved in any form of pain that appears to be exacerbated by psychologic factors is complicated because the clinician must account for secondary gain or reinforcement. Psychologic tests, most commonly the Minnesota Multiphasic Personality Inventory, are used routinely to identify psychologic factors.

A7. **e.** The treatment of choice for this patient is treatment in a multidisciplinary pain clinic. Such treatment has several objectives. Often patients must first be detoxified from analgesics and sedative hypnotics. Other nonpharmacologic treatments for pain control, including transcutaneous nerve stimulation, biofeedback, and other forms of behavioral psychotherapy are substituted. The therapeutic emphasis must be shifted from elimination of all pain to management of pain and its consequences. Both psychologic and physical therapies are used to minimize the functional limita-

tions caused by the pain. Patients are encouraged to increase their social, occupational, and physical activities. These techniques are similar to those employed in management of patients with chronic pain caused by general medical conditions. Specialized pain clinics are often the optimal treatment setting.

Depressive symptoms must also be addressed in pain management. Antidepressants are indicated when MDD is present in these patients.

A8. **b.** This patient has a conversion disorder. Conversion disorders represent a type of somatoform disorder in which there is a loss or alteration in physical functioning during a period of psychologic stress that suggests a physical disorder but that cannot be explained on the basis of known physiologic mechanisms. Conversion disorders are usually seen in ambulatory care settings or emergency departments. Conversion symptoms are exceedingly common; estimates of 20% to 25% prevalence are given for patients admitted to a general medical setting. General hospital patients have consistently shown conversion symptoms in 5% to 14% of all psychiatric consultations.

The Diagnostic and Statistical Manual of Mental Disorders, fourth edition (DSM-IV) criteria for conversion disorder are as follows:

a. The symptom(s) or deficit(s) are under voluntary control, affecting motor or sensory function. This suggests a medical condition.

b. The initiation or exacerbation of the symptom(s) or deficit(s) is preceded by conflicts or stressors; psychologic factors are prominent.

c. The symptom(s) or deficit(s) are not consciously or intentionally produced.

d. The symptom(s) or deficit(s) are not fully explained after clinical assessment as a medical condition or culturally sanctioned phenomenon.

e. The symptom(s) or deficit(s) impair social or occupational functioning, create significant distress, or require medical intervention.

f. The symptom(s) or deficit(s) are not limited to pain or sexual dysfunction and are not a component of somatization disorder or other psychiatric syndrome.

Common examples of conversion symptoms include paralysis, abnormal movements, aphonia, blindness, deafness, or pseudoseizures.

In this patient the possibility of domestic violence should be considered as a potential cause of stress leading to conversion symptoms. Although spousal abuse should always be considered, the somewhat peculiar demeanor of the husband in this case raises the index of suspicion. When spousal abuse is present, clinicians are often obligated to take necessary steps to notify civil or law enforcement authorities and to protect the victim.

A9. **e.** A wide variety of treatment techniques have been successfully used for the treatment of conversion disorder. The initial step in the management of acute symptoms is to quickly decrease the psychologic stress. Brief psychotherapy focusing on stress and coping and suggestive therapy and sometimes hypnosis may be extremely effective. Pharmacologic interventions, including the acute use of benzodiazepines, may also be useful. Brief hospitalization may sometimes be indicated, particularly when symptoms are disabling or alarming. Hospitalization may serve to remove the patient from the stressful situation and to assess for possible underlying general medical conditions.

A10. **b.** This patient has the disorder known as hypochondriasis, which is defined as a preoccupation with having a serious illness based on misinterpretation of physical symptoms that does not respond to physician reassurance after an appropriate evaluation. Individuals with hypochondriasis often have a profound fear of disease and an intense focus on multiple physical complaints. On presentation, the medical history is often related in great detail. There is commonly a history of assessment by multiple physicians, deteriorating doctor-patient relationships, and associated feelings of frustration and anger. The clinical course is chronic, with waxing and waning of symptoms.

The DSM-IV diagnostic criteria for hypochondriasis include the following:

a. The patient is preoccupied or afraid of serious disease with misinterpretation of bodily symptoms for 6 months or longer
b. Medical evaluation and reassurance are not effective in allaying the preoccupation.
c. The preoccupation is not delusional, is not consistent with body dysmorphic disorder, and is not a component of another psychiatric disorder.
d. Significant social, occupational, and functional impairment occurs together with clinically significant distress.

The differential diagnosis of hypochondriasis includes somatization disorder, anxiety disorders, MDD, factitious disorders, malingering, and psychotic disorders manifesting hypochondriacal delusions.

Hypochondriasis may be distinguished from somatization disorder by the patient's source of concern. In hypochondriasis the concern is that the symptoms imply a serious illness. In somatization disorder, the concern is with discomfort of the symptoms themselves.

Factitious disorder is another important differential diagnosis. It is less likely in this case because there is no evidence of pathologic lying or recurrent, feigned, or simulated illness.

A11. **d.** A crucial management technique in caring for the hypochondriacal patient is assessment and management of psychologic stressors and clear documentation in the medical record of the contribution of these factors. Psychologic stress is often associated with the onset and maintenance of hypochondriasis. The general principles in caring for patients with somatization disorders should be followed.

Generally, the most effective treatment takes place in the context of collaboration with a family physician, a psychiatrist, and other health care workers such as a psychologist and a social worker. Regular visits are essential to monitor symptoms, monitor anxiety or depression associated with the hypochondriacal symptoms, and help the patient come to terms with the condition.

A12. **d.** The term *somatothymia* denotes the use of physical complaints to convey emotional discomfort. Alexithymia denotes the inability or the limited capacity of some individuals to be aware of their own emotions or to articulate their feelings.

SOLUTION TO THE SHORT ANSWER MANAGEMENT PROBLEM

Pain is a prominent symptom in somatoform disorders and must be completely evaluated. The symptom of pain must be considered in both physiologic and psychologic contexts. The symptom of pain cannot and should not be dismissed; neither must it be misinterpreted as something it is not. The most fundamental question requiring an answer is whether the symptom of pain is primarily caused by a physical condition or is predominantly mediated by psychologic factors?

SUMMARY OF THE DIAGNOSIS AND TREATMENT OF SOMATOFORM DISORDERS

1. Somatization disorder:
   Diagnostic clues: Multiple physical complaints with onset before the age of 30. Tendency of these complaints is to be both chronic and long-standing. The complaints involve each of the following: pain symptoms, GI symptoms, sexual dysfunction symptoms, and pseudoneurologic symptoms. There is impairment of social or occupational functioning associated with these symptoms.

2. Conversion disorder:

Diagnostic clues: Physical symptoms primarily involving loss of motor or sensory function that are produced because of psychologic conflicts or stressors. They cannot be fully explained on an anatomic basis and result in impairment in social or occupational functioning. Conversion disorder is more common among medically unsophisticated groups; it may also be a manifestation of a disturbed family or marital situation.

3. Pain disorder:

Diagnostic clues: Pain is the prominent clinical presentation, and it results in social, occupational, or functional impairment. This diagnosis is made when psychologic factors are believed by the physician to have a significant role in the outset, severity, exacerbation, or perpetuation of the pain syndrome. Major depression or anxiety are often present and may be a component of the pain syndrome. The best therapeutic strategy is to limit inappropriate use of analgesics and other medical resources and to modify the patient's therapeutic expectations from cure to management of the pain while attempting to appreciate the role of psychosocial or psychologic factors, as well as stress. A multidisciplinary pain clinic is, in many or most of such patients, the treatment of choice.

4. Hypochondriasis:

Diagnostic clues: Hypochondriasis is characterized by a worry about having a serious disease that is based on a misinterpretation of physical symptoms and is not alleviated with appropriate physician reassurance. As with pain, the possibility of comorbid anxiety or depression should be strongly considered, and physical disease should be excluded. Treatment is most effective when there is collaboration between a primary care physician who continues regular appointments and a consulting psychiatrist. Again, the diagnosis requires significant social, occupational, or functional impairment.

5. Body dysmorphic disorder:

Diagnostic clues: The fundamental diagnostic feature is a pervasive feeling of ugliness or physical defect based on a grossly exaggerated perception of a minor (or even absent) physical anomaly. Patients frequently consult multiple primary care physicians, dermatologists, and plastic surgeons. Depressive symptoms, anxiety symptoms, social phobia, obsessive personality traits, and psychosocial distress frequently coexist. Intervention includes group or family therapy and, occasionally, the use

of SSRIs or other medication to decrease obsessive concerns and depression.

6. Malingering:

Diagnostic clues: The essential feature of malingering is the intentional production of illness consciously motivated by external incentives such as avoiding military duty, obtaining financial compensation through litigation or disability, evading criminal prosecution, obtaining drugs, or securing better living conditions. Malingering is more likely when medical and legal context overshadows the presentation, marked discrepancy exists between the clinical presentation and objective findings, and a lack of cooperation is experienced with the patient. Confrontation in a confidential and empathic but firm manner that allows an opportunity for constructive dialogue and appreciation of any psychologic or psychosocial problems is imperative.

SUGGESTED READINGS

American Psychiatric Association: *Diagnostic and statistical manual of mental disorders*, ed 4, Washington, DC, 1994, American Psychiatric Association Press.

Folks D, Ford CV, Houck CA: Somatoform disorders, factitious disorders, and malingering. In Stoudemire A, ed: *Clinical psychiatry for medical students*, ed 3, Philadelphia, 1998, JB Lippincott.

Kaplan HI, Sadock BJ: Somatoform disorders. In Kaplan HI, Sadock BJ, eds: *Kaplan and Sadock's synopsis of psychiatry: Behavioral sciences/clinical psychiatry*, ed 8, Baltimore, 1998, Williams & Wilkins.

Shaner R: *Psychiatry*, Baltimore, 1997, Williams & Wilkins.

PROBLEM·69

PANIC DISORDER

"I Just Can't Do It! I Think I Will Die If I Try."

Case 1 ■ A 29-Year-Old Female with a Pounding Heart, Shortness of Breath, Chest Pain, Dizziness, and Feelings That She Is Losing Her Mind

A 29-year-old female elementary school teacher comes to your office with recurrent attacks of anxiety associated with what she describes as a "pounding heart," "shortness of breath," "chest pain," "dizziness," and feels that she is losing her mind. These attacks have been ongoing for at least 8 months and only seem to occur during school days. She tells you that these symptoms begin when she gets up in front of the class in the morning. When you question her carefully, you learn that she also develops what she describes as "fear" when she gets into crowded stores or shopping malls.

Her history includes what a child psychiatrist diagnosed as separation anxiety. She states that her mother ran away with another man when she was 5 years old, and she was raised by her father.

Her physical examination is essentially unremarkable. Her blood pressure is 130/70 mm Hg and the examination of the cardiovascular system and the respiratory system is normal, as is the rest of the examination.

SELECT THE BEST ANSWER
TO THE FOLLOWING QUESTIONS

Q1. What is the most likely diagnosis in this patient?
   a. pheochromocytoma
   b. hyperthyroidism
   c. panic disorder
   d. paroxysmal atrial fibrillation
   e. generalized anxiety disorder (GAD)

Q2. The symptom that this patient displays in relationship to her expressed fear of crowded stores or shopping malls is known as:
   a. social phobia
   b. specific phobia
   c. claustrophobia
   d. agoraphobia
   e. generalized phobia

Q3. Which of the following is (are) characteristic of this disorder?
   a. smothering sensations
   b. fear of going crazy
   c. fear of not being able to control a particular situation
   d. fear of dying
   e. all of the above

Q4. The "phobia" that is described in Case 1 and that is specified in Question 2 is characterized by which of the following?
   a. an intense fear of being in public places
   b. acute bursts of terrifying levels of anxiety
   c. avoidance of places where help may be unavailable or escape is difficult
   d. a loss of contact with reality, including hallucinations and delusions
   e. a, b, and c
   f. all of the above

Q5. Which of the following is (are) true of the disorder described in the case history?
   a. it is more common in males
   b. it usually begins in middle age
   c. it is rarely confused with coronary artery disease

   d. none of the above
   e. all of the above

Q6. Which of the following statements regarding the pharmacologic treatment of the disorder described in Case 1 is (are) true?
   a. pharmacologic therapy is effective in blocking the symptoms of the disorder described
   b. pharmacologic therapy is effective in treating the "avoidance" of the specific situation
   c. a combination of pharmacologic therapy, psychoeducation, and biofeedback may be most helpful in the treatment of this disorder
   d. all of the above
   e. a and c only

Q7. Which of the following is the pharmacologic treatment of choice for this disorder?
   a. alprazolam
   b. phenelzine
   c. paroxetine
   d. imipramine
   e. atenolol

Q8. Which of the following drugs has the greatest potential for causing dependency during treatment of this condition?
   a. alprazolam
   b. phenelzine
   c. paroxetine
   d. imipramine
   e. atenolol

Case 2 ■ A 29-Year-Old Musician with an Intense Fear before Performing

A 29-year-old musician consults with you regarding what he describes as "an intense fear" before he begins his nightly performance with a civic orchestra. He tells you that it is only a question of time before he "makes a real major mistake."

Q9. What is the most likely diagnosis in this patient?
   a. a specific phobia
   b. a social phobia
   c. a mixed phobia
   d. panic disorder without agoraphobia
   e. panic disorder with agoraphobia

Q10. Which of the following is the treatment of choice for the patient described in Case 2?
   a. alprazolam before his nightly music performance
   b. phenelzine before his nightly performance

c. atenolol before his nightly performance
d. clomipramine before his nightly performance
e. paroxetine before his nightly performance

SHORT ANSWER MANAGEMENT PROBLEM
List four psychiatric disorders with which the condition described in Case 1 is associated?

ANSWERS

A1. **c.** The most likely diagnosis in this patient is panic disorder. Panic disorder is defined as recurrent episodes of panic attacks (discrete periods of intense fear or discomfort) associated with other symptoms including dyspnea, dizziness, trembling, palpitations, choking sensations, nausea, feelings of depersonalization, numbness, hot flushes, chest pain, a fear of dying, a fear of going crazy, or a fear of not being able to control a situation to which the patient may be exposed.

Although organic disease must be considered (including tachyarrhythmias and thyroid dysfunction), the constellation of symptoms is almost diagnostic of panic disorder.

A2. **d.** Agoraphobia is characterized by an intense fear of becoming helpless during a panic attack in a public place. This fear often leads to chronic anxiety and restriction of activities, often to the point of becoming housebound. The patient with agoraphobia avoids supermarkets, shopping malls, church services, meetings, parties, elevators, tunnels, bridges, buses, subways, and other places where help is unavailable or where escape is difficult.

A3. **e.** Symptoms of a panic attack include a discrete period of intense fear or discomfort in which at least four of the following symptoms develop abruptly and reach a peak within 10 minutes:
   a. Palpitations, pounding heart, or accelerated heart rate
   b. Sweating
   c. Trembling or shaking
   d. Sensations of shortness of breath or smothering
   e. A feeling of choking
   f. Chest pain or discomfort
   g. Nausea or abdominal distress
   h. Feeling dizzy, unsteady, lightheaded, or faint
   i. Derealization (feelings of unreality or detachment from others) or depersonalization (becoming detached from oneself)
   j. Fear of losing control or going crazy
   k. Fear of dying
   l. Paresthesias (numbness or tingling sensations)
   m. Chills or hot flushes

A4. **e.** As discussed in Answer 2, agoraphobia is characterized by an intense fear of being in public places, acute bursts of terrifying levels of anxiety, and avoidance of places or where help may be unavailable or escape is difficult. Agoraphobia is not, however, characterized by a loss of contact with reality, although patients may complain of "being in a daze" or "being in a fog" (feelings of derealization or depersonalization).

A5. **d.** Panic disorder is a common medical illness. It usually begins in the second or third decade of life, although children and older adults may develop the disorder. It is twice as common in women as it is in men.

Genetic and epidemiologic studies have consistently demonstrated increased rates of panic disorder among first- and second-degree relatives of panic disorder patients. This could be a result of genetic factors, nongenetic biologic factors, or cultural factors shared by family members. Between 15% and 18% of first-degree relatives of patients with panic disorder develop the condition.

Chest pain is a common presenting complaint among patients with panic disorder. Some patients with chest pain have even been referred for coronary angiography. Other than cardiovascular symptoms, the two most common classes of symptoms are neurologic symptoms and gastrointestinal (GI) symptoms.

A6. **e.** Available pharmacologic treatments for panic disorder are often effective for treating the symptoms of acute panic attacks in panic disorder. Pharmacologic agents are less effective for treating the "avoidance" of the actual panic-inducing situation itself. For this component of panic disorder, cognitive behavioral treatments are most useful.

The most commonly accepted therapy for panic disorder is as follows:
   a. Pharmacologic treatment (discussed in Answer 7)
   b. Behavioral treatment including the following:
      1) Graduated exposure to the phobic situation
      2) Cognitive therapy (reduces irrational beliefs)
      3) Relaxation training and biofeedback
      4) Panic control treatment: Comprised of breathing retraining, cognitive restructuring, and exposure to somatic cues
      5) Assertiveness training (can help with dependency, passivity, and suppressed anger)
      6) Psychoeducation (a presentation of knowledge to the patient that includes symptoms, theories of causation, reassurance that what they believe will happen will actually not happen, and treatment strategies)
      7) Group therapy (helps confirm to individuals with panic disorder that they are not alone)

A7. **c.** Paroxetine and other selective serotonin re-uptake inhibitors (SSRIs) such as fluoxetine, sertraline, and fluvoxamine are the treatment of choice for panic disorder. They are as efficacious as previous first-line medications such as clomipramine and imipramine and have fewer side effects and less toxicity.

Other agents that have proven effective in patients with panic disorder include the following:

a. Serotonergic tricyclic antidepressants (TCAs): Clomipramine and imipramine may be as efficacious as SSRIs, but are more toxic in overdose and have more side effects.

b. High-potency benzodiazepines: the benzodiazepine of choice is alprazolam. Alprazolam is often used when SSRIs and TCAs are either contraindicated or poorly tolerated. It is highly effective for decreasing panic attacks. However, drug withdrawal symptoms are often evident several hours after the last dose, and development of drug dependency is common (see below). Clonazepam is another benzodiazepine that is frequently used for this indication because it is better tolerated by some individuals. Although the nonbenzodiazepine anxiolytic agent buspirone is effective in treating GAD, it is usually ineffective in treating panic disorder.

c. Monoamine oxidase inhibitors (MAOIs): MAOIs such as phenelzine and tranylcypromine are effective in reducing the anxiety associated with panic disorder. Necessary warnings regarding the need to maintain a low serum tyramine level may sometimes give panic disorder patients "one more thing to worry about."

d. Beta-blockers: Although the beta-blockers may block symptoms such as palpitations and tremor, they are generally not as effective in treating panic attacks as SSRIs, benzodiazepines, TCAs, or MAOIs.

A8. **a.** Alprazolam is a high-potency benzodiazepine that is very effective for treating panic disorder. Often, doses in the range of 2 mg PO qid are required. The frequent daily doses are necessitated by the short half-life of the drug. Even with this dose frequency, withdrawal symptoms may develop after the most recent dose. These symptoms include anxiety and tremulousness and may be especially disturbing to patients with panic disorder. Drug dependency may develop, and it may be difficult to decrease the dose without using a very gradual taper. Clonazepam causes fewer problems with dependency but is associated with more sedation. Other benzodiazepines are not as effective.

A9. **b.** This patient has what is referred to as performance anxiety, which is classified as a social phobia, circumscribed type. This social phobia is really specific and is not at all uncommon. Most commonly, symptoms develop only in the situation of performance of the particular activity in question.

A10. **c.** The treatment of choice in this patient is a beta-adrenergic blocking agent. The most commonly used agents include atenolol, oxprenolol, and metoprolol. Although propranolol is considered "the gold standard," a more selective beta-blocker (selective in not crossing the blood-brain barrier) will not produce the side effects of lightheadedness or dizziness.

SOLUTION TO THE SHORT ANSWER MANAGEMENT PROBLEM

Attempts to decrease the anxiety may in fact cause individuals to self-medicate. This leads to a possible association between panic attacks and alcoholism or substance abuse.

Because of the nature of the symptoms, individuals with panic attacks and panic disorder commonly develop other associated psychiatric conditions. These include GAD and MMD. Anticipatory anxiety, defined as anxiety associated with worry about having panic attacks, sometimes causes individuals to avoid traveling and develop agoraphobia.

SUMMARY OF THE DIAGNOSIS AND TREATMENT OF PANIC DISORDER

1. Prevalence:
   a. Lifetime prevalence: Approximately 1.5%
   b. Lifetime prevalence: 2.5 to 4 times greater for females than males

2. Genetics: Risk of panic disorder in first-degree relatives of patients is about 15%.

3. Biochemistry: A wide range of substances are more likely to produce panic attacks in research subjects with panic disorder than in normal controls, leading to speculation as to biochemical causes. Panic-inducing substances include carbon dioxide, sodium lactate, yohimbine, and caffeine. Abnormalities in noradrenergic, serotonergic, and gamma aminobutyric acid-dependent neurotransmitter systems have been implicated in panic disorder.

   It is likely that panic disorder may result from multiple biochemical causes.

4. Symptoms:
  a. A panic attack is diagnosed when there is intense fear or discomfort associated with at least four of the following:
     1) Palpitations, pounding heart, tachycardia
     2) Sweating
     3) Trembling or shaking
     4) Shortness of breath, smothering
     5) Choking
     6) Chest pain or discomfort
     7) Nausea, abdominal distress
     8) Derealization, depersonalization
     9) Fear of dying
     10) Fear of losing control or going crazy
     11) Paresthesias
     12) Dizzy, unsteady, lightheaded
     13) Chills or hot flushes
  b. Recurrent panic attacks as described previously.
  c. Panic disorder is subclassified according to whether or not it is accompanied by agoraphobia. Agoraphobia is defined as anxiety about being in places or situations in which escape might be difficult (or embarrassing) or in which help may or may not be available in the event of having an unexpected or situationally predisposed panic attack. Agoraphobia may involve travel, driving, public places, or other situations such as sitting in a meeting or waiting in line.

5. Comorbid psychiatric conditions: Panic disorder is associated with alcoholism, substance abuse, GAD, separation anxiety disorder, and major depressive disorder.

6. Treatment:
  a. Nonpharmacologic:
     1) Behavioral therapy: Systematic desensitization through gradually increasing exposure
     2) Cognitive therapy: Reduces mistaken beliefs that serve to increase anxiety (e.g., "I am going crazy," "I will have a heart attack," and "I will smother.")
     3) Biofeedback/relaxation therapy: Training that counteracts anxiety, including breathing exercises, muscle relaxation techniques, and guided imagery
     4) Psychoeducation: Education about all aspects of the condition, especially the fact that it is common
     5) Group therapy: Sharing of experiences reinforces psychoeducation.
  b. Pharmacologic:
     1) SSRIs, including paroxetine, fluoxetine, sertraline, and fluvoxamine, are drugs of first choice but may be associated with GI distress, increased anxiety, or sedation.
     2) High-potency benzodiazepines, especially alprazolam and clonazepam, are highly effective but may be associated with sedation and dependency.
     3) Clomipramine and imipramine are effective, but they are associated with anticholinergic effects, sedation, and toxicity in overdose.
     4) Beta-blockers are useful when circumscribed social phobia (performance anxiety) is present.
     5) MAOIs are sometimes used when other medications are ineffective or contraindicated.

SUGGESTED READINGS

American Psychiatric Association: *Diagnostic and statistical manual of mental disorders*, ed 4, Washington, DC, 1994, American Psychiatric Association Press.

Kaplan HI, Sadock BJ: Anxiety disorders. In Kaplan HI, Sadock BJ, eds: *Kaplan and Sadock's synopsis of psychiatry: Behavioral sciences/clinical psychiatry*, ed 8, Baltimore, 1998, Williams & Wilkins.

Nagy L et al: Anxiety disorders. In Stoudemire A, ed: *Clinical psychiatry for medical students*, ed 3, Philadelphia, 1998, JB Lippincott.

Shaner R: *Psychiatry*, Baltimore, 1997, Williams & Wilkins.

PROBLEM · 70

SOCIAL PHOBIA, POSTTRAUMATIC STRESS DISORDER, AND OBSESSIVE-COMPULSIVE DISORDER

"Sometimes I Just Can't Do What I Should, Other Times I Must Do What I Shouldn't."

Case 1 ■ A 22-Year-Old Law Student Who Is Unable to Answer Questions in Class

A 22-year-old law student comes to your office in a state of anxiety. He is currently taking a law class in which 50% of the class grade is based on class participation. Although he knows the material well, he is unable to answer the questions when posed to him by the professor. He has now gone through 2 months of the 6-month class and has not been able to answer one of the 14 questions that the professor has asked him in class.

The professor asked him to make an appointment for a "little chat" the other day. At that time, he was told that he would (in the professor's words) "fail the class" unless he began to participate.

The student describes himself as a loner. He tells you that he has always been shy, but this is the first time the shyness has really threatened to have a major impact on him. His family history is significant for what he terms "this shyness."

His mother has the same characteristics, but for her it doesn't seem to be causing the kind of life difficulties it is causing him.

His mental status examination is essentially normal.

SELECT THE BEST ANSWER
TO THE FOLLOWING QUESTIONS

Q1. What is the most likely diagnosis in this patient?
   a. panic disorder with agoraphobia
   b. panic disorder without agoraphobia
   c. panic disorder with social phobia
   d. social phobia
   e. specific phobia

Q2. Which of the following is not a characteristic of the disorder described?
   a. persistent fear of humiliation
   b. exaggerated fear of humiliation
   c. embarrassment in social situations
   d. high levels of distress in particular situations
   e. fear of crowds or fear of closed-in spaces

Q3. Which of the following physiologic symptoms is not characteristic of the disorder described?
   a. blushing
   b. trembling
   c. bradycardia
   d. sweating
   e. elevated blood pressure

Q4. The neurochemical basis of the disorder described has been associated with which of the following neurotransmitters?
   a. epinephrine
   b. norepinephrine
   c. serotonin
   d. a and b only
   e. all of the above

Q5. Which of the following pharmacologic agents is most commonly used to treat this disorder?
   a. benzodiazepines
   b. monoamine oxidase inhibitors (MAOIs)
   c. tricyclic antidepressants (TCAs)
   d. newer antipsychotic medications
   e. beta-blockers

Q6. With respect to this disorder, which of the following psychotherapies is most effective?
   a. assertiveness training
   b. brief psychodynamic therapy
   c. psychoanalysis
   d. biofeedback
   e. all of the above

Case 2 ■ A 27-Year-Old Woman Who Is Terrified of Flying

A 27-year-old woman is terrified of flying in airplanes and avoids all travel in them. As a result, she has lost promotional opportunities in her work and rarely sees her family who lives in a distant city.

Q7. Which of the following disorders is the most likely diagnosis?
   a. panic disorder
   b. social phobia
   c. generalized anxiety disorder
   d. specific phobia
   e. obsessive compulsive disorder (OCD)

Case 3 ■ A 73-Year-Old Male Who Is Anxious and Withdrawn

A 73-year-old male is brought to your office by his wife. His wife states that for the last 2 months her husband has been anxious and withdrawn. He was robbed at gunpoint in a shopping mall parking structure just before his symptoms began. Since that time, her husband refuses to enter parking structures or drive alone. He sleeps poorly and has complained of nightmares about the robbery. The patient himself says only that he feels unhappy but does not want to talk about the robbery. He says, "I just want to put it behind me."

Q8. What is the most likely diagnosis in this patient?
   a. primary insomnia
   b. adjustment disorder with anxious mood
   c. major depressive disorder (MDD)
   d. borderline personality disorder
   e. posttraumatic stress disorder (PTSD)

Q9. Characteristics of this disorder include which of the following?
   a. recurrent and intrusive recollections of disturbing events
   b. efforts to avoid thinking about what has happened in the past
   c. irritability or outbursts of anger
   d. a and b only
   e. all of the above

Q10. Regarding the treatment of the disorder described in Case 3, which of the following statements is (are) true?
   a. treatment relies on a combination of nonpharmacologic and pharmacologic treatments

b. nonpharmacologic treatment centers on the learning of behaviors to avoid anxiety from the conditioned stimulus
c. TCAs have been used with some success in the treatment of this disorder
d. MAOIs have been used with some success in the treatment of this disorder
e. all of the above statements are true

Q11. Which of the following drugs has the most potential for abuse in the treatment of the disorder described in Case 3?
a. lithium carbonate
b. phenelzine
c. fluoxetine
d. alprazolam
e. desipramine

Q12. Which of the following medications would generally be considered the best initial choice for treatment of an acute episode of this disorder?
a. lithium carbonate
b. phenelzine
c. sertraline
d. alprazolam
e. desipramine

Case 4 ■ A Compulsive 26-Year-Old Male Who Is Newly Married

A 26-year-old male, recently married, comes to your office with his new wife. They have been married for 3 months, and she tells you that she is very concerned about some of his behaviors. Apparently, when they go out the door in the morning and close the garage door, he goes around the block "at least eight times to make sure it is closed." Also, when he washes his hands before a meal, he will often go back and wash them at least three or four times during the meal itself "just to make sure they are clean."

The husband sits quietly and volunteers no information. He lived with his parents until he was married and his wife tells you that apparently he was always very well protected by his mother.

When the patient finally begins to talk, he admits that everything his wife has just told you is true; he goes on to add, however, that his behaviors are simply "a way of protecting her."

His history is fairly unremarkable except for his "being a loner." Several family members, including his mother, have a history compatible with depression.

Q13. What is the most likely diagnosis in this patient?
a. atypical depression

b. schizophreniform disorder
c. OCD
d. spousal protective phobia
e. specific phobia

Q14. Which of the following medications is the best initial choice for the treatment of this disorder?
a. clomipramine
b. phenelzine
c. risperidone
d. fluvoxamine
e. pimozide

Q15. Which of the following psychotherapies is most useful for treatment of this disorder?
a. psychodynamic psychotherapy
b. humanistic psychotherapy
c. supportive psychotherapy
d. crisis counseling
e. behavioral psychotherapy

SHORT ANSWER MANAGEMENT PROBLEM
List five common obsessions and five common compulsions associated with OCD.

ANSWERS

A1. **d.** This patient has a social phobia, which is characterized by a marked and persistent fear of one or more social or performance situations in which the person is exposed to unfamiliar people or to possible scrutiny by others. They fear that they may act in a manner that will be humiliating or embarrassing. Examples include (as in this patient) not being able to talk when asked to speak in public, choking on food when eating in front of others, being unable to urinate in a public lavatory, hand-trembling when writing in the presence of others, and saying foolish things or not being able to answer questions (as in this patient) in social situations.

In addition, exposure to the feared social situation almost invariably provokes anxiety. The individual realizes that his or her behavior is abnormal and unreasonable. The feared social or performance situation is either avoided or endured with intense anxiety; and the avoidance, anxious participation, or distress in the feared social or performance situation interfere significantly with the person's normal routine, occupational (or, in this case, academic) functioning, or social activities and relationships with others.

A2. **e.** Fear of crowds, in which escape may not be possible, is known as agoraphobia. Fear of closed spaces is known as claustrophobia.

A3. **c.** The fear of speaking, meeting people, eating, or writing in public is related to the fear of "appearing nervous or foolish," making mistakes, being criticized, or being laughed at. Physical symptoms include blushing, trembling, sweating, elevated blood pressure, and tachycardia.

A4. **e.** Symptoms reported by social phobia patients in phobic situations suggest heightened autonomic arousal. When placed in a phobic situation, social phobics experience significant increases in heart rate that are highly correlated with self-perceived physiologic arousal (in contrast to claustrophobics, who experience less heart rate increase and negative correlations between perceived and actual physiologic arousal). Stressful public speaking situations result in twofold or threefold increases in plasma epinephrine levels. Norepinephrine increases are also seen.

Until recently, only epinephrine and norepinephrine were the neurotransmitters associated with the neurochemical basis of this disorder. However, now that the new selective serotonin reuptake inhibitors (SSRI) agents have been shown to be effective in social phobic situations, serotonin is recognized as likely to also be involved. In this case, it would seem that social phobics would demonstrate a relative deficiency of serotonin-mediated activity rather than an excess as seen with epinephrine and norepinephrine.

A5. **e.** Beta-blockers (such as atenolol 50 to 100 mg/day) are commonly used to treat circumscribed forms of social phobia such as fears of public speaking or performances.

Generalized social phobia is often less responsive to pharmacologic interventions. MAOIs, specifically phenelzine (45 to 90 mg/day), buspirone, SSRIs, and benzodiazepines, have all been reported to be occasionally effective.

A6. **a.** Assertiveness training is a cognitive-behavioral treatment that is particularly effective for treating social phobia. It consists of graduated exposure to social situations, education, and role-playing.

A7. **d.** The most likely diagnosis in this patient is specific phobia. Specific phobias involve intense fear and avoidance of specific objects or situations. The individual recognizes the fear and avoidance as excessive, and the symptoms result in occupational or social impairment. Common specific phobias include animals, heights, closed spaces, darkness, and blood.

A8. **e.** The most likely diagnosis in this patient is PTSD. The essential features of this disorder involve the presence of intrusive recollections, emotional numbing and avoidance, and anxiety, all occurring after an event that causes feelings of danger, helplessness, and horror.

A9. **e.** There are five major categories of criteria for the diagnosis of PTSD listed in the DSM-IV:
  a. Experiencing or witnessing an event that involves death, threat to life, or serious injury to himself or others that was experienced with intense fear, helplessness, or horror
  b. A traumatic event that is persistently experienced in ways such as recurrent and intrusive distressing recollections, dreams, feelings or thoughts that the event is recurring, psychologic distress at exposure to symbolic events of that time, and physiologic reactivity upon exposure to cues of that event
  c. Persistent avoidance of stimuli associated with the trauma or numbing of general responsiveness, including efforts to avoid thoughts or feelings of the event; efforts to avoid activities, situations, or people associated with the event; inability to recall some aspect of the event (psychologic amnesia); feelings of detachment or distance from others; diminished ability to have "affective feelings" and a sense of a foreshortened future
  d. Persistent symptoms of increased arousal (this is very common in war veterans) indicated by difficulty falling or staying asleep, irritability or outbursts of anger, difficulty concentrating, hypervigilance, and exaggerated startle response
  e. Duration of symptoms of at least 1 month
  f. Marked distress or significant impairment in social or occupational functioning caused by the disturbance

A10. **e.** As with other anxiety disorders, treatment for PTSD often is best accomplished with a combination of pharmacologic and nonpharmacologic therapies. SSRIs, including sertraline, are often used as medications of first choice for treating PTSD. However, many other medications have been used, and there are few controlled trials confirming the superiority of one class of drugs over another in the treatment of this disorder. Phenelzine (an MAOI) and imipramine (a TCA) have often been used. Other drugs that have shown some efficacy include clonidine, propranolol, lithium, and buspirone.

A11. **d.** Alprazolam and other benzodiazepines are relatively contraindicated in this patient because of their increased potential for substance abuse and dependence in patients with PTSD.

A12. **d.** Acute stress reactions associated with PTSD are best treated on a short-term basis with a benzodiazepine such as alprazolam or clonazepam, the latter having a lower incidence of dependency and a longer duration of action. This initial pharmacologic treatment should be supplemented by supportive or expressive psychotherapy.

However, the chronic, recurrent nature of PTSD requires a more complex treatment including drugs and cognitive-behavioral therapy. Drugs used to reduce anxiety, symptoms of intrusion, or avoidance behavior include TCAs such as imipramine, desipramine, or amitriptyline; MAOIs such as phenelzine; and SSRIs such as fluoxetine and sertraline. Trazodone, a sedating antidepressant, is often used to treat insomnia.

Cognitive-behavioral therapies (including relaxation training, systematic desensitization, flooding, and cognitive reframing) are most effective for decreasing symptoms of reexperiencing and hyperarousal. Hypnotherapy has also been useful.

A13. **c.** This patient has OCD, which consists of either recurrent obsessions or recurrent compulsions, or both. The recurrent obsessions include persistent thoughts, impulses, or images that the patient attempts to ignore but cannot. Additionally, the obsessions are not just excessive worries about real-life problems; the patient also recognizes that these obsessions are, in fact, the product of his or her own mind.

Common obsessions include obsessions regarding contamination or illness; violent images; fear of harming others or harming oneself; perverse or forbidden sexual thoughts, images, or impulses; symmetry or exactness; somatic situations; and religious thoughts.

Compulsions are repetitive behaviors or mental acts that the individual feels driven to perform in response to an obsession or according to rigid rules. The behavior or mental act is aimed at preventing or reducing distress or preventing a dreaded event or situation. These behaviors, however, are not connected in a realistic manner with what they are designed to neutralize or prevent and are clearly excessive.

The individual realizes that the compulsions are excessive and unreasonable. They cause marked distress in the person's life or significantly interfere with the person's normal routine, occupation, or social activities.

Common compulsions include checking things (e.g., door locks, water taps, and the oven), cleaning or washing articles or parts of the body, counting objects or things, hoarding or collecting articles or things, ordering or arranging articles or things, or repeating things (such as tapping).

A14. **d.** Fluvoxamine and other SSRIs have become the drugs of choice for treatment of OCD and have re-

placed clomipramine as the first-line medications for this indication.

A15. **e.** In addition to pharmacotherapy, behavioral psychotherapeutic techniques are also often effective. These techniques include relaxation training, guided imagery and stimulus exposure, paradoxic intent, response prevention and thought-stopping techniques, and modeling.

SOLUTION TO THE SHORT ANSWER MANAGEMENT PROBLEM

Some common obsessions are as follows:
   a. Contamination and illness
   b. Fear of harming others or self
   c. Perverse or forbidden sexual thoughts, images, or impulses
   d. Violent images
   e. Symmetry or exactness
   f. Somatic complaints or conditions
   g. Religious thoughts
Some common compulsions are as follows:
   a. Checking things (e.g., doors, locks, water taps)
   b. Cleaning or washing
   c. Counting objects of various types
   d. Hoarding or collecting objects of various types
   e. Ordering or arranging articles of various types
   f. Repeating things (speech, tapping)

SUMMARY OF THE DIAGNOSIS AND TREATMENT OF SOCIAL PHOBIA, PTSD, AND OCD

1. Social phobia:
   a. Epidemiology: Estimated 6-month prevalence rate of social phobia is 1.2% to 2.2%.
   b. Definition: Social phobia is a persistent and overwhelming fear of one or more social or performance situations in which the individual is exposed to unfamiliar people or to possible scrutiny by others. Fear of speaking in public, hand trembling, and answering questions are particular examples. The fear is one of not being able to perform the particular activity and of being humiliated in public because of this. It produces both embarrassment and high levels of distress.

   The individual either avoids the situation or endures it with intense anxiety. The individual also realizes that the fear is unreasonable but is powerless to do anything about it. Also, the individual experiences occupational, social, or academic interference with normal life schedule and/or goals because of it.

c. Symptoms: Not only are intense anxiety and fear produced but also symptoms of autonomic hyperactivity such as blushing, trembling, tachycardia, and elevated blood pressure.

d. Neurochemistry: Probable increased noradrenergic and adrenergic activity related to autonomic hyperarousal. Serotonin systems may also be involved, given the therapeutic effects of SSRIs in this disorder.

e. Treatment:
   1) Nonpharmacologic: Behavioral techniques and cognitive restructuring
   2) Pharmacologic: Drug class of choice is the SSRIs: fluoxetine and sertraline. Other drug classes of benefit are MAOIs (particularly phenelzine) and beta-blockers (particularly atenolol, oxprenolol, and propranolol)

f. Concomitant disorders: One third of patients with social phobia report a history of MDD.

2. PTSD:
   a. Epidemiology: Particularly important and common in war veterans. Lifetime prevalence rates as high as 30% in war veterans have been reported.
   b. Definition: PTSD is defined as specific constellation of symptoms that are an immediate or a delayed response to a catastrophic life event. The symptoms include recurrent or intrusive distressing recollections or dreams of the event, psychologic distress at exposure to events that symbolize or resemble the event, and physiologic reactivity on exposure to internal or external cues. As well, there is persistent avoidance of stimuli associated with the trauma or numbing of general responsiveness and persistent symptoms of increased arousal (such as being unable to fall asleep or stay asleep).
   c. Examples of typical traumatic events that can generate PTSD:
      1) Combat or war experiences
      2) Serious accidents (automobile, bus, plane, or train crashes)
      3) Natural disasters (tornado, hurricane, flood, or earthquake)
      4) Physical assault (rape, physical or sexual abuse, mugging, or torture)
      5) Other serious danger of death or severe injury to oneself
      6) Witnessing the mutilation, serious injury, or violent death of another person
   d. Nonpharmacologic therapy:
      1) Behavioral therapy
      2) Psychodynamic therapy
      3) Hypnotherapy
      4) Cognitive therapy
   e. Pharmacologic therapy: Drug classes that have been shown to be effective for various symptom include SSRIs, other antidepressants, beta-blockers, mood stabilizers, and buspirone. Long-term use of benzodiazepines is avoided when treating this disorder because of the increased association with substance dependence.
   f. Risk factors for development of PTSD: The risk factors for development of PTSD include separation from parents during childhood, family history of anxiety, preexisting anxiety or depression, family history of antisocial behavior, female sex, and neuroticism.

3. OCD:
   a. Epidemiology: The measured 6-month prevalence rate has been estimated at 2% to 3%.
   b. Definition: OCD is a mental disorder in which either obsessions (recurrent distressing thoughts, ideas, or impulses) are experienced as both unwanted and senseless but at the same time irresistible. Compulsions are repetitive, purposeful, intentional behaviors, usually performed in response to an obsession, and are recognized as unrealistic and unreasonable but are irresistible.
   c. Common obsessions and compulsions: See the Solution to the Short Answer Management Problem.
   d. Treatment:
      1) Nonpharmacologic: Prolonged exposure to ritual-eliciting stimuli together with prevention of the compulsive response.
      2) Pharmacologic: SSRIs are the drugs of choice; clomipramine is also effective but has more untoward effects. MAOIs and alprazolam or other high-potency benzodiazepines can also be used.
   e. Coexisting disorders:
      1) Other anxiety disorders
      2) Eating disorders
      3) Gilles de la Tourette's syndrome
      4) Schizophrenia
      5) Separation anxiety in childhood

SUGGESTED READINGS

American Psychiatric Association: *Diagnostic and statistical manual,* ed 4, Washington, DC, 1994, American Psychiatric Association Press.

Kaplan HI, Sadock BJ: Mood Disorders. In Kaplan HI, Sadock BJ, eds: *Kaplan and Sadock's synopsis of psychiatry: Behavioral sciences/ clinical psychiatry,* ed 8, Baltimore, 1998, Williams & Wilkins.

Nagy L et al: Anxiety disorders. In Stoudemire A, ed: *Clinical psychiatry for medical students,* ed 3, Philadelphia, 1998, JB Lippincott.

Shaner R: *Psychiatry,* Baltimore, 1997, Williams & Wilkins.

PROBLEM · 71

SEXUAL DYSFUNCTION DISORDERS

"Sex Is Not Wonderful Anymore."

Case 1 ■ A 65-Year-Old Hypertensive Male with Impotence

A 65-year-old male with hypertension, congestive heart failure, and peptic ulcer disease comes to your office for his regular blood pressure check. You have managed to effectively control his blood pressure. Although his blood pressure is now under control, he complains of an inability to maintain an erection. He is currently taking alpha-methyldopa, propranolol, verapamil, hydrochlorothiazide, and cimetidine.

On examination, his blood pressure is 140/70 mm Hg. His pulse is 56 and regular. The rest of the cardiovascular examination and the rest of the physical examination are normal.

SELECT THE BEST ANSWER TO THE FOLLOWING QUESTIONS

Q1. Which of the medications listed is the least likely to be the cause of this man's sexual dysfunction?
a. alpha-methyldopa
b. propranolol
c. verapamil
d. hydrochlorothiazide
e. cimetidine

Q2. Which of the following is generally considered to be the most common cause of sexual dysfunction in both males and females?
a. pharmacologic agents
b. panic disorder
c. generalized anxiety disorder (GAD)
d. major depressive disorder (MDD)
e. dysthymic disorder

Q3. Which of the following agents is not associated with sexual dysfunction?
a. captopril
b. labetalol
c. hydralazine
d. methadone
e. all of the above have been implicated as a cause of sexual dysfunction

Q4. Which of the following is the most common sexual complaint in younger males?
a. hypoactive sexual desire disorder
b. male erectile disorder

c. orgasmic disorder
d. premature ejaculation
e. none of the above

Q5. Which of the following is the most common sexual complaint in older males?
a. hypoactive sexual desire disorder
b. male erectile disorder
c. orgasmic disorder
d. premature ejaculation
e. none of the above

Q6. Which of the following statements regarding the cause of male sexual dysfunction is most accurate?
a. male sexual dysfunction is almost always psychologic in origin
b. male sexual dysfunction is almost always organic in origin
c. psychologic factors seem to predominate in male sexual dysfunction, both in primary and secondary forms
d. male sexual dysfunction in a younger patient has a greater probability of being organic in origin
e. male sexual dysfunction in an older patient has a greater probability of being psychologic in origin

Q7. Which of the following organic disorders is the most common cause of organic male sexual dysfunction?
a. benign prostatic hypertrophy
b. hyperthyroidism
c. Parkinson's disease
d. diabetes mellitus
e. atherosclerosis of the abdominal aorta

Q8. What is the single most important aspect of the evaluation of male sexual dysfunction?
a. the history
b. the physical examination
c. nocturnal penile tumescence measurement
d. ratio of penile/brachial blood pressure
e. serum testosterone measurement

Q9. Which of the following investigations is (are) indicated in a male patient with sexual dysfunction?
a. complete blood count (CBC)
b. blood urea nitrogen (BUN) and serum creatinine
c. thyroid function studies
d. serum testosterone level
e. all of the above

Q10. Which of the following is (are) important in the treatment of male sexual dysfunction?
   a. reducing performance anxiety by prohibiting intercourse
   b. anxiety reductions by identification and verbalization
   c. instruction in "sensate focus" techniques
   d. instruction in interpersonal communication skills
   e. all of the above

Q11. Which of the following is specifically indicated as a treatment for premature ejaculation?
   a. the penile squeeze technique
   b. the injection of testosterone
   c. structured behavior modification programs
   d. the intermittent injection of medroxyprogesterone
   e. interarterial penile injection of local vasoconstrictors

---

Case 2 ■ A 24-Year-Old Female Who Is Unable to Have Sexual Intercourse

A 24-year-old female who has been married for 6 months comes to your office in tears. She and her husband have been unable to have sexual intercourse. She says that when he tries to penetrate her she "tenses up" and is "unable to go any further."

Her significant history includes being raped at the age of 12. The patient has vivid memories of this event. Her general physical examination is normal. You do not attempt a vaginal examination.

Q12. Which of the following statements regarding vaginismus is false?
   a. most women with vaginismus also have difficulty with sexual arousal
   b. there is a strong association between vaginismus and an intense childhood and adolescent exposure to religious orthodoxy
   c. there is a strong association between vaginismus and a traumatic sexual experience
   d. vaginismus is a condition of involuntary spasm or constriction of the musculature surrounding the vaginal outlet
   e. vaginismus may begin with a poorly healed episiotomy following childbirth

Q13. Regarding the diagnosis and treatment of vaginismus, which of the following statements is false?
   a. throughout the diagnostic examination the woman must feel that she is in control and may terminate the examination at any time

   b. the diagnosis of vaginismus can often be made without inserting a speculum
   c. the sexual partner should be involved in all aspects of the treatment process
   d. the insertion of vaginal dilators is not a recognized part of the treatment protocol
   e. "sensate focus" techniques are an important part of the treatment protocol

Q14. Which of the following is the most common female sexual dysfunction disorder?
   a. anorgasmy
   b. delayed orgasm
   c. hypoactive sexual desire disorder
   d. sexual aversion disorder
   e. none of the above

Q15. Which of the following statements regarding female sexual arousal disorder is false?
   a. it is more common in women than in men
   b. the diagnosis takes into account the focus, intensity, and duration of the sexual activity
   c. if sexual stimulation is inadequate in focus, intensity, or duration, the diagnosis cannot be made
   d. in women it is not associated with inadequate vaginal lubrication
   e. in women it is often associated with inhibited female orgasm

Q16. Of the following listed causes, which is the most common cause of hypoactive sexual desire disorder in women?
   a. major psychiatric illness
   b. major psychiatric illness in the woman's partner
   c. dual-career families, with increased responsibilities on the woman both at work and in the home
   d. major physical illness in the woman
   e. alcoholism in the woman's partner

Q17. Which of the following statements regarding inhibited female orgasm is false?
   a. it is the most common female sexual dysfunction
   b. primary anorgasmia is more common among unmarried women than among married women
   c. women over the age of 35 years have increased orgasm potential
   d. women may have more than one orgasm without a refractory period
   e. fear of impregnation is a common cause

Q18. Which of the following statements regarding dyspareunia is (are) true?
a. it may be caused by endometriosis
b. it may be caused by vaginitis or cervicitis
c. it may be caused by an episiotomy scar
d. all of the above
e. none of the above

Q19. Which of the following methods is (are) useful in the treatment of female sexual dysfunction?
a. sexual anatomy and physiology education
b. "sensate focus" exercises
c. treatment of underlying anxiety and depression
d. none of the above methods are useful
e. all of the above methods are useful

Q20. Which of the following medications is most effective in treatment of male erectile disorder?
a. alprazolam
b. alprostadil
c. amphetamine
d. sildenafil
e. yohimbine

Q21. Which of the following major psychiatric conditions is most closely linked to sexual dysfunction?
a. panic attacks/panic disorder
b. GAD
c. MDD
d. schizoaffective disorder
e. schizophrenia

SHORT ANSWER MANAGEMENT PROBLEM
Describe the goal, selection, types, and duration of sexual dysfunction psychotherapies most commonly practiced today.

ANSWERS

A1. **c.** Of medications described for the patient in Case 1, the only antihypertensive agent that has not been associated with sexual dysfunction is verapamil (a calcium-channel blocker).

A2. **a.** Recreational and medicinal substances are the most common cause of sexual dysfunction. Although drugs are more of a problem in males than in females, they have certainly been shown to have a major effect in women as well as men.

A3. **e.** Many different classes of drugs have been implicated in sexual dysfunction, with the main offenders being the antihypertensive drugs, antidepressants, antipsychotics, psychostimulants, and other miscellaneous drugs including lithium, digoxin, indomethacin, antiparkinsonian drugs, and cimetidine.

Always consider the role of substances in the assessment of sexual dysfunction. Antihypertensive medications from a variety of classes, most recently angiotensin-converting enzyme inhibitors (particularly captopril), have been associated with sexual dysfunction. One recent study has confirmed that 19% of males taking captopril have worsening of their sexual function.

A4. **d.** Estimated prevalence rates for sexual dysfunctions vary greatly, depending on the surveyed population and the survey method. The most common sexual complaint in younger males is premature ejaculation. This dysfunction tends to lessen with age.

A5. **b.** The most common sexual complaint in older males is erectile dysfunction. This may reflect both normal aging changes and an increase in general medical conditions as well as the concomitant increased use of medications that interfere with erection.

A6. **c.** The cause of male sexual dysfunction may be psychologic, physiologic, or a combination of both. Psychologic problems often complicate male sexual dysfunction, even when the original cause is physiologic. As well, male organic sexual dysfunction is complicated by the relationship of the male with his partner. In young men, most cases of male sexual dysfunction are psychologic in origin. In older men, as the incidence of concurrent disease rises, so does the prevalence of organic sexual dysfunction.

A7. **d.** Diabetes mellitus is the most common organic cause of male sexual dysfunction. The pathophysiology of diabetes-induced male sexual dysfunction is diabetic neuropathy.

Other common causes of organic male sexual dysfunction include the following:
a. Atherosclerotic vascular disease
b. Congestive heart failure
c. Renal failure
d. Hepatic failure
e. Respiratory failure
f. Genetic causes (Klinefelter's syndrome)
g. Hypothyroidism
h. Hyperthyroidism
i. Multiple sclerosis
j. Parkinson's disease
k. Surgical procedures including: Radical prostatectomy, orchidectomy, and abdominal-perineal colon resection
l. Radiation therapy

A8. **a.** The single most important aspect in the evaluation of male (and female) sexual dysfunction is the history. For example, in a patient with male erectile disorder, if erections are achieved under certain conditions but not others, the likelihood is high that the dysfunction is psychogenic. Normal erectile function during masturbation, extramarital sex, and in response to erotic material suggests a psychologic cause. Similarly, if a normal erection is lost during vaginal insertion, a psychologic cause is suspected. A complete drug history is essential.

The history should include present and previous birth control, a complete past psychiatric history, a complete family history; a history of surgical procedures, a history of the marital relationship, and a history of present job satisfaction and hours of work. The recurrence or persistence of the presenting sexual problem should be sought.

A complete physical examination should be performed. The physical examination will determine whether there is any evidence of organic pathologic condition associated with the sexual dysfunction.

Measurement of nocturnal penile tumescence (most simply done using a strain gauge), the ratio of penile/brachial blood pressure, and the serum testosterone are investigations that have an important role to play in the overall evaluation of impotence, but they do not take the place of a good history.

A9. **e.** Based on the organic causes discussed in Answer 7, baseline screening blood work is indicated. This should include a CBC, BUN and serum creatinine, fasting blood sugar, fasting cholesterol, thyroid function studies, liver function tests, and a serum testosterone level.

A10. **e.** Most cases of sexual dysfunction have, as discussed previously, a significant psychologic component. After a complete history, a complete physical examination, screening blood work, and discontinuation of offending medications, the treatment of male sexual dysfunction (and female sexual dysfunction) is comprised of several important steps:

a. Reduction or, hopefully, elimination of performance anxiety by prohibiting intercourse during the initial treatment period

b. Anxiety reduction by identification and verbalization of the problem

c. Introduction of the process of "sensate focus" (semistructured touching that will permit focus on sensory awareness without any need to perform sexually)

d. Instruction to interpersonal communication skills

e. Physiologic treatment of sexual dysfunction must also be useful. Erectile dysfunction may be treated with sildenafil (Viagra) or alprostadil. Premature ejaculation may be ameliorated with selective serotonin reuptake inhibitors (SSRIs). Although no reliable aphrodisiacs exist, some patients with hypoactive sexual desire disorder may respond to androgenic steroids or yohimbine.

A11. **a.** The initial treatment of premature ejaculation is the same as other therapies described here. In addition, an exercise known as the "penile squeeze technique" is used to raise the threshold of penile excitability. The penis is stimulated until impending ejaculation is perceived. At this time, the partner squeezes the coronal ridge of the glans penis, resulting in diminished erection and inhibited ejaculation. Eventually, with repeated practice, the threshold for ejaculation is raised.

A12. **a.** Vaginismus is defined as recurrent or persistent involuntary spasm of the musculature of the outer third of the vagina that interferes with coitus. There is an association between vaginismus and an intense childhood and adolescent exposure to strong condemnation of sexual behavior based on some religious beliefs. Vaginismus may occur when an episiotomy fails to properly heal following childbirth. Most women with vaginismus have normal sexual arousal.

In this patient, the cause of vaginismus is most likely from the traumatic sexual experience that took place during her childhood.

A13. **d.** The evaluation and treatment of vaginismus begins with a carefully performed physical examination in which the patient is always in full control. She may terminate the examination at any time.

On inspection of the external genitalia, spasm and rigidity of the perineal muscles are often felt. In this case the diagnosis can be made even without inserting a speculum. From inspection, the examination may proceed to the insertion of one or more of the examiner's fingers.

The use of vaginal dilators in gradually increasing sizes has proved helpful in the treatment of vaginismus. Beginning with the smallest size, the woman inserts these herself until she becomes both comfortable and relaxed with their insertion. When the largest plastic dilator can be inserted, the couple can proceed to intercourse.

The partner must be involved in all aspects of assessment and treatment. Ideally, the partner should be present to observe the entire evaluation and treatment. Together with anatomy and physiology education, the couple learns the concept of sensate focus exercises, which play a major part in the therapy of any sexual dysfunction.

A14. **c.** The most commonly reported female sexual dysfunction disorder is hypoactive sexual desire disorder, present in up to one third of women in some studies. Orgasmic disorder, on the other hand, is present in 5% to 10%. The prevalence of female arousal disorder, dyspareunia, and vaginismus is less clear.

A15. **d.** Female sexual arousal disorder is defined as persistent or recurrent partial or complete failure to attain or maintain the lubrication-swelling response of sexual excitement until completion of the sexual activity. The diagnosis includes the subjective sense of sexual excitement and pleasure and requires the focus, the intensity, and the duration of stimulation to be adequate. Sexual arousal disorder is often associated with inhibited female orgasm.

A16. **c.** Hypoactive sexual desire disorder is defined as persistent or recurrent deficient or absent desire for sexual activity. The definition includes a lack of sexual fantasies. The major reasons for hypoactive sexual desire disorder are marital dysfunction, mismatched activity schedules, and exhaustion from work and family responsibilities.

A17. **a.** Inhibited female orgasm is defined as persistent or recurrent delay in, or absence of, orgasm in a female following a normal sexual excitement phase during sexual activity. The definition takes into account the adequacy of focus, intensity, and duration of the sexual activity.

Inhibited female orgasm (as one of the orgasmic disorders) is not the most common disorder of female sexual dysfunction (5% to 10%). It is surpassed by hypoactive sexual desire disorder (33%).

Primary anorgasmia (never having had an orgasm) is more common in unmarried women than in married women. Women over the age of 35 appear to have an increased orgasmic potential.

Women may have more than one orgasm without a refractory period.

Causes for inhibited female orgasm include fear of impregnation, rejection by the woman's sexual partner, hostility, and feelings of guilt regarding sexual impulses.

A18. **d.** Dyspareunia is defined as recurrent or persistent genital pain before, during, or after sexual intercourse. This dyspareunia cannot be caused exclusively by lack of lubrication or by vaginismus.

In many cases, however, vaginismus and dyspareunia are closely associated. Other causes of dyspareunia include episiotomy scars, vaginitis, cervicitis, endometriosis, postmenopausal vaginal atrophy, and anxiety regarding the sexual act itself.

A19. **e.**

A20. **d.** Sildenafil (Viagra) has been used extensively for treatment of male erectile disorder and has been effective when either psychologic or physiologic causes are of primary etiologic significance. Alprostadil is also efficacious but must be administered through penile injection (Caverject) or intraurethral insertion via a cannula (MUSE), and has therefore achieved less acceptance. Yohimbine may have some effect on libido but has not been demonstrated to be efficacious in male erectile disorder. Alprazolam may reduce anxiety about sexual performance. Use of amphetamines for male erectile disorder is controversial.

A21. **c.** The most common psychiatric condition associated with sexual dysfunction is major depressive illness in one or both mates.

In the absence of a psychiatric pathologic condition, dual sex therapy is the most accepted approach to the treatment of sexual dysfunction. One approach often used in the therapy of sexual dysfunction in couples is called the LEDO approach. The LEDO approach centers on the following:

 a. **L**owering stress, tension, and anxiety levels through discussion, examination, and observation

 b. **E**nsuring that both parties understand each other's desires, pleasures, and difficulties

 c. **D**etermining the partner's genuine awareness and knowledge of their own and each other's sexual autonomy and the process of intercourse

 d. **O**utlining, drawing, and explaining alternative approaches to arousal and excitation and intercourse techniques

The sexual problem often reflects other areas of marital disharmony or marital misunderstanding. The marital relationship as a whole is treated, with emphasis on sexual functioning as a part of that relationship. Both a female and a male therapist should be involved in the treatment of the couple's sexual problem. The therapy is short-term and behaviorally oriented. The goal is to reestablish communication within the marital unit. Information regarding anatomy and physiology are given. Specific sensate focus exercises are prescribed. The couple proceeds from nongenital touching and sensory awareness to genital touching and sensory awareness, to genital touching, and finally to intercourse. The couple learns to communicate with each other through these graded exercises.

If underlying MDD, dysthymic disorder, GAD, or other anxiety disorders are present, they must be treated concurrently.

SOLUTION TO THE SHORT ANSWER MANAGEMENT PROBLEM

The answer to this question is really a refinement of, reinforcement of, and expansion of the LEDO approach to sexual dysfunction psychotherapies.

a. Goal: Resolution of specific sexual dysfunctions
b. Selection:
1) Couples: All sexual dysfunction psychotherapy should ideally be performed with both partners.
2) Sexual dysfunction most suited for psychotherapy:
a) Male erectile disorder (impotence)
b) Premature ejaculation
c) Vaginismus
d) Orgasmic dysfunction
3) Make sure all medical causes are ruled out.
4) Types of psychotherapies employed:
a) Behavior modification techniques (including systemic desensitization), homework, and education
b) Psychodynamic approaches
c) Hypnotherapy
d) Group therapy
e) Couples therapy as needed to deal with system dynamics
5) Duration: Weeks to months

SUMMARY OF THE DIAGNOSIS AND TREATMENT OF SEXUAL DYSFUNCTION DISORDERS

1. Prevalence: It is extremely difficult to estimate the prevalence of sexual dysfunction disorders. However, estimates have stated that 40% of American couples at one time or another have sexual dysfunction of some type. The estimated prevalence of certain disorders are as follows:
a. Males:
1) Premature ejaculation: 37%
2) Hypoactive sexual desire disorder: 16%
3) Orgasmic disorder: 6%
4) Male erectile disorder: 7%
b. Females:
1) Hypoactive sexual desire disorder: 33%
2) Dyspareunia or vaginismus: Not applicable
3) Orgasmic disorder: 7%

2. Most common causes:
a. Pharmaceutical agents appear to be the most common cause of sexual dysfunction. Antihypertensives and mood-modifying drugs are especially important.

b. Diabetes mellitus is the single most common organic disorder responsible for sexual dysfunction. (See the complete list in the Answer 7.)
c. Remember that psychologic factors, even if not the predominant cause, accompany most sexual dysfunction disorders.

3. Approach to sexual dysfunction in couples:
a. Always begin by treating this relationship in reference to the couple.
b. Get complete histories from both partners
c. Do complete physical examinations
d. Laboratory testing must include CBC, renal function, liver function, thyroid function, blood glucose, serum cholesterol, and hormone levels (testosterone, follicle-stimulating hormone, luteinizing hormone, estrogen, and progesterone).
e. Remember association between dyspareunia or vaginismus and previous sexual abuse.
f. Remember the possibility of family violence in the present (such as wife abuse leading to rape).
g. Use the LEDO general approach.
h. Consider use of pharmacologic agents for male erectile disorder, including sildenafil and alprostadil.
i. Consider use of SSRIs for premature ejaculation.
j. Utilize the guidelines described in the Solution to the Short Answer Management Problem.

SUGGESTED READINGS

American Psychiatric Association: *Diagnostic and statistical manual of mental disorders*, ed 4, Washington, DC, 1994, American Psychiatric Association Press.

Fagan PJ, Schmidt CW: Psychosexual disorders. In Stoudemire A, ed: *Clinical psychiatry for medical students*, ed 3, Philadelphia, 1998, JB Lippincott.

Kaplan HI, Sadock BJ: Human sexuality. In Kaplan HI, Sadock BJ, eds: *Kaplan and Sadock's synopsis of psychiatry: Behavioral sciences/clinical psychiatry*, ed 8, Baltimore, 1998, Williams & Wilkins.

Shaner R: *Psychiatry*, Baltimore, 1997, Williams & Wilkins.

PROBLEM·72

PSYCHOTHERAPY IN FAMILY MEDICINE

"Stop the World, I Want to Get Off!"

Case 1 ■ A 29-Year-Old Working Mother with Three Children Who Is Unable to Cope

A 29-year-old mother who holds a full-time out-of-the-home job has just gone back to work after the birth of her third child. The child is currently 6 weeks old. She works as an accountant in a large company. Her company is currently restructuring and she worries that her job is not secure. Her husband has just lost his job as an assembly line worker at an automobile assembly plant.

When she returned to work, she sensed that the upper management was trying to make her feel guilty for "taking so much time off to have a baby." She is now waking up at 3 AM to 4 AM every morning to get her work done. On this schedule, she is too tired to spend quality time with her children. She is crying, fatigued, and absolutely exhausted after 10 days back on the job. She finds herself becoming "very sleepy every day at work," and the management has commented on that as well. She tells you, "I just can't take it any longer. I have to work to pay the mortgage and put food on the table. There are no other jobs available. What am I going to do? I just can't go on this way."

She has no history of psychiatric problems or sleep disorders. She has no family history of psychiatric disorders or personal or family history of drug or alcohol use. She is not taking any drugs at present.

**SELECT THE BEST ANSWER
TO THE FOLLOWING QUESTIONS**

Q1. What is the most likely diagnosis in this patient at this time?
   a. major depressive disorder (MDD)
   b. generalized anxiety disorder (GAD)
   c. adjustment disorder
   d. dysthymic disorder
   e. panic disorder

Q2. How is the "sleep disorder" that this patient exhibits most properly labeled?
   a. psychophysiologic insomnia
   b. adjustment sleep disorder
   c. inadequate sleep hygiene
   d. insufficient sleep syndrome
   e. idiopathic hypersomnolence

Q3. You decide to initiate psychotherapy. At this time, in this patient, and given this diagnosis, what is the single best psychotherapy to initiate in a primary care setting?
   a. cognitive psychotherapy
   b. brief psychodynamic psychotherapy
   c. behavioral psychotherapy (behavior modification)
   d. supportive psychotherapy
   e. intensive psychoanalytically oriented psychotherapy

Q4. What is the major goal of the psychotherapy in this patient's situation?
   a. to identify and alter cognitive distortions
   b. to understand the conflict area and the particular defense mechanisms used
   c. to maintain or reestablish the best level of functioning
   d. to eliminate involuntary disruptive behavior patterns and substitute appropriate behaviors
   e. to resolve symptoms and rework major personality structures related to childhood conflicts

Q5. What is the first priority at this time?
   a. foster a good working relationship with the patient
   b. approach the patient as a "blank screen"
   c. develop a "therapeutic alliance" with the patient
   d. begin the assignment of tasks for the patient to complete
   e. develop "free association" with the patient

Q6. What is the therapeutic method at this time?
   a. validate and explore the patient's concerns, provide advice, and help her deal with the stressors
   b. have the patient express her anger in the "here and now"
   c. prescribe a hypnotic to "get things under control"
   d. have the patient "intellectualize" her concerns
   e. have the patient discuss her dreams and free associations

Q7. Which of the following is (are) a technique(s) of supportive psychotherapy?
   a. support problem-solving techniques and behaviors
   b. develop a short-term "mentoring" relationship
   c. develop a short-term "guiding" relationship
   d. suggest, reinforce, advise, and reality test
   e. all of the above

Q8. Which of the following psychotherapies has been shown to be most efficacious in the treatment of psychiatric conditions encountered in primary health care settings?
   a. intensive analytically oriented psychotherapy
   b. psychoanalysis
   c. cognitive psychotherapy
   d. brief psychodynamic psychotherapy
   e. behavioral psychotherapy

Case 2 ■ A 39-Year-Old Female with a 4-Month History of Depression

A 39-year-old female comes to your office with a 4-month history of depression. She meets the DSM-IV criteria for MDD. She was started on sertraline 6 weeks ago and it appears to be helping significantly.

Q9. Which of the following statements is true regarding the therapeutic approach to this patient?
a. most primary care physicians treat MDD only with antidepressant medication
b. supportive psychotherapy is the ideal psychotherapy for this patient
c. there is little evidence to support a combination of medication and psychotherapy in preference to psychotherapy alone
d. brief psychodynamic psychotherapy has been shown to be the most effective psychotherapy when used with a selective serotonin reuptake inhibitor (SSRI)
e. none of the above statements is true

Q10. Which of the following statements regarding cognitive psychotherapy is (are) true?
a. the cognitive psychotherapist views the interpretations that depressed patients make about life as different than those of nondepressed patients
b. cognitive psychotherapy is best suited to patients who have depressive disorders without psychotic features
c. cognitive psychotherapy is generally conducted over a period of 15 to 25 weeks in weekly sessions
d. cognitive psychotherapy may be useful in patients who refuse to take, fail to respond to, or are unable to tolerate antidepressant medications
e. all of the above statements are true

Q11. What is the major goal of cognitive psychotherapy?
a. to help patients "pick themselves up by the bootstraps" and change their lives
b. to reestablish their previous best level of functioning
c. to understand the major conflict area and the particular defense mechanisms they are currently using
d. to identify and alter cognitive distortions
e. to clarify and resolve the focal area of conflict that interferes with current functioning

Q12. At this time, what is the ideal therapy for a patient with MDD?
a. cognitive psychotherapy and a tricyclic antidepressant (TCA)
b. cognitive psychotherapy and an SSRI
c. supportive psychotherapy and a TCA
d. supportive psychotherapy and an SSRI
e. brief dynamic psychotherapy alone

SHORT ANSWER MANAGEMENT PROBLEM
Describe the forms of psychotherapy and their appropriate use by primary care physicians.

ANSWERS

A1. **c.** This patient has an adjustment disorder. Although this condition is detailed in Problem 60, the basic characteristics of adjustment disorder are as follows:
a. The development of a psychologic reaction to identifiable stressors or events
b. The reaction reflects a change in the individual's normal personality and is different from the person's usual style of functioning.
c. The psychologic reaction is either "maladaptive," in that normal functioning (including social and occupational functioning) is markedly impaired, or greater than normally expected of others in similar circumstances.
d. The psychologic reaction does not represent an exacerbation of another psychiatric disorder.

A2. **d.** The sleep disorder that this patient has developed secondary to the "work demands" is known as insufficient sleep syndrome. Persons affected with this disorder voluntarily curtail their time in bed, usually in response to social and occupational demands. This results in daytime hypersomnolence and impairment.

A3. **d.** The type of psychotherapy that best fits treatment of this patient's life situation in a primary care setting is supportive psychotherapy. Supportive psychotherapy is discussed in detail in Answers 4, 5, 6, and 7.

A4. **c.** The major goal of supportive psychotherapy is to reestablish the best possible level of functioning given the limitations of the illness, personality, native ability, and life circumstances. In general, this distinguishes supportive psychotherapy from the change-oriented psychotherapies that aim to either reverse primary disease processes and symptoms or restructure personality.

A5. **a.** There is unanimous agreement among clinicians that the first priority of supportive psychotherapy is to foster a good working relationship with the patient.

A6. **a.** Once a working relationship is established between the patient and the therapist, a skilled supportive psychotherapist helps the patient explore her concerns and validates realistic worries. The therapist may give both advice and assistance. In the case in question, supporting a request for short-term disability or sick leave may be appropriate. During that time the patient's goals might be to refocus her life, attempt to negotiate a more realistic working relationship with her employers, and research other employment.

The prescription of a hypnotic risks compounding her problem.

A7. **e.** Some of the specific techniques employed in supportive psychotherapy include the following:
   a. Regular, weekly sessions where therapy for the patient is consistently available
   b. The support by the therapist of problem-solving by the patient
   c. Guiding or mentoring on the part of the therapist
   d. The concomitant use of medication (especially antidepressant medication)
   e. The specific techniques of suggestion, reinforcement, advice, teaching, reality testing, cognitive restructuring, reassurance, an active stance on the part of the therapist, the discussion of alternative behaviors, and the discussion of social and interpersonal skills

A8. **c.** There is an increasing amount of literature that supports the efficacy of cognitive psychotherapy in primary care settings. Studies examining the outcome of cognitive psychotherapy have found it to be an effective treatment in ambulatory outpatients with mild to moderate degrees of depression. One advantage of cognitive psychotherapy is that the therapeutic techniques can often be more easily learned and integrated into primary care treatment than can psychodynamic or behavioral techniques. Cognitive techniques include the questioning of maladaptive assumptions about problems, provision of information, and assignments for dealing with specific situations. There is a trend to combine these techniques with behavioral techniques such as relaxation training and desensitization. Cognitive behavioral therapy is widely studied and used.

A9. **a.** The most accurate statement in the series of choices offered is that most primary care physicians treat major depressive illness with antidepressant medicine. If psychotherapy is used at all, it is most commonly very brief supportive psychotherapy.

The other important aspects of treatment for MDD are as follows:
   a. A combination of psychotherapy and pharmacotherapy is more effective than either method alone in patients with MDD without psychotic features.
   b. The psychotherapy of choice in the treatment of major depressive illness is cognitive psychotherapy, not supportive psychotherapy.

Studies suggest that there is about a 70% to 75% success rate with each modality; if these are combined, the success rate is increased to somewhere between 85% and 90%.

A10. **e.**

A11. **d.** Cognitive psychotherapy is a method of brief psychotherapy developed over the last 25 years primarily for the treatment of mild to moderate depression and for patients with low self-esteem.

Cognitive psychotherapists see the conclusions about life that nondepressed patients reach as different from those of depressed patients. Depressed persons tend to have negative interpretations of the world, themselves, and the future. As well, depressed patients interpret events as reflecting defeat, deprivation, or disparagement and see their lives as being filled with obstacles and burdens. They also view themselves as unworthy, deficient, undesirable, or worthless and see the future as bringing a continuation of the miseries of the past.

Cognitive therapy is best suited to nonpsychotic patients with depressive disorders and is usually conducted over 15 to 25 weekly sessions.

Cognitive therapy can also be used in patients who refuse to take antidepressant medication, fail to respond to antidepressant medication, or are unable to tolerate antidepressant medications.

The major goal of cognitive psychotherapy is to identify and alter cognitive distortions and thoughts. The techniques that are used include behavioral assignments, reading materials, and teaching that helps these patients recognize the difference between positively and negatively biased automatic thoughts. It may seem, at first glance, completely straightforward, but it is sometimes difficult for the patient to tell the difference between the two. It also helps patients identify negative schemes, beliefs, and attitudes.

A12. **b.** At this time, the best combination of therapies for MDD is a combination of an SSRI and cognitive psychotherapy.

SOLUTION TO THE SHORT ANSWER MANAGEMENT PROBLEM

Primary care presents an opportunity to provide significant relief to patients through psychotherapy. There are many different forms of psychotherapy:

a. Psychoanalysis
b. Intensive (long-term) psychoanalytically oriented psychotherapy
c. Brief psychodynamic psychotherapy
d. Cognitive psychotherapy
e. Supportive psychotherapy
f. Behavioral psychotherapy

The goals of the various psychotherapies are:

a. Psychoanalysis: To resolve symptoms and perform major reworking of personality structures related to childhood conflicts
b. Psychoanalytically oriented psychotherapy: To understand a conflict area and the particular defense mechanisms used to defend it
c. Brief psychodynamic psychotherapy: To clarify and resolve focal areas of conflict that interfere with current functioning
d. Cognitive psychotherapy: To identify and alter cognitive distortions
e. Supportive psychotherapy: To reestablish through encouragement and empathy the most optimal level of functioning possible in the patient
f. Behavioral therapy (behavioral modification): To change disruptive behavior patterns through altering conditioned responses and through the use of environmental reinforcers

The two most important types of psychotherapy in primary care are cognitive psychotherapy and supportive psychotherapy.

a. Cognitive psychotherapy in primary care is useful in the treatment of nonpsychotic depressive disorders.
b. Supportive psychotherapy in primary care has a much broader scope, and its use is indicated in GAD and other anxiety disorders, family dysfunction, marital therapy, and any condition to which importance is attached by the patient.

In addition, group psychotherapy provides significant support to groups of primary care patients in certain situations such as dealing with serious general medical conditions, smoking cessation, stress reduction, and specific phobias including panic disorder.

SUMMARY OF THE DIAGNOSIS AND TREATMENT OF PRIMARY CARE PATIENTS WITH PSYCHOTHERAPIES

The do's and the don'ts of psychotherapy in family medicine:

1. **Do** consider the use of supportive psychotherapy in any condition, recognizing the biopsychosocial model of illness.

2. **Do** consider the increased efficacy of treating depressive disorders with a combination of SSRIs and cognitive psychotherapy.

3. **Do** realize that good results with psychotherapy require time: cognitive psychotherapy, 15 to 25 weekly sessions, and supportive psychotherapy, weekly sessions for various lengths of time.

4. **Do** realize that some studies point to significant cost-effectiveness of psychotherapy in relationship to other interventions.

5. **Do** realize that to properly perform any type of psychotherapy other than brief supportive psychotherapy you will require extra training.

6. **Do** not underestimate the effect of both transference and countertransference on both patient and therapist.

7. **Don't** underestimate the difficulty of changing patients' behaviors. Recognize the prevalence of somatoform disorders in family medicine and the relative difficulty of treating them successfully.

8. **Don't** routinely prescribe narcotic analgesics for patients that are receiving intensive psychotherapy in your clinic. If you do, the drugs you prescribe rather than the condition itself will often become the focus of the therapy.

9. **Don't** be afraid to refer a patient to qualified psychotherapy specialists after several sessions of psychotherapy in which it is apparent that no progress in being made.

10. **Do** be extremely careful in deciding what conditions you treat with psychotherapy. The more complicated the condition, the longer the duration of the condition, and the larger the number of coexisting factors, the more difficult the task you face and the more training you need.

SUGGESTED READINGS

American Psychiatric Association: *Diagnostic and statistical manual,* ed 4, Washington, DC, 1994, American Psychiatric Association Press.

Kaplan HI, Sadock BJ: Psychotherapies. In Kaplan HI, Sadock BJ, eds: *Kaplan and Sadock's synopsis of psychiatry: Behavioral sciences/ clinical psychiatry,* ed 8, Baltimore, 1998, Williams & Wilkins.

Shaner R: *Psychiatry,* Baltimore, 1997, Williams & Wilkins.

Ursano R et al: The psychotherapies: Basic theoretical principles and techniques. In Stoudemire A, ed: *Clinical psychiatry for medical students,* ed 2, Philadelphia, 1994, JB Lippincott.

PROBLEM · 73

PATIENT USE OF ALTERNATIVE COMPLEMENTARY CARE

"Doctor, I Know It Is a Long Shot, but It Seems to Be My Only Chance."

Case 1 ■ A 35-Year-Old Female with Metastatic Cancer of the Cervix

A 35-year-old female, a new patient to your practice, comes to your office to seek help in obtaining a referral to the Mexican Cancer Cure Center in a small town near Mexico City. She has metastatic carcinoma of the cervix, which has been treated with chemotherapy and radiation therapy but has now spread to her entire axial skeleton. The patient excitedly shows you the brochure that describes the brand-new facility. She tells you that she has contacted the facility and has been accepted for treatment even though there is an extremely long waiting list and it is very difficult to get in. You need to formally refer her, she tells you, to the chief of staff in the center.

SELECT THE BEST ANSWER TO THE FOLLOWING QUESTIONS

Q1. At this time what should you do?
   a. telephone the chief of staff at the center and make the necessary arrangements
   b. ask the patient to provide you with more information so that you can study it and make an informed decision on her behalf
   c. tell the patient that there is no way that you will have anything to do with "quack" medicine; if she wants a referral she will have to see another physician
   d. ask the patient to reconsider her request and come back to see you in 6 weeks; by that time you will have had time to discuss her case with the oncologists and will have been

able to determine more reasonable therapy for her
   e. none of the above

Q2. Regarding alternative/complementary (AC) therapy, which one of the following statements is true?
   a. AC therapy consumption is on the increase in North America
   b. AC therapy is unlikely to produce any significant adverse effects
   c. AC therapy clinics almost always provide their services at nominal cost to patients and their families
   d. AC therapy clinics are rarely, if ever, covered by most forms of health insurance
   e. AC therapy is almost always harmful to patients

Q3. Regarding patients who attend AC therapy clinics, which of the following is not a common characteristic?
   a. high education level
   b. high income level
   c. common coexistent psychiatric disorder
   d. previous or current conventional therapy
   e. Caucasian race

Q4. Regarding the total cost to patients and their families for AC therapy in North America, which of the following statements is true?
   a. the national cost may be as high as $27 billion annually
   b. the cost is likely to reflect only the cost of the products associated with AC therapies
   c. AC therapy costs are not funded by many major health care plans
   d. AC therapy costs are easy to quantify because of the careful tracking of expenditures by government and private insurance
   e. health care costs associated with AC therapies have decreased over time

Q5. Regarding AC therapies, which of the following statements is true?
   a. a major advantage of AC therapies over conventional therapies is their lack of side effects
   b. all AC therapies have been shown, in randomized controlled trials, to decrease longevity in cancer patients
   c. the U.S. Congress has decided not to fund any research trials involving AC therapies or other unconventional medical practices
   d. the simultaneous use of AC therapies and conventional therapies is extremely uncommon
   e. none of the above statements is true

Q6. Which of the following statements regarding alternative cancer therapy and conventional cancer therapy is true?
 a. Most patients who seek treatment with AC cancer therapies abandon conventional cancer therapies when alternative therapy begins
 b. Most patients who seek treatment with AC therapies continue conventional cancer therapies
 c. Most patients who seek treatment with AC cancer therapies never return to their primary physician
 d. Most patients who seek treatment with AC cancer therapies believe that conventional cancer therapies have irreversibly poisoned their organ systems
 e. Most patients who seek treatment with AC cancer therapies have developed a confusional state

Q7. What is the single most important difference between AC cancer therapies and conventional cancer therapies from the point of view of the patient?
 a. AC cancer therapies are directed at the symptoms of the cancer, whereas conventional cancer therapies are directed at the root cause of the cancer
 b. AC cancer therapies are much more likely to be successful in actual cure than conventional cancer therapies
 c. AC cancer therapies are less likely to produce fatigue than conventional cancer therapies
 d. In contrast to conventional therapies, AC cancer therapies are usually accompanied by a significant decision-making role on the part of the patient
 e. AC cancer therapies are more carefully administered than conventional cancer therapies

Q8. Which of the following statements regarding patients seeking treatment with AC treatments is (are) true?
 a. It is always wrong for a physician to prevent a patient who wishes to use AC therapies from doing so
 b. The probability of a patient using AC therapies bears a significant relationship to the belief system of his or her primary care physician
 c. Some AC therapies appear attractive to patients because of the patient's sense that the treatment is more "natural" and "nontoxic"
 d. b and c
 e. all of the above statements are true

SHORT ANSWER MANAGEMENT PROBLEM
A 56-year-old male diagnosed with carcinoma of the pancreas comes to your office for review of his narcotic pain medications. There is no doubt that this patient is palliative. He tells you that he has begun to take "shark's cartilage" as a chemotherapeutic agent. He explains to you that "sharks don't get cancer and it seems that shark's cartilage works by zeroing in on the cancer cells in the pancreas." Describe how you would respond to the news that this patient of yours is taking shark's cartilage.

ANSWERS

A1. **e.** You, as the patient's family physician, should carefully discuss with the patient the following:
 a. Her previous therapy and her feelings about its benefit and its effect on her quality of life
 b. Her relationship and feeling regarding the other physicians involved in her care
 c. Her current condition including pain control, symptom control, fears, and feelings about the future
 d. Her reason for wanting to go to Mexico, her hopes and thoughts for what can be accomplished, and want she thinks will be the result of her visit
 e. Her thoughts and wishes regarding further conventional therapy
 f. The need for someone to "coordinate her care" and act as her "advocate" from this point on, no matter what

It would be preferable to indicate to the patient that you, as her new family physician, are willing to do this. You are willing to discuss any and all options and to direct her in a way that you feel is in her best interest. By doing this you have the best chance of gaining the confidence of the patient and being able to influence her in a manner that may have her reconsider her decision.

A2. **a.** The use of AC therapies is a growing trend. The National Institutes of Health has developed a center for the study of potentially beneficial treatments. Some AC treatments are of benefit, even if only in terms of providing the patient with the comfort of an intervention that maintains hope.

The primary care physician should help the patient discern between harmful therapies and those that are not. The physician should also try to see that AC therapies do not keep patients away from proven curative or palliative therapies that may improve the quality of life. Conversely, the primary care physician should not try to prevent patients from obtaining AC therapies that might prove beneficial.

A3. **c.** Patients who seek AC therapies are generally well-educated patients with a relatively high income. They most commonly have been in or are currently in conventional therapy. Most are Caucasian and do not have any serious psychiatric disorder.

A4. **a.** We do not know precisely the total cost of AC therapies in the United States. The most recent estimates, however, have put the estimated cost at $27 billion annually. There were 630 million documented visits to AC providers in 1997, compared with only 430 million visits to primary care allopathic physicians. Undoubtedly, many visits to AC providers are not documented.

A recent study has shown that 67% of health maintenance organizations (HMOs) offer at least one form of alternative medicine. Chiropractic care is most commonly covered by 65% of HMOs, but massage, bodywork (yoga, tai chi, etc.), acupuncture, homeopathy, naturopathy, stress management, biofeedback, specific diet programs, and herbal therapies are rapidly becoming more significant offerings. These AC therapies share a commonality of being relatively low-cost and low-tech processes that are popular with the general population, in large part because they are also high-touch. It is the low cost and high index of popularity factors that make HMOs think they also may be profitable.

From the primary care physician's point of view, most, if not all, of the therapies mentioned in the previous paragraph should be thought of as "complementary" practices that the physician should be willing to work with and, in many cases, even encourage their patients to try. However, there still remain "alternative" therapies that are dangerous and even outright quackery.

There have been relatively few studies on the use of alternative cancer therapies, but the best data available suggest some 9% of patients diagnosed with cancer use such therapy. Some of those therapies that were popular a decade or two ago, such as laetrile therapy, have been proven ineffective and even dangerous. Today most alternative cancer treatments probably involve a mix in different proportions of diets, dietary supplements, and spiritual or psychologic support. Some of these modalities may be helpful, some innocuous, and some harmful. Many are expensive and not covered by any form of medical insurance. Probably a small fraction of these treatments are "high pseudotech" and very expensive. Physicians in charge or working in such expensive clinics appear to demonstrate the complete antithesis of altruism.

Because these therapies are not covered by insurance and are outside of the main stream of medicine, they are not effectively tracked by government or private insurance. Hard data relating to their use and ef-

fectiveness are difficult to obtain. However, undoubtedly, the cost of AC therapies will continue to increase parallel to that of conventional medicine.

A5. **e.** AC therapies are not necessarily free of side effects. AC therapies are increasingly being subjected to randomized controlled trials. They have clearly at least provided palliative relief to a variety of conditions, and even longevity in some patients with certain cancers has been improved. The U.S. Congress in 1992 established the Office of Alternative Medicine and in 1998 established the National Center for Complementary and Alternative Medicine (NCCAM). In 1999 the NCCAM had a budget of $50 million. Many patients undergo conventional therapy and AC therapies at the same time.

A6. **b.** Most cancer patients who seek treatment with alternative cancer therapies continue to receive either chemotherapy or radiotherapy following their return from an AC therapy clinic.

A7. **d.** One important difference between AC cancer therapies and conventional cancer therapies has nothing to do with the therapies themselves. Rather, it has much more to do with patient control and input into decision making. In contrast to treatment plans in AC therapies, many patients feel a loss of control when going through conventional cancer therapies.

A8. **d.** AC therapies appear attractive to patients at least in part because of the perception that they are natural and nontoxic. However, many of these therapies are, in fact, extremely toxic and cause multiple complications. It is not always wrong for a physician to dissuade a patient who wishes to use AC therapies from doing so. Some therapies may be of benefit; others, as long as they are not harmful, may be a source of comfort to the patient. The probability of a patient using AC therapies bears a significant relationship to the belief system of his or her primary care physician

SOLUTION TO THE SHORT ANSWER MANAGEMENT PROBLEM

Many patients with cancer or other life-threatening illnesses will decide, at one point or another, to try an AC therapy. You, as the attending physician, have two basic responsibilities in this situation:

  a. Reassure the patient and family that you will continue support throughout.
  b. After investigating the available information regarding the AC therapy, clearly indicate to the patient and family what your judgment is regarding the therapy that has been decided on.

This should be done in a nonjudgmental but informative manner. In addition, it is extremely important that the patient's family physician facilitate hope, not unrealistic hope or hope for a cure, but rather hope for minimization or elimination of pain and symptoms leading to an improved quality of life however short.

SUMMARY OF AC THERAPIES IN PATIENTS WITH CANCER AND OTHER LIFE-THREATENING DISEASES

1. Many cancer patients will avail themselves of one or more kinds of AC therapy at some time.

2. AC therapies vary from those that have the potential to produce very significant side effects to those that are unlikely to produce any harm.

3. Discuss honestly and openly your feeling about AC therapy and make every effort to become knowledgeable about the types of therapies that your patient is considering.

4. Indicate your concern about unfounded claims, false promises, toxic side effects, and the costs of some AC therapies.

5. Remind the patient that no matter what, you will remain his or her advocate and physician.

6. Encourage the patient to maintain regular contact with you if he or she decides to pursue an alternative therapy in a distant location.

7. AC therapy in the United States is a multibillion-dollar industry. There is every reason to believe that it will increase, not decrease.

8. Decide what you, as a family physician, can ethically accept regarding the various alternative therapies. Communicate this to your patients.

9. Remind your patients that your primary concern is their quality of life and that you are interested in pain and symptom control to maximize that quality of life.

10. Never leave the patient without hope!

SUGGESTED READINGS

American Psychiatric Association: *Diagnostic and statistical manual of mental disorders*, ed 4, Washington, DC, 1994, American Psychiatric Association Press.

Cassileth B, Brown H: Unorthodox cancer medicine, *Ca-A J Clin* 38(3):176-186, 1988.

Cassileth B et al: Contemporary unorthodox treatments in cancer medicine, *Ann Intern Med* 101:105-112, 1984.

Daily L: More HMOs covering alternative treatments and complementary care, *Physician's Financial News* 17(9):S1-S6, 1999.

DiPaola RS et al: Clinical and biologic activity of an estrogen herbal combination (PC-SPES) in prostate cancer, *N Engl J Med* 339(12):785-791, 1998.

Hauser S: Unproven methods in cancer treatment, *Curr Opin Oncol* 5:646-654, 1993.

McGinnis L: Alternative therapies, 1990, *Cancer* 67:1788-1792, 1992.

National Center for Complementary and Alternative Medicine *http://www.nccam.nih.gov.*

PROBLEM·74

SPOUSAL ABUSE

"A Useless Nothing Like Me Is Lucky to Have Any Man."

Case 1 ■ A 25-Year-Old Female with Pelvic Discomfort, Low Back Pain, Insomnia, and Fatigue

A 25-year-old female comes to the Emergency Room (ER) with a 6-month history of pelvic discomfort, low back pain, and generalized bone pain, lethargy, and fatigue. On direct questioning, she also notes some dryness of her hair and her nails. These problems have been getting progressively worse over 3 months.

She tells you that she "fell down the stairs last night" when she lost her balance.

Her husband who seems irritable and uncommunicative accompanies her. He implies that she exaggerates her symptoms.

On examination, she has a bruise on her left eye and a number of bruises on her arms and legs that are in various stages of healing. Her blood pressure is 130/85 mm Hg. Her pulse is 108 and regular. She looks very anxious and apprehensive. Examination of the cardiovascular system and the respiratory system is normal. Examination of the abdomen reveals deep lower abdominal and pelvic tenderness.

SELECT THE BEST ANSWER TO THE FOLLOWING QUESTIONS

Q1. Which of the following should be considered to be part of the differential diagnosis in this patient?
    a. acute leukemia
    b. hypothyroidism
    c. a bleeding disorder
    d. spousal abuse
    e. all of the above

Q2. Based on the constellation of findings and the relative probabilities of the various disease enti-

ties, which of the following is the most likely diagnosis?
a. acute leukemia
b. hypothyroidism
c. a bleeding disorder
d. spousal abuse
e. none of the above

Q3. What is the estimated prevalence of spousal abuse in North America?
a. 1 in 100 women
b. 1 in 50 women
c. 1 in 25 women
d. 1 in 10 women
e. 1 in 2 women

Q4. Which of the following is not a characteristic of the disorder described?
a. the association of violence with alcohol intake by the batterer
b. violent behavior in the family of origin of both victim and batterer
c. high risk of suicide attempt or gesture in the victim
d. high incidence of psychotropic drug use in the victim
e. association of this disorder mainly with the lower socioeconomic classes

Q5. What is the psychologic term or phrase that is most commonly used to describe the profile of women who are abused?
a. intense interpersonal conflict status
b. learned helplessness
c. inadequate psychologic functioning in general
d. uninhibited anger focus
e. inadequate personality disorder or thought process

Q6. Which of the following is the least common presenting symptom or complaint in a victim of spousal abuse?
a. back pain
b. headache
c. dyspareunia
d. spousal abuse itself
e. abdominal pain

Q7. Which of the following terms best describes the relationship that must develop between the patient and physician in this disorder?
a. understanding
b. active listening
c. active sharing
d. trust
e. collaboration

Q8. What is (are) the main fear(s) that women express concerning the condition described?
a. a fear of escalation of the process
b. a fear of being unable to function independently
c. a fear of not being believed when they tell their story
d. a fear of not being able to support themselves and their children
e. all of the above

Q9. What is the most common site for diagnosis of the condition described?
a. the ER
b. the gynecologist's office
c. the family doctor's office
d. the internist's office
e. all of the above are equally common

Q10. A woman who has been abused seeks medical help and receives it. She and her children are removed from a violent home environment and placed in a transition house where intensive counseling takes place. She leaves the transition house in 6 weeks. What is the most likely next step in this scenario?
a. the woman and her children will establish a new life on their own
b. the woman and her children will soon enter into another abusive relationship
c. the woman will be unable to cope on her own and will go on to welfare; she and her children, however, will keep living independently
d. the woman and her children will go back to their original violent home with the husband
e. c or d

Q11. It is currently estimated that what percentage of husbands or partners that abuse their wives also abuse their children?
a. 5% to 10%
b. 10% to 15%
c. 15% to 20%
d. 20% to 25%
e. 25% to 50%

Q12. Following an episode of spousal abuse, the husband will usually be in what frame of mind?
a. anger
b. confused
c. conciliatory
d. silent
e. unrepentant

Q13. A husband physically abuses his wife for the first time on their honeymoon. Following the episode of violence he "promises that it will never happen again." What is the most likely outcome in this situation?
   a. he is right; it will never happen again
   b. it will happen again but the intensity of the violence will be less
   c. it will happen again but the intensity of the violence will be greater
   d. it will happen again and the intensity of the violence will be the same
   e. nobody really knows for sure; it depends on the situation

Q14. The state of learned helplessness usually evolves from which of the following?
   a. the upbringing of the victim
   b. the upbringing of the abuser
   c. repeated and escalating psychological abuse of the victim
   d. the economic environment (unemployment most often) that the abuser finds himself in
   e. none of the above

Q15. Which pharmacologic drug class is most commonly prescribed to victims of abuse when they present to physicians?
   a. tricyclic antidepressants
   b. sedative-hypnotics
   c. beta-blockers
   d. antipsychotic agents
   e. antimanic agents

SHORT ANSWER MANAGEMENT PROBLEM

Discuss the interventions and the order of those interventions that should take place for the victim, the victim's children, and the victim's mate in a situation similar to the one described in Case 1.

ANSWERS

A1. **e.** All of the diagnostic entities listed in the question are possibilities.

Although unlikely, the low back pain, generalized pain, bruising, and fatigue and lethargy could represent the signs and symptoms of an acute leukemia. The symptoms of fatigue and lethargy, along with the dry skin and dry nails, could certainly represent hypothyroidism. Similar to the explanation for acute leukemia, the signs and symptoms could represent a bleeding disorder. Although not listed as possible responses for the question, some of the symptoms could represent a depression with somatic complaints or a somatoform disorder.

A2. **d.** Spousal abuse is the most likely diagnostic entity. The common failure to diagnose spousal abuse may be explained by the fact that the profile presented to the clinician in cases of spousal abuse is vague. Women who are victims of spousal abuse visit physicians often, usually with somatic or conversion symptoms or psychophysiologic reactions. The most frequent complaints include headache, insomnia, a choking sensation, hyperventilation, gastrointestinal pain, chest pain, pelvic pain, and back pain. As well, the patient may show signs of suicidal behavior, drug abuse, and noncompliance with medication.

Spousal abuse is one of a number of diagnoses in medicine that is best described as follows: if you do not think of the diagnosis, you will not make the diagnosis.

A3. **d.** The estimated prevalence of spousal abuse in North America is 1 in 10 women. One study suggests that up to 12 million families in the United States are affected by spousal abuse. *The Diagnostic Statistical Manual of Mental Disorders, fourth edition* (DSM-IV) specifies five problems related to abuse or neglect: (1) physical abuse of a child, (2) sexual abuse of a child, (3) neglect of a child, (4) physical abuse of an adult, and (5) sexual abuse of an adult. The first three are covered in other chapters of this book, but remember from this that abuse is a family affair. When abuse occurs between two members of a family, it is very likely to occur between another two members. This will be discussed in detail later.

A4. **e.** Alcohol intake by the perpetrator is associated with spousal abuse. The majority of men who batter their spouses have an alcohol abuse problem. Sometimes, the batterer uses alcohol as an excuse to disavow his behavior and convince others that "I was not responsible for my actions at the time." The most important point to be made in this regard, however, is that alcohol does not cause spousal abuse. The two problems must be dealt with individually. As well as alcohol abuse, other drug abuse, including the use of crack cocaine, is frequently associated with spousal abuse.

A nuclear family of origin in which violence occurred is common in victims and batterers.

Spousal abuse occurs in families of every racial and religious background and in all socioeconomic strata of society. Every race and religious background and all socioeconomic groups are represented. It may well be true that psychosocial stressors such as chronic unemployment, welfare status, and other financial problems increase the probability of abuse.

A5. **b.** The psychological term that is most often used to describe women who are abused is *learned* *helplessness,* a situation in which a woman who has been abused and continually told that she is worthless eventually comes to believe just that. Not only do the victims often see themselves as worthless, but they also believe that everything that has happened and is happening is, indeed, their fault. As the abuse (both psychologic and physical) continues, this pattern becomes more and more deeply ingrained into the psyche of abuse victims.

A6. **d.** Women who are abused visit physicians frequently. Those visits, however, consist mainly of complaints or concerns regarding various "body pains" (back pain, headache, abdominal pain, pelvic pain, and dyspareunia), as well as anxiety and depression. Very rarely, however, do the victims go to a physician's office complaining of being abused. Usually this information has to be carefully sought, initially through the asking of general, open-ended questions, and later by a more close-ended, direct approach. If you suspect spousal abuse as the cause of the patient's presenting complaints, you could begin with an open-ended question such as, "Describe your marital relationship." After obtaining either verbal or nonverbal cues that indicate another agenda you could switch to a direct question regarding abuse such as, "Does your husband ever hit you?" This questioning approach provides the best opportunity for open dialogue and sharing of the essential information between patient and physician.

A7. **d.** The single most important aspect of the patient-physician communication process that must occur when a woman who has been abused comes to a physician is the development of a trusting relationship between herself and the physician. Without trust, essential information will not be revealed and no significant progress will be made. Although active listening and understanding on the part of the physician are important, they can never take the place of trust.

A8. **e.** All of the fears listed are reasons for victims choosing to stay in abusive relationships. Fear of escalation of violence and even of murder is a common reason for staying in the relationship. A significant percentage of the total homicides in the United States are committed by husbands who kill their wives. In fact, this is the single most common type of homicide in this country.

Fear of being unable to function independently and support both herself and her children is an almost universal fear.

Perhaps the greatest fear, and the fear that is linked to nondisclosure of spousal abuse, is the fear on the part of the victim that they will not be believed.

A9. **a.** The most common site for the diagnosis of spousal abuse is the ER. The reason for this is the cycle of violence in which there are three distinct phases:
  a. Escalating tension
  b. Erupting violence
  c. Reconciliation
The victim almost always seeks help immediately after the eruption of violence. At this time the individual is most vulnerable to suggestions for therapy. Because the abuse often involves significant physical injuries, the ER is the most likely place that the initial contact with health care professionals will take place. This does not mean, however, that the other medical facilities listed are not important; it simply puts the ER at the top of the list. As well, it illustrates the point that the most cost-effective screening with the highest rate of pickup will occur in the ER.

A10. **d.** Leaving an abusive relationship is difficult for many reasons, including fears of the victim that have already been discussed. On average, a woman will return four times to her residence of origin (that is, go back to her husband) before she permanently separates.

Many abused women seek financial assistance because inadequate child care resources make full-time work almost impossible. Recent federal welfare-to-work legislation has recognized that availability of child care is an essential component of any plan to move single-parent families off of welfare rolls.

We would hope the woman and her children would establish a new and independent life on their own.

Choice b unfortunately occurs all too often. Victims of spousal abuse who leave the original abusive relationship commonly enter into new abusive relationships. Unfortunately, this occurs all too often. Reasons for this are probably related to both environmental and psychologic factors.

Another outcome of an abusive relationship may be rehabilitation of the abuser. Current estimates suggest that approximately 25% of abusers can and do seek help to correct their behavior. Treatment often involves substance rehabilitation and individual, marital, and group counseling. Court mandates for treatment may also play a role.

A11. **e.** It is important to recognize that 25% to 50% of husbands and mates who physically abuse their wives also physically abuse their children. Thus family violence is a family affair. From this, the obvious follows: whenever one form of family violence exists in a family, all other potential types must be considered and evaluated.

Family violence can take many forms:
a. Husband abuses wife
b. Wife abuses husband (uncommon, but it does occur)
c. Husband abuses children
d. Wife abuses children (particularly when the husband has instigated the abuse)
e. Husband abuses grandmother or grandfather (elder abuse)
f. Wife abuses grandmother or grandfather
g. Older children abuse grandmother or grandfather (especially when father or mother has set the example)

A12. **c.** Going back to the cycle of violence described in the Answer 9, the husband is often in a very conciliatory mood after the episode of violence. He will seek the forgiveness of his wife with apparently heartfelt words such as, "It will never happen again, Honey; it was just a mistake and a misunderstanding. I'm sorry." Along with this apology will often come gifts and tokens. The wife, wanting desperately to believe this, will often go back at that time or shortly thereafter. Although in medicine we say "never say never and never say always", spousal abuse has a serious prognosis: without counseling and help, the abuse will almost surely recur.

A13. **c.** As stated previously, the violence will recur in increasingly severe episodes. It may culminate in murder. As mentioned earlier, spousal abuse is the single most important and prevalent category of homicide in the United States. In some of these cases an abuser also kills his children and then himself. This is obviously a very tragic end to a situation that might have been averted with proper diagnosis, assistance for both victim and abuser, and the provision of an ongoing safe environment for the children.

A14. **c.** Learned helplessness is characterized by a deep belief on the part of the victim that she can do nothing to change her environment. Additionally, a victim may believe that it is she who is ultimately responsible for all the violence that has occurred in the relationship. The abuser almost always encourages this belief.

A15. **a.** Frequently, physicians misidentify the anxiety and depression associated with abuse as resulting from an underlying psychiatric disorder. Victims are commonly given prescriptions for anxiolytics and antidepressants without having been adequately assessed.

SOLUTION TO THE SHORT ANSWER MANAGEMENT PROBLEM

The interventions that should take place include the following:
a. Victim and children:
1) Establish the diagnosis by asking open-ended questions followed by more direct, closed-ended questions.
2) Explain the importance of the removal of both the spouse and her children to a safe environment (preferably a transition house where peer counseling and other specific therapy is available).
3) Facilitate the placement of the victim and the children in this safe environment.
4) Use supportive psychotherapy in the safe environment to reestablish the victim's self-esteem and to reverse the ingrained feeling in the victim of learned helplessness.
5) After a period of approximately 6 weeks, facilitate the victim's and the children's assumption of new roles and relationships.
6) Continue contact and supportive psychotherapy for the victim and assist the children with any difficulties that they are having (such as school problems).
b. Abuser (husband or mate):
1) Group psychotherapy appears to work best for abusers. This facilitates the sharing of experiences with other individuals who have had the same experience.
2) Treatment of concurrent psychiatric problems (especially alcoholism and drug abuse) is essential.
3) Reuniting families should be done gradually and with caution.

SUMMARY OF THE DIAGNOSIS AND MANAGEMENT OF SPOUSAL ABUSE

1. Definition of wife abuse: The physical or psychologic abuse directed by a man against his female partner in an attempt to control her behavior or intimidate her

2. Prevalence: Current prevalence estimated as 10% of American women

3. Presenting symptoms: Usually vague somatic or psychophysiologic symptoms

4. Diagnosis: First, think of the diagnosis. Proceed from open-ended questions to more direct closed-ended questions.

5. Treatment:
   a. Victim or children: Removal to a safe environment and supportive psychotherapy for the victim to reestablish self-esteem and reverse learned helplessness
   b. Abuser: Group psychotherapy to help the abuser accept responsibility for his actions, to help him learn to express anger and frustration in other ways, and to treat concomitant psychiatric problems (especially alcoholism and drug abuse)
   c. Remember, one form of abuse begets another: where spousal abuse is present, consider the very high probability of child abuse and elder abuse.

SUGGESTED READINGS

American Psychiatric Association: *Diagnostic and statistical manual of mental disorders,* ed 4, Washington, DC, 1994, American Psychiatric Association Press.

Kaplan HI, Sadock BJ: Problems related to abuse or neglect. In Kaplan HI, Sadock BJ, eds: *Kaplan and Sadock's synopsis of psychiatry: Behavioral sciences/clinical psychiatry,* ed 8, Baltimore, 1998, Williams & Wilkins.

Shaner R: *Psychiatry,* Baltimore, 1997, Williams & Wilkins.

Swanson R: Battered wife syndrome, *Can Med Assoc J* 130:709-713, 1984.

Swanson R: Recognizing battered wife syndrome, *Can Fam Physician* 31:823-825, 1985.

PROBLEM·75

ETHICS AND RESPONSIBILITIES ASSOCIATED WITH REFERRALS AND CONSULTATIONS

"I Think I Should Get a Second Opinion!"

Case 1 ■ A 35-Year-Old Female with a 4-Year History of Chronic Abdominal Pain

A 35-year-old female, a well-known patient of yours who has a 4-year history of chronic abdominal pain (diagnosed by you as irritable bowel syndrome), comes to your office for a periodic health examination. During the encounter she mentions that she would like to see a specialist about her condition; although you have completely investigated her symptoms, she continues to have intermittent abdominal pain. She states that she really is not sure that her complaints have been sufficiently investigated and asks you to make a referral to a gastroenterologist that has been recommended to her.

SELECT THE BEST ANSWER TO THE FOLLOWING QUESTIONS

Q1. Considering the case cited, what should you do now?
   a. explain to the patient that you have completely investigated the condition and that there is no need for a referral
   b. tell the patient that if that is the way she feels she should probably find another family physician
   c. empathize with the patient about her symptoms and refer her to a gastroenterologist of your choice
   d. empathize with the patient about her symptoms and refer her to the gastroenterologist that she mentions unless there is a specific reason not to
   e. tell the patient that you are deeply offended by her request; she has no right to question your competence

Q2. Considering a patient's request for a second opinion, which of the following statements is true?
   a. a patient does not have the right to ask for a second opinion
   b. a patient who asks for a second opinion is demonstrating lack of trust in you as a family physician
   c. a patient has the right to ask for a second opinion
   d. the request for a second opinion should be granted only if you have some uncertainty about either diagnosis or therapy
   e. it is difficult to answer this question; some patients do have the right to ask for a second opinion, and others do not

Q3. In considering the relationship of the health care team to the patient, which of the following statements is true?
   a. the health care team must coordinate all patient care; there is no true leader or head
   b. the family physician is the head of the health care team
   c. the attending physician in whatever circumstance is being dealt with at the time is the head of the health care team
   d. the leadership or headship of the health care team depends on the individual situation, the patient, and many other factors
   e. none of the above statements is true

Q4. What is the primary purpose of consultation or referral to a specialist?
   a. to validate the findings of the family physician
   b. to make sure that you, the family physician, haven't missed anything
   c. to provide reassurance to your patient that you are concerned about his or her welfare
   d. to improve the quality of health care by making available to patients and referring physicians the knowledge and skills of specialist or consultant at appropriate times
   e. to provide protection for you, the family physician, against a malpractice suit

Q5. It is generally agreed that family physicians, given the proper training, can adequately care for what percentage of the patients they see in their practices without the aid of consultation or referral?
   a. 50%
   b. 60%
   c. 75%
   d. 85%
   e. 95%

Q6. Which of the following is (are) the responsibility(ies) of the physician making the referral to a specialist or consultant?
   a. to ensure that patients understand the need for and purpose of referral and consultation
   b. to demonstrate courtesy and respect for patients and specialists or consultants during the consultation and referral process
   c. to communicate clearly to the specialist or consultant the purpose and problems for which help is needed
   d. to send specialists or consultants (when necessary and possible) the results of findings and investigations, including copies of radiologic films, so that they will be available at the time of the consultation
   e. all of the above

Q7. In which of the five following situations is a referral made in an inappropriate manner?
   a. A family physician has carefully worked up a patient with multiple joint pains by careful history, physical examination, and laboratory testing. He is unable to find any abnormalities and refers his patient to a rheumatologist. His referral letter contains the essence of the patient's history, his physical examination, copies of the laboratory investigations, and his differential diagnosis and opinion.
   b. A family physician sees an elderly woman with multiple medical problems who is on multiple medications. The physician decides to refer the patient to a general internist and writes her a brief note stating: "Elderly patient with congestive heart failure, hypertension, diabetes, and osteoarthritis on multiple medications. PLEASE ASSESS. Thank you."
   c. A family physician sees a middle-aged man with what appears to be a chronic fatigue syndrome. She takes a complete history, does a complete physical examination, and does laboratory work to exclude anemia, other blood abnormalities, and hypothyroidism. She also rules out major depression. She refers the patient to an infectious disease specialist for a second opinion.
   d. A family physician sees a patient who has the signs and symptoms of a major depressive illness. The patient, however, does not accept this diagnosis and asks to be referred to a general internist for a second opinion. The family physician agrees to this referral.
   e. A family physician sees a new patient who has been to four other physicians with complaints of chronic lumbar pain. She requests a referral to a pain clinic. The family physician takes a complete history, does a complete physical examination, and agrees to the patient's request.

Q8. Regarding the responsibilities of patients in referral to a consultant or specialist, which of the following statements is (are) true?
   a. the patient should understand the need for and purpose of the consultation or referral
   b. the patient should demonstrate respect and courtesy for both the referring and the consulting physician
   c. the patient should understand that, after the consultation or referral, returning to the referring physician for continuing care and advice as a result of the consultation is the preferred practice
   d. the patient should understand the importance of keeping the appointment and make every effort to do so
   e. all of the above

Q9. Regarding the responsibilities of specialists or consultants in the referral process, which of the following statements is false?
   a. the consultant has the responsibility to provide his or her services in a timely manner depending on the urgency of the condition
   b. the consultant has the responsibility to communicate his or her findings in a timely manner to the referring physician

c. the consultant has the responsibility of deciding whether or not the patient should continue to be seen on an ongoing basis by himself or herself or should return to the family physician for ongoing care

d. the consultant has the responsibility to advise referring physicians promptly of their patients' admission to hospital

e. the consultant has the responsibility to participate in peer and system review of the consultation and referral process

---

Case 2 ■ A 28-Year-Old Female Seeking Referral to a Neurologist

A 28-year-old female with chronic headaches comes to your office for the specific purpose of seeking referral to a neurologist. She has seen five neurologists already but is not satisfied with what any of them have told her.

Q10. What is the most appropriate action for you to take at this time?
   a. agree to refer her to another neurologist and get out of the room as quickly as possible
   b. refuse to refer the patient to another neurologist
   c. ask the patient to come back in a few weeks; you have to think carefully about this request
   d. tell the patient that although you will refer her to another neurologist, this is a complete waste of everyone's time and money; there is obviously nothing wrong with her
   e. none of the above

Q11. Which of the following statements is true regarding the future number of family physicians in the United States relative to specialists or consultants?
   a. the relative proportion of family physicians to specialists is likely to remain the same
   b. the relative proportion of family physicians to specialists is likely to decrease
   c. the relative proportion of family physicians to specialists is likely to increase
   d. it is difficult to predict which way the trend will develop over the next several years
   e. there are likely to be decreases in both the number of family physicians and the number of specialists relative to other health care professionals

Q12. Regarding the definition of lateral referrals and the ethical implications of the same, which of the following statements is true?

   a. lateral referrals are referrals in which a family physician refers a patient from one specialist to another; lateral referrals are completely ethical
   b. lateral referrals are referrals in which a specialist who has been consulted refers the patient to another specialist without the knowledge or consent of the family physician; lateral referrals are completely ethical
   c. lateral referrals are referrals in which a specialist who has been consulted refers the patient to another specialist without knowledge of the family physician; lateral referrals without the knowledge of the referring family physician may not be in the patient's best interest and should be discouraged
   d. lateral referrals are referrals in which a family physician refers a patient to another family physician with expertise in the particular area; lateral referrals may not be in the best interest of the patient
   e. lateral referrals are referrals in which a family physician refers a patient to another family physician with expertise in the particular area; lateral referrals are always ethical and in the best interest of the patient

Q13. Regarding referrals from one family physician to another, which of the following statements is true?
   a. family physicians rarely develop expertise in a specific area; thus referrals from one family physician to another are rarely appropriate
   b. family physicians may develop significant expertise in a specific area; referrals from one family physician to another may well be in the best interest of the patient
   c. family physicians who develop specific areas of interest are really straying away from the foundations of their specialty
   d. family physicians should always consider referral to a specialist or consultant rather than to another family physician
   e. family physicians are not in a position to identify each other's areas of expertise with any degree of knowledge

---

Case 3 ■ A 35-Year-Old Female Who Is Admitted to a Hospital by a Surgeon

A 35-year-old female with colon cancer is admitted for surgery to her local hospital by the surgeon who is going to perform her hemicolectomy.

Q14. How should the patient's family physician be notified regarding the admission?
    a. via an admitting slip from the hospital once the patient is admitted
    b. through the ward clerk in charge of the ward to which the patient is admitted
    c. through the charge nurse who is looking after the patient on the day of the admission
    d. through the resident on the surgery service
    e. none of the above

Q15. A patient who was originally seen by an obstetrician for care during pregnancy is subsequently referred to an internist, a neurologist, a dermatologist, and a gastroenterologist for multiple other problems. No family physician is involved in the patient's care. Regarding this type of referral pattern, which of the following statements is true?
    a. this pattern of referral is likely to lead to optimal patient care
    b. this pattern of referral is likely to be followed by close communication among the various specialists
    c. this pattern of referral, without the coordinating role of a family physician, may create significant problems in the care of this patient and her family
    d. this pattern of referral is extremely uncommon
    e. none of the above statements is true

SHORT ANSWER MANAGEMENT PROBLEM
Your 28-year-old female patient is hospitalized for repair and reconstruction of a left anterior collateral knee ligament, removal of a left lateral meniscus, and partially torn left medial meniscus. After the surgery the patient is in severe pain, but the surgeon tells her that the pain is not severe enough to warrant a strong analgesic. As her family physician, you do not have admitting or order-writing privileges on the surgical floor. You are called by a close friend and informed of the patient's condition. Discuss your approach to help solving this problem.

ANSWERS

A1. **d.** Unless there is a specific reason not to, you should refer the patient to the gastroenterologist of her choice. Although the family physician may feel offended by the patient's request, he or she should not be. Patients with chronic symptoms are difficult to manage. You may very well find that a second opinion not only validates your findings, but also improves the relationship between you and the patient. She may in fact find the chronic abdominal pain to be less of a problem. In this case, it would prove to be less of a problem for both you and her.

A2. **c.** A patient has the right to ask for a second opinion. In this case, you should look on her request as an opportunity to confirm your findings and as an opportunity for the patient to receive the reassurance she needs to manage the abdominal pain more effectively. In the long term, this will turn out to be beneficial to you as well; the patient will likely complain less of the problem and the doctor-patient relationship will likely improve.

A3. **e.** The patient is the head of the health care team. The patient must be fully informed on all matters relating to his or her health and have the opportunity to make decisions with all pertinent information available. The responsibilities of the physicians (both family physicians and other specialists or consultants) and the patient will be discussed in subsequent questions.

A4. **d.** The primary purpose of consultation or referral is to improve the quality of health care by making available to patients and referring physicians the knowledge and skills of specialists or consultants at appropriate times.
    There may be situations in complicated cases in which you wish to validate your findings or make sure that nothing has been overlooked. There may also be times when additional reassurance is needed that only a specialist can provide.
    To refer to specialists for the sole purpose of protecting yourself against malpractice (especially on a regular basis) should give you cause for concern. Perhaps you need to upgrade your skills in one or more areas to help build confidence in your own abilities. Also, in this situation, perhaps you should reconsider the type of practice you are in and make adjustments that will decrease your anxiety level.

A5. **e.** Most authorities have stated that family physicians can well look after the vast majority of patient problems that cross their office doors. A well-trained family physician should be able to look after at least 95% of the patients seen in routine visits without referral to a specialist or consultant.

A6. **e.** In addition to the four responsibilities listed in the question choices, the other important responsibility of the referring physician is to participate in peer and system review of the consultation and referral process.

A7. **b.** This is not an infrequent occurrence and is really a situation of a family physician "dumping" a complicated patient on a consultant or specialist with little significant information given to the consultant. This type of referral is expensive and time-consuming (the specialist will no doubt have to start from the beginning) and certainly could be labeled as unprofessional.

All of the other situations described are appropriate referrals.

A8. **e.** The important point in this question is that patients, as well as their physicians, have a responsibility to make the consultation process work in an efficient, timely, and cost-effective manner.

A9. **c.** The major responsibilities of a consultant or specialist are as follows:
  a. To provide his or her services in a timely manner depending on the urgency of the condition. If the family physician believes that the condition is urgent, he or she should communicate this to the consultant, and the consultant should see the patient as quickly as possible. If he or she cannot personally see the patient, then appropriate arrangements should be made for the patient to be seen by someone else.
  b. To communicate clearly and promptly the results of the consultation process to both referring physicians and patients
  c. To communicate clearly and promptly the results of laboratory tests to the referring physician; the results can be explained to the patient.
  d. To participate in peer and system review of the consultation process in an effort to improve it
  e. To notify the referring physician at once when his or her patient has been admitted to the hospital

The consultant or specialist should return the patient to the referring physician once the consultation is complete. A consultation is just that: a consultation. It is inappropriate for consultants to take over the care of patients referred from family physicians unless they have been specifically asked to do so. Having said that, it may take a consultant or specialist a number of visits to feel that he or she has adequately dealt with the problem. Also, it may be totally appropriate for the consultant (with the family physician's permission) to see the patient on a periodic basis to maximize quality of care.

A10. **e.** This situation is not as uncommon as may initially be thought. There are many situations in which patients (for various reasons) request to see a number of specialists.

The most appropriate actions to take at this time are to perform a complete history, do a complete physical examination, and attempt to determine why the patient has been unsatisfied with the advice she has obtained previously. It may be that what this patient needs is someone to listen and help her deal with her chronic headaches in a different manner. Conversely, it may be that there is something else causing the headaches that has not yet been discovered.

Most likely, however, no matter what the case, it would appear that this patient needs a good family physician much more than referral to another neurologist.

A11. **d.** Although there is a need in the United States at this time for well-trained family physicians to balance the number of specialists, many factors affect the proportion including medical student choice, availability of residency programs, demographic trends of the physician population, and immigration, to name just a few.

A12. **c.** Lateral referrals are referrals that take place from one specialist or consultant to another. If the original referring family physician is not notified, the ethics of such process is questionable. If a consultant believes that a patient requires another specialist or consultant, the referral should be done with the knowledge, input, and involvement of the initial referring family physician.

A13. **b.** Family physicians may well develop areas of expertise in which it is in the best interest of the patient to consider referral to another family physician rather than to another consultant or specialist. This acquisition of knowledge and skills on the part of the family physicians involved is especially useful in regional centers where specialists are not always available. The patient, rather than having to travel significant distances and wait a significant length of time to see a consultant, may be served as well or better by a family physician with knowledge and skill in the specific area.

A14. **e.** The surgeon who is going to perform the operation should inform the patient's family physician and seek input and help from him or her. At a time when a patient is about to undergo a major cancer operation, the patient's family physician, whether or not he or she has formal hospital admitting privileges, is still able to make a significant contribution to the care of the patient. One of the most frequent errors is that the family physician of record is not notified at all or is notified in a way in which a significant delay occurs. The patient, meanwhile, is often left wondering where his or her family physician is and who to turn to for the answers to the many questions that may arise during a significant medical or surgical procedure.

As a principle, miscommunication is often avoided if the contact and communication is direct from attending physician to attending physician. In most cases, this route of communication will optimize patient care.

A15. **c.** This particular scenario is not at all uncommon and in many cases leads not only to a breakdown in communication among the various specialists but also to a lower overall quality of patient care. The role of the family physician in treating patients with multiple medical problems is even more critical than in a patient without such problems. The family physician understands the patient and the patient's family and is likely to be able to significantly improve the overall care delivered because of this knowledge.

SOLUTION TO THE SHORT ANSWER MANAGEMENT PROBLEM

One of the family physician's roles is to be a patient's advocate. In the case presented, it is reasonable to believe that your patient is in severe pain. Therefore the family physician should express his or her concerns directly to the surgeon and offer to undertake the responsibility of managing the patient's pain. Should the issue of hospital privileges create difficulties, it may be possible to transfer the patient's care to the family physician. If not possible, the family physician could offer to write analgesics suggestions on the chart, which could be followed by the nurse if the surgeon agrees. Because the referral to the surgeon was most likely made via the family physician, it seems probable that the surgeon would permit the family physician to participate in the patient's care.

SUMMARY OF THE ETHICS AND RESPONSIBILITIES ASSOCIATED WITH REFERRALS AND CONSULTATIONS

1. The referral or consultation process requires the participation and commitment of the family physician, the specialist or consultant, and the patient. All three have responsibilities.

2. Patients are ethically entitled to a second opinion; a physician should not feel offended when one is asked for.

3. The patient is the head of the health care team.

4. The primary purpose of referral or consultation is to improve the quality of care delivered to patients by making available the knowledge, skills, and experience of someone skilled in the management of a particular problem.

5. Family physicians can manage the vast majority of patient care problems without the need for consultation with specialist colleagues.

6. Family physicians who refer a patient to a specialist have the responsibility of providing a detailed summary of the patient's history, physical findings, and laboratory investigations. To refer a patient to a specialist with a brief one- or two-sentence note is completely inappropriate.

7. Specialists or consultants have the responsibility of seeing patients in a timely fashion; in an urgent situation if they are unable to see the patient, they should make arrangements for someone else to do so.

8. Specialists or consultants who admit a patient to a hospital should personally inform the patient's family physician and invite the family physician to participate in the care of the patient in whatever way is possible.

9. Lateral referrals from specialist to specialist without the involvement of the original referring family physician should be discouraged.

10. Patients who go from one consultant to another looking for answers should be listened to and cared for by a compassionate family physician.

11. Patient advocacy is a major responsibility of the family physician.

SUGGESTED READING
Report of a Joint Task Force of The College of Family Physicians of Canada and The Royal College of Physicians and Surgeons of Canada: Relationship between family physicians and specialists/consultants in the provision of patient care, *Can Fam Physician* 39:1309-1312, 1993.

PROBLEM · 76

HOW TO BREAK BAD NEWS

"Well, Doc, How Did the Tests Come Out?"

Case 1 ■ A 34-Year-Old Female Just Diagnosed with Metastatic Malignant Melanoma

You have just received the computed tomography (CT) scan report on a 34-year-old mother of three who had a malignant melanoma removed 3 years ago. Originally, it was a Clark's level I and the prognosis was excellent. The patient presented to your office 1 week ago complaining of chest pain and abdominal pain. A CT scan of the chest and abdomen revealed metastatic lesions throughout the lungs and the abdomen. She is in your office and you have to deliver the bad news of the significant spread of the cancer.

SELECT THE BEST ANSWER TO THE FOLLOWING QUESTIONS

Q1. Regarding the delivery of bad news to patients who are unsupported during the visit, which of the following statements is true?
   a. the fact that the patient is alone is insignificant
   b. you have no right to interfere with her decision to come alone to the office
   c. you should go into the consultation room and explain that the news you are about to deliver is complex; you would feel better if her husband or significant other were present when the test results were explained
   d. patients don't remember much of anything from the first visit, at which this type of news is delivered, so it does not really matter whether someone else is present or not
   e. having a significant other present will only complicate an already difficult situation

Q2. Which of the following settings is not acceptable for the delivery of bad news?
   a. a private physician's office
   b. a quiet room in a hospital setting
   c. the patient's home
   d. a private hospital room
   e. a multibed hospital room

Q3. Following the first step (getting started), what is the next step in breaking bad news?
   a. deliver the bad news all in one blow; get it over with as quickly as is humanly possible
   b. fire a "warning shot" that some bad news is coming
   c. find out how much the patient knows
   d. find out how much the patient wants to know
   e. it doesn't really matter what you do next; the end result will be the same

Q4. Which of the following statements regarding finding out how much the patient wants to know is true?
   a. it is not very important to find out how much the patient wants to know; everyone really should be told everything

   b. most patients would rather not know all of the details of their illness
   c. most patients can't really make up their minds at the first interview how much they want to know
   d. most patients will want to know the whole truth
   e. in some instances patients shouldn't be told anyway

Q5. In beginning to deliver bad news we frequently suggest that you "fire a warning shot" first. What would be an appropriate warning shot?
   a. "you have cancer, and unfortunately it is a very bad cancer"
   b. "you have a cancer but we'll do our best to 'zap-zap' it with radiation"
   c. "you have a very aggressive malignancy; fortunately, that means we may be able to kill more cells with the chemotherapy"
   d. "unfortunately, the situation appears to be more serious than we would have hoped for"
   e. "unfortunately, the cancer has spread all over your body; I think it's time you called your lawyer and started to get things wrapped up"

Q6. There are two languages that physicians use in talking to patients: English and "medispeak." Unfortunately, patients usually only understand English. Which of the following is an example of "medispeak"?
   a. blast cells
   b. multiple sclerosis
   c. tumor
   d. cancer
   e. leukemia

Q7. Which of the following statements is false regarding the involvement of family physicians in the care of a patient with cancer?
   a. ideally, the family physician should be present when the patient is told of a bad diagnosis or prognosis
   b. the family physician and the primary consultant should be in constant contact and should be certain that the same message is delivered
   c. family physicians have a limited role to play once the patient is enrolled in a tertiary care cancer treatment center
   d. the family physician has a responsibility to follow up on the care of his or her patients whether or not he or she is actively involved in all aspects of care
   e. as cancer becomes more common with an aging population, more and more of the care that

is traditionally delivered in a specialty center may be transferred to the family physician

Q8. Which of the following is a (are) descriptive role(s) played by family physicians in the care of patients with cancer?
   a. coordinating
   b. compassionate
   c. continuous
   d. comprehensive
   e. all of the above

Q9. Which of the following is (are) true regarding the delivery of bad news to patients with a serious disease?
   a. check the reception of the news frequently
   b. reinforce and clarify the information you are giving frequently
   c. check your communication level frequently
   d. listen for the patient's concerns
   e. all of the above are true

Q10. In an interview in which news of a serious disease is presented, which of the following is the thing to do before the patient leaves the office?
   a. make sure the patient understands every word
   b. make sure the patient understands that you are doing everything you can
   c. make sure you leave the patient with a follow-up plan and provide the patient with some hope
   d. make sure the patient understands the dismal prognosis
   e. make sure that you have left no question unanswered

Q11. The physician who is also a patient goes back to his home university to continue the pursuit of his academic career to the best of his ability after having received bad news about his medical condition. He purposefully does not tell his colleagues the truth about his condition and continues to teach, write, receive grants, publish, and practice medicine. As his condition deteriorates and he becomes more and more physically disabled, which of the following scenarios is (are) most likely to occur?
   a. he will likely receive more phone calls from concerned colleagues and more inquiries as to whether or not they can be of assistance to him
   b. when his colleagues see him in the hall, they will likely go out of their way to talk to him and offer any assistance they can

   c. once his colleagues are aware of the full extent of his illness they will likely offer not only moral support but support in terms of assistance in teaching, assistance in looking after his patients, and assistance in keeping his research programs viable
   d. all of the above are likely to occur
   e. none of the above is likely to occur

SHORT ANSWER MANAGEMENT PROBLEM
You are the physician in charge of the care of an 85-year-old woman who you have just diagnosed as having breast cancer. Before you have an opportunity to talk to the patient, the patient's son and daughter come to your office to advise you that they do not wish you to tell their mother anything about her diagnosis. Describe how you would respond to the request.

ANSWERS

A1. **c.** You should go into the patient's room and explain that the news you are about to deliver is complex; you would feel better if her husband or significant other were present when the test results were explained. To have devastating news delivered to a patient in an unsupported environment is absolutely unacceptable. If a spouse, son, daughter, brother, sister or other significant other cannot be present during the delivery of the news, a social worker, psychologist, or member of the clergy should be present for patient support.

A2. **e.** A multibed hospital room is not an acceptable location for the delivery of bad news. Patients in beds next to your patient will obviously be able to hear all or most of the conversation. Just pulling the hospital curtains is not an acceptable alternative.
   The first rule in breaking bad news is getting started, which includes getting the physical context right and starting off the discussion in the presence of a significant other.
   The other alternatives in the question are all acceptable.

A3. **c.** The next step is to find out how much the patient knows. The following are questions that may be of help in this regard:
   a. What have you made of the illness so far?
   b. What have you been thinking about this nausea, unsteadiness, and breast lump?
   c. Have you been worried about this illness or these symptoms?
   d. What did the previous doctors tell you about the illness or operation?

e. Have you been thinking that this illness might be serious?

f. Have you been worried about yourself?

g. When you first had symptom X, what did you think it might be?

h. What did Doctor X tell you when he sent you here?

i. Did you think something serious was going on then?

A4. **d.** Most patients will want to be told the whole truth, but there are some exceptions. Questions that can be asked to determine how much the patient wants to know include the following:

a. If this condition turns out to be something serious, are you the kind of person who likes to know exactly what's going on?

b. Would you like me to tell you the full details of the diagnosis?

c. Are you the kind of person who likes the full details of what's wrong, or would you prefer just to hear about the treatment plan?

d. Do you like to know exactly what's going on or would you prefer me to give you just a brief outline?

e. If your condition is serious, how much would you like to know about it?

f. Would you like me to tell you the full details of your condition, or is there somebody else that you'd like me to talk to?

A5. **d.** A "warning shot" tells the patient that there is going to be more bad news. The most appropriate warning shot in a situation like this would be something like one of the following:

a. "Unfortunately, the situation is more serious than we would have hoped for."

b. "The chest x-ray shows that there is a tumor on the lung. Does that make you think of anything?"

c. "When you had those bruises, your blood test showed that you weren't making some components in the blood called platelets. They're made in the bone marrow and that's why your doctor ordered a bone marrow test to see what was wrong. It was that test that showed the problem."

A6. **a.** Most health care professionals are justifiably proud of their own esoteric language. Unfortunately, this understanding does not extend to patients. Using "medispeak" to explain something to a patient makes it less likely that the patient will be able to ask difficult questions. As well, it isolates and alienates the patient who finds it unfamiliar. A comparison of English and "medispeak" is shown in the following list (Buckman R, 1992).

English	Medispeak
Leukemia	Blast cells
Multiple sclerosis	Demyelination
Cancer	Abnormal growth
Cancer	Space-occupying lesion
The situation is serious	The prognosis is guarded

A7. **c.** Family physicians must assume and maintain a coordinating role in the care of the cancer patient at all times. Although at a certain time a patient may be receiving treatment in a tertiary care treatment center, the family physician must be seen as coordinating that care. It is the family physician's responsibility to ensure that constant communication between himself or herself and the specialist(s) involved is maintained. As the population ages and more and more patients develop cancer, the care of patients with cancer will be transferred to the family physician.

A8. **e.** The family physician's role can best be described in terms of the 5 Cs: continuous, comprehensive, compassionate, coordinated, and competent care.

A9. **e.** While providing information to the patient, it is imperative that the physician keep the following principles in mind:

a. Provide the information in small chunks—remember the "warning shot."

b. Use English, not "medispeak."

c. Check reception frequently.

d. Reinforce and clarify information frequently.

e. Check communication level frequently.

f. Listen to your patient's concerns.

g. Blend your agenda with the patient's agenda.

A10. **c.** Make sure before the patient leaves your office that you provide him or her with a follow-up plan. This will reinforce the belief that you are indeed in charge of his or her care and will ensure that the care plan is implemented. In addition, be sure to leave the patient with some hope for the future. That hope must be realistic hope, but hope nevertheless.

A11. **e.** None of the above is likely to occur.

This case is a true story, and was eloquently told by a physician in the New England Journal of Medicine (Rabin, 1982). The observations made of both the consultation with the neurologist and the reaction and treatment that the physician patient received when he returned to his home university have been summarized.

My first reaction to the neurologist was one of deep disappointment from his impersonal manner. The neurologist exhibited no interest in me as a person and did not make even a perfunctory inquiry about my work. He gave me no guidelines about what I should do, either concretely—in terms of daily activities—or, what was more important, psychologically, to muster the emotional strength to cope with a progressive degenerative disease. The only thing my doctor did offer me was a pamphlet setting out in grim detail the future that I already knew about too well.

The reaction of colleagues is illustrated very well in the following description:

By early 1980, however, the limp was worse, and I now held a cane in my right hand. The inquiries ceased and were replaced by a very obvious desire to avoid me. When I arrived at work in the morning I could see, from the corner of my eye, colleagues changing their pace or stopping in their tracks to spare themselves the embarrassment of bumping into me. As the cane became inadequate and was replaced by a walker, so my isolation from my colleagues intensified.

One has to ask why this happened. The author suggests the following (Rabin D, 1982):

Perhaps it is because we, as physicians, are the healers. We dispense treatment, counsel, and support; and we represent strength. The dichotomy of being both doctor and patient threatens the integrity of the club. To this fraternity of healers, becoming ill is tantamount to treachery. Furthermore, the sick physician makes us uncomfortable. He reminds us of our own vulnerability and mortality, and this is frightening for those of us who deal with disease every day while arming ourselves with an imaginary cloak of immunity against personal illness. This account is meant to draw attention to our frequent inability as physicians to deal with members of our profession who no longer fit the mold of complete healer.

The author suggests some very simple steps that we can take to support our colleagues in time of illness, stress, trouble, or other difficulty. First, do not ignore your ill colleagues. Greet them, inquire about their health, and visit them. Offer them support if they are physically handicapped. Second, be conscious of the physician patient's family and extend support to them. The spouse and children are suffering at least as much as the physician and need support, encouragement, and acknowledgment of their difficulties. Third, remember that the absence of a magic potion against the disease does not render you impotent. No one can assume the burden, but the patient knowing that he or she has not forgotten does ease the pain.

This special type of communication and caring among physicians (or any other professional group) is essential as we enter an era of change unlike any other era health care has ever seen. Remember that the word *doctor* is translated from the Latin "doktor," meaning teacher. As physicians we are all teachers, some in more diverse ways than others. Medical students, residents, patients, other health care professionals, and most of all students play the role at one time or another.

When the student is ready, the teacher will appear.

Confucius

SOLUTION TO THE SHORT ANSWER MANAGEMENT PROBLEM

This is not an infrequent occurrence. In this situation, it is extremely important to remember who the patient is and what rights the patient has and does not have. Proceed in the following manner:

a. First, remember who the patient is—the mother, not the son or the daughter.

b. Second, attempt to sit down with the son and daughter and explain that as their mother's physician you have an ethical responsibility to talk to her about her disease. Offer to do it in such a way that their mother had an opportunity to communicate how much information about the disease that she wanted. As described earlier, ask the mother (in the presence of her son and daughter) if she was the kind of person who would like to know what the entire picture was or whether she would just as soon get on with treatment. This will usually be as far as you have to go. If the mother says she wants to know (and the son and daughter hear this), they will usually understand that she has that right. If, on the other hand, she states that she does not wish to know, then the problem is also solved.

c. In the very occasional circumstance, you will have to resort to other procedures such as a hospital ethics committee if the son and daughter still do not agree. This, however, is very unusual.

SUMMARY OF HOW TO BREAK BAD NEWS

1. The six-step protocol to breaking bad news:
   a. Getting started:
      1) Get the physical setting right.
      2) Ensure family support at the time of breaking the news.
   b. Find out how much the patient knows.
   c. Find out how much the patient wants to know.
   d. Share the information:
      1) Decide on objectives.
      2) Give the information in small chunks—start with the "warning shot."
      3) Use English, not "medispeak."

4) Reinforce and clarify the information frequently.

5) Listen for the patient's concerns.

6) Blend your agenda with the patient's agenda.

e. Respond to the patient's feelings.

f. Plan and follow through.

2. Remember your colleagues: physicians as patients are just as vulnerable if not more vulnerable than patients who are not physicians and need our friendship, encouragement, help, and hope.

3. Guidelines and suggestions:

a. Always leave the patient with realistic hope.

b. Realize that the patient will not absorb all the information on the first visit; schedule follow-up visits frequently.

c. Facilitate and coordinate all care from this point on.

d. Remember the 5 Cs of the family physician: **c**ontinuous, **c**omprehensive, **c**ompassionate, **c**oordinated, and **c**ompetent care.

e. Try to unlearn "medispeak."

SUGGESTED READINGS

American Psychiatric Association: *Diagnostic and statistical manual of mental disorders,* ed 4, Washington, DC, 1994, American Psychiatric Association Press.

Buckman R: *How to break bad news: A guide for health care professionals,* Toronto, 1992, University of Toronto Press.

Rabin D: Compounding the ordeal of ALS: Isolation from my fellow physicians, *N Engl J Med* 307(8):506-509, 1982.

Swanson RW: The role of the family physician in the treatment of cancer, *Can Fam Physician* 36:839, 1990.

Tierney LM, McPhee SJ, Papadakis MA, eds: *Current medical diagnosis and treatment, 2000,* Stamford, Conn, 1999, Appleton & Lange.

Children and Adolescents

ATTENTION-DEFICIT HYPERACTIVITY DISORDER, CONDUCT DISORDER, AND OPPOSITIONAL DEFIANT DISORDER

The Riddle of Ritalin

Case 1 ■ A 6-Year-Old Child Who Is "Always on the Go," "Into Everything," and "Easily Distractible"

A mother brings her 6-year-old boy to the office for a complete assessment. She states that "there is something very wrong with him." He just sprinkled baby powder all over the house, and last night he opened a bottle of ink and threw it on the floor. He is unable to sit still at school, is easily distracted, has difficulty waiting his turn in games, has difficulty in sustaining attention in play situations, talks all the time, always interrupts others, does not listen when talked to, and is constantly shifting from one activity to another.

As you enter the examining room, the child is in the process of destroying it. On examination (what examination you can manage), you discover that there are no physical abnormalities demonstrated.

SELECT THE BEST ANSWER TO THE FOLLOWING QUESTIONS:

Q1. What is the most likely diagnosis in this patient?
   a. mental retardation
   b. childhood depression
   c. attention-deficit hyperactivity disorder (ADHD)
   d. maternal deprivation
   e. childhood schizophrenia

Q2. Which of the following is (are) associated with the disorder described?
   a. feelings of low self-esteem
   b. feelings of depression
   c. feelings of demoralization
   d. propensity to sustain severe injuries
   e. all of the above

Q3. Who is the person who usually makes this diagnosis?
   a. the child psychiatrist
   b. the family physician
   c. the mother or father
   d. the schoolteacher
   e. the grandparents

Q4. The differential diagnosis of this disorder includes which of the following?
   a. adjustment disorder
   b. bipolar disorder
   c. anxiety disorder
   d. childhood schizophrenia
   e. a, b, and c
   f. all of the above

Q5. Which of the following is (are) true regarding the prevalence of the disorder?
   a. prevalence rates are higher in preschool children than in school-age children
   b. affected boys outnumber girls in surveys of school age children
   c. prevalence rates fall as a cohort of children ages into adulthood
   d. a, b, and c
   e. none of the above

Q6. This disorder is most closely linked to which of the following disorders?
   a. childhood depression
   b. childhood anxiety
   c. conduct disorder
   d. oppositional defiant disorder (ODD)
   e. c and d

Q7. The diagnosis of conduct disorder is made when which of the following criteria is (are) fulfilled?
   a. repetitive and persistent patterns of behavior that violate the rights of others
   b. stealing
   c. lying
   d. vandalism
   e. a and any two of b, c, and d

Q8. What is the best definition of the term *ODD*?
  a. chronic behavior patterns in children and adolescents that are more severe than those in conduct disorder
  b. chronic behavior patterns in children and adolescents that result in serious violation of the law and incarceration
  c. chronic behavior patterns in children and adolescents that are less severe than those seen in conduct disorder
  d. a and b
  e. none of the above

Q9. Which of the following disorders often appear together in the same individual at various life stages?
  a. mental retardation, ADHD, and learning disability
  b. childhood depression, ADHD, and early-onset adult schizophrenia
  c. ADHD, conduct disorder, and antisocial personality disorder
  d. adjustment disorder, ADHD, and major depression
  e. ADHD, bipolar disorder, and conduct disorder

Q10. Conduct disorder appears to result from an interaction of which of the following factors?
  a. temperament
  b. attention to problem behavior and ignoring good behavior
  c. association with a delinquent peer group
  d. a and c only
  e. a, b, and c

Q11. What is the pharmacologic treatment of choice for ADHD?
  a. methylphenidate
  b. dextroamphetamine
  c. magnesium pemoline
  d. all of the above
  e. a or b only

Q12. What is the pharmacologic treatment of choice for ADHD in patients who do not respond to stimulants?
  a. desipramine
  b. fluoxetine
  c. phenelzine
  d. clonidine
  e. a or d

Q13. Regarding the comparison between the effects of stimulants on children, adolescents, and adults, which of the following statements is (are) correct?
  a. in children and adolescents the use of stimulants has a paradoxic effect: they are "slowed down," as opposed to adults, in whom stimulants increase activity and awareness
  b. normal and hyperactive children, adolescents, and adults have similar cognitive responses to comparable doses of stimulants
  c. normal and hyperactive children, adolescents, and adults have similar behavioral responses to comparable doses of stimulants
  d. b and c
  e. nobody really knows for sure; it depends on the patient

Q14. A given child who is being treated with methylphenidate does not respond well to the medication; there is essentially no change in this behavior after 3 months of therapy. At this time, what would you do?
  a. continue methylphenidate at one and one-half times the dose (for another 3 months)
  b. switch the child to dextroamphetamine
  c. switch the child to magnesium pemoline
  d. discontinue stimulants altogether and prescribe desipramine
  e. b or c

Q15. What is the most appropriate time to give methylphenidate to a child with ADHD?
  a. twice per day (early morning and noon)
  b. three times per day (early morning, noon, and evening)
  c. once per day (early morning)
  d. four times per day (every 6 hours)
  e. it does not matter

Q16. What is the most common reason for referral to either a child psychiatry service or an adolescent psychiatry service?
  a. conduct disorder
  b. ADHD
  c. ODD
  d. childhood-adolescent depression
  e. childhood-adolescent schizophrenia

SHORT ANSWER MANAGEMENT PROBLEM
Part A: List four psychiatric disorders that are associated with ADHD.
Part B: List five parental behaviors, disorders, or situations that may be associated with ADHD.
Part C: Comment on the association between ADHD and the schoolteachers.

ANSWERS

A1. c. This child has ADHD. Diagnostic criteria for ADHD require a pattern of behavior that appears no later than the age of 7 years, has been present for at least 6 months, and is excessive for age and intelligence. The symptoms of the disorder are divided into inattention and hyperactivity/impulsivity; they must be present often, although not necessarily all of the time or in every situation. Possible symptoms are listed, but all are not required in a specific child:

a. Fidgety or restless
b. Difficulty staying seated
c. Easily distracted
d. Difficulty waiting in lines or awaiting his or her turn
e. Impulsive speech
f. Difficulty following instructions
g. Short attention span at work and at play
h. Difficulty playing quietly
i. Doesn't seem to listen
j. Loses things
k. Makes careless mistakes
l. Difficulty organizing
m. Avoids engaging in mental activities that require much effort, particularly when not interested
n. Forgetful
o. Runs about or climbs excessively in situations where these activities are inappropriate

Hyperactive behavior per se is no longer considered the key or even a necessary feature of this disorder, although the term is often used as shorthand for ADHD. Other examples of primary deficits include the following:

a. Lack of investment, organization, and maintenance of attention and effort in completing tasks
b. Inability to inhibit impulsive action
c. Lack of modulation of arousal levels to meet the demands of the situation
d. Unusually strong inclination to seek immediate reinforcement

A2. e. Commonly associated features of ADHD are low self-esteem, feelings of depression, feelings of demoralization, and lack of ability to take responsibility for one's actions. In social situations these young children are immature, bossy, intrusive, loud, uncooperative, out of synchrony with situational expectations, and irritating to both adults and peers. Children with ADHD are more likely to sustain severe injuries than those without ADHD.

A3. d. The most common person to make the diagnosis of ADHD is the schoolteacher. There is considerable controversy concerning the fact that many hyperactive children take Ritalin because of the remarks or diagnosis of the schoolteacher. There certainly is some truth to this statement. Inexperienced or overly critical teachers may in fact confuse normal age-appropriate overactivity with ADHD.

A4. e. The differential diagnosis of ADHD includes the following:

a. Adjustment disorder (an identifiable stressor is identified at home and the duration of symptoms is less than 6 months)
b. An anxiety disorder (instead of or in addition to the diagnosis of ADHD)
c. Bipolar disorder (bipolar disorder in children may manifest as a chronic mixed affective state marked by irritability, overactivity, and difficulty concentrating)
d. Mental retardation
e. A specific developmental disorder
f. Drugs (phenobarbital is prescribed for children as an anticonvulsant, and theophylline is prescribed for asthma)
g. Systemic disorders (hyperthyroidism)
h. Other disruptive behavioral disorders including ODD and conduct disorder

A5. d. Some studies suggest between 14% and 20% of preschool and kindergarten boys and approximately a third as many girls have ADHD. In elementary school studies, 3% to 10% of students have ADHD symptoms. Affected boys outnumber girls until young adulthood, where women predominate.

A6. e. In clinical settings, at least two thirds of patients with ADHD also have either ODD or conduct disorder. The characteristics of these two disorders will be discussed in subsequent questions.

A7. e. The diagnosis of conduct disorder requires a repetitive and persistent pattern of behavior that violates the basic rights of others or age-appropriate rules of society, manifested by at least three of the following behaviors:

a. Stealing
b. Running away from home
c. Staying out after dark without permission
d. Lying to "con" people
e. Deliberately setting fires
f. Repeated truancy (beginning before the age of 13)
g. Vandalism
h. Cruelty to animals
i. Bullying
j. Physical aggression
k. Forcing someone else into sexual activity

Conduct disorder is a purely descriptive label for a heterogenous group of children and adolescents. Many of these individuals also lack appropriate feelings of guilt or remorse, empathy for others, and a feeling of responsibility for their own behavior.

A8. **c.** ODD is best described as a milder form of conduct disorder. Children who are diagnosed as having ODD are certainly at risk for developing conduct disorder.

A9. **c.** ADHD commonly leads to conduct disorder. Adolescents who develop conduct disorder are predisposed to develop antisocial personality disorder or alcoholism as adults.

A10. **e.** Conduct disorder appears to result from an interaction among the following factors:
   a. Temperament
   b. Parents who provide attention to problem behavior and ignore good behavior
   c. Association with a delinquent peer group
   d. A parent "role model" of impulsivity and rule-breaking behavior
   e. Genetic predisposition
   f. Marital disharmony in the family
   g. Placement outside of the home as an infant or toddler
   h. Poverty
   i. Low intelligence quotient or brain damage

A11. **d.** The pharmacologic agents of choice for the management of ADHD are the following stimulant medications:
   a. Methylphenidate
   b. Dextroamphetamine
   c. Magnesium pemoline
Up to 96% of children with ADHD have at least some positive behavioral response to methylphenidate or dextroamphetamine, although side effects may limit efficacy or require discontinuation of medication in some children. Both preschool children and adolescents may require lower weight-adjusted doses than school-aged children and manifest a greater likelihood of side effects and somewhat lower therapeutic efficacy.

A12. **e.** Desipramine is the drug of choice in patients who do not respond to stimulants, who develop significant depression on stimulants, who have a personal or family history of tics, or who develop tics when on a stimulant.
   The other choice is clonidine. The alpha-adrenergic agent clonidine, when given either in pill form or transdermal form, is useful for a subgroup of children

with ADHD, including those with tics or a family history of Tourette's syndrome or those in whom a stimulant is only partially effective.

A13. **d.** Contrary to previous belief, normal and hyperactive children, adolescents, and adults have similar cognitive and behavioral responses to comparable doses of stimulants. Stimulants do not have a paradoxic sedative action; they do not lead to drug abuse or addiction, and many adolescents with ADHD continue to require and benefit from their use.

A14. **e.** Up to 25% of children who respond poorly to one stimulant have a positive response to another stimulant. Stimulants reliably decrease physical activity, especially during times when children are expected to be less active (such as during school but not during free time). They also decrease vocalization, noise, and disruption in the classroom to the level of normal peers and improve handwriting. Stimulants consistently improve compliance to adult commands.
   Stimulants also produce improvement on cognitive laboratory tasks measuring sustained attention, distractibility, impulsivity, and short-term memory. Stimulants increase productivity and decrease errors in tests of arithmetic, reading comprehension, sight vocabulary, and spelling and increase the percentage of assigned work completed.
   Because of these benefits, it is strongly suggested that if one of the stimulants is not effective, try another one before switching to a drug of another class.

A15. **a.** The best dosing schedule for stimulant medications used to treat ADHD is twice per day: (early morning and noon). By giving the stimulants at this time, the maximal effectiveness will be during school hours when needed most. A "drug holiday" should be considered on the weekends and vacations.

A16. **a.** The single most common reason for referral to a child or adolescent psychiatry clinic or hospital is conduct disorder.

SOLUTION TO THE SHORT ANSWER MANAGEMENT PROBLEM

Part A: Four psychiatric disorders associated with ADHD are as follows:
   a. Childhood depression
   b. Conduct disorder
   c. ODD
   d. Alcoholism

Part B: Five parental behaviors, disorders, or situations that may be associated with ADHD are as follows:

   a. Providing attention to problem behavior and ignoring good behavior

   b. Parental modeling (impulsivity and rule-breaking)

   c. Parental marital conflict

   d. Family poverty

   e. Inheritance (genetic predisposition)

These factors are more often associated with ODD than with true ADHD. However, as just mentioned, ADHD is related to ODD.

Part C: The relationship between ADHD and schoolteacher input in many cases is that the diagnosis of ADHD is made by the teacher, not by the physician. Instead of carefully considering the diagnostic criteria elaborated by *The Diagnostic Statistical Manual of Mental Disorders, fourth edition* (DSM-IV), the physician may simply accept the word of the schoolteacher and begin treatment with stimulant medication. The basic problem is the inability, in some cases on the part of the schoolteacher and ultimately on the part of the physician, to distinguish between ADHD and normal appropriate-for-age overactivity.

SUMMARY OF THE DIAGNOSIS AND TREATMENT OF ADHD, CONDUCT DISORDER, AND ODD

1. ADHD:
   a. Prevalence: Highest prevalence in preschoolers; decreases with age, males predominate
   b. Signs and symptoms: See the diagnostic criteria just described
   c. Treatment:
      1) Nonpharmacologic: Behavior modification can improve both academic achievement and behavioral compliance if they are specifically targeted.
      2) Pharmacologic:
         a) First choice: Methylphenidate, dextroamphetamine, or magnesium pemoline
         b) Second choice: Desipramine for cases of stimulant failure, but clonidine may also be considered
   d. Stepwise therapy:
      1) Begin first stimulant (usually methylphenidate).
      2) Increase dose gradually.
      3) End of dose failure: Consider another one of the two recommended stimulants.
      4) Failure: Switch to desipramine.
   e. Length of time and dosing:
      1) Consider early morning and noon dosing.
      2) Consider "drug holidays" on weekends and vacations.
      3) Use for as long as is needed.

2. Conduct disorder:
   a. Prevalence: The prevalence of conduct disorder has been estimated at 3% to 7%; males predominate.
   b. Signs and symptoms: See the criteria listed earlier. Conduct disorder is the most common reason for referral to a child or adolescent psychiatry service.
   c. Treatment:
      1) Nonpharmacologic: Cognitive-behavior modification (when used together) is the single most effective nonpharmacologic therapy.
      2) Pharmacologic: Lithium is the choice for severe impulse aggression. Carbamazepine is the choice for severe impulse aggression accompanied by emotional lability and irritability. One can also use propranolol for uncontrollable rage reactions, especially when associated with impulse aggression. In addition neuroleptics (e.g., haloperidol) may reduce aggression, hostility, negativism, and explosiveness in severely aggressive children, and antidepressants may help if the conduct disorder is secondary to major depression.

3. ODD:
   a. Prevalence: 6% to 10%; males predominate
   b. Differential diagnosis: "Stubbornness"
   c. Signs and symptoms: Best described simply as a less severe form of conduct disorder
   d. Treatment:
      1) Nonpharmacologic: An operant approach using environmental positive and negative contingencies to increase or decrease the frequency of behaviors is most useful.
      2) Pharmacologic: If ADHD and ODD coexist, treat with stimulant medication.

4. Order of progression: ADHD to conduct disorder or ODD to antisocial personality disorder to alcoholism.

5. Major differential diagnosis of disruptive behavior disorders:
   a. Major depressive illness
   b. Bipolar affective disorder
   c. Anxiety disorder
   d. Mental retardation
   e. Specific developmental disorder
   f. Adjustment disorder
   g. Pharmacotherapy (phenobarbital, theophylline)
   h. Systemic disorders (hyperthyroidism)

SUGGESTED READINGS

American Psychiatric Association: *Diagnostic and statistical manual of mental disorders*, ed 4, Washington, DC, 1994, American Psychiatric Association Press.

DiScala C et al: Injuries to children with attention-deficit hyperactivity disorder, *Pediatrics* 102(6):1415-1421, 1998.

Elia J et al: Treatment of attention-deficit hyperactivity disorder, *N Engl J Med* 340(10):780-787, 1999.

Zametkin AJ, Ernst M: Problems in the management of attention-deficit hyperactivity disorder, *N Engl J Med* 340:4-6, 1999.

PROBLEM · 78

CHILD ABUSE

"My Baby Cries Constantly; All I Want to Do Is to Shut Him Up!"

Case 1 ■ A 6-Month-Old Infant Who Fell Off a Sofa and Fractured His Humerus

A 6-month-old infant is brought to the hospital Emergency Room (ER) by his mother. She says that he fell off the sofa this evening and injured his right arm.

On examination, the infant has a swollen, bruised right arm. An x-ray reveals a spiral fracture of the right humerus. There are also a number of old abrasions and old bruises that appear to be in various stages of healing and evidence of recent trauma to his right eye and also to the right side of his face. The remainder of the physical examination is normal. The mother says that the child has been well since birth. He has not had any significant medical illnesses.

SELECT THE BEST ANSWER TO THE FOLLOWING QUESTIONS:

Q1. Given the history, the physical examination, and the x-ray report, what should you do now?
   a. obtain an orthopedic consultation
   b. prescribe a sling for the child's arm
   c. investigate the child for possible osteogenesis imperfecta
   d. suggest that the mother purchase a walker instead of laying her child on a sofa
   e. discuss the details of the incident more fully with the mother and contact the hospital social worker

Q2. After your initial intervention or recommendation, what is the next step you should take?
   a. ask the mother to return with the child for follow-up in 3 weeks
   b. ask the mother to return with the child for follow-up in 1 week
   c. arrange for the family physician to see the child at home the following day
   d. hospitalize the child
   e. none of the above

Case 2 ■ A Scared 1-Year-Old Male Whose Weight Is Below the 5th Percentile for His Age

A 1-year-old male child is admitted to the hospital for investigation of failure to thrive. The child's weight is below the 5th percentile for age. He appears scared and clings to anyone who is present in the room. His mother states that there is something wrong with him, and she can't understand why she had to get a kid like this.

Apart from the child being below the 5th percentile for weight, no other abnormalities are found on physical examination.

A complete blood count, a complete urinalysis, and serum electrolytes are within normal limits.

Q3. What is the most likely diagnosis for this child's behavior?
   a. the "white-coat" syndrome
   b. psychotic depression
   c. child abuse or neglect
   d. childhood schizophrenia
   e. acute paranoia of childhood

Q4. Which of the following statements regarding the parent(s) of a child with the disorder described in Case 2 is (are) true?
   a. the parent(s) may be overwhelmed
   b. the parent(s) may be depressed
   c. the parent(s) may be isolated
   d. the parent(s) may be impoverished
   e. all of the above statements may be true

Q5. You make the proper diagnosis for the child described in Case 2 and hospitalize him. You would expect that the child will:
   a. not gain significant weight during the initial hospitalization period
   b. gain weight during the initial hospitalization period only if put on a significant antipsychotic agent
   c. gain weight quickly during the initial hospitalization period
   d. lose weight during the initial hospitalization period
   e. none of the above

Q6. Which one of the following statements most accurately reflects the situation in a family in which there has been documented child abuse?

a. in most cases the child has to be permanently removed from the family and placed in a foster home

b. rehabilitation of parents that have been involved in child abuse is almost always unsuccessful

c. with comprehensive and intensive treatment of the entire family, 80% to 90% of families involved in child abuse or neglect can be successfully rehabilitated

d. in most cases child abuse will leave a permanent scar on the child's personality

e. in a situation in which one child in a family has been abused, there is usually no increased risk to other children in the same family

Q7. Which of the following statements concerning child abuse in relation to spousal abuse is true?

a. women who are abused are unlikely to abuse their children

b. men who abuse their wives or partners are unlikely to abuse their children

c. men who abuse their wives are much more likely to abuse their children than are men who do not abuse their wives

d. there is no correlation between the various forms of family violence

e. parents who abuse their children are unlikely to have come from families in which they themselves were abused or their mother was abused

Q8. Regarding the epidemiology of child abuse, which of the following statements is (are) true?

a. in 1997 the National Committee for the Prevention of Child Abuse estimated that over 3 million cases of child abuse and neglect were reported to public social service agencies in the United States

b. approximately 1000 deaths are caused by child abuse and neglect each year in the United States

c. each year over 200,000 new cases of child sexual abuse are reported in the United States

d. it is estimated that by the age of 18 years one out of every three or four girls will be sexually assaulted and one out of every six to eight boys will be sexually assaulted

e. all of the above are true

Case 3 ■ A Blistered 8-Month-Old Baby

An 8-month-old child is brought to the hospital ER with a large blistering burn in the shape of an iron on his buttocks. The child's father states that the child dropped the iron on himself approximately 20 minutes ago as he was reaching for his toys.

Q9. As the ER doctor in charge, what is your next step?

a. treat the burn and move on to the next patient: time is money!

b. call the police and have the hospital security guards detain and restrain the father

c. obtain a more detailed history of the child's present injury and his previous health; at the same time immerse the child's buttocks in cold water in an attempt to minimize damage from the burn

d. obtain a more detailed history of the child's present injury and his previous health; try to make the child comfortable with analgesics and apply a burn dressing as soon as possible

e. use a confrontational approach and accuse the father of concealing information and abusing the child; have your resident deal with the immediate burn injury

Q10. What is the most common form of childhood sexual abuse in the United States?

a. father-son

b. father-daughter

c. mother-son

d. mother-daughter

e. uncle or close relative-female child

SHORT ANSWER MANAGEMENT PROBLEM

Consider the following 10 environmental, family, or genetic factors and situations. Indicate whether each one is or is not related to child abuse and is or is not a risk factor for child abuse.

a. Parents brought up in harsh family environment

b. A single mother who is socially isolated and unemployed outside the home

c. Alcohol abuse in the father

d. Major depressive disorder in the mother

e. The child himself or herself is mentally retarded

f. The child himself or herself has attention-deficit hyperactivity disorder

g. The family lives below the poverty line

h. Both father and mother have inappropriately high expectations of their children

i. Father was brought up in a strictly religious home where lack of immediate obedience meant corporal punishment

j. Mother has just recently lost her job as a waitress

ANSWERS

A1. **e.** Such a child is almost always a victim of child abuse. Child abuse is defined as any maltreatment of children or adolescents by their parents, guardians, or other caretakers. The definition includes physical abuse, sexual abuse, physical neglect, medical neglect, emotional abuse, and emotional neglect.

The physician must be able to distinguish accidental from nonaccidental injury. Clues to nonaccidental injury include the following:

a. A discrepant history: The explanation given by the parents or significant other does not fit the pattern and severity of the medical findings. Thus the "baby rolling off the sofa" is a totally inadequate explanation for a fractured humerus.

b. A delay in seeking care

c. A current family crisis

d. A triggering behavior such as excessive crying

e. Unrealistic expectations of the child on the part of the parents or guardians

f. Increasing severity of injuries

g. A history of the parent(s) being abused as children

h. Families that are socially isolated

The treatment of the fracture itself, although it must be treated, should not be the focus of attention. An orthopedic consultation may be appropriate depending on the severity of the fracture.

It would be inappropriate to suggest the purchase of a walker at the best of times because this is associated with an increased incidence of falls and injuries.

Although not all children with osteogenesis imperfecta have blue sclera or multiple fractures, there are no associated findings to suggest the diagnosis of osteogenesis imperfecta when the old abrasions and bruises directly point to abuse.

A2. **d.** The most appropriate action at this time is to hospitalize the child. This removes the child to a safe environment and permits time for a complete evaluation.

The complete evaluation must include a complete physical evaluation, a complete laboratory evaluation, a complete radiologic evaluation (of which the most important element is a skeletal survey), a complete evaluation by a child psychiatrist, and a complete evaluation of family dynamics including any other problems that are evident in other family members, such as alcohol or drug abuse in the father or mother, other psychiatric problems in either mother or father, and problems in other siblings (such as truancy).

A3. **c.** The most likely diagnosis in this child is failure to thrive as a result of child abuse or neglect. A maltreated child often demonstrates no obvious evidence of being battered but has multiple signs of minor deprivation, neglect, and abuse. Such a child is often taken to a hospital or a private physician and has a history of failure to thrive, malnutrition, poor skin hygiene, irritability, withdrawal, and other signs of psychologic and physical neglect.

Children who have been neglected may show overt failure to thrive at less than 1 year of age, and their physical and emotional development is drastically impaired. The child may be physically small and not able to show appropriate social interaction. Hunger, chronic infection, poor hygiene, and inappropriate dress may be present. Malnutrition is common.

These chronically neglected children may be indiscriminately affectionate, even with strangers, or they may be socially unresponsive. Child abuse or neglect is one of the most common causes of failure to thrive, even in familiar social situations. Older neglected children may present either as runaways or as children with a conduct disorder.

A4. **e.** Parents who neglect their children are often overwhelmed, depressed, isolated, or impoverished. Unemployment, lack of a two-parent family, and substance abuse may exacerbate the situation.

There are several prototypes of neglectful mothers that have been suggested. Again, the term *neglect* seems to be somewhat disparaging and some may object to it. Some mothers are young, some are inexperienced, some are socially isolated, and some cannot comprehend what is going on around them. Others have been portrayed as chronically passive and withdrawn; these women often have been raised in chaotic, abusive, and neglectful homes.

A5. **c.** Once the neglected child is hospitalized and in a safe environment, the child should gain weight rapidly if given unlimited feedings.

A6. **c.** With comprehensive and intensive treatment of the entire family, 80% to 90% of families involved in child abuse or neglect (excluding incest) can be rehabilitated to provide adequate and appropriate care for their children. Approximately 10% to 15% of such families can only be stabilized and will require an indefinite continuation of support services until the children in the family become independent. In only 2% to 3% of cases is termination of parental rights or continued foster care necessary (again excluding incest).

A7. **c.** Men who abuse their wives are more likely to abuse their children than men who do not abuse their wives. In fact, the abuse of a spouse is an absolute red flag to inquire about child abuse. It is estimated that approximately 25% to 50% of men who abuse their wives also abuse their children.

Women who are currently abused (as spouses) or who have been abused in the past (as children) are also more likely to abuse their children than women who are not abused or who have not been abused (either as a spouse or as a child).

Parents who abuse their children are much more likely than not to have come from nuclear families in which abuse occurred. Most commonly they were abused themselves as children, although the witnessing of abuse as a child is also a common characteristic.

Thus abuse is very much a family affair and moves not only from generation to generation at different times, but also occurs among different generations at the same time. That is, it may well be that child abuse, spousal abuse, and elder abuse are occurring at the same time in the same family.

A8. **e.** According to the National Committee to Prevent Child Abuse and The National Clearing House on Child Abuse Information, in 1997 almost 3.2 million cases of child abuse and neglect were reported to public social service agencies; 33% of that number were substantiated. Neglect accounts for some 52% of the reports, physical abuse for some 24% to 26% , sexual abuse for some 7% to 13%, emotional maltreatment for about 6%, and medical neglect for about 3%. Each year in America about 1000 children die as the result of fatal physical injuries from beatings or other physical trauma. It is estimated that one in every three or four girls will be sexually assaulted by the age of 18 years, and one out of every six to eight boys will be sexually assaulted. It should be remembered that the actual occurrence rates are likely to be higher than those estimates because many maltreated children go unrecognized and many are reluctant to report the abuse, particularly sexual abuse.

A9. **d.** The most appropriate next steps at this time are as follows:
   a. Treat the child's burn injury: use analgesics and apply an appropriate sterile dressing. Cold-water immersion is inappropriate and may actually extend the injury and trauma.
   b. Obtain a more detailed history of the child's present injury and his previous health: Even though it seems obvious what has actually happened here, it is important that as complete a history as possible be taken and documented for legal purposes.

A10. **b.** Incest is defined as the occurrence of sexual relations between close blood relatives. A broader definition describes incest as intercourse between partici-

pants who are related to one another by some formal or informal bond of kinship that is culturally regarded as a barrier to sexual relations. As an example of the latter, sexual relations between stepparents and stepchildren or among step siblings are usually considered incestuous even though no blood relationship exists.

The most common forms of incest include father or stepfather abusing his daughter or son, mother abusing her daughter or son, uncle or other relative abusing their niece or nephew, or a close friend abusing the daughter or son.

Of the relationships cited previously, the most common relationship involved in sexual abuse is father-daughter. Father-daughter incest accounts for 75% of the total of reported cases.

A few general rules:
   a. Mothers abuse their children more often than fathers. Roughly two thirds of the perpetrators are women who are responsible for some 75% of neglect and medical neglect cases. However, men were responsible for about 75% of the sexual abuse cases.
   b. Girls are abused more often than boys. The overall ratio being about 53%:46%. However, girls are subjected to sexual abuse at almost twice the rate as boys. For both sexes some 22% to 23% of the incidents of sexual abuse occurred before the age of 8.
   c. Strangers are seldom the perpetrators of the child abuse. Of the abusers, 77% were a parent and another 11% were a close relative.
   d. One parent is usually the active perpetrator, while the other parent passively accepts the abuse.

SOLUTION TO THE SHORT ANSWER MANAGEMENT PROBLEM

The answer to all 10 scenarios or situations is yes. All of the scenarios and situations cited are associated with an increased risk of child abuse.

SUMMARY OF THE DIAGNOSIS AND TREATMENT OF CHILD ABUSE

1. Prevalence: 3 million cases reported each year in the United States; over 1000 children die every year of injuries incurred from child abuse in the United States.

2. Definition: Child abuse can be defined as any short-term, intermediate-term, or long-term situation in a family in which a child is
   a. Physically abused

b. Sexually abused
c. Emotionally or psychologically abused
d. Physically neglected
e. Emotionally neglected
f. Medically neglected by any other member of that family

3. Characteristics: Most commonly child abuse is perpetrated by a close relative, usually the parent. Mothers abuse their children more often than fathers; girls are abused more often than boys; one parent is usually the "active perpetrator" and the other parent is the "passive perpetrator." Strangers are rarely involved in child abuse.

4. "Red lights" for child abuse: Suspect child abuse if:
a. There is a discrepant history (what is said to have happened does not match the injury pattern).
b. There is a delay in seeking care.
c. There was a recent family crisis.
d. There are unrealistic expectations put on the child by the parents.
e. There is a pattern of increasing severity of so-called accidents.
f. Families are living under stressful living conditions including overcrowding and poverty.
g. There is a real lack of a support system for the family and the family members, and aggressive behavior is displayed by the child.
h. You are aware of underlying psychiatric disease in either the father or the mother.
i. There is either alcohol abuse or drug abuse in the father or the mother.

5. Acute treatment: The acute treatment (no matter what type of child abuse is being dealt with) is hospitalization of the child. This allows time to subcategorize the type of child abuse that has occurred (often more than one type); observe the child and the child's behavior in a safe environment; investigate the child from a physical, psychologic, and social perspective; obtain all details necessary to clearly understand this episode of abuse and any others that have taken place before this; and interview the parents, grandparents, and other family members.

6. Immediate and long-term treatment: The ultimate goal in a situation in which child abuse has occurred is to eventually return the child to the home. However, first it is necessary to do the following:
a. Restore the child to a healthy state.
b. Identify and understand the reason for the abuse.

c. Provide individual and family counseling to the parents and the family.
d. Treat coexisting psychiatric conditions in both parents (alcoholism, drug abuse, depression).
e. Set up an ongoing counseling program for the individuals in the family.
f. Establish a contract with the abusing parents ("I will call if I get to a stage where I think I can no longer handle it"). Remember that family violence begets family violence. Where you find one type you will likely find another type (child abuse, spousal abuse, or elder abuse).

SUGGESTED READINGS

American Psychiatric Association: *Diagnostic and statistical manual of mental disorders*, ed 4, Washington, DC, 1994, American Psychiatric Association Press.

Bethea L: Primary prevention of child abuse, *Am Fam Physician* 59(6):1577-1585, 1591-1592, 1999.

Finkelhorn D et al: Sexual abuse in a national survey of adult men and women: Prevalence, characteristics, and risk factors, *Child Abuse Negl* 14:19-28, 1990.

Forjuoh SN, Zwi AB: Violence against children and adolescents: International perspectives, *Pediatr Clin North Am* 45(2):415-26, 1998.

Freitag R et al: Psychosocial aspects of child abuse for primary care pediatricians, *Pediatr Clin North Am* 45(2):391-402, 1998.

Holmes WC, Slap GB: Sexual abuse of boys: definition, prevalence, correlates, sequelae, and management, *JAMA* 280(21):1855-1862, 1998.

Kaplan HI et al: Problems related to abuse or neglect. In Kaplan HI, Sadock BJ, eds: *Kaplan and Sadock's synopsis of psychiatry: Behavioral sciences/clinical psychiatry*, ed 7, Baltimore, 1997, Williams & Wilkins.

The National Clearing House on Child Abuse Information: 330 C Street, SW, Washington, DC, 20447, *http://www.nccanch@calib.com*.

Wang C, Daro D: *Current trends in child abuse reporting and fatalities: The results of the 1997 annual fifty state survey*, Working Paper 808, Chicago, 1998, National Committee to Prevent Child Abuse.

PROBLEM · 79

NEONATAL JAUNDICE

"Oh My! My Baby Is Yellow."

Case 1 ▪ A Full-Term Neonate with Jaundice

A 3750-g male infant was delivered by you at 40 ³/₇ weeks' gestation. The prenatal course was unremarkable. The mother's blood type is group A and Rh positive. The neonate's blood type is the same. At approximately 36 hours of age the neonate begins to develop visible jaundice. The baby is being breast fed and is feeding well, approximately every 2 hours. The baby's hemoglobin is 175 g/L. His total bilirubin is 171 mmol/L (10 mg/dl), and his indirect bilirubin is 154 mmol/L (9 mg/dl). His direct and indirect Coombs' test results are negative.

On physical examination, the infant looks healthy and happy. There is no lethargy, no difficulties with feeding, and no significant abnormalities apart from the yellow color of his skin and the whites of his eyes. There is no organomegaly.

SELECT THE BEST ANSWER TO THE FOLLOWING QUESTIONS

Q1. What is the most likely diagnosis in this infant?
  a. undiagnosed neonatal sepsis
  b. breast milk jaundice
  c. normal physiologic jaundice
  d. jaundice caused by a minor antigen blood group incompatibility
  e. ABO blood group incompatibility

Q2. Which of the following characteristics would suggest that the diagnosis established in Question 1 is incorrect?
  a. jaundice beginning in the first 24 hours of life
  b. an increase in the serum bilirubin level of greater than 86 mmol/L (5 mg/dl/day or 24 hours)
  c. the total serum bilirubin exceeds 256 mmol/L (15 mg/dl) at any time
  d. all of the above suggests that the correct diagnosis in Question 1 is, in fact, incorrect
  e. none of the above suggest that the diagnosis in Question 1 is, in fact, incorrect

Q3. Which of the following causes of jaundice is the least common cause of jaundice in the newborn?
  a. ABO mother-neonate blood group incompatibility
  b. neonatal sepsis
  c. physiologic jaundice
  d. breast milk jaundice
  e. a and b are equally unlikely causes of jaundice in the newborn

Q4. What is the treatment of choice for the neonate described in Case 1?
  a. grab the neonate from his mother and immediately transfer him to the nearest neonatal intensive care unit for emergency exchange transfusions; this is a serious medical situation, and we have no time for this biopsychosocial stuff and explanations to the parents as to what is going on
  b. intensive phototherapy; this neonate has to be zapped with ultraviolet (UV) light right away

  c. grab the infant from the mother, tell the mother that "breast feeding is out", and take the baby to make sure that she does not disobey your orders
  d. gently explain to the mother the need for stopping breast feeding; however, let the infant have "one more feeding"
  e. none of the above

Q5. What is the major pathophysiologic basis for normal physiologic jaundice in the newborn?
  a. the presence of a substance in human breast milk that inhibits glucuronyl transferase activity
  b. glucuronyl transferase deficiency (immaturity basis) in the liver and the breakdown of fetal red blood cells (RBCs) into bilirubin and bilirubin metabolites
  c. gamma glutamyl transferase deficiency (immaturity basis) in the liver
  d. dehydration caused by lack of sufficient fluid intake in the first 48 hours of life
  e. none of the above

Q6. Which of the following is (are) associated with exaggerated physiologic jaundice in the newborn?
  a. prematurity
  b. Asian race
  c. Caucasian race
  d. a and b
  e. a and c

Case 2 ■ A Full-Term Infant Who Develops Jaundice on the Fourth Day of His Life

A full-term infant weighing 3640 g develops jaundice on the fourth day of life. He is being breast fed and is feeding extremely well (every 2 hours).

On examination, the child is not lethargic, his temperature is normal, and he is not irritable, nor does he have any other signs or symptoms that would suggest significant disease.

The mother is blood group A and Rh positive. The baby is blood group A and Rh positive as well. The infant's hemoglobin is 160 g/L. The direct and indirect Coombs' tests are negative.

The total serum bilirubin is 256 mmol/L (15 mg/dl). The indirect serum bilirubin is 242 mmol/L (14.15 mg/dl).

Q7. What is the most likely diagnosis in this neonate?
  a. undiagnosed and unsuspected neonatal sepsis
  b. breast milk jaundice
  c. physiologic jaundice

d. jaundice caused by minor antigen blood group incompatibility
e. exaggerated physiologic jaundice

Q8. What is the treatment of choice for the neonate described?
a. phototherapy
b. exchange transfusions
c. withdrawal of breast feeding for 2 to 4 days
d. supplementation of breast feeding with D_5W
e. none of the above

Case 3 ■ An Infant Born at Term Who Develops Jaundice at 18 Hours of Life

A 2900-g infant born at term develops jaundice at approximately 18 hours of life. The infant appears generally well, is not lethargic, and is breast feeding well. Vital signs are normal, and examination of all systems reveals no abnormalities.

The infant's bilirubin at 24 hours is 220 mmol/L (12.9 mg/dl). The direct bilirubin is 205 mmol/L (12 mg/dl). The neonate is blood group B and Rh positive. The mother is blood group O and Rh positive. The neonate's hemoglobin is 135 g/L, and the reticulocyte count is 10%.

Q9. What is the most likely cause of jaundice in this neonate?
a. neonatal sepsis
b. breast milk jaundice
c. physiologic jaundice
d. jaundice caused by minor antigen blood group incompatibility
e. ABO blood group incompatibility

Q10. What is the treatment of choice for the neonate described in Case 3?
a. phototherapy
b. exchange transfusion
c. cessation of breast feeding for 2 to 4 days
d. supplementation of breast feeding with D_5W
e. none of the above

Q11. When is blood group ABO incompatibility in the neonate most common?
a. when the mother is blood group O and the infant is blood group O
b. when the mother is blood group A and the infant is blood group A
c. when the mother is blood group O and the infant is blood group A or blood group B
d. when the mother is blood group A and the infant is blood group B

e. it doesn't really matter; this ABO business has been overdone

Q12. Jaundice develops in approximately what percentage of full-term neonates?
a. 20%
b. 40%
c. 60%
d. 80%
e. 95%

Q13. Which of the following statements most accurately reflects the association between physiologic jaundice and kernicterus?
a. kernicterus is a serious problem and can result from failure to treat physiologic jaundice in the newborn with phototherapy
b. kernicterus is a serious problem and can result from failure to treat exaggerated physiologic jaundice in the newborn with phototherapy
c. kernicterus is a serious problem and can result from failure to treat breast milk jaundice in the newborn with phototherapy
d. all of the above statements are true
e. none of the above statements is true

Q14. What is the mechanism of action of phototherapy in treating neonatal jaundice?
a. hemolysis of the fetal RBCs remaining in the circulation
b. hemolysis of the fetal hemoglobin F blood cells remaining in the circulation
c. increase in the activity of the liver enzyme glucuronyl transferase
d. increase in the activity of the liver enzyme gamma glutamyl transferase
e. none of the above

Q15. Which of the following is (are) associated with breast milk jaundice?
a. a qualitative deficiency in gamma glutamyl transferase in the neonatal liver
b. a qualitative deficiency in glucuronyl transferase in the neonatal liver
c. a nonesterified long-chain fatty acid(s) containing 5-beta-pregnane-3-alpha-20-beta-diol in the breast milk of the mother
d. all of the above
e. none of the above

Q16. Neonatal jaundice that appears after what day of neonatal life should suggest the possibility of neonatal sepsis?
a. the fifth day

b. the second day

c. the third day

d. the eighth day

e. the tenth day

Q17. With respect to breast-fed and bottle-fed neonates, which of the following statements is (are) true?

a. neonatal jaundice is more common in bottle-fed babies

b. neonatal jaundice is more common in breast-fed babies

c. supplementation of breast-fed babies with D_5W will reduce the serum bilirubin level

d. a and c

e. b and c

Q18. Which of the following statements best explains the bronze baby syndrome? The bronze baby syndrome is

a. associated with Asian babies whose mothers breast feed and do not supplement feedings with D_5W

b. associated with Asian babies whose mothers breast feed and supplement feedings with D_5W

c. associated with Caucasian babies whose mothers breast feed and do not supplement feedings with D_5W

d. associated with Caucasian babies whose mothers breast feed and supplement feedings with D_5W

e. none of the above

Q19. What is the lowest level at which kernicterus has been seen to develop in uncomplicated neonates?

a. 10 mg/dl (171 mmol/L)

b. 20 mg/dl (342 mmol/L)

c. 30 mg/dl (511 mmol/L)

d. 40 mg/dl (684 mmol/L)

e. nobody really knows for sure

SHORT ANSWER MANAGEMENT PROBLEM

Part A: Discuss the current recommended guidelines for the use of phototherapy in the treatment of jaundice in the newborn.

Part B: List five complications of phototherapy in the treatment of neonatal jaundice.

ANSWERS

A1. **c.** The most likely cause of jaundice in the neonate described in Case 1 is normal physiologic jaundice. Physiologic jaundice usually begins on the second or third day of life. It is caused by the breakdown of fetal RBCs into bilirubin and transient limitation in the conjugation of bilirubin. This pathophysiologic mechanism differs from the pathophysiologic mechanism involved in exaggerated physiologic jaundice, which will be discussed later.

A2. **d.** Physiologic jaundice would not be the explanation for this neonate's jaundice if any of the following factors were present:

a. the jaundice appears in the first 24 hours of life

b. serum bilirubin is rising at a rate greater than 5 mg/dl in the first 24 hours of life

c. the serum bilirubin reaches a value of greater than 12 mg/dl in full-term infants (especially in the absence of risk factors) or 14 mg/dl in preterm infants

d. jaundice persists after the first week of life

e. direct-reacting bilirubin is greater than 1 mg/dl at any time

A3. **b.** The differential diagnosis of neonatal jaundice (presented in order of prevalence) is as follows:

a. normal physiologic jaundice

b. exaggerated physiologic jaundice

c. breast milk jaundice

d. jaundice caused by ABO incompatibility (mother/neonate)

e. jaundice caused by Rh and other blood group antigens (such as Anti-Kell or Anti-Duffy)

f. neonatal sepsis

There may be some dispute about the order of items e and f on the previous list; the prevalence of neonatal sepsis will very much depend on the particular facility's capabilities so a high-risk neonatal nursery will have a substantially higher prevalence of neonatal sepsis.

A4. **e.** For this neonate, no treatment should be instituted at this time. First, the levels at which phototherapy should be instituted are controversial (a guideline will be provided later on in this problem). Second, to the best of our knowledge kernicterus has never developed in the absence of at least one other cause for jaundice.

A5. **b.** The terms *exaggerated physiologic jaundice* and *hyperbilirubinemia of the newborn* are used for those infants whose primary pathophysiologic mechanism for hyperbilirubinemia is a deficiency in or inactivity of the enzyme bilirubin glucuronyl transferase rather than an excessive load of bilirubin for excretion.

A6. **d.** Exaggerated physiologic jaundice is associated with the following risk factors:

   a. Asian race

   b. Prematurity

   c. Breast feeding or excessive weight loss

Note that there is a distinct difference between exaggerated physiologic jaundice caused by breast feeding and breast milk jaundice. The former is much more common than the latter. The two are very frequently confused.

A7. **b.** The most likely diagnosis in this neonate is breast milk jaundice. Breast milk jaundice usually begins between the fourth and the fourteenth days of life. Bilirubin levels range between 171 mmol/L (10 mg/dl) to 520 mmol/L (30.4 mg/dl). If breast feeding is continued, the maximum concentration of bilirubin is reached during the third week of life and then gradually decreases (but persists) between 3 weeks and 10 weeks.

If breast feeding is discontinued, however, the serum bilirubin falls rapidly, usually reaching normal levels within a few days. Cessation of breast feeding for 2 to 4 days and substitution with formula (not glucose in water) will result in the rapid decline. Following the 2- to 4-day period, breast feeding can be resumed; there should not be any difficulties in reestablishing breast feeding.

As with physiologic jaundice, there are no other signs of illness in these infants and kernicterus has not been reported. There used to be a differentiation that classified breast milk jaundice into early breast milk and late breast milk jaundice. It appears that early breast milk jaundice (thought to be caused by caloric restriction) is really part of what we now call *exaggerated physiologic jaundice.* Late breast milk jaundice, on the other hand, is thought to be caused by the 5-beta-pregnane-3-alpha, 20-beta-diol or nonesterified long-chain fatty acids that competitively inhibit the enzyme glucuronyl transferase conjugating activity.

A8. **e.** The treatment of this neonate should consist of careful consideration as to whether or not you would suggest that the mother stop breast feeding.

The infant has a total bilirubin of 256 mmol/L (15 mg/dl). As stated earlier, bilirubin levels secondary to breast milk jaundice may reach levels as high as 520 mmol/L. Although interruption of breast feeding will definitely improve the jaundice, the risk of prematurely terminating breast feeding is theoretically present, even though it usually does not happen. Water supplementation usually does not help.

Although phototherapy would be initiated by some clinicians at this level, it is not necessary. As well as with physiologic jaundice and exaggerated physiologic jaundice, breast milk jaundice does not lead to kernicterus.

A9. **e.** This neonate's jaundice is caused by an ABO blood group incompatibility.

A10. **a.** The treatment of choice for this neonate is phototherapy. Even though the bilirubin has not reached a critically high level, this only represents jaundice in the first 24 hours of life; it will obviously rise without therapy. It is generally accepted that if a neonate with ABO incompatibility develops a significant hemolytic anemia, he or she should be treated with phototherapy (this has already occurred in this patient; the hemoglobin is 135 g/L and the reticulocyte count is 10%). If phototherapy is unsuccessful in keeping the serum bilirubin below 342 mmol/L (20 mg/dl), exchange transfusions should be considered. Kernicterus can result from untreated hemolytic anemia secondary to blood group incompatibility.

A11. **c.** In cases of ABO blood group incompatibility, the most likely scenario is as follows:

   a. the mother is blood group O

   b. the neonate is blood group A or blood group B

Possible ABO blood group incompatibility develops in approximately 20% to 25% of all pregnancies; however, in only 10% of these pregnancies does hemolytic disease actually develop.

The factors suggesting ABO blood group incompatibility in this case are as follows:

   a. the correct match-up: Mother is group O, infant is group A or group B

   b. that jaundice develops within the first 24 hours of life, therefore this is not physiologic jaundice, exaggerated physiologic jaundice, or breast milk jaundice.

Also, because of the compatible Rh factors, it is not Rh incompatibility.

The only other serious consideration at this time is neonatal sepsis; there is, however, no indication that this is a serious consideration from the physical signs and symptoms.

Pathophysiologically, maternal antibody may be formed against B cells if the mother is type A or against A cells if the mother is type B; usually, however, as mentioned, we have a mother who is type O and an infant who is type A or type B.

A12. **c.** Jaundice is extremely common in newborn infants. Under normal nursery conditions, jaundice is observed during the first week in approximately 60% of full-term infants and 80% of preterm infants.

A13. **e.** Kernicterus is a neurologic syndrome resulting from the deposition of unconjugated bilirubin in the brain cells and does not occur from the following syndromes:
  a. Physiologic jaundice
  b. Exaggerated physiologic jaundice
  c. Breast milk jaundice
  It is related to the following:
  a. ABO blood group incompatibility
  b. Rh blood group incompatibility
  c. Other blood group antigen incompatibility
  d. Under conditions of prematurity: the less mature the infant, the greater susceptibility to kernicterus
  e. Associated with neonatal sepsis, perinatal hypoxia, neonatal hypoglycemia, and intracranial hemorrhage

To the best of our knowledge, kernicterus has never resulted from a simple case of physiologic jaundice, exaggerated physiologic jaundice, or breast milk jaundice.

A14. **e.** Clinical jaundice and indirect hyperbilirubinemia are reduced on exposure to a high intensity of light in the visible spectrum. Bilirubin absorbs light maximally in the blue range (from 420 to 470 nm). Bilirubin in the skin absorbs light energy, which by photoisomerization coverts the toxic native 4Z, 15Z-bilirubin into the unconjugated configurational isomer, 4Z, 15E-bilirubin. The latter is the product of a reversible reaction and is excreted in the bile without the need for conjugation. Phototherapy also converts native bilirubin, by an irreversible reaction, to the structural isomer, which is excreted by the kidney in the unconjugated state.

Phototherapy is indicated only after the presence of pathologic hyperbilirubinemia has been established. The basic cause(s) of the jaundice should be treated concomitantly.

A15. **c.** See Answer 7 and Answer 8.

A16. **a.** Jaundice appearing after the fifth day should be highly suspect for neonatal sepsis as a cause. Causes of neonatal sepsis include the following:
  a. Neonatal pneumonia
  b. Neonatal meningitis
  c. Neonatal urinary tract infection
  d. Necrotizing enterocolitis
  e. *Streptococcal/staphylococcal* skin infections
  f. Herpes simplex viremia
  g. Toxoplasmosis

A17. **b.** Neonatal jaundice is more common in breast-fed babies than in bottle-fed babies. Supplementation with D_5W increases neonatal jaundice rather than decreases it. The increased incidence of neonatal jaundice in breast-fed babies is thought to be mainly caused by decreased intake during the first few days and subsequent weight loss.

A18. **e.** The bronze baby syndrome refers to a dark, grayish, brown discoloration of the skin of neonates sometimes noted in infants undergoing phototherapy. Almost all infants observed with this syndrome have had a mixed type of hyperbilirubinemia with other evidence of obstructive liver disease. The discoloration may last for months.

A19. **b.** The precise blood level above which indirect-reacting bilirubin or free bilirubin will be toxic for an individual infant is unpredictable, but kernicterus is rare in term infants with serum levels under 20 mg/dl (342 mmol/L). The duration of exposure necessary to produce toxic effects is also unknown. There is some evidence that motor disturbances in later childhood are more common among newborn infants whose total serum bilirubin raises above 15 mg/dl. The less mature the infant, the greater is the susceptibility to kernicterus.

SOLUTION TO THE SHORT ANSWER MANAGEMENT PROBLEM

Part A: Guidelines for maximal permissible total serum bilirubin concentrations:

Birth Weight	Uncomplicated Course (Complicated Course)
1250 g	13 mg/dl (10 mg/dl)
1250 to 1499 g	15 mg/dl (13 mg/dl)
1500 to 1999 g	17 mg/dl (15 mg/dl)
2000 to 2499 g	18 mg/dl (17 mg/dl)
>2500 g	20 mg/dl (18 mg/dl)

Part B: Complications of phototherapy in treating jaundice in the newborn include the following:
  a. Loose stools
  b. Skin rashes
  c. Overheating
  d. Dehydration (insensible water loss, diarrhea); may be associated with electrolyte disturbances, particularly hyponatremia and hypokalemia
  e. Chilling from exposure of the infant
  f. The bronze baby syndrome

SUMMARY OF THE DIAGNOSIS AND MANAGEMENT OF NEONATAL JAUNDICE

1. Prevalence:
  a. Full-term: 60% of infants
  b. Preterm: 80% of infants

2. Differential diagnosis of neonatal jaundice:
   a. Physiologic jaundice (most common)
   b. Exaggerated physiologic jaundice
   c. Breast milk jaundice
   d. ABO blood group incompatibility jaundice (hemolytic)
   e. Neonatal sepsis
   f. Minor blood group antigen incompatibility and Rh disease of the newborn

3. Pathophysiology:
   a. Physiologic jaundice: Breakdown of fetal RBCs and transient inability to conjugate bilirubin. Onset on day 2 or 3; disappears by day 4 or 5
   b. Exaggerated physiologic jaundice: Breakdown of fetal RBCs and transient inability to conjugate bilirubin and a risk factor (Asian race, prematurity, breast feeding, or excessive neonatal weight loss). Onset on day 3 or 4; disappears by day 7 to 9
   c. Breast milk jaundice: Mother's milk contains 5-beta-pregnane-3-alpha, 20-beta-diol. Onset between day 4 and 14; persists for 3 to 10 weeks
   d. ABO incompatibility: Usually arises when mother is type O and neonate is type A or type B; may appear within first 24 hours
   e. Neonatal sepsis: The infective process itself with certain associated risk factors: prematurity and hypoglycemia; suspect if neonatal jaundice appears after day 5
   f. Minor blood group incompatibility and Rh disease: Remember that there are over 60 different blood group antigens, as well as the Rh system.

4. Treatment:
   a. Physiologic jaundice/exaggerated physiologic jaundice: Phototherapy is usually not indicated unless bilirubin exceeds 20 mg/dl (342 mmol/L).
   b. Breast milk jaundice: Phototherapy is usually not indicated unless bilirubin exceeds 20 mg/dl (342 mmol/L). Consider cessation of breast feeding for 2 to 4 days.
   c. ABO incompatibility and other blood group incompatibilities: Level at which phototherapy is begun is not agreed on. Suggest initiating phototherapy as soon as the diagnosis is made.

5. Neonatal hyperbilirubinemia diagnosis and treatment:
   a. Remember that phototherapy has its risks: Always balance risk against benefit. Remember that physiologic jaundice, exaggerated physiologic jaundice, and breast milk jaundice are not associated with kernicterus.
   b. Remember the differentiation between exaggerated physiologic jaundice caused by breast feeding and breast milk jaundice.
   c. Jaundice after day 5 of life causes neonatal sepsis, until proven otherwise.
   d. Jaundice within the first 24 hours of life causes pathologic jaundice.
   e. Remember that ABO incompatibility can cause kernicterus. Treat with phototherapy earlier rather than later (follow the guidelines outlined in the Short Answer Management Problem).
   f. When considering discontinuation of breast feeding in breast milk jaundice, consider risk vs benefit of discontinuing breast feeding.

SUGGESTED READINGS

Behrman RE et al, eds: *Nelson: Textbook of pediatrics,* ed 15, Philadelphia, 1996, WB Saunders.

Bland HE: Jaundice in the healthy term neonate: when is treatment indicated? *Curr Probl Pediatr* 26(10):355-63, 1996.

Gourley GR: Bilirubin metabolism and kernicterus, *Adv Pediatr* 44:173-229, 1997.

Johnson L, Bhutani VK: Guidelines for management of the jaundiced term and near-term infant, *Clin Perinatol* 25(3):555-74, viii, 1998.

Lasker MR, Holzman IR: Neonatal jaundice: When to treat, when to watch and wait, *Postgrad Med* 99(3):187-193, 197-198, 1996.

PROBLEM·80

INFANTILE COLIC

"My Baby Cries Constantly. Can't You Do Something to Help Her?"

Case 1 ■ An 8-Week-Old Infant with Inconsolable Crying for Many Hours and Days

A 28-year-old mother of two comes to your office with her 8-week-old infant. Her baby has been "crying constantly" for the last 4 weeks, and she is at her "wit's end." She is bottle feeding her baby and is having no significant feeding problems apart from what may be "excessive" gas and burping following feeding. No other symptoms have been identified. The mother also states that her first child had "some crying" spells but it was "nothing like this." The baby has had no other problems, specifically no constipation or diarrhea.

On examination, the infant is afebrile and has no abnormalities of the ears, throat, and lungs. The abdomen is soft, and there are no palpable masses.

SELECT THE BEST ANSWER
TO THE FOLLOWING QUESTIONS

Q1. What is the most likely diagnosis in this infant?
a. infantile colic
b. excessive spasm syndrome of infancy
c. early Crohn's disease
d. psychosocial stress syndrome of infancy
e. urinary tract infection

Q2. Investigations that should be undertaken in the infant described include which of the following?
a. complete blood count (CBC)
b. CBC/differential white cell count/erythrocyte sedimentation rate (ESR)
c. CBC/differential white cell count/ESR/ urinalysis
d. urinalysis
e. none of the above; no investigations need be done

Q3. What is the most likely underlying cause of the infant's symptom of excessive crying?
a. bottle feeding
b. hormone abnormalities produced by the newly diagnosed psychiatric condition labeled "baby stress"
c. gastrointestinal hyperperistalsis
d. maternal stress
e. none of the above; the cause of these symptoms is unknown

Q4. Which of the following definitions correctly identifies infants with the syndrome described?
a. unexplained fussiness or crying lasting longer than 3 hr/day, 3 days/wk, and continuing for more than 3 weeks in infants younger than 3 months old
b. unexplained fussiness or crying lasting longer than 6 hr/day, 3 days/wk, and continuing for more than 2 weeks in an infant younger than 4 months old
c. unexplained fussiness or crying lasting longer than 4 hours, 3 days/wk, and continuing for longer than 2 weeks in an infant younger than 6 months old
d. unexplained fussiness or crying lasting longer than 6 hr/day, 5 days/wk, and continuing for more than 3 weeks in an infant younger than 8 months old
e. unexplained fussiness or crying lasting longer than 7 hr/day, 6 days/wk, and continuing for more than 7 weeks in an infant younger than 6 months old

Q5. At this time, what should you do?
a. tell the mother to relax and to call you in 4 weeks if the crying has not improved
b. set up an appointment for the baby with the infant psychiatrist
c. do nothing
d. discontinue cow's milk and begin soy formula
e. none of the above

Q6. Which of the following statements regarding treatment of the condition described is true?
a. treatment should begin and should continued until the condition improves
b. treatment is ineffective; it is not worth the bother
c. the most effective treatment is reassuring the mother about the benign nature of the condition
d. treatment with oral analgesics appears to be the most effective therapy that can be offered
e. treatment with antibiotics should be started

Q7. Which of the following statements regarding drug therapy for the condition described is true?
a. antispasmodics are safe and effective
b. antihistamines given to the infant may be beneficial in sedating the baby and settling everybody down
c. antispasmodics and antihistamines together offer the best form of drug therapy
d. aspirin should be considered as a first-line option
e. none of the above statements is true

SHORT ANSWER MANAGEMENT PROBLEM
Describe the educational approach you would attempt with the mother.

ANSWERS

A1. **a.** This infant most likely has infantile colic, which is defined as spells of unexplained fussiness or crying lasting longer than 3 hr/day, 3 days/wk, and continuing for more than 3 weeks in infants younger than 3 months old. "Unexplained fussiness or crying" implies that other causes (particularly infection) have been ruled out.

Excessive spasm syndrome of infancy and psychosocial stress syndrome of infancy do not exist. Early Crohn's disease is not possible.

Urinary tract infection, along with otitis media, pharyngitis, pneumonitis, and other infections, should be carefully considered before labeling the child as having infantile colic.

A2. **d.** A urinary tract infection is the first infection that should be ruled out by performing a urinalysis. In addition, a complete physical examination should be performed to rule out any other causes. At this age otitis media, pharyngitis, pneumonia, meningitis, intussusception, or volvulus may present initially only with excessive crying. If your index of suspicion is raised following a physical examination, particularly in the presence of a fever, a more complete laboratory workup and hospitalization is indicated.

A3. **e.** The cause of excessive crying in infancy is unknown. Although gastrointestinal hyperperistalsis, cow's milk protein allergy, lactose intolerance, disturbances in the parent-infant relationship, and a neurophysiologic response of the immature newborn to external and internal stimuli have all been proposed as potential underlying causes of infantile colic, nobody really knows for sure.

The newly diagnosed psychiatric condition known as "baby stress" does not exist.

A4. **a.** Although you may correctly argue that the only type of person who would ask a question like this is one who was really strapped for good questions in the first place, it does reinforce the Wessel criteria for the diagnosis of infantile colic: unexplained fussiness or crying lasting longer than 3 hr/day, 3 days/wk, and continuing for longer than 3 weeks in an infant younger than 3 months old.

A5. **e.** The most reasonable course of action in this case (after you have ruled out other causes) is as follows:
a. Describe the condition to the mother.
b. Explain that the cause is unknown.
c. Reassure the mother that the colic will pass by the age of 3 months, or shortly thereafter, and if it does continue longer it will certainly continue to improve.
d. Discuss maternal coping strategies with the mother.
e. Ask the mother to call you in 2 weeks if the symptoms have not improved, or sooner if any other symptoms develop.

A6. **c.** The most effective and important treatment is reassurance, stressing the benign nature of the condition and the assurance of resolution of the condition.

Reassure the mother that there is nothing that she is doing wrong and that there is no reason to switch to a soy-based formula. Although infantile colic is less frequent in breast-fed babies than in bottle-fed babies, it is not less common in soy-based feeding compared with ordinary infant formula.

To simply tell the mother to relax is not particularly helpful to anyone and indicates your lack of sensitivity to a very difficult problem.

As with the "baby stress" syndrome, the infant psychiatrist option does not exist.

A7. **e.** Many different pharmacologic treatments have frequently been used to treat infantile colic, including dicyclomine (Bentyl), phenergan (an antihistamine), "grippe water" (which is basically a watered-down alcoholic drink), aspirin, acetaminophen, and codeine. Dicyclomine has been associated with apnea and respiratory difficulties and antihistamines may cause significant central nervous system difficulties.

An "alcoholic mixture" speaks for itself. Aspirin, because of the potential association with Reye's syndrome, should not be used.

Although you may consider using simple acetaminophen, even with this drug there are no good data to indicate its safety in very young infants.

SOLUTION TO THE SHORT ANSWER MANAGEMENT PROBLEM

The most important points to be made in discussing the infant's condition with the mother are as follows:
a. There is nothing the mother could have done to prevent the condition, and there is nothing that she is doing wrong at present.
b. There is no association between infantile colic and other, more serious problems in the future.
c. Although bottle-fed babies get colic somewhat more frequently than breast-fed babies, this is no reason to change her current feeding pattern.
d. No specific therapy is more effective than explanation to the parent of the benign, self-limited nature of the condition.
e. The condition will resolve spontaneously and will probably resolve by the age of 3 months.
f. If anything changes or any other symptoms appear or if the mother is worried about anything else, urge her to call you.

SUMMARY OF DIAGNOSIS AND TREATMENT OF INFANTILE COLIC

1. Infantile colic is extremely common; it occurs in up to 25% of infants.

2. Although there are a number of theories as to its cause, the cause at this time is idiopathic.

3. The most important differential diagnosis is infection: if the ears, throat, and lungs are clear and if no abnormalities are detected on abdominal examination, a urinalysis is the only investigation that is necessary.

4. Diagnosis of infantile colic is based on Wessel criteria: 3,3,3, and 3 (see Answer 4).

5. Reassurance of the parent is as effective as any other therapy and is the treatment of choice.

6. Medications including dicyclomine (Bretylol), antihistamines, watered down alcohol, and aspirin should not be used. If anything is going to be used it should be acetaminophen.

SUGGESTED READINGS

Balon AJ: Management of infantile colic, *Am Fam Physician* 55(1):235-242, 245-246, 1997.

Berkowitz CD: Management of the colicky infant, *Comp Ther* 23(4):277-280, 1997.

Crowcroft N: Effectiveness of treatments for infantile colic, *Br Med J* 317(7170):1451, 1998.

Parkin P et al: Randomized controlled trial interventions in the management of persistent crying of infancy, *Pediatrics* 92:197-201, 1993.

PROBLEM·81

GUIDELINE FOR NEWBORN, INFANT, AND CHILDHOOD IMMUNIZATIONS

"That Shot Made My Baby Ill."

Case 1 ■ A 2-Month-Old-Infant with a High Fever 8 Hours after Receiving Her First Set of Immunizations

A 2-month-old-infant is brought to your office by his mother following his first set of immunizations at age 2 months. His mother states that approximately 8 hours after being immunized, the infant developed a temperature of 39.9° C. The child is screaming and irritable. On physical examination, no localizing signs of infection are found. Examination of the ears shows hyperemia of both tympanic membranes. You realize, of course, that this is probably caused by the crying itself. The throat is normal. The lungs are clear. The cardiovascular system and abdomen are normal. Skin is without rash.

SELECT THE BEST ANSWER TO THE FOLLOWING QUESTIONS

Q1. Which immunization(s) is (are) the most likely cause of the fever and the irritability in this child?
   a. poliomyelitis
   b. pertussis
   c. diphtheria
   d. tetanus
   e. any of the above

Q2. Considering this an adverse reaction that appears to be related to the immunization, what would you do?
   a. hospitalize the child
   b. advise the mother to give the child aspirin to bring down the fever
   c. advice the mother to give the child acetaminophen to bring down the fever
   d. obtain immediate blood cultures, complete blood count, and urine for analysis and culture and perform a lumbar puncture
   e. none of the above

Q3. Which of the following statements regarding future immunizations is (are) true?
   a. all future diphtheria-tetanus-pertussis (DTaP) and polio immunizations should be canceled
   b. irritability seen in this child is a contraindication to future immunization
   c. future immunizations should omit tetanus toxoid
   d. future immunizations should not be affected; DTaP and polio immunizations should be given as before
   e. none of the above statements is true

Q4. Which of the following statements regarding vaccination against poliomyelitis is (are) true?
   a. at this time, although two forms of vaccination against poliomyelitis exist, only one is licensed for use in the United States
   b. oral polio vaccine (OPV) is a live, attenuated, trivalent vaccine known as the Salk vaccine
   c. inactivated poliomyelitis vaccine (IPV) is an inactivated (killed), trivalent vaccine known as Sabin vaccine
   d. all of the above statements are true
   e. none of the above statements is true

Q5. Which of the following statements is (are) true regarding hepatitis B vaccine in children?
   a. it is not recommended as a routine immunization
   b. it is recommended as a routine immunization, and the first dose should be given at 8 months

c. it is recommended as a routine immunization, and the first dose should be given at 6 months
d. it is recommended as a routine immunization, and the first dose should be given at 4 months
e. none of the above statements is true

Q6. Which of the following statements is (are) true regarding reactions that follow the immunization of infants and children with whole cell DTP?
a. there are three different types of adverse reactions that may occur
b. the fever that may develop from one type of reaction often reaches 40.5° C
c. this vaccine is no longer recommended
d. a, b, and c
e. none of the above statements is true

Q7. Which of the following is (are) true contraindications to immunization?
a. prematurity
b. recent exposure to an infectious disease
c. current antimicrobial therapy
d. moderate or severe illness with or without a fever
e. history of penicillin or other allergies

Q8. Which of the following statements regarding immunization against *Haemophilus influenzae* type b is (are) true?
a. the vaccine is known as the Hib vaccine
b. the first dose of *H. influenzae* type b vaccine should be given at age 2 months
c. the *H. influenzae* type b vaccine is given to protect the infant only from *H. influenzae* type b infections that lead to meningitis
d. all of the above statements are true
e. a and b only

Q9. Which of the following vaccines is (are) recommended for first administration at age 12 to 15 months?
a. hepatitis B
b. *H. influenzae* type b vaccine
c. measles-mumps-rubella (MMR) vaccine
d. all of the above
e. a and b only

Q10. By the time a child born today reaches 7 years old, how many doses of OPV should have been administered?
a. 1 dose
b. 2 doses
c. 3 doses
d. 4 doses
e. none of the above

SHORT ANSWER MANAGEMENT PROBLEM
Discuss some of the important causes for the reduction in neonatal, infant, and childhood mortality that have occurred during the last century. Indicate whether or not these causes are still a concern in certain parts of the world.

ANSWERS

A1. **e.** Although in the past pertussis was most frequently associated with fever, the new recommendations for use of acellular pertussis in place of whole cell DTP makes any of these vaccines equally culpable. Nonimmunization causes should be considered.

A2. **c.** Hospitalization and an intensive septic workup are unnecessary. Acetaminophen is the analgesic of choice for the treatment of fever in children. Aspirin should not be given because of its possible link with Reye's syndrome. This child should be reassessed within 24 hours if the symptoms (especially the fever) do not improve with the administration of the antipyretic acetaminophen or if any other symptoms or signs develop.

A3. **d.** Much progress has been made in reducing the incidence of adverse reactions to vaccines. Although all vaccines may produce minor reactions, particularly local soreness, redness, swelling following the administration of an injectable antigen, these are not absolute contraindications to further immunizations.

A4. **e.** Two types of vaccine are licensed in the United States for prevention of polio: OPV, a live, attenuated, trivalent poliovirus vaccine known as Sabin; and an IPV, an inactivated (killed) trivalent vaccine known as Salk. Both are available, but Salk inactivated vaccine is now recommended for all routine polio immunizations see Table on p. 380 for special use of Sabin oral vaccine).

A5. **e.** Vaccination against hepatitis B is routinely recommended for all children born in the United States. The easiest schedule for hepatitis B immunization is birth, 2 months, and 4 months. Thimerosal-free vaccines are recommended.

A6. **d.**

A7. **d.** There are three true contraindications to the administration of childhood immunizations:
a. an anaphylactic reaction to a vaccine contraindicates further doses of that vaccine
b. an anaphylactic reaction to a vaccine constituent

contraindicates the use of vaccines containing that substance

    c. moderate or severe illness with or without a fever is a true contraindication

Mild acute illness with or without a fever is not a contraindication. Convulsions, encephalopathy, collapse, or shocklike state within 48 hours of receipt of any vaccine is a cause for concern and may be considered a contraindication to further vaccination. Such episodes, which had been related to the whole cell DTP vaccine, are extremely rare with the acellular DTaP vaccine.

A8. **e.** Vaccination against *H. influenzae* type b is recommended in three doses: at 2, 4, and 12 to 15 months of age. *H. influenzae* vaccine is given at these times because of the age at which *H. influenzae* meningitis affects infants and children. Meningitis caused by this organism usually occurs between the ages of 1 month and 4 years. Other significant infections caused by *H. influenzae* are acute epiglottis; pneumonia; septic arthritis; cellulitis; osteomyelitis; pericarditis; bacteremia without an associated focus; neonatal disease; and miscellaneous infections such as urinary tract infection, cervical adenitis, uvulitis, endocarditis, primary peritonitis, periappendiceal abscess, and otitis media. The Hib immunization should, theoretically, be effective against all of these infections.

A9. **c.** Only two vaccinations are given for the first time at 12 to 15 months of age: MMR and varicella.

A10. **d.** By the time a child born today reaches 7 years old, four doses of IPV should have been administered, one at each of 2 months, 4 months, between 6 and 18 months, and between 4 and 6 years of age.

SOLUTION TO THE SHORT ANSWER MANAGEMENT PROBLEM

The reductions in neonatal, infant, and childhood mortality in the developed world during the last century are truly remarkable. These reductions are a result of better prenatal care and prenatal assessment of high-risk status; improved perinatal care; immunizations; antibiotics; other diagnostic and therapeutic tools; and public health measures including filtration and chlorination of water, hygienic food handling (especially of milk), mosquito control, and isolation of individuals infected with a communicable disease.

    In addition, the health of children has been directly affected by improvements in social conditions, economic conditions, and educational advances in the developed world. Little more can be done to further reduce mortality rates apart from a paradigm shift from acute episodic care of children to primary preventive care on visits that occur for a different reason. For example, if a 6-month-old child is brought to your office by his mother for assessment of fever and irritability, it is a perfect opportunity to discuss the inadvisability of walkers near stairs, the use of child safety seats in automobiles, and locations of potential toxic substances and medicines in the home.

    There is, however, a startling contrast between neonatal, infant, and childhood health in the developed world and the health of the same-aged population in the developing world, especially in areas of continual war and strife. In some areas of the developing world neonatal, infant, and childhood mortality is significantly higher today than it was in the United States in the eighteenth century.

SUMMARY OF THE CENTER FOR DISEASE CONTROL AND PREVENTION'S GUIDELINES FOR NEWBORN, INFANT, AND CHILDHOOD IMMUNIZATIONS (see Table, p. 380)

SUGGESTED READING

Zimmerman RK: ACIP recommended immunization schedule. Centers for Disease Control and Prevention, Atlanta, updated annually, *http://www.aafp.org*.

PROBLEM · 82

INFANT FEEDING

"I Just Know My Milk Is Inadequate."

Case 1 ■ An Anxious Mother with a 3-Week-Old Infant and Many Questions Concerning Feeding

A mother who just delivered her first baby 3 weeks ago comes to your office for her first neonatal visit. She has many questions concerning breast feeding and has been getting much advice from her friends and especially her mother-in-law.

    The infant appears to be growing well and, according to her mother, is happy and content. The mother-in-law has suggested that her daughter-in-law change from breast feeding to cow's milk because she feels the infant's crying is waking up her son (the baby's father) and preventing him from getting "the rest that the poor boy needs."

    The mother appears somewhat tired herself. The child is at the 50th percentile for weight and the 50th percentile for length. More importantly, the child has gained an average of 50 g/day since discharge from hospital. The child is feeding every 2 hours at this time.

Vaccines[1] are listed under routinely recommended ages. | Bars | indicate range of recommended ages for immunization. Any dose not given at the recommended age should be given as a "catch-up" immunization at any subsequent visit when indicated and feasible. (Ovals) indicate vaccines to be given if previously recommended doses were missed or given earlier than the recommended minimum age.

Age→ Vaccine↓	Birth	1 mo	2 mos	4 mos	6 mos	12 mos	15 mos	18 mos	24 mos	4-6 yrs	11-12 yrs	14-16 yrs
Hepatitis B[2]		Hep B									(Hep B)	
			Hep B			Hep B						
Diphtheria, Tetanus, Pertussis[3]		DTaP	DTaP	DTaP		DTaP[3]				DTaP	Td	
H. influenzae type b[4]		Hib	Hib	Hib	Hib							
Polio[5]		IPV	IPV		IPV[5]					IPV[5]		
Measles, Mumps, Rubella[6]						MMR				MMR[6]	(MMR[6])	
Varicella[7]						Var					(Var[7])	
Hepatitis A[8]										Hep A[8] in selected areas		

From Zimmerman RK: *Am Fam Physician* 61(1):232-239, 2000.

Approved by the Advisory Committee on Immunization Practices (ACIP), the American Academy of Pediatrics (AAP), and the American Academy of Family Physicians (AAFP).

NOTE: On October 22, 1999, the Advisory Committee on Immunization Practices (ACIP) recommended that Rotashield (RRV-TV), the only U.S.-licensed rotavirus vaccine, no longer be used in the United States (*MMWR,* Vol 48, No 43, Nov. 5, 1999). Parents should be reassured that their children who received rotavirus vaccine before July are not at increased risk for intussusception now.

[1]This schedule indicates the recommended ages for routine administration of currently licensed childhood vaccines as of 11/1/99. Additional vaccines may be licensed and recommended during the year. Licensed combination vaccines may be used whenever any components of the combination are indicated and its other components are not contraindicated. Providers should consult the manufacturers' package inserts for detailed recommendations.

[2]*Infants born to HBsAg-negative mothers* should receive the first dose of hepatitis B (*Hep B*) vaccine by age 2 months. The second dose should be at least 1 month after the first dose. The third dose should be administered at least 4 months after the first dose and at least 2 months after the second dose but not before 6 months of age for infants.

Infants born to HBsAg-positive mothers should receive the hepatitis B vaccine and 0.5 ml hepatitis B immune globulin (HBIG) within 12 hours of birth at separate sites. The second dose is recommended at 1 to 2 months of age and the third dose at 6 months of age.

Infants born to mothers whose HBsAg status is unknown should receive the hepatitis B vaccine within 12 hours of birth. Maternal blood should be drawn at the time of delivery to determine the mother's HBsAg status; if the HBsAg test is positive, the infant should receive HBIG as soon as possible (no later than 1 week of age).

All children and adolescents (through 18 years of age) who have not been immunized against hepatitis B may begin the series during any visit. Special efforts should be made to immunize children who were born in or whose parents were born in areas of the world with moderate or high endemicity of hepatitis B virus infection.

[3]The fourth dose of diphtheria and tetanus toxoids and acellular pertussis vaccine (DTaP) may be administered as early as 12 months of age, provided 6 months have elapsed since the third dose and the child is unlikely to return at age 15 to 18 months. Tetanus-diphtheria toxoid (Td) is recommended at 11 to 12 years of age if at least 5 years have elapsed since the last dose of DTP, DTaP, or DT. Subsequent routine Td boosters are recommended every 10 years.

[4]Three *H. influenzae* type b (Hib) conjugate vaccines are licensed for infant use. If PRP-OMP (PedvaxHIB or ComVax [Merck]) is administered at 2 and 4 months of age, a dose at 6 months is not required. Because clinical studies in infants have demonstrated that using some combination products may induce a lower immune response to the Hib vaccine component, DTaP/Hib combination products should not be used for primary immunization in infants at 2, 4, or 6 months of age, unless FDA-approved for these ages.

[5]To eliminate the risk of vaccine-associated paralytic polio (VAPP), an all-IPV schedule is now recommended for routine childhood polio vaccination in the United States. All children should receive four doses of IPV at 2 months, 4 months, 6 to 18 months, and 4 to 6 years. OPV (if available) may be used only for the following special circumstances:

1. Mass vaccination campaigns to control outbreaks of paralytic polio
2. Unvaccinated children who will be traveling in <4 weeks to areas where polio is endemic or epidemic
3. Children of parents who do not accept the recommended number of vaccine injections. These children may receive OPV only for the third or fourth dose or both; in this situation, health care providers should administer OPV only after discussing the risk for VAPP with parents or caregivers.
4. During the transition to an all-IPV schedule, recommendations for the use of remaining OPV supplies in physicians' offices and clinics have been issued by the American Academy of Pediatrics (Committee on Infection Disease, American Academy of Pediatrics: *Pediatrics,* 104[6]:1404-1406, 1999).

[6]The second dose of the measles, mumps, and rubella (MMR) vaccine is recommended routinely at 4 to 6 years of age but may be administered during any visit, provided at least 4 weeks have elapsed since receipt of the first dose and that both doses are administered beginning at or after 12 months of age. Those who have not previously received the second dose should complete the schedule by the 11- to 12-year-old visit.

[7]Varicella (Var) vaccine is recommended at any visit on or after the first birthday for susceptible children (i.e., those who lack a reliable history of chickenpox as judged by a health care provider and who have not been immunized). Susceptible persons 13 years of age or older should receive 2 doses, given at least 4 weeks apart.

[8]Hepatitis A (Hep A) is shaded to indicate its recommended use in selected states and/or regions; consult your local public health authority (*MMWR* [RR12]:1-37, 1999).

SELECT THE BEST ANSWER
TO THE FOLLOWING QUESTIONS

Q1. What is the minimal appropriate weight gain (and a sign of both infant health and maternal-infant bonding with breast feeding) following discharge from hospital?
   a. 15 g/day
   b. 20 g/day
   c. 30 g/day
   d. 50 g/day
   e. 75 g/day

Q2. What would be your suggestion to the mother in terms of feeding her infant?
   a. ask her mother-in-law; she seems to know all the answers
   b. to decrease the feeds of the infant to every 3 hours
   c. to feed the infant on demand
   d. to switch from breast feeding to bottle feeding; it will end up being less hassle for everyone
   e. a and c

Q3. Common mistakes in the feeding of infants (especially with first-time mothers) include which of the following?
   a. feeding the infant too little
   b. feeding the infant too much
   c. feeding the infant on a fixed schedule
   d. feeding the infant whole cow's milk
   e. all of the above

Q4. Regarding the feeding of infants when they cry, which of the following offers the best advice to the mother?
   a. feed the baby; no ifs, and, or buts
   b. let the infant cry for at least 37.5 minutes; if the infant is still crying, check things out, it's likely to be either one of a diaper problem or a food problem
   c. stop breast feeding; it is too much hassle and much easier just to stick a bottle in the infant's mouth
   d. crying may or may not indicate hunger; infants need not be fed every time they cry
   e. crying almost always indicates hunger; assume that the baby needs to be fed until proven otherwise (that will eliminate the potential problem of underfeeding)

Q5. Which of the following statements regarding breast milk flow and maternal anxiety is (are) true?
   a. there is little correlation between breast milk flow and maternal anxiety

   b. maternal anxiety may significantly increase the quantity of breast milk in breast milk flow
   c. maternal anxiety may significantly decrease the quantity of breast milk in breast milk flow
   d. maternal anxiety may significantly decrease the quality of breast milk in breast milk flow
   e. c and d

Q6. Human colostrum is the precursor to good-quality human breast milk. What is (are) the major components found in colostrum that offer a significant advantage to breast-fed infants?
   a. macrophages that synthesize complement, lysozyme, and lactoferrin
   b. bacterial antibodies that protect the infant against bacterial organisms entering through the gastrointestinal (GI) tract
   c. antibodies that protect the infant against viral organisms entering through GI tract
   d. b and c
   e. all of the above

Q7. One substance of importance described in Answer 6 is of what subtype?
   a. IgA
   b. IgG
   c. IgM
   d. IgE
   e. none of the above

Case 2 ■ A 28-Year-Old Primigravida with Mastitis

A 28-year-old primigravida develops an erythematous skin discoloration in the upper outer quadrant of the left breast. You suspect bacterial mastitis.

Q8. At this time, what would you do?
   a. stop breast feeding; have the mother express her breast milk until the infection is cleared up
   b. continue breast feeding and treat the mother with hot compresses and antibiotics
   c. continue breast feeding and treat both the mother and the infant with antibiotics
   d. forget breast feeding for now; provide the "big gun" antibiotics (quadruple therapy) just to make sure you "snow" the bacteria
   e. operate immediately; you never know what you may find underneath that inflamed tissue

Q9. What is the organism most likely responsible for the condition described in Case 2?
   a. *Streptococcus pneumoniae*
   b. *Staphylococcus aureus*
   c. *Escherichia coli*: subtype H-57

d. *Bacteroides fragilis*
e. b and d

Q10. Which of the following statements comparing human breast milk with cow's milk is false?
  a. cow's milk may be responsible for diarrhea, intestinal bleeding, and occult melena
  b. spitting up, infantile colic, and atopic dermatitis are more common in infants fed with cow's milk (or infant formula)
  c. human breast milk contains bacterial and viral antibodies, antibodies mainly of the IgA class
  d. breast-fed babies do not require iron supplementation until the age of 1 year
  e. human breast milk has an adequate amount of vitamin C

Q11. The mother described in Case 1 has been told that she should be "giving the baby lots of every vitamin under the sun." Her mother-in-law even offers to purchase the 37 different vitamins for the baby.
  Although it is difficult to acknowledge, the mother-in-law may be right with respect to which of the following vitamins?
  a. vitamin A
  b. vitamin C
  c. vitamin D
  d. b and c
  e. all of the above

Q12. Fluoride supplementation for both breast-fed babies and bottle-fed babies should not be required if the fluoride concentration in the water supply of the community exceeds which of the following?
  a. 1.0 ppm
  b. 2.0 ppm
  c. 5.0 ppm
  d. 10.0 ppm
  e. 100.0 ppm

Q13. Human breast milk, in comparison to cow's milk, has which of the following?
  a. a higher fat content
  b. a lower carbohydrate content
  c. a lower protein content
  d. a greater concentration of the protein casein
  e. a greater number of kilocalories per gram of milk

Q14. Which of the following statements is false regarding infant feeding?
  a. infants establish their own feeding pattern; there is considerable variation from one infant to another
  b. for the first 1 to 2 months of life, feedings are regularly taken throughout the 24-hour period
  c. breast-fed babies should be fed on an established schedule
  d. during the first month of life, feedings average 8 to 10/24 hours
  e. by 8 months of age, the average number of feedings is 3 to 4/24 hours

Q15. The mother-in-law in Case 1 recommends that solids be introduced on day 8 and that one new solid food be introduced every 4 days until a total of 28 different solids are being regularly consumed.
  You have a slightly different recommendation. Your recommendation is that solid foods do not have to be introduced into the infant's diet until what age?
  a. 1 month of age
  b. 2 to 3 months of age
  c. 6 months of age
  d. 9 months of age
  e. 12 months of age

Six weeks later, you see the same mother presented in Case 1. She has switched from breast feeding to infant formula feeding because she had to go back to her full-time job as an accountant. She tells you that her infant is now constipated. On careful questioning, you determine that the infant is having one hard bowel movement every 4 days. The physical examination is completely normal, including anal sphincter tone.

Q16. What should you do now?
  a. tell the mother to go home, take a Valium, and relax
  b. suggest supplementation with extra fluids, extra foods, and prune juice
  c. suggest the use of milk of magnesia at bedtime
  d. suggest the addition of two teaspoons of bran to the pablum and force-feed the pablum every 3 hours
  e. pull out the "old glycerine suppositories" and suggest their regular use four times a day for 6 weeks

---

Case 3 ■ A Mother with a Baby Who Spits Up Her Formula

A mother comes to your office with her infant. Her baby is 6 weeks of age and has been "spitting up" all of her formula for the last 3 weeks. She believes the infant is malnourished and has been told so by another very helpful mother-in-law.

You weigh the baby; she is 11 pounds, 3 ounces. Her birth weight was 7 pounds, 6 ounces.

Q17. At this time, you should advise the mother to do which of the following:
   a. go home and relax; the child will grow out of it
   b. increase the time spent burping the infant and put the infant on her abdomen for a nap immediately after the feeding
   c. investigate the child for pyloric stenosis
   d. suggest the use of a GI tract motility modifier such as metoclopramide intravenous push q4h
   e. immediately refer the child to a pediatric gastroenterologist

Case 4 ■ A Mother Trying to Breast Feed

A mother comes to your office with her 8-week-old infant girl. The mother is tearful and depressed. She has been trying to breast feed but she tells you that "I'm obviously inadequate; I'm not producing enough milk and the baby is fussy all of the time."

On examination, the infant looks thin. Since her last checkup 3 weeks ago, she has gained only 90 g. The rest of the physical examination is normal.

Q18. At this time, what should you do?
   a. ask some very direct questions about the mother's feeding technique
   b. refer the mother to a lactation consultant
   c. include the husband or significant other in feeding expressed breast milk to the infant
   d. suggest a temporary supplementation with infant formula after breast feeding
   e. all of the above

Q19. Which of the following statements regarding breast feeding is (are) true?
   a. most breast-fed babies lose weight in the first week of life
   b. infants should be encouraged to empty both breasts at each feeding during the first few weeks of life
   c. maternal fatigue may impair breast feeding
   d. 80% to 90% of the breast milk obtained is obtained in the first 4 minutes of breast feeding on a particular breast
   e. all of the above statements are true

SHORT ANSWER MANAGEMENT PROBLEM
Compare the composition of human breast milk with infant formula or cow's milk.

ANSWERS

A1. **c.** The minimal acceptable weight gain in the neonatal period and infancy is 30 g/day. If weight gain equals or exceeds that, you can be reasonably confident that the infant is thriving.

A2. **c.** It is well accepted that especially during the first few weeks and months of life the ideal feeding schedule is feeding on demand. This will vary from infant to infant but will eventually settle into a reasonable schedule averaging 8 to 10 feedings per day.

A3. **e.** Mistakes that are made frequently in the neonatal and infant period regarding feeding include the following:
   a. Feeding the infant too much
   b. Feeding the infant too little
   c. Feeding the infant on a fixed schedule (rather than on demand)
   d. Feeding the infant cow's milk rather than breast milk or formula (cow's milk tends to be more allergenic and less digestible)

A4. **d.** It is important to appreciate that infants cry for other reasons besides hunger and that they need not be fed every time they cry. Some infants are placid, some are unusually active, and some are irritable. Sick infants are often uninterested in food. Infants who awaken and cry consistently at short intervals may not be receiving enough milk at each feeding or may have discomfort from some other cause (wearing too much clothing, a soiled or wet diaper or clothing, an uncomfortable diaper or clothing, swallowing air ["gas"]; being in an uncomfortably hot or cold environment; or being ill). Some infants cry to gain sufficient attention, whereas other infants deprived of adequate mothering become indifferent. Some infants simply need to be held. Those who stop crying when they are picked up or held do not usually need food, but those who continue to cry when held and when food is offered should be carefully evaluated for other causes of distress.

A5. **c.** Maternal anxiety, fatigue, postpartum depression, or stress from other causes are candidates for a decreased quantity of milk that may further compound the problem. It is conceivable that mothers may find themselves in a situation where they are in a vicious cycle: maternal stress leads to maternal fatigue, which results in decreased quantity of breast milk, which causes further maternal stress, and so on. It appears that only the quantity and not the quality of breast milk is affected.

A6. **e.**

A7. **a.** Human colostrum contains macrophages that are able to synthesize complement, lysozyme, lactoferrin, and the iron-binding whey protein that is normally about one-third saturated with iron. In addition, human colostrum contains antibodies of the IgA class that protect the infant from bacterial species such as *E. coli* and certain viruses.

A8. **b.** See Answer 9.

A9. **b.** Unless exceptional circumstances dictate otherwise, the recommended course of action with maternal mastitis is to continue breast feeding and treat the mother with both symptomatic treatments such as hot compresses and antibiotics effective against *S. aureus* (including coagulase-positive *Staphylococcus*). The antibiotic of choice in this case is either cloxacillin or methicillin.

A10. **d.** Breast milk has many advantages over cow's milk for the feeding of infants. These advantages are that it is easier to digest; it has the bacterial and viral antibodies mentioned in Answer 7; it does not produce allergic manifestations such as diarrhea, GI tract bleeding, and atopic dermatitis; it has a lower incidence of feeding problems including regurgitation and constipation; it has a lower incidence of infantile colic; and it is the most important method of establishing maternal-infant bonding. Breast milk usually contains adequate supplies of all vitamins, with the possible exception of vitamin D. Vitamin C is not required for supplementation.

Although breast milk contains some iron and the iron that is present is well absorbed, the child will need iron-fortified pablum or foods by 6 months of age to prevent iron-deficiency anemia.

A11. **c.** Vitamin D is the only vitamin that may be required for supplementation in a breast-fed baby. If a baby is not exposed to adequate sunlight or has dark skin, the quantity of vitamin D may not be sufficient. The daily recommended vitamin D intake is 400 IU/day.

A12. **a.** Fluoride supplementation for infants (both breast-fed and bottle-fed) is not required if the fluoride concentration of the water supply exceeds 1.0 ppm. Additional fluoride given to formula-fed babies in a community with a fluoridated water supply could result in fluorosis.

A13. **c.** In comparison to cow's milk, human breast milk has a higher carbohydrate concentration, a lower protein concentration, different protein composition (lactalbumin and lactoglobulin), a higher percentage of polyunsaturated fat (qualitative difference), and the same caloric content (20 kcal/oz).

A14. **c.** The following statements concerning infant feeding are true:
   a. There is considerable variation in feeding patterns from infant to infant.
   b. During the first month or two of life, feedings are taken regularly during the 24-hour period.
   c. During the first few months of life, feedings average 8 to 10/24-hour period.
   d. By 8 months of age, feedings have settled down to an average of 3 to 4/24-hour period.
As stated previously, neonates and infants should be fed on demand, not on a strictly imposed schedule.

A15. **c.** Solid foods do not have to be introduced into an infant's diet until 6 months of age. Infant pablum is usually the first food to be introduced. Infant pablum should be followed by vegetables, fruits, and finally meats. New foods should not be introduced more often than one every 1 to 2 weeks. The order of food introduction appears relatively unimportant. The introduction of one food at a time will allow you to establish an allergic or atopic reaction to any particular newly introduced food.

A16. **b.** Constipation is a common problem in formula-fed infants. It is extremely rare in a breast-fed baby. Constipation in a formula-fed baby may be caused by an insufficient amount of food or fluid, a diet too high in fat or protein, or a diet deficient in bulk. Constipation may be alleviated by increasing the amount of fluid or sugar in the formula or by adding or increasing the amounts of cereal, vegetables, or fruit; prune juice (0.5 to 1 ounce) may also be helpful.

The use of milk of magnesia and glycerine suppositories as anything but a temporary measure is inappropriate. The addition of 2 teaspoons of bran to the pablum, although theoretically sound as a measure of increasing the bulk in the infant's diet, would be somewhat unpalatable and would result in an irate infant!

Telling the mother to go home and relax is not appropriate.

A17. **b.** Regurgitation, or spitting up, is a common problem in infants. The mechanism appears to be an incompetent gastroesophageal sphincter. Regurgitation can be reduced by adequate eructation of swallowed air during and after eating, by gentle handling, by avoidance of emotional conflicts, and by placing the infant on the right side or abdomen for a nap immediately after eating. The head should not be lower than the rest of the body during rest periods. Unless the child (especially a male) demonstrates projectile vomiting and has a palpable mass in the pylorus, pyloric stenosis is not likely.

A18. **e.** This is a very common scenario in family practice. The mother should be carefully questioned regarding feeding technique. Before assuming that the mother has insufficient milk, three possibilities should be excluded: errors in feeding technique responsible for the infant's inadequate progress; remediable maternal factors related to diet, rest, or emotional distress; or physical disturbances in the infant that interfere with eating or with weight gain.

Occasionally infants who seem to be nursing well may not thrive because of milk insufficiency; in this case increased frequency of feedings may be indicated.

Referral to the La Leche League is an alternative that can be recommended to this mother. The La Leche League is a volunteer organization composed of successfully nursing mothers willing to assist other mothers desiring to nurse.

If the mother is able to successfully express sufficient milk, the husband or significant other may be able to assist the mother in feeding. This alternative is attractive because it gives the mother time to rest and recover her strength.

Supplementation with an infant formula is an alternative that should be considered in some cases. In this case the mother is encouraged to breast feed and supplement her baby with formula following each feeding. As long as the nipple in the bottle does not have too big a hole in it (making it too easy for the infant to obtain the formula), the infant will probably continue to suck vigorously at the breast. This will allow the mother to continue breast feeding while ensuring adequate infant nutrition.

Infant formulas provide satisfactory nutrition for the infant. They all combine milk, sugar, water, and modification of a digestible curd protein. As with breast milk, infant formulas provide 20 kcal/oz. Although "breast is best," a dogmatic approach to breast feeding should be avoided.

A19. **e.** Important characteristics of breast feeding include the following:
  a. Most breast-fed babies lose weight in the first week.
  b. Infants should be encouraged to empty both breasts at each feeding.
  c. Maternal fatigue may impair breast feeding.
  d. 80% to 90% of breast milk is obtained by the infant during the first 4 minutes of the feeding.

SOLUTION TO THE SHORT ANSWER MANAGEMENT PROBLEM

A succinct comparison between human breast milk and formula or cow's milk follows:
  a. Breast milk has a higher carbohydrate content than formula or cow's milk.
  b. Breast milk has a lower protein content than cow's milk.
  c. Breast milk has qualitatively different proteins.
  d. Breast milk has lactalbumin and lactoglobulin.
  e. Formula or cow's milk has casein as a major protein.
  f. Breast milk has a different composition of fats; it has a higher percentage of polyunsaturated fat.
  g. Breast milk and cow's milk or formula have equivalent caloric content (20 kcal/oz).

SUMMARY OF INFANT FEEDING

1. Preference of infant feeding: Breast feeding is preferable. Advantages of breast feeding include convenience, digestibility, transfer of antiviral and antibacterial antibodies, lack of allergic phenomena, maternal-infant bonding, low incidence of regurgitation, and no constipation.

   Breast feeding should be encouraged: Before assuming that milk production is insufficient for the infant you should consider errors in feeding techniques, remediable maternal factors, and physical disturbances in the infant.

   Feeding should be on demand: Although erratic in the first few months, infants tend to regulate themselves after short periods of time.

   Supplementation with formula and formula feeding provide excellent nutrition; a dogmatic approach to breast feeding should be avoided.

2. Vitamin, fluoride, and iron supplements: Vitamins are unnecessary in all formula-fed infants and probably in most breast-fed babies. If the baby is not exposed to sufficient sunlight or is darkly pigmented, supplemental vitamin D is recommended. Fluoride supplementation is unnecessary if the community water supply contains 1.0 ppm or more fluoride; this applies to breast-fed and bottle-fed babies.

   Iron supplements (in the manner of iron-fortified food) should be begun at the age of 6 months in breast-fed babies because breast milk contains an inadequate supply.

3. Solid foods: Solid foods need not be introduced until 6 months of age; after that time introduce one new food every 1 to 2 weeks.

4. Unwarranted assumptions: Do not assume that a crying infant is a hungry infant. Consider all causes of infant crying before making that assumption. Do not assume that information received from other sources (including well-meaning family members) is valid information.

5. Advantages of human colostrum:
   a. Macrophages
   b. Viral antibodies
   c. Bacterial antibodies
   d. Antibody class: IgA

6. Growth and development: The minimum standard for the neonate is a weight gain of 30 g/day.

7. Comparison of human milk and formula or cow's milk:
   a. Carbohydrate: Higher in human milk
   b. Protein content: Lower in human milk
   c. Protein quality: Lactalbumin and lactoglobulin in human milk versus casein in formula or cow's milk
   d. Fat: Quality and distribution: polyunsaturated fat content is higher in breast milk; saturated fat content is lower
   e. Caloric content: Identical: 20 kcal/oz

SUGGESTED READING
Barness LA, Curran JS: Nutrition. In Behrman R, ed: *Nelson textbook of pediatrics*, ed 15, Philadelphia, 1998, WB Saunders.

PROBLEM·83

FAILURE TO THRIVE AND SHORT STATURE

"How Come He Seems So Skinny and Small?"

Case 1 ■ An 8-Month-Old Infant Who Appears Malnourished

An 8-month-old infant is brought to the Emergency Department by his mother for an assessment of an upper respiratory tract infection. He has been coughing for the past 3 days and has had a runny nose.

On examination, his temperature is 37.5° C. He appears malnourished and has thin extremities, a narrow face, prominent ribs, and wasted buttocks. He has a prominent diaper rash, unwashed skin, a skin rash that resembles the skin infection impetigo contagiosum on his face, uncut fingernails, and dirty clothing. His weight is below the 3rd percentile for his age, his length is at the 25th percentile, and his head circumference at the 50th percentile.

SELECT THE BEST ANSWER TO THE FOLLOWING QUESTIONS

Q1. What is the most likely diagnosis in the infant described?
   a. nonorganic failure to thrive (FTT)
   b. organic FTT
   c. child neglect
   d. a and c
   e. b and c

Q2. What is the most likely cause of this child's condition?
   a. maternal deprivation
   b. cystic fibrosis
   c. constitutionally small for age
   d. infantile autism
   e. congenital bilateral sensorineural hearing loss

Q3. What is (are) the procedure(s) of choice for this infant at this time?
   a. provision of a high-calorie formula; reassessment of the infant in 1 week
   b. initiation of outpatient investigations in the child to exclude serious organic disease
   c. treatment of the respiratory tract infection and instruction to the mother in correct feeding practices
   d. all of the above
   e. none of the above

Q4. Where is follow-up of this child best performed?
   a. in the hospital outpatient department
   b. in the hospital Emergency Room
   c. in the family physician's office
   d. in the home by the public health nurse
   e. in the social worker's office

Q5. The initial follow-up plan suggests the frequency of visits for the child to be which of the following?
   a. every month
   b. every 3 months
   c. every week
   d. every 6 weeks
   e. every 6 months

Q6. The environment that exists for this child should be thoroughly assessed for which of the following?
   a. child abuse or potential for child abuse
   b. spousal abuse or potential for spousal abuse
   c. level of family income
   d. inappropriate parental coping mechanisms: alcohol and drug use
   e. all of the above

Case 2 ■ A 13-Year-Old Female with a Short, Webbed Neck

A 13-year-old female is brought to your office for assessment of her short stature. On examination the child has a height and weight below the 5th percentile, a webbed neck, lack of breast bud development, a high-arched palate, and a low-set posterior hairline.

Q7. What is the most likely diagnosis in this child?
   a. Noonan's syndrome
   b. trisomy 21
   c. Turner's syndrome
   d. fragile X syndrome
   e. constitutional delay of growth

Q8. What is the most common cause of short stature in children?
   a. familial short stature
   b. chromosomal abnormality
   c. constitutional delay of growth
   d. hypothyroidism
   e. psychosocial dwarfism

Q9. Bone age can sometimes be used to differentiate certain causes of short stature in children. With respect to bone age, which of the following statements is true?
   a. bone age is normal in both familial short stature and in constitutional delay of growth
   b. bone age is normal in familial short stature and delayed in constitutional delay of growth
   c. bone age is normal in constitutional delay of growth and delayed in growth hormone deficiency
   d. bone age is delayed in both familial short stature and in short stature caused by hypothyroidism
   e. bone age is variable and cannot be used to differentiate familial short stature and constitutional delay

Psychosocial dwarfism is a situation in which poor physical growth may be associated with an unfavorable psychosocial situation.

Q10. With respect to psychosocial dwarfism, which of the following statements is (are) true?
   a. sleep and eating aberrations occur in these children
   b. growth usually returns to normal when the stress is removed
   c. behavioral problems are common in these children
   d. all of the above are true
   e. none of the above statements is true

Q11. Which of the following investigations should be performed in a child with FTT or a child in which short stature is unlikely to be familial in nature?
   a. complete blood count (CBC)
   b. complete urinalysis
   c. serum blood urea nitrogen (BUN) and creatinine
   d. T4 and thyroid-stimulating hormone (TSH)
   e. all of the above

SHORT ANSWER MANAGEMENT PROBLEM
List 10 physical disorders that may manifest themselves as FTT in infants and children.

ANSWERS

A1. **d.** This child most likely has nonorganic FTT, secondary to child neglect.

A2. **a.** FTT may be a result of organic causes, nonorganic causes, or both. Nonorganic causes predominate. Nonorganic FTT includes psychologic FTT (maternal deprivation), child neglect, lack of education regarding feeding, and errors in feeding.

Nonorganic FTT is most often attributable to maternal deprivation (as in this case) or lack of a nurturing environment at home.

Organic FTT is most commonly caused by a medical condition impairing the child's ability to take in, absorb, or metabolize adequate calories.

A3. **e.** The treatment of choice at this time is to hospitalize the child and to give the child unlimited feedings for a minimum period of 1 week. At the same time, a careful physical examination and certain routine investigations including CBC, complete urinalysis, renal function testing, and serum TSH level can be completed. If the child lives in a poor inner-city neighborhood in the United States, a serum lead level test should also be done.

The family physician can and should involve social services and should also initiate a detailed assessment of the child's home environment.

Before the child is discharged home, the home environment must be assessed and the parents of the child must be given explicit instructions in feeding practices.

A4. **d.** If the child begins to gain weight rapidly and reestablish his health in the hospital (which is very likely), reassessment should ideally be done in the environment that allowed the development of the problem in the first place (at least on some occasions). This is obviously the home, and the health care professional in the best position to do this is probably the public health nurse or the community health nurse.

A5. **c.** The initial follow-up supervision should be close and frequent; every week for the first 6 weeks following discharge from the hospital is reasonable.

A6. **e.** Maternal neglect resulting in nonorganic FTT should not be just left at that: the reasons need to be investigated. A mother who neglects her child (a form of child abuse) is also at risk for other forms of child abuse. In addition, she herself is at greater-than-average risk of being abused by her husband or partner. Remember that family violence begets family violence, and in this case we already have established that a form of family violence (child abuse [neglect]) exists.

A7. **c.** The most likely cause of this child's short stature is Turner's syndrome. Noonan's syndrome (an autosomal dominant trait with widely variable expressivity) also has short stature and neck webbing as its most common presentation. It can be easily distinguished from Turner's syndrome, however, by its normal chromosome complement and characteristic facies including hypertelorism and ptosis. Patients with Turner's syndrome will have either a 45 XO chromosome complement or a mosaic involving loss of sex chromosomal material.

Trisomy 21 will usually be recognized long before the age of 13 years. The fragile X syndrome is a syndrome associated with mental retardation and macroorchidism in males.

A8. **a.** The most common cause of short stature in children is short parents. When a short child who is growing at a normal rate and has a normal bone age is found to have a strong family history of short stature, familial short stature is the most likely cause. Other causes of short stature include constitutional delay of growth, chromosomal abnormalities, intrauterine growth retardation, chronic diseases such as renal disease or inflammatory bowel disease, hypothyroidism, adrenal hyperplasia, growth hormone deficiency or resistance, and psychosocial dwarfism.

A9. **b.** Bone age determination can distinguish between the two most common causes of short stature: familial short stature and constitutional delay of growth. Children with familial short stature have normal bone ages. Constitutional delay of growth, which is really a delay in reaching ultimate height and sexual maturation, presents with delayed bone age and delayed sexual maturation. Hypothyroidism and growth hormone deficiency usually present with a delayed bone age.

A10. **d.** Inadequate growth in children may be associated with an unfavorable psychologic environment. In this situation the child may show transiently low human growth hormone levels during periods of stress. He or she may also have behavioral, sleep, and eating disturbances. Both growth and growth hormone levels return to normal when the psychologic stressors are removed.

A11. **e.** Recommended investigations in a child with FTT or a child in which short stature is unlikely to be familial in nature should include CBC, complete urinalysis, serum BUN and creatinine, erythrocyte sedimentation rate (ESR), serum thyroxine, TSH, and bone age hand x-ray. Serum lead level, stool for ova and parasites, and liver enzymes (serum bilirubin, alanine aminotransferase, and aspartate aminotransferase) may be considered when the clinical history is suggestive.

SOLUTION TO THE SHORT ANSWER MANAGEMENT PROBLEM

Ten disorders that may manifest themselves as FTT in infants and children include:
   a. Emotional/psychologic factors
   b. Central nervous system (CNS) abnormality
   c. Gastrointestinal (GI) malformation or disease (cleft palate, Hirschsprung's disease, gastroesophageal reflux, cardiac failure, inflammatory bowel disease, liver disease, parasites)
   d. Congenital heart disease
   e. Chronic renal disease (anomalies, renal failure)
   f. Chromosomal disorders (Down syndrome, Turner's syndrome)
   g. Chronic infection (GI system, kidney, pulmonary system, CNS, tuberculosis, human immunodeficiency virus)
   h. Inborn error of metabolism/hypothyroidism
   i. Malignancies (neuroblastoma, nephroblastoma, glioma)
   j. Congenital low birth weight syndrome (fetal alcohol or drug exposure)

SUMMARY OF THE DIAGNOSIS AND TREATMENT OF FTT AND SHORT STATURE IN INFANTS AND CHILDREN

1. FTT:
   a. Nonorganic: Psychologic FTT; maternal deprivation; child neglect; lack of education regarding feeding; errors in feeding. Suspect family dysfunction and monitor carefully in these cases.

b. Organic FTT: See the Solution to the Short Answer Management Problem.
c. Treatment:
   1) An initial period of hospitalization is indicated in most cases. Unlimited feedings (especially to any infant) should be given in these cases, and a complete investigation should be performed to attempt to elucidate the cause.
   2) When the child goes home, careful and frequent observation is indicated, especially in the initial period. Some of these observations should take place in the environment (the home) in which the problems began (for nonorganic FTT). Weekly observation is indicated initially.

2. Short stature:
   a. Familial short stature is the most common cause.
   b. Familial short stature can be differentiated from constitutional delay of growth (the second most common cause) by bone age.
   c. Other causes of short stature include chromosomal abnormalities, intrauterine growth retardation, hypothyroidism, psychosocial dwarfism, Turner's syndrome, and growth hormone deficiency.
   d. Investigations of a child with short stature should include CBC, complete urinalysis, serum BUN/creatinine, liver enzymes and bilirubin, ESR, serum thyroxine, TSH, and x-ray of the hands and wrist for bone age.

SUGGESTED READING

Needleman RD: Growth and development. In Behrman R, ed: *Nelson textbook of pediatrics*, ed 15, Philadelphia, 1998, WB Saunders.

PROBLEM·84

DIAGNOSIS AND TREATMENT OF SERIOUS RESPIRATORY SYNDROMES IN INFANTS AND CHILDREN

"Do Something! My Baby Can't Breathe."

Case 1 ■ An 18-Month-Old Infant with an Upper Respiratory Tract Infection

An 18-month-old infant is brought to the Emergency Department by his mother. He developed an upper respiratory tract infection 2 days ago and suddenly this evening developed a harsh, barky cough and difficulty breathing.

On examination, the child is coughing. His respiratory rate is 40 breaths per minute and he is in some respiratory distress. The breath sounds that are heard appear to be transmitted from the upper airway. There are nasal flaring and suprasternal, infrasternal, and intercostal retractions. The child's temperature is 38.5° C.

SELECT THE BEST ANSWER TO THE FOLLOWING QUESTIONS

Q1. What is the most likely diagnosis in this child?
   a. viral pneumonia
   b. acute epiglottis
   c. bronchiolitis
   d. croup
   e. bacterial pneumonia

Q2. The causative agent responsible for this child's condition is most likely which of the following?
   a. adenovirus
   b. *Pneumococcus*
   c. parainfluenza virus
   d. *Haemophilus influenzae*
   e. respiratory syncytial virus (RSV)

Q3. What is the treatment of choice for moderate cases of the disorder described?
   a. racemic epinephrine
   b. aerosolized budesonide
   c. humidification
   d. dexamethasone intravenously
   e. a, b and c

Case 2 ■ A 19-Month-Old Male with a Cough, Wheezing, Dyspnea, and Irritability

A 19-month-old boy with an acute onset of rhinorrhea and cough, which has progressed to wheezing, dyspnea, and irritability is brought to the Emergency Department by his mother. On examination, the child's temperature is 38° C. There are rhonchi heard in all lobes. His respiratory rate is 50 breaths per minute, and he exhibits flaring of the alae nasi and use of the accessory muscles of respiration resulting in intercostal and subcostal retractions. Widespread fine rales are heard at the end of inspiration and in early expiration. The expiratory phase is prolonged, and wheezing is audible throughout the lung fields.

Q4. What is the most likely diagnosis in this patient?
   a. viral pneumonia
   b. acute epiglottis
   c. bronchiolitis
   d. croup
   e. bacterial pneumonia

Q5. The treatment of this child at this time may include which of the following?
  a. humidified oxygen
  b. nebulized bronchodilators
  c. ribavirin
  d. all of the above
  e. none of the above

Q6. What is the causative agent most likely responsible for this child's condition?
  a. adenovirus
  b. *Pneumococcus*
  c. rhinovirus
  d. *H. influenzae*
  e. RSV

Case 3 ■ A 5-Year-Old Child Who Has Been Talking Strangely and Is Anorexic

A 5-year-old child is brought to the Emergency Department by his mother. The mother tells you that for the past 24 hours the child has been "talking strangely" and drooling. He has had no appetite and has not been drinking.

Q7. Based on this history, what is the diagnosis of major concern?
  a. viral pneumonia
  b. acute epiglottis
  c. bronchiolitis
  d. croup
  e. bacterial pneumonia

Q8. What is the diagnostic procedure that can substantiate the diagnosis you made in response to Question 7 for the patient described in Case 3?
  a. a white blood cell count (WBC)
  b. an erythrocyte sedimentation rate
  c. a chest x-ray
  d. a lateral x-ray of the neck
  e. a computed tomography scan of the head and neck

Q9. What is the antibiotic treatment of choice for the patient described in Case 3?
  a. intravenous (IV) ampicillin
  b. oral (PO) ampicillin
  c. IV/intramuscular (IM) ceftriaxone
  d. IV ciprofloxacin
  e. PO ciprofloxacin

Q10. What is the causative organism most often responsible for the condition described in Case 3?
  a. parainfluenza virus

  b. RSV
  c. *H. influenzae*
  d. rhinovirus
  e. *Pneumococcus*

Q11. Which of the following statement(s) concerning wheezing in infancy is (are) true?
  a. it is sometimes difficult to differentiate bronchial asthma from bronchiolitis by clinical assessment
  b. children with bronchiolitis who do not develop asthma may be inappropriately labeled as asthmatics
  c. the relationship between bronchiolitis and ongoing airway hyperreactivity is unclear; ongoing bronchial hyperreactivity or asthma may be precipitated by an acute episode of bronchiolitis
  d. none of the above statements is true
  e. all of the above statements are true

Case 4 ■ A 6-Year-Old Male in Severe Respiratory Distress

A 6-year-old male is brought to the Emergency Department with an acute asthmatic attack. He developed a respiratory tract infection 3 days ago and began wheezing 24 hours ago. He had his first asthma attack 2 years ago and usually has one attack per month. He is on no prophylactic medications.

On examination, the child is in severe respiratory distress. His respiratory rate is 48 breaths per minute. He has marked indrawing of the accessory muscles of respiration. Generalized wheezes are heard throughout the lung fields.

Q12. What is the treatment of choice in this patient at this time?
  a. IV sodium cromoglycate
  b. IV corticosteroids
  c. nebulized beta-agonist with or without ipratropium bromide
  d. humidified oxygen
  e. b, c, and d

Q13. Pulmonary function tests are performed on the patient described in Case 4. Which of the following parameters of pulmonary function would be expected to increase after administration of a bronchodilator?
  a. forced vital capacity (FVC)
  b. forced expiratory volume in 1 second (FEV_1)
  c. maximum expiratory flow between 25% and 75% of the vital capacity (MEF 25-75)

d. total lung capacity (TLC)
e. b and c

Q14. The patient described in Case 4 is treated and eventually discharged. You learn his attacks are primarily allergic in origin and decide to begin prophylactic therapy. Which of the following is the prophylactic agent of choice?
a. an inhaled beta-agonist
b. PO theophylline
c. an inhaled corticosteroid
d. sodium cromoglycate
e. a PO corticosteroid

Case 5 ■ A 12-Year-Old Male
with Exercise-Induced Asthma

A 12-year-old boy comes to your office for assessment of exercise-induced asthma. The child is fine when at rest but develops shortness of breath and wheezing at the end of or during a vigorous exercise session.

Q15. What is the treatment of first choice in this child?
a. sodium cromoglycate
b. an inhaled beta-agonist
c. PO theophylline
d. an inhaled corticosteroid
e. a PO corticosteroid

SHORT ANSWER MANAGEMENT PROBLEM
Defend the statement, "All that wheezes is not asthma."

ANSWERS

A1. **d.** This child has croup. A child with croup (the most common form being acute laryngotracheobronchitis) usually has a typical upper respiratory tract infection for several days before the brassy cough, inspiratory stridor, and respiratory distress become apparent. As the infection extends downward involving the bronchi and the bronchioles, respiratory difficulty increases and the expiratory phase of respiration becomes labored and prolonged.

The child often appears restless, agitated, and frightened. The child's temperature may be only slightly elevated, or it may be as high as 39° to 40° C (102° to 104° F).

Croup can be characterized based on the severity of symptoms. In mild croup, stridor is present with excitement only or is present at rest without signs of respiratory distress. In moderate croup, stridor occurs at rest and there is intercostal, suprasternal, or subcostal retractions. In severe croup, there is severe respiratory distress, decreased air entry, and an altered level of consciousness. Children with severe croup should be hospitalized and intubated under controlled conditions.

A2. **c.** Most cases of croup (the most common form being acute laryngotracheobronchitis) are caused by the parainfluenza group of viruses. RSV, influenza, and adenoviruses may be implicated in some cases.

A3. **e.** Until recently, the treatment of choice for mild to moderate cases of croup was simple humidification. However, it has clearly established that nebulized budesonide (an inhaled glucosteroid) or PO dexamethasone are of significant benefit in young children with mild to moderate croup. In moderate or severe cases, nebulized racemic epinephrine has been proven to be of value.

A4. **c.** This child has bronchiolitis. The signs and symptoms of bronchiolitis have been well described in the clinical history just noted.

Roentgenographic examination reveals hyperinflation of the lungs and an increased anteroposterior diameter of the chest on lateral view. Scattered areas of consolidation are found in about one third of patients and are caused by either atelectasis secondary to obstruction or to inflammation of the alveoli. The WBC and the differential are usually within normal limits.

A5. **d.** Humidified oxygen is of benefit in the treatment of infants and children with bronchiolitis.

Ribavirin (Virazole), an antiviral agent, is effective in reducing the severity of bronchiolitis caused by RSV infection when administered early in the course of the illness. Its use is indicated in children under 2 years of age who have severe infection documented by fluorescent antibodies or culture or strongly suspected on epidemiologic grounds and whose hospitalization is likely to exceed 3 days. It should also be administered to patients with milder bronchiolitis caused by RSV infection who have underlying severe chronic illness as a result of cardiac disease.

Bronchodilating aerosolized drugs are frequently used empirically. Epinephrine or alpha-adrenergic agents have a theoretic basis for use but have not been adequately tested.

Antibiotics have no therapeutic value unless there is a secondary bacterial infection.

A6. **e.** The agent responsible for most cases of bronchiolitis is the RSV. Other causes include the parainfluenza 3 virus, mycoplasma, some adenoviruses, and occasionally other viruses. Adenovirus-caused bronchiolitis may be responsible for long-term complications including bronchiolitis obliterans and unilateral hyperlucent lung syndrome.

A7. **b.** This child must be suspected of having acute epiglottitis until proven otherwise.

Acute epiglottitis, a potentially lethal condition, occurs in children ages 2 to 7 years old and peaks at the age of 3.5 years. The incidence of this disease has dropped dramatically thanks to routine immunization against *H. influenzae.* Acute epiglottitis is characterized by a fulminating course of fever, sore throat, dyspnea, rapidly progressive respiratory obstruction, and prostration. In hours epiglottitis can lead to complete obstruction of the airway and death unless adequate treatment is administered.

Respiratory distress is the first symptom. The child may be well at bedtime but awakens later in the evening with a high fever, aphonia, drooling, and moderate to severe respiratory distress with stridor. An older child will often complain of a "sore throat."

Severe respiratory distress may ensue within minutes or hours of the onset with inspiratory stridor, hoarseness, a brassy cough, irritability, and restlessness. Drooling and dyspnea are common.

A8. **d.** On physical examination, the child is noted as having moderate to severe respiratory distress with inspiratory and, at times, expiratory stridor; flaring of the alae nasi; and inspiratory retractions of the suprasternal notch, the supraclavicular and intercostal spaces, and the subcostal area. The pharynx is inflamed, and there is often an abundance of mucus and saliva, which may also result in rhonchi. With progression, stridor and breath sounds may become diminished as the patient tires. There may be a brief period of air hunger with restlessness and agitation, which may progress to cyanosis, coma, and death. The other presentation is that of only mild hoarseness and a large, shiny, cherry-red epiglottis.

The child's pharynx should not be examined with a tongue depressor. The diagnosis requires direct visualization by laryngoscopy with the ability to intubate immediately at hand. The diagnosis can be made by a lateral x-ray of the neck, which will clearly show the swollen epiglottitis.

A9. **c.** See Answer 10.

A10. **c.** The treatment of choice for a child with acute epiglottitis is as follows:
   a. An artificial airway must be immediately established. Untreated patients have a substantial

mortality even when observed in the hospital with appropriate intubation equipment nearby.
   b. Ceftriaxone (100 mg/kg/24 hr) or ampicillin (200 mg/kg/24 hr) and chloramphenicol (100 mg/kg/24 hr) should be given pending culture and susceptibility reports because of the increasing possibility of ampicillin-resistant strains of *H. influenzae* being the cause of the condition.
   c. Supplemental oxygen: The causative organism associated with acute epiglottitis is *H. influenzae.* As mentioned, there are increasing problems with ampicillin-resistant *Haemophilus* species.

A11. **e.** All of the statements are true. It is sometimes difficult to differentiate bronchial asthma from bronchiolitis by clinical assessment. Thus an inappropriate diagnosis of asthma may be made, and the child may be labeled as having this disease. The relationship, however, between bronchiolitis and asthma is unclear; young infants with bronchiolitis may be at an increased risk of developing asthma later in childhood. Bronchial asthma may be precipitated by an acute episode of bronchiolitis.

A12. **e.** This child is in severe respiratory distress from the current asthmatic attack and should be treated with a combination of an IV corticosteroid (determined on a milligram-per-kilogram basis) and a nebulized beta-agonist with or without ipratropium bromide. Oxygen and fluids should also be administered. Early and aggressive treatment will prevent deterioration and possibly even death.

A13. **e.** Pulmonary function testing before and after administration of an aerosol bronchodilator will assess the degree of reversibility of airway obstruction. Normally the administration of a bronchodilator will result in an increase in FEV_1 and MEF 25-75. FVC and TLC, which may already be increased in patients with bronchial asthma, will not increase further after administration of a bronchodilator.

A14. **d.** In mild chronic asthma, sodium cromolyn is an effective prophylaxis agent. It is particularly effective in allergic conditions and is more desirable than the use of chronic steroids. However, an inhaled beta-agonist remains the drug of choice in acute exacerbation.

A15. **b.** Exercise-induced asthma may be manifested by both an early (in terms of time following exercise) and late bronchoconstriction. Early bronchoconstriction begins 3 to 8 minutes following exercise and late bronchoconstriction occurs 4 to 6 hours after exercise. Inhaled sodium cromoglycate will block both early and late bronchoconstriction, but is less effective than inhaled beta-agonists. Inhaled beta-agonists will block only early bronchoconstriction but are extremely effective. Corticosteroids will block only late bronchoconstriction. Leukotriene modifiers and long-acting beta-agonists have also been found to be effective in exercise-induced asthma.

SOLUTION TO THE SHORT ANSWER MANAGEMENT PROBLEM

It is important to realize that there are causes for wheezing in infancy and childhood other than asthma. Although asthma remains the most common cause of wheezing, it is by no means the only cause. The second most common cause is bronchiolitis. As described earlier, the association between asthma and bronchiolitis remains unclear. It may very well be the case that an attack of acute bronchiolitis actually predisposes a child to develop asthma at a later date.

In addition to asthma and bronchiolitis as causes of wheezing, remember airway obstruction. This would most commonly be caused by the lodging of a foreign body in the trachea or in one of its branches.

As a corollary to "all that wheezes is not asthma" we can add "all asthma does not wheeze." This is particularly true with the so-called cough variant asthma, in which the principal manifestation is cough. It is estimated that up to one third of children with asthma exhibits this variation, a variation that unfortunately all too often goes unnoticed or undiagnosed.

SUMMARY OF THE DIAGNOSIS AND TREATMENT OF SERIOUS RESPIRATORY SYNDROMES IN INFANTS AND CHILDREN

1. Major worrisome symptoms:
   a. Harsh, barky cough
   b. Stridor and respiratory distress
   c. Drooling
   d. Wheezing

2. Croup: Most common form is acute laryngotracheobronchitis. A harsh, barky cough in a young infant is almost pathognomonic of croup. Respiratory distress can be pronounced.
   a. Causative agent: Parainfluenza virus
   b. Treatment, which used to consist of humidified oxygen almost exclusively: Croup now has been shown to be effectively treated with PO or nebulized corticosteroids even in mild to moderate cases. Racemic epinephrine is effective in moderate to severe cases.

3. Bronchiolitis: May produce very significant respiratory distress and stridor, rales, and wheezing—expiratory phase prolonged.
   a. Causative agent: RSV
   b. Treatment: Humidified oxygen and ribavirin

4. Acute epiglottitis: Drooling, very sore throat, and difficulty swallowing liquids (this can be used as a diagnostic test). Do not attempt visualization of the epiglottis unless you are prepared to intubate.
   A lateral x-ray of the neck will help substantiate the diagnosis (swollen epiglottis seen on lateral x-ray of the neck).
   a. Causative agent: *H. influenzae*
   b. Treatment: IV/IM intubation and ceftriaxone

5. Asthma: Most common cause of wheezing in infants and children
   a. Causative agent: Often familial; often associated with some extrinsic allergen in children
   b. Treatment:
      1) For acute, severe cases, use IV steroids, nebulized beta-agonists, and oxygen.
      2) Chronic cases: Inhaled corticosteroids are added in more severe cases. Inhaled beta-agonists are used in mild cases.
      3) Exercise-induced: Beta-agonists should be used.
   c. Other information:
      1) Asthma still kills. Asthma should be treated aggressively.
      2) Not all that wheezes is asthma.
      3) Not all asthma wheezes.

SUGGESTED READINGS

Adelman A: Treatment of croup with nebulized dexamethasone, *J Fam Pract* 43(1):19-20, 1996.

Belfer RA: Group A beta-hemolytic streptococcal epiglottitis as a complication of varicella infection, *Pediatr Emerg Care* 12(3):203-204, 1996.

Geelhoed GC: Croup, *Pediatr Pulmonol* 23(5):370-374, 1997.

Hickerson SL et al: Epiglottitis, *South Med J* 89(5):487-490, 1996.

Johnson DW et al: A comparison of nebulized budesonide, intramuscular dexamethasone, and placebo for moderately severe croup, *N Engl J Med* 339(8):498-503, 1998.

Kaditis AG, Wald ER: Viral croup: current diagnosis and treatment, *Pediatr Infect Dis J* 17(9): 827-834, 1998.

Klassen TP et al: Nebulized budesonide and oral dexamethasone for treatment of croup: a randomized controlled trial, *JAMA* 279(20):1629-1632, 1998.

Orenstein DM: Brochiolitis. In Behrman R, ed: *Nelson textbook of pediatrics*, ed 15, Philadelphia, 1998, WB Saunders.

PROBLEM · 85

OTITIS MEDIA

"My Child Won't Become Deaf, Will He?"

Case 1 ■ A 24-Month-Old Child Who Is Constantly Crying and Who Complains of a Right-Sided Earache

A mother comes to your office with her 24-month-old daughter. The child developed an upper respiratory tract infection approximately 1 week ago. The infection started with cough, congestion, and rhinorrhea. Two days ago the child began complaining of pain in the right ear.

On examination, the child has nasal congestion and a hyperemic throat. The left tympanic membrane is normal and the right tympanic membrane is bulging and red. There appears to be fluid behind it. The lungs are clear. The child's temperature is 39.5° C.

SELECT THE BEST ANSWER TO THE FOLLOWING QUESTIONS

Q1. What is the most likely diagnosis in this child?
a. acute otitis media
b. otitis media without effusion
c. chronic otitis media (COM)
d. otitis media with effusion (OME)
e. none of the above

Case 2 ■ An 8-Month-Old Male with an Upper Respiratory Tract Infection but No External Signs of Acute Ear Infection

An 8-month-old male is brought to your office the same day as the child in Case 1. He, too, has had an upper respiratory tract infection but has no signs of acute ear infection such as pain, pulling at his ears, or fever.

On examination, there is a middle-ear effusion, confirmed by pneumatic otoscopy and the tympanic membrane is dull but not red.

Q2. What is the most likely diagnosis in this child?
a. acute otitis media
b. otitis media without effusion
c. COM
d. OME
e. none of the above

Case 3 ■ A 7-Month-Old Child with an Upper Respiratory Infection and Erythema of the Tympanic Membrane

A 7-month-old child is brought to your office by his mother the same day as you saw the children in Cases 1 and 2. He has had an upper respiratory tract infection for the past 3 days.

On examination, there is erythema of the left tympanic membrane with opacification. There are no other signs or symptoms.

Q3. What is the most likely diagnosis in this patient?
a. acute otitis media
b. otitis media without effusion
c. COM
d. OME
e. none of the above

Case 4 ■ A 9-Month-Old Child with a Discharge from His Ear

This is obviously "ear day" in your practice. A fourth child, 9 months of age, is brought to your office with a discharge from the left ear that has been present for the last 4 days. The child has a history of frequent ear infections, all of which have been treated with antibiotics.

Q4. What is the most likely diagnosis in this patient?
a. acute otitis media
b. otitis media without effusion
c. COM with perforation
d. OME
e. none of the above

Q5. Referring again to the patient you saw in Case 1, which of the following statements regarding her condition described is false?
a. this condition usually begins a few days after the onset of an upper respiratory tract infection
b. this condition is usually associated with eustachian tube dysfunction
c. environmental factors such as pollen, dusts, molds, and cigarette smoke are unlikely to be associated with an increase in the incidence of this condition
d. many cases of this condition are considered to be bacterial in origin
e. none of the above statements is false

Q6. What are the three most common bacterial organisms, in order of frequency, that are responsible for the condition described in the patient in Case 1?

a. pneumococcus, group A streptococci, *Haemophilus influenzae*

b. pneumococcus, *H. influenzae*, staphylococcus

c. pneumococcus, *H. influenzae*, *Moraxella catarrhalis*

d. *H. influenzae*, pneumococcus, group A streptococcus

e. *H. influenzae*, pneumococcus, *M. catarrhalis*

Q7. What is the drug of choice for the condition described in Case 1?

a. penicillin

b. amoxicillin

c. erythromycin-sulfamethoxazole

d. cefaclor

e. amoxicillin-clavulanic acid

Q8. A family practice resident who is working with you describes the condition of a child he has just seen. He describes a normal tympanic membrane behind which is significant fluid. He tells you, however, that there are no other symptoms associated with this effusion. He asks you what he should do. You should tell him to do which of the following?

a. forget about it; it's not bothering him

b. perform a myringotomy and suck out all the fluid that is present

c. perform a pneumatic otoscopy to assess the movement of the tympanic membrane

d. refer the child to an ear, nose, and throat (ENT) surgeon for myringotomy, tubes, and an adenoidectomy (you might as well suggest a tonsillectomy at the same time and get everything over at once)

e. none of the above

Q9. Which of the following statements regarding treatment of the condition described in Case 1 is (are) false?

a. earache and fever should be treated with aspirin

b. topical decongestants are useful in improving eustachian tube dysfunction

c. eardrops provide significant relief in children with the condition described in Case 1

d. systemic antihistamine-decongestants have been shown to improve the symptoms and shorten the course of the condition described in Case 1

e. all of the above statements are false

Q10. The condition described in the patient in Case 1 has occurred at least once in what percentage of children by 18 months of age?

a. 10%

b. 35%

c. 74%

d. 18%

e. 29%

Q11. How is *recurrent otitis media* defined?

a. three or more episodes of acute otitis media that occur within 6 months, or four episodes that occur within a year

b. four or more episodes of acute otitis media that occur within 6 months, or five episodes that occur within a year

c. five or more episodes of acute otitis media that occur within 6 months, or six episodes that occur within a year

d. six or more episodes of acute otitis media that occur within 6 months, or eight episodes within a year

e. two or more episodes of acute otitis media that occur within 6 months, or three or more episodes that occur within a year

Q12. Which of the following statements regarding recurrent otitis media is true?

a. recurrent bouts of acute otitis media usually occur in the winter or early spring

b. recurrent bouts of acute otitis media should be managed by myringotomy and the insertion of ventilation tubes

c. medical management appears to be less effective and is not as safe as myringotomy and tubes in children with recurrent acute otitis media

d. amoxicillin does not have a major role to play in the management of recurrent acute otitis media

e. none of the above statements is true

Q13. Which of the following is (are) possible intracranial complications of otitis media?

a. meningitis

b. subdural empyema

c. brain abscess

d. all of the above

e. none of the above

Q14. Which of the following is (are) possible extracranial complications of otitis media?

a. mastoiditis

b. cholesteatoma

c. labyrinthitis

d. all of the above

e. none of the above

SHORT ANSWER MANAGEMENT PROBLEM

A mother comes to your office with her 18-month-old child following the treatment of an episode of acute otitis media. She states that the child was in considerable pain despite analgesics and antibiotics and asks you to refer her child to an ENT surgeon. She wishes to have "tubes" inserted in her child's ears. She has a number of friends who have had this done to their children following the first episode of acute otitis media and it has been extremely successful. Discuss how you would approach this problem.

ANSWERS

A1. **a.** Acute otitis media: This is also known as *acute suppurative, acute purulent,* or *acute bacterial otitis media.* pathophysiology is basically an effusion of the middle ear that becomes infected with viruses and/or bacteria. There is often a rapid onset of signs and symptoms such as fever; ear pain; a red, bulging, tympanic membrane; and fluid behind the middle ear.

A2. **d.** OME: This is also known as nonsuppurative, serous, or mucoid otitis media. This is manifested as otitis media without signs or symptoms of acute disease but with a middle-ear effusion. OME may be subdivided into acute, subacute, and chronic based on the duration of the effusion.

A3. **b.** Otitis media without effusion: This is also known as *myringitis.* It indicates the presence of erythema (redness) and opacification of the tympanic membranes without the presence of an effusion. This may be seen in the early stages of acute otitis media or as otitis media resolves.

A4. **c.** COM: This is synonymous with chronic suppurative, purulent, or intractable otitis media. There is a pronounced, intractable middle-ear pathologic condition with or without suppurative otorrhea. *Suppurative* refers to an active infection, and *otorrhea* refers to a discharge through a perforated tympanic membrane.

A5. **c.** Acute otitis media usually begins a few days after the onset of an upper respiratory tract infection. The upper respiratory tract infection usually produces eustachian tube dysfunction and obstruction. This subsequently leads to the accumulation of fluid in the middle ear. This fluid then becomes infected with a virus, a bacteria, or a virus followed by bacteria.

Environmental factors such as exposure to respiratory tract irritants (cigarette smoke, pollen, dust, molds) may increase the incidence of upper respiratory tract infection and acute otitis media. Supine nursing (habitually putting the infant to bed with a bottle) may also contribute to the incidence of otitis media.

A6. **c.** The bacteriology of acute otitis media suggests that the following bacterial organisms (in this order) are responsible for most cases of acute otitis media:
   a. *Pneumococcus*
   b. *H. influenzae*
   c. *M. catarrhalis*
   d. Group A streptococci
   e. *Staphylococcus aureus*

As mentioned previously, viruses have also been implicated as primary causative agents. Also, if a virus produces the primary infection, many of these cases will become secondarily infected with a bacterium.

A7. **b.** The drug of choice for acute otitis media in primary care practice is still amoxicillin. The usual length of treatment is 7 to 10 days. Although this has been challenged and does not apply to those patients with recurrent otitis, it is true for primary cases of acute infection.

A patient who does not improve on amoxicillin most likely has an infection with a beta-lactamase-producing organism. In this case, second-line agents including trimethoprim-sulfamethoxazole, erythromycin-sulfamethoxazole, or cefaclor can be used.

A8. **c.** The most reasonable maneuver to perform at this time is pneumatic otoscopy to assess the movement of the tympanic membrane. This will provide an accurate indication of whether or not there is fluid present in the middle-ear cavity. This easily performed maneuver is often omitted in primary care. Tympanometry is an acceptable alternative.

Referral to an ENT surgeon for myringotomy, tubes, adenoidectomy, and tonsillectomy is not indicated at this time. Similarly, the performance of a myringotomy in the office is an invasive and painful procedure. Observation or antibiotic treatment are options for therapy. See the Agency for Health Care Policy and Research guidelines.

A9. **e.** Symptoms of earache or fever should be treated with acetaminophen. Aspirin should be avoided because of the possible link to Reye's syndrome. Ear drops do not provide any symptomatic relief in otitis media and interfere with otoscopic examination and follow up.

Topical decongestants (sympathomimetic nose drops and sprays), used to relieve obstruction in the eustachian tube, and systemic antihistamine-decongestant combinations have not been shown to be effective in the treatment of otitis media. They affect neither the duration nor the severity of symptoms.

A10. **c.** Studies suggest that 35% of children have at least one episode of acute otitis media by 6 months of age; 74% have at least one episode between the ages of 6 months and 18 months.

A11. **a.** Recurrent otitis media is defined as three or more episodes of acute otitis media that occur within 6 months or four episodes within a year.

A12. **a.** Recurrent bouts of acute otitis usually occur in the winter or early spring. Such recurrent episodes can be managed to some extent with prophylactic antibiotics. Although a myringotomy and the insertion of ventilation tubes may ultimately have to be performed, it is not the first-line option. Medical management with antibiotics has been shown, in most studies, to be just as effective. Half-strength amoxicillin or sulfamethizole is reasonable prophylactic therapy.

A13. **d.** Otitis media is not always an innocuous diagnosis. Intracranial complications associated with otitis media include meningitis, subdural empyema, brain abscess, lateral sinus thrombosis, and focal otitis encephalitis.

A14. **d.** Extracranial complications and sequelae associated with otitis media include hearing loss, tympanic membrane perforation, chronic suppurative otitis media, mastoiditis, cholesteatoma, facial paralysis, tympanosclerosis, and labyrinthitis.

SOLUTION TO THE SHORT ANSWER MANAGEMENT PROBLEM

This is a difficult issue because the mother has come to your office expecting and wanting a referral to an ENT surgeon. At this time, we suggest you do the following:
a. Discuss the incidence of acute otitis media and point out to the mother that more children have had it than have not had it.
b. Emphasize that in most cases the symptoms resolve with simple antibiotic therapy.
c. Describe briefly the anatomy of the eustachian tube and point out that as her child grows, the probability of infections will continue to decrease.
d. Try to establish why she is so concerned and wants a referral at this time. Often (referring back to the biopsychosocial model) there are other issues that need to be addressed with the mother.
e. If the mother, despite all of your reassurance, insists on a referral, give her one. However, point out to the mother that the ENT surgeon is unlikely to want to put in tubes at this time.
f. Offer to discuss the issue of her child's otitis media or any other issues at any time. Provide for

the mother a framework in which she can begin to view you, the family physician, as her advocate in health care. She probably needs this more than anything else.

SUMMARY OF THE DIAGNOSIS AND TREATMENT OF OTITIS MEDIA

1. Acute otitis media is common in childhood. By 18 months of age, 74% of children have had at least one infection.

2. When discussing otitis media, use the right terminology. The Panel for the Definition and Classification of Otitis Media suggests the following:
   a. Otitis media without effusion
   b. Acute otitis media
   c. OME
   d. COM

3. Most common bacterial causative agents in order of frequency are *Pneumococci, H. influenzae, M. catarrhalis*, and group A streptococci.

4. Treatment of choice for acute otitis media in the primary care setting is still amoxicillin.

5. The definition of acute otitis is otalgia, fever, and irritability associated with a full or bulging tympanic membrane with effusion.

6. Decongestants-antihistamines and ear drops have not been shown to influence either the severity or duration of the symptoms.

7. Consider prophylactic antibiotics before considering myringotomy and tubes for the treatment of recurrent otitis media.

8. Remember that otitis media can produce complications. Treat otitis media with an antibiotic for at least 7 full days.

SUGGESTED READINGS

Dowell SF et al: Appropriate use of antibiotics for URIs in children. Part I. Otitis media and acute sinusitis, *Am Fam Physician* 58(5):1113-1118, 1998.

Dowell SF et al: Otitis media-principles of judicious use of antimicrobial agents, *Pediatrics* 101:165-171, 1998.

Hoppe HL, Johnson CE: Otitis media: focus on antimicrobial resistance and new treatment options, *Am J Health Syst Pharm* 55(18):1881-1897; quiz 1932-1933, 1998.

Otitis Media Guideline Panel and Consortium: *Otitis media with effusion in young children*, AHCPR pub no 940622, Rockville, Md, 1994, Department of Health and Human Services, Public Health Service, Agency for Health Care Policy and Research, *http://www.ahcpr.gov.*

PROBLEM·86

THE COMMON COLD

"Since My Youngest Started Nursery School, All I Do Is Wipe His Runny Nose."

Case 1 ■ A 4-Year-Old Child with a Runny Nose, a Sore Throat, and a Nonproductive Cough

A 4-year-old child with a runny nose, a sore throat, a feeling of "fullness" in his ears, and a nonproductive cough comes to your office with his mother. He has had these symptoms for the last 4 days and is not improving. He has had no fever, no chills, or any other symptoms.

On examination, the child's temperature is 37.6° C. His ears are clear, his throat is slightly hyperemic, and both sides of his nose look congested and red. His lung fields are clear, there is no significant cervical lymphadenopathy and no other localizing signs are present.

The child's history is unremarkable, and he has had no significant medical illnesses.

SELECT THE BEST ANSWER TO THE FOLLOWING QUESTIONS

Q1. What is the most likely diagnosis in this child?
   a. early streptococcal pharyngitis
   b. early mycoplasma pneumonia
   c. early acute otitis media
   d. early viral pneumonia
   e. none of the above

Q2. What is the most likely pathogen responsible for this condition?
   a. *Streptococcus pneumoniae*
   b. rhinovirus
   c. parainfluenza A
   d. adenovirus
   e. respiratory syncytial virus (RSV)

Q3. Investigations at this time should include which of the following?
   a. complete blood count (CBC)
   b. throat swab
   c. rapid antigen test for *Streptococcus* (ELISA)
   d. all of the above
   e. none of the above

Q4. Which of the following statements regarding the common cold is false?
   a. adults are affected less than children
   b. the highest incidence of the common cold is among children of kindergarten age

   c. adults with young children at home have an increased number of colds
   d. infants with older siblings have an increased incidence of colds
   e. none of the above is false; all of the above are true

Q5. Which of the following statements regarding treatment of the condition described is true?
   a. the use of antibiotics in the condition described in Case 1 has been shown to decrease the probability of complications; their routine use is reasonable
   b. vitamin C has definitely shown to decrease the frequency of occurrences of the condition described in Case 1
   c. interferon shows promise for the treatment of rhinovirus-caused upper respiratory tract infections
   d. rhinoviruses associated with the condition described in Case 1 have not been shown to be temperature sensitive
   e. antihistamines have not been shown to be effective in reducing symptoms in the condition described in Case 1

Q6. Children of kindergarten age are subject to how many colds on an average yearly basis?
   a. 12
   b. 7
   c. 3
   d. 6
   e. 8

Q7. What is the most effective preventive measure against the common cold?
   a. megadoses of vitamin C
   b. meticulous hand-washing
   c. extra sleep
   d. avoiding all contact with children and adults who have a cold
   e. none of the above

SHORT ANSWER MANAGEMENT PROBLEM

A 28-year-old male comes to your office with "a cold." He has had the cold for approximately 10 days and his rhinorrhea, cough, and congestion continue. He tells you that his wife has just seen her family doctor for the same symptoms. An antibiotic was prescribed for his wife, and he asks you to prescribe the same for him. On examination, he has nasal congestion and a hyperemic throat. No other abnormalities are found. Discuss your approach to this patient's request.

ANSWERS

A1. **e.** This child most likely has the common cold. Although the fullness in his ears may be associated with fluid in the middle-ear cavity, the absence of fever, pain, and hyperemia on the tympanic membranes makes acute otitis media unlikely. Movement of the tympanic membranes would further clarify the likelihood of fluid collection in the middle ear.

The presence of a runny nose and a cough significantly diminishes the probability of streptococcal pharyngitis.

Although viral pneumonia or mycoplasma pneumonia may develop, there is no evidence of either of these now.

A2. **b.** The most common cause of the common cold is a rhinovirus. Rhinoviruses are responsible for approximately 25% of all cases of the common cold. Influenza viruses; parainfluenzae types A, B, and C; RSVs; and mumps and measles viruses are responsible for many others. Other viruses that cause coldlike symptoms include coronaviruses, adenoviruses, certain enteric cytopathic human orphan viruses, and coxsackievirus.

More than 100 serospecific rhinovirus types have been established, and many viruses remain untyped.

The absence of significant fever, cervical lymphadenopathy, and exudates along with the presence of rhinorrhea and cough significantly decrease the probability of *S. pneumoniae* as a cause of this patient's symptoms.

A3. **e.** At the present time no investigations should be initiated. As the pretest probability of a streptococcal pharyngitis is very low, it is inappropriate to order a CBC, a throat swab, a rapid antigen test for streptococcus, or any other investigations at the present time.

A4. **e.** In general, the common cold affects children significantly more frequently than adults. The highest incidence is among children of kindergarten age. Adults with young children in the home do themselves have an increased number of colds, as do infants with older siblings. At times parents often notice the latter (the "second sibling syndrome") and sometimes need reassurance that their children do not have some other constitutional weakness.

A5. **c.** Interferon has been used experimentally as a nasal spray and, when studied, has been shown to prevent 75% of rhinovirus-caused colds. It may hold promise as a future prophylactic measure.

Antibiotics have not been shown to reduce the incidence of complications and thus should not be used in a prophylactic fashion.

Vitamin C, although extremely controversial, has not been shown to be effective in reducing the frequency or severity of symptoms. This is, however, a difficult area to study objectively because of problems associated with measuring improvement in symptoms.

Rhinoviruses are temperature sensitive. A controlled study testing warm (30° C) humidified air against hot (45° C) humidified air to provide nasal hyperthermia for 20 to 30 minutes has demonstrated a significant reduction in the severity and duration of common cold symptoms. Thus it may be that this "old-fashioned" remedy has some basis in fact.

Antihistamines have been found to be helpful in reducing symptoms of the common cold. Antihistamines act through nonspecific sedating or anticholinergic mechanisms rather than through any histamine-releasing action of the virus. As well, pseudoephedrine, alone or in combination with antihistamines, is also effective in reducing symptoms. Analgesics, such as acetylsalicylic acid or acetaminophen, have not been shown to have any significant effect on the duration or the severity of the common cold.

A6. **a.** Children of kindergarten age are subject to an average of 12 colds annually, whereas school-aged children are subject to an average of 7 colds annually. Adolescents and adults are subject to an average of 3 colds annually.

A7. **b.** The most effective preventive measure against the common cold is meticulous hand-washing and avoidance of contact with the face or nose. There is increasing evidence that aerosol spread of the cold viruses is less important than indirect spread. Experiments suggest that cold-causing viruses can be spread by self-inoculation from deposits of virus on such surfaces as plastics to the surface of the finger, and then transferred to mucous membranes of the nose and eye. This is particularly true if the inoculum is still moist.

Extra sleep and megadoses of vitamin C have not been shown to be at all effective.

It is unrealistic to suggest avoiding all contact with children and adults who have colds. Cold viruses are everywhere and will continue to be everywhere.

SOLUTION TO THE SHORT ANSWER MANAGEMENT PROBLEM

The prescription of antibiotics for an obviously viral infection (the common cold is probably the best example) is likely the most frequent "mistake" made by family physicians. It is obviously a lot easier to prescribe an antibiotic for the child than to explain to the parent why one is not needed. Considering that upper respiratory tract infections are the most frequent presenting complaint to a family physician's office, this "mistake" may actually happen several times a day in an average practice. A reasonable approach to take to this patient's request may be as follows:

a. Explain the viral nature of the symptoms and your certainty in coming to that conclusion in the patient.

b. Explain the side effects of antibiotics including drug intolerance, drug allergy, and the possibility of creating an environment in the patient's body that promotes the growth of resistant organisms.

c. Carefully go over some alternatives to antibiotic therapy that the patient may pursue. These include the use of steam, the use of antihistamines for symptomatic relief, and the importance of adequate rest.

d. Take the opportunity to discuss how meticulous hand-washing and related hygienic measures can significantly decrease spread of the common cold among family members.

e. Repeat the following age-old edict to the patient: "The symptoms will abate in a week with antibiotics and in 7 days without" (Having said that, remember that 30% of patients with common cold symptoms who had visited a physician still had a cough and a runny nose by the eighth day.)

f. Do not compromise your principles and prescribe an antibiotic when you know it is, at best, not indicated and possibly harmful. If the patient insists on an antibiotic, consider this an opportunity to discuss your philosophy of care with the patient: have the patient consider whether or not he is comfortable with the advice you are giving. If not, you should ask the patient if he really wishes to continue as a patient in your practice.

This can actually be done in a very pleasant manner. There is rarely a problem in reaching a mutually agreeable position. It really comes down to a question of trust between the patient and the physician.

SUMMARY OF THE DIAGNOSIS AND TREATMENT OF THE COMMON COLD

1. As the most common presentation of an upper respiratory tract infection, it is the most common problem presenting to the family physician.

2. Viral infections are the major, if not the only, cause of common colds.

3. Rhinovirus is the most common pathogen (25%); influenza; parainfluenza A, B, and C; and RSV make up another 15%.

4. No laboratory investigations are necessary: The combination of rhinorrhea, cough, congestion, sneezing, and a sore throat (or some reasonable combination) in the absence of significant fever, cervical nodes, or an exudate virtually rules out streptococcal pharyngitis.

5. Prevention of spread to family members is best accomplished by meticulous hygiene. Self-inoculation is more important than aerosol spread.

6. Treatment is symptomatic: Steam and antihistamines. Interferon given prophylactically may hold some hope for the future.

7. Resist the temptation to prescribe antibiotics. Remember, "a week with antibiotics, 7 days without."

SUGGESTED READINGS

Dowell SF et al: Appropriate use of antibiotics for URIs in children. Part II. Cough, pharyngitis and the common cold: The pediatric URI consensus team, *Am Fam Physician* 58(6):1335-1342, 1345, 1998.

Maltinski G: Nasal disorders and sinusitis, *Prim Care* 25(3):663-683, 1998.

Marshall S: Zinc gluconate and the common cold: Review of randomized control trials, *Can Fam Physician* 1037-1042, 1998.

Mossad SB: Treatment of the common cold, *Br Med J* 317(7150):33-36, 1998.

Saroea HG: Common colds: Causes, potential cures, and treatment, *Can Fam Physician* 39:2215-2220, 1993.

PROBLEM·87

STREPTOCOCCAL INFECTIONS IN CHILDREN

"You Mean My Little Boy's Sore Throat Can Cause Heart Problems?"

Case 1 ■ A 4-Year-Old Male with an Extremely Sore Throat

A 4-year-old male is brought to your office by his mother. The child has had a fever, chills, pain on swallowing, and pain in both ears for the past 3 days.

On examination, the child has a temperature of 39.5° C. He has tender anterior cervical lymphadenopathy and exudates on both tonsils. There is no hepatomegaly or splenomegaly present. He has no rhinorrhea, no cough, and no other respiratory tract symptoms. He is developing a fine macular-papular rash over his body.

He had a similar episode of sore throat 6 months ago, and another episode 15 months ago. He has had no other significant illnesses. He has no allergies.

SELECT THE BEST ANSWER
TO THE FOLLOWING QUESTIONS

Q1. What is the most likely diagnosis in this child?
a. bilateral otitis media
b. non-beta-hemolytic streptococcal pharyngitis
c. group A beta-hemolytic streptococcal pharyngitis
d. infectious mononucleosis
e. none of the above

Q2. At this time, what would you do?
a. perform a throat culture; wait before treating
b. perform a rapid *Streptococcus* test and begin treatment with penicillin
c. begin treatment with penicillin; no throat culture
d. do not test and do not treat
e. nobody really knows for sure

Q3. Regarding culture-confirmed streptococcal pharyngitis in childhood, which of the following statements is (are) true?
a. 80% of children with culture-confirmed streptococcal pharyngitis have tonsillar exudates
b. if pharyngitis is accompanied by exudates, 80% have culture-confirmed streptococcal pharyngitis
c. of all children with clinically documented pharyngitis, only 15% have culture-proven streptococcal pharyngitis
d. all of the above statements are true
e. none of the above statements is true

Q4. Scarlet fever is caused by which of the following organisms?
a. non-beta-hemolytic *Streptococcus*
b. group A beta-hemolytic *Streptococcus*
c. group B beta-hemolytic *Streptococcus*
d. group D *Streptococcus*
e. Lancefield group G *Streptococcus*

Q5. What percentage of children has group A *Streptococci* as part of the normal flora of the mouth and pharynx?
a. 5% to 10%
b. 10% to 15%
c. 15% to 20%
d. 25% to 35%
e. 35% to 50%

Q6. What is the most common organism responsible for bacterial endocarditis in children?
a. group A beta-hemolytic *Streptococcus*
b. group B beta-hemolytic *Streptococcus*
c. group D *Streptococcus* (*Enterococcus*)

d. *Streptococcus viridans*
e. group A non-beta-hemolytic *Streptococcus*

Q7. What is the most common cause of neonatal septicemia and meningitis?
a. group B *Streptococcus*
b. group A beta-hemolytic *Streptococcus*
c. group D *Streptococcus* (*Enterococci*)
d. *Streptococcus viridans*
e. group A non-beta-hemolytic *Streptococcus*

Q8. Erysipelas is most commonly caused by which of the following?
a. group A beta-hemolytic *Streptococcus*
b. *Streptococcus pneumoniae*
c. group B *Streptococcus*
d. *S. viridans*
e. Lancefield group G *Streptococcus*

Q9. Which of the following statements concerning impetigo (pyoderma) is (are) true?
a. deeper skin infections (cellulitis) may complicate impetigo
b. impetigo is most frequently caused by group A beta-hemolytic *Streptococcus*
c. colonization of unbroken skin usually precedes impetigo by 7 to 10 days
d. all of the above statements are true
e. none of the above statements is true

Q10. Which of the following statements concerning rapid strep test is (are) true?
a. the rapid strep test has a very high sensitivity
b. the rapid strep test has a very high specificity
c. the rapid strep test has a very low false positive rate
d. the rapid strep test has a very low false negative rate
e. b and c
f. a and d

Q11. Recurrent tonsillitis is usually caused by which of the following?
a. group A beta-hemolytic *Streptococcus*
b. parainfluenzae virus
c. rhinovirus
d. adenovirus
e. Epstein-Barr virus

Q12. Which of the following statements regarding tonsillitis and recurrent sore throat is (are) correct?
a. tonsillectomy often decreases the frequency of recurrent sore throat in young children
b. in many cases children who have not undergone a tonsillectomy experience a similar decrease in recurrent sore throat

c. tonsillectomy often decreases the frequency of recurrent upper respiratory tract infection (colds) in young children

d. a and b

e. all of the above statements are true

f. none of the above

Q13. Regarding tonsillar size and the frequency of tonsillitis, which of the following statements is (are) true?

a. most hypertrophic tonsils are actually normal in size

b. in children, tonsils are relatively larger in younger children than in older children

c. hypertrophic (larger) tonsils are more likely to become infected than nonhypertrophic (smaller) tonsils

d. a and b

e. all of the above

Q14. Which of the following is (are) complications of tonsillectomy?

a. hemorrhage

b. postoperative throat infection

c. pulmonary edema

d. a and b

e. all of the above

Q15. Which of the following is (are) manifestations of adenoidal hypertrophy?

a. mouth breathing

b. persistent rhinitis

c. snoring

d. a and c

e. all of the above

SHORT ANSWER MANAGEMENT PROBLEM
List the definite indications for performance of a tonsillectomy.

ANSWERS

A1. **c.** The most likely diagnosis in this child is group A beta-hemolytic streptococcal pharyngitis. The ear pain that the boy is experiencing is most likely referred pain from the throat. The absence of other symptoms (rhinorrhea and cough) favors bacterial pharyngitis over viral pharyngitis, although this is by no means certain.

A2. **b.** At this time you should do the following:

a. Make a provisional diagnosis of group A beta-hemolytic streptococcal infection.

b. Perform a rapid *Streptococcus* test, if negative (highly unlikely) culture the exudates bilaterally.

c. Begin the child on penicillin V in a milligram-per-kilogram dose three or four times per day.

d. Await the results of the throat culture.

There are a number of advantages to performing a rapid *Streptococcus* test and starting the child on penicillin if the test results are positive:

a. Early treatment with penicillin reduces the severity of symptoms from group A beta-hemolytic *Streptococcus* and decreases the time to resolution of symptoms.

b. Early treatment of group A beta-hemolytic *Streptococcus* infections reduces the incidence of subsequent rheumatic fever; it does not, however, reduce the incidence of poststreptococcal glomerulonephritis.

c. Early treatment of group A beta-hemolytic *Streptococcus* decreases the incidence of sibling and family colonization, subsequent infection, and the so-called ping-pong effect of colonization and recolonization.

A3. **c.** During winter months, the prevalence of group A beta hemolytic streptococcal pharyngitis in children is 15%. Streptococcal pharyngitis is suggested by age greater than 5 years, tender anterior cervical lymphadenopathy, scarlatiniform rash, and a history of exposure. Only 15% of children with pharyngitis and 25% of children with exudates have streptococcal infection; as well, 30% of those with streptococcal pharyngitis do not have tonsillar exudates.

A rapid *Streptococcus* test is the most convenient and accurate laboratory aid in making a diagnosis of acute tonsillitis or pharyngitis. In instances where a false negative rapid *Streptococcus* test is suspected, a throat culture may be performed.

A4. **b.** Scarlet fever is caused by group A beta-hemolytic *Streptococcus*. The patient described in Case 1 has the characteristic features of scarlet fever, which is described in detail in Problem 88.

A5. **c.** In 15% to 20% of children with group A beta-hemolytic *Streptococcus,* the group A beta-hemolytic *Streptococcus* is a normal commensal organism. This makes the interpretation of the throat swab difficult because of the false positives produced.

A6. **d.** The causative organism of bacterial endocarditis in children is *S. viridans*. Bacterial endocarditis caused by *S. viridans* may follow one of three patterns:

a. A protracted course featuring prolonged fever (often the only manifestation for several months)

b. An acute course with high fever and prostration

c. Symptoms that are nonspecific and consist of low-grade fever with afternoon elevations, fatigue, myalgias, arthralgia, headache, chills, nausea, and vomiting

A7. **a.** Group B *Streptococcus* is the most common cause of neonatal septicemia and neonatal meningitis. Group B *Streptococcus* is the organism cultured for in the last trimester of pregnancy. It is usually acquired by the neonate as he or she passes through the birth canal. To significantly decrease the probability of neonatal group B streptococcal infection, it is recommended that all pregnant women have a cervical culture performed at 34 to 36 weeks, and those who test positive be treated.

A8. **a.** Erysipelas is caused by group A beta-hemolytic *Streptococcus*. It is an acute, well-demarcated infection of the skin involving the face (associated with pharyngitis) and extremities (associated with wounds). With erysipelas the skin is erythematous and indurated; the margins of the lesions have a raised, firm, border. Associated symptoms include fever, vomiting, and irritability.

A9. **d.** Impetigo (pyoderma) is the most common form of skin infection caused by group A beta-hemolytic *Streptococcus*. Colonization of unbroken skin precedes pyoderma by 7 to 10 days. Skin lesions including impetigo and cellulitis develop following intradermal inoculation by insect bites, scabies, or minor trauma. Deeper soft tissue infections may occur secondary to impetigo. Streptococcal cellulitis is a painful, erythematous, indurated infection of the skin and subcutaneous tissues. Lymphangitis and regional lymphadenitis are common.

The other major causative organism of impetigo and other skin infections is *Staphylococcus aureus*.

A10. **e.** The rapid *Streptococcus* test is an enzyme-linked immunosorbent assay (ELISA) test designed to detect antibodies against multiple streptococcal extracellular antigens. It has a very high specificity and a very low false positive rate. The sensitivity of the test ranges from 75% to 87%, and the specificity ranges from 90% to 96%. The sensitivity of the test is lower, and therefore the false negative rate can be somewhat high. In clinical terms, therefore, if a test is positive, it can be assumed that the patient has the disease; if it is negative, on the other hand, it cannot be assumed that the patient does not have *Streptococcus*, particularly if signs and symptoms are suggestive.

The "gold standard" for the diagnosis of streptococcal pharyngitis is the throat culture. It should be performed in most patients suspected of having streptococcal pharyngitis who have a negative rapid *Streptococcus* test.

A11. **a.** Recurrent tonsillitis is almost always caused by group A beta-hemolytic *Streptococci*. We must, however, differentiate between cases of clinically suspected streptococcal tonsillitis and culture-proven streptococcal tonsillitis.

Often, a parent will come to your office with a child, complaining that the child has "continual tonsillitis" or "recurrent tonsillitis." It is very important to document whether or not these cases of tonsillitis are laboratory group A streptococcal tonsillitis or simply recurrent pharyngitis assumed to be streptococcal. This is especially important when the issue of tonsillectomy for recurrent tonsillitis is raised.

A12. **d.** Tonsillectomy often decreases the frequency of recurrent sore throats in young children. However, a similar rate of decrease in the frequency of recurrent sore throats occurs in children as they grow older, in spite of not having had a tonsillectomy. It is difficult, therefore, to suggest a "relative value" of tonsillectomy in this age group and for this reason.

Tonsillectomy, does not, however, decrease the incidence of recurrent upper respiratory tract infections (colds) in young children. Thus an important distinction exists between recurrent sore throats and recurrent upper respiratory tract infections in relationship to the efficacy (or lack of efficacy) of tonsillectomy.

A13. **d.** Most hypertrophic tonsils are actually normal in size; the misinterpretation results from failure to appreciate that normal tonsils are relatively larger in young children than in older children. There is no evidence that hypertrophic (or larger) tonsils become infected any more frequently than nonhypertrophic (or smaller) tonsils.

A14. **e.** Complications of tonsillectomy include minor hemorrhage, postoperative throat infection, severe postoperative hemorrhage, and pulmonary edema.

Pulmonary edema is not uncommon after the relief of upper airway obstruction with tonsillectomy or adenoidectomy. It seems to be directly related to the relief of airway obstruction.

The possibility of severe postoperative hemorrhage also makes this operation a risky procedure. The indications for the procedure (that are discussed in the Solution to the Short Answer Management Problem) should be followed closely.

A15. **e.** Reasons for adenoidectomy include persistent mouth breathing, persistent rhinitis, chronic otitis, and persistent snoring.

SOLUTION TO THE SHORT ANSWER MANAGEMENT PROBLEM

The relative indications for the performance of a tonsillectomy include the following:
  a. One episode of peritonsillar abscess (quinsy)
  b. Airway obstruction (as a result of markedly hypertrophied tonsils)
  c. Seven episodes of throat-culture-proven streptococcal tonsillitis in 1 year; five episodes of throat-culture-proven streptococcal tonsillitis per year in 2 successive years.

SUMMARY OF THE DIAGNOSIS AND TREATMENT OF STREPTOCOCCAL INFECTIONS IN CHILDREN

1. Neonates: Group B *Streptococcus* is now the most frequent cause of neonatal septicemia and meningitis.

2. Streptococcal pharyngitis:
   a. Only 15% of pharyngitis cases in children have group A beta-hemolytic *Streptococcus* as the cause.
   b. Streptococcal pharyngitis is suggested by the following:
      1) Age greater than 5 years
      2) High fever
      3) Tonsillar exudates
      4) Tender anterior cervical lymphadenopathy
      5) Scarlatiniform rash
      6) History of exposure
      7) Absence of cough
      8) Absence of rhinitis
   c. Only 25% of patients with exudates have streptococcal pharyngitis.
   d. Although some authorities believe that the predictive value of physicians in distinguishing streptococcal pharyngitis from viral pharyngitis is at best 50%, in the presence of either cough or rhinitis, the probability of streptococcal pharyngitis is very low.
   e. Of children, 15% to 20% carry group A beta-hemolytic *Streptococcus* as a normal commensal organism.

3. Erysipelas: Acute, well-demarcated infection of the skin caused by group A beta-hemolytic *Streptococcus*

4. Impetigo: Caused primarily by a group A beta-hemolytic *Streptococcus;* may lead to more serious conditions such as cellulitis; also significantly caused by *S. aureus*.

5. Bacterial endocarditis: In children, typically caused by *S. viridans*.

6. Tonsillitis and tonsillectomy: Tonsillectomy should be performed only if there is one episode of peritonsillar abscess (quinsy), a history of airway obstruction, or seven documented episodes of group A beta-hemolytic *Streptococcus* infections in a 12-month period, or 5 documented episodes in each of 2 successive years. Remember the following:
   a. Most hypertrophied tonsils are normal tonsils.
   b. Tonsils grow smaller as the child grows older.
   c. Large tonsils are no more prone to tonsillitis than small tonsils.
   d. Not all tonsillitis is caused by beta-hemolytic *Streptococcus* (approximately 25%; the other 75% of causes are viral in origin).

7. Adenoids and adenoidectomy:
   a. The only indication that is similar for both tonsillectomy and adenoidectomy is airway obstruction.
   b. The other indications for adenoidectomy are chronic otitis media and chronic rhinitis.

8. Other streptococcal infections: Human infection with streptococci of groups C, D, E, F, G, H, K, L, M, N, and O has been reported in normal infants and children. Penicillin G provides effective therapy for non-group-A streptococci except for group D *(Enterococci)*. This organism is generally susceptible to ampicillin.

9. Treatment for streptococcal infections:
   a. Group A beta-hemolytic streptococcal pharyngitis: Laboratory diagnosis and begin treatment with penicillin V for 10 days. In unreliable patients use benzathine penicillin G.
   b. *S. viridans:* Bacterial endocarditis: use ampicillin and an aminoglycoside.
   c. Infection with Lancefield group G streptococci has been recognized as an increasingly serious and frequent cause of human disease. This group can cause endovascular infection, endocarditis, and septic arthritis.
   d. Early treatment of group A beta-hemolytic streptococcal pharyngitis:
      1) Decreases the virulence and severity of the infection

2) Decreases the length of symptoms of the infection.

3) Protects against rheumatic fever, an increasing problem once again in the United States. It does not, however, protect against post-streptococcal glomerulonephritis.

SUGGESTED READINGS

Pinchichera ME: Group A beta-hemolytic streptococcal infections, *Pediatr Rev* 19(9):291-302, 1998.

Todd J: Streptococcal infections. In Behrman R, ed: *Nelson textbook of pediatrics*, ed 15, Philadelphia, 1998, WB Saunders.

Todd J: Rheumatic fever. In Behrman R, ed: *Nelson textbook of pediatrics*, ed 15, Philadelphia, 1998, WB Saunders.

PROBLEM · 88

THE "BIG FIVE" VIRAL EXANTHEMS IN CHILDREN

Don't Judge a Rash Too Rashly.

Case 1 ■ A 1-Year-Old Male with a Rash and a Fever

A 1-year-old boy is brought to your office by his mother. The child was well until 3 days ago when he developed a fever of 40° C. The child's mother has been trying to keep the fever down with acetaminophen. Today the child's temperature suddenly dropped, and at the same time he developed a skin rash.

On physical examination, the child does not look ill. His temperature has come down to 38° C. He has a fine (in texture) erythematous maculopapular eruption over his entire body. His nose is running and his throat is slightly hyperemic. His lungs are clear. His blood pressure is 75/50 mm Hg and his pulse is 124 bpm and regular. The results from his abdominal, musculoskeletal, and neurologic examinations are normal.

SELECT THE BEST ANSWER TO THE FOLLOWING QUESTIONS

Q1. What is the most likely diagnosis in this child at this time?
   a. exanthem subitum
   b. erythema infectiosum
   c. adenoviral exanthem
   d. rubella
   e. rubeola

Q2. What is the most outstanding feature of this illness?
   a. the rapid fall in the temperature
   b. the rapid rise in the temperature

   c. the appearance of the rash at the same time as the temperature falls
   d. the absence of physical signs to explain the (usually) extremely high temperature
   e. the complication of Reye's syndrome that is directly linked to the causative agent

Q3. What is the causative agent of the condition described?
   a. human parvovirus
   b. human papillomavirus
   c. human herpesvirus 6
   d. adenovirus
   e. rhinovirus

Case 2 ■ A 5-Year-Old Male with a Bright Red Rash on Both Cheeks

A 5-year-old boy is brought to your office by his father. The child has been running a low-grade fever for the past 24 hours. This afternoon he suddenly developed a bright red rash on both cheeks.

On physical examination, the child has erythema of the cheeks, as well as the beginning of a maculopapular rash on the trunk and the extremities. No other abnormalities are noted on examination.

Q4. What is the most likely diagnosis in this child?
   a. exanthem subitum
   b. erythema infectiosum
   c. adenoviral exanthem
   d. rubella
   e. rubeola

Q5. What is the causative agent of the condition described in Case 2?
   a. human papillomavirus
   b. adenovirus
   c. human parvovirus
   d. human herpesvirus 6
   e. rhinovirus

Q6. The characteristic rash of the condition described in Case 2 is morphologically best linked to which of the following descriptions of facial rash appearance and appearance of the rash on the trunk?
   a. circumoral pallor and sandpaper-like appearance of the trunk
   b. slapped-cheek appearance and lacy reticular pattern
   c. fine pustular appearance and a bright red maculopapular rash with central clearing
   d. coalesced erythema-like appearance and solid macular rash
   e. none of the above

Case 3 ■ A 4-Year-Old Female with Pain behind Her Ears and a Maculopapular Rash

A 4-year-old female is brought to your busy office by her mother for assessment and treatment of a fever and a skin rash.

The child's present illness began with very mild upper respiratory tract symptoms approximately 1 week ago. Then last night the child complained to her father of pain behind her ears. This morning a maculopapular rash that began on the face appears to be spreading distally.

This child has not seen a physician, a nurse practitioner, or a public health nurse or clinic since birth. Her mother basically does not believe in anything the medical profession has to offer. She brought the child in to see you today only because her teacher threatened to keep her out of school until she had a doctor's note that authorized her return.

On examination, the child's temperature is 38.8° C. Examination of the head and neck reveals a moderately infected pharynx, a "flushed face," a slight reddening of the conjunctiva bilaterally, and coryza. The child appears what you would term *slightly ill.*

Q7. What is the most likely diagnosis in this child?
   a. exanthem subitum
   b. erythema infectiosum
   c. adenoviral exanthem
   d. rubella
   e. rubeola

Q8. Which of the following statements is true concerning the condition described in Case 3?
   a. this condition is a self-limiting condition that poses no significant risk to anyone
   b. this condition is caused by human parvovirus B27
   c. this condition is likely to reoccur several times during childhood
   d. there is no protection available for the prevention of this condition
   e. none of the above statements is true

Q9. The American Academy of Pediatrics recommends which of the following for the treatment or prevention of this condition?
   a. no antibiotics; no vaccination in childhood
   b. no antibiotics; yearly vaccination in childhood
   c. no antibiotics; an antiviral agent to prevent complications
   d. no antibiotics; two vaccinations in childhood
   e. antibiotics; no vaccinations in childhood

Case 4 ■ A Pregnant Woman Exposed to Rubella

A pregnant woman comes to your office for her first prenatal visit at 8 weeks' gestation. She has her routine blood work done and you determine her rubella titer to be ⅛. Three weeks later her 18-month-old son (who has not received any immunizations to date) develops rubella. She is aware of the risk of congenital rubella syndrome developing in the fetus but indicates to you that under no conditions would she consider a therapeutic abortion (TA).

Q10. At this time, what should you do?
   a. immunize her with live rubella virus vaccine
   b. immunize her with attenuated rubella virus vaccine
   c. immunize her with inactivated rubella virus vaccine
   d. provide passive protection to her with an injection of immune serum globulin (ISG)
   e. inform her that, under the circumstances, "your hands are tied"

Case 5 ■ A 4-Year-Old Male with a Dry Hacking Cough, Coryza, Conjunctivitis, a Temperature of 40° C, and a Fine Maculopapular Rash

A 4-year-old male, previously unimmunized, is brought to your office with a 5-day history of fever, a dry hacking cough, coryza, and conjunctivitis. This morning the child's temperature rose to 40° C and a fine maculopapular rash appeared on his face, his upper arms, and the upper part of his chest. The other significant symptom is photophobia.

On examination, there is significant posterior cervical lymphadenopathy. There is marked conjunctival injection bilaterally. There is a diffuse maculopapular eruption over the face, arms, and chest that appears to be spreading onto the back and the thighs.

Q11. What is the most likely diagnosis in this patient?
   a. exanthem subitum
   b. erythema infectiosum
   c. adenoviral exanthem
   d. rubella
   e. rubeola

Q12. Which of the following is (are) characteristic of the disease described in Case 5?
   a. Koplik's spots
   b. coryza
   c. conjunctivitis
   d. cough
   e. all of the above

Case 6 ■ An 8-Year-Old Male with a Fever of 39° C, Chills, Vomiting, and a Headache

An 8-year-old male is brought to your office by his father. The child has been ill for 3 days. The illness began as a fever that reached 39° C. Associated with the fever have been chills, vomiting, and headache.

On physical examination, the child has a hyperemic pharynx and tonsillar areas. The tonsils are covered with exudate. The dorsum of the tongue has a white coat and also appears edematous. There is a generalized, fine maculopapular rash that has the consistency of sandpaper. The child has a flushed forehead and flushed cheeks, and the area around the child's mouth is pale (circumoral pallor).

Q13. What is the most likely diagnosis?
a. erythema infectiosum
b. adenoviral exanthem
c. rubella
d. rubeola
e. none of the above

Q14. What is the causative agent in this child's illness?
a. human parvovirus
b. human adenovirus
c. *Paramyxoviridae*: genus *Morbillivirus*
d. group A beta-hemolytic *Streptococcus*
e. *Togaviridae*: genus *Rubivirus*

Questions 15 to 25 are matching questions. Eleven disease-producing pathogens or disease entities are listed in the left-hand column, and 11 disease-defining characteristics are listed in the right-hand column. Beside each disease-producing pathogen or disease entity, put the letter of the disease-defining characteristic to which it corresponds.

15. Herpes varicella
16. Herpes simplex
17. Coxsackievirus A16
18. Kawasaki disease
19. Adenovirus
20. Lyme disease
21. Parainfluenza virus
22. Tinea versicolor
23. Tinea corporis
24. Pityriasis rosea
25. Molluscum contagiosum

a. discrete, dome-shaped papules
b. herald patch
c. erythema chronicum migrans
d. hand-foot-and-mouth disease
e. acute gingivostomatitis
f. ringworm
g. primary cause of conjunctivitis
h. primary cause of infectious croup
i. hyperpigmented or hypopigmented lesions
j. coronary vasculitis
k. "crops of lesions": vesicles

SHORT ANSWER MANAGEMENT PROBLEM
Define the following primary skin lesions seen in children: *macule, bullae, papule, pustule, nodule, wheal, vesicle,* and *cyst.*

ANSWERS

A1. **a.** The most likely diagnosis in this child is exanthem subitum (roseola infantum).

A2. **d.** The most outstanding feature of exanthem subitum is the inability to explain to any degree the very high fever that this condition produces. The rapid fall of the temperature and the appearance of the rash at the same time that the fever falls are not as "outstanding" as the inability to explain the high fever. There are sometimes very minor physical signs such as slight reddening of the throat, but nowhere near the degree of signs or symptoms that would explain the high fever.

A3. **c.** Exanthem subitum is a viral illness of infants and young children that initially presents with a high fever that typically lasts for 3 or 4 days. Usually there are no physical findings to explain the fever, and the child looks generally well. As the child's temperature falls (often rapidly), a fine maculopapular rash appears over the entire body that lasts for approximately 24 hours.

The causative agent of exanthem subitum is human herpesvirus 6. The treatment of exanthem subitum is symptomatic only. Acetaminophen should be administered if the temperature exceeds 40° C.

A4. **b.** The most likely diagnosis in this child is erythema infectiosum (fifth disease).

A5. **c.** Erythema infectiosum is caused by a human parvovirus B19.

A6. **b.** Erythema infectiosum begins as a low-grade fever and produces a "slapped-cheek" rash appearance on the face associated with a lacy, reticular-like maculopapular rash pattern on the trunk and extremities. The rash may last from a few days to several weeks. It is frequently pruritic. Recurrences after exercise or after application of heat or emotional upset are not uncommon.

Constitutional symptoms of this infection include headache, pharyngitis, myalgia, arthritis, gastrointestinal upset, and coryza. There are no diagnostic tests for this condition.

The differential diagnosis of erythema infectiosum includes rubella, atypical rubeola, drug-induced rashes, and other viral exanthems.

A7. **d.** This child has rubella, or German measles, as it is commonly known. Rubella is caused by a pleomorphic, RNA-containing virus currently listed in the family of viruses named Togaviridae, genus Rubivirus. Rubella usually begins with symptoms of a mild upper respiratory tract infection. There is significant tender retroauricular, posterior cervical, and postoccipital lymphadenopathy. In some cases of rubella, an enanthem covering the soft palate and fauces may appear before the onset of the rash.

The exanthem usually begins on the face and spreads to cover the trunk. The rash is maculopapular, with areas of confluence and flushing. Mild pruritus is common. The rash usually clears by the third day. There is no associated photophobia and few complications; unusual complications include neuritis, arthritis, and encephalitis.

A8. **e.** The statements given in Question 8 are all false, for the following reasons:
a. Pregnant women are at moderately severe risk for rubella if they have no antibodies against it.
b. This condition is caused by Togaviridae virus, genus Rubivirus.
c. Once rubella has been contacted for sure on one occasion, active immune status is produced. The condition can occur again in the same individual, but it is extremely unlikely.
d. A rubella live virus vaccine, RA 27/3, is used extensively in the United States as an immunization against rubella.

A9. **d.** The American Academy of Pediatrics recommends immunization against rubella twice in childhood: first at 12 to 15 months and then again at 4 to 6 years. Antibiotics are not recommended.

A10. **d.** Pregnant women, especially early in pregnancy but also during the entire gestational period, should avoid exposure to rubella regardless of either history of the disease during childhood or history of active immunization. Exposure of pregnant women to infants with congenital rubella syndrome should be especially guarded against because of prolonged shedding of the virus.

Because TA has been rejected by this mother-to-be (you should certainly not advocate TA, but you should inform her of the risk of exposure of congenital rubella syndrome in her infant if she were to acquire the infection with a nonimmune status), you should provide passive protection to her with an intramuscular injection of ISG given in a large dose (0.25 to 0.50 ml/kg or 0.12 or 0.20 ml/lb) within the first 7 to 8 days of exposure.

Pregnant women should not be given live rubella virus vaccine (live viral vaccine is the only rubella vaccine available).

A11. **e.** This child has rubeola.

A12. **e.** The prodromal phase of rubeola (red measles) is characterized by a low-grade to moderate fever, a dry hacking cough, coryza, and conjunctivitis. Koplik spots are grayish-white dots, usually as small as grains of sand, with slight, reddish areolae that are occasionally hemorrhagic. Their location tends to be opposite the lower molars, but they may spread irregularly over the rest of the buccal mucosa. Thus rubeola can be remembered by the following mnemonic, which refers to a copy of a letter sent to CPK (cc-CPK): **c**ough, **c**oryza, **C**onjunctivitis, **P**hotophobia, **K**oplik spots.

The temperature in rubeola rises as the rash appears. The maculopapular rash usually begins on the face and neck and spreads over the entire body from the neck down. By the time the rash reaches the feet, clinical improvement has begun. Cervical lymphadenopathy may be prominent.

The major complications of rubeola are otitis media, bronchopneumonia, and gastrointestinal symptoms including vomiting and diarrhea. Patients with rubeola are ill appearing. Prevention against rubeola can be achieved with active immunization at 12 to 15 months. This is preferable to passive immunization (with gamma globulin) for disease attenuation.

A13. **e.** This child has scarlet fever.

A14. **d.** Scarlet fever, which is caused by group A beta-hemolytic streptococcus, usually begins with the abrupt onset of fever, vomiting, headaches, pharyngitis, and chills. The temperature usually peaks on the second day and gradually returns to normal within 5 to 7 days.

The tonsils are hyperemic and edematous and may be covered with an exudate. The throat is inflamed and may be covered by a membrane. The dorsum of the tongue often initially has a white coat, with projecting edematous papillae.

The exanthem usually consists of a finely papular or punctate group of lesions. It is sometimes described as having the consistency of sandpaper. The rash generally begins in the axillae, the groin, and the neck; within 24 hours it becomes generalized. The forehead and the cheeks may appear to be flushed and the area around the mouth (circumoral) is pale.

Desquamation usually begins on the face and proceeds to the hands and feet and may continue for up to 6 weeks.

The treatment of choice for all group A beta-hemolytic streptococcus is penicillin. Amoxicillin is a better-tasting and acceptable alternative for children. If an allergy to penicillin exists, the drug of choice is erythromycin.

Of the other choices listed for causative agents, remember that *Morbillivirus* is the cause of rubeola and *Rubivirus* is the cause of rubella.

A15. **k.** Viral agent: Herpes varicella (chicken pox). Disease-defining characteristics are crops of small, red, papules that develop into oval vesicles on an erythematous base.

A16. **e.** Viral agent: Herpes simplex virus. Disease-defining characteristic: acute herpetic gingivostomatitis, which is the most common cause of stomatitis in children ages 1 to 3 years.

A17. **d.** Viral agent: Coxsackievirus A16. Disease-defining characteristics are hand-foot-mouth disease and an enteroviral exanthem-enanthem with the distribution portrayed by the name.

A18. **j.** Disease entity: Kawasaki disease. The disease-defining characteristic is coronary vasculitis, also known as mucocutaneous lymph node syndrome or infantile polyarteritis. Cardiac involvement is the most important manifestation of Kawasaki disease (10% to 40% of children within the first 2 weeks of illness). The causal agent is unknown.

A19. **g.** Viral agent: Adenovirus. The disease-defining characteristic is adenovirus, the single most common cause of conjunctivitis.

A20. **c.** Disease entity: Lyme disease. The disease-defining characteristic is erythema chronicum migrans, which begins as an erythematous macule or papule at the site of a tick bite. The causative organism is *Borrelia burgdorferi,* which develops into an expanding erythematous annular lesion with central clearing and often reaches a diameter of 16 cm.

A21. **h.** Viral agent: Parainfluenza virus. The disease-defining characteristic is that it is the most common cause of infectious croup.

A22. **i.** Disease entity: Tinea versicolor. The disease-defining characteristic is hypopigmented or hyperpigmented macules covered with a fine scale. Lesions begin in a perifollicular location, enlarge, and form confluent patches, most commonly on the neck, upper chest, back, and upper arms. The causative organism is dimorphic yeast (*Pityrosporon orbiculare* [*Malassezia furfur*]).

A23. **f.** Disease entity: Tinea corporis. The disease-defining characteristic is ringworm, the common name for a group of disorders known as dermatophytoses. The three principal genera responsible for dermatophyte infections are *Trichophyton, Microsporum,* and *Epidermophyton.* Classical lesion begins as a dry, mildly erythematous, elevated, scaly papule or plaque and spreads centrifugally as it clears centrally to form the characteristic annular lesion responsible for the designation ringworm.

A24. **b.** Disease entity: Pityriasis rosea. The disease-defining characteristic is the herald patch, a solitary, round or oval lesion that may occur anywhere on the body and is often but not always identifiable by its large size. The herald patch usually precedes the generalized maculopapular eruption of oval or round lesions that crop. The rash can assume a characteristic Christmas-tree appearance on the back.

A25. **a.** Disease entity: Molluscum contagiosum. The disease-defining characteristic describes a disorder characterized by discrete, dome-shaped papules varying in size from 1 to 5 mm. Typically these lesions have a central umbilication from which a cheesy material can be expressed. The papules may occur anywhere on the body, but the face, eyelids, neck, axillae, and thighs are sites of predilection. Causative agent is a DNA virus, the largest member of the poxvirus group.

SOLUTION TO THE SHORT ANSWER MANAGEMENT PROBLEM

a. Macule: An alteration in skin color that cannot be felt
b. Papule: Palpable solid lesions smaller than 1.0 cm
c. Nodule: Palpable solid lesions larger than 1.0 cm
d. Vesicle: Raised, fluid-filled lesions less than 0.5 cm in diameter
e. Bullae: Raised, fluid-filled lesions larger than 0.5 cm in diameter
f. Pustules: Raised lesions that contain pustular material
g. Wheals: Flat-topped, palpable lesions of variable size and configuration that represent dermal collections of edema fluid
h. Cyst: Circumscribed, thick-walled lesions that are located deep in the skin; are covered by a normal epidermis; and contain fluid or semisolid material

SUMMARY OF THE "BIG FIVE" VIRAL EXANTHEMS IN CHILDREN

Because so many conditions were described in this chapter, the summary will be limited to a discussion of what are termed the *big five* viral exanthems in children. (Note that erythema infectiosum is also known as fifth disease.)

1. Exanthem subitum (roseola infantum): High fever followed by defervescence with the appearance of an erythematous maculopapular rash at the same time

2. Erythema infectiosum: Low-grade fever followed by the appearance of a rash: "slapped-cheek" appearance followed by a generalized lacy-reticular pattern rash

3. Rubella: Mild fever; significant tender retroauricular, posterior, and postoccipital lymphadenopathy

4. Rubeola: Prodromal symptoms include the 3 Cs: **c**ough, **c**oryza, and **c**onjunctivitis. Koplik spots are pathognomonic. Photophobia is common. The temperature rises abruptly as the rash appears. The severity of the disease is directly related to the extent and confluence of the rash. The mnemonic is *cc-CPK*: **c**ough, **c**oryza, **C**onjunctivitis, **P**hotophobia, **K**oplik's spots.

5. Scarlet fever: Group A beta-hemolytic streptococcal infection that presents as fever, chills, headache, vomiting, and pharyngitis. Exanthem has texture of coarse sandpaper. Circumoral pallor is common. Penicillin V is the drug of choice.

SUGGESTED READINGS

Kock WC: Parvovirus B19. In Behrman R, ed: *Nelson textbook of pediatrics*, ed 15, Philadelphia, 1998, WB Saunders.

Kohl S: Human herpesvirus 6. In Behrman R, ed: *Nelson textbook of pediatrics*, ed 15, Philadelphia, 1998, WB Saunders.

Maldonado Y: Measles. In Behrman R, ed: *Nelson textbook of pediatrics*, ed 15, Philadelphia, 1998, WB Saunders.

Maldonado Y: Rubella. In Behrman R, ed: *Nelson textbook of pediatrics*, ed 15, Philadelphia, 1998, WB Saunders.

Todd J: Streptococcal Infection. In Behrman R, ed: *Nelson textbook of pediatrics*, ed 15, Philadelphia, 1998, WB Saunders.

PROBLEM·89

CHILDHOOD PNEUMONIA

"My Baby Has Water in His Lungs?"

Case 1 ■ A 2-Day-Old Infant with Pneumonia

A 4000-g infant born at 39½ weeks' gestation appeared healthy at birth. His Apgar scores were 7 and 9. On the second day of life he begins to cough, his temperature increases to 40.5° C, his breathing becomes labored, and he appears ill.

His chest x-ray shows a reticulogranular pattern, a pattern that appears exactly like hyaline membrane disease. On physical examination, you also note apnea, tachypnea, grunting, flaring of the nares, and subcostal retractions. There are adventitious breath sounds heard in all lobes of the lungs.

SELECT THE BEST ANSWER TO THE FOLLOWING QUESTIONS

Q1. Based on the information provided to this point, what is the most likely diagnosis?
   a. group A streptococcal pneumonia
   b. *Klebsiella* pneumonia
   c. adenoviral pneumonia
   d. group B streptococcal pneumonia
   e. staphylococcal pneumonia

Q2. What is the most likely source of this infant's infection?
   a. airborne droplets
   b. oral-fecal transmission
   c. direct spread from the mother
   d. intrauterine colonization
   e. none of the above

Q3. What is the treatment of choice in this child at this time?
   a. penicillin G
   b. amoxicillin
   c. trimethoprim-sulfamethoxazole
   d. clavulanic acid
   e. penicillin G and metronidazole

Case 2 ■ A 3-Year-Old Female with Fever, Chills, Nasal Flaring, Subcostal Indrawing, and a Harsh Cough

A 3-year-old female is brought to your office with a 4-day history of fever, chills, nasal flaring, subcostal indrawing, and a harsh cough. The child is in respiratory distress.

Before the onset of the present symptoms, the child had a recent respiratory tract infection. The child's symptoms were bilateral conjunctivitis, rhinorrhea, nonproductive cough, and sore throat.

On physical examination, the child's temperature is 39° C. Her respiratory rate is 32 per minute. There are rales and rhonchi in all lobes. The child is using her accessory muscles of respiration, especially her intercostal muscles and sternocleidomastoid muscles.

Q4. What is the most likely diagnosis in this case?
   a. *Mycoplasma pneumoniae*
   b. adenoviral pneumonia
   c. *Streptococcus pneumoniae*
   d. *Haemophilus influenzae* pneumonia
   e. group B streptococcal pneumonia

Q5. What is the most common causative agent responsible for pneumonia in children age 5 years and under?
   a. respiratory syncytial virus (RSV)
   b. *Mycoplasma pneumoniae*
   c. adenovirus
   d. *S. pneumoniae*
   e. *H. influenzae*

Q6. What is the most common bacterial causative agent responsible for pneumonia in children under the age of 5 years?
   a. *S. pneumoniae*
   b. *Staphylococcus aureus*
   c. group A beta-hemolytic *Streptococcus*
   d. *H. influenzae*
   e. *Klebsiella pneumoniae*

Q7. A child who is considered low risk for complications and who develops the clinical picture described in Case 2 should be treated with which of the following?
   a. ribavirin
   b. ampicillin
   c. erythromycin
   d. penicillin
   e. none of the above

Q8. A child who is considered high risk for complications and who develops the clinical picture described in Case 2 should be treated with which of the following?
   a. ribavirin
   b. ampicillin
   c. erythromycin
   d. hospitalization
   e. a and d

Q9. A high-risk child who develops a secondary pneumonia infection caused by the causative agent most likely responsible for bacterial pneumonia in children under the age of 5 years should be treated with which of the following?
   a. ribavirin
   b. ampicillin
   c. penicillin G
   d. hospitalization
   e. c and d

Q10. What is the most common nonviral pneumonia in children over the age of 5 years?
   a. *M. pneumonia*
   b. *S. pneumoniae*
   c. *Listeria monocytogenis* pneumonia
   d. *H. influenzae* pneumonia
   e. group B *S. pneumoniae*

Q11. What is the second most common bacterial agent responsible for pneumonia in children over the age of 4 years?
   a. *S. pneumoniae*
   b. *H. influenzae*
   c. *S. aureus*
   d. *K. pneumoniae*
   e. group B *S. pneumoniae*

Q12. Which of the following causative agents usually evolves into a pneumonia that often includes an empyema or a pleural effusion?
   a. *S. pneumoniae*
   b. *S. aureus*
   c. group B *S. pneumoniae*
   d. *H. influenzae*
   e. *K. pneumoniae*

SHORT ANSWER MANAGEMENT PROBLEM
With respect to viral, mycoplasmal, and bacterial pneumonias in neonates, infants, and children, list the following:
   a. The most common causative agent in the age group in question
   b. The most common bacterial causative agent in the age group in question
   c. The recommended treatment for each of the pneumonias in question

ANSWERS

A1. **d.** This neonate has group B streptococcal pneumonia.

A2. **c.** In newborns this is primarily a disease in which the organism is colonized by passage through the birth canal, thus a direct spread from the mother.

A3. **a.** The treatment of choice for group B *Streptococcus* is penicillin G. The recommended dose of penicillin G is 300,000 units/kg/24 hours.

The mortality rate from group B streptococcal pneumonia is still quite high: 10% to 40%. Thus early diagnosis and treatment are critical.

A4. **b.** The initial presentation of conjunctivitis, nonproductive cough, rhinorrhea, and sore throat is most compatible with adenoviral infection. The real clue in this case is the conjunctivitis, a symptom much more common with adenovirus infection than with any other viral infection.

The probable sequence of events is minor adenoviral upper respiratory tract infection proceeding to adenoviral pneumonia.

A5. **a.** The most common cause of pneumonia in children under the age of 5 years is RSV pneumonia.

The typical signs and symptoms of viral pneumonia in children include a dry, tight, and nonproductive cough; fever or chills absent as frequently as present; and auscultatory findings including rhonchi, fine rales, and audible wheezing.

In general, the younger the infant the more severe the disease symptoms, which may include significant respiratory distress, listlessness, and apnea.

Radiographic findings are more likely to include air trapping, bilateral fine/fluffy infiltrates, and atelectasis. Secondary bacterial invasion must be considered when consolidation is present.

The five most common viral agents causing pneumonia in infants and children are as follows:
  a. RSV
  b. Parainfluenza virus
  c. Influenza virus (in children mostly influenza B)
  d. Adenovirus
  e. Enterovirus

A6. **a.** The most common bacterial cause of pneumonia in a child under the age of 5 years is *S. pneumoniae*.

Bacterial pneumonias usually present with quite a different clinical picture. Signs and symptoms of bacterial pneumonias include fever, chills, cough productive of purulent sputum, pleuritic chest pain, and dyspnea and tachypnea. Also, the use of the accessory muscles of respiration is very common, especially in children.

The chest x-ray will frequently show lobar consolidation. The complete blood count will often reveal an extremely high white blood cell count with a shift to the left.

A7. **e.** The treatment of an infant or child with probable adenoviral pneumonia is symptomatic. No antibiotics or antiviral agents have been shown to be effective for the treatment of this infection. The major decision regarding this child will be whether or not hospitalization is necessary. This will depend on the child's clinical condition and, most importantly, on the degree of respiratory distress that the child demonstrates.

If you even think about hospitalizing a child with pneumonia, do it. You will not have made a mistake.

A8. **e.** A child with possible adenoviral pneumonia who is at high risk for complications (congenital heart disease, cystic fibrosis, malignancy, chronic immunosuppression, or any primary immune deficiency) should be hospitalized and given supplementary oxygen (with or without a mist tent). It also is reasonable to treat such high-risk children with ribavirin to reduce potential coinfection with RSV, the most common cause of viral pneumonia in this age group.

A9. **e.** The treatment of choice for a high-risk child who has a secondary streptococcal pneumonia includes antibiotic therapy (penicillin G is still the drug of first choice) as well as ribavirin and hospitalization with supplementary oxygen and close monitoring as described in Answer 8. As the child improves, it is not uncommon for the chest x-ray changes to lag significantly behind the clinical improvement. In a child with this picture, arterial blood gases or pulse oximetry are also a very good way of measuring response to treatment and improvement.

A10. **a.** The most common cause of nonviral pneumonia in children over the age of 5 years is *M. pneumoniae.* In a child with mycoplasma pneumonia there is often a significant discrepancy between the clinical findings and the radiologic findings. The most important clinical symptom is a persistent, hacking, nonproductive cough that is difficult to treat. Often auscultation of the lungs will be normal. The chest x-ray, on the other hand, may very well be quite revealing (with a significant bilateral infiltrate being the most common picture).

The treatment of choice for *M. pneumoniae* in a child is erythromycin.

A11. **a.** In children over the age of 4 years, streptococcal pneumonia is the most common cause of bacterial pneumonia after mycoplasma (see Answer 6).

A12. **b.** The answer is staphylococcal pneumonia. Most patients with staphylococcal pneumonia have roentgenographic evidence of nonspecific bronchopneumonia early in the course of the illness.

However, the infiltrate may soon become patchy and limited in extent or, on the other hand, dense and homogenous and involve an entire lobe or hemithorax. The right lung is involved in approximately 65% of cases; bilateral involvement occurs in fewer than 20% of cases. A pleural effusion or empyema is noted during the course of illness in most patients; pyopneumothorax occurs in approximately 25% of patients. Pneumatoceles occur frequently and vary considerably in size.

Although no x-ray change can be considered diagnostic, progression over a few hours from bronchopneumonia to effusion or pyopneumothorax with or without pneumatoceles is highly suggestive of staphylococcal pneumonia.

The treatment of choice for staphylococcal pneumonia is a semisynthetic, penicillinase-resistant penicillin (such as methicillin) given intravenously.

SOLUTION TO THE SHORT ANSWER MANAGEMENT PROBLEM

A reasonable approach to diagnosis includes an understanding of prevalence of different types of pneumonia based on age:
  a. Age <2 weeks:
    1) Most common organism: Group B streptococcus
    2) Treatment: Penicillin or ampicillin
  b. Age 2 weeks to 4 months:
    1) Most common organism: *Chlamydia trachomatis*
    2) Treatment: Erythromycin
  c. Age 4 months to 4 years:
    1) Most common organism: Viral
    2) Most common viruses causing pneumonia:
      a) RSV
      b) Parainfluenza viruses
      c) Influenza
      d) Adenovirus
      e) Enterovirus
    3) Treatment: Symptomatic (or Ribavirin for severe RSV)
    4) Most common type of bacterial pneumonia: *S. pneumoniae*
    5) Treatment: Penicillin
  d. Age > 4 years:
    1) Most common cause: Viral
    2) Most common bacterial cause: *M. pneumoniae*
    3) Treatment: Erythromycin
    4) Second most common type of bacterial pneumonia: *S. pneumoniae*
    5) Treatment: Penicillin

SUMMARY OF THE DIAGNOSIS AND TREATMENT OF CHILDHOOD PNEUMONIA

This is well summarized in the Solution to the Short Answer Management Problem.

SUGGESTED READINGS

Bassi O et al: Clinical and economic outcomes of empiric parenteral antibiotic therapy for pneumonia: A retrospective study of 1,032 hospitalized patients, *J Chemother* 10(5):369-374, 1998.

Klein JO: Role of nontypeable *Haemophilus influenzae* in pediatric respiratory tract infections, *Pediatr Infect Dis J* 16(2suppl):S5-8, 1997.

Marrie TJ: Community-acquired pneumonia: epidemiology, etiology, treatment. *Infect Dis Clin North Am* 12(3):723-740, 1998.

Tsarouhas N et al: Effectiveness of intramuscular penicillin versus oral amoxicillin in the early treatment of outpatient pediatric pneumonia, *Pediatr Emerg Care* 14(5):338-341, 1998.

Vuori E et al: Etiology of pneumonia and other common childhood infections requiring hospitalization and parenteral antimicrobial therapy. SE-TU Study Group, *Clin Infect Dis* 27(3):566-572, 1998.

PROBLEM · 90

FEVER WITHOUT FOCUS

"My Child Is Fine Except for His Fever."

Case 1 ■ A 9-Month-Old Infant with Fever and No Localized Signs

A 9-month-old infant is seen in the Emergency Department for evaluation of fever. His mother states that he has had an intermittent fever of 39° C for 24 hours. She has used acetaminophen to treat the fever and has brought the temperature down to 38° C. The child has not been ill and has had no symptoms of upper respiratory tract infection or other symptoms.

The child has no history of serious illnesses, allergies, or other problems. He is on no medications.

On examination, the child is actively playing with his toys. He does not look toxic. His rectal temperature is 39° C. The head and neck, lungs, cardiovascular system, abdomen, neurologic, and musculoskeletal system examination results are normal.

Your clinical judgment suggests that this child has no serious illness.

SELECT THE BEST ANSWER TO THE FOLLOWING QUESTIONS

Q1. What is the diagnosis in this child at this time?
  a. fever without a focus
  b. fever of unknown origin (FUO)
  c. infantile febrile response
  d. fever of occult bacteremia
  e. none of the above

Q2. FUO is strictly defined as which of the following?
  a. fever in a child that persists for a time that exceeds 1 week in duration
  b. fever that continues once a child is hospitalized
  c. fever that continues despite at least 1 week of ongoing investigations
  d. all of the above
  e. a and c only

Q3. What is the most important diagnostic entity to consider in the infant?
  a. drug fever
  b. occult bacteremia
  c. factitious fever
  d. occult viremia
  e. collagen vascular disease

Q4. What is the most appropriate next step in the treatment of the patient described in Case 1?
  a. obtain a more detailed history
  b. order a white blood cell count (WBC) and erythrocyte sedimentation rate (ESR)
  c. start the child on antibiotics
  d. send the child home on antipyretic therapy
  e. obtain an immediate consultation with a pediatrician

Q5. If you are unable to obtain the necessary information based on the most appropriate action taken in Question 4, what is the next step?
  a. to perform a WBC
  b. to perform a lumbar puncture
  c. to perform an ESR
  d. to send the child home on antipyretic therapy
  e. to obtain an immediate consultation with a pediatrician

Q6. In an infant between the ages of 3 months and 24 months, the probability of occult bacteremia is increased if
  a. the temperature is greater than 40° C
  b. the WBC is <5000/mm^3
  c. the WBC is >15,000/mm^3
  d. there is a positive exposure history
  e. all of the above increase probability

Q7. What is the most common organism responsible for occult bacteremia in infants?
  a. *Neisseria meningitidis*
  b. *Haemophilus influenzae*
  c. *Streptococcus pneumoniae*
  d. *Salmonella* species
  e. *Mycoplasma pneumoniae*

Q8. What is the most common condition in infants associated with occult bacteremia?
  a. pneumonia
  b. otitis media
  c. cellulitis
  d. gastroenteritis
  e. osteomyelitis

Q9. Which of the following statements regarding the presumptive use of antibiotic therapy in infants with fever without a focus is (are) true?
  a. presumptive use of oral antibiotics in infants with febrile illnesses decreases morbidity
  b. the earlier an antibiotic is used, the more significant the effect on morbidity
  c. presumptive oral antibiotics reliably prevent meningitis
  d. all of the above statements are true
  e. none of the above statements is true

Q10. A remittent fever pattern in an infant is defined as which of the following?
  a. a daily temperature elevation that returns neither to a baseline level nor to a normal level
  b. a daily temperature elevation that returns to a baseline level but not to a normal level at least once a day
  c. a daily temperature elevation that returns to both a baseline level and a normal level at least once a day
  d. a daily temperature elevation that returns to a baseline level but not to a normal level at least three times a day
  e. a daily temperature elevation that returns to both a baseline level and normal level three times a day

Q11. Which of the following statements regarding antipyretic therapy in infants and children is (are) true?
  a. all infants and children with pyrexia should be treated
  b. high-risk infants and children with pyrexia should be treated
  c. antipyretic therapy alters the course of common infectious diseases in children
  d. antipyretic therapy alters the course of common infectious diseases in children regardless of the temperature
  e. all of the above statements are true

Q12. Which of the following statements concerning antipyretic therapy in infants and children is (are) true?

a. acetaminophen, aspirin, and nonsteroidal antiinflammatory drugs (NSAIDs) are equally effective antipyretics in infants and children

b. tepid sponge bathing in warm water (not alcohol) is recommended for reducing body temperature in infants and children

c. aspirin and acetaminophen have an equal safety/efficacy ratio for reducing pyrexia in infants and children

d. a and b

e. all of the above statements are true

Q13. Fever, an elevation in body temperature, is mediated as a final common pathway by which of the following?

a. endotoxins produced by the invading agent

b. exotoxins produced by the invading agent

c. antiendotoxins produced by the body in response to the invading agent

d. antiexotoxins produced by the body in response to the invading agent

e. production of endogenous pyrogens, which directly alter the hypothalamic temperature set-point

Q14. The signal to the hypothalamus to reset the heat regulatory set point is mediated by which of the following?

a. endogenous-produced cytokines

b. exogenous-produced cytokines

c. endogenous macrophages

d. endogenous monocytes

e. type B lymphocytes

Case 2 ■ A 2-Year-Old Infant with a Temperature of 39° C, a Sore Ear, and a Convulsion

A 2-year-old infant develops a temperature of 39° C. He began complaining of a sore right ear this afternoon. His mother called you and you asked her to meet you at the hospital this evening. On the way to the hospital, the child had a convulsion.

When the mother arrived at the hospital, the ictal phase was over. The infant appeared slightly lethargic. His rectal temperature was 39.5° C. His right tympanic membrane was red and bulging. The rest of the physical examination was normal.

Q15. Which of the following is (are) characteristic(s) of febrile convulsions in infants and children?

a. the onset is usually between the ages of 6 months and 5 years

b. the convulsion is usually of short duration (<15 minutes)

c. the convulsion is usually a generalized tonic-clonic pattern

d. there are usually no focal or lateralizing features

e. all of the above

SHORT ANSWER MANAGEMENT PROBLEM
Describe a reasonable approach to the diagnosis and management of a fever without a focus in a 1-year-old infant.

ANSWERS

A1. **a.** This infant has fever without a focus. Fever without localizing signs and symptoms is a common diagnostic dilemma for physicians caring for infants younger than 24 months old. Fever is usually of acute onset and present for less than 1 week. Age is a very significant risk factor; the younger the infant, the greater the risk.

Fever occurs when various infectious and noninfectious processes interact with the infant's defense mechanisms. In most children fever is either caused by an identifiable microbiologic agent or subsides after a short time.

A2. **d.** Fever in children is best classified in the following manner:

a. Fever of short duration with localizing signs in which the diagnosis can be established by clinical history and physical examination, with or without laboratory tests

b. Fever without localizing signs, in which the history and physical examination do not suggest a diagnosis but in which laboratory tests may establish a diagnosis

c. FUO, which by strict definition only applies to children who:

1) Have a fever exceeding 1 week in duration

2) Have a fever that is documented in the hospital

3) Have had all possible investigations performed during that week

A3. **b.** Fever without a focus is caused by an occult bacteremia until proven otherwise.

A4. **a.** The next step is to obtain a more detailed history, including the fever itself (remittent, intermittent, hectic, or sustained) and a history of exposure to infective agents such as siblings at home with a febrile illness, exposure to other children in a day care center, and other exposure to infectious diseases.

A5. **a.** The prevalence of occult bacteremia depends in part on the value of the WBC. Thus this is the most appropriate next step for infants who are 3 to 24 months old.

A6. **e.** The probability of occult bacteremia will be increased if any of the following criteria are met:
  a. The fever is higher than 40° C.
  b. The WBC is <5000/mm^3 or >15,000/mm^3.
  c. There is a positive exposure history.

A7. **c.** The most common organism causing occult bacteremia in children is *S. pneumoniae*. This organism is responsible for approximately 65% of cases of occult bacteremia. Other common causative agents include the following:
  a. *H. influenzae* type b (25%)
  b. *N. meningitidis*
  c. *Listeria monocytogenes*
  d. Group B *Streptococcus*

A8. **b.** The most common condition in infants and children associated with occult bacteremia is otitis media. This otitis media is most likely to be caused by *S. pneumoniae*. Remember that *S. pneumoniae* also causes pneumonia and meningitis in infants and children.
  H. influenzae type b is a very common cause of otitis media and is the second most common cause of occult bacteremia.

A9. **e.** The use of presumptive or prophylactic antibiotics in the prevention of morbidity associated with bacteremia is controversial. Although oral antibiotics may retard the emergence of some less serious focal bacterial disease (streptococcal pharyngitis, otitis media, and pneumonia), they do not reliably prevent meningitis. There is no solid evidence that the sooner a presumptive antibiotic is used, the greater it will affect morbidity and mortality from the disease.

A10. **b.** The diurnal variation of temperature is usually preserved in patients with febrile illnesses. When this circadian rhythm is associated with tachycardia, chills (rigors), and sweating, a true rather than a factitious fever should be suspected. Fever patterns are classified as follows:
  a. Remittent fever: daily elevated temperature returning to a baseline level but above the normal temperature
  b. Intermittent fever: daily elevated temperature returning not only to a baseline level but also to a normal level
  c. Hectic fever: daily elevated temperature of either an intermittent pattern or a remittent pattern with temperature excursion of 1.4° C (2.5° F)
  d. Sustained or continuous fever: daily elevated temperature with fluctuation of an elevated temperature of 0.3° C (0.5° F)

A11. **b.** Not all children with a fever need antipyretic treatment. In fact, antipyretics do not alter the natural history of the disease. The only children that should be treated with an antipyretic are those who are considered to be a high risk because of chronic cardiac disease, chronic respiratory disease, neurologic disease, febrile or nonfebrile convulsions, and metabolic disorders.

A12. **d.** Although acetaminophen, aspirin, and NSAIDs are equally efficacious antipyretics, they do not have an equal safety/efficacy ratio: aspirin has been associated with Reye's syndrome, and NSAIDs have been associated with gastric side effects and gastric bleeding. The antipyretic of choice is acetaminophen.
  Tepid sponge bathing may be just as effective as antipyretic therapy with drugs in reducing an infant's body temperature.

A13. **e.** Fever, defined as an elevation in body temperature, is mediated as a final common pathway by the production of exogenous pyrogens. This directly alters the hypothalamus temperature set point, resulting in heat generation and heat conservation.

A14. **b.** This hypothalamic set point is mediated by cytokine generation by exogenous pyrogens with subsequent hypothalamic prostaglandin E$_2$ production. This supports the drawing of blood for culture before fever elevation, when circulating bacteria (exogenous pyrogens) are more likely to be present.

A15. **e.** Febrile convulsions may accompany high fever in a child. Few children with febrile convulsions go on to develop epilepsy in later life.
  Febrile convulsions usually develop between the ages of 6 months and 5 years; occur with a rise in temperature above 39° C, last 15 minutes or less, are tonic-clonic in character, have no focal or lateralizing aspects, and do not manifest neurologic deficits postictally.
  Treatment of the fever and the underlying condition is usually sufficient.

SOLUTION TO THE SHORT ANSWER MANAGEMENT PROBLEM

A reasonable approach to the diagnosis and management of fever without a focus in a 1-year-old infant is as follows:
  a. Remember that a proper history and physical examination is both sensitive and specific in deter-

mining the prevalence of occult bacteremia. Does the child appear ill? If no, then reassure the parent. If yes, then consider this a serious sign and continue investigation. Consider the following in an infant:

1) Quality of cry
2) Reaction to parent stimulation
3) Color
4) Hydration
5) Response (talk, smile) to social overtones

b. Remember: the risks for occult bacteremia:
1) Fever higher than 40° C
2) WBC <5000/mm^3
3) WBC >15,000/mm^3
4) Positive exposure history

c. Remember the importance of repeated examinations and continuing contact with parents if fever without a focus is diagnosed and the child is allowed to go home.

d. Remember the most common organisms associated with occult bacteremia:
1) *S. pneumoniae*
2) *H. influenzae*
3) Group A beta-hemolytic *Streptococcus*
4) *N. meningitidis*

e. Remember the most common conditions associated with occult bacteremia:
1) Otitis media
2) Bacterial pneumonia
3) Streptococcal pharyngitis
4) Meningitis

f. Consider the possibility of febrile convulsions if the temperature is >40.0° C.

g. Remember that not all infants with fever have to be treated with antipyretics. Antipyretics do not speed the resolution of the condition. They may, in fact, hide certain symptoms.

h. Remember that symptomatic treatment (tepid sponge baths) may be just as effective as antipyretics.

i. Remember the importance of repeated reassessment of a child with fever without a focus until either the fever abates or the condition becomes overt.

j. Remember that if you are going to use an antipyretic to treat a child with a fever without a focus, the preferred agent is acetaminophen or ibuprofen.

k. Remember that blood cultures should be obtained before the rise in temperature.

SUMMARY TO THE MANAGEMENT OF INFANTS HAVING FEVER WITHOUT FOCUS

The Solution to the Short Answer Management Problem adequately summarizes this chapter.

SUGGESTED READINGS

Bonadio WA: The history and physical assessments of the febrile infant, *Pediatr Clin North Am* 45(1):65-77, 1998.

McCarthy PL et al: Fever without apparent source on clinical examination, infectious diseases, and low respiratory infections in children, *Office Pediatr* 10:101-116, 1998.

Schuchat A et al: Bacterial meningitis in the United States in 1995, *N Engl J Med* 337(14):970-976, 1997.

PROBLEM·91

PEDIATRIC GASTROENTERITIS

"I'm Sure Glad I Use Disposable Diapers."

Case 1 ■ An 18-Month-Old Infant with Diarrhea

A mother comes to your office with her 18-month-old infant son who has had diarrhea for the past 5 days. When asked about the diarrhea, the mother states that the infant has "six to eight loose bowel movements every day." There has been no blood in the stools. The infant has a mild fever (38.5° C) and appears to have some abdominal discomfort. The child vomited several times in the first 3 days of the illness, but this has since subsided. The infant has two siblings; neither one of them has any abnormal symptoms.

On physical examination, the child is active and does not appear to be significantly dehydrated. Examination results of the ears, throat, lungs, and abdomen are normal. There are no abdominal masses and no tenderness.

SELECT THE BEST ANSWER TO THE FOLLOWING QUESTIONS

Q1. What is the most likely cause of this infant's diarrhea?
   a. Norwalk agent
   b. rotavirus
   c. coxsackievirus
   d. echovirus
   e. *Shigella*

Q2. What is the treatment of choice in this infant at this time?
   a. admission to hospital for intravenous (IV) therapy
   b. observation in hospital and oral rehydration therapy
   c. treatment at home with fluids including fruit juices and noncarbonated beverages
   d. treatment at home with an oral rehydrating solution
   e. none of the above

Q3. Which of the following statements regarding rotavirus infection in children is (are) true?
  a. upper respiratory tract symptoms frequently precede the gastrointestinal symptoms of rotavirus
  b. upper respiratory tract symptoms of rotavirus include rhinorrhea, pharyngeal erythema, and cough
  c. otitis media frequently precedes the gastrointestinal symptoms of rotavirus
  d. a and b
  e. all of the above statements are true

Q4. Which of the following represents the composition of an ideal rehydrating solution for moderate dehydration (all numbers are represented in mEq/L except CHO, which is given in g/L)?
  a. Na^+, 23; K^+, 53; Cl^-, 15; CHO, 30
  b. Na^+, 40; K^+, 10; Cl^-, 20; CHO, 30
  c. Na^+, 90; K^+, 20; Cl^-, 80; CHO, 20
  d. Na^+, 140; K^+, 50; Cl^-, 80; CHO, 50
  e. Na^+, 100; K^+, 40; Cl^-, 100; CHO, 75

Q5. What is the most common bacterial cause of diarrhea in the pediatric age group?
  a. *Salmonella*
  b. *Shigella*
  c. *Campylobacter*
  d. *Escherichia coli*
  e. *Enterococcus*

Q6. Which of the following infectious agents may produce bloody diarrhea in infants and children?
  a. *Shigella*
  b. *Salmonella*
  c. enteroinvasive *E. coli*
  d. *Enterococcus*
  e. a, b, and c
  f. all of the above

Q7. Which of the following subtypes of *E. coli* cause(s) gastroenteritis in infants and children?
  a. enteropathogenic *E. coli*
  b. enteroinvasive *E. coli*
  c. enterohemorrhagic *E. coli*
  d. a and c
  e. all of the above

Q8. What is the most common cause of antibiotic-associated diarrhea in infants and children?
  a. ampicillin
  b. clindamycin
  c. erythromycin
  d. penicillin
  e. none of the above

Case 2 ■ A 23-Month-Old Infant with Sunken Eyeballs and Doughy Skin

An infant, age 23 months, is brought to the Emergency Department by his mother. He has had diarrhea and vomiting for the past 3 days and appears to be at least 15% dehydrated. His eyeballs are sunken and his skin is doughy. The child has no satisfactory veins in which to place an IV line.

Q9. What should you do now?
  a. attempt oral rehydration therapy
  b. perform a venous cutdown in the ankle
  c. begin an interosseous infusion
  d. begin a subcutaneous infusion
  e. any one of the above

Q10. Which of the following investigations should be performed on all children who have ongoing diarrhea?
  a. urine-specific gravity
  b. stool evaluation for blood
  c. stool evaluation for fecal leukocytes
  d. all of the above
  e. none of the above

Case 3 ■ A 3-Year-Old Male with Diarrhea Who Had Been Camping

A mother comes to your office with her 3-year-old boy who has developed severe crampy diarrhea and mild fever. The family has just returned from a camping trip in the Rocky Mountains; the child became sick on the third day. He was apparently drinking water from the local stream.

Q11. What is the most likely diagnosis in this patient?
  a. viral gastroenteritis
  b. *Shigella* gastroenteritis
  c. *Salmonella* gastroenteritis
  d. giardiasis
  e. amebiasis

Q12. Which of the following pediatric infections often present(s) with diarrhea as the initial symptoms?
  a. acute appendicitis
  b. otitis media
  c. urinary tract infections
  d. pneumonia
  e. all of the above

ANSWERS

A1. **b.** The most common cause of pediatric gastroenteritis is rotavirus. Symptoms of rotavirus infection include low-grade fever, anorexia, nausea, vomiting, diarrhea, and abdominal cramps. Dehydration may occur. The disease typically runs its course in a 4- to 10-day time frame.

Other causes of viral diarrhea in children include the following:

a. parvoviruses such as the Norwalk agent
b. coxsackievirus
c. echovirus
d. adenovirus
e. calicivirus

A2. **d.** Because this child does not appear to be significantly dehydrated, hospitalization is not required. The treatment of choice is home oral rehydration therapy. Fruit juices (undiluted) and commercial beverages are not recommended because of high osmolarity and the danger of hypernatremia or exacerbation of stool losses.

Details of oral rehydrating solutions are discussed in Answer 4.

A3. **e.** Viruses are the most common cause of wintertime diarrhea in infants. Rotavirus, as mentioned previously, is the most common agent. It is responsible for more than 50% of cases of acute diarrhea in children. The other viral causes are listed in Answer 1. The majority of infants and children who develop rotavirus develop an upper respiratory tract infection preceding the gastrointestinal symptoms. The respiratory tract symptoms include rhinorrhea, cough, pharyngeal erythema, and otitis media.

A4. **c.** Oral rehydration therapy effectively resolves most cases of pediatric gastroenteritis.

The World Health Organization recommended standard for oral rehydration therapy is Na^+, 90 mEq/L; K^+, 20 mEq/L; Cl^-, 80 mEq/L; HCO_3^-, 30 mEq/L; and, CHO 20 mEq/L.

Among the common oral rehydration solutions used, Gastrolyte has the identical composition to the World Health Organization's formula.

Clear liquids should not be given to infants with diarrhea because they have a low sodium content, a low potassium content, and a high carbohydrate content.

Examples of clear liquids include apple juice, carbonated beverages, and other liquids.

A5. **c.** The most common cause of bacterial gastroenteritis in both the pediatric and adult populations is *Campylobacter jejuni.*

Campylobacter gastroenteritis typically begins with fever and malaise, followed by nausea, vomiting, diarrhea, and abdominal pain. The diarrhea is often profuse and may contain blood. The illness is self-limited, lasting less than 1 week in 60% of cases. Recurrences and chronic symptoms can occur, especially in infants.

Symptoms caused by *C. jejuni* usually occur due to endotoxin production. Invasive strains also occur and produce disease. *Campylobacter* is effectively treated with erythromycin, although the infection is usually self-limiting and clears up when left untreated.

A6. **e.** *Salmonella* gastroenteritis begins with watery diarrhea and is accompanied by fever and nausea. As with *Campylobacter*, *Salmonella* produces disease both by mucosal invasion and endotoxin production, and the diarrhea may be bloody. Most cases of *Salmonella* gastroenteritis do not require antibiotic therapy.

Shigella gastroenteritis begins with watery diarrhea, high fever, and malaise; this is usually followed in 24 hours by tenesmus and frank dysentery. Mucosal invasion with frank ulceration and hemorrhage often occur. Dehydration is common. *Shigella* gastroenteritis should be treated with trimethoprim-sulfamethoxazole (TMP-SMX).

E. coli gastroenteritis may occur as an enteropathic infection, an enterohemorrhagic infection, an enterotoxigenic infection, or an enteroinvasive infection. Enteropathic *E. coli* usually produces a mild self-limited illness. Enterohemorrhagic *E. coli* produces diarrhea that is initially watery and later becomes bloody. Enterotoxigenic *E. coli* is the most common cause of traveler's diarrhea.

Enteroinvasive *E. coli* invades the mucosa and produces a dysentery-like illness with bloody stool.

In infants and children, *Yersinia enterocolitica* may produce acute and chronic gastroenteritis as well as mesenteric lymphadenitis. Mesenteric lymphadenitis is, at times, extremely difficult to distinguish from acute appendicitis. Diarrhea, fever, and crampy abdominal pain are the most common presenting symptoms. Treatment is symptomatic only; antibiotic therapy is unnecessary.

Enterococcus is not a cause of bacterial gastroenteritis in children.

A7. **e.** Enteropathic *E. coli* infection is seen primarily in infants. Enterotoxigenic *E. coli* infection is usually brief and self-limited. This is the most common cause of traveler's diarrhea. Enterohemorrhagic *E. coli* infection can progress to hemolytic uremic syndrome (especially O157:H7).

A8. **a.** The most common cause of antibiotic-associated diarrhea is ampicillin. Ampicillin and other antibiotic-associated diarrheas are common and generally self-limiting. Most cases resolve on discontinuation of the drug. However, on occasion a pseudomembranous colitis may develop because of an overgrowth of *Clostridium difficile* or release of its toxin. The prognosis of severe *C. difficile* induced pseudomembranous colitis cases is poor with a 20% to 30% fatality rate and a 10% to 20% relapse rate. Treatment of severe cases consists of oral vancomycin or metronidazole.

A9. **c.** In a young infant or child who presents with severe dehydration, it is often very difficult to establish good IV access. A skull vein is a possibility, but even that is difficult. An excellent alternative is an interosseous infusion (usually placed in the tibia). A large bore needle is used after local anesthesia has been infiltrated around the bone. This allows easy access and affords an excellent alternative to venous access.

A10. **d.** The investigations that should be performed on all children who have ongoing diarrhea include urine-specific gravity, stool analysis for blood, and stool analysis for fecal leukocytes. A urine-specific gravity below 1.015 suggests adequate hydration.

If a patient presents with bloody diarrhea, high fever, persistent symptoms, tenesmus, or a history of foreign travel, a stool culture and examination of the stool for ova and parasites should be performed. Routine stool culture, however, is not cost-effective.

Other investigations that should be considered in a toxic child include complete blood count, serum electrolytes, and serum osmolality.

A11. **d.** Gastroenteritis that begins while camping in the Rocky Mountains is most likely caused by giardiasis. Giardiasis needs a very low "organism load" to produce a very painful gastroenteritis. The recommended treatment is metronidazole and rehydration.

A12. **e.** Many nonenteric infections may produce diarrhea as the first and most prominent symptom. These include otitis media, urinary tract infection, acute appendicitis (from inflammation extending to involve the ureter on the right side of the body), lower lobe pneumonia, and mesenteric lymphadenitis *(Y. enterocolitica)*

SOLUTION TO THE SHORT ANSWER MANAGEMENT PROBLEM

The most common cause of gastroenteritis-produced death in infants and children is cholera. Cholera is both endemic and epidemic, and both have a seasonal pattern. Contaminated water is the major source of infectivity and transmission, and cholera becomes an epidemic when crowded conditions such as refugee camps are established.

The responsible organism is *Vibrio cholerae*. The resulting illness is sudden in onset and produces severe rice-water diarrhea and severe dehydration that can lead to death quickly.

SUMMARY OF THE DIAGNOSIS AND TREATMENT OF PEDIATRIC GASTROENTERITIS

1. Prevalence: During the first 3 years of life a child experiences an estimated one to three acute, severe episodes of diarrhea.

2. Most common causes: Rotavirus is the most common cause (50%). Rotavirus gastroenteritis is usually preceded by upper respiratory tract symptoms.
   C. jejuni is the most common bacterial cause. Other viral agents producing gastroenteritis include the following:
   a. Norwalk agent (parvovirus)
   b. Coxsackievirus
   c. Echovirus
   d. Adenovirus
   e. Calicivirus
   Other bacterial agents include the following:
   a. *Salmonella*
   b. *Shigella*
   c. *Yersinia*
   d. *E. coli*
   Parasites include the following:
   a. Giardiasis ("beaver fever") most common
   b. Amebiasis

3. Diagnosis: All children should be evaluated by having a complete urinalysis performed, including urine-specific gravity and a stool examination for blood and fecal leukocytes. Specific gravity, 1.015 suggests adequate hydration.
   If bloody diarrhea, persistent symptoms, fever, tenesmus, or recent foreign travel are present, a stool culture for ova and parasites should be done. In mild and self-limiting diarrhea, a stool culture is not cost-effective.

4. Treatment: Most children can be managed by oral rehydration therapy using a solution containing the following:
   a. Na^+ 90 mEq/L
   b. K^+ 20 mEq/L
   c. Cl^- 80 mEq/L
   d. HCO_3^- 30 mEq/L
   e. CHO 20g/L

   Antibiotic therapy should be initiated for *Shigella* (TMP-SMX) and *C. jejuni* (erythromycin).

SUGGESTED READINGS

Arnon SS: Anaerobic infections. In Behrman R, ed: *Nelson textbook of pediatrics*, ed 15, Philadelphia, 1998, WB Saunders.

Boyle JT: Chronic diarrhea. In Behrman R, ed: *Nelson textbook of pediatrics*, ed 15, Philadelphia, 1998, WB Saunders.

Lifschitz CH: Treatment of acute diarrhea in children, *Curr Opin Pediatr* 9(5):498-501, 1997.

McCarthy PL et al: Fever without apparent source on clinical examination, lower respiratory infections in children, other infectious diseases, and acute gastroenteritis of infancy and early childhood, *Curr Opin Pediatr* 9(1):105-126, 1997.

PROBLEM·92

RECURRENT ABDOMINAL PAIN IN CHILDHOOD

"I Just Can't Go to School, My Tummy Aches Again."

Case 1 ■ A 12-Year-Old Female with Recurrent Abdominal Pain

A 12-year-old female is brought to your office with a history of recurring abdominal pain. She is having episodes of abdominal pain once or twice a week. These episodes last approximately 8 hours. She has been seen on many occasions for the same problem and has been completely investigated. The investigations have included a complete blood count (CBC); urinalysis; stool for ova and parasites; an x-ray of the kidneys, ureter, and bladder (KUB); and an abdominal ultrasound. All investigations were normal. The pain is described as umbilical in location with a quality described as a "dull ache." She rates the pain at a baseline quantity of 6/10, with increases to 8/10 and decreases to 4/10. It is not associated with any food intake, and it is not associated with any diarrhea or constipation.

On physical examination, the young girl is in no apparent distress. Her vital signs, height, and weight are normal for age. On examination of the abdomen, there is slight tenderness in the area of the periumbilical region. There is no hepatosplenomegaly and no other masses.

SELECT THE BEST ANSWER TO THE FOLLOWING QUESTIONS

Q1. What is the most likely diagnosis in this patient?
   a. recurrent abdominal pain (RAP) syndrome
   b. lactose intolerance
   c. Crohn's disease
   d. mesenteric lymphadenitis
   e. chronic appendicitis

Q2. What is the prevalence of this condition in children?
   a. 1%
   b. 5%
   c. 10%
   d. 20%
   e. 25%

Q3. Regarding the physiologic basis for the pain that occurs in the condition described in Case 1, which of the following statements is (are) true?
   a. the pain can be conceptualized as a disorder that provokes pain pathways
   b. the pain can be conceptualized as an alteration in the patient's threshold to pain
   c. there is evidence that an abnormality in the autonomic nervous system is involved in this condition
   d. there is evidence that intestinal motility can be affected along with the occurrence of hyperalgesia
   e. all of the above statements are true

Q4. Which of the following statements regarding school attendance and the condition described in Case 1 is true?
   a. there is no association between school attendance and the condition described
   b. school phobia (reluctance to attend school) may be an important causative factor in this condition
   c. children with this condition usually achieve higher marks than their counterparts without this condition
   d. there is no association between stressful events at school and this condition
   e. none of the above statements is true

Q5. Which of the following investigations should be reordered in the patient described in Case 1 at this time?
   a. urinalysis
   b. CBC
   c. KUB x-ray
   d. abdominal ultrasound
   e. none of the above

Q6. Which of the following organisms is most commonly associated with organic recurring abdominal pain in children?
a. enterotoxigenic *E. coli*
b. enteropathogenic *E. coli*
c. *Giardia lamblia*
d. *Entamoeba histolytica*
e. *Salmonella*

Q7. Which of the following is the treatment of choice for the condition described?
a. muscle relaxants
b. tricyclic antidepressants
c. narcotic analgesics
d. nonsteroidal antiinflammatory agents
e. none of the above

SHORT ANSWER MANAGEMENT PROBLEM

List eight causes of acute abdominal pain for each of the following:
a. Infancy (<2 years)
b. Preschool (2 to 5 years)
c. School age (5 to 10 years)
d. Adolescence (11 to 15 years)
Rank these in decreasing order of prevalence.

ANSWERS

A1. **a.** The most likely diagnosis in this patient is RAP syndrome. The signs and symptoms of RAP syndrome are marked by their lack of specificity. The crucial separation of organic from nonorganic pain can be based on a few important findings, including the specificity and consistency of the pain and the relationship of the pain to meals and movement. The patient with nonspecific RAP tends to look well, to have pain that is inconsistent in relationship to meals and to movement, and to be free of the occurrence of additional symptoms such as nausea, vomiting, or dysuria.

Lactose intolerance is often confused with RAP syndrome in childhood and with irritable bowel syndrome in adults. In fact, these two syndromes can coexist. Lactose intolerance is usually associated with diarrhea.

Crohn's disease and mesenteric lymphadenitis are usually associated with systemic symptoms. The lack of systemic symptoms in this patient is strong evidence against these diagnoses.

Chronic appendicitis, if it exists, is more likely to be associated with pain in the right lower quadrant, as well as with nausea and vomiting.

A2. **c.** The prevalence of RAP syndrome in childhood is 10%.

A3. **e.** There are many theories related to RAP syndrome in children. Pain in children is conceptualized as a disorder that provokes pain pathways or an alteration in the patient's threshold to pain. A widely held plausible explanation in these cases is some abnormality in the functioning of the autonomic nervous system. This is thought to result in altered intestinal motility and the occurrence of hyperalgesia as well as altered secretory pathways.

A4. **b.** School phobia (reluctance to attend school) may be an important causative factor in RAP syndrome in childhood. There is a significant association between stressful events at school and RAP syndrome. Children with this condition, on average, achieve lower grades than their cohorts without this condition. This may actually be more associated with diminished school attendance than anything else. There is a significant association between stressful events at school and exacerbations of this condition.

A5. **e.** Because this child has already had numerous investigations, including all of the investigations described in Question 5, it is pointless to repeat them unless her condition is markedly different from previous episodes.

Because the possible mechanisms associated with abdominal pain are so numerous and not completely understood, the investigation and treatment of these cases of RAP in childhood test not only the physician's scientific acumen but also their skill in the practice of the art of medicine. There is a great temptation to "overdo" the testing and treatment when reliance on a careful clinical evaluation is the most important first step toward resolving the problem.

A6. **c.** *Giardia lamblia* is sometimes the cause of a recurrent pain syndrome in children. Thus every child with recurrent pain should have an examination of the stool for ova and parasites.

A7. **e.** Treatment for RAP syndrome in childhood should not be based on pharmacotherapy, especially pharmacotherapy that may do more harm than good. Therapy should emphasize the patient's response to the pain. In most cases, these efforts should involve the parents.

First, the patient and parents need to be reassured that the problem is not life threatening. Second, the physician should be realistic and frank and warn the patient and family that the problem may persist for an extended period. As mentioned, the physician should avoid prescribing medications and other therapies that may be harmful. Sedatives, antispasmodics, and analgesics are not only not beneficial, but also actually harmful. These agents, as well as having potentially deleterious effects on the intestinal motility and appetite, may also create dependency.

Laxatives and, at times, enemas may be beneficial. With some evidence of retained stool or, in difficult cases, even a suspicion of constipation, a trial of aggressive targeted treatment with mineral oil or lactulose with or without enemas can be effective in relieving the constipation that often goes along with RAP syndrome.

General measures such as the promotion of full activity and a sense of normal health are extremely important. A well-balanced diet, which is not excessive in fiber content, is recommended.

Every attempt should be made to maintain school attendance. In some otherwise physically well patients, a cycle of emotional turmoil, school absenteeism, and pain evolve. Identifying the stressors and breaking the cycle by ongoing counseling is the most important first step.

The prognosis for children with RAP is unclear. There is certainly no increased risk of intraabdominal disease, and in most cases symptoms improve before the age of 20 years. Some children with RAP syndrome do, however, go on to develop an irritable bowel syndrome as adults.

SOLUTION TO THE SHORT ANSWER MANAGEMENT PROBLEM

INFANCY
1. Colic
2. Gastroenteritis
3. Milk intolerance
4. Intussusception
5. Urinary tract infection
6. Trauma
7. Volvulus/intestinal anomaly
8. Incarcerated hernia

SCHOOL AGE
1. Gastroenteritis
2. Urinary tract infection
3. Appendicitis
4. Recurrent abdominal pain syndrome
5. Inflammatory bowel disease
6. Ingestion
7. Gonadal torsion
8. Lactose intolerance

PRESCHOOL
Gastroenteritis
Urinary tract infection
Trauma
Intussusception
Henoch-Schönlein purpura
Appendicitis
Hemolytic uremic syndrome

Meckel's diverticulum

ADOLESCENCE
Gastroenteritis
Urinary tract infection
Appendicitis
Pelvic inflammatory disease/ dysmenorrhea
Inflammatory bowel disease

Peptic ulcer disease
Ingestion
Gonadal torsion

Additional causes for all ages include mesenteric lymphadenitis, tumor, pneumonia, constipation, sickling syndrome, cystic fibrosis, diabetes mellitus, and celiac disease

SUMMARY OF THE DIAGNOSIS AND TREATMENT OF RAP IN CHILDHOOD

1. The diagnosis of RAP syndrome in childhood can usually be made from the history and physical examination, supplemented with a few investigations including CBC, urinalysis, ESR, stool for ova and parasites, occult blood, KUB x-ray, and abdominal ultrasound.

2. RAP in childhood is common; the prevalence is estimated at 10%.

3. Do not overinvestigate or overtreat patients with RAP in childhood. The vast majority of cases are nonorganic in origin.

4. Treatment should be supportive and should consist of reestablishing a healthy lifestyle, eating a well-balanced diet, exercising daily, and avoiding stress, especially at school.

5. There is a strong association between school phobia (school avoidance) and RAP syndrome. Take a careful history of school performance, school fears, and general feelings about attending school.

SUGGESTED READING
Ulshen M: Major symptoms and signs of digestive tract disorders. In Behrman RE et al, eds: *Nelson's textbook of pediatrics,* ed 15, Philadelphia, 1998, WB Saunders.

PROBLEM · 93

THE LIMPING CHILD

"Mom! Can You Rub My Legs? They Hurt So."

Case 1 ■ A 9-Year-Old Male with Leg Pain

A 9-year-old boy comes to your office with his mother. He complains of a recurrent (nightly) pain in both legs. The pain is so severe that it wakes him from sleep. It is described as a "deep pain." The pain is bilateral and is usually gone by morning. There is no associated fever, chills, limp, or other symptoms. Occasionally the pain may come on during the day; this usually occurs with excessive or strenuous exercise.

His history has been excellent. He has had no significant medical illnesses. On examination, the child has no limp and no leg length discrepancy.

**SELECT THE BEST ANSWER
TO THE FOLLOWING QUESTIONS**

Q1. What is the most likely diagnosis in this child?
   a. slipped capital femoral epiphysis (SCFE)
   b. Legg-Calvé-Perthes disease
   c. osteogenic sarcoma
   d. Ewing's sarcoma
   e. "growing pains"

Q2. What is the preferred treatment for this condition?
   a. surgical fixation
   b. bracing or traction
   c. amputation
   d. radiotherapy followed by chemotherapy
   e. none of the above

Q3. Regarding limb pain in children, which of the following statements is (are) true?
   a. limb pain is a common presenting complaint in children
   b. there is significant association between limb pain, headache, and abdominal pain
   c. there is frequently an association between limb pain in children and pain of other types in family members
   d. there is frequently an emotional component to limb pain in children
   e. all of the above statements are true

Q4. The following criteria describe which of the following pediatric orthopedic conditions listed?
   Criteria:
   1. The condition occurs as a result of acute trauma or in a more subtle fashion over time.
   2. The typical patient is a somewhat overweight and sedentary teenage boy.
   3. Pain is located either in the groin or on the medial side of the knee.
   4. The hip is held in abduction and external rotation, and there is marked limitation of internal rotation.
   5. Diagnosis is made by x-ray.
   Conditions:
   a. SCFE
   b. Legg-Calvé-Perthes disease
   c. osteogenic sarcoma
   d. Ewing's sarcoma
   e. "growing pains"

Q5. What is the preferred treatment for the condition chosen in response to Question 4?
   a. surgical fixation
   b. bracing or traction
   c. amputation

d. radiotherapy followed by chemotherapy
   e. none of the above

Q6. These following criteria describe which of the pediatric orthopedic conditions listed?
   Criteria:
   1. It is also known as *avascular necrosis* of the femoral head
   2. It is found mainly in children under the age of 10
   3. It is suggested by pain in the area of the hip or knee
   4. Demonstration of a limp and a decreased range of motion on physical examination is most likely
   Conditions:
   a. SCFE
   b. Legg-Calvé-Perthes disease
   c. femoral head abnormality
   d. hypermobile femur
   e. none of the above

Q7. What is the preferred treatment for the condition described in Question 6?
   a. surgical fixation
   b. bracing or traction
   c. casting
   d. any of the above may be indicated, depending on the case
   e. none of the above is indicated

Q8. The following criteria describe which of the following orthopedic pediatric conditions listed?
   Criteria:
   1. There is localized tenderness and swelling present over the tibial tubercle.
   2. The pain is aggravated by running, jumping, going up and down stairs, and kneeling.
   3. The condition is an overuse syndrome that occurs commonly in physically active males around puberty.
   4. Significant athletic activity and a recent growth spurt may result in detachment of cartilage fragments from the tibial tuberosity.
   Conditions:
   a. chondromalacia
   b. osteochondritis dissecans
   c. Osgood-Schlatter disease
   d. patellofemoral syndrome
   e. lateral diskitis

Q9. What is the preferred treatment for the condition described in Question 8?
   a. surgical removal
   b. casting

c. bracing or traction
d. splinting
e. none of the above

Q10. The following criteria describe which of the following pediatric orthopedic conditions?
Criteria:
1. The condition is characterized by subchondral bone necrosis and complete or partial separation of articular fragments.
2. The condition is usually caused by repeated trauma to a segment of the bone with tenuous vascularity.
3. The clinical manifestations may include episodic knee pain, aching after exercise, stiffness, clicking, muscle atrophy, mild joint swelling, and occasional locking.
4. The demarcated fragments of subchondral bone are best demonstrated radiographically by a "notch view" of the knee.
Conditions:
a. chondromalacia
b. osteochondritis dissecans
c. Osgood-Schlatter disease
d. patellofemoral syndrome
e. lateral diskitis

Q11. What is the usual preferred treatment for the condition described in Question 10?
a. surgical removal
b. casting
c. bracing and/or traction
d. splinting
e. none of the above

Case 2 ▪ A 13-Year-Old Female with Pain and a Grating Sensation in Her Knee

A 13-year-old female, a star on the junior high school basketball team, comes to your office with left anterior knee pain and a grating sensation aggravated by activities involving knee flexion such as climbing stairs and running.

On physical examination, you ask the patient to extend her knee while you compress the patella against the femoral condyle. The patient refuses to extend the femoral condyle because of pain.

Q12. What is the most likely diagnosis?
a. patellofemoral syndrome
b. osteochondritis dissecans
c. Osgood-Schlatter disease
d. soft patella syndrome
e. none of the above

Q13. What is the preferred treatment for most cases of this condition?
a. surgical removal
b. casting
c. bracing or traction
d. splinting
e. none of the above

Q14. The following criteria describe which of the following pediatric orthopedic conditions?
Criteria:
1. It is the most common cause of limb and hip pain in the 3- to 6-year-old age group.
2. It is characterized as an idiopathic, nonspecific, common, unilateral, inflammatory arthritis involving the hip joint.
3. Symptoms of upper respiratory tract infection often precede hip symptoms in this condition.
4. This condition is more common in boys than in girls.
Conditions:
a. toxic synovitis
b. Legg-Calvé-Perthes disease
c. SCFE
d. septic arthritis
e. osteomyelitis

Q15. What is the preferred treatment for the condition described in Question 14?
a. surgical decompression
b. casting
c. bracing or traction
d. splinting
e. none of the above

SHORT ANSWER MANAGEMENT PROBLEM
The differentiation between urgent versus nonurgent hip or leg pain often has to be made, which is sometimes difficult for the primary care physician.

Compare and contrast seven characteristics or distinguishing features of urgent limb pain or nonurgent limb pain that will help you, the family physician, distinguish serious illness from nonserious illness when presented in your office with a similar problem.

ANSWERS

A1. **e.** This child has typical "growing pains" or idiopathic limb pain.

Growing pains occur in 15% to 30% of otherwise normal children. It consists of deep pain often in the lower limbs that can be severe enough to wake the child from sleep. The pains occur intermittently, are always bilateral, are poorly localized, and are usually completely gone in the morning. The pains can, however, be aggravated by heavy exercise during the day and improved by nonpharmacologic therapies such as heat, massage, and physiotherapy. There is no limp or apparent disability and the cause is unknown.

There is often a psychologic component to growing pains. There seems to be a relationship between limb pain, abdominal pain, and headaches in children and an inherited or environmentally determined link between siblings with pain and parents with pain.

A2. **e.** Treatment consists of reassuring the family about the benign, self-limited course of the condition. Systematic treatment such as heat and an analgesic can be provided. Although avoidance of activities that aggravate the condition should be advised, this must be balanced against the positive benefits of maintaining some type of exercise program. Inform the family that if clinical features change, the child should be brought back to the office for reevaluation.

A3. **e.** Limb pain is a common presenting complaint in primary care practice. It is estimated to account for 7% of pediatric visits.

With limb pain in childhood, there is frequently an emotional component. There is a relationship between growing pains and headache and abdominal pain in children with these symptoms, who often come from "pain-prone" families. The parents have often had pain as children that has sometimes persisted into adulthood. In up to 33% of cases this "childhood pain syndrome" persists.

A4. **a.** This child has an SCFE, the characteristics of which are listed in the Question 4. Physiologically, SCFE occurs before the epiphyseal plate closes and usually at a time before and during the maximal pubertal growth spurt (13 to 15 years old in males; 11 to 13 years old in females). This condition is the most common adolescent hip disorder. Obesity is present in 80% of children with this disorder. It is more common in males. In nearly 50% of cases, both hips will ultimately be affected.

A5. **a.** An SCFE is an orthopedic emergency. Immediate hospitalization and operative fixation is indicated. Stabilization of the SCFE is essential if acute or gradual slipping is to be prevented. In severe chronic (and poorly aligned) SCFE, osteotomies are required to realign and stabilize the capital femoral epiphysis.

A6. **b.** These criteria describe Legg-Calvé-Perthes disease. The major criteria have been listed in Question 6. Perthes disease, in pathologic terms, is a juvenile idio-

pathic avascular necrosis of the femoral head. The cause is unknown, although repeated trauma, variation in the vascularity of the proximal femur, coagulation abnormalities, and other mechanisms have been suggested.

Legg-Calvé-Perthes disease occurs in about 1 of every 750 children. It primarily occurs between the ages of 4 and 10 years and affects primarily boys.

A7. **d.** Legg-Calvé-Perthes disease is difficult to treat because of the necessity for long-term treatment and the need to limit activities. The psychologic status of the child during treatment must be monitored. A biopsychosocial approach is often necessary to treat both the psychologic and orthopedic aspects of the problem. Braces and casting may be required for up to 1 to 2 years. Surgery, the other option, will allow the child to return to normal activity in 4 to 6 months.

The prognosis for Legg-Calvé-Perthes disease is, at best, fair. In the middle years, approximately 50% of patients go on to develop severe degenerative hip disease and require hip replacement.

A8. **c.** Osgood-Schlatter disease results from overuse of the lower extremity. It is a traction apophysitis of the tibial tubercle resulting from repetitive microtrauma. Athletic activity with or without a recent growth spurt may lead to cartilage detachment. The diagnosis is made by localizing the point of maximal tenderness over the tibial tuberosity.

A9. **e.** The preferred treatment for Osgood-Schlatter disease is a reduction in physical activity. The disease process itself is usually self-limited with complete remission when there is fusion of the tibial tubercle to the diaphysis. Resolution occurs over a period of months.

In a small percentage of cases the use of a knee immobilizer splint may be helpful. Rarely, excision of the ossicle may eventually be required. Local corticosteroid injections should not be used; injections of this nature may weaken the quadriceps tendon and produce local cutaneous thinning and depigmentation.

A10. **b.** Osteochondritis dissecans is a condition characterized by subchondral bone necrosis and, on occasion, by complete or partial separation of the articular fragments.

The most common site for osteochondritis dissecans is the lateral aspect of the medial femoral condyle. It may also occur in the patella and the lateral condyle of the femur.

Males are affected more often than females (3:1), and there appear to be two peaks of incidence: children younger than 12 years of age and young adults.

A11. **e.** In most cases of osteochondritis dissecans the treatment (in the patient with open growth plates) is conservative. Isometric quadriceps exercises, limitation of activities, and time lead to resolution of most lesions. Open arthrotomy or arthroscopic surgery is indicated when the fragments are greater than 1 cm in diameter, otherwise conservative treatment fails.

A12. **a.** Patellofemoral syndrome is a common cause of anterior knee pain in teenagers. It is an overuse syndrome. Most affected individuals show some degree of patellofemoral malalignment.

The principal symptoms (anterior knee pain and a grating sensation aggravated by activities involving knee flexion, such as climbing stairs or running) are reflected by a tender undersurface on the medial side of the patella and some crepitans.

A13. **e.** The treatment for patellofemoral syndrome includes an active isometric progressive resistance exercise program to strengthen the quadriceps. During the acute phase, nonsteroidal antiinflammatory drugs may be of benefit. In very few cases arthroscopy may be needed to remove bone or cartilaginous fragments, to shave the undersurface of the patella, or to release the lateral retinacular tethering structures.

A14. **a.** Toxic, or transient, synovitis is an idiopathic, transient, nonspecific, common, unilateral (5% bilateral) inflammatory arthritis involving the hip joint. It principally occurs in children between the ages of 3 and 6 years and is the most common cause of limp with hip pain in this age group.

Toxic synovitis usually follows a viral upper respiratory infection, and begins 3 to 6 days after the respiratory symptoms abate. In addition to guarded hip rotation, there is pain in the hip and pain in the anteromedial aspect of the thigh and knee. There also may be constitutional symptoms. These include a low-grade fever (less than or equal to 38° C [101° F]) and slight elevation of the erythrocyte sedimentation rate (ESR).

Aspirated fluid from the hip joint is clear, and x-ray demonstrates normal hips with an increased space between the medial acetabulum and the ossified femoral head. Because the bones are normal, the probability of aseptic necrosis, osteomyelitis, and other serious conditions is greatly diminished. Ultrasound of the hips usually demonstrates a joint effusion.

Note that it is extremely important to differentiate toxic synovitis from septic arthritis. In contradistinction to toxic synovitis, septic arthritis demonstrates higher fever, malaise, more pronounced spasm, guarding and fixed positioning, and a higher white blood cell count and ESR.

A15. **e.** The preferred treatment for toxic synovitis is conservative:
   a. Non-weight-bearing on the affected leg
   b. Rest in bed for a few days
   c. Analgesics or antiinflammatory drugs

SOLUTION TO THE SHORT ANSWER MANAGEMENT PROBLEM

The differentiation of disease in a child that limps is a critical skill for the family physician. The family physician must be able to differentiate disorders that require urgent versus nonurgent treatment. These differences are succinctly summarized in the following table:

Characteristic	Urgent	Nonurgent
Pain: Timing	Day and night	Only at night
Pain: Timing	Persistent pain	Intermittent pain
Pain: Severity	Interrupts play and normal activities	Child carries out other pleasant activities
Pain: Location	Located in joint or referred pain	Located between joints
Pain: Location	Usually unilateral	Usually bilateral
Limp	Child limps or refuses to walk	Child is able to walk normally
Pain description	Fits with logical anatomic explanation	Pattern does not fit with logical, recognizable, anatomic pattern

SUMMARY OF THE LIMPING CHILD (AGES 3 AND UP) IN FAMILY MEDICINE

1. A child with a limp is a common presentation in family medicine.

2. First priority of family physician: Distinguish urgent limp from nonurgent limp.

3. Second priority of family physician:
   a. If urgent comanage with specialist.
   b. If nonurgent, evaluate, treat, and reassure parent.

4. Common causes of childhood limp:
   a. Urgent
      1) Toxic or transient synovitis
      2) Septic arthritis

3) Osteomyelitis
4) Legg-Calvé-Perthes disease
5) SCFE
6) Malignancies (uncommon)
b. Nonurgent
1) Growing pains
2) School phobias
3) Osgood-Schlatter disease
4) Osteochondritis dissecans (consultation strongly suggested)
5) Chondromalacia patellae
6) Other patellofemoral disorders or syndromes

5. The most common cause of organic hip pain for each age group:
a. Toxic synovitis at age 3 to 6 years
b. Legg-Calvé-Perthes disease at 4 to 10 years
c. SCFE at 11 to 15 years

SUGGESTED READINGS

Eilert R, Georgopoulos G: Orthopedics. In Hathaway WE et al, eds: *Current pediatric diagnosis and treatment*, ed 11, Norwalk, Conn, 1993, Appleton & Lange.

Thompson GH, Scoles PV: Orthopedic problems. In Behrman R, ed: *Nelson textbook of pediatrics*, ed 15, Philadelphia, 1998, WB Saunders.

PROBLEM·94

FOOT AND LEG DEFORMITIES IN INFANTS AND CHILDREN

"I Would Just Die If I Had a Son with Crooked Legs."

Case 1 ■ An Anxious Mother with a 3-Month-Old Infant with Crooked Feet

A 3-month-old infant is brought to your office by his mother. She states that he has "crooked feet." She has been told by her friend that he will "need a number of casts to correct this."

On examination, the infant's feet are everted. The heel position as viewed from behind with his feet dorsiflexed is valgus. No other abnormalities are found on examination.

The mother's pregnancy was unremarkable. The birth weight of the infant was 10 pounds, 8 ounces.

SELECT THE BEST ANSWER TO THE FOLLOWING QUESTIONS

Q1. What is the most likely diagnosis in this infant?
a. congenital calcaneovalgus
b. metatarsus valgus
c. metatarsus varus
d. talipes equinovarus
e. clubfoot

Q2. What is the treatment of choice in this child?
a. serial casts
b. bilateral osteotomies
c. Denis-Browne splints
d. immediate referral to an orthopedic surgeon
e. reassurance and foot exercises

Case 2 ■ A 4-Week-Old Pigeon-Toed Infant

A mother brings her 4-week-old infant to the office for assessment of her child's "toeing in." She states that another physician has told her that this will probably require "serial casts" to correct.

On physical examination, both feet deviate medially. The feet dorsiflex easily and the heels are in a neutral position. The lateral borders of the feet are convex.

Q3. What is the most likely diagnosis in this patient?
a. calcaneovalgus
b. metatarsus varus
c. metatarsus valgus
d. talipes equinovarus
e. clubfoot

Q4. What is the most likely predisposing factor to the diagnosis described in Case 2?
a. abnormality at the embryo stage of development
b. hereditary susceptibility to the condition
c. position of the fetus in utero
d. abnormality in the shape of the maternal uterus
e. abnormality in the formation of the fetal legs and feet

Q5. What is the treatment of choice for the majority of patients with the condition described in Case 2?
a. serial casts
b. bilateral osteotomies
c. Denis-Browne splints
d. immediate referral to an orthopedic surgeon
e. reassurance and foot exercises

Case 3 ■ A 15-Month-Old Bowlegged Infant

A mother brings her 15-month-old infant into your office for an assessment of "his bowlegs." She states that he has been "bowlegged" since he began to walk 3 months ago.

On examination, the toddler's feet point inward while his knees point straight ahead.

Q6. On the basis of the information provided, what is the most likely diagnosis?
   a. internal tibial torsion
   b. internal femoral torsion
   c. metatarsus varus
   d. fixed tibia varum
   e. calcaneovalgus

Q7. What is the treatment of choice for the child described in Case 3?
   a. serial casts
   b. bilateral osteotomies
   c. Denis-Browne splints
   d. immediate referral to an orthopedic surgeon
   e. reassurance and leg exercises

Case 4 ■ An 18-Month-Old Infant with Twisted Legs

A mother comes to your office with her 18-month-old infant. She tells you that her child appears to have "both legs twisted inward from the hips." You examine the child and confirm that the mother's impression appears to be correct. The anterior aspect of the patellae is directed medially, and hip internal rotation is greater than external rotation.

Q8. What is the most likely diagnosis in this patient?
   a. internal tibial torsion
   b. excessive femoral anteversion
   c. flexible flat feet
   d. metatarsus adductus
   e. metatarsus varus

Q9. What is the most common cause of intoeing in children over the age of 3?
   a. internal tibial torsion
   b. excessive femoral anteversion
   c. metatarsus adductus
   d. metatarsus varus
   e. none of the above

Q10. What is the initial treatment of choice of the condition described in Case 4?
   a. serial casts
   b. bilateral osteotomies
   c. Denis-Browne splints
   d. immediate referral to an orthopedic surgeon
   e. watchful expectation

Q11. What is the most common method of measuring the degree of the condition described in Case 4?
   a. computed tomography scan of the lower leg
   b. ultrasonography of the lower leg
   c. biplanar radiography of the lower leg

   d. magnetic resonance imaging scan of the lower leg
   e. none of the above

Case 5 ■ A 6-Month-Old Infant with Crooked Feet

A mother brings her 6-month-old infant to your office for assessment. She tells you that her child's feet are "completely crooked" and that there is no way she can correct it.

On examination, you are unable to dorsiflex either foot. You notice that the heels are in the varus position (medial deviation) and the sole is kidney-shaped when viewed from the bottom.

Q12. What is the most likely diagnosis in this infant?
   a. talipes equinovarus
   b. metatarsus adductus
   c. internal tibial torsion
   d. excessive femoral anteversion
   e. none of the above

Q13. Which of the following treatments may be indicated for correction of the condition described in Case 5?
   a. posterior medial release of the heel cords
   b. series casts
   c. reassurance and foot exercises
   d. a and b
   e. all of the above

Q14. Which of the following may be associated with the condition described in Case 5?
   a. congenital dislocation of the hip
   b. spina bifida
   c. myotonic dystrophy
   d. a and b
   e. all of the above

Case 6 ■ A 21-Month-Old Infant with Flat Feet

A mother comes to your office with her 21-month-old infant. She tells you that he "slaps his feet when he walks." Her mother-in-law has informed her that he has "flat feet" and instructed her to "make darn sure the doctor does something about it." On examination, you observe the child walking. There certainly does seem to be a difference between the contour of the foot when weight bearing as compared to when not weight bearing.

Q15. Assuming that the abnormalities in this child's feet involve arch support and ligamentous laxity, what is the most likely diagnosis?

a. muscular dystrophy
b. cerebral palsy
c. flexible flatfeet
d. osteochondrosis
e. obesity

Q16. What is the most likely difference?
a. a difference in "heel lift"
b. a difference in "toe lift"
c. a difference in foot varus
d. a difference in foot valgus
e. a difference in sag versus nonsag weight bearing

Q17. Which of the following coexisting conditions is (are) associated with this condition?
a. muscular dystrophy
b. cerebral palsy
c. congenital heel cord tightness
d. a and c
e. all of the above

Q18. What is the treatment of choice for the primary condition described in Case 6?
a. corrective orthopedic shoes
b. orthotic inserts
c. flexible, well-fitted soft shoes
d. specially designed shoes
e. none of the above; watchful waiting is more appropriate

SHORT ANSWER MANAGEMENT PROBLEM
A mother comes to your office with her 6-month-old infant boy who is intoeing. Her mother-in-law has indicated that "a serious problem exists" that needs to be fixed now! Describe in detail how you would handle this situation.

ANSWERS

A1. **a.**

A2. **e.** The calcaneovalgus foot is a common neonatal foot deformity. It is the result of positional confinement in utero. The foot has a banana-shaped sole (lateral deviation); dorsiflexes quite easily because of a stretched, abnormally long heel cord; and has a heel that deviates laterally.

Prognosis is excellent; most cases improve spontaneously and rapidly. Parents who are uncomfortable with the prescription of observation alone should be encouraged to exercise the child's foot at each diaper change by stretching the ligaments and stretching the dorsal tendons.

Only in the rare instance that the foot remains severely deformed should corrective casts be applied. If the calcaneovalgus foot can be only partially corrected, a flexible flatfoot results.

This calcaneovalgus foot must be differentiated from a congenital vertical talus (congenital convex pes valgus), which is associated with neurologic disorders such as spina bifida or arthrogryposis in about 50% of cases. The vertical talus foot has a "rocker-bottom" appearance with a tight heel cord.

A3. **b.** This child has metatarsus adductus and metatarsus varus. They are used synonymously in practice, although they describe slightly different variations in the forefoot. In both cases, the sole is kidney bean–shaped (medial deviation), and the foot is easily dorsiflexed.

A4. **c.** Metatarsus adductus (varus) may be either bilateral or unilateral; it is probably secondary to in utero confinement. Two conditions associated with metatarsus adductus are muscular torticollis and congenital hip dysplasia.

A5. **e.** Metatarsus adductus usually improves spontaneously; this applies to at least 85% of cases. The severity of the metatarsus adductus, determined from the examination, should be documented. Severity is classified as follows:
Category A: mild/flexible
Category B: moderate/fixed
Category C: severe/rigid
The vast majority of cases fall into the mild/flexible group (Category A).

The parents can be taught to stretch the child's foot by firmly holding and stabilizing the heel and stretching the forefoot laterally, holding it to a count of five. The exercise can be performed five times at each diaper change.

Category B metatarsus adductus may need to be treated by serial casting. Category C: metatarsus adductus may need corrective surgery.

A6. **a.** Internal tibial torsion is a normal finding in the newborn. The mean tibial torsion at maturity is 15 degrees to 20 degrees. At birth, the mean tibial torsion is 5 degrees, that is, 10 to 15 degrees inward compared with adults. Internal tibial torsion usually presents at walking age, and affected children have an inward foot progression angle. When the child walks, it can be observed that the kneecaps point forward but the foot points inward.

Internal tibial torsion is thus a physiologic bowing of the lower extremities produced by the external rotation of the femur and internal rotation of the tibia.

A7. **e.** The natural history of internal tibial torsion is spontaneous resolution in more than 95% of children. Internal tibial torsion usually resolves by 7 or 8 years of age, at which time the rotatory conformation of the bones is largely established. Reassurance and leg exercises are the treatment of choice for the management of internal tibial torsion.

A8. **b.**

A9. **b.** The most common cause of intoeing in children over the age of 3 years is excessive femoral anteversion. The femoral neck is normally anteverted 10 to 15 degrees with respect to the axis of the femoral condyles in the knee of adults. The femoral neck is more anteverted in children. In one large study the average degree of anteversion of the femur in children between the ages of 3 months and 12 months was 39 degrees and 31 degrees in 1- to 2-year-old children.

A10. **e.** The treatment of choice in children with excessive femoral anteversion is "watchful waiting." In 90% to 95% of children, the degree of anteversion will progressively decrease to a level that is both within the normal range and completely acceptable.

A11. **c.** A number of techniques have been devised to accurately measure the degree of femoral anteversion. The most commonly used techniques involve biplanar radiography.

In children who have excessive femoral anteversion as the cause of their intoeing, the typical clinical finding is that the child is observed to walk with his or her patellae and feet pointing inward. The clinical diagnosis is made by having the child lie prone or supine with the hips extended and externally rotating the hip. In children with excess femoral anteversion, most of the arc of rotation of the hip will be inward.

A12. **a.** This child has talipes equinovarus, or clubfoot. When a child develops clubfoot, you notice the following:
   a. The inability to dorsiflex the clubfoot (heel equinus)
   b. The presence of heel varus (medial deviation)
   c. A sole that is kidney-shaped (forefoot and midfoot adductus)
Mild cases of clubfoot can be attributed to deformation caused by intrauterine compression, whereas more severe, fixed cases are usually secondary to underlying anatomic abnormalities such as an abnormal talus.

A13. **d.** Treatment options for talipes equinovarus include the following:
   a. Corrective serial casts
   b. Posterior medial release of the heel cords.
The proportion of children requiring corrective surgery varies from 75% if full anatomic, radiographic, and clinical correction is attempted to less than 50% if mild radiographic and clinical deformity is accepted.

A14. **e.** Accompanying deformities with talipes equinovarus include congenital dislocation of the hip, spina bifida, myotonic dystrophy, and arthrogryposis.

A15. **c.** This child has flexible flatfeet. The flexible flatfoot is extremely common, with an incidence ranging from 7% to 22%.

A16. **e.** The condition is often hidden by normal adipose tissue and usually becomes noticeable after a child begins to stand. The most common cause of the flexible flatfoot is ligamentous laxity, which allows the foot to sag with weight bearing. Children often present with accompanying hyperextension of fingers, elbows, and knees, as well as a family history of flatfeet and ligamentous laxity.

A child with flexible flatfeet secondary to ligamentous laxity can form a good arch when asked to stand on tiptoe. The heel rolls into a varus position (medial deviation) on tiptoe, and good strength of the ankle and foot muscles is assured.

When the child walks, the difference that can be seen immediately is that when the child is not bearing weight there is an arch. When the child is bearing weight, there is no arch.

A17. **e.** Although flexible flatfeet are usually not associated with any secondary conditions (that is, primary flexible flatfeet), it must be recognized that flexible flatfeet can be secondary to muscular dystrophy, mild cerebral palsy, or congenital tightness of the heel cords.

A18. **e.** Although many treatments have been advocated for flatfeet (corrective shoes, custom orthotics, corrective inserts, and flexible flatfoot wear), none of them has been shown to be better than "no treatment" or "watchful expectation."

SOLUTION TO THE SHORT ANSWER MANAGEMENT PROBLEM

The single most important aspect of management at this time is to establish a therapeutic alliance with the mother.

a. Begin with a complete history of the pregnancy and birth (pay particular attention to any complications).
b. Carry out a complete physical examination where the following are especially noted:
1) Foot varus versus foot valgus
2) Flexibility of varus or valgus deformity
3) Explain to the mother the various causes of intoeing and the very high frequency with which they self-correct (90% to 95%)
c. Have the patient return regularly for follow-up.
d. Refer to a specialists when indicated.

SUMMARY OF THE DIAGNOSIS AND TREATMENT OF FOOT AND LEG DEFORMITIES IN INFANTS AND CHILDREN

1. Prevalence of foot and leg deformities: Common (up to 10% of infants)

2. Foot deformities in infants and children:
a. Congenital calcaneovalgus foot: Very common neonatal foot deformity. It results from the fetal position in utero. The foot has a banana-shaped sole (lateral deviation) and dorsiflexes quite easily because of a stretched, abnormally long heel cord and a heel that deviates laterally. Treatment consists of watchful waiting.
b. Metatarsus adductus (metatarsus varus): The sole is kidney bean–shaped (medial deviation), and the foot is easily dorsiflexed. Treatment consists of foot exercises and watchful waiting.
c. Talipes equinovarus (clubfoot): This disorder is characterized by the inability to dorsiflex the foot, the presence of a heel varus (medial deviation), and a sole that is kidney-bean shaped when viewed from the bottom. The tarsal navicular position is abnormal. A tight heel cord is exceedingly common. Many cases are caused by intrauterine position. Treatment consists of serial casts or surgical posterior medial heel cord release.

3. Other causes of intoeing in young children:
a. Internal tibial torsion: In internal tibial torsion, the entire foot points inward and the patella points straight ahead (medial tibial torsion). Treatment consists of watchful waiting.
b. Excessive femoral anteversion: The entire leg turns in so that both the patella and the foot are facing medially (medial femoral torsion or increased anteversion of the hips). Treatment consists of watchful waiting.

4. Flexible flatfeet: In a child with flexible flatfeet, when the foot is not bearing weight, the arch of the foot is preserved. When the child is bearing weight, the arch of the foot is not preserved. Treatment consists of watchful waiting.

SUGGESTED READINGS

Churgay C: Diagnosis and treatment of pediatric foot deformities, *Am Fam Physician* 47(4):883-889, 1993.
Dietz F: Intoeing—fact, fiction, and opinion, *Am Fam Physician* 50(6):1249-1259, 1994.
Tolo VT, Wood B: *Pediatric orthopaedics in primary care*, Baltimore, 1993, Williams & Wilkins.

PROBLEM·95

ADOLESCENT DEVELOPMENT

"I'm Good. Just a Few Pimples."

Case 1 ■ A 16-Year-Old Male with Acne

A 16-year-old male comes to your office for assessment of "pimples." He tells you that he has had "a lot of pimples for the last 4 years" and "they really aren't getting much worse or much better." He has never seen a physician for this problem. You wonder why he has chosen to seek advice from a doctor at this time.

On examination, the patient appears to answer questions slowly, and he never makes eye contact with you. He has a mild case of acne with scattered whiteheads, blackheads, and a few papules.

SELECT THE BEST ANSWER TO THE FOLLOWING QUESTIONS

Q1. With respect to this young man's presentation, which of the following statements most likely best portrays the patient's situation and/or your response at this time?
a. acne is most likely the only problem this young man has
b. acne may very well be the "ticket of entry" to your office
c. acne is the problem; treat his acne and send him on his way
d. adolescents like this young man are more likely rather than less likely to present with minor problems
e. it is difficult to establish rapport with an adolescent patient like this young man

Q2. Regarding the patient described, you should now do which of the following?
a. attempt to identify an underlying agenda
b. call his mother and ask her if she thinks anything is wrong with him

c. call the social worker and ask that the patient be seen at once

d. refer the patient to a dermatologist

e. none of the above

Q3. To facilitate further discussion with this patient at this time, what should you say?

a. "We'll treat your acne; any other problems?"

b. "Acne is easily treated; don't worry."

c. "I have a feeling there is something else you'd like to talk about—I'm listening."

d. "Don't look so down; this is as easy as pie to treat."

e. "My nurse will give you your acne medications. I'll see you in a month."

Q4. In the United States the most common cause of death among people 15 to 24 year old is:

a. homicide

b. suicide

c. accidents

d. congenital malformations

e. acquired immunodeficiency syndrome (AIDS)

Q5. What is the psychiatric disorder most common in adolescents?

a. major depressive disorder

b. bipolar disorder

c. schizophrenia

d. adjustment disorder

e. antisocial personality disorder

Q6. What is the key ingredient to ensure healthy adolescent development?

a. early graded independence

b. a prolonged supportive environment

c. negotiating autonomy

d. prevention of consequences for failure to perform up to parental expectations

e. independence dependent on performance

Q7. Regarding exploratory behavior in adolescence, which of the following statements is (are) true?

a. exploratory behavior is unnecessary and should be discouraged

b. exploratory behavior is associated with some risks

c. much of adolescent exploratory behavior is developmentally appropriate

d. b and c

e. all of the above statements are true

Q8. Early adolescence is mostly concerned with which of the following?

a. a preoccupation with bodily changes

b. a preoccupation with independence

c. a preoccupation with becoming an adult

d. a preoccupation with conforming to the peer group

e. a preoccupation with distancing from parents

Q9. Which of the following is the third leading cause of death among people 15 to 24 years old in the United States?

a. motor vehicle accidents

b. cancer

c. alcohol-related disease

d. suicide

e. infectious disease (primarily AIDS)

Q10. Which of the following factors is (are) associated with an increased risk of early adolescent sexual intercourse?

a. divorce or separation of the parents

b. poor school grades or low future education plans

c. negative parental attitudes

d. none of the above

e. all of the above

Q11. Regarding the abuse of alcohol and other drugs by adolescents, which of the following statements is (are) true?

a. cigarette smoking is the "gateway"

b. the age at which children and adolescents begin experimenting with alcohol and other drugs is decreasing

c. alcohol is the principal substance of abuse

d. none of the above statements is true

e. all of the above statements are true

Q12. The risk of adolescent drug abuse is influenced by which of the following?

a. risky sexual behavior

b. school performance

c. physical activity

d. a and b only

e. all of the above

Q13. Regarding visits to family physicians by adolescents, which of the following is (are) true?

a. the acute episodic visit is often the only type of visit adolescents make to physicians

b. most adolescents making acute episodic visits to their family physicians have either an underlying behavior, an underlying social circumstance, or an underlying "myth" that should be explored at this opportunity

c. 10% of adolescents have chronic conditions necessitating frequent visits to physicians' offices

d. a and b only
e. all of the above

Q14. Which of the following statements regarding teenage pregnancy is (are) true?
a. teenage pregnancy is associated with poor prenatal care
b. teenage pregnancy is associated with poor nutrition
c. teenage pregnancy is associated with the use of illicit drugs
d. all of the above statements are true
e. none of the above statements is true

Q15. The central task of adolescence is generally considered to be which of the following:
a. the formation of a self-image of competency and strength
b. to develop a way of coping with the major adjustment disorder that goes along with adolescence
c. the ability to develop an independent ego
d. the ability to follow the cycle of dependence to interdependence to independence without significant problems
e. the ability to begin to think independently

SHORT ANSWER MANAGEMENT PROBLEM
Describe the preventative medicine strategies that should be incorporated into an office visit in which an adolescent comes to see his or her physician for acute episodic care.

ANSWERS

A1. **b.** The acne that this young man has may very well be the ticket of entry to your office. Although it is possible that acne is the major reason for attending your office at this time, it is unlikely. He states that his acne is "not much better or not much worse" than it has been for the last 4 years; therefore, more likely than not there is a second, or hidden, agenda.

A2. **a.**

A3. **c.** At this time you should attempt, if possible, to identify exactly what the likely hidden agenda is. An appropriate opener would be, "I have a feeling there is something else that you would like to talk about. I'm listening." An alternative would be, "Are there any other problems that you wish to discuss at this time with me?" More direct questions would include questions about school (problems at school), questions

about the relationship with his parents, questions about relationships (girlfriend problems and so on), and questions about sexual activity.

A4. **c.** In 1995 U.S. statistics showed that accidents were the leading cause of death among individuals who are 15 to 24 years old. Many of these deaths are preventable.

A5. **d.** Many youths have emotional symptoms. Unfortunately, some physicians feel uncomfortable or awkward with these patients, and others deal with them in an awkward manner. The majority of adolescents in this category is suffering from a minor adolescent adjustment disorder and requires little more than caring and reassurance. On the other hand, be on the lookout for more serious psychiatric conditions, conditions that would lead you to come up with a diagnosis of major depression, suicidal ideation, or a similar serious condition.

A6. **b.** Experts agree that the key ingredient to ensure healthy adolescent development is a prolonged supportive environment with graded steps toward autonomy. Healthy development is encouraged by a process of mutual positive engagement between adolescents, various adults, and peers. Schools and youth-serving community agencies can also play a major role by engaging youth in meaningful ways.

A7. **d.** Adolescence is characterized by exploratory behavior, much of which is developmentally appropriate and socially adaptive. The adolescent must experiment with new behaviors and relationships, inevitably courting some risks. There is a not a simple distinction between what is normal and what is abnormal in exploratory behavior. It is better to judge a particular behavior in the context of how the adolescent is developing in the family, at school, and among peers and friends.

A8. **a.** Early adolescence brings a preoccupation with body changes. Early adolescents feel uncertain about their appearance, and their interests are directed toward themselves. This is a period marked by high levels of physical activity and mood swings.

A9. **d.** Suicide is the third leading cause of death among people who are 15 to 24 years old in the United States; homicide is second.

A10. **e.** Factors associated with initiation of intercourse in adolescence include divorce or separation of parents, poor school grades and low future educational plans, negative parental attitudes (that is, if teens are taught that sex is not healthy or normal), and the use of drugs or alcohol.

A11. **e.** First, nicotine is definitely the "gateway drug"—the drug that leads to the use of other and more dangerous drugs, including alcohol, marijuana, and cocaine. Second, the age at which adolescents first begin experimenting with alcohol and other drugs is dropping. Third, alcohol is the principal substance of abuse. Marijuana, heroin, cocaine, crack cocaine, and other stimulant abuse are significant but not as common.

A12. **e.** The use of alcohol and other drugs is one of the many risk factors that contribute to the deterioration in the health of adolescents. Different risk factors are associated with each individual, and these risks vary in accordance with age and sex. The use of drugs and alcohol, risky sexual behavior, school performance, peer pressure, diet, physical activity, socioeconomic status, and parental relationships are all factors that influence and predict the likelihood of risky behavior.

A13. **e.** Acute episodic care or the acute episodic visit is the most frequent reason for an adolescent to visit a physician's office. These visits most frequently involve visits for respiratory tract infections, skin conditions, genitourinary tract concerns, musculoskeletal trauma, and emotional disorders.

First, an episodic care visit is often the only type of visit that a youth will make to a physician's office. Second, most youth have an underlying behavior, a social circumstance, or a myth that may or may not be affecting the presenting condition but has the potential to affect future health. Third, youths are establishing health habits for adult life.

Of adolescents, 10% have chronic medical conditions affecting them, including problems such as diabetes mellitus, asthma and respiratory allergies, epilepsy, inflammatory bowel disease, juvenile rheumatoid arthritis, various cancers (especially leukemia), congenital heart disease, cystic fibrosis, and hemophilia.

A14. **d.** Teenage pregnancy is associated with the following:
 a. Poor prenatal care because of reluctance to seek care
 b. Poor nutrition leading to intrauterine growth retardation
 c. Smoking (one third of pregnant teens)
 d. Use of illicit drugs
 e. Associated sexually transmitted diseases
 f. Poor parenting skills
 All of these may negatively affect the infant.

A15. **a.** It is development in the psychosocial area that gives adolescence its main distinctive characteristics. The adolescent is faced with the resolution of a number of developmental tasks. It is widely accepted that the central task of adolescence is the formation of a self-image of competency and strength. Adolescents who have difficulty establishing an identity are plagued by role confusion. They also have difficulty establishing long-lasting relationships and stable career opportunities. If they enter adulthood without a sense of identity, their further development may be in jeopardy.

SOLUTION TO THE SHORT ANSWER MANAGEMENT PROBLEM

1. Universal: Adolescence is a period of time when at least one health maintenance examination should be carried out. Episodic care visits are an ideal time to carry out these health screenings and assessments. Two mnemonics are available that are useful in screening adolescents:
 a. SAFE TIMES
  S Sexuality issues
  A Affect (depression) and abuse (drugs)
  F Family (function and medical history)
  E Examination (sensitive and appropriate)
  T Timing of development (body image)
  I Immunizations
  M Minerals (nutritional issues)
  E Education, employment (school and work issues)
  S Safety (vehicle)
 b. HEADS
  H Home
  E Education, employment (school and work issues)
  A Activities, affect, anxieties, ambitions
  D Drugs
  S Sex, stress, suicide, self-esteem
2. Phases of adolescent development:
 a. Early adolescence: Preoccupation with body changes. Early adolescents often feel uncertain about their appearance and their interests are directed toward themselves. This is a period marked by high levels of physical activity and mood swings.
 b. Mid-adolescence: In mid-adolescence the major concern is independence. The peer group dominates social life, and risk behaviors become more prevalent. This is the time when sexual matters receive much interest.
 c. Late adolescence: In many ways, youths in the late adolescence phase appear to be adults. They are more capable of future orien-

tation, mutual caring, and internal control. However, most late adolescents also have uncertainties about sexuality, future relationships, and future work possibilities. Allowing them to be adolescents is very important.

SUMMARY OF THE DIAGNOSIS AND TREATMENT OF ADOLESCENT DEVELOPMENT

The Solution to the Short Answer Management Problem is an excellent summary of adolescent development.

SUGGESTED READINGS

Bennett D: Understanding the adolescent patient, *Aust Fam Physician* 17(5):345-346, 1988.

DiClemente RJ: The psychological basis of health promotion for adolescents, *Adolesc Med* 10(1):13-22, v, 1999.

Juszczak L, Sadler L: Adolescent development: Setting the stage for influencing health behaviors, *Adolesc Med* 10(1):1-11, v, 1999.

Lammers C et al: Influences on adolescents' decision to postpone onset of sexual intercourse: a survival analysis of virginity among youths age 13 to 18 years, *J Adolesc Health* 26(1):42-48, 2000.

Patel DR et al: Adolescent growth, development, and psychosocial aspects of sports participation: an overview, *Adolesc Med* 9(3):425-440, v, 1998.

Resnick MD et al: The impact of caring and connectedness on adolescent health and well being, *J Paediatr Child Health* 29(suppl 1): S3-S9, 1993.

Schubiner HH: Preventive health screening in adolescent patients, *Prim Care* 16(1):211-230, 1998.

Story M, Neumark-Sztainer D: Promoting healthy eating and physical activity in adolescents, *Adolesc Med* 10(1):109-123, vi, 1999.

Windle M, Windle RC: Adolescent tobacco, alcohol, and drug use: current findings, *Adolesc Med* 10(1):153-63, vii, 1999.

PROBLEM·96

ENURESIS IN CHILDREN

"My 6-Year-Old Son Still Needs Diapers at Night."

Case 1 ■ A 6-Year-Old Male Who Still Wets the Bed

A mother brings her 6-year-old son to your office for a periodic health assessment. The child continues to wet his bed at night (an average is two to three times per week). He is dry during the day. The child has no history of significant medical problems. Specifically, he has had no urinary tract infections. Labor and delivery were normal, as was the neonatal period. His growth (both weight and height) has always been in the 10th percentile. He started school last year but did not do well. He had to repeat the first grade. His blood pressure measured today is 85/60 mm Hg. The examination of all other body systems is normal.

SELECT THE BEST ANSWER TO THE FOLLOWING QUESTIONS

Q1. What is the most likely diagnosis in this child?
a. separation anxiety, with or without school phobia
b. nocturnal enuresis
c. small bladder syndrome (SBS)
d. masked childhood depression
e. none of the above

Q2. With respect to this condition, which of the following statements is false?
a. by the 6th year some 7% of children have the condition
b. the condition is more common when one or both parents had the condition
c. the condition is more common in boys
d. the condition usually implies significant psychopathology in the child
e. urethral valves, neurogenic bladder, and ectopic ureter may be associated with the condition

Q3. A child is defined as enuretic if he or she has not attained full bladder control by what age?
a. 3 years
b. 4 years
c. 5 years
d. 6 years
e. 8 years

Q4. Which of the following investigations is the most important to be performed in a child with enuresis?
a. urinalysis
b. urine culture
c. complete blood count (CBC)
d. complete cystometric evaluation
e. intravenous pyelography (IVP)

Q5. Which of the following is not a consideration in the differential diagnosis of enuresis?
a. diabetes mellitus
b. diabetes insipidus
c. petit mal seizures
d. separation anxiety disorder
e. posterior urethral valve syndrome

Q6. Which of the following is the drug of choice in the pharmacologic treatment of this disorder?
a. oxybutynin chloride
b. imipramine
c. chlorpromazine
d. diazepam
e. none of the above

Q7. Which of the following statements most accurately reflect(s) the treatment of this condition?
  a. most nonpharmacologic therapies have been shown to be no more effective than placebo in the treatment of this condition
  b. behavior modification has been shown to be superior to other nonpharmacologic therapies
  c. pharmacologic therapy is recommended in enuretic children who do not respond to nonpharmacologic therapies
  d. b and c
  e. all of the above

Q8. What is the most effective form of behavior modification in the treatment of the disorder described?
  a. biofeedback
  b. electric shock treatment (spontaneously triggered when the child wets the bed)
  c. a bell or buzzer system
  d. the behavior modification theory of logical consequences
  e. all of the above are equally effective

Q9. Which of the following is (are) important in the treatment of this condition?
  a. enlisting the cooperation of the child in dealing with the problem
  b. establishing a rule that older children should be expected to launder their own soiled bedclothes and pajamas
  c. elimination of liquids before bedtime
  d. voiding just before bedtime
  e. all of the above

Q10. Which of the following should not be used in the treatment of this condition?
  a. punishing the child
  b. postponing bedtime in an effort to decrease the frequency of the problem
  c. providing the child with a feeling of inferiority for having the problem
  d. all of the above
  e. a and c

SHORT ANSWER MANAGEMENT PROBLEM

Discuss the possible relationship between enuresis in a child and psychologic or psychiatric problems in children.

ANSWERS

A1. **b.** Nocturnal enuresis is urinary leakage that occurs at night during sleep. Enuresis can be primary (if the individual has never been dry at night for any substantial time) or secondary (i.e., returning after having one or fewer wetting episodes per month for at least 1 month).

The *Diagnostic Statistical Manual of Mental Disorders, fourth edition* (DSM-IV) classification of enuresis (which this child has) is based on the following criteria:
  a. Repeated voiding of urine into bed or clothes (whether involuntary or intentional)
  b. The behavior is clinically significant as manifested by either frequency of twice a week for at least 3 consecutive weeks or the presence of clinically significant distress or impairment in social, academic (occupational), or other important areas of functioning.
  c. Age of at least 5 years
  d. Not caused by the direct physiologic effect of a substance (such as a diuretic) or a general medical condition (such as diabetes, spina bifida, or a seizure disorder). DSM-IV further subclassifies enuresis into the following categories:
    1) Nocturnal only
    2) Diurnal only
    3) Nocturnal and diurnal

This child does not meet the criteria for separation anxiety disorder, and there is no information that suggests a diagnosis of masked depression. SBS does not exist.

A2. **d.** It is estimated that mental disorders are present in only about 20% of enuretic children. They are most common in enuretic girls, in children with symptoms during both day and night, and in children who maintain the symptoms into older childhood. Thus mental disorders are the exception rather than the rule.

A3. **c.** Enuresis is usually defined as the involuntary discharge of urine after the age at which bladder control should usually have been established (age 5). As just classified, this child has nocturnal enuresis (only at night).

The prevalence of enuresis decreases with increasing age. Thus 82% of 2-year-old children, 49% of 3-year-old children, 26% of 4-year-old children, and by the end of the 5th year 7% of children still wet beds or clothes on a regular basis.

Enuresis is definitely more common in children when one or both parents were enuretic as children.

There appears to be a developmental immaturity leading to a decreased functional bladder capacity in enuretic children. Uropathies may be associated with enuresis. Urethral valves, neurogenic bladder, and ectopic ureter may occasionally be the cause of primary enuresis. Urinary tract infections are a common organic cause of enuresis, especially secondary enuresis, in girls.

A4. **a.** The only mandatory laboratory evaluation for enuretic children is a urinalysis. The presence of white blood cells in the urine caused by a urinary tract infection; low urine-specific gravity caused by diabetes insipidus, proteinuria, or hematuria caused by renal disease; and glucosuria caused by diabetes mellitus are all important abnormalities that may be associated with enuresis.

Urine culture, CBC, IVP, and cystometric evaluation should be performed only if specific indications suggest the need. Posterior urethral valves (especially in boys) may be associated with enuresis.

A5. **d.** The only disorder listed in Question 5 that is not part of the differential diagnosis of enuresis is separation anxiety disorder.

A6. **e.** At one time the pharmacologic therapy of choice for enuresis was imipramine. However, because its administration is generally effective only briefly and drug tolerance, exacerbation of symptoms after the discontinuation of the drug, and medication side effects are common, recommendations presently discourage its use in children with enuresis. Use of the antidiuretic hormone analogue desopressin acetate nasal spray (DDAVP) for treatment of nocturnal enuresis has been increasing. Although DDAVP can lessen the number of wet nights in many children, it is not curative. Relapses occur commonly on cessation of the drug.

A7. **b.**

A8. **c.**

A9. **e.**

A10. **d.** Because there is usually no identifiable cause of enuresis and the disorder tends to remit spontaneously even if not treated, treatment should be conservative. The methods approved for the treatment of enuresis include the following:
   a. Appropriate toilet training (scheduled voiding times especially in the evening; wake up to urinate in the middle of the night)
   b. Behavior modification (bell or buzzer) and pad
   c. Positive reinforcement system that charts the child's progress. Although all of the approved methods are effective and should be used together, it appears that the most effective behavior modification method is the buzzer or bell and pad system.

Here are some general recommendations that may prove helpful in the treatment of enuresis:
   a. Enlisting the support and cooperation of the child in treating the condition
   b. Having older children launder their own soiled bedclothes and pajamas (not as a punishment but rather as participation in their own illness)
   c. Prohibiting liquids after dinner
   d. Making sure the child voids before retiring
Here are some general recommendations to avoid in the treatment of enuresis:
   a. Waking the child repeatedly during the night to take him or her to the bathroom; this has negative consequences in most children for the following reasons:
      1) It disturbs sleep
      2) It may further engender or aggravate anger in the child or the parent.
   b. Punishing the child for wetting the bed
   c. Intimidating the child or lowering his self-esteem
   d. Postponing the child's bedtime in an effort to decrease the frequency of bed-wetting

SOLUTION TO THE SHORT ANSWER MANAGEMENT PROBLEM

The key points to consider in discussing the relationship between enuresis and psychologic or psychiatric problems in children are as follows:
   a. The vast majority of enuretic children have no associated psychologic or psychiatric pathologic condition.
   b. Chronic psychologic stress (unrelated to toilet training experiences) can impair the child's ability to achieve bladder control.
   c. A situation in which the child becomes enuretic after a period of dryness is called secondary, or regressive, enuresis. This type of enuresis is precipitated by stressful environmental events such as a move to a new home, marital conflict, birth of a sibling, or a death in the family. Such bed-wetting is intermittent and transitory; the prognosis is better, and management is less difficult than in a child with primary enuresis.

SUMMARY OF THE DIAGNOSIS AND TREATMENT OF ENURESIS IN CHILDREN

1. Prevalence: 7% at the age when bladder control should have been fully achieved (that is, after 5 years of age)

2. Subtypes of enuresis:
   a. Classification based on whether or not child has ever achieved bladder control
      1) Primary enuresis: Child has never been dry.
      2) Secondary enuresis: Child has been dry for a period but becomes enuretic later.
   b. Classification based on period when child does not have bladder control
      1) Nocturnal enuresis: Enuresis at night only
      2) Diurnal enuresis: Enuresis during the day only
      3) Nocturnal and diurnal enuresis: Enuresis during both day and night

3. Pathophysiology: Immaturity of the part of the autonomic nervous system that controls the bladder in the vast majority of cases. Infrequently, enuresis is associated with organic problems such as congenital urinary tract system abnormality or urinary tract infection.
   a. Only 20% of children with enuresis have a psychodevelopmental disorder (lower intelligence quotient or behavioral disorder).
   b. Regressive enuresis is usually associated with some stressful environmental event.

4. Investigations: Urinalysis is the only mandatory investigation for nocturnal enuresis. If enuresis occurs also in the daytime or if urinary flow is small or interrupted, a renal ultrasound and a careful neurologic examination (including inspection of the sacral area for structural abnormalities) are indicated.

5. Treatment:
   a. Pharmacologic: Imipramine is no longer recommended for the treatment of enuresis in most children.
   b. Nonpharmacologic: A behavior modification program is the treatment of choice.
      1) Buzzer or bell system and a pad
      2) Positive reinforcement
      3) Charting progress to increase confidence and self-esteem of the child
      4) Urinating before bed
      5) Avoiding liquids after supper
      6) Relationship to psychopathology

SUGGESTED READINGS

American Psychiatric Association: *Diagnostic and statistical manual of mental disorders*, ed 4, Washington, DC, 1994, American Psychiatric Association Press.
Dalton R: Enuresis (bedwetting). In Behrman R et al, eds: *Nelson's textbook of pediatrics*, ed 15, Philadelphia, 1998, WB Saunders.
Gonzalez R: Voiding dysfunction. In Behrman R et al, eds: *Nelson's textbook of pediatrics*, ed 15, Philadelphia, 1998, WB Saunders.

PROBLEM · 97

ALLERGIC RHINITIS

"I Don't Want to Play; You're a Stupid Snot Nose!"

Case 1 ■ A 6-Year-Old Male with a Constantly Running Nose

A mother comes to your office with her 6-year-old son. She states that for the past 15 months the child has been "constantly rubbing his nose and his eyes." She adds that "his nose is constantly running." He has had no significant upper respiratory tract infections, nor is there any history of wheezing or coughing that might suggest asthma.

There is, however, a family history of both asthma and hay fever. There appears to be a temporal association between the onset of the symptoms the mother describes and the acquisition of "Boots," a black cat with white paws.

On examination, there is obvious nasal congestion, hyperemia, and clear discharge bilaterally. There also appear to be bluish-purple rings around both eyes. On examination of the respiratory system, there are a few rhonchi heard, especially on expiration.

SELECT THE BEST ANSWER TO THE FOLLOWING QUESTIONS

Q1. What is the most likely diagnosis in this child?
   a. vasomotor rhinitis
   b. chronic infectious rhinitis
   c. allergic rhinitis
   d. primary atrophic rhinitis
   e. nonallergic rhinitis with eosinophilia syndrome (NARES)

Q2. The bluish-purple rings around both eyes are best described as which of the following?
   a. abnormal: the diagnosis is most likely a serious coagulation defect
   b. normal: the diagnosis is most likely a mild coagulation defect
   c. normal: the rings are known as allergic shiners
   d. normal: the rings are known as eosinophilic eye syndrome
   e. nobody really knows for sure; we know the rings have something to do with allergy, but not much more

Q3. Which of the following immunoglobulins are associated with the condition described in Case 1?
   a. IgA
   b. IgE
   c. IgG

d. IgM

e. none of the above

Q4. Which of the following statements regarding the cause of this child's symptoms is true?

a. there is likely no association between this child's symptoms and "Boots"

b. although there is a temporal relationship between the acquisition of the cat and the symptoms, it is unlikely to be a true cause-and-effect relationship

c. the temporal relationship between the acquisition of "Boots" and the symptoms suggests a cause-and-effect relationship

d. although the cat may be a small part of the answer, there is likely to be some other underlying reason for this child's symptoms

e. there is likely to be no significance to this child's symptoms and the family history of allergy

Q5. What is the single most common cause of seasonal allergic rhinitis in children in the United States?

a. grass

b. tree pollens

c. tumbleweed

d. ragweed pollen

e. mold spores

Q6. What is the single most common cause of perennial allergic rhinitis in children in the United States?

a. house dust mite

b. cat dander

c. cat saliva

d. feathers

e. mold spores

Q7. What is the single most important part of the treatment protocol in the condition described?

a. the use of intranasal corticosteroids

b. the use of intranasal sodium cromoglycate

c. the use of systemic antihistamines

d. the use of systemic adrenergic drugs

e. none of the above

Q8. What is the pharmacologic agent of first choice in the treatment of the condition described?

a. intranasal corticosteroids

b. intranasal sodium cromoglycate

c. systemic antihistamines

d. systemic adrenergic drugs

e. a or b

Q9. What is the single best pharmacologic treatment for the condition described?

a. intranasal corticosteroids

b. intranasal sodium cromoglycate

c. systemic antihistamines

d. systemic adrenergic drugs

e. none of the above

Q10. What is the mechanism of action of sodium cromoglycate as a treatment for the condition described?

a. a decongestant

b. a vasoconstrictor

c. an antigen-induced mediator inhibitor

d. an IgE inhibitor

e. none of the above

Q11. What is the diagnostic test of choice for the condition described?

a. serum IgE determination

b. a nasal smear for eosinophil count

c. RAST

d. skin prick testing

e. computed tomography scan of the nose

Q12. Vasomotor rhinitis is best distinguished from allergic rhinitis by which of the following?

a. the absence of sneezing, itching, or rhinorrhea in vasomotor rhinitis

b. the absence of eosinophils on nasal smear in vasomotor rhinitis

c. the predominance of nasal obstruction as the primary symptom in vasomotor rhinitis

d. all of the above

e. none of the above

Q13. Which of the following systemic disorders is most closely associated with nasal obstruction?

a. diabetes mellitus

b. hyperthyroidism

c. hyperparathyroidism

d. hypothyroidism

e. systemic lupus erythematosus

Q14. The condition Saint's triad includes all of the following except:

a. nasal polyps

b. asthma

c. aspirin intolerance

d. persistent nasal rhinorrhea

e. all of the above are included

Q15. Allergic conjunctivitis associated with the condition described is best treated with which of the following?

a. corticosteroid eye drops
b. sodium cromoglycate eye drops
c. silver nitrate eye drops
d. erythromycin eye ointment
e. chloramphenicol eye drops

SHORT ANSWER MANAGEMENT PROBLEM
Define and describe the disorder *rhinitis medicamentosa.*

ANSWERS

A1. **c.** This child most likely has allergic rhinitis. Allergic rhinitis affects about 10% of children and up to 20% of teenagers. Most patients with this condition develop symptoms before age 20.

A2. **c.** The symptoms of allergic rhinitis include nasal congestion (stuffy nose), sneezing, pruritus, rhinorrhea, clear nasal discharge, mouth breathing, snoring, and bluish-purple rings around the eyes that are often referred to as *allergic shiners.*

Exposure to cigarette smoke, paint fumes, strong odors, and allergens may precipitate the symptoms.

Physical examination may show an "allergic salute" (rubbing and dorsal manipulation of the nose resulting in a transverse wrinkle externally over the lower portion of the nose), edematous and congested nasal mucosa, obstruction of venous drainage in the periorbital region (the allergic shiners just mentioned), hypertrophy of the tonsils, and hypertrophy of the adenoids. Serous otitis media is commonly observed in association with allergic rhinitis. As well, allergic rhinitis is more common in children who have either atopic dermatitis or asthma.

A small subset of patients may have NARES. Patients may manifest the same symptoms as allergic rhinitis, but this is much less common and may be distinguished by the absence of positive skin tests or radioallergosorbent tests (RASTs).

Vasomotor rhinitis is a nonallergic, noninfectious rhinitis caused by an imbalance of autonomic nervous system control.

Chronic infectious rhinitis results in mucopurulent rhinorrhea, often associated with low-grade fever, cough, sore throat, and malaise. Sinusitis and recurrent purulent otitis media may be present.

Primary atrophic rhinitis, with autosomal dominant inheritance, rarely occurs in children.

A3. **b.** Allergic rhinitis is an inflammatory disorder of the nasal mucosa initiated by an IgE-mediated hypersensitivity. It is the most common disease of the nasal passages.

A4. **c.** Because this child did not have symptoms before the acquisition of the cat, the temporal relationship certainly is very suspicious and, unfortunately, the most likely cause of this child's symptoms. The actual allergen may be either cat dander or cat saliva.

A5. **d.** Approximately 75% of seasonal allergic rhinitis symptoms are caused by ragweed. Ragweed is found most frequently in the eastern and central parts of North America, often growing in grain fields and construction areas.

A6. **a.** The symptom of a constantly running nose suggests the subtype of allergic rhinitis classified as perennial allergic rhinitis. The causative agents, when identified, are usually allergens to which the patient is exposed more or less continually, although exposure may vary during the year. Indoor inhalant allergens are implicated most often. These include the following:
   a. Components of house dust (house dust and house dust mites are the most common cause)
   b. Feathers
   c. Allergens or danders of household pets
   d. Mold spores
Seasonal allergic rhinitis, on the other hand, is also known as hay fever. This is most commonly seen in children who have been exposed to wind-borne pollens of trees, grass, and weeds. The single most common cause of seasonal allergic rhinitis is ragweed pollen.

A7. **e.** The single most important part of the treatment protocol for allergic rhinitis is removing, whenever possible, the environmental source responsible for the condition.

Although it is often difficult or impractical to avoid exposure to seasonal pollens, much can be done to avoid indoor inhalant factors such as house dust, house dust mites, animal danders, and molds. Control of house dust, with special attention to the child's bedroom, often significantly improves symptoms. Elimination of exposure to danders and feathers is mandatory for a child with perennial allergic rhinitis when these factors are responsible for the symptoms. Thus, after confirmation by prick testing, Boots will have to go.

A8. **e.** Sodium cromoglycate is often the drug of first choice in the treatment of allergic rhinitis. It is administered by intranasal inhalation, 1 or 2 inhalations 3 to 6 times/day.

Intranasal corticosteroids are considered to be by most authorities the drugs of second choice. Although they have superior efficacy, the possibility of systemic absorption does exist.

A9. **a.** Intranasal corticosteroids are by far the most effective treatment for allergic rhinitis. Beclomethasone or flunisolide should be used in children whose nasal symptoms are resistant to sodium cromoglycate. The usual dose of metered inhaler is 1 to 2 inhalations 2 or 3 times/day.

A10. **c.** Sodium cromoglycate is a mast cell stabilizer.

Systemic antihistamines also are useful in the treatment of allergic rhinitis, especially in the seasonal subtype. Nonsedating receptor blocking H1 antihistamines, such as loratadine, eliminate the major sedative side effects of older antihistamines such as hydroxyzine. All antihistamines are more effective in treatment of seasonal allergic rhinitis than in perennial allergic rhinitis.

Inhaled or systemic adrenergic agents such as the decongestant pseudoephedrine or phenylpropanolamine are best avoided, especially in perennial allergic rhinitis. Nasal sprays containing these agents should be used sparingly if at all because of the possibility of rebound congestion.

A11. **b.**

A12. **d.** Vasomotor rhinitis is a very poorly understood diagnostic entity that is related somehow to autonomic nervous system dysfunction. In this condition, symptoms are increased or triggered by temperature changes, odors, and spicy foods. Vasomotor rhinitis has the following features:
   a. Nasal obstruction is the primary symptom.
   b. There is an absence of sneezing, itching, and rhinorrhea.
   c. No eosinophils are seen on nasal smear.

A13. **d.** The systemic disease most closely associated with nasal obstruction is hypothyroidism.

The drug most closely associated with nasal congestion in the past was reserpine, a drug almost unheard of for pediatric use.

A14. **d.** The Saint's triad, or triad asthma, includes nasal polyps, asthma, and aspirin intolerance. On examination, this child demonstrates audible expiratory rhonchi; these rhonchi may well be a sign of bronchial asthma.

Persistent nasal rhinorrhea is not part of the symptom complex triad asthma.

A15. **b.** Allergic conjunctivitis goes along with allergic rhinitis. The treatment of choice for allergic conjunctivitis at this time is sodium cromoglycate. If severe, corticosteroid eye drops can be temporarily used

with caution. A consultation with an ophthalmologist would be advisable.

SOLUTION TO THE SHORT ANSWER MANAGEMENT PROBLEM

Rhinitis medicamentosa is a disorder of chronic nasal congestion and obstruction produced by a rebound effect from the excessive use of vasoconstrictor nose drops. It is imperative to educate patients regarding the use of nasal decongestant nose drops for a time not to exceed a few days.

Rebound congestion works in much the same manner as rebound headaches from the too-frequent use of analgesics.

SUMMARY OF THE DIAGNOSIS AND TREATMENT OF ALLERGIC RHINITIS

1. Classification:
   a. Seasonal allergic rhinitis (also known as seasonal pollinosis and hay fever): Causes include tree pollen, weed pollen, and grass. The most common cause is ragweed.
   b. Perennial allergic rhinitis: The patient has symptoms year-round. The causative agents include house dust and house dust mites (most common), animal saliva, animal dander, feathers, and molds.

2. Symptoms:
   a. Nasal congestion
   b. Sneezing
   c. Itching
   d. Rhinorrhea
   e. Nasal discharge

3. Clues:
   a. Allergic shiners: Caused by venous stasis resulting from interference with blood flow through edematous nasal mucous membranes
   b. Allergic salute: Rubbing hand in an upward direction

4. Diagnosis:
   a. Nasal smear to demonstrate eosinophils
   b. Allergy testing to identify specific allergen

5. Associated disorders:
   a. Serous otitis media (acute and chronic)
   b. Adenoid hypertrophy
   c. Tonsillar hypertrophy
   d. Asthma

6. Treatment:
    a. Avoidance:
        1) It is difficult to avoid seasonal allergic pollens in seasonal allergic rhinitis.
        2) In perennial allergic rhinitis, the causative agent should be minimized wherever possible. Special attention should be paid to the child's bedroom and an electronic air filter installed if possible.
    b. Pharmacologic agents:
        1) Inhaled sodium cromoglycate (drug of first choice)
        2) Inhaled corticosteroids (best and most effective drug)
        3) Systemic (nonsedating antihistamines)
        4) Sparing use of decongestants and local vasoconstrictors

7. Differential diagnosis of rhinitis:
    a. Allergic rhinitis
    b. NARES
    c. Infectious rhinitis: Viral or bacterial
    d. Vasomotor rhinitis
    e. Rhinitis medicamentosa

SUGGESTED READING

Sly RM: Allergic disorders. In Behrman R, ed: *Nelson textbook of pediatrics*, ed 15, Philadelphia, 1998, WB Saunders.

PROBLEM · 98

DIAPER DERMATITIS

"Doctor, His Cheeks Are Too Red."

Case 1 ■ A 2-Month-Old Infant with a Rash on His Cheeks

A 2-month-old infant is brought to your office by his mother. He developed an erythematous, dry skin rash on both cheeks approximately 1 week ago. Although the rash is always present, the mother states that it seems to be worse after I feed him.

The mother breast fed for the first 4 weeks of life but returned to work 4 weeks ago and switched the baby from breast feeding to bottle feeding. In addition, she decided to feed him with "whole milk" rather than with infant formula.

On examination, the child appears healthy. He has an erythematous maculopapular eruption that covers his cheeks, and he appears to be developing an erythematous rash on his neck, both wrists, and both hands. The rest of the physical examination is within normal limits.

SELECT THE BEST ANSWER TO THE FOLLOWING QUESTIONS

Q1. What is the most likely cause of this infant's skin rash?
    a. atopic dermatitis
    b. allergic contact dermatitis
    c. seborrheic dermatitis
    d. infectious eczematoid dermatitis
    e. none of the above

Q2. What is (are) the recommended treatment(s) of the skin rash in the infant presented?
    a. skin hydration
    b. local corticosteroid therapy
    c. systemic antihistamines
    d. avoidance of precipitant
    e. all of the above

Q3. With which of the following antibodies is the described disorder associated?
    a. IgA
    b. IgG-viral capsid antigen (VCA)
    c. IgM-VCA
    d. IgE
    e. none of the above

Q4. Regarding this child's feeding, what would be the best course of action at this time?
    a. continue feeding the infant with cow's milk
    b. switch from whole milk to a soy-based formula as the first step
    c. switch from whole milk to a non-soy-based formula as the first step
    d. switch from whole cow's milk to 1% cow's milk
    e. switch from whole cow's milk to skimmed cow's milk

Case 2 ■ A 1-Month-Old Infant with a 2-Week-Old Diaper Rash

A 1-month-old infant is brought to your office by his mother. She states that the infant has had a diaper rash for the past 2 weeks that has not cleared up with the use of zinc oxide three times a day. She tells you that she must be doing something wrong and she is extremely upset.

On examination, the infant has an erythematous, weeping, oily eruption in the diaper area. He also has a scaly eruption on the scalp, the ear, the sides of the nose, and the eyebrows and eyelids. The rest of the physical examination is normal.

Q5. What is the most likely diagnosis in this infant?
   a. atopic dermatitis
   b. allergic contact dermatitis
   c. seborrheic dermatitis
   d. infectious eczematoid dermatitis
   e. none of the above

Q6. What is (are) the treatment(s) of choice for the condition described in Case 2?
   a. wet compresses
   b. topical corticosteroids
   c. topical ketoconazole
   d. a and b
   e. all of the above

Case 3 ■ An 8-Month-Old Infant with a Long-Term Persistent Diaper Rash

An 8-month-old infant is brought to your office by his mother for assessment of a diaper rash. His mother has tried cornstarch, talcum powder, vitamin E cream, zinc oxide, and three different prescribed corticosteroid creams from three different physicians as remedies. She tells you that she went to three doctors because the first two said, "Oh, don't worry dear, just a little diaper rash, it will go away; don't worry your pretty little head about it."

On examination, the infant has an intensely erythematous diaper dermatitis that has a scalloped border and a sharply demarcated edge. There are numerous "satellite lesions" present on the lower abdomen and thighs.

Q7. What is the most likely diagnosis in this infant?
   a. atopic dermatitis
   b. allergic contact dermatitis
   c. seborrheic dermatitis
   d. infectious eczematoid dermatitis
   e. candidal diaper dermatitis

Q8. What is the treatment of choice for the diaper rash of the infant described in Case 3?
   a. a topical corticosteroid
   b. a topical antibiotic
   c. a systemic antibiotic
   d. a topical antifungal agent
   e. none of the above

Case 4 ■ A 4-Month-Old Infant with a Diaper Rash Caused by Dirty Diapers

A 4-month-old infant is brought to your office by her mother. Her mother complains that the child has a diaper rash that is probably related to her "lack of changing by the babysitter." Apparently, the infant went for long periods of time while the babysitter sat on the couch watching television. Needless to say, the babysitter is no longer in the employ of the mother.

On examination, the infant has an erythematous, scaly, papulovesicular diaper dermatitis with numerous bullous lesions, fissures, and erosions.

Q9. What is the most likely diagnosis in this infant?
   a. atopic dermatitis
   b. primary irritant contact dermatitis
   c. seborrheic dermatitis
   d. fungal dermatitis
   e. allergic contact dermatitis

Q10. What is (are) the treatment(s) of choice for the infant described in Case 4?
   a. zinc oxide paste
   b. topical hydrocortisone
   c. systemic antibiotics
   d. a and b
   e. all of the above

SHORT ANSWER MANAGEMENT PROBLEM
For each of the following four types of diaper dermatitis, provide a "diagnostic clue" that will help distinguish one from another.
   a. Atopic dermatitis
   b. Seborrheic dermatitis
   c. Candidal dermatitis
   d. Primary irritant dermatitis

ANSWERS

A1. **a.** This child has atopic dermatitis. Atopic dermatitis is an inflammatory skin disease characterized by erythema, edema, pruritus, exudation, crusting, and scaling.

Atopic dermatitis usually begins in infancy. The areas most commonly affected include the cheeks, neck, wrists, hands, and extensor aspects of the extremities. Spread often occurs from extensor to flexor. Pruritus may lead to intense scratching and secondary infection.

Atopic dermatitis is usually precipitated by or exacerbated by the introduction of certain foods to the infant's diet, particularly cow's milk, wheat, or eggs. Environmental factors such as dust, mold, and cat dander may also trigger the condition.

A2. **e.** The treatment of atopic dermatitis begins with the avoidance of any environmental factors that precipitate the condition.

Smooth-textured cotton garments help reduce added irritation in this disorder. The use of soaps and detergents, abstract lipids from the skin, and bathing without bath oil should be avoided when possible. Ideally, the child should be in the tub for at least 15 minutes before the bath oil is added to the water.

Atopic dermatitis is best managed with local therapy. Flare-ups of the condition are treated with topical corticosteroid creams or lotions. To further prevent scratching, the fingernails should be cut short. Percutaneous absorption of corticosteroid does occur, and atrophy of the skin should be watched for. This can be avoided by using a moderate potency topical corticosteroid for 7 days followed by a low-potency topical hydrocortisone preparation (0.5% hydrocortisone) for 2 to 3 weeks until the lesions have resolved.

Systemic antihistamines such as diphenhydramine, promethazine, and hydroxyzine may have to be used to control pruritus (use with caution). Nonsedating antihistamines such as loratadine or cetirizine also can provide relief.

Infected atopic dermatitis is best managed by antibiotic therapy. Systemic antibiotics are the mainstays of treatment for infected atopic dermatitis. However, the newer, nonsensitizing local antibiotic preparations such as mupirocin may be used for local infections.

A3. **d.** Atopic dermatitis is mediated and regulated by an IgE antibody response and by antigen-specific T cells that secrete IgE antibody binding factors. It usually remits by the age of 3 to 5 years. There is often a family history of allergies, asthma, hay fever, or atopic dermatitis.

A4. **c.** This child should be taken off cow's milk and, as a first step, put onto a regular infant formula. If the atopic dermatitis persists despite the regular infant formula, it would then be reasonable to consider switching to a soy-based formula.

A5. **c.** This infant has seborrheic dermatitis, an inflammatory disorder that often begins in the first month of life. The initial manifestation of seborrheic dermatitis is often a diffuse or focal scaling and crusting of the scalp, a condition known as *cradle cap*. A dry scaly, erythematous, papular dermatitis, which is usually nonpruritic, may develop, involving the face, neck, retroauricular areas, axillae, and diaper area. The dermatitis may be patchy or focal or may spread to involve the entire body.

A6. **e.** Wet compresses (saline) are an effective first treatment for seborrheic dermatitis. A soft brush can be used to remove some of the scales associated with cradle cap. Scalp lesions may also be controlled with an antiseborrheic shampoo such as selenium sulfide.

Topical corticosteroids (hydrocortisone 0.5% to 1%) may be applied to inflammatory lesions. The use of topical ketoconazole (2%) has been found to be of benefit in the treatment of seborrheic dermatitis.

A7. **e.** This infant has candidal diaper dermatitis, which presents as an erythematous confluent plaque formed by papules and vesiculopustules, with a scalloped border and a sharply demarcated edge. Candidal diaper dermatitis can usually be distinguished from other childhood diaper dermatoses by the presence of "satellite lesions" produced at some distance from the primary eruption.

A8. **d.** The treatment of choice in candidal diaper dermatitis is a topical antifungal agent. Topical miconazole, clotrimazole, or ketoconazole can be used after soaking the inflamed area with wet aluminum acetate compresses. In an infant with a severe inflammatory reaction, a topical corticosteroid may be mixed 50/50 with a topical antifungal agent and applied on a regular basis for a few days to a week.

The attitude displayed by the first two physicians (condescending and arrogant) is not as uncommon as we think. Doctor-patient communication in something as simple as a diaper dermatitis can significantly affect not only the efficacy of treatment, but also compliance and postdiagnostic attitudes.

A9. **b.** This child has a primary irritant contact dermatitis. Irritant contact dermatitis is a reaction to friction, maceration, and prolonged contact with urine and feces. It usually presents as an erythematous, scaly dermatitis with papulovesicular or bullous lesions, fissures, and erosions. The eruption can be either patchy or confluent. The genitocrural folds are often spared.

Secondary infection with either bacteria or yeast can occur. The infant can be in considerable discomfort because of the marked inflammation that is sometimes associated with this type of diaper rash.

Primary irritant diaper dermatitis should be managed by frequent changing of diapers and thorough washing of the genitalia with warm water and a mild soap. Occlusive plastic pants that promote maceration should be avoided. Disposable diapers should be used instead of cloth diapers.

A10. **d.** An occlusive topical agent such as zinc oxide can be applied until healing occurs. Systemic antibiotics are not indicated in the treatment of primary irritant diaper dermatitis.

SOLUTION TO THE SHORT ANSWER MANAGEMENT PROBLEM AND SUMMARY TO DIAPER DERMATITIS

a. Atopic dermatitis:
  1) Diagnostic clue: Usually begins and is more prominent on the cheeks of infants
  2) Treatment: Moisturization, mild topical corticosteroids, systemic antihistamines (with caution), systemic or topical antibiotics for secondary infection
b. Seborrheic dermatitis:
  1) Diagnostic clue: Cradle cap often associated with this type of diaper dermatitis
  2) Treatment: Wet compresses (saline), mild topical corticosteroids, topical ketoconazole
c. Candidal dermatitis:
  1) Diagnostic clue: Satellite lesions around the peripheral area of the main area of dermatitis
  2) Treatment: Topical miconazole, topical ketoconazole, mild topical hydrocortisone mixed 50/50 when severe inflammation is present
d. Primary irritant dermatitis:
  1) Diagnostic clue: Maceration, often a history of the use of cloth diapers or plastic pants
  2) Treatment: Occlusive topical agent such as zinc oxide or petroleum jelly or zinc oxide applied over hydrocortisone base when severe inflammation is present

SUGGESTED READING

Sly RM: Allergic disorders. In Behrman R, ed: *Nelson textbook of pediatrics*, ed 15, Philadelphia, 1998, WB Saunders.

PROBLEM · 99

CARDIAC MURMURS IN CHILDREN

"My Baby Has Heart Problems?"

Case 1 ■ A 3-Year-Old Child with a Cardiac Murmur

A 3-year-old child is brought to your office by his mother for a periodic health examination. The child has been well and has no history of significant medical illness. He has reached all of his developmental milestones.

On physical examination, the child is in the 50th percentile for weight and height. His blood pressure is 90/70 mm Hg. He has a grade II/VI short ejection systolic murmur heard maximally along the left sternal edge from the midsternum to the lower end of the sternum. There is no radiation of the murmur to either the neck or back. There is no associated thrill with this murmur. The child's pulse is 84 per minute and regular. The femoral artery pulses are normal and are not delayed. The rest of the physical examination is normal.

SELECT THE BEST ANSWER TO THE FOLLOWING QUESTIONS

Q1. Which of the following statement(s) best reflect(s) the character of this heart murmur?
  a. the location of the heart murmur (mid to low sternum) increases the probability of this murmur being pathologic
  b. the systolic timing of the heart murmur increases the probability of this murmur being pathologic
  c. the grade of the murmur (II/VI rather than I/VI) increases the probability of this murmur being pathologic
  d. all of the above
  e. none of the above

Q2. This murmur is best referred to as which of the following?
  a. Mustard's murmur
  b. Fallot's murmur
  c. Still's murmur
  d. De Bakey's murmur
  e. Framingham's murmur

Q3. Which of the following signs or symptoms is not associated with "innocent" cardiac murmurs?
  a. low frequency
  b. an associated thrill
  c. short ejection systolic in timing
  d. grade I or grade II in audibility
  e. a and b

Q4. The murmur described is intensified by which of the following?
  a. the sitting position
  b. increasing the heart rate
  c. fever
  d. anxiety
  e. all of the above

Q5. At this time, which of the following investigations should be performed on the child?
  a. a chest x-ray
  b. an electrocardiogram (ECG)
  c. an echocardiogram
  d. none of the above
  e. all of the above

Q6. At this time, what should you do?
  a. call the pediatric cardiologist immediately
  b. tell the child's mother that the child has a heart

murmur but "not to worry, it probably isn't anything important"

c. tell the mother that all heart murmurs need to be taken very seriously; therefore, it is probably best to have the pediatric cardiologist do "every test he can"

d. tell the mother that the heart sound you hear (a very soft murmur) is very common and occurs in at least half of all children

e. tell the mother nothing; there is no need to cause her unnecessary worry

---

Case 2 ■ A 6-Month-Old Infant with a Harsh Grade III/VI Pansystolic Heart Murmur

A 6-month-old infant is brought to your office by his mother. She came in for a periodic health assessment. You have not seen the child before. The mother states that the child has been well and has had no medical problems.

On examination, the child has a grade III/VI harsh pansystolic heart murmur heard along the lower left sternal edge. There is no radiation of the murmur. The heart rate is 72 beats per minute and regular. There is no thrill. The blood pressure is 80/60 mm Hg.

No other abnormalities are found on examination. Most importantly, the child is in the 50th percentile for weight and length.

Q7. What is the most likely cardiac diagnosis in this infant?
   a. innocent cardiac murmur
   b. tetralogy of Fallot
   c. pulmonary atresia
   d. ventricular septal defect (VSD)
   e. coarctation of the aorta

Q8. At this time, the child described in Case 2 should
   a. have immediate surgery
   b. be managed with digoxin and diuretics
   c. be managed with digoxin, diuretics, and an angiotensin-converting enzyme inhibitor
   d. have an immediate cardiac catheterization performed followed by surgical closure within 3 months
   e. none of the above

Q9. What preventative health practices should be followed for the child described in Case 2?
   a. prophylaxis against bacterial endocarditis if dental work is to be done
   b. cardiac catheterizations every 3 months until resolution
   c. echocardiograms every 3 months until resolution

   d. a and c
   e. none of the above

Q10. What is the prevalence of cardiac murmurs in childhood?
   a. 5%
   b. 10%
   c. 20%
   d. 50%
   e. 90%

Q11. What is the most common pathologic cardiac murmur in childhood?
   a. atrial septal defect
   b. tetralogy of Fallot
   c. VSD
   d. transposition of the great arteries
   e. aortic stenosis

Q12. Which of the following is (are) common innocent cardiac murmurs in childhood?
   a. neonatal pulmonary artery branch murmur
   b. "venous hum" of late infancy
   c. "Still's aortic vibratory" murmur
   d. pulmonary valve area "flow" murmur
   e. all of the above

SHORT ANSWER MANAGEMENT PROBLEM
Discuss the relative sensitivity and specificity of an experienced clinician's clinical diagnosis of a childhood cardiac murmur compared to the findings or diagnosis suggested by echocardiography.

ANSWERS

A1. **e.** This murmur has all the characteristics of an innocent murmur:
   a. It is located at the mid to low sternal border.
   b. It is systolic in timing.
   c. It has no associated thrill.

A2. **c.** This murmur, which is described as "vibratory" or "musical" in nature, is known as Still's murmur. Still's murmur is safely diagnosed clinically, and laboratory studies add nothing to its assessment.

A3. **b.** There is no such thing as an innocent thrill.

A4. **e.** Other characteristics of an innocent cardiac murmur (such as a Still's murmur) include the following:
   a. It is low in frequency and localized
   b. It is seldom greater than grade II/VI in intensity
   c. It is accentuated by the sitting position, anxiety, fever, and increasing heart rate. Note that an in-

nocent cardiac murmur in a child is never associated with a thrill.
d. Heart sounds are always normal

A5. **d.** This Still's murmur is safely diagnosed clinically, and laboratory and diagnostic imaging studies add nothing to its assessment.

A6. **d.** In explaining heart murmurs to parents, not just what you say but how you say it is very important. It is important to be reassuring in your tone and to point out that 50% of children have cardiac murmurs. Make sure that you provide an opportunity for the mother to ask any questions that she may have.

It is extremely unwise not to tell the parents when you detect a heart murmur in a young child. Sooner or later someone is going to hear it and mention it. At that time it will come back to haunt you. It is far better to tell the parent(s) that a heart murmur exists but that you are positive (if you are) that it is innocent. If you are not positive, an elective referral to a pediatric cardiologist would be reasonable.

A7. **d.** The most likely cardiac diagnosis in this infant is VSD. The typical heart murmur associated with a VSD is harsh, pansystolic, and best heard at the lower left sternal edge. Even as the VSD becomes smaller, it maintains its regurgitant characteristic of starting off with the first heart sound (holosystolic timing).

A8. **e.** The treatment recommended at this time is none of the above. Rather, watchful expectation should be pursued. The prognosis is excellent, and the defect will likely close spontaneously. As the VSD becomes smaller, the murmur becomes shorter and (as mentioned) maintains its regurgitant characteristics (that is, it starts off with the first heart sound). At least 50% of VSDs will close by the end of the first year or shortly thereafter. Pediatric cardiology referral is appropriate.

A9. **a.** The only prophylaxis that needs to be followed in this child is protection with antibiotic therapy (penicillin) before any dental procedure or any other procedure that would increase the probability of bacterial endocarditis. This can obviously be discontinued when the defect closes.

A10. **d.** The prevalence of cardiac murmurs in the pediatric population is at least 50%, probably considerably higher to the sensitive ear. The vast majority of these murmurs is innocent in nature and does not reflect any cardiac pathologic condition.

A11. **c.** The most common pathologic cardiac murmur in childhood is VSD. With a VSD, the cardiac murmur is often not present at birth but is first heard at the 2- to 4-week well-baby checkup. As discussed previously, the most common outcome of this congenital heart defect is spontaneous closure. In some cases, however, surgical closure is indicated. The most uncommon scenario is the development of congestive cardiac failure secondary to VSD.

The relative frequency of pathologic cardiac murmurs in childhood are: VSD, 38%; atrial septal defect, 18%; pulmonary valve stenosis, 13%; pulmonary artery stenosis, 7%; aortic valve stenosis, 4%; patent ductus arteriosis, 4%; mitral valve prolapse, 4%; and all others, 11%.

A12. **e.** The common functional or common innocent murmurs of infancy and childhood include the following:
a. Neonatal pulmonary artery branch murmur
b. Venous hum of late infancy and early childhood
c. Still's aortic vibratory systolic murmur
d. Pulmonary valve area "flow" murmur of late adolescence and childhood

SOLUTION TO THE SHORT ANSWER MANAGEMENT PROBLEM

As our health care dollars become stretched to the limit, we need to take a critical look at exactly how much more certain diagnostic tests add to the diagnosis and treatment arrived at by an experienced clinician in all aspects of medicine. The diagnosis of childhood cardiac murmurs is no exception.

A recent study of experienced pediatric cardiologists yielded the following results with respect to their diagnostic acumen.
a. Sensitivity of clinical examination of all childhood cardiac murmurs is 96%
b. Specificity of clinical examination of all childhood cardiac murmurs is 95%
c. Positive predictive value of clinical examination of all childhood cardiac murmurs is 88%
d. Negative predictive value of clinical examination of all childhood cardiac murmurs is 98%

Thus this study showed that the clinical examination by a pediatric cardiologist is the most useful means of initial evaluation of referred pediatric cardiac murmurs.

As supplementary screening tools, the ECG and the echocardiogram were unlikely to reveal clinically unsuspected cardiac disease. Thus there is every reason (clinically and cost-effectively) to go back to the evaluation of patients by physicians rather than by machines. Remember, as doctors we treat patients, not laboratory results.

SUMMARY OF THE DIAGNOSIS AND TREATMENT OF CHILDHOOD CARDIAC MURMURS

1. Prevalence of murmurs:
   a. Overall prevalence: ~50% of all children
   b. Innocent/pathologic: 10/1

2. Epidemiology: Experienced clinical assessment is just as sensitive and specific as echocardiography and more sensitive and specific than electrocardiography.

3. Innocent murmurs:
   a. Still's murmur (most common)
   b. Venous hum (second most common)
   c. Pulmonary flow murmur
   d. Neonatal pulmonary artery branch murmur

4. Pathologic murmurs:
   a. VSD (most common)
   b. Atrial septal defect (second most common)
   c. Pulmonary valve stenosis

5. Clinical signs and symptoms that are reassuring for the family physician as he or she evaluates a childhood cardiac murmur. The following are 10 questions a family physician should ask himself or herself about a cardiac murmur:
   a. Is there any evidence of failure to thrive in the child? If no, this suggests an innocent murmur.
   b. Are there any symptoms (shortness of breath, blue lips, lethargy) or signs (cyanosis, diastolic murmur, parasternal heave, thrill, loud murmur II/VI, holosystolic murmur) to suggest pathologic murmur? If no, this suggests an innocent murmur.
   c. Is the murmur accentuated by sitting forward? If yes, this suggests an innocent murmur.
   d. Is the murmur accentuated by exercise or increased heart rate resulting from another cause? If yes, this suggests an innocent murmur.
   e. Is the murmur accentuated by fever? If yes, this suggests an innocent murmur.
   f. Is the murmur accentuated by anxiety, restlessness, or crying? If yes, this suggests an innocent murmur.
   g. Is the murmur a murmur without any radiation (that is, to the neck or to the back)? If yes, this suggests an innocent murmur.
   h. Is the murmur present lower (rather than higher) along the left sternal edge? If yes, this suggests an innocent murmur.
   i. Did the mother bring the child in for a specific reason that may be associated with cardiac disease (such as having to stop and rest while playing)? If no, this suggests an innocent murmur.
   j. Do you, an experienced clinician, think this is an innocent murmur? If yes, this suggests an innocent murmur.

SUGGESTED READINGS

Bernstein D: The cardiovascular system. In Behrman R, ed: *Nelson textbook of pediatrics*, ed 15, Philadelphia, 1998, WB Saunders.

Symthe J et al: Initial evaluation of heart murmurs: Are laboratory tests necessary? *Pediatrics* 86(4):497-500, 1990.

PROBLEM·100

USE AND ABUSE OF OVER-THE-COUNTER DRUGS FOR INFANTS AND YOUNG CHILDREN

"You Mean That Medicine from the Drug Store Can Be Bad for My Baby?"

Case 1 ■ A 6-Month-Old Infant with an Upper Respiratory Tract Infection

A 6-month-old infant is brought to your office by his mother. He has had an upper respiratory tract infection (URI) consisting of a runny nose, cough, and a mild fever for the last 4 days. The infant's mother is concerned because his temperature reached 39° C last evening.

On physical examination, the child looks well. He has nasal congestion as well as a hyperemic pharynx. His lungs are clear; no adventitious breath sounds are heard.

SELECT THE BEST ANSWER TO THE FOLLOWING QUESTIONS

Q1. Regarding the child's fever, what should you tell the mother?
   a. treat the fever with baby aspirin if it reaches 39° C again
   b. treat the fever with elixir of acetaminophen if it reaches 39° C again
   c. treat the fever with a combination of baby aspirin and elixir of acetaminophen if it reaches 39° C again
   d. use only symptomatic treatment (cool clothes, fan in the room)
   e. tell the mother that everyone has a different opinion; as far as you are concerned, she can do whatever she wants

Q2. What is the analgesic agent of choice in the treatment of childhood fever and mild childhood pain?
 a. elixir of naproxen
 b. elixir of hydromorphone
 c. elixir of acetaminophen
 d. children's aspirin: 75 mg
 e. elixir of acetaminophen and codeine

Q3. Regarding the use of aspirin and acetaminophen in pediatric analgesia, which of the following statements most accurately reflects current recommended practice?
 a. aspirin is still the analgesic of choice in the treatment of infant and childhood pain
 b. aspirin is not contraindicated in the treatment of infant and childhood pain associated with URIs
 c. aspirin is a more potent analgesic than acetaminophen
 d. acetaminophen is the drug of choice for the treatment of infant and childhood pain
 e. acetaminophen should be used in all infants and children

Q4. Regarding the use of antihistamines in pediatric patients, which of the following statements is true?
 a. antihistamines shorten the duration of respiratory tract illness in children
 b. antihistamines reduce the incidence of otitis media following the beginning of an URI in a young child
 c. the prescription of an antihistamine in a child with a viral URI is considered good practice
 d. antihistamines may produce seizures in young children who are given antihistamine doses (tablets or suppositories) that are meant for older children (on a milligram-per-kilogram basis)
 e. none of the above statements is true

Q5. Regarding the relief of nasal congestion in infants and children, which of the following statements is true?
 a. antihistamines produce excellent relief of pediatric nasal congestion
 b. antihistamines, when compared to cool or warm steam, produce superior relief of nasal congestion in pediatric patients
 c. cool or warm steam, when compared to antihistamines, produce superior relief of nasal congestion in pediatric patients
 d. antihistamines and cool or warm steam are equally efficacious in providing relief of nasal congestion
 e. nobody really knows for sure

The child described in Case 1 returns in 3 days with his mother. She states that despite your treatment the child has not improved. He now has significantly greater nasal congestion and is having a difficult time breathing at night.

On examination, the ears and throat remain clear. You do not really notice any change in the state of the nasal congestion.

Q6. With respect to treatment of this infant at this time, which of the following statements is true?
 a. a decongestant to relieve nasal congestion is a reasonable therapeutic maneuver now
 b. decongestants have been shown to reduce the duration of viral URI symptoms
 c. topical sympathomimetic agents are unlikely to be systemically absorbed
 d. overstimulation is a common side effect when decongestant preparations are given to children
 e. none of the above statements is true

Case 2 ■ A 6-Month-Old Infant with a Persistent Cough

A mother brings her 6-month-old infant daughter to your office for assessment of a persistent cough. The cough has been present for the past 10 days. It is nonproductive, and the mother believes it is interfering significantly with the child's sleep. You are considering prescribing an antitussive or an expectorant.

Q7. Which of the following statements regarding the use of antitussives or expectorants in infants and children is true?
 a. dextromethorphan suppresses cough and is unlikely to produce any significant adverse reactions in infants and children
 b. the combination of a cough suppressant and an expectorant is a logical combination to try in a child with a persistent cough
 c. dextromethorphan has been shown to significantly decrease the duration of respiratory tract infection symptoms in children
 d. respiratory depression in children has been reported with dextromethorphan
 e. none of the above is true

Case 3 ■ A 13-Month-Old Infant with Nausea
      and Vomiting

A mother brings her 13-month-old infant to the office for assessment of nausea and vomiting. She stopped in at the local Emergency Department 24 hours previously and was told to purchase childhood dimenhydrinate suppositories for the nausea. Apparently, the Emergency Department physician did a complete workup and there were no other significant findings.

However, the nausea and vomiting continued. At this time the child appears to be approximately 5% dehydrated. On physical examination, there are no other abnormalities found. The child appears somewhat sedated and lethargic.

You decide to admit the child for observation, reevaluation, and rehydration.

Q8. Which of the following statements regarding the use of antiemetics in children is (are) true?
   a. dimenhydrinate is effective for the treatment of nausea and vomiting associated with gastrointestinal infection and is devoid of significant side effects
   b. the sedation that is seen in this infant may be secondary to the dimenhydrinate
   c. dimenhydrinate toxicity may be difficult to distinguish from worsening of the illness
   d. b and c
   e. all of the above statements are true

Case 4 ■ An 8-Month-Old Infant with Fever, Diarrhea, and Red Cheeks

A mother brings her 8-month-old infant to your office for assessment of fever, diarrhea, and red cheeks that she attributes to teething. She was advised by her neighbor to purchase a preparation of topical benzocaine. This has not helped.

On examination, the infant has a temperature of 39° C. There are no other abnormalities on physical examination.

Q9. Which of the following statements regarding this infant is (are) true?
   a. the symptoms described are probably caused by teething
   b. topical benzocaine preparations are virtually devoid of side effects
   c. acetaminophen is a reasonable treatment for a child that is teething
   d. teething often begins at 4 to 6 months of age and carries on intermittently up to the age of 2 years
   e. c and d
   f. all of the above statements are true

Q10. Adolescents have recently adopted the use of a common over-the-counter (OTC) drug for its central nervous system (CNS) properties as a favorite drug of abuse. This has caused many pharmacies to move this drug from the drug store shelf to behind the counter. Which drug is this?
   a. chlorothiazide
   b. diphenylhydramine
   c. dimenhydrinate
   d. terfenadine
   e. dextromethorphan

SHORT ANSWER MANAGEMENT PROBLEM
Describe a general rule of thumb for the use of OTC drugs in infants and children

---

ANSWERS

A1. **d.** The basic axiom relevant to this question is that "not all fever has to be treated with drugs." In fact, there are good reasons for suggesting that fever per se only be treated when it reaches a level of 39.5° C. Fever is a normal body response mechanism. In children, the major concern with very high fever is the possibility of a febrile convulsion.

A2. **c.** The analgesic agent of choice in the treatment of childhood fever and mild to moderate childhood pain is acetaminophen. Hydromorphone is a strong narcotic. Naproxen is a nonsteroidal antiinflammatory agent, and aspirin is contraindicated (see Answer 3).

Acetaminophen with codeine elixir is available and may be indicated in more severe pain syndromes in childhood.

A3. **d.** Acetaminophen is the analgesic of choice for the treatment of infant and childhood pain. Aspirin use should basically be discouraged; this is by far the safest policy. Aspirin use has been linked to Reye's syndrome (influenza and Reye's syndrome) and it seems wise to avoid this drug in any children with infections of any kind. Not all childhood pain needs to be treated with drugs. Many children will do just as well and feel just as well without drug use.

A4. **d.** Most cough and cold remedies contain antihistamines. Antihistamines, however, have never been shown to be of value in the treatment of viral URIs (contrary to many authorities, including ear, nose, and throat specialists). Antihistamines do not shorten the duration of respiratory tract illness in children and do not reduce the subsequent incidence of otitis media following the onset of a viral upper respiratory illness. They may, however, produce seizures in children if given in toxic amounts. The younger the child, the easier it is to inadvertently produce antihistamine toxicity.

Treatment of a viral URI in an infant or young child should consist of reassurance and cool steam (if nasal congestion is present).

A5. **c.** Cool or warm steam is actually superior to antihistamines in producing relief of nasal congestion in infants and young children. If steam is being used in a humidifier in the child's room, it is safer to use a humidifier that emits cool steam, due to the risk of burns. However, the use of warm steam (as from turning on the shower in the bathroom) does, as well, produce significant symptomatic relief of nasal congestion.

A6. **d.** Decongestants have not been shown to shorten the duration of viral URI symptoms. Topical sympathomimetic agents are systemically absorbed and may result in elevation of blood pressure, tachycardia, and overstimulation of the CNS leading to irritability, insomnia, and sometimes even frank psychosis. Overstimulation is a particularly common side effect in children. Thus, as with antihistamines, the risks of using decongestants in children outweigh any potential benefits.

It may be reasonable to use a very dilute nasal sympathomimetic for a short period in this child if all else fails; however, it is still preferable to stick to steam if possible.

A7. **d.** Dextromethorphan is the most common ingredient in OTC cough medicines. As well as producing drowsiness, it has been reported to produce respiratory depression in infants and children. As with antihistamines and decongestants, dextromethorphan has not been shown to shorten the duration of respiratory tract illness in children or adults.

Many cough preparations also contain an expectorant. The combination of a cough suppressant and an expectorant in one preparation is beyond comprehension.

Time remains the best cure for the viral URI symptoms. The use of a nasal aspirator (bulb syringe) will help to clear a young infant's nasal secretions and make feeding easier. Saline nasal drops may also be used. In infants who are irritable and feverish from viral symptoms, the use of acetaminophen is the safest OTC drug to use.

A8. **d.** Dimenhydrinate should not be used for the treatment of nausea and vomiting secondary to gastroenteritis in children (especially very young children). Even in adults the use of this agent is questionable; it has been demonstrated to be of value only in the treatment of motion sickness in adults. Dimenhydrinate may produce significant sedation (and even a semicomatose state) in children. The pediatric

suppository contains 25 or 50 mg of dimenhydrinate (half the adult oral dose or the full oral adult dose, respectively).

It may be difficult for the physician to differentiate dimenhydrinate toxicity from a worsening of the illness itself. This makes the use of this agent in children dangerous.

A9. **e.** Teething usually begins at 4 to 6 months and continues until the age of 2 years. Although often blamed on teething, there is no good evidence that rash, fever, diarrhea, vomiting, nasal congestion, irritability, or sleeplessness are related to teething.

Although topical benzocaine usually does not produce any side effects, cases of methemoglobinemia have been reported in children who have been treated with this agent.

Teething is best treated with reassurance and appropriate doses of acetaminophen.

A10. **c.** An OTC drug that has recently been adopted by adolescents as a drug of abuse is dimenhydrinate. The CNS side effects that the adolescent is looking for are the sedation, drowsiness, and perhaps euphoria. This has caused many pharmacists to move the drug from the drug store shelf to behind the counter.

SOLUTION TO THE SHORT ANSWER MANAGEMENT PROBLEM

A good general rule of thumb for treating infants and children with OTC drugs is to avoid their use in almost all cases, especially in young infants and children. The only safe drug that can be routinely used without significant concern (as long as the directions are followed as per dose) is acetaminophen.

SUMMARY OF THE ABUSE OF OTC DRUGS IN INFANTS AND YOUNG CHILDREN

1. URIs: There is no evidence to suggest that antihistamines, decongestants, cough suppressants, or expectorants are of any value in the treatment of viral URI symptoms in infants and young children. Potential toxicity is present with all of these agents.

2. Nausea and vomiting: Dimenhydrinate is not useful and is potentially toxic.

3. Diarrhea: kaolin or pectin may change the appearance of stools slightly but has no effect on water loss, the major hazard of protracted diarrhea.

4. Teething: There is no evidence to suggest that rash, diarrhea, vomiting, nasal congestion, irritability, and sleeplessness are associated with teething. Benzocaine preparations should be avoided. Reassurance and judicious use of acetaminophen may be indicated.

SUGGESTED READING

English JA, Bauman KA: Evidence-based management of upper respiratory infection in a family practice teaching clinic, *Fam Med* 29(1):38-41, 1997.

PROBLEM · 1 0 1

SICKLE-CELL DISEASE

"Mom, Why Should I Have This Disease? I'm Never Going to See a Malaria Mosquito."

Case 1 ■ An 8-Year-Old Female with Acute Skeletal Pain

An 8-year-old female comes to your office with an acute attack of pain in the back, ribs, sternum, and extremities. The child, of African-American descent, has had previous episodes of the same type of pain in the same areas. On physical examination, the child is in acute distress and is clutching both lower extremities.

Examination of the head and neck, the respiratory system, the cardiovascular system, and the abdomen is normal. Examination of the musculoskeletal system demonstrates acute tenderness in the areas in which the pain is presently located.

SELECT THE BEST ANSWER
TO THE FOLLOWING QUESTIONS

Q1. Based on the findings described, what is the most likely diagnosis in this patient?
   a. sickle-cell trait
   b. sickle-cell disease
   c. metastatic carcinoma
   d. malingering
   e. none of the above

Q2. What is the pathophysiology of this condition?
   a. replacement of normal hemoglobin A by hemoglobin S
   b. replacement of normal hemoglobin A by hemoglobin C
   c. replacement of normal hemoglobin A by hemoglobin F
   d. osteolytic bone lesions produced by an undifferentiated carcinoma
   e. none of the above

Q3. An aplastic crisis is often associated with this condition. Which of the following infections is often associated with an aplastic crisis?
   a. human papillomavirus
   b. human parvovirus
   c. Herpes zoster
   d. Pneumococcus
   e. *Haemophilus influenzae*

Q4. Which of the following immunizations or vaccines should be given to this patient?
   a. hepatitis B vaccine
   b. *H. influenzae* immunization
   c. Pneumococcal vaccine
   d. a and c
   e. all of the above

Q5. A 4-year-old girl of African-American descent presents to the Emergency Department with painful swelling of both hands and feet. What is the most likely cause of this symptom?
   a. the hand-foot syndrome
   b. acute gout
   c. acute juvenile rheumatoid arthritis
   d. bilateral hand and foot osteomyelitis
   e. none of the above

Q6. What is the pathophysiologic reason for the patient presented in Question 5?
   a. an autoimmune process
   b. an osseous infection
   c. an acute bacterial infection
   d. a viral infection
   e. none of the above

Q7. What is the most frequent complication of sickle-cell trait?
   a. splenic rupture
   b. painless hematuria
   c. splenic sequestration
   d. stroke
   e. none of the above

Q8. In which of the following races is the disease state discussed least common?
   a. African-Americans
   b. Italians
   c. Greeks
   d. Saudi Arabians
   e. Caucasian North Americans

Q9. Which of the following statements regarding this disease and priapism is false?
   a. priapism is a recognized complication of this condition

b. priapism in this disorder usually presents in younger men

c. priapism, when it occurs, is generally self-limited

d. nifedipine or nitroglycerine is the treatment of choice for this priapism

e. hospitalization is rarely indicated

Q10. Which of the following is a (are) recognized complication(s) of this disorder?

a. a stroke, a stroke in evolution, or a transient ischemic attack

b. avascular necrosis primarily affecting the hips

c. acute vasoocclusion

d. splenic sequestration and splenic enlargement

e. all of the above

SHORT ANSWER MANAGEMENT PROBLEM

List the major complications of the disorder described.

ANSWERS

A1. **b.** This child has sickle-cell disease, which is an inherited hemolytic anemia that results when the normal hemoglobin A (HbA) is replaced by the mutant hemoglobin S (HbS), that is they are homozygous (S/S). About 1 in 12 people of African descent in the Americas carry the sickle-cell trait; that is they are heterozygous (A/S). HbS is also expressed in significant numbers among subpopulations of Greeks, Italians, Turks, Saudi Arabians, and certain tribes on the Indian subcontinent, all of whom share a history of having lived for many generations in regions where *Plasmodium falciparum* malaria is endemic.

Subjects who have the sickle-cell trait (A/S heterozygous) are not anemic and have a normal life expectancy. Between 25% and 40% of their hemoglobin is HbA and, therefore, under normal circumstances their red blood cells do not sickle and then hemolyze.

Sickle-cell anemia (S/S), as this child has, is caused by the inheritance of two HbS genes, one from each parent. At birth, the red blood cells of the S/S infant contain mainly fetal hemoglobin (HbF). However, within a few months these red cells are replaced by cells containing mainly HbS. The solubility of HbS decreases when it is deoxygenated. The precipitated HbS molecules form aggregates that, when present in sufficient volume, deform the red cells forcing them to take a sicklelike shape. These sickled cells may become entangled and thereby frequently block the flow of blood in small diameter blood vessels.

The acute pain that this child is experiencing at this time is caused by such a vasoocclusive phenomenon. Throughout their lives, sickle-cell patients are plagued by recurrent painful crises. These episodes may occur with explosive suddenness and may attack various parts of the body, particularly the abdomen, chest, back, and joints. Approximately 25% of these painful crises are preceded by a viral or a bacterial infection. A given patient may have months or even years without a crisis and then have a cluster of frequent, severe attacks. In some patients these crises occur more frequently in cold weather; this may be a result of reflex vasospasm. In others the attacks occur in warm weather and are presumably caused by dehydration.

When a sickle-cell crisis is localized to the extremities, as in this case, it may induce acute synovitis and joint effusion.

A2. **a.** As mentioned, sickle-cell disease is genetically inherited from both parents, with HbA being replaced by HbS. HbS may be distinguished from HbA by electrophoresis because of the substitution of an uncharged valine for a negatively charged glutamic acid at the sixth position of the beta-chain.

A3. **b.** In patients with sickle-cell disease, aplastic crises are often precipitated by viral infections, particularly viral infection with the human parvovirus B19. An aplastic crisis usually occurs in a child under the age of 18 who may be recovering from an infection. The child presents with profound anemia and a fall in the reticulocyte count to below 1%.

Treatment consists of blood transfusions. The child usually recovers spontaneously within 7 to 10 days.

A4. **e.** Patients with sickle-cell disease should be given the usual course of immunizations as described in Problem 81. In addition, however, it is imperative that the child receive Haemophilus B conjugate and pneumococcal vaccine.

A5. **a.** This presentation, designated hand-foot syndrome (or acute sickle cell dactylitis), presents as a painful swelling of either the hand or foot and is caused by infarction of bone marrow in metacarpal or metatarsal bones and phalanges. It resolves spontaneously in approximately 1 week.

As the patient with sickle-cell disease grows older, infarcts in the long bones can cause pain or swelling of an arm or leg. In these cases osteomyelitis, usually caused by *Salmonella*, should be ruled out.

A6. **e.** The pathophysiology of the hand-foot syndrome is basically a vasoocclusive process, a process that occurs as a result of the sickle shape of the red blood cells themselves, a shape that predisposes to vasoocclusion in the bone marrow.

A7. **b.** The most frequent complication of sickle-cell trait is painless hematuria. The hematuria, which is usually gross hematuria, is produced by necrosis of the tip of the renal papilla and is prolonged by the action of urokinase in the urine. Although the hematuria may continue for several weeks, it seldom requires hospitalization and may cease spontaneously.

Even considering the frequency of painless hematuria (approximately 20% of patients with sickle-cell trait), it is obviously important to rule out other causes and not automatically assume that it is caused by the sickle-cell disease every time it occurs.

A8. **e.** Sickle-cell disease and sickle-cell trait, as discussed in Answer 1, occur among African-Americans, Greeks, Italians, Turks, Saudi Arabians, and certain tribes on the Indian subcontinent. They do not, however, occur in white North Americans.

A9. **e.** Attacks of priapism in boys and young men are not uncommon complications. These attacks are distressing but can usually be managed conservatively. The attacks, which are self-limited, may occur frequently, often during erection, which increases the proportion of deoxyhemoglobin in the corpora spongiosa.

Priapism sometimes responds to nifedipine (10 mg in repeated doses) and to a nitroglycerine patch, 0.2 to 0.4 mg/hr applied at bedtime, to prevent nocturnal attacks. If an attack persists for more than 6 hours, the patient should be admitted to a hospital. If it continues for more than 24 hours despite conservative treatment measures, a urologist should be consulted.

Many of the patients who develop attacks of priapism have relatively high hemoglobin and hematocrit levels.

A corpora spongiosa or cavernosa shunt through the glans penis is often effective and may need to be repeated. Subsequent erectile function is usually not affected.

Repeated attacks of priapism can result in thickening and gross enlargement of the penis, which may remain semierect. Impotence can be effectively treated by penile implants.

A10. **e.** Cerebrovascular accidents (CVAs [stroke]) resulting from blockage of the internal carotid artery or its branches affect approximately 5% of S/S children. The treatment for same is a program of exchange transfusions to lower the proportion of HbS to less than 50% and maintain it at that level throughout childhood. This facilitates prevention of a recurrence as well as neurologic recovery.

Avascular necrosis, particularly of the head of the femur, is very common in patients with sickle-cell disease and can lead to significant disability. Some patients benefit from surgical intervention; this ranges from core decompression to total hip replacement. Like infarcts in other organs, infection is much more common as a complication of these surgical interventions.

Acute vasoocclusion, as discussed, is the basic pathophysiologic process underlying many of the complications of sickle-cell disease. Specifically, it is responsible for osseous complications such as the hand-foot syndrome and acute pain crises, which have been discussed previously.

The spleen is usually palpable in infants and small children but may become acutely enlarged due to rapid sequestration of sickled blood. As the acute anemia can be rapidly fatal, this is an emergency requiring admission to the hospital and rapid blood transfusion.

SOLUTION TO THE SHORT ANSWER MANAGEMENT PROBLEM

Sickle-cell disease is characterized by the following complications (although not required for the answer, a detailed explanation of each complication is provided):

a. Hemolytic anemia: Sickle-cell disease (genotype S/S) is associated with a severe hemolytic anemia with hematocrit values varying between 18% and 30%. The mean red blood cell survival is between 10 and 15 days.
b. Acute pain crises and chronic organ damage: the morbidity and mortality of sickle-cell disease are primarily a result of recurrent vasoocclusive phenomena. This vasoocclusive damage can be divided into microinfarcts that produce the painful crisis and macroinfarcts that produce organ damage. Although almost any organ can be involved, the most common organs involved are the lungs, kidneys, liver, skeleton, and skin.
c. Pulmonary function restriction: impairment of pulmonary function is a common complication of sickle-cell disease. Resting arterial PO_2 is reduced in part because of the intrapulmonary arterial-venous shunting. Since S/S red blood cells have decreased oxygen affinity, arterial blood is significantly undersaturated. This creates an increased tendency for red blood cells to sickle when they reach the peripheral circulation.
d. Congestive cardiac failure: S/S homozygotes frequently develop overt congestive heart failure (CHF). The pathophysiology of this CHF is associated with the severe chronic anemia and hypoxemia (high-output cardiac failure).

e. CVAs: The primary cause of a CVA in patients with sickle-cell disease is cerebral thrombosis. The other cause, however, is subarachnoid hemorrhage. A sickle-cell disease patient has approximately a 25% lifetime chance of developing some type of neurologic complication. Hemiplegia is encountered more frequently than are coma, convulsions, or other visual disturbances.

Patients generally make a full recovery, particularly after only one CVA.

f. Ophthalmologic complications: A variety of ocular abnormalities are encountered in patients with S/S disease. These include retinal infarcts, peripheral vessel disease, arteriovenous anomalies, vitreous hemorrhage, proliferative retinopathy, and retinal detachment.

g. Genitourinary complications: Patients with sickle-cell disease develop significant and prolonged painless hematuria as a result of papillary infarcts. The amount of blood loss can be so significant that iron deficiency develops.

Longer surviving S/S patients (patients living into their fourth or fifth decade) develop progressive renal failure. Boys and young men with sickle-cell disease occasionally develop priapism. The treatment of this condition was discussed in Answer 8.

h. Hepatobiliary complications: Patients with sickle-cell disease are icteric because of the hemolytic anemia discussed previously. The hyperbilirubinemia that is associated with sickle-cell disease is nonconjugated hyperbilirubinemia. Patients with sickle-cell disease are also at increased risk of gallstone formation.

i. Skeletal complications: The skeletal complications associated with S/S disease develop as a result of expansion of the red marrow, bony infarcts, and avascular necrosis of joints in hip and shoulder. The biconcave, or "fishmouth," vertebrae are virtually pathognomonic for sickle-cell disease. The previously mentioned hand-foot syndrome is a painful swelling of the hand or foot caused by infarction of the bone marrow in metacarpal or metatarsal bones and phalanges.

j. Skin disease: Chronic skin ulcers often occur in the lower extremities. These skin ulcers appear to be associated with S/S patients that have more severe hemolytic anemia.

k. Splenic sequestration: The spleen becomes enlarged as a result of the rapid sequestration of sickled blood. The acute anemia that results may be rapidly fatal and should be treated with emergency blood transfusions.

l. Aplastic crises: The previously mentioned aplastic crises, which usually occur when a child is recovering from an infection, are caused by human parvovirus B19. Profound anemia occurs, and blood transfusions are necessary to treat it.

SUMMARY OF THE DIAGNOSIS AND TREATMENT OF SICKLE-CELL DISEASE

1. Population at greatest risk: African-Americans
   a. 1 in 12 carry the sickle-cell trait A/S (are heterozygous for sickle-cell trait)
   b. Homozygous genotype S/S

2. Diagnosis:
   a. Blood smear: Red blood cells sickle and hemolyze
   b. Hemoglobin electrophoresis

3. Clinical manifestations: Prominent and frequent clinical manifestations include the following:
   a. Severe hemolytic anemia
   b. Recurrent bouts of acute pain crises that arise from vasoocclusion and microinfarction also associated with hand-foot syndrome
   c. Chronic organ damage from same pathophysiologic condition: Lungs, kidneys, liver, skeleton, skin
   d. CHF
   e. CVAs
   f. Eye complications: Proliferative retinopathy, retinal infarcts, retinal detachment, vitreous hemorrhage
   g. Chronic renal failure, painless hematuria, priapism
   h. Jaundice (unconjugated hyperbilirubinemia), cholelithiasis
   i. Systemic skeletal microinfarction, avascular necrosis
   j. Skin ulcers
   k. Splenic sequestration
   l. Aplastic crises
   m. Sepsis in association with asplenia

4. Treatment:
   a. Treatment and, whenever possible, prevention of complications (recurrent CVA may be prevented by starting the child on a chronic transfusion program)
   b. Nutritional supplements: Folic acid, 1 mg/day
   c. Immunizations or vaccines: *H. influenzae* B, pneumococcal vaccine, and all other routine vaccinations recommended for other children as summarized in Problem 81.
   d. Prophylactic antibiotics: Penicillin V 125 mg bid up to age 3; then 250 mg bid up to age 5.

e. Pain control for acute pain crises and other painful events: intravenous fluids and analgesics as needed; do not be afraid to use narcotic analgesics
f. Painless hematuria: Aminocaproic acid
g. Transfusion: Indicated for symptomatic episodes of acute anemia, severe symptomatic episodes of acute anemia, severe symptomatic chronic anemia, prevention of recurrent strokes in children, acute chest syndromes with hypoxia, surgery with general anesthesia
h. Hydroxyurea: Indicated for adolescents or adults with frequent episodes of pain, a history of the acute chest syndrome, or other severe va-soocclusive complications, or severe symptomatic anemia.
i. Transplantation: Bone marrow transplantation successful; a consideration in children and adolescents under 16 years old who have severe complications and an HLA-matched donor available

SUGGESTED READINGS

Honig GR: Hemoglobin disorders. In Behrman RE et al, eds: *Nelson textbook of pediatrics*, ed 15, Philadelphia, 1998, WB Saunders.

Steinberg MH: Drug therapy: Management of sickle cell disease, *N Engl J Med* 340(13):1021-1030, 1999.

CHAPTER VI

GENERAL SURGERY AND SURGICAL SPECIALTIES

ACUTE APPENDICITIS

The Great Imitator

Case 1 ■ A 29-Year-Old Female with Nausea, Vomiting, and Central Abdominal Pain

A 29-year-old female comes to your office with a 2-day history of nausea, some vomiting, and vague central abdominal pain. The pain has begun to move down and to the right. She also describes mild dysuria. Anorexia began 24 hours ago and the patient also has "felt warm." Her last menstrual period was 2 weeks ago.

Her past health has been excellent. She has no drug allergies and is on no medication. On physical examination, the patient looks ill. Her temperature is 38.1° C. She has tenderness in both the right and left lower quadrants, but tenderness is greatest in the right lower quadrant. Rebound tenderness is present. The rectal examination discloses tenderness on the right side. There is no costovertebral angle tenderness.

SELECT THE BEST ANSWER
TO THE FOLLOWING QUESTIONS

Q1. What is the most likely diagnosis in this patient?
   a. pelvic inflammatory disease (PID)
   b. twisted ovarian cyst
   c. acute appendicitis
   d. acute cholecystitis
   e. acute pyelonephritis

Q2. At this time, what would be the most reasonable course of action?
   a. advise the patient to go home and return for follow-up in 24 hours
   b. hospitalize the patient for observation, evaluation, and possible operation
   c. begin outpatient oral antibiotic therapy and see the patient in 48 hours
   d. advise the patient to go home and call you if no improvement occurs within the next 72 hours
   e. none of the above

Q3. The investigations you perform heighten your suspicion of the primary diagnosis. The white blood cell count is elevated and there is a definite abnormality seen on the abdominal x-ray. At this time, you, the family physician, should do which of the following?
   a. continue to observe the patient for improvement or deterioration
   b. arrange for a computed tomography (CT) scan to definitely establish the diagnosis
   c. arrange for an ultrasound to definitely establish the diagnosis
   d. arrange for a barium enema to definitely establish the diagnosis
   e. none of the above

Q4. A consultant sees your patient and makes an appropriate suggestion. Which of the following is the suggestion likely to be?
   a. perform an abdominal laparoscopy or laparotomy
   b. begin intensive triple-drug intravenous antibiotics
   c. continue the period of observation
   d. perform further diagnostic tests
   e. none of the above

Q5. Which of the following is a (are) complication(s) of the definitive therapy and the original condition?
   a. wound infection
   b. subphrenic abscess
   c. pelvic abscess
   d. appendiceal abscess
   e. all of the above

Q6. In which of the following age groups are the signs and symptoms of the condition described likely not to be classic?
   a. infants
   b. young children
   c. elderly
   d. all of the above
   e. none of the above

Q7. In which of the following age groups is the diagnosis of the condition described in Case 1 most likely to be confused with another serious intra-abdominal inflammatory condition?
a. infants
b. young children
c. young adult males
d. young adult females
e. elderly males and females

Q8. The condition described has been called which of the following?
a. the "great imitator"
b. the "typical condition"
c. a diagnosis "unable to miss"
d. a diagnosis "unable to make under the best of conditions"
e. none of the above

Q9. Regarding the pathophysiology of the condition described, which of the following is a (are) usual component(s) of the pathologic process?
a. obstruction of the organ accounting for early symptoms and signs
b. rapid invasion of the wall of the organ by bacteria leading to inflammation
c. spreading of the inflammation to involve the whole wall of the organ
d. perforation of the organ
e. all of the above

Q10. Which of the following is the most important sequelae of delayed treatment of this condition in young women?
a. tuboovarian abscess formation
b. chronic low-grade pelvic infection
c. infertility caused by peritonitis and subsequent adhesion formation
d. chronic inflammatory bowel disease
e. endometriosis

SHORT ANSWER CLINICAL MANAGEMENT PROBLEM
Discuss the use of antibiotics in patients with signs and symptoms suggesting peritonitis.

ANSWERS

A1. **c.** The most likely diagnosis in this patient is acute appendicitis. The typical history of acute appendicitis is vague central abdominal discomfort followed by anorexia, nausea, and some vomiting. The pain, which is continuous but often not severe, usually moves into the right lower quadrant.

The pain is aggravated by movement, walking, or coughing.

In patients with retrocecal appendicitis (which this description fits) there may be dysuria and hematuria with rectal tenderness because of the proximity of the appendix to the ureter and bladder. With perforation (as in this patient) there is generalized abdominal tenderness and rebound tenderness. Retrocecal appendicitis often produces poorly localized epigastric pain and only mild nausea and vomiting. Thus retrocecal appendicitis can be significantly more difficult to diagnosis than classic appendicitis. Peritonitis can develop very rapidly. Temperature elevation is usually mild in appendicitis.

The most important differential diagnosis in this case is acute pain. The constellation of signs and symptoms, however, favors appendicitis. Acute cholecystitis, acute pyelonephritis, and acute PID will be discussed in separate problems.

A2. **b.** This patient has an acute abdomen and therefore should be hospitalized for further evaluation and possible operation. A white blood cell count, a urinalysis, and three views of the abdomen are all investigations that should be performed in this patient.

In acute appendicitis the average leukocyte count is $15,000/mm^3$, and 90% of patients have a leukocyte count greater than $10,000/mm^3$. In 75% of patients the differential count will show greater than 75% neutrophils.

Three views of the abdomen may show localized air-fluid levels, localized ileus, and an increased soft tissue density in the right lower quadrant. In addition, an altered right psoas shadow or an abnormal right flank stripe may be seen. On the other hand, they may show nothing specific.

With an acute abdomen, definitive treatment, as described in Answer 3, should not be delayed.

Antibiotics should not be given to this patient because they may mask the signs of peritonitis by reducing the inflammation of the peritoneum without treating the underlying pathologic condition.

A3. **e.** At this time the probability of the diagnosis of acute appendicitis with perforation and peritonitis is very high, and the most important intervention is a surgical consult as soon as possible.

A4. **a.** The most appropriate action at this time would be an abdominal laparoscopy or laparotomy to confirm the diagnosis and treat the condition. The laparoscope is now being used for the removal of appendices by some surgeons. Advantages to laparoscopy include the ability to examine the entire abdomen without the need for extending the operative incision. In addition, there are significantly fewer infectious wound complications. Once the decision to operate has been made, it is appropriate to consider starting the patient on broad-spectrum antibiotics that are effective against both aerobic and anaerobic organisms. The probability of an anaerobic organism as part of the bacterial process is extremely high.

A5. **e.** Complications of appendectomy include the following:
  a. Wound infection. This complication occurs in less than 1% of patients with unperforated appendicitis but rises to 20% with perforation. With perforation, delayed primary closure of the wound may be a good strategy. Treatment is directed at drainage of the infection followed by the administration of appropriate antibiotics.
  b. Subphrenic abscess. The persistence of spiking fevers beginning on day 4 or day 5 without obvious cause should raise the suspicion of an intra-abdominal collection of pus. The diagnosis is established by physical examination demonstrating an elevated diaphragm and a pleural effusion. There is often tenderness over the seventh and eighth ribs laterally and edema or erythema of the lower chest wall.
  c. Pelvic abscess. Recurrent fever and diarrhea in a patient after an appendectomy suggest the formation of a pelvic abscess. Diagnosis is made by rectal examination and is confirmed by ultrasonography or a CT scan.
  d. Appendiceal abscess. Although uncommon, a small percentage of patients seek treatment after the acute infection has become walled off. Under these conditions, it may be preferable to delay appendectomy until the inflammation has settled down.

A6. **d.** Infants, young children, and elderly and frail patients may all have symptoms that are not classic, making the diagnosis of appendicitis difficult. In infants and young children the presenting symptoms may be nonspecific and include only lethargy and irritability, especially in the early stages. In elderly patients the same situation applies. Moreover, in elderly patients the probability of rupture increases from 20% to 70%.

A7. **d.** This question is meant to reiterate both the difficult issue raised previously and the importance of distinguishing acute appendicitis from acute PID and its complications such as tuboovarian abscess. Laparoscopy is definitely indicated in this circumstance.

A8. **a.** Acute appendicitis is often called the "great imitator." This name arises from the different presentations of the disease that are possible, especially at the extremes of life. Elderly patients, infants, and children will often have signs and symptoms that may not be "classic textbook." Thus appendicitis is one of those conditions in which you often will not make the diagnosis unless you think about the diagnosis and have a high level of suspicion.

A9. **e.** The small size of the appendix accounts for its ability to produce symptoms quickly. The pathologic process can be divided into the following stages:
  Stage 1 involves the obstruction of the appendix by a fecalith, a mucous plug, a foreign body, a parasite, or a tumor. This obstruction is associated with the early signs of periumbilical cramping and vomiting caused by distention of the appendix.
  Stage 2 involves the rapid invasion of the wall of the organ by bacteria with secondary inflammation. Gradual onset of systemic signs such as anorexia and malaise, low-grade fever, and leukocytosis then occur.
  Stage 3 involves spreading of the infection or inflammation to involve the entire wall of the organ and neighboring peritoneum, leading to a change in character of the pain to constant and localized. At this stage this differential diagnosis may include pyelonephritis, cholecystitis, or tuboovarian abscess.
  Young women with right-sided ovarian disease are particularly difficult to differentiate from young women with acute appendicitis. One clue may lie in the point of maximal tenderness. In appendicitis the point of maximal tenderness is McBurney's point (two thirds of the distance from the umbilicus to the anterior superior iliac spine). In right-sided ovarian disease the point of maximal tenderness is 2 to 3 cm below this point.
  Stage 4 is the last stage and involves perforation of the appendix. All four stages may develop within a short period (24 to 48 hours).

A10. **c.** The most significant complication of peritonitis following a ruptured appendix in young women is the development of pelvic adhesions and scar tissue. This may significantly decrease the fertility of a young woman. Chronic pelvic pain may also develop.

SOLUTION TO THE SHORT ANSWER MANAGEMENT PROBLEM

Antibiotics should not be used initially in patients with signs and symptoms suggesting peritonitis. The antibiotic may mask the infectious or inflammatory process that is ongoing in the patient and thus prolong definitive diagnosis and therapy. The patient should be observed, placed on nothing-by-mouth status and intravenous fluids, and observed and monitored both clinically and by laboratory evaluation.

SUMMARY OF THE DIAGNOSIS AND TREATMENT OF ACUTE APPENDICITIS

1. Acute appendicitis is the "great imitator." If you don't think of appendicitis, you won't make the diagnosis. Maintain a high index of suspicion, especially in the young and in the elderly.

2. Classic symptoms of appendicitis: Central abdominal pain, initially vague, but later localized to the right lower quadrant; anorexia; nausea and some vomiting; localized abdominal tenderness; low-grade fever; and leukocytosis

3. Retrocecal or retroileal appendicitis: Poorly localized abdominal pain, mild nausea and vomiting, mild diarrhea, urinary frequency, and hematuria

4. Diagnostic tests: Whole blood cell count, urinalysis, three views of the abdomen, ultrasonography, and CT scan

5. Definitive therapy: Laparoscopic appendectomy or laparotomy and open removal. (Laparoscopic appendectomy is being performed more and more commonly; the procedure itself is associated with fewer postoperative complications.)

6. Complications: Wound infection, subphrenic abscess, pelvic abscess (leading to adhesions and fertility problems), and appendiceal abscess (with appendix walled off)

SUGGESTED READINGS

Graffeo CS, Counselman FL: Appendicitis, *Emerg Med Clin North Am* 14(4):653-671, 1996.

Hale DA et al: Appendectomy: A contemporary appraisal, *Ann Surg* 225(3):252-261, 1997.

Irish MS et al: The approach to common abdominal diagnosis in infants and children, *Pediatr Clin North Am* 45(4):729-772, 1998.

Memon MA, Fitztgibbons RJ, Jr: The role of minimal access surgery in the acute abdomen, *Surg Clin North Am* 77(6):1333-1353, 1997.

Snyder BK, Hayden SR: Accuracy of leukocyte count in the diagnosis of acute appendicitis, *Ann Emerg Med* 33(5):565-574, 1999.

Wilcox RT, Traverso LW: Have the evaluation and treatment of acute appendicitis changed with new technology? *Surg Clin North Am* 77(6):1355-1370, 1997.

PROBLEM · 1 0 3

BILIARY TRACT DISEASE

Stones and Groans but Not Bones

Case 1 ■ A 43-Year-Old Female with Recurrent Right Upper Quadrant Pain

A 43-year-old female comes to your office with a 3-hour history of right upper quadrant pain. The pain is described as spasmodic and sharp. It radiates through to the back. The patient describes several episodes of this pain within the past 6 months. Nausea and vomiting accompany most of these episodes. Fever and chills are usually absent. The pain usually comes on after a meal.

On examination, there are no abdominal masses or tenderness. The chest is clear and the cardiovascular system is normal. The patient's blood pressure is 140/70 mm Hg. The patient has no drug allergies and is on no medications at the present time.

SELECT THE BEST ANSWER TO THE FOLLOWING QUESTIONS

Q1. What is the most likely diagnosis in this patient?
   a. acute cholecystitis
   b. biliary colic
   c. acute pancreatitis
   d. ileocecal appendicitis
   e. Crohn's disease

The patient's symptoms subside before your consultation is complete. You elect a wait-and-see policy. In 3 weeks the patient returns. On this occasion the patient's symptoms have been present for the last 24 hours. The patient is nauseated and has vomited three times since this pain began. The pain, as well as radiating to the back, is also radiating to the right shoulder.

On examination, there is tenderness in the right upper quadrant. On deep inspiration and palpation the patient's pain is accentuated and actually interrupts inspiration. The patient also has a mild fever.

Q2. What is the most likely diagnosis at this time?
   a. acute cholecystitis
   b. biliary colic
   c. acute pancreatitis
   d. ileocecal appendicitis
   e. Crohn's disease

Q3. Given this patient's signs and symptoms, which of the following investigative procedure is likely to yield the best information?

a. a white blood cell count
b. an oral cholecystogram
c. an abdominal ultrasound
d. an electrocardiogram
e. three views of the abdomen

Q4. What is (are) the treatment(s) of choice for the patient at this time?
a. intravenous fluids
b. parenteral antibiotics
c. nasogastric suction
d. all of the above
e. none of the above

Q5. Regarding the definite procedure to correct this condition, which of the following statements is true?
a. a definite procedure should not be contemplated at this time; if required it should be performed several months later
b. a definitive procedure should not be contemplated at this time; if symptoms continue to recur, you can reconsider
c. a definitive surgical procedure should be performed at this time
d. a definitive procedure is contraindicated given the signs and symptoms with which this patient presents
e. a definitive procedure should not be considered until all other methods of treatment have failed

Q6. Which of the following statements about gallbladder disease in the United States is (are) true?
a. more than 20 million Americans have gallstones
b. in the United States more than 300,000 cholecystectomies are performed annually
c. most gallstones are composed predominantly of cholesterol
d. all of the above statements are true
e. none of the above statements is true

Q7. Regarding the use of oral dissolution therapy in gallstone disease, which of the following statements is (are) true?
a. oral dissolution therapy is an excellent option for most patients
b. few if any gallstones that are dissolved with oral dissolution therapy recur
c. the preferred agent for oral dissolution therapy is ursodiol
d. oral dissolution therapy should not be combined with extracorporeal shock wave lithotripsy (ESWL)

e. oral dissolution therapy works best in patients with large gallstones

Q8. Which of the following statements regarding the treatment of asymptomatic gallstones is most accurate?
a. asymptomatic gallstones should be treated with cholecystectomy
b. asymptomatic gallstones should not be treated
c. whether or not asymptomatic gallstones should be treated depends on the presence or absence of comorbid conditions
d. asymptomatic gallstones should or should not be treated; it all depends on who you talk to
e. asymptomatic gallstone treatment has radically changed since the introduction of laparoscopic cholecystectomy

Q9. What is the most common complication during laparoscopic cholecystectomy?
a. excessive bleeding
b. small bowel perforation
c. injury to the biliary tract system
d. inability to remove the gallbladder through the laparoscope
e. liver laceration

Q10. Which of the following statements is (are) true of laparoscopic cholecystectomy?
a. laparoscopic cholecystectomy provides a safe and effective treatment for most patients with symptomatic gallstones; it is the treatment of choice
b. laparoscopic cholecystectomy provides distinct advantages over open cholecystectomy
c. laparoscopic cholecystectomy can be performed at a treatment cost equal to or slightly less than that for open cholecystectomy
d. during laparoscopic cholecystectomy, when the anatomy is obscured because of excessive bleeding or other problems, the operation should be converted promptly to open cholecystectomy
e. all of the above statements are true

SHORT ANSWER MANAGEMENT PROBLEM
The two most common diagnostic conditions associated with gallbladder disease are biliary colic and acute cholecystitis. Describe the differences in presentation and pathophysiology between biliary colic and acute cholecystitis.

ANSWERS

A1. **b.** This patient exhibits a typical presentation of biliary colic, which is characterized by transient obstruction of the cystic duct. The pain, located in the right upper quadrant, lasts from minutes to several hours. The pain is best described as spasmodic and constant. Postprandial presentation is common. Nausea and vomiting usually accompany the pain.

A2. **a.** The persistent nature of the pain in acute cholecystitis is a major clinical symptom that differentiates it from biliary colic. In addition, there is right upper quadrant (RUQ) abdominal tenderness and voluntary guarding as well as continuation of other signs. The pain is sometimes referred to the right scapula, and the gallbladder may be palpable. Moreover, mild jaundice may occur.

Acute cholecystitis is manifested pathologically by gallbladder distention (hydrops), serosal edema, and infection secondary to obstruction of the cystic duct. Although the other choices presented can sometimes present atypically with RUQ pain only, the probability is low.

A3. **c.** The diagnostic procedure of choice in this patient is an abdominal ultrasound. Gallstones will be demonstrated in approximately 95% of cases, and the specificity of the procedure is very high.

A4. **d.** In a patient with acute cholecystitis, intravenous fluids should be given to correct dehydration and possible electrolyte imbalance and a nasogastric (NG) tube should be inserted if the patient has protracted vomiting. For acute cholecystitis, appropriate parenteral antibiotics should be given.

A5. **c.** In years past, acute cholecystitis was managed either aggressively or conservatively. Since the disease resolves spontaneously in approximately 60% of cases, the conservative approach was to manage the patient expectantly, with a plan to perform elective cholecystectomy after recovery, reserving early surgery for those patients with severe or worsening disease.

The preferred treatment plan at this time, however, is to perform cholecystectomy in all patients following an episode of acute cholecystitis unless there are specific contraindications to performing the operation. The most common contraindication is severe concomitant disease. The reasoning for this approach is as follows:

a. The incidence of technical complications is no greater with early surgery.
b. Early surgery reduces the total duration of illness by approximately 30 days, the length of

hospitalization by 5 to 7 days, and direct medical costs by several thousand dollars.
c. In the absence of surgery, recurrent episodes are not uncommon, which may increase morbidity.

In addition, the following factors affect the decision as to when to operate:

a. The diagnostic certainty
b. The general health of the patient
c. Signs of local complications of acute cholecystitis such as gangrene or empyema

A6. **d.** More than 20 million Americans have cholelithiasis; approximately 300,000 operations are performed annually for the disease. The incidence of cholelithiasis increases with age.

Most gallstones (70% to 95%) are comprised predominantly of cholesterol. The remainder are pigment stones. The composition of the gallstone affects neither the symptoms associated with biliary colic nor the symptoms associated with acute cholecystitis.

A7. **c.** Oral dissolution therapy with bile acids was first introduced in the early 1970s. The first agent available was chenodiol, which has been replaced by ursodiol. Oral dissolution therapy is indicated only in a small minority of patients. The most effective use of bile acids occurs with small gallstones (50 mm in diameter or less) that are floating, cholesterol in nature, and within a functioning gallbladder. This represents approximately 15% of patients. Patients must be treated between 6 and 12 months, and monitoring is necessary until dissolution is achieved. In such patients 60% to 90% of gallstones will dissolve. Unfortunately, at least 50% of these stones reoccur within 5 years.

Dissolution rates are higher and recurrence rates are lower in patients with single stones, in nonobese individuals, and in young patients. Unfortunately, many patients suffer distressing side effects such as nausea from this treatment. Indications for bile acid therapy are limited to patients with a comorbid condition that precludes safe operation and patients who choose to avoid operation.

ESWL is not commonly used by itself but along with oral dissolution therapy. This technique may be successful in up to 95% of patients with a functioning gallbladder and solitary noncalcified stones 20 mm in diameter or less. Recurrence is infrequent following therapy with ESWL for a single small stone, but it is more common in patients with multiple stones. Again, the gallbladder remains and the probability of further stone formation is high.

A8. **b.** Current opinion suggests that asymptomatic gallstones should not be treated. The vast majority of gallstones remain silent throughout life. Only 1% to 4% per year of asymptomatic patients will develop symptoms or complications of gallstone disease. Existing data suggest that 10% of patients will develop symptoms within the first 5 years following diagnosis and approximately 20% within 10 years. Almost all patients will experience symptoms for a period of time before they develop a complication. Therefore, with few exceptions, prophylactic treatment of asymptomatic patients cannot be justified.

A9. **c.** All of the complications listed are possible, but the most common complication of laparoscopic cholecystectomy is bile duct injury. The frequency of bile duct injury is dependent on the skills of the surgeon and has been consistently decreasing as more experience with this procedure has been gained.

A10. **e.** Laparoscopic cholecystectomy provides a safe and effective treatment for most patients with symptomatic gallstones. It appears to be the treatment of choice for most patients at this time providing distinct advantages over open cholecystectomy. It decreases pain and disability without increasing mortality or overall morbidity. Although the rate of common bile duct injury is slightly increased, this rate is still sufficiently low to justify the use of this procedure.

Laparoscopic cholecystectomy can be performed at a treatment cost that is equal to or slightly less than that of open cholecystectomy and will result in substantial cost savings to the patient and society because of reduced loss of time from work.

The outcome of laparoscopic cholecystectomy is influenced greatly by the training, experience, skill, and judgment of the surgeon performing the procedure. During laparoscopic cholecystectomy, when anatomy is obscured, excessive bleeding occurs, or other problems arise, the operation should be converted promptly to open cholecystectomy. Conversion under these circumstances reflects sound surgical judgment and should not be considered a complication of laparoscopic cholecystectomy.

SOLUTION TO THE SHORT ANSWER MANAGEMENT PROBLEM

Biliary colic results from transient obstruction of the cystic duct with a gallstone. The pain associated with biliary colic usually begins abruptly after a meal and subsides gradually, lasting from a few minutes to several hours. It is located in the upper right quadrant and may or may not be associated with abdominal tenderness. There is no associated inflammation of the gallbladder with biliary colic because of the transient nature of the condition.

Acute cholecystitis, on the other hand, is associated pathophysiologically with inflammation of the gallbladder wall, with secondary infection in the gallbladder caused by blockage of the cystic duct. The first symptom is abdominal pain in the RUQ, with referral of the pain to right scapula. The pain persists and becomes associated with abdominal tenderness. There is nausea, vomiting, and a positive Murphy's sign (arrest of inspiration with palpation in the right upper quadrant). The pain does not resolve spontaneously. There may be fever.

SUMMARY OF THE DIAGNOSIS AND TREATMENT OF BILIARY TRACT DISEASE

1. Acute cholecystitis:
   a. Symptoms and signs:
      1) Acute RUQ pain and tenderness
      2) Mild fever and leukocytosis
      3) Nausea and vomiting
      4) Palpable gallbladder
      5) Gallstones on ultrasound scan
   b. Treatment:
      1) Nasogastric suction
      2) Parenteral fluids
      3) Analgesics
      4) Intravenous antibiotics
      5) Laparoscopic cholecystectomy as soon as possible

2. Biliary colic:
   a. Symptoms and signs:
      1) Recurrent abdominal pain (usually RUQ)
      2) Dyspepsia
      3) Gallstones on ultrasound
   b. Treatment: Laparoscopic cholecystectomy when recurrent episodes occur

3. Choledocholithiasis/cholangitis: choledocholithiasis occurs in 15% of patients with gallstones. Preoperative endoscopic retrograde cholangiography with sphincterotomy or intraoperative common duct exploration is options in concert with cholecystectomy.
   Choledocholithiasis is the major cause of cholangitis. Symptoms of cholangitis include biliary colic, jaundice, fever, and chills. Treatment of cholangitis includes intravenous antibiotics, cholecystectomy and intervention to the common duct.

4. Laparoscopic cholecystectomy: Laparoscopic cholecystectomy is now the treatment of choice for the vast majority of patients with biliary tract disease. It is a much more conservative operation, causes much less postoperative pain, and is associated with a much earlier return to work.

5. Asymptomatic gallstones: Asymptomatic gall-stones should be left where they are: do not create a problem where one does not exist.

SUGGESTED READINGS

Giurgiu DI, Roslyn JJ: Treatment of gallstones in the 1990s, *Prim Care Clin Office Pract* 23(3):497-513, 1996.

Hashizume M, Sugimachi K, MacFadyen BV: The clinical management and results of surgery for acute cholecystitis, *Semin Laparosc Surg* 5(2):69-80, 1998.

Martin RF, Flynn P: The acute abdomen in the critically ill patient, *Surg Clin North Am* 77(6):1455-1464, 1997.

Moscati RM: Cholelithiasis, cholecystitis, and pancreatitis, *Emerg Med Clin North Am* 14(4):719-737, 1996.

NIH Consensus Conference: Gallstones and laparoscopic cholecystectomy, *JAMA* 269:1018, 1993.

Rescorla FJ: Cholelithiasis, cholecystitis, and common bile duct stones, *Curr Opin Pediatr* 9(3):276-282, 1997.

Rosenthal RJ et al: Options and strategies for the management of choledocholithiasis, *World J Surg* 22(11):1125-1132, 1998.

Sanson TG, O'Keefe KP: Evaluation of abdominal pain in the elderly, *Emerg Med Clin North Am* 14(3):615-627, 1996.

Way L: Biliary tract. In Way L, ed: *Current surgical diagnosis and treatment: General surgery and surgical specialists*, ed 10, Norwalk, Conn, 1993, Appleton & Lange.

PROBLEM·104

COMMON PROCEDURES IN OFFICE SURGERY

"Are You Sure You Can Cut It Out, Right Here in Your Office?"

Case 1 ■ A 37-Year-Old Female with a Skin Lesion on Her Back

A 37-year-old female comes to your office for assessment of a skin lesion on her back that has been present for the last 3 years. It has recently increased in size, and the patient is concerned about it. The lesion is pigmented, raised, and dark brown. It is approximately 1.5 cm in greatest diameter. There are other, smaller lesions that have a similar appearance on the patient's back, but they have neither increased in size nor changed color.

You decide to remove the skin lesion in your office.

SELECT THE BEST ANSWER TO THE FOLLOWING QUESTIONS

Q1. In removing the skin lesion from your patient's back, what should you do?
a. follow Langer's lines
b. use silk sutures for skin closure
c. use catgut sutures for subcutaneous tissue closure
d. all of the above
e. none of the above

Q2. In considering the deep subcutaneous tissue on your patient's back and your selection of suture material, you should be aware that it takes approximately how many days for fibroblasts to grow across the wound line and develop enough strength to hold together the deep portion of the wound?
a. 10 days
b. 15 days
c. 21 days
d. 28 days
e. 35 days

Q3. In deciding on the use of needles for suture placement on skin surfaces in deep layers, which of the following statements is true?
a. a cutting needle should be used for skin closure; a taper needle should be used for deeper tissues
b. a taper needle should be used for skin closure; a cutting needle should be used for deep tissue
c. a cutting needle should be used for both skin closure and deep tissue closure
d. a taper needle should be used for both skin closure and deep tissue closure
e. both cutting and taper needles may be used for either skin or deep tissue closure

Q4. What is the local anesthetic of choice for the patient described?
a. lidocaine with epinephrine
b. lidocaine plain
c. bupivacaine plain
d. bupivacaine with epinephrine
e. none of the above

Q5. Which of the following is (are) useful in controlling bleeding from a skin lesion base?
a. application of pressure
b. electrocautery
c. a pressure dressing
d. hemostatic sutures
e. all of the above

Q6. Which of the following techniques is (are) recommended for the removal of pigmented skin lesions?
a. punch biopsy
b. shave biopsy
c. electrocautery
d. a or b
e. any of the above

Q7. What is (are) the treatment(s) of choice for the removal of plantar warts?
a. cryosurgery
b. electrocautery
c. surgical excision
d. podophyllin application
e. any of the above

Q8. The treatment(s) of choice for the removal of venereal warts include which of the following?
a. electrocautery
b. cryosurgery
c. surgical excision
d. podophyllin application
e. all of the above

Case 2 ■ A 5-Year-Old Child with a Second-Degree Burn on Her Right Hand

A 5-year-old child is brought to your office with a small second-degree burn on her right hand. The burn was sustained when she put her hand in a kettle of boiling water. On examination, there is an area of 3 cm × 5 cm on the right hand that has undergone blister formation. Her mother wrapped the burn in a gauze dressing.

Q9. At this time, what would be the most appropriate first course of action?
a. debride the wound
b. cool the burn site by immediately immersing the hand in cold water
c. aspirate the fluid underneath the blister
d. clean the area and redress it with gauze
e. debride the wound, aspirate the fluid, and apply an antibiotic cream

Q10. Following the initial step described in Question 9, what should be the next step(s)?
a. arrange for a revisit in 48 hours
b. debride the burn site
c. provide tetanus prophylaxis
d. a and c
e. all of the above

Case 3 ■ A 4-Year-Old Male Who Banged His Thumb

A 4-year-old boy is brought to your office by his mother after having banged his thumb in a door. He is crying and irritated. His left thumb has a purplish discoloration under the nail.

Q11. At this time, what should you do?
a. reassure the mother and send the child home with a pat on the head

b. reassure the mother and give the child some plain acetaminophen
c. under local anesthetic remove the nail
d. under local anesthetic perform a wedge resection
e. none of the above

Case 4 ■ A 25-Year-Old Female with a Sore Big Toe

A 25-year-old female has had a sore left great toe for the past 4 weeks. On examination, the lateral aspect of the left toe is erythematous and puffy, with pus oozing from the corner between the nail and the skin tissue surrounding the nail. This is the first occurrence of this condition in this patient.

Q12. At this time, what should you do?
a. do nothing
b. have the patient soak her toe in hydrogen peroxide three times daily
c. have the patient apply a local antibiotic cream and prescribe system antibiotics for 7 to 10 days
d. under local anesthesia, remove the whole toenail
e. b and c

Q13. If the treatment advocated in Question 12 is unsuccessful, what should you do then?
a. still do nothing; these things have a habit of going away if you wait long enough; tell the patient she will only be in pain for another 3 or 4 months at the most
b. have the patient continue to soak her toe in hydrogen peroxide; tell the pharmacist to mix up a double-strength mixture for her
c. change both the local and the systemic antibiotics to the big, all-inclusive, all-pervasive, kill-everything-in-sight guns
d. under local anesthesia, remove the whole toenail
e. none of the above

Case 5 ■ A 45-Year-Old Male with Rectal Pain

A 45-year-old male comes to your office with a 4-day history of rectal pain. The pain is dull, constant, and made worse by defecation. On examination, there is a 3 cm × 2 cm thrombosed mass present at the 3 o'clock position in the anal area.

Q14. At this time, what should you do?
a. advise the patient to take five sitz baths per day

b. advise the patient to apply a local antiinflammatory cream three times a day
c. under local anesthesia, remove the contents of the mass with a straight incision
d. under local anesthesia, remove the contents of the mass with an elliptical incision
e. apply a band to this mass and wait for it to fall off

Case 6 ■ A 28-Year-Old Male with Rectal Bleeding

A 28-year-old male comes to your office with rectal bleeding and local burning and searing pain in the rectal area. The patient describes a small amount of bright red blood on the toilet paper. The pain is maximal at defecation and following defecation. The burning and searing pain that occurs at defecation is replaced by a spasmodic pain after defecation that lasts approximately 30 minutes.

Q15. What is the most likely diagnosis in this patient?
a. adenocarcinoma of the rectum
b. squamous cell carcinoma of the rectum
c. internal hemorrhoids
d. anal fissure
e. an external thrombosed hemorrhoid

Q16. What is (are) the treatment(s) of choice for large prolapsing internal hemorrhoids?
a. excision and drainage
b. sclerotherapy
c. internal banding
d. all of the above are equally effective
e. none of the above

SHORT ANSWER MANAGEMENT PROBLEM
Discuss the classification of burns and how that classification affects office or hospital treatment.

ANSWERS

A1. **a.** For skin incision, it is extremely important that the skin lines of tension be followed (Langer's lines). This is especially important on areas such as the face where Langer's lines tend to run horizontally on the upper face and vertically on the lower face.

A2. **c.** It takes approximately 21 days for fibroblasts to grow across a wound line and for the wound to develop enough strength to hold deep portions of a wound together. If deep portions of a wound pull apart, a depression on the skin surface may develop, which represents a poor cosmetic outcome.

A3. **a.** Cutting needles should always be used on the skin. Almost all cutting needles now have a reverse cutting design (flat surface is on the inside of the curve). For deeper layers, taper needles are less likely to cut through a blood vessel and start bleeding that is difficult to control.

A4. **a.** The anesthetic agent of choice for this patient is lidocaine with epinephrine. The epinephrine will decrease the amount of bleeding from the incision site. The prepackaged solution of lidocaine with epinephrine has a very low pH (pH 4.05) and produces much more pain on injection than lidocaine plain. The pain reaction can be avoided by buffering the lidocaine with sodium bicarbonate in a combination of 10 parts of lidocaine to 1 part of sodium bicarbonate. When this combination is used, the pH is near neutral and the stinging sensation is eliminated.

Other measures that lessen the pain of injection include warming the solution to body temperature, injecting the solution extremely slowly, and cooling the injection site with ice or ethyl chloride before injection. In addition, very small caliber needles can be used for the initial injection (such as a #30½ inch needle) or a local anesthetic such as tetracaine, epinephrine, and cocaine (TAC) or 20% benzocaine liquid or gel can be used.

A5. **e.** Common methods for controlling bleeding after incision include the following:
a. Application of pressure with a sponge held firmly against the bleeding areas
b. Electrocautery
c. Use of local anesthesia containing epinephrine
d. Topical epinephrine or lidocaine containing epinephrine
e. Drysol solution (aluminum chloride, 20% in alcohol)
f. Hemostatic sutures
g. Elevation
h. Pressure dressings
i. Various methods of cooling

A6. **d.** A pigmented skin lesion should be removed intact to ensure an "unharmed" specimen for pathologic evaluation. If electrocautery is used to remove the lesion, the lesion will obviously be destroyed in the process.

A7. **a.** The treatment of choice for the removal of plantar warts is cryosurgery with liquid nitrogen. This combined with paring down the callus has been shown to be the most effective method of removal.

The first step is to pare down the excess callus in the area of the wart. This is best done by shaving off thin layers of the callus with a straightedge razor blade held by hand or a scalpel with a #10 blade. This process should be continued until most of the callus is gone and normal-appearing pliable skin is seen.

The shaving is kept superficial to any bleeding or sensation of pain. The circular plantar wart then becomes much clearer and more evident. Some of the keratin plug can then be excised with the corner of the razor blade or the tip of the scalpel blade. Following that, cryosurgery is performed with liquid nitrogen. A donut-shaped felt pad should be applied. This pad transfers the patient's weight off the hard wart and provides immediate relief of pain during walking. After adequate cryosurgery, the wart should peel off in 1 to 3 weeks. On occasion, a second or third treatment is necessary to ensure complete removal.

A8. **d.** The treatment of choice for venereal warts is 25% podophyllum in tincture of benzoin. Care must be taken to apply the agent only to the wart to avoid damaging the surrounding normal skin. This can be accomplished with the application of petroleum jelly to the surrounding tissue. The patient should be instructed to wash off the podophyllin in 2 to 4 hours to avoid a chemical burn. Pregnant patients should not be treated with podophyllin.

A9. **d.** The burn should be cleaned and dressed with a nonadherent dressing. Cooling runs the risk of compromising circulation to marginally surviving areas of the burn and should not be done for serious burns. If the blister is intact, the burn should not be debrided. Oral analgesia should be provided.

The pain associated with minor first-degree burns will be alleviated to some degree by cooling. Moreover, since tissue damage is minimal it will do no harm.

A10. **d.** Cleaning the burn site with a surgical soap to remove dirt, oil, or other foreign matter is the first step. The use of 4 × 4 gauze sponges or cotton balls can facilitate cleansing. If cleansing is done gently and the burn site is properly cooled, minimal pain should result.

Tetanus prophylaxis is important in all patients with serious burns. If this child's tetanus is not up to date, it must be brought up to date.

For a second-degree burn as in this child, expert opinion is divided on whether or not debridement should take place. Most experts elect to leave the blister intact for several days. The skin of a natural blister may act as a natural dressing, protecting the wound against infection and reducing the amount of pain.

After the initial cleansing, the blistered area may be covered with a layer of silver sulfadiazine ointment (Silvadene) or, in patients who are allergic to sulfa,

Polysporin. A nonadherent dressing should then be applied. Following that, a conforming protective material, such as Kling or Kerlix, should be applied. The wound should be rechecked within 48 hours.

A11. **e.** This patient has a subungual hematoma that needs to be released. The best method of release is to heat a wire (a paper clip), reassure the patient that this is not going to hurt, and gently press the hot metal tip directly over the central portion of the hematoma. As soon as penetration is complete, blood flows through the opening and relief of pain is immediate. An antibiotic ointment will help protect against infection.

A12. **e.**

A13. **e.** This patient has an ingrown toenail. It is perfectly reasonable to try a conservative approach first. The conservative approach consists of topical and oral antibiotics for infection, hot soaks or hydrogen peroxide soaks, good nail care (make sure that the nail is cut straight across), and wearing wider shoes. The corner of the nail that is causing the problem (that is, the corner of the nail that is infected) can often be encouraged to grow out over the skin at the end of the toe by elevation. The corner may be held up by some articles such as a wisp of cotton, a folded piece of Telfa, or a Vaseline gauze or other dressing.

This first attempt at conservative treatment has the additional advantage of decreasing the swelling and inflammation and facilitating injections of the local anesthetic if wedge resection does, in the end, have to be performed. Wedge resection of the nail (the next step) is a procedure whereby the offending curve is cut off at an angle of approximately 30 degrees. Only in recurrent cases is it necessary to completely remove the nail.

A14. **d.** This patient has a thrombosed external hemorrhoid. This condition is painful and causes the patient a great deal of discomfort. Treatment consists of removal of the contents (a clot) using an elliptic incision with a #15 scalpel under local anesthetic. The area should be cleansed and, once bleeding is controlled, an antibiotic ointment and 4 × 4 gauze pads applied.

A15. **d.** This patient has an anal fissure, which is a common cause of rectal bleeding. A crack or a fissure in the skin of the anal canal results from the passage of large, hard boluses of stool. A small amount of bright red blood is noted on the toilet paper. The bleeding most often occurs after defecation. Pain is an important symptom; it is usually a local burning or searing pain and is often very severe.

Examination reveals a semielliptical defect or crack in the anal skin running in a radial direction.

Initially, treatment of anal fissures involves the application of a local steroid cream applied twice daily for 2 or 3 weeks. The use of stool softeners and daily hot sitz baths are recommended. In most cases this treatment will promote complete healing.

A16. **c.** The treatment of choice for internal hemorrhoids is banding. This office procedure should be performed with no more than two hemorrhoids at once. If there are three or more hemorrhoids, wait 3 or 4 weeks before repeating the procedure.

SOLUTION TO THE SHORT ANSWER MANAGEMENT PROBLEM

Burns are classified as follows:
   a. First-degree: Symptoms and signs include pain and redness but no blistering. Dressing is unnecessary. Pain from small burn areas can be relieved by cooling or application of topical creams, ointments, and lotions containing a "caine" medication.

   In areas of clothing, the burn can be covered and a medicated ointment followed by the application of a nonadherent dressing is recommended. Pain can be treated with either acetaminophen, aspirin, or another nonsteroidal antiinflammatory drug.
   b. Second-degree: The hallmark of a second-degree burn is blister formation. Second-degree burns may be either superficial or deep. Treatment options include cleaning and application of a topical antibiotic and dressing. In most cases, leave the blister intact.
   c. Third-degree: These are full-thickness skin burns. Referral to a plastic surgeon as soon as possible is mandatory. Third-degree burns are much more likely to be more serious, be more extensive, have a much greater chance of developing sepsis, and often require an intensive care unit situation if the burn covers a significant portion of the body.

SUMMARY OF COMMON PROCEDURES IN OFFICE SURGERY

1. Remember the ABCs: Always have an emergency cart available if you are planning on doing office surgery.

2. Skin lesion removal:
   a. Follow Langer's lines.
   b. Use an elliptic incision (long enough to avoid puckering at the ends).
   c. Local: Lidocaine with epinephrine except on the fingers and toes
   d. Sutures: Skin: monofilament nylon 3-0, 4-0, 5-0, 6-0; Deep: Dexon needle, cutting needle for a skin suture, taper needle for deep suture
   e. Do not use electrocautery on anything that should rightly go for biopsy.
   f. Small skin lesion removal: Punch biopsy
   If you are not absolutely 100% sure of what a skin lesion is, then biopsy it.

3. Sebaceous cysts: These are most frequent on the scalp and back and can be a cause of significant irritation. Try wherever possible to shell out the whole cyst. If you are unable to remove the entire cyst, there is a significant chance of recurrence.

4. Incision and drainage of abscesses: Make sure you know exactly what you are incising and draining and why you are doing it. Be very careful of both the vascular supply and the nerve supply if you go deep.

5. Common warts: Cryosurgery with liquid nitrogen. Be careful on the digits not to disturb blood flow.

6. Plantar warts:
   a. Pare down excess callus to bleeding point.
   b. Remove keratin plug if possible.
   c. Perform cryosurgery with liquid nitrogen.

7. Burns: Described in the Solution to the Short Answer Management Problem

8. Paronychia:
   a. Try conservative management first.
   b. Remove proximal segment of fingernail and dress.

9. Subungual hematoma: The old, wise, worn, and true heated paper clip

10. Thrombosed external hemorrhoids:
   a. Local anesthesia
   b. Elliptic incision and clot removal

11. Lacerations: Use rules as stated for skin lesion removal.

12. Anal fissures:
   a. Mandatory prevention of further episodes; prevention best achieved by preventing constipation
   b. Conservative treatment using sitz baths and local steroid cream

13. Internal hemorrhoids:
   a. Make sure you know what you're banding before you band it.
   b. Banding is the preferred method of treatment.

SUGGESTED READINGS

AAFP Home Study Self-Assessment: *Office surgery,* Monograph #174, Leawood, Ks, 1993, American Academy of Family Physicians.

Cunningham SJ: Surgical office procedures, *Pediatr Ann* 25(12):699-704, 1996.

PROBLEM·105

PANCREATITIS

"Another Drink Will Settle My Stomach."

Case 1 ■ A 44-Year-Old Male with a History of Very Heavy Alcohol Intake

A 44-year-male with a 20-year history of heavy drinking comes to your office with his wife. His wife is very concerned about her husband's condition and, specifically, about an abdominal pain that began 4 days ago. The pain has been so severe that her husband has been crying at night. Despite this severe pain, the patient managed to make it to his local bar last evening and straggled home at 3 AM.

On examination, you observe a stoic, overweight male who looks much older than his stated years. When you ask him what is wrong, he says, "Nothing, just a little indigestion." As you examine him you clearly smell alcohol on his breath. The patient's blood pressure is 90/70 mm Hg. He has a marked tenderness in the epigastric region along with "bruising" in the epigastric area. There is also a sensation of a mass present in the epigastric area. When questioned about the bruising, the patient states that he fell down the stairs yesterday. No other abnormalities are present.

SELECT THE BEST ANSWER
TO THE FOLLOWING QUESTIONS

Q1. Following the history and physical examination, which of the following is the next step?
   a. send the patient for blood work
   b. send the patient for x-rays
   c. send the patient for both blood work and x-rays
   d. consult a psychiatrist to assess his alcohol intake and subsequent family problems
   e. none of the above

Q2. Following the step taken in Question 1, what would you do now?
   a. order additional blood tests and x-rays if any abnormalities were found
   b. order an ultrasound of the abdomen
   c. call a colleague who specializes on the gastrointestinal system and ask him to see the patient within a few days
   d. do a complete mental status examination to determine suicidal ideation
   e. none of the above

Q3. What is the most likely diagnosis in this patient?
   a. alcoholic esophagitis
   b. severe alcoholic gastritis
   c. acute pancreatitis
   d. perforated duodenal ulcer
   e. early alcoholic encephalopathy with underlying alcoholic gastritis

Q4. The "bruising" present in the epigastrium is most likely the result of which of the following?
   a. the patient's wife's floor wax
   b. trauma secondary to a barroom brawl
   c. retroperitoneal bleeding
   d. superior mesenteric artery erosion
   e. disseminated intravascular coagulation

Q5. What is the most likely disease complication associated with the "bruising?"
   a. a defect in the intrinsic coagulation pathway
   b. a defect in the extrinsic coagulation pathway
   c. diffuse intravascular coagulation as a result of the alcohol intake
   d. pseudocyst formation
   e. hemorrhagic abscess formation

Q6. What is (are) the essential diagnostic feature(s) of the condition of the patient described in Case 1?
   a. abrupt onset of epigastric pain with radiation to the back
   b. nausea and vomiting
   c. elevated serum amylase
   d. all of the above
   e. none of the above

Q7. The treatment of this condition must include all except which of the following?
   a. gastric suction
   b. fluid replacement
   c. calcium replacement
   d. oxygen
   e. an H2 receptor blocker

Q8. Which of the following statements about the disease discussed is (are) true?
   a. many cases of this disease are associated with a pathologic condition of the biliary tract
   b. strong evidence suggests a link between this disease and alcohol
   c. the chronic condition of this disease is more likely to be associated with alcohol abuse rather than biliary tract disease
   d. all of the above statements are true
   e. none of the above statements is true

Q9. In approximately two thirds of cases of this disease, a plain film of the abdomen is abnormal. Which of the following abnormalities is this plain film most likely to show?
   a. a "sentinel loop"
   b. the "colon cutoff sign"
   c. air under the diaphragm
   d. distention in both the small bowel and the large bowel
   e. feces throughout the colon

Q10. Complications of the condition described in Case 1 include which of the following?
   a. ascites
   b. pleural effusion
   c. abscess formation
   d. all of the above
   e. none of the above

SHORT ANSWER MANAGEMENT PROBLEM

Describe the four essential features of the diagnosis of chronic pancreatitis.

ANSWERS

A1. **e.** This patient is extremely ill and should be hospitalized now.

A2. **e.** The combination of low blood pressure, abdominal pain, and a history of heavy alcohol intake strongly suggest the diagnosis of an acute abdomen. No time should be taken for doing laboratory investigations or x-rays at this time; that can wait until the patient has been assessed and is hemodynamically stabilized.

A3. **c.** This patient has acute pancreatitis. His admission to an intensive care unit (ICU) would be the best course of action. His blood pressure should be stabilized and input and output measurements begun immediately.

A4. **c.** This patient has Cullen's sign, an ecchymosis in the periumbilical area caused by the dissection of blood retroperitoneally. This also confirms the diagnosis of hemorrhagic pancreatitis. Another sign that can sometimes be found in patients with acute pancreatitis is called Grey-Turner's sign. In Grey-Turner's sign there is the same ecchymosis, only the location is the flank area rather than the periumbilical area.

A5. **d.** The most likely complication is bleeding into a pancreatic pseudocyst that has formed as a complication of acute pancreatitis. Such bleeding must be stopped. This may be accomplished by embolization of the artery. If the bleeding cannot be stopped by embolization, emergency surgery should be performed. In this patient it may be necessary to open the pseudocyst, ligate the bleeding vessel in the cyst wall, and drain the cyst.

A6. **d.** The essential diagnostic features of acute pancreatitis include abrupt onset of epigastric pain with radiation to the lower lumbar spine, nausea and vomiting, and elevated serum or urinary amylase. Acute pancreatitis usually is caused by cholecystitis or alcoholism.

The essential diagnostic features of pancreatic pseudocyst include an epigastric mass and pain, mild fever and leukocytosis, persistent serum amylase or serum lipase elevation, and demonstration of pseudocyst by computed tomography (CT) scan.

A7. **e.** The essentials of treatment of acute pancreatitis include the following:
   a. Gastric suction to eliminate gastric secretions and decompression
   b. Fluid replacement to replace sequestered fluid in the retroperitoneal space
   c. Replacement of calcium and magnesium: In severe attacks of pancreatitis both hypocalcemia and hypomagnesemia may occur and need to be treated
   d. Oxygen therapy: Severe hypoxemia develops in 30% of patients; the onset is often insidious and can result in adult respiratory distress syndrome
   e. Peritoneal lavage in severe cases to remove toxins
   f. Nutrition: nothing by mouth (NPO) and total parenteral nutrition (TPN)
   g. Blood transfusion: when hemorrhage into either the pancreas or a pancreatic pseudocyst occurs

Although the use of H2 receptor blockers, anticholinergic drugs, glucagon, and antibiotics is reasonably common, their efficacy has not been demonstrated.

A8. **d.** Gallstone disease and alcohol abuse are responsible for approximately 80% of cases of acute pancreatitis. Other causes include hyperparathyroidism, hyperlipidemia, familial pancreatitis, postoperative (iatrogenic) pancreatitis, protein deficiency, use of certain drugs, obstruction of the pancreatic duct, and trauma.

Chronic pancreatitis is much more likely to be associated with alcoholism than with biliary tract disease. In fact, an alcoholic patient who presents with one attack of acute pancreatitis is very likely to go on to subsequent attacks and to chronic disease.

A9. **a.** In approximately two thirds of cases, a plain film of the abdomen is abnormal. The most frequent finding is isolated dilatation of a segment of gut (the sentinel loop) consisting of jejunum, transverse colon, or duodenum adjacent to the pancreas.

Gas distending the right colon that abruptly stops in the mid or left transverse colon is called the colon cutoff sign. This is caused by colonic spasm adjacent to the pancreatic inflammation.

Air under the diaphragm is suggestive of a perforated peptic ulcer.

A completely distended small and large bowel suggests a distal bowel obstruction.

Constipation is not associated with acute pancreatitis.

A10. **d.** In addition to chronic pancreatitis and pancreatic pseudocyst formation, acute pancreatitis may also be associated with pancreatic abscess (fatal if not treated surgically), pancreatic ascites, and pancreatic pleural effusion.

SOLUTION TO THE SHORT ANSWER MANAGEMENT PROBLEM

The four essential features of chronic pancreatitis are as follows:
   a. Persistent or recurrent abdominal pain in almost all cases
   b. Pancreatic calcification on x-ray in 50% of cases
   c. Pancreatic insufficiency in 30% of cases; this may lead to either steatorrhea or diabetes mellitus.
   d. Most often caused by alcoholism

SUMMARY OF THE DIAGNOSIS AND TREATMENT OF PANCREATITIS

1. Acute pancreatitis is usually caused by either alcohol abuse or biliary tract disease (40% biliary tract-gallstone associated; 40% alcohol intake).

2. Essential features of diagnosis: abrupt onset of epigastric pain radiating through to the back; nausea and vomiting; and elevated serum amylase, serum lipase, or urinary amylase.

3. Laboratory investigations: complete blood count; serum amylase and urine amylase; serum lipase; serum glucose; serum lactate dehydrogenase (LDH), serum bilirubin, serum aspartate aminotransferase (AST)/alanine aminotransferase (ALT); serum calcium, serum magnesium, electrolytes, cholesterol and triglycerides, blood gases, plain film of abdomen, abdominal ultrasound, CT scan

4. Ranson's criteria of severity of acute pancreatitis:
   a. Criteria initially present:
      1) Age >55 years
      2) WBC >16,000/mm^3
      3) Blood glucose >200 mg%
      4) Serum lactate dehydrogenase >350 IU/L
      5) aspartate aminotransferase (serum glutamate oxaloacetate transaminase) >250 IU/L
   b. Criteria developing within 48 hours of admission:
      1) Hematocrit decreases more than 10%
      2) BUN increases more than 5 mg/dl
      3) Serum Ca: 8 mg/dl or less
      4) Arterial PO$_2$ <60 mm Hg
      5) Base deficit >4 mEq/L
      6) Estimated fluid sequestration ≥600 ml (volume requirement)
   c. Morbidity and mortality rates correlate with number of criteria present:
      1) 0 to 2 criteria 1% mortality
      2) 3 or 4 criteria 15% mortality
      3) 5 or 6 criteria 40% mortality
      4) 7 or 8 criteria 50% or greater mortality

5. Essentials of management: NPO, nasogastric suction; urine output (a measure of fluid sequestration), fluid replacement of sequestered fluid, replacement of calcium and magnesium if low; oxygen, peritoneal lavage, TPN

6. Resolution within a week in most cases.

7. Complications: Pseudocyst formation, abscess formation, hemorrhage, ascites, pleural effusion, chronic pancreatitis

8. Chronic pancreatitis almost always associated with alcohol-induced cases; complications of chronic pancreatitis: malabsorption (steatorrhea), diabetes mellitus, and chronic pain.

SUGGESTED READINGS

Alridge MC et al: Colonic complications of severe acute pancreatitis, *Br J Surg* 76:362, 1988.

Berry SH, Fink AS: Acute pancreatitis. In Rakel R, ed: *Conn's current therapy*, Philadelphia, 1995, WB Saunders.

Garder B, Stone HH: Acute abdominal pain. In Polk HC et al, eds: *Basic surgery*, ed 4, St Louis, 1993, Quality Medical Publishing.

Way L, ed: *Current surgical diagnosis and treatment: General surgery and surgical specialties*, ed 10, Norwalk, Conn, 1994, Appleton & Lange.

PROBLEM·106

COLONIC DISORDERS

"Doctor, I Think the Idea of Having a Tube Stuck Up My Rear Is Disgusting."

Case 1 ■ A 48-Year-Old Male with Weakness, Fatigue, and Lower Right-Sided Abdominal Fullness

A 48-year-old male comes to your office with a vague lower right-sided abdominal fullness (not pain). He describes to you a general feeling of "not feeling well," fatigue, and a somewhat tender area "down near my appendix." He states "I have no energy; I'm tired all the time." He also suspects that his skin has changed color, first to a pale color and then to a slightly yellow color.

On direct questioning he admits to anorexia, weight loss of 30 pounds in 6 months, nausea most of the time, vomiting twice, some diarrhea that seems to be mucus, and blood in the stool almost every day for the past 3 months. When you ask him what he makes of all this he tells you, "Maybe a very bad flu."

On examination, the patient looks very pale. Examination of the abdomen reveals abdominal distention. You record the abdominal girth as a baseline. There is a sensation of "fullness" in the right lower quadrant of the abdomen. This area also is dull to percussion and is slightly tender. There is definite percussion of tympany on both sides of the area of dullness. The liver span is approximately 20 cm. The sclerae are yellow.

SELECT THE BEST ANSWER TO THE FOLLOWING QUESTIONS

Q1. At this time, what would you do?
 a. tell the patient to relax and recheck with your office in 6 months
 b. diagnose the irritable bowel syndrome and start the patient on dietary therapy
 c. tell that patient that he probably is going through a viral illness; relax and come back in 2 months if the symptoms have not improved
 d. order a complete workup on the patient; the good old shotgun approach (every test known to man and then some)
 e. none of the above

Q2. What is the definitive diagnostic procedure of choice in this patient?
 a. complete blood count (CBC)
 b. fecal occult blood samples
 c. air-contrast barium enema
 d. colonoscopy
 e. three views of the abdomen

Q3. What is the most likely diagnosis in this patient?
 a. irritable bowel syndrome
 b. lactose intolerance
 c. adenocarcinoma of the pancreas
 d. adenocarcinoma of the colon
 e. ruptured appendix

Q4. Having made a correct diagnosis from Question 3, what is the definitive treatment of choice?
 a. colonic segmental resection
 b. total colectomy
 c. removal of the appendix
 d. abdominoperineal resection of the rectum
 e. neodymium:yttrium-aluminum garnet (Nd: YAG) laser photocoagulation of the identified lesion

Q5. Carcinoma of the colon most commonly originates in which of the following?
 a. an adenomatous polyp
 b. an inflammatory polyp
 c. a hyperplastic polyp
 d. a benign lymphoid polyp
 e. a leiomyoma

Q6. Adenomatous polyps are found in approximately what percentage of asymptomatic patients who undergo screening?
 a. 5%
 b. 10%
 c. 15%
 d. 20%
 e. 25%

Q7. A barium enema is performed on a patient with a suspected carcinoma of the descending colon following an unsuccessful colonoscopy. What is the best radiologic description that fits the probable diagnosis in this patient?
 a. a "strawberry cutout" lesion
 b. an "orange dimpled" lesion
 c. an "apple core" lesion

d. a "cabbage fulgurating" lesion
e. a "banana peel" lesion

Q8. Colorectal polyps are thought to be the origin of most colorectal cancers. Which of the following statements regarding colorectal polyps is false?
a. the larger the colorectal polyps, the greater the chance of malignancy
b. hyperplastic polyps have the highest malignant potential of all colorectal polyps
c. adenomatous polyps increase in incidence with each decade after the age of 30 years
d. routine removal of adenomas from the colon reduces the incidence of subsequent adenocarcinoma
e. villous adenomas carry the highest malignant potential of all adenomas

Q9. Which of the following statements best describes the current evidence for fecal occult blood screening as a measure to reduce the morbidity and mortality from colorectal cancer?
a. there is excellent evidence to include fecal occult blood testing in screening asymptomatic patients over the age of 50 years for colorectal carcinoma
b. there is fair evidence to include fecal occult blood testing in screening asymptomatic patients over the age of 50 years for colorectal carcinoma
c. there is insufficient evidence to include or exclude fecal occult blood testing as an effective screening test for colorectal cancer in asymptomatic patients over the age of 50 years
d. none of the above

Q10. Which of the following statements regarding carcinoembryonic antigen (CEA) and colorectal cancer is true?
a. CEA is a cost-effective screening test for colorectal cancer
b. elevated preoperative CEA levels correlate well with postoperative recurrence rate in colorectal cancer
c. CEA is a sensitive test for colorectal cancer
d. CEA is a specific test for colorectal cancer
e. CEA has no value in predicting recurrence in colorectal cancer

Case 2 ■ A 78-Year-Old Male with Acute and Severe Abdominal Pain

A 78-year-old male comes to your office with acute and severe abdominal pain, left lower-quadrant tenderness, a left lower quadrant mass, and a temperature of 39° C. The patient has had no significant illnesses in the past. He is very healthy. He sees his physician once a year and has had a normal heart, normal blood pressure, and normal "everything else," as he says, for many years.

On examination, the patient's temperature is 39.5° C. His pulse is 96 and regular. His blood pressure is 210/105 mm Hg. There is significant tenderness in the left lower quadrant. Rebound tenderness is not present. There is a definite sensation of a mass present.

Q11. What is the most likely diagnosis in this patient?
a. adenocarcinoma of the colon
b. diverticulitis
c. diverticulosis
d. colorectal carcinoma
e. atypical appendicitis

Q12. What is the treatment of choice for the patient described in Case 2?
a. primary resection of the diseased segment with anastomosis
b. primary resection of the diseased segment without anastomosis
c. colectomy
d. abdominal perineal resection
e. none of the above

Q13. Which of the following is a (are) component(s) of the acute treatment of this patient's condition?
a. intravenous (IV) fluids
b. IV (broad-spectrum) antibiotics
c. nasogastric (NG) suction, if abdominal distention or vomiting is present
d. all of the above
e. a and c only

Q14. Which of the following investigations is contraindicated at this time in the patient described in Case 2?
a. computed tomography (CT) scan of the abdomen and pelvis
b. magnetic resonance imaging scan of the abdomen and pelvis
c. three views of the abdomen
d. air-contrast barium enema
e. none of the above is contraindicated

Q15. Which of the following statements regarding this patient's blood pressure elevation is true?
a. this patient most likely has essential hypertension
b. this patient's abdominal pain is most likely related to his hypertension
c. this elevation of blood pressure could be caused by the pain he is experiencing

d. this patient's physician (the one he has been seeing every year) obviously has made a very serious mistake in labeling this patient as normotensive

e. none of the above statements is true

Q16. What is the analgesic of choice for control of pain in this patient?

a. morphine
b. hydromorphone
c. methadone
d. pentazocine
e. codeine

Q17. Which of the following organisms is (are) the most likely cause(s) of the condition described?

a. *Escherichia coli*
b. *Bacteroides fragilis*
c. *Streptococcus pneumoniae*
d. a and b only
e. all of the above

Case 3 ■ A 35-Year-Old Male with Rectal Bleeding and Mucoid Discharge from the Rectum

A 35-year-old male comes to your office with rectal bleeding, mucoid discharge from the rectum, and protrusion of certain structures through the anal canal. On proctoscopic examination, large internal hemorrhoids are seen.

Q18. What is the best next step in the management of this patient?

a. proceed with definitive treatment
b. proceed with further investigations
c. prescribe a hemorrhoidal cream
d. do nothing; ask the patient to return in 6 months for review
e. none of the above

Q19. What is the treatment of choice for the patient described in Case 3?

a. a hemorrhoidal cream
b. a hemorrhoidal ointment
c. hemorrhoidectomy
d. injection of phenol into the hemorrhoidal tissue
e. rubber band ligation of the internal hemorrhoids

Q20. Which of the following statements regarding angiodysplasia is (are) true?

a. angiodysplasia is an acquired condition most often affecting individuals over the age of 60 years

b. angiodysplasia is a focal submucosal vascular ectasis that has the propensity to bleed profusely

c. most angiodysplastic lesions are located in the cecum and proximal ascending colon

d. multiple lesions occur in 25% of cases

e. all of the above statements are true

SHORT ANSWER MANAGEMENT PROBLEM
Discuss the evidence for dietary modification to reduce the risk of developing colorectal cancer.

ANSWERS

A1. **e.** None of the answers are appropriate or sufficiently focused.

A2. **d.** The colonoscopy will allow for a tissue biopsy and diagnosis as well

A3. **d.** In this patient the problem list at this point is as follows:

a. Middle-aged male: Nonspecific feelings of "ill health"
b. Right lower-quadrant mass on physical examination: Query carcinoma
c. Enlarged liver: Query metastases
d. Pale appearance: Query anemia
e. Icterus: Query conjugated hyperbilirubinemia
f. Clinically apparent abdominal distention: Query ascites

With this constellation of symptoms and signs, the working diagnosis is adenocarcinoma of the cecum with liver metastases.

The investigations that must be performed at this time include the following:

a. Laboratory:
 1) CBC
 2) Serum bilirubin
 3) Liver enzymes: aspartate aminotransferase, alanine aminotransferase, gamma-glucuronosyltransferase
 4) Alkaline phosphatase
 5) Serum calcium
 6) Serum electrolytes
 7) CEA

b. Radiology:
 1) Chest x-ray
 2) Three views of the abdomen
 3) Abdominal ultrasound

c. The diagnostic procedure of choice in this patient is a total colonoscopy to confirm a mass lesion, to determine the location of that lesion, and to obtain a biopsy of the lesion if possible.

d. For colon carcinoma the essentials of diagnosis are as follows:
1) Right colon:
   a) Unexplained weakness or anemia
   b) Occult blood in feces, diarrhea with mucus
   c) Dyspeptic symptoms
   d) Persistent right abdominal discomfort
   e) Palpable abdominal mass
   f) Characteristic x-ray findings
   g) Characteristic colonoscopic findings
2) Left colon:
   a) Change in bowel habits with thin stools
   b) Gross blood in stool
   c) Obstructive symptoms
   d) Characteristic x-ray findings
   e) Characteristic colonoscopic or sigmoidoscopic findings
3) Rectum:
   a) Rectal bleeding
   b) Alteration in bowel habits
   c) Sensation of incomplete evacuation
   d) Intrarectal palpable tumor
   e) Sigmoidoscopic findings

A4. **a.** The definitive surgical treatment of choice in this patient (if feasible) is colonic resection. The preliminary location of the lesion based on physical examination is in the area of the cecum. If this proves to be correct, the colonic resection will involve the removal of the area from the vermiform appendix to the junction of the ascending and transverse colons. With the presence of liver metastasis, this procedure is palliative.

A5. **a.** The vast majority of colonic adenocarcinomas evolve from adenomas. Adenomas are a premalignant lesion, and in the large bowel the sequence is: adenoma-dysplasia in the adenomas, and adenocarcinoma.

A6. **e.** Both adenomas and the subsequent evolved adenocarcinomas increase in incidence with age, and the distribution of adenomas and cancer in the bowel is similar. Overall, adenomatous polyps are found in approximately 25% of asymptomatic patients who undergo screening colonoscopy. The age-related prevalence of adenomatous polyps is 30% at age 50 years, 40% age 60 years, 50% at age 70 years, and 55% at age 80 years. The mean age of patients with adenomas is 55 years, approximately 5 to 10 years earlier than the mean age for patients with adenocarcinoma of the colon. Approximately 50% of polyps occur in the sigmoid colon or in the rectum. About 50% of patients with adenomas have more than one adenoma, and

15% have more than two adenomas. There is an interesting correlation between patients with breast cancer and adenomatous polyps in the colon and rectum. Those patients with breast cancer have an increased risk of adenomatous polyps.

The malignant potential of the adenoma depends on the growth pattern, the size of the polyp, and the degree of atypia or dysplasia. Adenocarcinoma of the colon is found in approximately 1% of adenomas less than 1.0 cm in diameter, in approximately 10% of adenomas between 1.0 cm and 2.0 cm in diameter, and in approximately 45% of adenomas with a diameter greater than 2.0 cm.

The potential for cancerous transformations rises with increasing degrees of dysplasia.

Sessile lesions are more apt to be malignant than pedunculated ones. The time it takes an adenoma to proceed through the process to frank adenocarcinoma is between 10 and 15 years.

The following is a summary of the types of adenomas and their malignant potential:
a. Villous adenoma: 40% become malignant
b. Tubulovillous adenoma: 22% become malignant
c. Tubular adenoma: 5% become malignant

A7. **c.** This patient most likely suffers from a constricting carcinoma of the descending colon. A barium enema (preferably an air-contrast barium enema) of a constricting carcinoma of the descending colon presents what is best described as an "apple core" lesion. On the barium enema you will note the loss of mucosal patterns, the "hooks" at the margins of the lesion, the relatively short length of the lesion, and the abrupt ending of the lesion.

A8. **b.** Hyperplastic polyps are polyps that are designated as "unclassified" but are totally benign. The highest malignant potential is carried by villous adenomas.

A9. **a.** The current United States Preventive Services Task Force recommendation for screening colorectal cancer is for all persons aged 50 or older to be screened by annual fecal occult blood testing. We now know that annual fecal occult blood testing reduces mortality.

A10. **b.** CEA is a glycoprotein found in the cell membranes of a number of tissues, a number of body fluids, and a number of secretions including urine and feces. It is also found in malignancies of the colon and rectum. Since some of the CEA antigen enters the bloodstream, it can be detected by the use of a radioimmunoassay technique of serum.

Elevated CEA is not specifically associated with colorectal cancer; abnormally high levels of CEA are also found in patients with other gastrointestinal (GI) malignancies and non-GI malignancies. CEA levels are elevated in 70% of patients with an adenocarcinoma of the large bowel, but less than 50% of patients with localized disease are CEA-positive. Thus because of these difficulties with sensitivity and specificity, CEA does not serve as a useful screening procedure, nor is it an accurate diagnostic test for colorectal cancer at a curable stage. However, elevated preoperative CEA levels correlate with postoperative recurrence rate, and failure of CEA to fall to normal levels after resection implies a poor prognosis. CEA is helpful in detecting recurrence after curative surgical resection; if high CEA levels return to normal after operation and then rise progressively during the follow-up period, recurrence of cancer is likely.

A11. **b.** This patient has diverticulitis, an infection and inflammation of one or more diverticula that, in its noninflammatory state, is known as *diverticulosis*. In the United States and Canada approximately 50% of patients have diverticula, 10% by age 40 and 65% by age 80. The prevalence of diverticula varies tremendously around the world.

Cultural factors, especially diet, play an important causative role. Among dietary factors, the most important one is the fiber content of ingested food.

The essentials of diagnosis of diverticulitis are:
a. Acute abdominal pain (usually left lower)
b. Left lower quadrant tenderness with or without a mass in the same area
c. Fever and leukocytosis
d. Imaging findings:
   1) Plain films: If inflammation is localized: ileus, partial colonic obstruction, small bowel obstruction, or left lower-quadrant mass.
   2) CT scans: No perforation: effacement of pericolic fat with or without abscess or fistulas
   3) Barium enema: Contraindicated during an acute attack of diverticulitis; the risk of perforation and barium escape into the peritoneal cavity is high

A12. **e.** The treatment of choice for diverticulitis is expectant unless surgical treatment is necessary because of rupture and subsequent peritonitis or multiple recurrences. The natural history of the disease includes the following:
a. Approximately 10% to 20% of patients with diverticulosis develop diverticulitis.
b. Approximately 75% of complications of diverticular disease develop in patients with no prior colonic symptoms.
c. Approximately 25% of patients hospitalized with acute diverticulitis require surgical treatment; the operative mortality of primary resection has dropped from 25% to less than 5%.

A13. **d.** Treatment includes the following:
a. Nothing by mouth
b. IV fluids with potassium
c. NG suction if abdominal distension or vomiting is present
d. IV antibiotics

A14. **d.** See Answer 11.

A15. **c.** The elevation of blood pressure in this patient is almost certainly directly associated with the pain that he is experiencing. Acute and chronic pain (but especially acute pain) increases the release of the "pressor hormones" such as norepinephrine. This produces vasoconstriction that ultimately results in elevated blood pressure. The patient thus experiences a vicious pain cycle that is circular in dimension: more pain, pressor hormone release, elevated blood pressure, increase in pressor hormone release, more pain, and so on.

A16. **a.** Morphine will readily relieve the pain, decrease anxiety, and lower the elevated blood pressure.

A17. **d.** The most common organisms involved in the development of diverticulitis are *E. coli* and *B. fragilis*.

A18. **a.**

A19. **e.** This patient has internal hemorrhoids. The treatment of choice for the protruding internal hemorrhoids that this patient has is rubber band ligation. Rubber band ligation is especially useful in situations in which the hemorrhoids are enlarged or prolapsing.

To accomplish this procedure, the anoscope is used and the redundant mucosa above the hemorrhoid is grasped with forceps and advanced through the barrel of a special ligator. The rubber band is then placed snugly around the mucosa and the hemorrhoidal plexus. Ischemic necrosis occurs over several days, with eventual slough, fibrosis, and fixation of the tissues. One hemorrhoidal complex at a time is treated, with repeat ligations done at 2- and 4-week intervals as needed.

The major, but uncommon, complication of this procedure is pain severe enough to require removal of the band. To avoid this, the band must be placed high and well above the junction of the mucocutaneous region (dentate line). In this location the innervation is autonomic, not somatic. If pain begins and does not resolve, infection should be suspected and investigated immediately. At the time the dead tissue falls off, there may be significant bleeding; the patient should be aware of this.

A20. **e.** Angiodysplasia is an acquired colonic condition that mainly affects elderly individuals. Pathophysiologically, angiodysplasia can be described as a focal submucosal vascular ectasis that has a high probability of producing significant bleeding. The vast majority of angiodysplastic lesions occur in the cecum and in the proximal ascending colon. In at least 25% of patients, multiple lesions are present.

The primary symptom is bright red rectal bleeding that can be extensive and that may require transfusion.

Diagnosis is made by colonoscopy. The diagnosis is made when two of the following three features are present:
   a. An early-filling vein (within 4 to 5 seconds after injection)
   b. A vascular tuft
   c. A delayed-emptying vein

If searched for carefully, as many as 25% of individuals over the age of 60 have angiodysplasia. In many cases expectant management or colonoscopic cauterization is all that is needed. If surgery is required, the operative procedure of choice appears to be hemicolectomy.

SOLUTION TO THE SHORT ANSWER MANAGEMENT PROBLEM

Recently there has been increasing interest in dietary therapy to reduce the risk of developing colonic cancer. The recommendations of the National Cancer Institute include the following:
   1. Drink alcohol only in moderation, if at all.
   2. Reduce dietary fat from 40% to 30% of total calories.
   3. Include whole grains and vegetables high in carotenoids in the diet.
   4. Limit ingestion of smoked, pickled, and cured meats.
   5. Increase fiber consumption.
   6. Increase vitamin C consumption.
   7. Limit consumption of nitrates and nitrites.
The recommendations of the American Cancer Society include the following:
   1. Avoid obesity.
   2. Reduce total fat intake.
   3. Eat high-fiber foods, including foods that are rich in vitamins A and C.
   4. Include cruciferous vegetables in the diet such as cabbage.

   5. Drink alcohol moderately, if at all.
   6. Consume only moderate (at most) amounts of salted, smoked, or nitrate-cured foods.
There appears to be almost universal support for the following:
   1. Decreasing the amount of fat in the diet, especially saturated fat (this will also lead to decreased body mass index or total body weight)
   2. Increasing the amount of fiber in the diet
   3. Increasing the intake of cruciferous vegetables and fiber
   4. Decreasing alcohol intake
   5. Decreasing the intake of salted, smoked, and nitrate-based foods

SUMMARY OF THE DIAGNOSIS AND TREATMENT OF COLORECTAL CANCER AND OTHER COLONIC DISORDERS

1. Colorectal cancer:
   a. Incidence: In North America cancer of the colon and rectum ranks second after cancer of the lung in incidence and death rates. In the United States the number of new cases has been increasing since 1990, but mortality has been decreasing.
   b. Age and sex:
      1) Age: The incidence of carcinoma of the colon increases with age, from 0.39/1000 persons per year at age 50 to 4.5/1000 persons at age 80.
      2) Sex: Carcinoma of the colon, particularly the right colon, is more common in women, and carcinoma of the rectum is more common in men.
   c. Genetic predisposition: Genetic predisposition to cancer of the large bowel is well recognized in persons with familial adenomatous polyposis.
   d. Risk factors for carcinoma of the colon:
      1) Ulcerative colitis
      2) Crohn's disease
      3) Exposure to radiation
      4) Colorectal polyps
   e. Essentials of diagnosis: See Answer 3.
   f. Distribution of cancer of the colon and rectum:
      1) Rectum: 30% of all colorectal cancers
      2) Sigmoid: 20% of all colorectal cancers
      3) Descending colon: 15% of all colorectal cancers
      4) Transverse colon: 10% of all colorectal cancers
      5) Ascending colon: 25% of all colorectal cancers
   g. Pathophysiology: The vast majority of colorectal cancers originate in colonic polyps. Tubular adenomas (tubulovillous adenoma) and villous adenomas are both premalignant.

h. Treatment of colorectal cancer:
   1) Basic treatment for cancer of the colon consists of wide surgical resection of the lesion and its regional lymphatic drainage after preparation of the bowel.
   2) Basic treatment for cancer of the rectum consists of abdominoperineal resection of the rectum or a low anterior resection of the rectum.
   3) Adjuvant therapy includes radiotherapy and combination chemotherapy.

2. Polyps of the colon and rectum:
   a. Prevalence: Adenomatous polyps are found in approximately 25% of asymptomatic adults who undergo screening colonoscopy. The prevalence of adenomatous polyps is 30% at age 50 years, 40% at age 60 years, 50% at age 70 years, and 55% at age 80 years.
   b. Malignant potential: Adenomas are a premalignant lesion, and most authorities believe that the majority of adenocarcinomas of the large bowel evolve from adenomas (adenoma-to-carcinoma sequence). The mean age of patients with polyps is 5 to 10 years younger than the mean age of patients with colorectal cancer.
   c. Benign polyps include hematomas, inflammatory polyps, and hyperplastic polyps.
   d. Essentials of diagnosis: The essentials of diagnosis of polyps of the colon and rectum include the passage of blood per rectum and sigmoidoscopic, colonoscopic, or radiologic discovery of polyps.
   e. Treatment: Adenomatous polyps should be removed by methods that include electrocautery, Nd:YAG laser therapy, and laparotomy if removal through the colonoscope is unsuccessful.
   f. Prevention: High-fiber diet

3. Diverticulosis and diverticulitis:
   a. Prevalence: Approximately 50% of individuals in the United States develop diverticula. Diverticular disease is much more common in the United States than in Japan or other Eastern countries.
   b. Symptomatic versus asymptomatic: Diverticulosis probably remains asymptomatic in 80% of individuals.
   c. Essentials of diagnosis of diverticulitis:
      1) Acute abdominal pain
      2) Left lower quadrant tenderness with or without a mass
      3) Fever and leukocytosis
      4) Characteristic radiologic signs showing diverticula

d. Treatment:
   1) Conservative: Some patients can be treated at home with oral antibiotics and analgesics.
   2) In-hospital treatment consists of NPO, insertion of an NG tube, and administration of IV fluids, antibiotics, and pentazocine for analgesia.
   3) Surgical: Surgical treatment is necessary when there is a diverticula rupture or when abscess and peritonitis ensue. Approximately 25% of hospitalized patients need surgery.
e. The "DO NOT" of diverticulitis: DO NOT do a barium enema in the acute phase (potential rupture and peritonitis).
f. Organisms associated with diverticulitis:
   1) *E. coli*
   2) *B. fragilis*
g. Prevention: High-fiber diet

4. Other conditions of note:
   a. Internal hemorrhoids with prolapse: Treatment consists of rubber band ligation
   b. Angiodysplasia: Consider angiodysplasia as another cause of rectal bleeding in elderly patients.

SUGGESTED READINGS

Guide to Clinical Preventive Services: 1996, *http://www.ahcpr.gov.*
Prevention of Colorectal Cancer: 1999, *http://www.cancernet.nci.nih.gov.*
Schrock TR: Large intestine. In Way LW, ed: *Current surgical diagnosis and treatment: General surgery and surgical specialties,* ed 10, Norwalk, Conn, 1994, Appleton & Lange.

PROBLEM·107

BREAST DISEASE

"A Lump! Does That Mean Mastectomy?"

Case 1 ■ A 41-Year-Old Female with a Painless Breast Lump

A 41-year-old female comes to your office after finding a breast lump during a routine self-examination. She has been examining her breasts regularly for the past 5 years; this is the first lump she has found.

On examination, there is a lump located in the right breast. The lump's anatomic location is in the upper outer quadrant. It is approximately 3 cm in diameter and is not fixed to skin or muscle. It has a hard consistency. There are three axillary nodes present on the right side; each node is approximately 1 cm in diameter. No lymph nodes are present on the left.

SELECT THE BEST ANSWER
TO THE FOLLOWING QUESTIONS

Q1. At this time, what would you do?
   a. tell the patient that she has fibrocystic breast disease; ask her to return in one month—preferably 10 days after the next period for a recheck
   b. tell the patient to see her lawyer and update her will; death is imminent
   c. tell the patient to go home and relax—we generally get too worked up about breast lumps
   d. order an ultrasound of the area
   e. none of the above

Q2. What is the first diagnostic procedure that should be performed in this patient?
   a. ultrasound of the breast
   b. mammography
   c. fine-needle biopsy
   d. all of the above
   e. none of the above

Q3. What is the definitive procedure that should be performed in this patient?
   a. ultrasound of the breast
   b. mammography
   c. biopsy
   d. all of the above
   e. none of the above

Case 2 ■ A 49-Year-Old Female with a Suspicious Lesion Discovered with Mammography

A mammographic examination uncovered a very suspicious lesion in the right breast of a 49-year-old female. Clinically, the lesion is a 3-cm mass present in the left upper outer quadrant. No axillary lymph nodes are palpable. You refer her to a surgeon who books her for a surgical procedure.

Q4. What surgical procedure should be used for this case?
   a. a lumpectomy
   b. a modified radical mastectomy
   c. a lumpectomy plus axillary lymph node dissection
   d. modified radical mastectomy plus axillary lymph node dissection
   e. none of the above

Q5. The risk factors for carcinoma of the breast include which of the following?
   a. a first-degree relative with breast cancer
   b. nulliparity

   c. birth of a first child after age 35
   d. early menarche
   e. all of the above

Q6. Current estimates by the American Cancer Society suggest that one out of every how many women will eventually develop breast cancer?
   a. 1 out of 8
   b. 1 out of 15
   c. 1 out of 25
   d. 1 out of 50
   e. 1 out of 100

Q7. The U.S. Preventive Services Task Force on the Periodic Health Examination recommends which of the following as the preferred mammographic screening protocol for breast cancer in women?
   a. screen all women over the age of 40 years every year
   b. screen all women over the age of 40 years every 2 years
   c. screen all women over the age of 50 every 1 or 2 years
   d. screen all women over the age of 40 every 1 to 2 years
   e. screen all women between the ages of 35 and 40 with a baseline mammogram and screen all women over the age of 40 every 1 to 2 years

Q8. Which of the following statements regarding breast-conserving surgery or lumpectomy is (are) correct?
   a. lumpectomy and breast irradiation is just as effective as modified radical mastectomy for patients with stage I or stage II disease
   b. lumpectomy has not undergone enough testing to predict its efficacy relative to modified radical mastectomy
   c. most American surgeons are following the National Institutes of Health (NIH) recommendations concerning lumpectomy
   d. modified radical mastectomy remains the treatment of choice for most women with breast cancer
   e. nobody really knows for sure

Q9. What is the most common histologic type of breast cancer?
   a. infiltrating ductal carcinoma
   b. medullary carcinoma
   c. invasive lobular carcinoma
   d. noninvasive intraductal carcinoma
   e. papillary ductal carcinoma

Questions 10 to 16 consist of seven case histories describing seven patients with seven different combinations of breast cancer, estrogen-receptor status, and axillary lymph nodes. Match the numbered case history to the preferred treatment option. Each preferred treatment option may be used once, more than once, or not at all.

   a. tamoxifen
   b. adjuvant combination chemotherapy
   c. neither tamoxifen nor combination chemotherapy

Q10. A 37-year-old premenopausal woman with an estrogen receptor-positive breast cancer and positive axillary lymph nodes

Q11. A 34-year-old premenopausal women with an estrogen receptor-positive breast cancer with negative axillary lymph nodes

Q12. A 42-year-old premenopausal woman with a 1.5-cm estrogen receptor-negative breast cancer with negative axillary lymph nodes

Q13. A 61-year-old postmenopausal woman with a 3-cm estrogen receptor-positive breast cancer with positive axillary lymph nodes

Q14. A 63-year-old postmenopausal woman with a 2-cm estrogen receptor-negative breast cancer with positive axillary lymph nodes

Q15. A 58-year-old postmenopausal woman with a 2-cm estrogen receptor-positive breast cancer and negative axillary lymph nodes

Q16. A 72-year-old postmenopausal woman with a 3-cm estrogen receptor-negative breast cancer with negative axillary lymph nodes

Case 3 ■ A 42-Year-Old Female with Painful Bilateral Breast Masses That Wax and Wane with Her Period

A 42-year-old female comes to your office with bilateral breast masses that are painful and seem to "come and go" depending on the stage of the menstrual cycle. There is significant pain with these masses during menstruation.

On examination, there are two areas of dense tissue, one in each breast, each approximately 4 cm in diameter. No axillary lymph nodes are palpable.

Q17. What is the most likely diagnosis in this patient?
   a. carcinoma of the breast
   b. mammary dysplasia (fibrocystic disease)

   c. fibroadenoma
   d. Paget's disease of the breast
   e. none of the above

Q18. If medical treatment is indicated and prescribed for the condition described in Case 3, which of the following should be considered as the therapeutic agent of first choice?
   a. hormone therapy: the oral contraceptive pill
   b. hormone therapy: danazol
   c. a thiazide diuretic
   d. vitamin E
   e. none of the above

Case 4 ■ A 23-Year-Old Female with a Firm but Mobile Mass

A 23-year-old female consults her physician because of a breast mass; the mass is mobile, firm, and approximately 1 cm in diameter. It is located in the upper outer quadrant of the right breast. No axillary lymph nodes are present.

Q19. What is the most likely diagnosis in this patient?
   a. carcinoma of the breast
   b. mammary dysplasia (fibrocystic disease)
   c. fibroadenoma
   d. Paget's disease of the breast
   e. none of the above

Q20. What is the treatment of choice for the condition described in Case 4?
   a. modified radical mastectomy
   b. lumpectomy
   c. biopsy
   d. radical mastectomy
   e. watchful waiting

Case 5 ■ A 33-Year-Old Female with a Small Lump and a Bloody Nipple Discharge

A 33-year-old female comes to your office with a 2-month history of a bloody unilateral left nipple discharge. She has also noted a small and soft lump just beneath the areola on the left side.

On examination, there is a 4-mm soft mass located just inferior to the left areola. No other abnormalities are present in either breast.

Q21. What is the most likely diagnosis in this patient?
   a. carcinoma of the breast
   b. fibroadenoma

c. intraductal papilloma
d. fibrocystic breast disease
e. none of the above

SHORT ANSWER MANAGEMENT PROBLEM
Discuss the recommendations of the U.S. Preventive Services Task Force on (1) breast self-examination, (2) physical examination of the breast, (3) ultrasound of the breast, and (4) mammography.

ANSWERS

A1. **e.** The most likely diagnosis in this patient is carcinoma of the breast. Therefore delay is not appropriate. On the other hand, even if that were the diagnosis, it is not a death sentence. The most common presenting symptom in breast cancer is a painless lump. Most breast lumps are discovered by patients themselves. Other symptoms that may occur in patients with breast cancer (usually at a more advanced stage) are breast pain, nipple discharge, erosions, retraction, enlargement or itching of the nipple, redness, generalized hardness of the breast, and enlargement or shrinking of the breast.

A2. **b.** The first diagnostic procedure that should be performed in this patient is a mammogram. A mammogram will more clearly outline the characteristics of the mass but must be followed by biopsy, either open or fine needle. Use of the latter has improved greatly, and presently has a very low level of false-negative diagnoses.

A3. **c.** Biopsy, either open or needle, is the surgical procedure of choice in this patient.

A4. **e.** The important choice of the type of surgery as well as the local and regional treatment needs to be made if this is a breast cancer. This is often a difficult decision and requires considerable thought on the part of both the patient and the doctor as well as information (education) and time.

A5. **e.** Factors associated with an increased risk of breast cancer include the following:
   a. Race: white
   b. Age: older
   c. Family history: breast cancer in mother or sister (especially high risk if breast cancer was bilateral or premenopausal)
   d. Previous medical history:
      1) Endometrial cancer
      2) Some forms of mammary dysplasia
      3) Cancer in the other breast

e. Menstrual history:
   1) Early menarche (younger than age 12)
   2) Late menopause (older than age 50)
   f. Pregnancy: late first pregnancy (especially after 35)

A6. **a.** Current estimates indicate that among North American women, approximately one woman in eight will, at some time in her life, develop breast cancer.

A7. **c.** Mammographic screening is recommended for all women age 50 years and older on a time interval basis of one mammogram every 1 to 2 years. However, some studies recommend mammography beginning at age 40.

A8. **a.** The National Surgical Adjunctive Breast Project has concluded that segmental mastectomy (lumpectomy) followed by breast irradiation in all patients and adjunctive chemotherapy in women with positive nodes is appropriate therapy and is just as effective (that is, no difference in mortality rates) as modified radical mastectomy in patients with stage I and stage II breast cancer with tumors less than 4 cm in diameter.

A9. **a.** The most common histologic type of breast cancer is an infiltrating ductal carcinoma. This type comprises 70% to 80% of all breast cancers. The subtypes of infiltrating ductal carcinoma include medullary, colloid (mucinous), tubular, and papillary carcinoma.

A10 through A16: Matching Questions

The current recommendations for the use of tamoxifen and adjuvant combination chemotherapy based on menopausal status (premenopausal or postmenopausal), estrogen receptor (ER) status, and axillary lymph node involvement are summarized as follows:
   a. Premenopausal women with positive axillary lymph nodes and either ER-positive or ER-negative tumors should be treated with adjuvant combination chemotherapy.
   b. Premenopausal women with negative axillary lymph nodes whose tumors are ER positive benefit from tamoxifen; premenopausal women with negative axillary lymph nodes whose tumors are ER negative should be treated with combination chemotherapy.
   c. Postmenopausal women with positive axillary lymph nodes and positive hormone receptors should be treated with tamoxifen.
   d. Postmenopausal women with positive axillary lymph nodes whose tumors are ER- negative should be treated with adjuvant combination chemotherapy.

e. Postmenopausal women with negative axillary lymph nodes whose tumors are ER positive should be treated with tamoxifen; however, postmenopausal women with negative axillary lymph nodes whose tumors are ER-negative should be treated with combination chemotherapy.

In addition, the NIH has issued the following statement concerning women with early-stage breast cancer: "All patients who are candidates for clinical trials should be offered the opportunity to participate in such trials [and] all node-negative patients who are not candidates for clinical trials should be made aware of the benefits and risks of adjuvant systemic therapy."

A10. **b.**; A11. **a.**; A12. **b.**; A13. **a.**; A14. **b.**; A15. **a.**; and A16. **b.**

A17. **b.** The patient in Case 3 almost certainly has fibrocystic breast changes also known as mammary dysplasia. All breast tissue contains cysts, and thus the term *fibrocystic breast disease*, as the condition was previously called, is confusing and inappropriate. The most common scenario following this label is that a woman with fibrocystic breast changes believes, in fact, that she has a serious breast disease.

Fibrocystic breast changes are most likely hormonal in origin. This may be either an estrogen or progesterone imbalance or a prolactin excess.

The most common presenting symptom of fibrocystic breast change is pain. The pain usually begins 1 week before menstruation and is relieved following menstruation. The pain is usually bilateral and is most commonly located in the upper outer quadrants. It may be associated with breast swelling and yellow-green breast discharge.

A18. **a.** In most women, fibrocystic breast changes do not have to be treated. If they do, the most effective treatments are a low-dose oral contraceptive pill that contains a potent progestational agent (such as Loestrin 1/20) or medroxyprogesterone acetate 5 to 10 mg/day from days 15 to 25 of the calendar month.

Danazol may be used to induce a pseudomenopause in patients with severe fibrocystic breast changes. It is expensive, however, and has significant side effects.

Thiazide diuretics are useful in reducing total body fluid volume and edema. In the case of the type of "localized swelling in an enclosed cyst" that is seen in fibrocystic breast change, they are not useful.

Vitamin E has not been shown to be of value in the treatment of fibrocystic breast changes.

A19. **c.** This patient has a fibroadenoma, or *breast mouse*. Fibroadenomas are the most common type of solid benign breast tumors. They are most prevalent in women younger than 25 years old. They are usually painless, well circumscribed, completely round, and freely mobile. The classic description with respect to consistency is "rubbery."

A20. **c.** The treatment of choice for a suspected fibroadenoma is either a fine-needle biopsy or an excisional biopsy. Although rare, malignancies have occasionally been found in fibroadenomas.

A21. **c.** This patient has an intraductal papilloma, which is a small, soft, tumor that is found just below the areola. If a patient has a bloody nipple discharge associated with a small, soft mass, there is a 95% probability that this is an intraductal papilloma. If physical examination reveals no mass, Paget's disease of the nipple, an adenoma of the nipple, or a breast carcinoma with ductal invasion must be considered in the differential diagnosis.

The treatment of choice is surgical removal. This is often facilitated by mammography or a ductogram.

SOLUTION TO THE SHORT ANSWER MANAGEMENT PROBLEM

The recommendations of the U.S. Preventive Services Task Force regarding screening for carcinoma of the breast include the following:

a. Breast self-examination: There is not enough evidence to either include or exclude breast self-examination in the periodic health examination, but it is clear that most breast lumps are discovered by the patients themselves. Therefore self-examination of the breasts should be encouraged.

b. Physical examination of the breast: All women over the age of 40 should receive an annual clinical breast examination.

c. Ultrasound of the breast: There is no evidence to suggest that breast ultrasound is a useful screening tool for women in the early detection of cancer of the breast.

d. Mammography: Mammography screening should be performed every 1 to 2 years beginning at age 50. Some recommend having at least a base line study at the age of 40. The only exception is a woman in whom a previous pathologic condition has been demonstrated.

SUMMARY OF THE DIAGNOSIS AND TREATMENT OF BREAST DISEASE

1. Fibrocystic breast changes:
   a. Cause: Hormonal factors
   b. Symptoms: Breast pain and fullness premenstrually, with or without discharge

c. Diagnosis: Breast cyst aspiration supplemented by mammography and ultrasound
d. Treatment: Supportive measures, oral contraceptives with low estrogenic activity and potent progestin, medroxyprogesterone acetate

2. Fibroadenoma:
   a. Prevalence: Most frequent solid benign tumor of breast; painless, well circumscribed, round, rubbery, freely mobile lesion; common in young women
   b. Treatment: Biopsy

3. Intraductal papilloma:
   a. Bloody, unilateral nipple discharge with a soft mass
   b. Treatment: Surgical removal

4. Carcinoma of the breast:
   a. Most common symptom: Painless lump diagnosed by the patient herself
   b. Treatment: Lumpectomy with radiation for stage I or stage II or modified radical mastectomy; adjuvant combination chemotherapy or tamoxifen for both premenopausal and postmenopausal patients (see Questions 10 to 16)
   c. Screening: Mammography every 1 to 2 years for women age 50 to 75 years old; clinical breast examination every year for all women.

All women between the ages of 50 and 75 years old should have a screening mammogram performed every 1 to 2 years (depending on risk factor status).

There is controversy regarding the recommendations for screening mammography beginning at age 40. Some evidence suggests that women in the 40- to 49-year-old age group may benefit from mammography as much as, or more than, women over age 50.

SUGGESTED READINGS

Giuliano A: Breast. In Way L, ed: *Current surgical diagnosis and treatment General surgery and surgical specialties*, ed 10, Norwalk, Conn, 1994, Appleton & Lange.

Hortobagyi GN: Treatment of breast cancer, *New Engl J Med* 339(14):974-984, 1998.

PROBLEM·108

PANCREATIC CARCINOMA

A Little Organ; Big Problems

Case 1 ■ A 62-Year-Old Male with Abdominal Pain

A 62-year-old male comes to your office for a third opinion. He has seen two other physicians during the last 3 months regarding an abdominal pain that is, according to the patient, "getting worse and worse." It is unrelated in any way to food intake except that the patient has become significantly anorexic since developing the pain. The first physician told him that he had irritable bowel syndrome; the second physician told him that the pain was a psychoneurotic pain: "Basically, sir, that means it is all in your head." The patient tells you that he was very disappointed with the two physicians, especially since the first one had been his family doctor for over 15 years.

You decide to spend your time today on a very focused history. The most important information you gather is the following:

1. The patient has lost 20 pounds in 3 months.
2. The pain is constant.
3. The patient has never had abdominal pain before.
4. The patient's mood has definitely changed over this period of time. In fact, the very first symptom was depression (even before the pain started).
5. The pain is central abdominal, radiating through to the back, dull and aching in character, and described as a 10/10 in terms of severity.

On examination, the patient looks "unwell." You cannot describe it any more clearly than that. He just looks unwell. There is no clinical evidence of anemia, jaundice, or cyanosis. Examination of the abdomen reveals some tenderness in the midabdominal region. The liver edge is felt 2 cm below the left costal margin.

SELECT THE BEST ANSWER TO THE FOLLOWING QUESTIONS

Q1. The differential diagnosis in this patient would include all except which of the following?
   a. inflammatory bowel disease
   b. carcinoma of the stomach
   c. carcinoma of the pancreas
   d. irritable bowel syndrome
   e. none of the above can be excluded

Q2. If you could order only one investigation at this time, which one of the following would you order?
   a. a magnetic resonance imaging (MRI) scan of the abdomen
   b. gastroscopy
   c. a computed tomography (CT) scan of the abdomen
   d. a colonoscopy
   e. serum amylase or serum lipase

Q3. Which of the following statements regarding the relationship between this patient's depressive symptoms and his abdominal symptoms is correct?

a. the abdominal symptoms are unrelated to the depression

b. the abdominal symptoms are indirectly related to the depression

c. the abdominal symptoms are directly related to the depression

d. the abdominal symptoms and the depressive symptoms usually do not coexist in this disorder

e. nobody really knows for sure

Q4. The appropriate investigation is ordered. What is the sensitivity of this investigation in the disorder described?

a. 70%

b. 80%

c. 90%

d. 95%

e. 100%

Q5. The patient had planned a vacation for the week after the investigation was performed. You persuaded him to return to your office when he gets back from his vacation in 6 weeks for further evaluation. You encourage him to take his vacation because of your suspicions regarding his disease. Before he leaves for his vacation, however, you must provide the patient with one other treatment. What is the single most important treatment to be undertaken at this time?

a. begin the patient on an antiinflammatory

b. begin the patient on an oral corticosteroid

c. begin the patient on an antidepressant

d. begin the patient on an oral chemotherapeutic agent

e. none of the above

Q6. Cancer pain is an extremely important medical problem. Which of the following statements regarding the management of cancer pain in the United States is true?

a. cancer pain is extremely well managed by most American physicians

b. the overtreatment of cancer pain is much more of a problem than the undertreatment of cancer pain in the United States

c. the undertreatment of cancer pain is much more of a problem than the overtreatment of cancer pain in the United States

d. most Americans with cancer pain die in very good control; few have cancer pain that is not well controlled

e. none of the above statements is true

Q7. The patient returns to your office in 6 weeks following an overseas tour. Because of your therapy, he was able to enjoy most of his holiday. Three days ago, his pain began to become acutely worse. The patient now appears jaundiced. He has lost another 15 pounds, and there is a palpable mass in the periumbilical region. The investigation performed earlier is repeated, and a mass measuring 6 cm × 5 cm is now seen in the appropriate region. At this time, what should you do?

a. explore with a surgeon the possibility of a Whipple's procedure

b. begin aggressive radiotherapy and chemotherapy

c. begin high-dose prednisone to increase his weight

d. explore with a surgeon the possibility of the total removal of the organ in question

e. none of the above

Q8. What is the most clearly established risk factor for the disease described?

a. alcohol consumption

b. cigarette smoking

c. high fat intake

d. environmental toxins

e. previous exposure to radiation

Q9. With respect to the molecular biology of this disease, which of the following statements is true?

a. no genetic mutations have been established for this disease

b. the CK-Ras gene mutates to become the CK-Ras oncogene in 25% of patients with this disease

c. the CK-Ras oncogene is present in 50% of patients with this disease

d. the CK-Ras oncogene is present in 75% of patients with this disease

e. the CK-Ras oncogene is present in 90% of patients with this disease

Q10. A patient with this disease will demonstrate which of the following physical findings?

a. decreased pain when assuming the supine position

b. increased pain when assuming the supine position

c. decreased pain with flexion of the spine

d. increase pain with flexion of the spine

e. b and c

f. a and d

SHORT ANSWER MANAGEMENT PROBLEM
Discuss the impact of this disease on the American population under the following headings:
- a. Disease prevalence over last 30 years (increase or decrease)
- b. Place as a killer of Americans (among all cancers)
- c. Risk factors
- d. Symptoms and signs
- e. Treatment
- f. Prognosis

ANSWERS

A1. **d.** From the history and the physical examination, you determine that the patient has a serious disease. In forming a differential diagnosis, you should consider diagnostic possibilities in the following categories:
- a. Infectious/inflammatory
- b. Neoplastic
- c. Circulatory
- d. Traumatic

From the history, the following are diagnostic possibilities:
- a. Infectious/inflammatory:
  - 1) Inflammatory bowel disease:
    - a) Crohn's disease
    - b) Ulcerative colitis
  - 2) Pancreatitis
  - 3) Cholecystitis
- b. Neoplastic:
  - 1) Carcinoma of the stomach (linitis plastica)
  - 2) Carcinoma of the head of the pancreas
  - 3) Carcinoma of the colon
- c. Circulatory
  - 1) Aortic aneurysm (leaking)
  - 2) Mesenteric ischemia
- d. Traumatic: Pancreatic pseudocyst

A2. **c.** Obviously, before you decide on which investigation to order, you have to make a commitment to your primary diagnosis. The most likely diagnosis is adenocarcinoma of the pancreas. The reasons are as follows:
- a. The abdominal pain is constant and unrelated to food.
- b. The patient has experienced a 20-pound weight loss.
- c. The patient has a depression.

Therefore the investigation of choice is a CT scan of the abdomen.

A3. **c.** There is a significant correlation between carcinoma of the pancreas and depression. In many cases, as in this case, the depression actually precedes the abdominal pain.

A4. **d.** The sensitivity of the CT scan in the diagnosis of adenocarcinoma of the pancreas is 95% That is, only one out of every 20 patients with adenocarcinoma will have a falsely negative CT scan.

A5. **e.** Although it is reasonable to start the patient on an antidepressant, it is the second most important treatment. The most important treatment is to start the patient on an adequate pain relief program. It would seem that, because of the severity of the pain, an oral narcotic analgesic would be the drug of first choice. You suggest that while he is on vacation he telephone on a regular basis so you can advise medication changes.

A6. **c.** Cancer pain is an enormous medical problem in the United States and Canada. It is likely to become even more of a problem in the future because the population is aging. It is estimated that close to 50% of patients in North America with cancer die in moderately severe to severe pain. The reason appears to be multifactorial and related to inadequate education in medical school, in residency, and in continuing medical education; reluctance to use narcotic analgesics when they need to be used; and fear of licensure difficulties if "too many narcotics" are prescribed.

A7. **e.** You should do the following:
- a. Break the news to the patient with his spouse or significant other present, if possible.
- b. Discuss with the patient his treatment options, including palliative radiotherapy, palliative chemotherapy, and palliative radiotherapy and chemotherapy.
- c. Suggest an aggressive pain control program. You could consider the following:
  - 1) a celiac plexus block
  - 2) changing narcotic analgesics
  - 3) continuing to increase his dosage of narcotics.
- d. In terms of symptoms, you should:
  - 1) maintain control of nausea or vomiting
  - 2) maintain control of constipation
  - 3) consider an appetite stimulant (Megace)

A8. **b.** The most likely established risk factor for adenocarcinoma of the pancreas is cigarette smoking. There is some controversy regarding alcohol intake, but most authorities consider it a significant risk factor as well.

A9. **e.** There is insufficient evidence to suggest a particular genetic predisposition for adenocarcinoma of the pancreas. However, over 90% of patients who develop adenocarcinoma of the pancreas have a mutation of the Ki-ras gene on codon 12. This is simply an example of the powerful influence of genetics on cancer and the explosion of new knowledge that will eventually result in more effective, more precise, and more targeted treatments for most or all cancers in the future.

A10. **e.** One of the most important tests in the physical examination of a patient suspected of having a malignancy is known as a provocative maneuver. A provocative maneuver attempts to reproduce the pain (gently). An example of a provocative maneuver for somatic pain caused by bony metastatic disease is to put pressure on the bone in question. The provocative maneuver for a patient with a tumor that is retroperitoneal is to have the patient lie flat or lie with a pillow or other object underneath the small of his or her back. This will reproduce the pain. The same patient will obtain relief from their pain when leaning forward.

SOLUTION TO THE SHORT ANSWER MANAGEMENT PROBLEM

Adenocarcinoma of the pancreas:
1. Prevalence over last 30 years: The prevalence of adenocarcinoma of the pancreas among Americans has been rising rapidly. Until recently, the incidence of the disease was increasing in the United States at an annual rate of 15%. It now appears to have leveled off.
2. Mortality from adenocarcinoma: Approximately 28,000 new cases of adenocarcinoma of the pancreas occur each year. After squamous cell carcinoma of the lung and adenocarcinoma of the colon, adenocarcinoma of the pancreas is the third leading cause of death caused by cancer in men between the ages of 35 and 54 years old.
3. Risk factors for adenocarcinoma of the pancreas:
   a. Cigarette smoking (number one risk factor)
   b. High dietary consumption of fat and meat (especially fried meat)
   c. History of gastrectomy (more than 20 years ago)
   d. Alcohol intake
   e. African-American or Caucasian race
   f. Diabetes mellitus

High intake of fruits and vegetables appears to have a protective effect.
4. Symptoms and signs:
   a. Abdominal symptoms and signs:
      1) Central abdominal pain radiating through to the back; dull, aching and steady in character; most commonly described as a "deep" pain
      2) Weight loss
      3) Hepatomegaly (50% of patients)
      4) Palpable abdominal mass (indicates inoperability)
      5) A palpable gall bladder. A palpable nontender gall bladder in a jaundiced patient suggests neoplastic obstruction of the common bile duct (Courvoisier's law)
   b. Nonabdominal symptoms and signs: Depression as a result of the patient's general medical condition (DSM-IV) is often the initial symptom appearing before any of the abdominal symptoms or painless jaundice.
5. Treatments:
   a. Surgical: Carcinoma of the pancreas is resectable in only 20% of patients (Whipple's procedure).
   b. Chemotherapy/radiotherapy: Palliative chemotherapy or radiotherapy can be offered.
   c. Pain control: Pain control appears to be the single most important part of therapy.
      1) Celiac plexus block
      2) Narcotic analgesics
   d. Symptom control
      1) Nausea and vomiting: Control with combination antiemetics
      2) Constipation: Control with lactulose or stool softener and a peristaltic stimulant
6. Prognosis: The prognosis for adenocarcinoma of the pancreas is dismal. A 5-year survival rate is approximately 5%.

SUMMARY OF THE DIAGNOSIS AND TREATMENT OF PANCREATIC CARCINOMA

See the Solution to the Short Answer Management Problem.

SUGGESTED READINGS
Hoffman JP et al: Management of exocrine carcinoma of the pancreas, *Cancer Treat Res* 98:65-82, 1998.

Madura JA et al: Adenosquamous carcinoma of the pancreas, *Arch Surg* 134(6):599-603, 1999.

Reber HA, Way L: Pancreas. In Way L, ed: *Current surgical diagnosis and treatment: General surgery and surgical specialties*, ed 10, Norwalk, Conn, 1994, Appleton & Lange.

PROBLEM·109

DIAGNOSIS AND TREATMENT OF OPHTHALMOLOGIC PROBLEMS

"Doc, I Can Hardly See."

Case 1 ■ A 32-Year-Old Female with Bilateral Red Eyes, a Sore Throat, and a Cough

A 32-year-old female comes to your office with a 1-week history of bilateral red eyes associated with tearing and crusting, a sore throat with difficulty swallowing, and a cough that was initially nonproductive but has become productive over the last few days. The patient displays significant fatigue and lethargy and is having great difficulty performing any of her routine daily chores.

On physical examination, there is bilateral conjunctival infection. There is significant pharyngeal erythema but no exudate of membrane. Cervical lymphadenopathy is not present. Examination of the chest reveals a few expiratory crackles bilaterally.

SELECT THE BEST ANSWER TO THE FOLLOWING QUESTIONS

Q1. What is the most likely cause of this patient's "red eye" condition?
a. an autoimmune reaction secondary to the beginning of a severe systemic illness
b. bacterial conjunctivitis related to her other symptoms
c. bacterial conjunctivitis unrelated to her other symptoms
d. allergic conjunctivitis secondary to a severe eosinophilic pneumonia
e. none of the above

Q2. Concerning this patient's sore throat and in relation to the case scenario described and the physical findings provided, what would you do?
a. perform a throat culture and order antibiotics
b. perform a throat culture and a rapid enzyme-linked immunosorbent assay (ELISA) *Streptococcus* test and treat with an antibiotic if the ELISA test is positive
c. perform a throat culture and await the results
d. order a complete blood count and total eosinophil count
e. none of the above

Q3. What is the most likely (organism or condition) responsible for the constellation of symptoms in this patient?

a. endotoxin-producing *Staphylococcus*
b. endotoxin-producing *Streptococcus*
c. exotoxin-producing *Staphylococcus*
d. activation of the autoimmune system
e. none of the above

Case 2 ■ A 17-Year-Old Female With a 1-Day History of Red Eye

A 17-year-old female comes to your office with a 1-day history of red eye. She describes a sensation of not being able to open her right eye in the morning because of the discharge. The right eye feels uncomfortable, although there is no pain.

On examination, she has a significant infection of the right conjunctiva. There is a mucopurulent discharge present. No other abnormalities are present on physical examination.

Q4. What is the most likely diagnosis in this patient?
a. bacterial conjunctivitis
b. viral conjunctivitis
c. allergic conjunctivitis
d. autoimmune conjunctivitis
e. none of the above

Q5. Which of the following agents is (are) a common cause(s) of bacterial conjunctivitis?
a. *Haemophilus influenzae*
b. *Staphylococcus aureus*
c. *Streptococcus pneumoniae*
d. a and b
e. a, b, and c

Case 3 ■ A 29-Year-Old Male with Bilateral Red Eyes

A 29-year-old male comes to your office with bilateral red eyes. This symptom came on quite suddenly 2 hours ago while visiting a friend's home. He describes itching and a clear discharge from both eyes. The patient mentions one previous episode that also began while visiting the same friend.

On examination, the conjunctiva are diffusely injected and edematous. On eversion of the eyelids, there are large papillae present.

Q6. What is the most likely diagnosis in this patient?
a. chemical conjunctivitis
b. toxic conjunctivitis
c. allergic conjunctivitis
d. bacterial conjunctivitis
e. none of the above

Case 4 ■ A 29-Year-Old Female with a Tender, Painful, and Sore Red Eye

A 29-year-old female comes to your office for assessment of a red eye. She describes a tender, painful, and sore right eye that began yesterday. She has had no other symptoms.

On examination, the patient has a localized area of inflammation and infection in the area of the right conjunctiva. The inflammation appears to lie beneath the conjunctival surface.

Q7. What is the most likely diagnosis in this patient?
 a. localized bacterial conjunctivitis
 b. acute iritis
 c. acute angle closure glaucoma
 d. acute episcleritis
 e. none of the above

Case 5 ■ A 35-Year-Old Female with an Acutely Inflamed and Painful Eye

A 35-year-old female comes to your office with an acutely inflamed and painful left eye. Her symptoms began 2 days ago. There is some visual blurring associated with the symptoms. The patient wears contact lenses.

On examination, there is a diffuse inflammation of the left conjunctiva. On fluorescein staining, there is a dendritic ulcer seen in the center of the cornea.

Q8. What is the most likely diagnosis in this patient?
 a. corneal abrasion
 b. herpetic corneal ulcer
 c. contact lens stress ulcer
 d. adenoviral ulcer
 e. foreign body complicated by a viral ulcer

Case 6 ■ A 36-Year-Old Male with Ankylosing Spondylitis and a Painful Red Eye

A 36-year-old male with ankylosing spondylitis comes to your office for assessment of a painful, red left eye. The pain is associated with photophobia.

On examination, the redness is more pronounced around the area of the cornea. His visual acuity in the left eye has decreased to 20/60.

Q9. What is the most likely diagnosis in this patient?
 a. bacterial conjunctivitis
 b. viral conjunctivitis
 c. acute iridocyclitis
 d. acute episcleritis
 e. acute angle closure glaucoma

Case 7 ■ A 61-Year-Old Male with an Extremely Painful Eye

A 61-year-old male comes to your office with a 12-hour history of an extremely painful and red left eye. The patient complains that his vision is blurred and he is seeing halos around lights. He states that he has had similar but milder attacks in the past.

On examination, the eye is tender and inflamed. The cornea is hazy and the pupil is semi-dilated and fixed. On palpation, the left eye is significantly harder than the right.

Q10. What is the most likely diagnosis in this patient?
 a. bacterial conjunctivitis
 b. viral conjunctivitis
 c. acute iridocyclitis
 d. acute episcleritis
 e. acute angle closure glaucoma

Case 8 ■ A 23-Year-Old Female with a Painful Eye and Blurred Vision

A 23-year-old female comes to your office with a painful left eye, conjunctival infection, and blurred vision. The conjunctival infection is primarily circumcorneal.

Q11. What is the most likely diagnosis in this patient?
 a. acute conjunctivitis
 b. acute iritis
 c. acute episcleritis
 d. acute angle closure glaucoma
 e. acute corneal abrasion

Q12. In the patient described in Case 8, what will the size of the left pupil be, relative to that of the right pupil?
 a. larger than the right pupil
 b. smaller than the right pupil
 c. the same size as the right pupil
 d. indeterminate
 e. nobody really knows for sure

SHORT ANSWER MANAGEMENT PROBLEM
Part A: Summarize the major causes of a red eye and how they can be distinguished from one another.
Part B: Summarize the treatment of each of the conditions you described in Part A

ANSWERS

A1. **e.**

A2. **e.**

A3. **e.** This picture is completely consistent with adenovirus infection and a primary viral conjunctivitis. Viral agents, especially adenovirus, produce signs and symptoms of upper respiratory tract infection, with the presence of the red eye being prominent among those symptoms.

With adenovirus there is often associated conjunctival hyperemia, eyelid edema, and a serous or seropurulent discharge. Viral conjunctivitis is self-limiting, lasting 1 to 3 weeks. If the conjunctivitis is definitely caused by a virus, no antibiotic treatment is necessary.

There is no indication for performing a throat culture or any other test at this time. The only theoretical concern are the "rales" that present in both lung bases; you could argue that if the patient is sick enough, a chest x-ray may be indicated.

A4. **a.** This patient has a primary bacterial conjunctivitis. Unlike in viral conjunctivitis, bacterial conjunctivitis will produce a mucopurulent discharge from the beginning. Symptoms are more often unilateral and associated eye discomfort is common.

In bacterial conjunctivitis, normal visual acuity is always maintained. There is usually uniform engorgement of all the conjunctival blood vessels. There is no staining of the cornea with fluorescein.

Bacterial conjunctivitis should be treated with antibiotic drops such as sodium sulfacetamide or Garamycin.

A5. **e.** The most common organisms responsible for bacterial conjunctivitis are *Staphylococcus*, *Streptococcus*, and *Haemophilus*. *Pseudomonas* and *Moraxella* are other common bacterial isolates.

A6. **c.** The most likely diagnosis in this patient is allergic conjunctivitis. The most common complaint with allergic conjunctivitis is itchy, red eyes. Both eyes are affected, and there is usually a clear discharge.

Examination reveals diffusely infected conjunctiva, which may be edematous (chemosis). The discharge is usually clear and stringy.

Treatment can include: avoidance of allergens, immunotherapy, oral antihistamine, topical antihistamine, topical nonsteroidal antiinflammatory drugs (NSAIDs), topical mast cell stabilizer, and topical corticosteroids (use with caution).

The culprit, in this case, is most likely something in his friend's home.

A7. **d.** This patient has episcleritis, which differs from conjunctivitis in that it usually presents as a localized area of inflammation. Although episcleritis may occur secondary to autoimmune disease such as rheumatoid arthritis, most cases of episcleritis are idiopathic. Episcleritis is almost always self-limiting; scleritis, on the other hand, may lead to serious complications such as loss of visual acuity and perforation of the globe.

Patients with episcleritis usually have a sore, red, and tender eye. Although there may be reflex lacrimation, there is usually no discharge. Scleritis is much more painful than episcleritis, and the signs of inflammation are usually more prominent.

In episcleritis there is episcleral infection, which can be nodular, sectoral, or diffuse. There is no palpebral conjunctival infection or discharge like that seen in conjunctivitis.

The symptoms of episcleritis usually resolve spontaneously in 1 to 2 weeks. Chilled artificial tears can be given until the redness resolves. Cases associated with systemic disease are treated appropriately.

A8. **b.** This patient has a dendritic ulcer, which is almost always caused by a herpetic infection, although other viral agents, bacterial agents, or fungal agents may also be responsible. These infections may be primary or secondary to excessive contact lens wear, a corneal abrasion, or the use of corticosteroid eye drops.

The patient with a herpetic dendritic ulcer usually has an acutely painful eye associated with conjunctival infection, discharge, and visual blurring. Visual acuity, however, depends on the location and the size of the corneal ulcer. The discharge may be watery (reflex lacrimation) or purulent (bacterial). Conjunctival infection may be generalized or localized depending on the location of the ulcer.

Treatment consists of specific antiinfective therapy (vidarabine or trifluridine for herpes simplex ulcers and topical antibiotics for ulcers suspected of being primarily or secondarily infected by bacteria) and cycloplegic drops to relieve pain caused by ciliary muscle spasm. Topical corticosteroids are absolutely contraindicated in patients with a dendritic herpetic ulcer.

In a patient with a dendritic ulcer, referral to an ophthalmologist is recommended.

A9. **c.** This patient has an acute iridocyclitis or anterior uveitis. Patients at risk for anterior uveitis are those patients with a history of a seronegative arthropathy—particularly if they are positive for HLA-B27. Children with seronegative arthritis are also at high risk.

Symptoms of acute iridocyclitis include a painful red eye, often associated with photophobia, and decreased visual acuity.

On examination, the affected eye is red; the inflammation is particularly prominent over the area of the inflamed ciliary body (circumcorneal). The pupil is small because of spasm of the sphincter or irregular because of adhesions of the iris to the lens (posterior synechiae). Inflammatory cells may be seen on the back of the cornea (keratitic precipitates) or may settle to form a collection of cells in the anterior chamber of the eye (hypopyon).

Treatment of anterior uveitis should include topical corticosteroids to reduce the inflammation and prevent adhesions within the eye. Mydriatics should be used to paralyze the ciliary body to relieve pain.

As with episcleritis and dendritic ulcers, a patient with iridocyclitis should be referred to an ophthalmologist.

A10. **e.** This patient has acute angle closure glaucoma. Acute glaucoma should always be suspected in a patient who, over the age of 50 years old, has a painful red eye.

Acute glaucoma usually comes on rapidly. The most common symptom is severe pain in one eye, which may or may not be accompanied by other symptoms such as nausea and vomiting. The patient complains of impaired vision and halos around lights. This is caused by edema of the cornea.

On examination, the eye is tender and inflamed. The cornea is hazy and the pupil is partially dilated and fixed. Vision is impaired because of edema of the cornea. On palpation, the involved eye often feels significantly harder than the uninvolved eye.

Initial emergent treatment to reduce intraocular pressure includes topical beta-blockers, intravenous and oral carbonic anhydrase inhibitors (such as acetazolamide), and hyperosmotic agents. Once intraocular pressure is under control a peripheral laser iridectomy is performed.

The other eye should be treated prophylactically with a laser iridotomy.

A11. **b.** This patient has an acute iritis.

A12. **b.** Acute iritis is characterized by incidence, common; eye discharge, none; visual acuity, slightly blurred; pain, moderate; conjunctival injection, mainly circumcorneal; cornea, usually clear; pupil size, smaller than unaffected eye; pupillary light response, poor; intraocular pressure, normal; and Gram's stain and smear, no organisms.

The treatment of acute iritis is a mydriatic to relieve ciliary spasm and a corticosteroid to decrease inflammation. Again, this patient should be referred to an ophthalmologist.

SOLUTION TO THE SHORT ANSWER MANAGEMENT PROBLEM

There are four major conditions that should be considered when a patient comes to the physician's office with a red eye: acute conjunctivitis, acute iritis, acute glaucoma, and corneal trauma or infection. Their differentiation and treatment are as follows:

a. Incidence:
1) Acute conjunctivitis: Extremely common
2) Acute iritis: Common
3) Acute glaucoma: Uncommon
4) Corneal trauma or infection: Common

b. Discharge:
1) Acute conjunctivitis: Moderate to copious
2) Acute iritis: None
3) Acute glaucoma: None
4) Corneal trauma or infection: Watery or purulent

c. Vision:
1) Acute conjunctivitis: No effect on vision
2) Acute iritis: Slightly blurred
3) Acute glaucoma: Markedly blurred
4) Corneal trauma or infection: Usually blurred

d. Pain:
1) Acute conjunctivitis: None
2) Acute iritis: Moderate
3) Acute glaucoma: Severe
4) Corneal trauma or infection: Moderate to severe

e. Conjunctival infection:
1) Acute conjunctivitis: Diffuse, more toward fornices
2) Acute iritis: Mainly circumcorneal
3) Acute glaucoma: Diffuse
4) Corneal trauma or infection: Diffuse

f. Cornea:
1) Acute conjunctivitis: Clear
2) Acute iritis: Usually clear
3) Acute glaucoma: Steamy
4) Corneal trauma or infection: Change in clarity related to cause

g. Pupil size:
1) Acute conjunctivitis: Normal
2) Acute iritis: Small
3) Acute glaucoma: Moderately dilated and fixed
4) Corneal trauma or infection: Normal

h. Pupillary light response:
1) Acute conjunctivitis: Normal
2) Acute iritis: Poor
3) Acute glaucoma: None
4) Corneal trauma or infection: Normal

i. Intraocular pressure:
1) Acute conjunctivitis: Normal
2) Acute iritis: Normal
3) Acute glaucoma: Elevated
4) Corneal trauma or infection: Normal

j. Smear:
1) Acute conjunctivitis: Causative organisms
2) Acute iritis: No organisms
3) Acute glaucoma: No organisms

4) Corneal trauma or infection: Organisms found only in corneal ulcers caused by infection

SUMMARY OF DIAGNOSIS AND TREATMENT OF RED EYE

1. Infectious conjunctivitis:
   a. Etiologic agents:
      1) Adenovirus is the most common cause of conjunctivitis.
      2) Bacterial conjunctivitis: Most commonly caused by *Staphylococcus aureus*, *Streptococcus pneumoniae*, and *Haemophilus influenzae*
   b. Symptoms:
      1) Discharge: Watery discharge with viral infection; mucopurulent discharge with bacterial infection
      2) Other symptoms as described in the Short Answer Management Problem
   c. Treatment: Sulfacetamide or gentamicin drops

2. Allergic conjunctivitis:
   a. Symptoms: Itching and clear discharge are the main symptoms; conjunctiva are diffusely injected and may be associated with swelling (chemosis).
   b. Treatment: Avoidance of allergens, immunotherapy, topical antihistamines, topical NSAIDs, topical mast cell stabilizers, oral antihistamines, topical corticosteroids (use with caution).

3. Corneal ulcers:
   a. May be bacterial, viral, or fungal in origin or may also be secondary to a corneal abrasion, contact lens wear, etc.
   b. Visual acuity depends on the location and size of the ulcer. Conjunctival infection may be generalized or localized. Fluorescein must be used to stain the cornea.
   c. Treatment: Cycloplegic eye drops are used to relieve ciliary muscle spasm. Trifluridine or Vidarabine is used for dendritic (herpetic) ulcer; antibiotic drops are used for suspected bacterial infection. Corticosteroid eye drops are absolutely contraindicated in herpetic ulcers.

4. Iridocyclitis (anterior uveitis):
   a. Iridocyclitis is often associated with seronegative arthropathy.
   b. Inflammation of the iris (iritis) and inflammation of the ciliary body (cyclitis) occur together.
   c. The inflammation of anterior uveitis is circumcorneal in location, and the pupil is usually small because of associated spasm.

d. Treatment: Mydriatics are used to relieve ciliary spasm; corticosteroid drops are used to decrease inflammation.

5. Acute angle closure glaucoma:
   a. Acute, unilateral, painful red eye in a patient over the age of 50 years
   b. The attack usually comes on quickly, characteristically in the evening.
   c. Impaired vision caused by corneal edema and halos around lights are common.
   d. Palpation reveals a hard eye.
   e. Emergent treatment: Topical beta-blocker, intravenous and oral carbonic anhydrase inhibitors, and hyperosmotic agents. Once intraocular pressure is under control, a peripheral laser iridectomy is performed.

SUGGESTED READING
Vaughan D et al: *General ophthalmology*, Stamford, Conn, 1999, Appleton & Lange.

PROBLEM · 110

LOW BACK PAIN AND WHIPLASH INJURIES

"Do You Think I'm Hurt Bad Enough for Me to Sue?"

Case 1 ■ A 28-Year-Old Male with Chronic Low Back Pain

A 28-year-old male with chronic low back pain (LBP) comes to your office for renewal of his medication. He was injured at work 5 years ago while attempting to lift a box of heavy tools. Since that time, he has been off work and has not been able to find a job that does not aggravate his back.

On physical examination, the patient demonstrates some vague tenderness in the paravertebral area around L3 to L5. He has some limitations on both flexion and extension.

SELECT THE BEST ANSWER TO THE FOLLOWING QUESTIONS

Q1. Which of the following statements regarding the epidemiology of acute LBP is (are) true?
   a. the annual incidence of acute LBP is 5%
   b. approximately 2% of all workers injure their backs each year
   c. the lifetime prevalence of LBP is 80% to 85%
   d. all of the above are true
   e. none of the above is true

Q2. Which of the following statements regarding chronic LBP is (are) true?
 a. chronic LBP is the most common cause of disability among people younger than 45 years
 b. back injuries account for the majority of claims to compensation boards
 c. in terms of expense to society, LBP peaks at approximately 40 years of age
 d. all of the above statements are true
 e. none of the above statements is true

Q3. Regarding the pathogenesis of chronic LBP, which of the following statements is (are) true?
 a. in up to 85% of cases of chronic LBP, a definite anatomic or pathophysiologic diagnosis cannot be made
 b. approximately 10% of patients with acute LBP will eventually require surgery
 c. patients with acute LBP and no previous surgical procedures have a 20% to 25% chance of recovering after 6 weeks regardless of the treatment employed
 d. the anatomic structures causing LBP are clearly identified
 e. none of the above statements is true

Q4. Regarding the pathogenesis of chronic LBP, which of the following statements is (are) true?
 a. researchers continue to debate whether the pain originates from the spine or from soft tissues
 b. no diagnostic test can definitely distinguish among pain generated from discs, facet joints, or supporting muscles and ligaments
 c. ordinary radiographs, computed tomography (CT) scans, and magnetic resonance imaging (MRI) scans of the lumbar spine have low specificity
 d. all of the above statements are true
 e. none of the above statements is true

Q5. Which of the following is the most common cause of LBP?
 a. metastatic bone disease
 b. inflammatory back pain
 c. lumbosacral sprain or strain
 d. posterior facet strain
 e. none of the above

Q6. Which of the following is not indicative of inflammatory back pain?
 a. insidious onset
 b. onset before the age of 40 years
 c. pain for more than 3 months

 d. morning stiffness
 e. aggravation of pain with activity

Q7. Which of the following statements regarding the history and physical examination of a patient with LBP is (are) true?
 a. the positive predictive value of the history in LBP is high
 b. the positive predictive value of the physical examination in LBP is high
 c. the positive predictive value of the radiographic investigations for patients with LBP is high
 d. the positive predictive value of serum blood and chemistry for LBP is high
 e. none of the above statements is true

Q8. Which of the following is (are) characteristic of a history of mechanical LBP?
 a. relatively acute onset
 b. a history of overuse or a precipitating injury
 c. pain worse during the day
 d. a and b only
 e. all of the above

Q9. Which of the following is a danger signal relative to the diagnosis of LBP?
 a. bowel or bladder dysfunction
 b. impotence
 c. weight loss
 d. significant pain at night
 e. all of the above

Q10. Which of the following statements regarding plain spinal x-rays of patients with LBP is false?
 a. osteophyte formation in the intervertebral space is predictive of discogenic disease
 b. there is little justification for the extensive use of radiography in LBP
 c. there is a poor relationship between most radiographic abnormalities and symptoms of LBP
 d. x-rays of the lumbar spine are associated with gonadal radiation exposure
 e. there is a low yield of findings that alter management from plain x-rays of the lumbar spine

Q11. Which of the following statements regarding the use of CT or MRI scanning in the diagnosis of disc herniations and spinal stenosis is (are) false?
 a. CT and MRI scanning have largely replaced myelography in the diagnosis of disc herniations
 b. the sensitivity of CT scanning for disc herniations is 95%

c. the specificity of CT scanning for disc herniations is 95%

d. if CT or MRI scanning is to be employed in the diagnosis of disc herniations or spinal stenosis, surgery should be a serious pretest consideration

e. all the above statements are true

Q12. What is the most cost-effective and crucial aspect of the treatment of chronic LBP?
a. patient education
b. physiotherapy
c. bed rest
d. muscle relaxants
e. nonsteroidal antiinflammatory drugs (NSAIDs)

Q13. Regarding exercise for treatment of chronic LBP (LBP), which of the following statements is (are) true?
a. exercise allows patients to participate in their treatment program
b. any exercise should follow a graduated progression
c. following the beginning of an exercise program for LBP, a temporary increase in pain may occur
d. stretching exercises are recommended in the initial exercise program; isometric strengthening exercises follow
e. all of the above statements are true

Q14. Which of the following treatment modalities has (have) been used in the treatment of chronic LBP?
a. physical therapy
b. spinal manipulation
c. epidural injections
d. psychologic counseling
e. all of the above

Q15. Which of the following drugs have been shown to has (have) the best cost/benefit ratio in the treatment of chronic LBP?
a. NSAIDs
b. muscle relaxants
c. narcotic analgesics
d. tricyclic antidepressants
e. acetaminophen

Q16. What is the most common injury cited for personal litigation in the United States?
a. work environment–related headaches
b. whiplash injury
c. chronic LBP

d. physical assault injury claims
e. chronic thoracic back strain

Q17. Whiplash injury pathophysiologically is equated to which of the following?
a. cervical sprain
b. cervical strain
c. cervical facet joint dysfunction
d. cervical flexion injury
e. cervical rotation injury

Q18. The relationship between the physiologic time predicted for a whiplash injury to heal and the actual real time required to heal should be 1:1. In whiplash injury, what is that ratio (when considering the totality of cases)?
a. 1 to 25
b. 1 to 5
c. 1 to 1
d. 5 to 1
e. 25 to 1

Q19. Which of the following has (have) been found to prolong whiplash symptoms?
a. emotional instability or psychologic pathologic condition
b. overtreatment by physicians
c. previous illnesses, especially psychophysiologic illness
d. litigation
e. all of the above

Q20. Which of the following statements about whiplash symptomatology is (are) true?
a. whiplash injury is an artificial disease
b. we have allowed the notion that whiplash is a debilitating condition to become part of our unchallenged belief system
c. by believing that whiplash is a debilitating condition, we frequently manage to make it so
d. none of the above statements is true
e. all the above statements are true

SHORT ANSWER MANAGEMENT PROBLEM
Compensation benefits have been alleged to prolong disability from LBP. Describe reasons that may be responsible for this phenomenon.

ANSWERS

A1. **d.** The annual incidence of acute LBP is 5%. Approximately 2% of all workers injure their backs each year. The lifetime prevalence of LBP is 80% to 85%. Back pain is considered to be one of the most expensive ailments occurring in advanced industrial societies. Costs are estimated to be at least $16 billion each year in the United States alone. About 80% of these costs are incurred by those 7% to 10% of patients who go on to develop chronic LBP.

A2. **d.** There is increasing concern (and frustration) expressed about the epidemic of LBP disability in Western industrialized countries, where approximately 1% of the population is considered totally disabled as a result of back problems. Back injuries account for the vast majority of Worker's Compensation Board claims and the highest dollar amount paid out to injured workers. Chronic LBP is the most common cause of disability among people younger than 45 years old and the third most common cause of disability among people 45 to 64 years old. In terms of its expense to society, it peaks at about 40 years of age.

A3. **a.** For up to 85% of cases of LBP a definite anatomic or pathophysiologic diagnosis cannot be made. Only 1% of patients with acute LBP will eventually require surgery. Patients with acute LBP and no previous surgical procedure have an 80% to 90% chance of recovering after 6 weeks no matter what treatment is prescribed.

A4. **d.** The anatomic structures causing LBP are not clearly identified. Researchers continue to debate whether the pain originates from the spine (facet joints and discs) or soft tissues (supporting muscles and ligaments). The well-entrenched axiom that pain on flexion originates in the disc and pain on extension in the facet joints is difficult to prove and does not necessarily hold true. In many of these cases, several spinal conditions may coexist.

No diagnostic test can definitively distinguish among pain generated from discs, facet joints, or supporting muscles and ligaments. Physicians should focus on injured musculoligamentous structures as common causes of chronic LBP. Despite improved radiographic diagnostic techniques, there are still significant limitations correlating clinical symptoms with radiologic interpretations. Radiographs, CT scans, and MRIs suffer from poor specificity (many false positives).

Often the debate over musculoligamentous or spinal LBP is resolved with the diagnosis of "mechanical LBP." This does not suggest a pathologic source but does indicate that back pain is aggravated by the effects of activity or sustained postures on already injured but unidentified structures.

A5. **c.** The most common diagnosis in LBP is lumbosacral sprain or strain, or, (as discussed in Answer 4) me-

chanical LBP. Although some experts would argue that these terms are unacceptable diagnostic realities, they do reflect current diagnostic realities. Injury is thought to result from abnormal stress on normal tissues or normal stress on damaged or degenerated tissues.

A6. **e.** Inflammatory back pain (ankylosing spondylitis) is an important subset of chronic LBP, although it accounts for very few cases of acute or chronic LBP. Diagnostic clues to inflammatory LBP include the following:

1. Insidious onset of back pain
2. Onset before the age of 40 years
3. Pain 3 months in duration
4. Morning stiffness (longer than 30 minutes)
5. Pain relief with activity
6. Pain forcing patient from bed
7. History of psoriasis, Reiter's disease, colitis, or ankylosing spondylitis
8. Limitation of lumbar spine in sagittal and frontal planes
9. Chest inspiratory expansion less than 2 cm
10. Evidence of sacroiliitis during physical examination
11. Evidence of peripheral inflammatory joint disease

A7. **e.** One of the problems with the diagnosis, physical examination, laboratory investigation, and radiographic investigation of chronic LBP is that the sensitivity, specificity, and positive predictive value of the assessments, procedures, and other diagnostic modalities produce false positives and many false negatives. From that follows that the patient ends up with misinformation that may actually "create" disease (anxiety, worry, and increased pain) where none existed before.

A8. **e.** The history of mechanical back pain is typically one of relatively acute onset of pain, often with known precipitating injury or history of overuse. The pain is worse during the day, is relieved by rest (although the pain may worsen with prolonged rest), and is made worse with activity.

In contrast, the history of inflammatory back pain classically presents with an insidious onset of pain and stiffness that is worse at rest and improved with activity and often worse at night and in the morning. Many patients need to get up at night to find a comfortable position to partially relieve the pain and stiffness.

A9. **e.** Danger signals in patients with acute or chronic LBP include the following:
a. Bowel or bladder dysfunction
b. Impotence
c. Ankle clonus

d. Color change in extremities
e. Considerable night pain
f. Constant and progressive symptoms
g. Fever and chills
h. Weight loss
i. Lymphadenopathy
j. Distended abdominal veins
k. Buttock claudication
l. New onset LBP in children and adolescents and individuals over age 50

A10. **a.** Plain x-rays of the lumbar spine are frequently ordered for LBP. More than 3 million lumbar spine films are ordered annually in the United States. There is, however, little justification for such extensive use of radiography. A much more cost-effective and selective approach should be undertaken.

Apart from the cost factor, routine radiographs of the lumbar spine have three important drawbacks: a very low yield of findings that alter management in any way, a poor relationship between most radiographic abnormalities and signs and symptoms of LBP, and gonadal irradiation. Abnormalities seen on x-ray, particularly changes such as degenerative osteoarthritis, spondylolysis, and congenital abnormalities seen on the radiographs of the lumbosacral spine are often as common in asymptomatic individuals as they are in symptomatic individuals. As well, many patients who have chronic LBP have normal x-ray examination results. There is no direct correlation between intervertebral osteophyte formation and discogenic disease. Most importantly, radiographs rarely alter treatment plans.

Specific indications for radiographic studies include the following:
a. Ruling out an infectious or malignant process
b. Assessing a patient with objective evidence of neurologic abnormalities in the lower extremities, with loss of bowel or bladder control or loss of sexual function unexplained by another cause
c. Identifying a compression fracture
d. Chronic sacroiliitis

A11. **c.** CT and MRI scanning have largely replaced myelography and are valuable for diagnosing disc herniations and spinal stenosis. If the test is to influence management, then surgery must be considered a serious option before the test is performed (that is, there should be sciatica potentially caused by intraspinal disease, such as suspected disc herniation or spinal stenosis, that is intractable to conservative management. Myelography has a sensitivity of 92% and a specificity of 64% to 87%. The sensitivity of a CT for disc herniations is 95% (only 5% are false negatives), whereas the specificity is between 68%

and 88% (12% to 32% false positives). The major potential problem with CT scanning in disc herniations and spinal stenosis is the relatively lower specificity.

A12. **a.** Patient education is the most crucial and cost effective aspect of the treatment protocol for LBP. Many patients are very worried that they have a "serious illness" that is causing their pain and are dissatisfied by what they perceive as an inadequate explanation of their symptoms.

Most patients with mild to moderate LBP do not even consult physicians, and many symptomatic patients are more interested in seeking information and reassurance (the diagnosis and prognosis) than they are in "finding a cure." It is extremely important to reassure patients that "hurt is not equal to harm" in almost all cases. Older treatment regimens recommended bed rest, but studies have shown that early activity as tolerated leads to better outcome.

A13. **e.** A cornerstone of treating LBP is physical exercise. Scientific information about the method of action exerted by physical exercise is limited, which reflects the uncertainty regarding the pathophysiology of LBP. Exercise allows patients to participate in the treatment program and as well serve to prevent contractures, deconditioning, and weakness. Contrary to popular belief, exercise programs can safely begin within hours of developing LBP or an exacerbation of chronic LBP, even with the persisting muscle spasm.

The exercise programs that have been developed tend to emphasize repeated flexion and extension exercises and abdominal and lumbar strengthening exercises.

Any exercise program that is developed and begun should follow a graduated course. Patients need to be warned about a temporary increase in pain; otherwise they will tend to stop the program when it occurs. Stretching exercises are recommended first, followed by isometric strengthening exercises. One of the most important aspects of any exercise program is regularity.

A14. **e.** Physical therapy and spinal manipulation are used in the treatment of LBP. Functional status after 6 months demonstrates no difference regardless of the type of therapy used. Patient satisfaction, however, is higher with hands-on types of therapy.

Epidural corticosteroid injections deliver corticosteroids to the level of the nerve root and alleviate any nerve root inflammation that is contributing to pain or sciatica. Epidural corticosteroids appear to be useful for cases of nerve root compression since improvement is usually noted within days. With respect to a pathologic condition of the facet joint, epidural corticosteroids appear to be no more effective than placebo. Epidural corticosteroids are most effective in relieving radicular symptoms. Usually a series of up to three injections are given.

Chronic pain and the disability that accompanies chronic pain always have a significant psychologic component. The psychologic problems certainly add to the complexity of a problem that even under optimal circumstances often proves intractable to medical intervention. At times, patients may exaggerate their symptoms as a plea for help. Individual reactions and clinical responses vary depending on coping skills, the environment, and the culture. In many cases, patients feel absolutely overwhelmed, and they react with anxiety, depression, and desperation. This often results in maladaptive coping mechanisms and strategies. For these reasons supportive psychotherapy and cognitive psychotherapy may have prominent roles to play in the treatment of chronic LBP.

A15. **d.** Pharmacologic treatment is certainly of some value in treating LBP, both acute and chronic. NSAIDs appear to have some value, but the benefit must be weighed against the side effects, particularly gastric side effects and detrimental effects on hepatic and renal function.

Antidepressant medications, particularly desipramine, nortriptyline, and amitriptyline, often given in subtherapeutic doses are the most commonly used drugs for chronic pain and appear to have the highest benefit/cost ratio. They have both analgesic and antidepressant effects and may also improve sleep.

Muscle relaxants have shown little efficacy in the treatment of chronic LBP. Narcotic analgesics should be used with extreme caution and monitored constantly. For chronic pain, it is best to avoid them completely.

A16. **b.** Currently, alleged "whiplash" injury is by far the most common grounds for personal injury litigation in the United States. More than 1 million whiplash injuries occur each year in the United States; whiplash is the cause of much ongoing disability. In one study, 6% of whiplash patients were off work after 1 year, and in another study 9.6% were permanently disabled.

A17. **b.** Whiplash injury is physiologically equated to cervical strain, which, like strains in other parts of the body, can be painful.

A18. **b.** Most strains heal within a few days, weeks, or at most months, with the pain gradually subsiding. However, in spite of normal findings, the symptoms of whiplash frequently do not remit. In the United States and Canada a medicolegal industry has mushroomed around whiplash injury; this situation undoubtedly fosters disability.

The average actual time to heal for whiplash injuries is approximately five times the normal physiologic time to heal would be. Thus, on average, if a normal strain injury would take 3 weeks to heal, the average whiplash strain injury will take 15 weeks to heal (especially if associated with either a motor vehicle accident or a work-related accident).

A19. **e.** The delay in recovery of whiplash injury patients is multifactorial. Reasons include the following:
a. Emotional instability
b. Psychologic pathologic condition
c. Previous illnesses, especially illnesses involving chronic pain
d. Overtreatment by physicians; failure to recognize that a whiplash injury can be equated to a cervical strain and, as such, should heal within the average length of time for a strain injury
e. Medical-legal action or litigation: it has been shown in a number of studies that the injury improves when the legal claim is settled

A20. **e.** Whiplash is indeed an artificial disease and is so because we have allowed the notion that whiplash is a debilitating condition to become part of our unchallenged belief system. In believing that whiplash is disabling, we frequently manage to make it so. Unfortunately, physicians are often at fault; they have often reinforced this idea by helping their patients make this into a truly remarkable chronic disease state not linked in any way to the reality of the physiologic basis of strain injuries and strain injury healing.

SOLUTION TO THE SHORT ANSWER MANAGEMENT PROBLEM

Current compensation schemes often prolong disability from LBP for many reasons, including the following:
a. Patients must convince doctors that injuries are serious enough to deserve compensation.
b. Medical disbelief hardens patients' defensive attitudes and increases the need to prove pain and disability.
c. Compensation represents a personal vindication for patients who blame third parties (that is, employers) for the injury.
d. Patients perceive that return to work would compromise their safety.

e. Patients sometimes prolong disability to avoid a difficult or boring job or the threat of being laid off or fired.

f. Insecurity about finances results in anxiety and muscle tension that may increase pain.

g. Disability with compensation may be a patient's solution to a variety of difficult situations.

SUMMARY OF THE DIAGNOSIS AND TREATMENT OF LBP AND WHIPLASH INJURIES

1. LBP:
   a. Incidence: 5%/year. Lifetime prevalence is 80% to 85%.
   b. Importance: Back pain (especially LBP) is considered one of the most expensive ailments in advanced industrial societies. LBP in industrialized countries can be labeled an epidemic.
   c. History/physical examination: Both the history and the physical examination lack both sensitivity and specificity.
   d. Pathophysiology: LBP has been described as "an illness in search of a disease." Specific medical diagnosis and specific medical therapy are seldom possible. It is difficult to specifically identify if chronic LBP is muscular, arises from the muscles, ligaments, tendons, facet joints, discs, or some combination thereof.
   e. Investigations: Radiographs and CT and MRI scans, the most commonly used tests, are over-utilized and suffer from a lack of specificity. Plain spine x-rays in most cases are virtually useless.
   f. Nomenclature: The debate over musculoligamentous or spinal LBP is resolved with the diagnosis of "mechanical" LBP.
   g. Education of patient and prevention: Education is the most crucial and cost-effective treatment. This often alleviates the patient's worry that the pain is caused by a "serious illness."
   h. Treatment:
      1) Rest: For cases of acute nonspecific LBP, a short period of rest will decrease time lost from work by up to 40% to 50% and reduce the level of discomfort by 60%. This should not extend past 2 or 3 days.
      2) Drugs: In general, pharmacologic treatment is somewhat beneficial in LBP.
         a) Muscle relaxants are of little efficacy.
         b) NSAIDs have some value early in the course.
         c) Antidepressants are the most commonly used drugs for chronic pain, including chronic LBP.
      3) Physical treatments: Physical therapy and manipulation do not change outcome but improve patient satisfaction
      4) Exercise is an effective treatment modality and may be started early in the course of illness.
      5) Supports (including lumbar braces and corsets)
      6) Epidural corticosteroids: There is no evidence of any long-term benefit.
      7) Surgery: Surgery is the final resort. It is indicated only for intractable discogenic pain, progressive neurologic deficits, and advanced symptoms and signs of spinal stenosis unresponsive to other modalities.
   i. Psychologic sequelae, disability, and compensation: These are major problems that are often compounded, rather than helped, by the physician. Always try to determine whether or not an injury is taking longer to heal than it normally should. In other words, is there a significant difference between predicted physiologic healing time and actual healing time? If the answer is yes, do not become part of the problem. Attempt to help the patient understand the problem, and mobilize the patient in an effort to return to a normal lifestyle as soon as possible.

2. Whiplash injuries:
   a. Incidence: More than 1 million whiplash injuries occur per year in the United States.
   b. Importance: By far the most common grounds for personal injury litigation. Chronic LBP can be regarded as an epidemic in North America.
   c. Pathophysiology: Essentially, whiplash is a cervical strain.
   d. Treatment:
      1) Pharmacologic: NSAIDS, acetaminophen
      2) Physical: Exercises, physical therapy, manipulation

SUGGESTED READINGS

Borenstein DG: Epidemiology, etiology, diagnostic evaluation, and treatment of low back pain, *Curr Opin Rheumatol* 11(2):151-157, 1999.

Daniels JM: Treatment of occupationally acquired low back pain, *Am Fam Physician* 55(2):587-596, 601-602, 1997.

Nordin M, Campello M: Physical therapy: exercises and the modalities: when, what, and why? *Neurol Clin* 17(1):75-89, 1999.

Rose-Innes AP, Engstrom JW: Low back pain: an algorithmic approach to diagnosis and management, *Geriatrics* 53(10):26-28, 33-36, 39-40, 1998.

Rosomoff HL, Rosomoff RS: Low back pain: Evaluation and management in the primary care setting, *Med Clin North Am* 83(3):643-662, 1999.

Samanta A, Beardsley J: Low back pain: Which is the best way forward? *BMJ* 318(7191):1122-1123, 1999.

PROBLEM·111

RENAL STONES

Stones and Groans and, on Occasion, Bones

Case 1 ■ A 30-Year-Old Male with Flank Pain

A 30-year-old male comes to the Emergency Department with acute onset of severe right-side flank pain. The pain radiates down into the groin and testicle and is associated with hematuria, urinary frequency, urgency, and dysuria.

On examination, the patient is in acute distress. He has significant right costovertebral angle tenderness. The rest of the abdominal examination is normal. The patient is afebrile.

SELECT THE BEST ANSWER TO THE FOLLOWING QUESTIONS

Q1. What is the most likely diagnosis in this patient?
   a. renal colic
   b. acute pyelonephritis
   c. acute pyelitis
   d. atypical appendicitis
   e. none of the above

Q2. What is the most common composition of a kidney stone?
   a. calcium oxalate
   b. mixed calcium oxalate/calcium phosphate
   c. calcium phosphate
   d. struvite
   e. uric acid

Q3. Which of the following abnormalities is (are) usually associated with calcium oxalate stones?
   a. hypercalciuria
   b. hyperuricuria
   c. hypocitraturia
   d. all of the above
   e. none of the above

Q4. What is the drug of choice for the management of idiopathic hypercalciuria?
   a. cellulose sodium phosphate
   b. an orthophosphate
   c. potassium citrate
   d. hydrochlorothiazide
   e. pyridoxine

Q5. What is the most important component of the diagnostic workup in a patient with a kidney stone?
   a. serum calcium/serum uric acid
   b. serum creatinine
   c. intravenous pyelography
   d. 24-hour urine for volume, calcium, uric acid, citrate, oxalate, sodium, creatinine, and pH
   e. serum parathyroid hormone

Q6. Which of the following statements regarding uric acid stones is (are) correct?
   a. uric acid stones are formed in patients who are found to have acidic urine
   b. uric acid stones are formed in patients with increased uric acid secretion
   c. the initial treatment for patients with uric acid stones is alkalinization of the urine
   d. patients with recalcitrant uric acid stones should be treated with allopurinol
   e. all of the above statements are correct

Q7. Which of the following statements regarding the treatment of nephrolithiasis is (are) true?
   a. extracorporeal shock wave lithotripsy (ESWL) has become widely used for the treatment of renal stones
   b. ureteral stones, unless large, are best managed by awaiting their spontaneous passage
   c. ESWL has shown its greatest benefit in patients with stones less than 2 cm in diameter
   d. all of the above statements are true
   e. none of the above statements is true

Q8. Which of the following is (are) part of the differential diagnosis of renal colic?
   a. acute pyelonephritis
   b. renal adenocarcinoma
   c. papillary necrosis
   d. all of the above
   e. none of the above

Q9. What is the treatment of choice for metabolic stone formation?
   a. hydrochlorothiazide
   b. sodium potassium citrate
   c. pyridoxine
   d. an organophosphate
   e. none of the above

Q10. Magnesium-ammonium phosphate stones are usually secondary to urinary tract infection with which of the following?
   a. *Escherichia coli*
   b. *Proteus* species
   c. *Klebsiella*
   d. Enterococcus
   e. Enterobacter

SHORT ANSWER MANAGEMENT PROBLEM

A 45-year-old male comes to the Emergency Department with left-sided flank pain. An x-ray of the kidneys, ureter, and bladder (KUB) suggests a ureteric stone. While straining his urine, the patient discovers a stone. The pain subsides. The stone is analyzed and found to be a calcium oxalate stone.

Describe the general treatment measures that you would use to prevent further stone formation in this patient.

ANSWERS

A1. **a.** This patient has renal colic. Renal colic is characterized by the sudden onset of severe flank pain radiating toward the groin. It is usually associated with hematuria, urinary frequency, urgency, and dysuria and is relieved immediately following the passage of the stone. Acute pyelonephritis, which may be associated with similar symptoms, is usually accompanied by fever and chills.

The sudden onset of severe flank pain is not typical of appendiceal disease.

A2. **a.** Calcium oxalate stones are the most common type of renal stones; they constitute 60% of all stones. They are most commonly idiopathic. Other stones in order of frequency of occurrence are uric acid, mixed calcium oxalate/calcium phosphate, struvite, and cystine stones.

A3. **d.** Calcium oxalate stones may be associated with hypercalciuria, hyperuricosuria, and hypocitraturia. Hypercalciuria is most common.

A4. **d.** A thiazide diuretic, such as hydrochlorothiazide, is the agent of choice for the treatment of idiopathic hypercalciuria. Thiazide diuretics work by lowering urine calcium excretion. Other measures include increasing total daily fluid intake and decreasing total daily calcium intake.

A5. **d.** The basic laboratory evaluation of a patient with renal colic includes urinalysis; urine culture; and blood chemistry profile including serum calcium, phosphorus, uric acid, electrolytes, and creatinine; x-ray examination of the KUB; and intravenous pyelogram. The most sensitive test, however, for the diagnosis of metabolic abnormalities associated with nephrolithiasis is the 24-hour urine collection. The 24-hour specimen should be analyzed for calcium, uric acid, citrate, oxalate, sodium, creatinine, and urine pH.

When stone composition is unknown, urine should also be obtained for qualitative cystine screening. Se-

rum parathyroid hormone assay should be performed when hypercalcemia is present.

A6. **e.** Uric acid stones, the second most common type of renal stone, are formed in patients with persistent acidic urine or a high uric acid secretion (exceeding 1000 mg/day). The initial treatment of a patient with a uric acid stone involves alkalinization of the urine with either sodium bicarbonate or citrate. Patients with uric acid stones should be treated with allopurinol. A decreased purine intake (that is decreased consumption of red meat and, in particular, animal organs such as liver, sweetbreads, and kidney) is also recommended.

A7. **d.** ESWL is widely used in the treatment of nephrolithiasis to break up renal stones with shock waves, permitting them to pass spontaneously.

Lithotripsy is most effective when the stone is less than 2 cm in diameter. For patients with stones larger than 2 cm, a combination of ESWL and percutaneous lithotripsy produces superior results. Initial percutaneous nephrolithotomy followed by ESWL and a "second look" percutaneous nephrolithotomy gives the best results.

Patients with staghorn calculi, obstruction, or complex anatomy should be treated with open surgery.

Ureteral stones are best managed by awaiting spontaneous passage. If spontaneous passage is unlikely or delayed, ESWL is the first choice for stones in the upper two thirds of the ureter; endoscopic surgery is the best alternative for lower ureteral stones.

A ureteropelvic or other obstruction, as well as stones deposited in diverticula, should be managed by endourologic techniques.

A8. **d.** The major differential diagnosis of renal colic includes infection of the upper urinary tract (acute pyelonephritis or acute pyelitis), renal adenocarcinoma, and papillary necrosis. Papillary necrosis (ischemic necrosis of the renal papillae or of the entire renal pyramid) is usually secondary to excessive ingestion of analgesics, sickle-cell trait (associated with hematuria), diabetes mellitus, obstruction with infection, or vesicoureteral reflux with infection.

A9. **b.** Metabolic stones, including cystine stones, are best treated by giving the patient a sodium-potassium citrate solution, 4 to 8 ml qid. In this case the urine pH should be monitored.

A10. **b.** Magnesium-ammonium-phosphate stones are usually secondary to urinary tract infection with bacteria that produce urease (primarily *Proteus* species). The urease hydrolyzes the urea producing ammonia and thereby raising the pH as well as providing the source of ammonia. Eradication of the infection prevents further stone formation. After calculi removal, prevention of stone growth is best accomplished by urinary acidification, long-term use of antibiotics, and the use of acetohydroxamic acid (a urease inhibitor that maintains an acid urinary pH).

SOLUTION TO THE SHORT ANSWER MANAGEMENT PROBLEM

The treatment of calcium oxalate stones includes the following:
- a. Maintain normal calcium intake with meals. This binds the oxalate that forms stones increasing its loss from the gastrointestinal tract.
- b. Restrict dietary sodium to 2000 mg/day (6 g of salt per day).
- c. Limit intake of proteins and carbohydrates.
- d. Use oral orthophosphates to decrease stone-forming potential.
- e. Use thiazide diuretics to decrease urine calcium content.
- f. Use allopurinol and urinary alkalinization to reduce the formation of urate crystals.

SUMMARY OF THE DIAGNOSIS AND TREATMENT OF RENAL STONES

1. Classic symptoms of renal colic: Sudden, severe, flank pain with radiation to the groin; associated with hematuria, frequency, urgency, dysuria, and relief following stone passage.

2. Types of stones:
   a. Calcium oxalate stones:
      1) Most frequent type of stone
      2) Usually idiopathic and associated with hypercalciuria, hyperuricuria, and hypocitraturia
   b. Uric acid stones:
      1) Second most frequent type of stone
      2) Associated with urine that is persistently acidic and in conjunction with massively increased urinary uric acid secretion (greater than 1000 mg/day)
      3) Prevention with alkalinization of urine with bicarbonate or citrate; may have to use allopurinol.
   c. Infective stones:
      1) Caused by urea-splitting organisms (*Proteus* species)
      2) Stone should be completely removed and antibiotic therapy prescribed

   d. Cystine stones: Occur with the inherited transport disorder cystinuria

3. Stone treatment:
   a. Ureteral stones: Await spontaneous passage. If not forthcoming, then use ESWL (upper two thirds of ureter) and endoscopic techniques (lower one third of ureter).
   b. Renal stones: ESWL is the treatment of choice for stones less than 2 cm and located in the upper pole of the kidney. If stones larger than 1 cm are located in the lower pole of the kidney, a combination of ESWL and percutaneous nephrolithotomy is preferred.

SUGGESTED READINGS

Dawson C, Whitfield H: ABC of urology: Urinary stone disease, *BMJ* 312(7040):1219-1221, 1996.

Donovan JF, Williams RD: Urology. In Way L, ed: *Current surgical diagnosis and treatment*, ed 10, Norwalk, Conn, 1994, Appleton & Lange.

Goldfarb DS et al: Renal stone disease in older adults, *Clin Geriatr Med* 14(2):367-381, 1998.

Pak CY: Kidney stones, *Lancet* 351(9118):1797-801, 1998.

Santos-Victoriano M et al: Renal stone disease in children, *Clin Pediatr* 37(10):583-599, 1998.

Sundaram CP, Saltzman B: Extracorporeal shock wave lithotripsy: a comprehensive review, *Compr Ther* 24(6-7):332-335, 1998.

Trivedi BK: Nephrolithiasis: How it happens and what to do about it, *Postgrad Med* 100(6):63-67, 71-72, 77-78, 1996.

PROBLEM·112

DISORDERS OF THE PROSTATE

"Doc, I Can Hardly Pee."

Case 1 ■ A 75-Year-Old Male with Nocturia, Hesitancy, and a Slow Flow of Urine

A 75-year-old male comes to your office with a 6-month history of nocturia, hesitancy, a slow flow of urine, and terminal dribbling. The symptoms have been progressing. Otherwise, he is well and has had no significant medical illnesses.

On examination, his abdomen is normal. He has an enlarged prostate gland, which is smooth in contour and firm and has no nodules or irregularities.

SELECT THE BEST ANSWER TO THE FOLLOWING QUESTIONS

Q1. What is the most likely diagnosis in this patient?
   a. benign prostatic hypertrophy (BPH)
   b. carcinoma of the bladder

c. prostatic carcinoma
d. urethral stricture
e. chronic prostatitis

Q2. Which of the following symptoms is (are) associated with the condition described in Case 1?
a. dysuria
b. daytime frequency
c. incomplete voiding
d. urgency
e. all of the above

Q3. Which of the following pharmacologic treatments may be indicated in the treatment of the condition described in Case 1?
a. finasteride
b. prazosin
c. terazosin
d. all of the above
e. none of the above

Q4. Before the medical or surgical treatment of the condition described in Case 1, which of the following should be performed?
a. digital rectal examination
b. transrectal ultrasound
c. computed tomography (CT) scan of the pelvis
d. a and b
e. all of the above

Q5. Which of the following surgical procedures is the treatment of choice for severe cases of the condition described in Case 1?
a. transurethral resection of the prostate (TURP)
b. open prostatectomy
c. transurethral incision of the prostate
d. hyperthermia of the prostate
e. balloon dilatation of the prostate

Case 2 ■ A 58-Year-Old Male with Hesitancy
of the Urinary Stream and Bone Pain

A 58-year-old male comes to your office with a 3-month history of gradually worsening hesitancy of urinary stream, urgency, nocturia, and terminal dribbling. He also complains of lumbar and pelvic bone pain present for the past 3 weeks.

On physical examination, the prostate is enlarged and very hard. There is some tenderness over the pelvic ischium on the left side as well as the fourth and fifth lumbar vertebrae.

Q6. Which one of the following statements regarding this patient's condition is false?

a. the most likely diagnosis is prostatic carcinoma
b. radiotherapy is the most probable first line of therapy in the management of this patient
c. this patient most likely has metastatic disease
d. the evaluation of this patient should include a bone scan
e. combination chemotherapy may be indicated for the treatment of this condition

Q7. Which of the following statements regarding carcinoma of the prostate is (are) true?
a. prostatic cancer is a major public health problem in men
b. prostatic cancer is now the most commonly diagnosed cancer in men
c. bone is the most common site of metastatic disease
d. all of the above statements are true
e. none of the above statements is true

Q8. Which of the following is (are) risk factors for the disease described in the patient in Case 2?
a. increased age
b. African-American men
c. positive family history for the disease
d. dietary fat intake
e. all of the above

Q9. Which of the following statements is true regarding screening for this disorder according to the U.S. Preventive Services Task Force?
a. there is strong evidence to recommend the inclusion of the digital rectal examination in the periodic health examination
b. there is fair evidence to recommend the inclusion of the digital rectal examination in the periodic health examination
c. there is insufficient evidence to recommend for or against the digital rectal examination in the periodic health examination
d. there is fair evidence to recommend the exclusion of the digital rectal examination from the periodic health examination
e. there is strong evidence to recommend the exclusion of the digital rectal examination from the periodic health examination

Q10. Which of the following is the treatment of choice for stage A-1 of this disease in an 81-year-old male?
a. radiation therapy
b. radical prostatectomy
c. hormone therapy

d. combination chemotherapy
e. none of the above

Q11. What is the most common symptom with which a male with prostatic cancer presents?
a. a feeling of "hardness" in the rectal area
b. obstructive voiding symptoms
c. anorexia
d. weight loss
e. bone pain

Case 3 ■ A 24-Year-Old Male with Fever, Suprapubic Discomfort, and Inhibited Urinary Voiding

A 24-year-old male comes to your office with a 2-day history of fever, chills, perineal and suprapubic discomfort, dysuria, and inhibited urinary voiding.

On physical examination, the lower abdomen is tender. A digital rectal examination reveals a swollen, boggy, and tender prostate. Examination of the urine reveals pus cells and bacterial rods. The man has no history of similar symptoms.

Q12. What is the most likely diagnosis in this patient?
a. acute prostatitis
b. acute cystitis
c. chronic prostatitis
d. acute perineal pain syndrome
e. acute nongonococcal urethritis

Q13. What is the most likely organism responsible for the condition described in Case 3?
a. *Escherichia coli*
b. *Pseudomonas*
c. *Proteus*
d. *Serratia*
e. *Chlamydia trachomatis*

Q14. What is the pharmacologic agent of choice for the condition described in Case 3?
a. trimethoprim-sulfamethoxazole (TMP-SMX)
b. erythromycin
c. ampicillin
d. tetracycline
e. gentamicin

SHORT ANSWER MANAGEMENT PROBLEM
Describe the therapeutic mechanism and the therapeutic effects of the drug finasteride, recently marketed for the treatment of BPH.

ANSWERS

A1. **a.** The most likely diagnosis in this patient is BPH (hyperplasia). Hyperplasia of the prostate causes increased outflow resistance.

A2. **e.** The symptoms of BPH are described as either obstructive or irritative. Obstructive symptoms are attributed to the mechanical obstruction of the prostatic urethra by the hyperplastic tissue and include the following:
a. Hesitancy
b. Weakening of the urinary stream
c. Intermittent urinary stream
d. Feeling of residual urine (incomplete bladder emptying)
e. Urinary retention
f. Postmicturition urinary dribbling

Irritative symptoms are attributed to involuntary contractions of the vesical detrusor muscle (detrusor instability) and are associated with obstruction in approximately 50% of patients with prostatism. These symptoms include the following:
a. Nocturia
b. Daytime frequency
c. Urgency
d. Urge incontinence
e. Dysuria

Differential diagnosis includes carcinoma of the prostate, neuropathic bladder, chronic prostatitis, and urethral stricture.

A3. **d.** The pharmacologic treatment of BPH is directed toward relaxation of the prostatic smooth muscle fibers through inhibition of alpha-adrenergic receptors, as well as toward regression of the hyperplastic tissue by hormonal suppression.

The growth of BPH depends on the presence of the androgenic hormone testosterone and its derivative dihydrotestosterone (via conversion by the enzyme 5-alpha reductase). The strategy of antiandrogenic therapy in BPH is to interfere with dihydrotestosterone production. Many antiandrogenic drugs have been tried, but at present the most promising is the 5-alpha reductase inhibitor, finasteride. Finasteride (Proscar) 5 mg/day results in a 20% reduction in prostatic size and a modest improvement of the urine's score and the symptom score. It also has a low incidence of adverse effects. Finasteride significantly decreases the prostate specific antigen (PSA) level, and detection of cancer of the prostate becomes difficult. Finasteride treatment should be considered in patients with moderate symptoms of prostatism. If the patient improves and side effects are minimal, continuation of therapy under careful urologic control is appropriate.

The tone of prostatic smooth muscle is mediated by the alpha$_1$, adrenoreceptor stimulation through selective or nonselective antagonists relaxing the smooth muscle, resulting in a diminution of urethral resistance, improvement of urine flow, and a significant improvement in symptoms. The results of double-blind, randomized controlled trials have demonstrated the short-term efficacy of selective alpha$_1$ blockade. Selective alpha$_1$-blocking drugs such as terazosin (Hytrin) and prazosin (Minipress) represent an option for patients with moderate symptoms. The long-term efficacy remains to be established.

A4. **d.** The following should be performed before any medical or surgical intervention for BPH:
   a. A complete history
   b. A complete physical examination
   c. A digital rectal examination
   d. Ultrasound (transrectal or abdominal)
   e. Determination of postvoiding residual urine
   f. Routine urinalysis and culture
   g. Electrolytes (especially urea and creatinine)
   h. PSA
   i. Cystoscopy

A5. **a.** In general, TURP remains both safe and efficacious and is the "gold standard" against which all other treatments, both medical and surgical, must be measured. More than 80% of patients experience subjective improvement, including a significant improvement in urine flow rate. Approximately 15%, however, report no benefit 1 year after surgery.

Other surgical treatment options include the following:
   a. Transurethral incision of the prostate
   b. Open surgery
   c. Transurethral laser-induced prostatectomy
   d. Transurethral balloon dilatation of the prostate
   e. Prostatic stents and coils

A6. **b.** This patient most likely has a prostatic carcinoma with osseous bone metastases. Evaluation of this patient should include a PSA level, a bone scan, plain x-rays of the pelvis and lumbar areas, and a CT scan of the pelvis. If these investigations confirm stage D carcinoma of the prostate (pelvic lymph node metastases or distant metastases), the patient should receive hormonal therapy. Although radiotherapy for stage D cancer is not entirely ruled out, it is not a first-line option.

Palliative treatment of cancer pain is discussed in Problem 18.

A7. **d.** Prostate cancer represents the most common tumor among men in the United States and is certainly a major public health problem; approximately 179,000 new cases were estimated to be diagnosed in 1999, and some 37,000 men were estimated to have died that year of their disease. The single most important risk factor for cancer of the prostate is age; the disease prevalence increases almost exponentially after age 50. The true prevalence is unknown, but estimates can be obtained from autopsy series or from a series of patients undergoing TURP. These series suggest that the prevalence of the disease is about 30% in men age 60 to 69 and about 67% in men age 80 to 89. It approaches 100% in men older than 90 years old. The incidence among various populations is similar in autopsy samples, but the clinical incidence varies considerably. This suggests that environmental/dietary differences among various cultural groups may be important determinants of the rate of cancer growth. It is suspected that growth is promoted by a high-fat diet and is inhibited by antioxidants.

The most common site of prostatic metastases is bone.

A8. **e.** As mentioned in Answer 7, increasing age is the most important risk factor for carcinoma of the prostate. Other risk factors include African-American race, dietary fat intake, positive family history for carcinoma of the prostate, and possible exposure to certain chemicals (herbicides and pesticides). Certain occupations such as farming and work in the industrial chemical industry may present an especially high risk.

A9. **c.** The U.S. Preventive Services Task Force on the Periodic Health Examination has indicated that "there is insufficient evidence to recommend for or against routine digital rectal examinations as an effective screening test for prostate cancer in asymptomatic men. Transrectal ultrasound and serum tumor markers are not recommended for routine screening in asymptomatic men." This is termed by the U.S. Task Force as a class C recommendation.

A10. **e.** Multiple treatment options exist for localized prostate cancer. Studies of the natural history of untreated stages A and B disease attest to the slow progression of these lesions with disease-specific survival rates in excess of 85% at 10 years. For this reason, a watch-and-wait policy for older patients and those with significant other comorbid conditions is a reasonable option. For younger patients with a long life expectancy ($\leq$10 years), treatment for cure can be accomplished with radical prostatectomy, radiotherapy, or interstitial radiotherapy (therapy) where the radiation source is placed close to the tumor.

A11. **b.** The diagnosis of prostate cancer is usually a serendipitous finding. Signs and symptoms of the disease are usually encountered only at an advanced stage. These signs and symptoms include anorexia, bone pain, neurologic deficits, obstructive voiding symptoms, and weight loss. Of these, the most common initial presenting symptom is obstruction to voiding.

A12. **a.** This patient's symptoms are classic for acute bacterial prostatitis. The symptoms include both systemic symptoms (fever and chills) as well as local urinary symptoms such as perineal and suprapubic discomfort, dysuria, and inhibited urinary voiding.

The digital rectal examination that reveals a swollen, tender, and boggy prostate is probably the most sensitive and specific diagnostic test for prostatitis. When performing the rectal examination in a patient with systemic symptoms, it is imperative that the prostate gland not be massaged; this may release a significant number of bacteria into the bloodstream. Only when systemic symptoms are absent can the prostate gland be safely massaged to obtain a prostatic specimen for culture.

A13. **a.** The two bacteria responsible for most cases of bacterial prostatitis are *E. coli* and *Klebsiella*. Nonbacterial prostatitis is most often caused by *Chlamydia trachomatis* or *Ureaplasma urealyticum*.

A14. **a.** The drugs of choice for the treatment of acute prostatitis are TMP-SMX, norfloxacin, and ciprofloxacin. Antibiotic treatment should continue for at least 4 weeks.

SOLUTION TO THE SHORT ANSWER MANAGEMENT PROBLEM

The medical treatment of BPH has been revolutionized. The growth of BPH depends on the presence of the androgenic hormone testosterone and its derivative dihydrotestosterone (via conversion by the enzyme 5-alpha reductase). The strategy of antiandrogenic therapy in BPH is to interfere with dihydrotestosterone production.

As mentioned in Answer 3, finasteride results in an approximately 20% reduction in prostatic size and a modest improvement of the flow rate of urine and symptom score and has a very low rate of adverse effects. The main adverse effects are a decrease in libido and/or erectile dysfunction.

Finasteride also significantly decreases the serum PSA level and thus reduces the ability to screen for carcinoma of the prostate.

The treatment of BPH with finasteride should be considered in patients with moderate symptoms of prostatism. If the patient improves on the drug and does not experience significant side effects, continuation of therapy under careful physician supervision is reasonable.

SUMMARY OF THE DIAGNOSIS AND MANAGEMENT OF BPH (HYPERPLASIA), PROSTATIC CANCER, AND PROSTATITIS

1. BPH:
   a. Symptoms: Both obstructive symptoms (hesitancy, weak stream, intermittent urinary stream, feeling of incomplete emptying, urinary retention, terminal dribbling) and irritative symptoms (nocturia, daytime frequency, urgency, urge incontinence, dysuria)
   b. Investigations: Complete history, physical examination, urinalysis, culture, transrectal ultrasound, residual urine, electrolytes, blood urea nitrogen, creatinine, serum PSA, cystoscopy
   c. Treatment: Pharmacologic treatment: 5-alpha reductase inhibitor (finasteride), alpha- receptor blocker (prazosin, terazosin); surgical treatment: TURP

2. Carcinoma of the prostate:
   a. Prevalence: Carcinoma of the prostate is now the most common malignancy in men and the second leading cause of death from cancer.
   b. Symptoms and signs: Symptoms and signs are the same as those of BPH except abnormalities are found on examination of the prostate.
   c. Treatment:
      1) Stages A and B-1 (younger than age 65): Prostatectomy or radiation
      2) Stages A and B-1 (older than age 65): Watchful waiting
      3) Stages B and C: Radiotherapy
      4) Stage D:
         a) Asymptomatic: Await the onset of symptoms or hormone therapy.
         b) Symptomatic: Hormone therapy [orchiectomy, antiandrogens, luteinizing hormone-releasing hormone analogues]. Combination chemotherapy can be used in hormone-resistant cases.

3. Prostatitis:
   a. Acute bacterial prostatitis:
      1) Symptoms: Fever, chills, perineal and suprapubic discomfort, dysuria, and inhibited urinary voiding
      2) Treatment: Septra, norfloxacin, ciprofloxacin

3) Organisms: *E. coli/Klebsiella* and *Chlamydia trachomatis* are thought to be the major causes of nonbacterial prostatitis.
   b. Chronic bacterial prostatitis:
      1) Symptoms: Either asymptomatic or symptoms are less prominent than in acute bacterial prostatitis
      2) Investigation: Three-part urine culture (third after prostatic massage)
      3) Treatment: Same drugs as those used to treat acute bacterial prostatitis

SUGGESTED READINGS

Anderson R: Prostatitis. In Rakel R, ed: *Conn's current therapy*, Philadelphia, 1994, WB Saunders.

Anonymous: Treating prostate cancer: An overview, *Harv Mens Health Watch* 4(1):1-4, 1999.

Godley PA: Prostate cancer screening: Promise and peril—a review, *Cancer Detect Prev* 23(4):316-324, 1999.

Henry RY, O'Mahony D: Treatment of prostate cancer, *J Clin Pharm Ther* 24(2):93-102, 1999.

Holtgrewe HL: The medical management of lower urinary tract symptoms and benign prostatic hyperplasia, *Urol Clin North Am* 25(4):555-569, vii, 1998.

Jepsen JV, Bruskewitz RC: Office evaluation of men with lower urinary tract symptoms, *Urol Clin North Am* 25(4):545-554, vii, 1998.

Madsen PO et al: Benign prostatic hyperplasia. In Rakel R, ed: *Conn's current therapy*, Philadelphia, 1994, WB Saunders.

Ramsey EW: Office treatment of benign prostatic hyperplasia, *Urol Clin North Am* 25(4):571-580, 1998.

Thompson I, Teague J: Genitourinary tumors. In Rakel R, ed: *Conn's current therapy*, Philadelphia, 1994, WB Saunders.

Tierney LM, Jr, McPhee SJ, Papadakis MA, eds: *Current medical diagnosis and treatment, 2000*, Stamford, Conn, 1999, Appleton & Lange.

Wilde MI, Goa KL: Finasteride: an update of its use in the management of symptomatic benign prostatic hyperplasia, *Drugs* 57(4):557-581, 1999.

Ziada A et al: Benign prostatic hyperplasia: An overview, *Urology* 53(3 Suppl 3a):1-6, 1999.

PROBLEM · 113

COMMON EAR, NOSE, AND THROAT PROBLEMS

"Doc, I Can Hardly Hear and My Head Is Spinning."

Case 1 ■ A 38-Year-Old Female with a Feeling of Dizziness and Imbalance

A 38-year-old female comes to your office with a 1-year history of episodic dizziness, ringing in both ears, a feeling of fullness, and hearing loss. The symptoms come on every 1 to 2 weeks and usually last for 12 hours. Nausea and vomiting are present. When asked to describe the dizziness, the patient says, "The world is spinning around me."

On physical examination, the patient has horizontal nystagmus. The slow phase of the nystagmus is to the left and the rapid phase is to the right. Audiograms reveal bilateral sensorineural hearing loss in the low frequencies.

SELECT THE BEST ANSWER TO THE FOLLOWING QUESTIONS

Q1. What is the most likely diagnosis in this patient?
   a. vestibular neuritis
   b. acute labyrinthitis
   c. benign positional vertigo
   d. orthostatic hypotension
   e. Meniere's disease

Q2. The treatment of this disorder includes which of the following:
   a. decrease caffeine intake
   b. decrease alcohol intake
   c. use of a thiazide diuretic
   d. use of an antiemetic for nausea and vomiting
   e. all of the above
   f. none of the above

Case 2 ■ A 23-Year-Old Female Who Is Dizzy

A 23-year-old female comes to your office with a 6-month history of dizziness. She "feels dizzy" when she stands up (as if she is going to faint). The sensation disappears within a minute.

She has a history of major depression. You placed her on doxepin 6 months ago, and she has improved much since that time.

The patient's blood pressure is 140/90 mm Hg sitting and drops to 90/70 mm Hg when she stands. There is no ataxia, no nystagmus, and no other symptoms.

Q3. What is the most likely diagnosis in this patient?
   a. vestibular neuronitis
   b. acute labyrinthitis
   c. benign positional vertigo
   d. orthostatic hypotension
   e. Meniere's disease

Q4. What is the best treatment for the patient described in Case 2?
   a. an antiemetic
   b. education and reassurance
   c. a thiazide diuretic
   d. a change in the antidepressant
   e. b and d

Case 3 ■ A 30-Year-Old Male Who Becomes Dizzy When He Rolls Over

A 30-year-old male comes to your office for assessment of "dizziness." The dizziness occurs when he rolls over from the lying position to either the left side or the right side. It also occurs when he is looking up. He describes a sensation of "the world spinning around" him. The episodes usually last for 10 to 15 seconds. They have been occurring for the past 6 months and occur on average 1 to 2 times per day.

Q5. What is the most likely diagnosis in this patient?
a. vestibular neuronitis
b. acute labyrinthitis
c. benign positional vertigo
d. orthostatic hypotension
e. Meniere's disease

Q6. What is the treatment of choice for the patient described in Case 3?
a. avoidance of alcohol and caffeine
b. dimenhydrinate
c. a thiazide diuretic
d. reassurance and simple exercises
e. endolymphatic surgery

Case 4 ■ A 29-Year-Old Female with Unrelenting Dizziness Associated with Nausea and Vomiting

A 29-year-old female comes to your office with a 4-day history of "unrelenting dizziness." The dizziness is associated with nausea and vomiting. There has been no hearing loss, no tinnitus, and no sensation of aural fullness. The patient has just recovered from an upper respiratory tract infection.

On examination, nystagmus is present. The slow phase of the nystagmus is toward the left, and the rapid phase of the nystagmus is toward the right. There is a significant ataxia present.

Q7. What is the most likely diagnosis in this patient?
a. vestibular neuronitis
b. acute labyrinthitis
c. benign positional vertigo
d. orthostatic hypotension
e. Meniere's disease

Q8. What is the treatment of choice for the patient described in Case 4?
a. avoidance of alcohol and caffeine
b. a thiazide diuretic
c. endolymphatic surgery
d. reassurance and antiemetics
e. none of the above

Case 5 ■ A 26-Year-Old Female with Severe Dizziness, Ataxia, and Hearing Loss

A 26-year-old female comes to your office with a 6-day history of severe dizziness associated with ataxia and right-sided hearing loss. She had an upper respiratory tract infection 1 week ago. At that time her right ear felt plugged.

On examination, there is fluid behind the right eardrum. There is horizontal nystagmus present with the slow component to the right and the quick component to the left. Ataxia is present.

Q9. What is the most likely diagnosis in this patient?
a. vestibular neuronitis
b. acute labyrinthitis
c. benign positional vertigo
d. orthostatic hypotension
e. Meniere's disease

Q10. What is the treatment of choice for the patient described in Case 5?
a. avoidance of caffeine and alcohol
b. a thiazide diuretic
c. endolymphatic surgery
d. rest, antiemetics, and antibiotics
e. none of the above

Q11. What is the most common cause of sensorineural hearing loss in the adult population?
a. Meniere's disease
b. chronic otitis media
c. presbycusis
d. otosclerosis
e. mastoiditis

Q12. What is the most common cause of conductive hearing loss in adults who have normal-appearing tympanic membranes?
a. Meniere's disease
b. chronic otitis media
c. presbycusis
d. otosclerosis
e. mastoiditis

Case 6 ■ A 37-Year-Old Female with Intermittent Hearing Loss

A 37-year-old female comes to your office for assessment of hearing loss. She has had problems intermittently for the past 12 months.

On examination, the Weber tuning fork test lateralizes to the right ear and the Rinne tuning fork test is negative in the right ear (bone conduction is greater than air conduction [BC>AC]).

Q13. This suggests which one of the following hearing losses?
a. a right-sided conductive hearing loss
b. a left-sided conductive hearing loss
c. a right-sided sensorineural hearing loss
d. a left-sided sensorineural hearing loss
e. a or d

Case 7 ■ A 43-Year-Old Male with Hearing Loss Lateralized to the Left Ear

A 43-year-old male comes to your office for assessment of hearing loss. He has had hearing difficulties for the past 4 years.

On examination, the Weber tuning fork test lateralizes to the left ear. The Rinne tuning fork test is positive (AC > BC).

Q14. This suggests which one of the following hearing losses?
a. a right-sided conductive hearing loss
b. a left-sided conductive hearing loss
c. a right-sided sensorineural hearing loss
d. a left-sided sensorineural hearing loss
e. b or c

Q15. Which of the following statements is (are) true regarding the condition of acute mastoiditis?
a. it is a complication of acute otitis media
b. it is most likely caused by *Streptococcus pneumoniae*
c. otalgia, aural discharge, and fever are characteristically seen 2 to 3 weeks after an episode of acute suppurative otitis media
d. none of the above statements is true
e. all of the above statements are true

Q16. Which of the following statements concerning sinusitis is (are) true?
a. the most common causes of sinusitis are allergic sinusitis and viral sinusitis
b. rhinovirus is the most common cause of viral sinusitis
c. viral sinusitis is often accompanied by fever, malaise, and systemic symptoms
d. a and b only
e. all of the above statements are true

Q17. Acute bacterial sinusitis is most commonly caused by which of the following organisms?
a. *Streptococcus pneumoniae*
b. *Haemophilus influenzae*
c. *Moraxella catarrhalis*
d. *Streptococcus pyogenes*
e. *Staphylococcus aureus*

Q18. Which of the following is the most predictive factor distinguishing viral sinusitis and bacterial sinusitis?
a. thick and greenish nasal discharge
b. facial pain
c. degree of fever
d. location of the pain
e. systemic symptoms

Q19. What is the antibacterial drug of first choice for acute bacterial sinusitis?
a. amoxicillin (10-day course)
b. Bactrim/Septra (10-day course)
c. cefuroxime (10-day course)
d. Augmentin (10-day course)
e. erythromycin (10-day course)

Q20. Which of the following anatomic forms of acute bacterial sinusitis is most serious?
a. maxillary sinusitis
b. ethmoidal sinusitis
c. frontal sinusitis
d. mandibular sinusitis
e. anterior sinusitis

SHORT ANSWER MANAGEMENT PROBLEM
Describe the long-term consequences of otitis media.

ANSWERS

A1. **e.** This patient has Meniere's disease. The classic features of Meniere's disease are recurrent episodes of vertigo, fluctuating sensorineural hearing loss, tinnitus (ringing or buzzing in the ears), and aural fullness in the affected ear.

Meniere's disease is associated with vertigo typically lasting hours, not minutes or days. Low-tone sensorineural hearing loss also occurs. The fluctuating hearing may not be related temporally to the vertigo. In many cases, the tinnitus and fullness become severe just before the vertigo attack begins.

To make the diagnosis of Meniere's disease, the characteristic pattern of vertigo lasting a matter of hours, as well as sensorineural hearing loss, must be present. One additional factor (low-frequency hearing loss, aural fullness, or buzzing tinnitus) should also be present.

A2. **e.** Some patients with Meniere's disease are acutely sensitive to alcohol, caffeine, or both. In these patients, alcohol and caffeine should obviously be avoided.

Meniere's disease is also known as endolymphatic hydrops. This suggests that a buildup of fluid in the endolymphatic system may be responsible for the development of the acute attack. Thus the use of a mild diuretic such as hydrochlorothiazide is a reasonable treatment (especially for patients that are having frequent attacks).

The use of an antinauseant such as droperidol IM, chlorpromazine IM, or dimenhydrinate IM or PO may be extremely effective in the treatment of the acute attack.

Surgery is reserved for patients who do not respond to medical management.

A3. **d.** This patient has orthostatic hypotension. This case description illustrates the importance of obtaining an accurate history in the patient who complains of "feeling dizzy." In any patient who has this complaint, it is important to ask four specific questions:
   a. Can you describe your dizziness?
   b. If you had "a dollar's worth of dizziness," how much would be a sensation of the "world spinning around you," and how much would be a sensation of "things going black in front of you and a feeling that you're about to pass out?"
   c. How long does the feeling of dizziness last: seconds, minutes, or hours?
   d. Are there any other symptoms present when you feel dizzy such as deafness, ear fullness, or ringing in the ears?

Orthostatic hypotension is typically initiated after standing up suddenly or, in many cases, is experienced after the patient has been up for a long time, often in closed quarters or crowded shopping malls. The feeling described is that of a subjective dizziness and is closely related to a simple faint or a syncopal episode. It is often accompanied by nausea. It is not associated with any other neurologic sensations or ear symptoms.

In this case the orthostatic hypotension is almost certainly associated with the beginning of the tricyclic antidepressant therapy 6 months ago.

A4. **e.** The most important treatment in this patient is to reassure the patient and explain how the symptom can be minimized by slowly assuming the upright position.

As the orthostatic hypotension developed after the initiation of the tricyclic antidepressant, doxepin, it would be reasonable to switch to an antidepressant with fewer alpha-adrenergic side effects. A good choice would be one of the new selective serotonin reuptake inhibitors such as sertraline, fluoxetine, or paroxetine.

A5. **c.** This patient has benign positional vertigo, a disorder that consists of brief episodes (lasting any-where from 2 to 10 seconds) usually caused by either rolling over toward either the right or the left when supine or looking up such as when searching for something on a shelf.

The cause of benign positional vertigo is unknown but is thought to be either idiopathic or caused by trauma.

A6. **d.** The treatment of choice for the patient discussed in Case 3 is reassurance and the prescription of the following simple exercises.
   Step 1:
      The patient lies on his back with his head hanging down and to the right. If this does not cause vertigo, proceed to Step 2. If it does cause vertigo, wait until it subsides. The patient then rotates his head and body slowly to the right (clockwise) until a complete 360 degree rotation is made. If further vertigo occurs, the rotation is halted until the vertigo subsides. Then the rotation is continued. If there is no vertigo after one rotation, proceed to Step 2. If vertigo reoccurs, repeat clockwise rotation until it is gone.
   Step 2:
      The patient lies on his back with his head hanging down and to the left. If this does not cause vertigo, the exercise is finished. If vertigo occurs, wait until it subsides. Then the patient slowly rotates his head and body 360 degrees to the left (counterclockwise). This maneuver is repeated until the vertigo is gone.
   Step 3:
      The patient should avoid the head dependent position for 24 hours. The exercises can be repeated at home if the positional vertigo reoccurs.

Performance of these exercises three or four times in a row (three or four times a day) often provides dramatic relief, but improvement in symptoms sometimes takes up to 10 days to occur.

Even if the exercises are not prescribed, the condition tends to resolve with time (usually several weeks to a few months).

A7. **a.** This patient has a left vestibular neuronitis. This disorder is most commonly associated with a viral infection (such as adenovirus) following a respiratory tract infection and involves some portion of the vestibular system but with total sparing of the cochlear area.

The disorder consists of severe vertigo with associated ataxia and nausea and vomiting. There is no hearing loss, no aural pain, and no other symptoms. Recovery usually takes 1 to 2 weeks.

A8. **d.** The treatment of choice for a patient with vestibular neuronitis is rest, reassurance, and antiemetics.

Antiemetics such as droperidol, chlorpromazine, or dimenhydrinate may be given for symptomatic relief of the vertigo. Rest and reassurance are sufficient in most cases.

A9. **b.** This patient has acute labyrinthitis. Acute labyrinthitis usually follows an upper respiratory tract infection accompanied by middle ear effusion. The disorder probably represents a chemical irritation of the inner ear from middle ear fluid. The features of acute labyrinthitis include significant sensorineural hearing loss (with a conductive component if a middle ear effusion is present) and severe vertigo that lasts several days.

A10. **d.** The treatment of choice for acute labyrinthitis includes rest, antiemetics, and antibiotics. Bacterial labyrinthitis may complicate serous labyrinthitis if antibiotics are not administered. Amoxicillin would be a good first-line agent for antibiotic prophylaxis. If symptoms do not improve, the addition of clavulanic acid to amoxicillin would be a reasonable second choice.

A11. **c.** Hearing loss can be divided into sensorineural hearing loss and conductive hearing loss. The most common cause of sensorineural hearing loss in adults is presbycusis, a gradual deterioration that begins after the age of 20 years in the highest frequencies and often involves all speech frequencies by the sixth and seventh decades of life. The impaired hearing associated with presbycusis stems from degenerative changes in the hair cells, auditory neurons, and cochlear nuclei. Tinnitus is a common complaint.

Sound amplification with an electrical hearing aid does benefit some patients with relatively good speech discrimination.

A12. **d.** The most common cause of conductive hearing loss in adults who have normal-appearing tympanic membranes is otosclerosis. Otosclerosis is a localized disease of the otic capsule, reducing ankylosis or fixation of the stapes footplate. The resulting conductive hearing loss starts insidiously in the third and fourth decades of life and progressively involves both ears in 80% of individuals. Otosclerosis, an inherited disease, is more common in whites.

A13. **a.** Facts for Question 13:
   a. BC > AC: This indicates that this is a conductive hearing loss.
   b. Weber test lateralizes to the right ear: In conductive hearing loss, the Weber test lateralizes to the affected ear. Therefore, this is a unilateral right-sided conductive hearing loss.

A14. **c.** The characterization of hearing loss can be localized by a combination of the Weber test and the Rinne test.

In the Weber test, placement of a 512-Hz tuning fork on the skull in the midline or on the teeth stimulates both cochleae simultaneously. If the patient has a conductive hearing loss in one ear, the sound will be perceived loudest in the affected ear (that is, it will lateralize). When a unilateral sensorineural hearing loss is present, the tone is heard in the unaffected ear.

The Rinne test compares AC with BC. Normally AC is greater than BC. Sound stimulation by air in front of the pinna is normally perceived twice as long as sound placed on the mastoid process (AC > BC). With conductive hearing loss, the duration of AC is less than BC (that is, negative Rinne test). In the presence of sensorineural hearing loss, the duration of both AC and BC are reduced; however, the 2:1 ratio remains the same (that is, a positive Rinne test).
   Facts for Question 14:
   a. AC is greater than BC. Therefore, this is a sensorineural hearing loss.
   b. Weber test lateralizes to the left ear: In sensorineural hearing loss the Weber test lateralizes to the unaffected ear. Therefore, the right ear is the affected ear. This is a unilateral right-sided sensorineural hearing loss.

A15. **e.** Acute mastoiditis is a complication of acute otitis media that develops as a result of the retention of pus in the mastoid area. Acute mastoiditis is most commonly caused by *Streptococcus pneumoniae*. *Streptococcus pyogenes* and *Staphylococcal aureus* are other recognized causes.

The inflammatory process in acute mastoiditis results in the destruction of bony septa (almost an osteomyelitis-like process) and, as a result, there is a coalescence of mastoid air cells. This leads to subsequent erosion of the mastoid process of the petrous temporal bone.

The symptoms of acute mastoiditis include otalgia, aural discharge, and fever. These symptoms usually appear 2 to 3 weeks after an episode of acute suppurative otitis media. Examination reveals severe mastoid tenderness, lateral displacement of the pinna, and postauricular mastoid swelling secondary to the periosteal abscess. The treatment of choice is ceftriaxone (with or without metronidazole) and surgical drainage (for a subperiosteal abscess).

A16. **e.** The most common causes of acute rhinosinusitis are allergic and viral. It is often extremely difficult to distinguish between the two types, although a seasonal sinusitis points to allergic sinusitis, as do symptoms such as itching and redness of the eyes.

Viral rhinitis and sinusitis may be accompanied by systemic systems including fever, chills, facial pain, malaise, and fatigue. The viruses most commonly responsible for viral sinusitis are (in order of frequency) rhinovirus, adenovirus, parainfluenzae, and influenzae.

A17. **a.** The organisms most commonly implicated in bacterial sinusitis include *Streptococcus pneumoniae* (the most common), *Haemophilus influenzae, Moraxella catarrhalis,* and *Streptococcus pyogenes.* Other organisms implicated include *Staphylococcus aureus* and anaerobic organisms.

Chronic sinusitis is most often associated with *Staphylococcus aureus, Haemophilus influenzae,* and anaerobic organisms.

A18. **a.** Bacterial sinusitis can be distinguished from viral sinusitis by the thick, greenish discharge that accompanies the congestion.

A19. **a.** The use of antibiotics in the treatment of acute sinusitis is controversial. Few well-designed, large, randomized controlled trials exist, particularly in primary care settings. A Chochran sinusitis study protocol is underway.

The 1996 Canadian Sinusitis Symposium recommended the following:
a. The antibiotic treatment of choice for acute bacterial sinusitis is at minimum a 10-day course of amoxicillin.
b. Second-line antibiotics include trimethoprim-sulfamethoxazole (Septra/Bactrim), cefaclor (Ceclor), cefuroxime (Ceftin), and amoxicillin-clavulanic acid (Augmentin).

A20. **c.** The most serious form of acute sinusitis is frontal sinusitis, which manifests as pain, tenderness, and edema of the anterior cortex of the frontal sinus. Acute frontal sinusitis usually necessitates high-dose intravenous antibiotics and decongestants.

Cases of chronic sinusitis not responsive to antibiotics require endoscopic sinus surgery.

SOLUTION TO THE SHORT ANSWER MANAGEMENT PROBLEM

The long-term complications of chronic otitis media include the following:
a. Seventh nerve paralysis
b. Labyrinthitis
c. Petrositis
d. Intracranial suppuration
e. Cholesteatoma

The major complication of acute otitis media is acute mastoiditis.

SUMMARY OF THE DIAGNOSIS AND TREATMENT OF COMMON EAR, NOSE, AND THROAT PROBLEMS

1. Vertigo:
   a. Meniere's disease:
      1) Symptoms: Vertigo (lasting hours), hearing loss, tinnitus, aural fullness
      2) Treatment: Avoidance of caffeine, avoidance of alcohol, low-dose hydrochlorothiazide, antiemetics
   b. Acute labyrinthitis:
      1) Symptoms: Vertigo (lasting days) and associated hearing loss usually follow an upper respiratory tract infection in which there is a middle ear effusion
      2) Treatment: Rest, antiemetics, antibiotics if middle ear fluid is infected
   c. Vestibular neuronitis:
      1) Symptoms: Vertigo (lasting days), no hearing loss, no ear pain, no other symptoms; may result from upper respiratory tract infection
      2) Treatment: Rest, reassurance, antiemetics
   d. Benign positional vertigo:
      1) Symptoms: Vertigo (lasting for seconds), also associated with rolling over toward the left or the right when supine or when looking up
      2) Treatment: Reassurance, simple exercises

2. Orthostatic hypotension:
   a. Symptoms: Not true vertigo (rather a sensation of lightheadedness or faintness) on assuming the upright position; often associated with antihypertensive and antidepressant medications
   b. Treatment: Reassurance, change in medications to one with fewer alpha-blockade properties and fewer orthostatic side effects

3. Hearing loss:
   a. Sensorineural hearing loss:
      1) Pathologic condition: Usually a disorder affecting the cochlea and auditory nerves with the perception of a "distorted sound." The deficit is usually greater in the higher frequencies. There are usually degenerative changes in the hair cells, auditory neurons, and cochlear nuclei.
      2) Causation: The most common cause is presbycusis, which is a gradual deterioration that starts with high-frequency loss and often involves all speech frequencies by the sixth or seventh decade.

3) Treatment: A hearing aid may benefit patients with relatively good speech discrimination.
b. Conductive hearing loss:
1) Pathologic condition/causation: Conductive hearing loss involves either chronic serous otitis media or otosclerosis. Otosclerosis results as a localized disease of the otic capsule where new spongy bone replaces normal bone, producing ankylosis or fixation of the stapes footplate.
2) Treatment: The treatments for the chronic causes of conductive hearing loss are usually surgical.
c. Interpretation of hearing loss:
1) Audiogram
2) Weber test or Rinne test

4. Sinusitis:
a. Pathologic condition:
1) Allergic
2) Viral
3) Bacterial

b. Organisms:
1) Rhinovirus is the most common viral cause, followed by adenovirus.
2) *Streptococcus pneumoniae* is most common bacterial cause, followed by *Haemophilus influenzae* and *Moraxella catarrhalis*.
c. Symptoms: Fever, chills, malaise, fatigue, facial pain
d. Bacterial sinusitis is distinguished from viral sinusitis mainly by the presence of thick, greenish nasal discharge.
e. Treatment: Amoxicillin (10 days) is the drug of choice for acute bacterial sinusitis.

SUGGESTED READINGS

Baloh RW: Vertigo, *Lancet* 352(9143):1841-1846, 1998.
Baloh RW: The dizzy patient, *Postgrad Med* 105(2):161-164, 167-172, 1999.
Derebery MJ: The diagnosis and treatment of dizziness, *Med Clin North Am* 83(1):163-177, 1999.
Guaderas JC: Rhinitis and sinusitis, *Mayo Clin Proc* 71(9):882-888, 1986.
Hotson JR, Baloh RW: Acute vestibular syndrome, *New Engl J Med* 339(10):680-685, 1998.

CHAPTER VII

Geriatric Medicine

PROBLEM·114

ELDERLY ABUSE

"I'm a Very Patient Person, but That Old Bitch Simply Will Not Do What She Should."

Case 1 ■ A 72-Year-Old Female with a Sore Right Shoulder and Multiple Bruises

A daughter brings her 72-year-old mother to the Emergency Department for assessment. The mother has Alzheimer's disease and is unable to communicate with you directly. The daughter tells you that her mother has had Alzheimer's disease for 5 years and has been living with her for the majority of that time.

The daughter tells you that her mother fell on her right shoulder approximately 3 hours ago. As you look at the patient you notice a large bruise in the area of the head of the right humerus.

On examination, there are multiple bruises on her arms, legs, and abdomen. The head of the humerus is tender. The resident who is with you tells you that he "has things pretty well squared away." He has made the diagnosis of a rare inherited bleeding disorder on the basis of (as the nurse that is caring for the patient says) "goodness knows what."

You decide that you are not satisfied with this diagnosis and need to investigate further. Meanwhile, the patient is complaining of pain and holding her shoulder. You order an x-ray of the shoulder and diagnose a fractured head of the humerus.

SELECT THE BEST ANSWER TO THE FOLLOWING QUESTIONS

Q1. At this time, what should you do?
   a. treat the patient's pain, provide a collar and cuff, and say good-bye to the patient and her daughter
   b. treat the patient's pain, provide a collar and cuff for the patient, and tell the patient that she really should be more careful
   c. treat the patient's pain and contact an orthopedic surgeon who you are sure will wish to manage this fracture with internal fixation

   d. order a complete blood count (CBC), clotting time, and all other laboratory tests vaguely associated with the hematologic and clotting system
   e. none of the above

Q2. What is the prevalence of elder abuse in the United States population?
   a. 4%
   b. 2%
   c. 10%
   d. 8%
   e. 15%

Q3. Regarding screening for the condition described in Case 1, which of the following statements is (are) true?
   a. screening for the condition described in Case 1 is recommended by the American Medical Association
   b. it is recommended that physicians incorporate routine questions related to the condition in Case 1 into their daily practice
   c. direct, concrete action should be taken when a situation is identified that confirms the diagnosis described in Case 1
   d. all of the above statements are true
   e. none of the above statements is true

Q4. When comparing the prevalence of this condition in the community setting with the prevalence of the same condition in long-term care institutions, which of the following statements is (are) true?
   a. the prevalence of this condition is much higher in institutionalized elderly patients compared to elders in the community setting
   b. the institutionalized elderly patient is at greater risk of this condition because of his (her) physical or psychological status
   c. one of the reasons for the high prevalence of this condition in the institutionalized elderly is lack of staff training and/or institutional under staffing
   d. all of the above statements are true
   e. none of the above statements is true

Q5. There are various forms of this condition. Which of the following would be placed in that category of forms?
   a. a physical form
   b. a psychologic form
   c. a financial form
   d. a neglect form
   e. all of the above

Q6. Which of the following is (are) associated with the condition described?
   a. excessive use of restraints
   b. pushing
   c. grabbing
   d. yelling
   e. all of the above

Q7. What is the most common manifestation of the condition described in Case 1?
   a. excessive use of restraints
   b. pushing
   c. grabbing
   d. yelling
   e. slapping or hitting

Q8. Which of the following is not a risk factor for the condition described?
   a. unsatisfactory living arrangements
   b. low educational level of staff
   c. physical or emotional dependence on the caregiver
   d. living apart from the victim
   e. older than 75 years old

Q9. Which of the following is false regarding the condition described?
   a. abusive events tend to be one-time-only events
   b. abusive events tend to escalate in the same manner in which spousal abuse escalates
   c. the situation rarely resolves spontaneously
   d. many victims refuse help
   e. serious illness, crisis, admission to an institution, or even death are all long-term sequelae of this condition

Q10. With respect to research priorities and the condition described, which of the following is (are) true?
   a. there should be a determination of the cause of the condition in different ethnic and cultural groups in North America
   b. there should be a comprehensive assessment of the prevalence of this condition in American long-term care institutions
   c. valid, reliable tools should be developed for use in settings such as primary care, hospital Emergency Departments, and long-term care institutions
   d. all of the above
   e. a and c only

Q11. In which of the following settings is the incidence (i.e., pick-up rate) of the condition described likely to be highest based on screening history and physical examination?
   a. in the family physician's office
   b. in the local Emergency Department facility
   c. in the referral-based specialist's office
   d. any of the above
   e. none of the above

SHORT ANSWER MANAGEMENT PROBLEM
Discuss a comprehensive plan to manage elder abuse in your community.

ANSWERS

A1. **e.** This patient is much more likely to have injuries inflicted as a result of abuse rather than to have a rare inherited clotting disorder or anything else.

Obviously, the patient's pain and her fractured arm have to be treated. This is not, however, the end of the treatment.

Elder abuse is extremely common and is one of those conditions that will not be diagnosed unless it is included in a differential diagnosis and thought of in all situations in which it may occur. In this case, a consult to social services is essential. With the history of physical injury, it would seem that the wisest course of action at this time is removal of the patient to a safe environment.

A2. **a.** The prevalence of elder abuse in North America is estimated at 4%. This represents 700,000 to 1.2 million cases per year in those over the age of 65. In many cases this abuse is long-term, repeated, or both. In one study 58% of elderly patients had suffered previous incidents of abuse.

Some studies have estimated the prevalence of elder abuse to be much higher than 4%; 10% appears to be a more realistic figure.

A3. **d.** When a situation arises that confirms elder abuse, direct action should be taken to rectify, improve, or resolve the situation.

The American Medical Association recommends that physicians screen for elder abuse in their practices and that they incorporate routine questions related to elder abuse and neglect when seeing elderly patients. For example, the physician may ask, "Is there any violence in your family that you want to tell me about?" or "Has anyone tried to hurt or harm you?" or "Did anyone take anything from you or force you to do anything that you did not want to do?"

A4. **d.** The prevalence of elder abuse is much higher in institutionalized elderly patients than in elderly patients who live in the community. In one study of nursing home staff, 36% had witnessed physical abuse of residents in the preceding year.

A5. **e.** The simplest definition of elder abuse is "any act of commission or omission that results in harm to an elderly person."

Elder abuse is distinguished from other crimes against elderly people by the perpetrator's occupying a position of trust. The following definition of elder abuse and neglect is proposed:
  a. Physical abuse: Assault, rough handling, sexual abuse, or the withholding of physical necessities such as food or other items of personal, hygienic, or medical care
  b. Psychosocial abuse: Verbal assault, social isolation, lack of affection, or denial of the person's participation in decisions affecting his or her life
  c. Financial abuse: The misuse of money or property, including fraud or use of funds for purposes contrary to the needs, interests, or desires of the elderly person
  d. Neglect: In active neglect, the caregiver consciously fails to meet the needs of the elderly person; in passive neglect the caregiver does not intend to injure the dependent person. Neglect can lead to any of the three types of abuse.

A6. **e.** Other categories of abuse have been proposed, such as violation of rights and medical abuse (inappropriate treatment, excessive use of restraints, and withholding of treatment). Abuse may be intentional or unintentional.

A7. **a.** As mentioned previously, a figure of 36% has been quoted as the percentage of institutionalized elderly that have been abused. In this study, the most common forms of abuse were excessive use of restraints (witnessed in the quoted study by 21% of staff), pushing, grabbing, shoving, or pinching (17%), and slapping or hitting (15%).

Psychologic abuse was observed by 81% of the staff; 70% had witnessed a staff member yelling at a patient in anger; 50% had seen someone insulting or swearing at a patient; and 23% had seen a patient isolated inappropriately.

A8. **d.** Living apart from the victim is not a risk factor for elder abuse. The risk factors for elder abuse are as follows:
  a. Situational factors:
    1) Community situational factors:
      a) Isolation
      b) Lack of money
      c) Lack of community resources for additional care
      d) Unsatisfactory living arrangements
    2) Institutions:
      a) Shortage of beds
      b) Surplus of patients
      c) Low staff-to-patient ratio
      d) Low staff compensation
      e) Staff burnout
  b. Characteristics of the victim:
    1) Physical or emotional dependence on caregiver
    2) Lack of close family ties
    3) History of family violence
    4) Older than 75 years old
    5) Recent deterioration in health
  c. Characteristics of the perpetrator:
    1) Stress caused by financial, marital, or occupational factors
    2) Deterioration in health
    3) Bereavement
    4) Substance abuse
    5) Psychopathologic illness
    6) Related to victim
    7) Living with victim
    8) Long duration of care for victim (mean 9.5 years)

A9. **a.** Elder abuse rarely resolves spontaneously; it tends to escalate in the same way as spousal abuse. Abusive events tend to be repeated and will almost always continue unless there is a major change in the environment. Such an environmental change may not occur because, in 25% to 75% of cases, victims or their families refuse help. This may subsequently result in serious illness, crisis, admission to an institution, or even death.

A10. **d.** The research priorities for elder abuse include the following:
  a. A determination of the causes of this condition in different ethnic and cultural groups in the United States and Canada
  b. A determination of the prevalence of abuse in American and Canadian institutions
  c. The development of valid and reliable assessment tools for use in such settings as primary care, hospital Emergency Departments, and long-term care institutions

d. An evaluation of the effectiveness of interventions on the prevalence of this condition

A11. **b.** The highest incidence is likely to be at the local Emergency Department facility. The reason is that the time that elders are most likely to come to the Emergency Department is at the time of, or shortly after, an event of abuse. This does not imply that screening should not occur at the other facilities; it should occur in all health care settings all of the time.

SOLUTION TO THE SHORT ANSWER MANAGEMENT PROBLEM

A comprehensive plan to manage elder abuse should include recognition of the condition, comprehensive treatment of the condition, and a significant education component aimed at the following:
  a. Increasing public awareness of the magnitude of the problem
  b. Increasing public awareness of the signs and symptoms of elder abuse
  c. Increasing public awareness of the treatment options available
The actual components of the management of elder abuse include the following:
  a. Detection and risk assessment:
    1) Documentation of the type of abuse, the frequency and severity of abuse, the danger to the victim, and the perpetrator's intent and level of stress
    2) Involvement of other health care professionals (social worker, visiting nurse, and geriatric assessment team)
    3) Documentation of the injuries (take photographs if possible)
    4) Assessment of the victim's overall health status, the victim's functional status, and the victim's social and financial status
  b. Assessment of decision-making capacity of the victim: Assess the cognitive state and the emotional state of the victim.
  c. Measures to take if the victim is competent:
    1) Provide information to the victim.
    2) In providing information, outline the choices or possible choices that the victim has such as temporary relocation, home support, community agencies, and criminal charges
    3) Support the victim's decision.
  d. Measures to take if the victim is not competent:
    1) Separate the victim and the perpetrator.
    2) Relocate the victim.
    3) Arrange advocacy services for the victim.
    4) Inform a protective service agency.
    5) Reduce caregiver stress.
    6) Treat all medical disorders.
    7) Minimize or simplify medications,
    8) Seek agencies to provide respite care, support for house cleaning, personal care, and transportation.
    9) Provide support groups for primary caregivers.
  e. Key questions to guide intervention:
    1) How safe is the patient if he or she is sent home?
    2) What services of resources are available to help a stressed family?
    3) Does the elderly person need to be removed to a safe environment?
    4) Does the situation need an unbiased advocate to monitor the care and finances for this patient?

SUMMARY OF ELDER ABUSE

See the Solution to the Short Answer Management Problem.

SUGGESTED READINGS

Butler RN: Warning signs of elder abuse, *Geriatrics* 54(3):3-4, 1999.
The Canadian Task Force on the Periodic Health Examination: Periodic health examination, 1994 update: 4. Secondary prevention of elder abuse and mistreatment, *Can Med Assoc J* 151(10):1413-1420, 1994.
Clark Me, Pierson W: Management of elder abuse in the emergency department, *Emerg Med Clin North Am* 17(3):631-644, 1999.
Marshall CE et al: Elder abuse: Using clinical tools to identify clues of mistreatment, *Geriatrics* 55(2):42-44, 2000.
Paris BE et al: Elder abuse and neglect: How to recognize warning signs and intervene, *Geriatrics* 50(4):47-51, 1995.
Swagerty DL, Jr, et al: Elder mistreatment, *Am Fam Physician* 59(10):2804-2808, 1999.

P R O B L E M · 1 1 5

ETHICAL DILEMMAS

"Don't Let Her Know, Doctor. It Will Just Kill Her."

Case 1 ■ An 87-Year-Old Female with a Terminal Malignancy Who Has Not Been Informed of Her Condition by Her Doctors

An 87-year-old female has just been diagnosed as having inoperable cancer of the colon. The biopsied lesion that was sent to Pathology following a flexible sigmoidoscopy came back as "anaplastic adenocarcinoma." A liver scan confirms metastatic disease.

A nurse on the patient's unit has told the patient's daughter and son that their mother has cancer. The daughter immediately telephones you and insists that her mother not be told. You have been the family physician to this patient for many years.

SELECT THE BEST ANSWER TO THE FOLLOWING QUESTIONS

Q1. On the basis of the information given, what would you do?
- a. tell the daughter not to interfere; you are the boss, and you will tell the mother as soon as possible
- b. tell the daughter that this is not her decision; you will decide how the whole affair will be settled
- c. tell the daughter quite firmly that you have every intention of telling her mother when the time is right
- d. call your lawyer
- e. none of the above

Case 2 ■ A Terminal 45-Year-Old Female Who Experiences a Cardiopulmonary Arrest

You are the resident in a ward where a 45-year-old female with metastatic breast cancer has just been admitted. The patient is cachectic and exhibits Cheyne-Stokes respirations upon admission. Your attending physician refuses to write a "Do Not Attempt Resuscitation" order on the chart. Three hours after admission the patient suffers a cardiopulmonary arrest and the attending physician stops the code 45 minutes after advanced cardiac life support (ACLS) has been instituted.

Q2. Which of the following statements concerning this case is true?
- a. this is an extremely unusual occurrence
- b. patients in the terminal phase of a malignant disease should rarely, if ever, be subjected to attempted resuscitation
- c. to not attempt resuscitation may be an ethically unacceptable decision
- d. cardiopulmonary resuscitation (CPR) has been shown to save lives in terminal cancer patients
- e. none of the above is true

Case 3 ■ A 44-Year-Old Female with Multiple Liver Metastases

You are the resident in charge of a 44-year-old female who was admitted with nausea and vomiting. The abdominal ultrasound you ordered shows multiple liver metastases from a primary pancreatic cancer. You call the attending physician and he instructs you to "say nothing; it's better that way." The patient questions you that evening about the results of her studies.

Q3. At this time, what should you do?
- a. tell the patient that you know nothing
- b. tell the patient that the ultrasound machine broke
- c. tell the patient that everything will be OK
- d. tell the patient that her attending physician will break the very bad news tomorrow
- e. none of the above

Case 4 ■ A 27-Year-Old Female Came Back with a Diagnosis of Malignant Melanoma

You are just completing your plastic surgery rotation. On the last day the results of a skin lesion biopsy on a 27-year-old female come back as "malignant melanoma—Clark's level IV." You also note that the patient's liver function tests are grossly elevated and conclude that she most likely already has significant metastatic disease.

You are with the attending surgeon as he sees the patient in his outpatient clinic in the afternoon. You accompany him into the room. He stands by the door flipping nervously through the chart for about 5 minutes while the patient stares at him hoping that he will eventually say something. He then looks up at the patient and says, "My dear, you have a very bad skin cancer that is probably going to kill you. It appears that it is already in your liver. If I were you I would get my affairs in order and do what you've always wanted to do as quickly as you can." You are speechless and try to console the patient after he quickly departs the room.

Q4. With respect to this case, which of the following statements is (are) true?
- a. this situation is not real in any way; doctors just do not do those sorts of things
- b. the remarks of the doctor described are entirely a reflection of the lack of training physicians receive in dealing with this type of scenario
- c. this situation is more common than we either admit or believe
- d. these remarks are not in any way unethical
- e. physicians are well trained in breaking bad news; something is very wrong in this circumstance

Case 5 ■ An Unmarried Pregnant 18-Year-Old Woman

You have just established a family practice in the suburban area of a large city. One of your first patients is an 18-year-old girl who comes to your office for a pregnancy test. The test is positive. When you present this result to the patient she bursts into tears and requests an abortion. She is not married, does not love her boyfriend, and is sure her parents will "just die" if they find out. You have very strong feelings against abortion and are planning on becoming actively involved in your local pro-life chapter.

Q5. Based on this information and assuming you hold the views stated previously, what should you do?
   a. tell the patient to leave your office; you are completely opposed to her request
   b. ask the patient to find another doctor as quickly as she can; you can have nothing more to do with her care
   c. discuss the three options that the patient has: carrying through with the pregnancy and keeping the baby, carrying through with the pregnancy and giving the baby up for adoption, and therapeutic abortion; refer her for counseling and ask her to see you again following that counseling
   d. tell the patient that your religious beliefs preclude further discussion of the matter
   e. none of the above

Case 6 ■ A "Brain Dead" Newborn Male

A male infant born at 26 weeks' gestation has been monitored in the intensive care unit for the last 8 weeks. Unfortunately, the infant suffers a severe intraventricular hemorrhage, and the electroencephalogram (EEG) demonstrates no electric activity. The infant is thought to be essentially "brain dead." When you, the attending physician, ask the parents for permission to consider discontinuing life support systems, you are accused of "just trying to get rid of our son to save money." The parents inform you that you will hear from their lawyer shortly.

Q6. At this time, what would you do?
   a. call your own lawyer
   b. express your displeasure at this "attitude" directly to the parents
   c. disconnect the life-support system anyway
   d. arrange a family conference with significant support people for the parents present
   e. continue the life-support system and promise yourself that you will not bring up the subject again

Q7. The right of the patient to express his or her desire for treatment following serious unforeseen complications arising out of a hospitalization is referred to as which of the following?
   a. the Patient Self-Determination Act
   b. the Desire to Live Act

   c. the Patient Emancipation Act
   d. the Patient Self-Care Act
   e. the Medical Profession Obligation Act

Q8. The term *advance directive* includes or is best described as which of the following?
   a. the legal instrument entitled "Directive to Physicians" in the Natural Death Acts enacted by various states
   b. the less formal living will
   c. the durable power of attorney
   d. all of the above
   e. none of the above

Q9. In the case analysis method of ethical decision making, which of the following categories must be considered?
   a. indications for medical intervention
   b. preferences of patients
   c. quality of life
   d. contextual features
   e. all of the above

Q10. In the case analysis method of ethical decision making, the category "Indications for Medical Intervention" includes which of the following?
   a. the concept of beneficence
   b. the concept of nonmaleficence
   c. the concept of clinical judgment
   d. the concept of realistic understanding of the goals of treatment
   e. all of the above

Q11. In the case analysis method of ethical decision making, the category "Preferences of Patients" includes which of the following?
   a. the concept of paternalism
   b. the concept of informed consent
   c. the concept of medical capacity
   d. all of the above
   e. none of the above

Q12. In the case analysis method of ethical decision making, the category "Quality of Life" includes which of the following?
   a. the concept of life-supporting interventions
   b. the concept of euthanasia
   c. the concept of physician-assisted suicide
   d. the concept of pain relief
   e. all of the above

Q13. In the case analysis method of ethical decision making, the category "Contextual Features" includes which of the following?
   a. the concept of ethical problems and public policies

b. the concept of family, friends, and relatives
c. the concept of the economics of care
d. the concept of managed care plans
e. all of the above

SHORT ANSWER MANAGEMENT PROBLEM

Using the case analysis approach to ethical decision making, consider the following case and attempt to arrive at an ethical solution.

A 71-year-old female in your care in the hospital has advanced ovarian cancer that is rapidly progressing to the point where the patient is extremely cachectic, taking almost nothing by mouth, and beginning to exhibit Cheyne-Stokes respiration. Her daughter comes to you and confronts you with the following statement: "Doctor, you are under no circumstances to offer my mother anything less than an all-out resuscitative effort in the event that she arrests while undergoing treatment in this hospital."

ANSWERS

A1. **e.** The best response to this kind of request from a member of the patient's immediate family is to ask to meet with the family as soon as possible. At that time you should gently point out the following:

a. Most patients who have a terminal disease know they have one; to refuse to discuss the patient's condition with the patient is in no one's best interest and in fact violates the Medical Code of Ethics.

b. Ask the family to be present when you discuss the results of the tests with the patient. Reassure the daughter and the rest of the family that one of the first questions you will ask of the patient is "How much do you know about your disease?" to be followed shortly by "Are you the kind of person who wants to know everything, or are you the kind of person who would rather just leave everything up to us?"

In most cases a response as described from a member of the immediate family indicates that there is some "unfinished business" that the family would rather not discuss. It is in everyone's best interest for this to be allowed to surface.

A2. **b.** Patients in the terminal phase of a malignant disease should rarely, if ever, be subjected to a CPR attempt. It is rare that a patient with a terminal malignancy is successfully resuscitated with basic life support and ACLS protocols.

A3. **e.** The patient has every right to ask about her results, and you have an ethical responsibility to provide her with as much information as she requests and can handle emotionally. The best plan in the case described is a call to the attending physician to let him know that the patient has "specifically asked you about the results." If the attending physician refuses to discuss the results the next day, you may have to take this to a higher level. Your best approach in this case is a telephone call to the chairman of your local hospital ethics committee for advice and action.

A4. **c.** This type of situation and the remarks associated with it are a lot more common than we admit or believe. This situation can be neither accepted nor condoned.

It is at least partially attributable to the physician's lack of training in breaking bad news. That, however, is not the entire picture. It is an example of a complete lack of compassion and understanding on the part of the attending physician. It is both unacceptable and unethical.

A5. **c.** This patient has come to you as a patient and because of the fiduciary doctor-patient relationship you have a responsibility to discuss her options with her. In this case, referral for counseling would be very appropriate and, depending on her subsequent decision, will allow you to decide how much personal involvement you wish to have. You must, however, separate your personal beliefs from your responsibilities as a physician. Even in cases in which ethical dilemmas are prominent, you can usually provide the medical care necessary for your patient's well being and at the same time not sacrifice your personal beliefs and convictions.

A6. **d.** The response of the parents to this request is quite typical and common. First, the parents have certainly not completed their grief work (especially if hope for a good outcome was put forward to them). Second, they may well have been exposed to the criticism of their son "taking up valuable resources" potentially usable for an infant with a better prognosis by some overt or inadvertent comment. Third, parents may misinterpret something that you said or the manner in which it was said. A family conference with significant support available for the parents is the preferred method for resolving this situation. Time will be a key that will enable the parents to see the logic of your arguments as well as the nature and reasons for your suggestions. It is important to recognize anticipatory grieving in situations like this. Anticipatory grieving is grieving that takes place before the actual death. It is important to recognize that this may "blunt" the response of the parents at the time of the death itself.

A7. **a.** Legislation written and passed by the United States Congress requires that patients be informed of their right to decide on life-supporting treatment in the event of a catastrophic complication resulting from hospitalization. This is known as the Patient Self-Determination Act.

A8. **d.** In recent years the concept of "advance directives" has emerged and has been widely promoted as a solution to the dilemma expressed by patients concerning their potential inability to make crucial decisions about their medical care when they become mentally incompetent. The general term *advance directive* covers the following:
  a. The legal instrument entitled "Directive to Physicians" enacted in the Natural Death Acts of various states in the union
  b. The less formal "living will"
  c. The Durable Power of Attorney for Health Care (which includes medical decision making capacity)

A9. **e.** Clinical ethics are an intrinsic aspect of medical practice. Like diagnosis, prognosis, and treatment, ethical considerations are essential in clinical care issues. The ethics of any particular case arise out of both the facts and the values embedded in the case itself. This is most easily accomplished by dividing the considerations of the case into four categories:
  a. Medical indications for interventions and treatment
  b. Patient preferences (also referred to as patient autonomy)
  c. Quality-of-life issues
  d. Contextual features
Details of these categories are considered later in this problem.

A10. **e.** Indications for medical intervention include the following:
  a. Beneficence: The duty to assist patients in need
  b. Nonmaleficence: The duty to "first do no harm"
  c. Clinical judgment: Judgment regarding the purely "clinical facts" of the case. Recognize that clinical judgments are made considering a matrix of facts and values that are susceptible to the influence of negative attitudes. Clinical judgments also reflect tacit inclinations about risk avoidance, skepticism about intervention, enthusiasm for innovation, peer esteem, and other personal values.
  d. Realistic understanding of the goals of treatment: What exactly are you attempting to accomplish, and why are you trying to accomplish it?

  e. Medical futility: A desire to define when a proposed treatment is, in fact, useless
  f. The moribund patient: Best defined as "eminent death"
  g. The terminally ill patient: Most commonly the considerations concerning palliative treatment in a patient with cancer or other irreversible disorder
  h. Medical indications and contraindications for the performance of CPR

A11. **d.** Patient preferences and patient autonomy must, by their very nature, include analysis and synthesis of the following concepts:
  a. Paternalism: Overriding or ignoring a person's preferences when you believe it will benefit them or enhance their welfare
  b. Informed consent: Informed consent is defined as the willing acceptance of a medical intervention by a patient after adequate disclosure by the physician of the nature of the intervention. Disclosure is judged "adequate" by two standards:
     1) Information that is commonly provided by competent practitioners in the community or in the specialty
     2) Information that would allow a reasonable person to make prudent choices on their own behalf
  c. Mental capacity: The ability to understand, on the basis of intelligence and comprehension, what is being said or asked of a patient on the part of that patient
  d. Refusal of treatment: Reasons for refusal of treatment
  e. Advance directives/living wills (discussed in Answer 8)

A12. **e.** Quality of life can best be defined as the subjective satisfaction expressed or experienced by an individual in his or her physical, mental, and social situation. Quality-of-life considerations include:
  a. The distinction between quality of life (as just defined) and sanctity of life (the concept that human life is so valuable that it must be preserved at all costs, under any conditions, and for as long as possible)
  b. Subjective versus objective considerations in quality of life: Who is defining quality in this case, and how does your (or someone else's) definition compare with the definition given by the patient? As well, how does a subjective determination of quality of life compare to objective criteria? These objective criteria include con-

sideration of "restricted quality of life" and "minimal quality of life."
  c. Mental retardation: Who defines quality here?
  d. Issues concerning nutrition and hydration
  e. Euthanasia with all its implications and definitions (active, passive, physician-assisted suicide, etc.)
  f. Pain and symptom relief (especially in terminal cancer)
  g. Suicide

A13. **e.** Contextual features in ethical decision making are diverse, complicated, and multiple. The most important considerations include the following:
  a. The possible conflict between physician responsibilities to the patient and physician responsibilities to the society. This is most clearly articulated in matters concerning cost.
  b. The multiple responsibilities of physicians and methods of resolving how to resolve conflict between those responsibilities: The responsibility to the patient (first and foremost); the responsibility to society; the responsibility to other health professionals; and the responsibility to self.
  c. The role of the patient's next of kin in ethical decision making
  d. The importance of confidentiality of patient information
  e. The importance of the public welfare; that is, is the patient a danger to others? If so, how can those "others" be identified without revealing confidential information?
  f. The concept of patient safety
  g. The economics of care, including ever-decreasing health care resources, health care rights versus privilege, emergency care, prospective payments and diagnostic related groups, and managed care plans
The term *contextual features* is also known as *distributive justice*.

SOLUTION TO THE SHORT ANSWER MANAGEMENT PROBLEM

  a. Medical intervention:
    1) Indications for medical intervention:
      a) Very serious and aggressive tumor
      b) Advanced state of cachexia at present
      c) No likelihood that patient will improve
      d) Symptoms objectively distressing
    2) Conclusion to indications for medical intervention issue:
      a) Very reasonable to offer interventions that

will increase the comfort and reduce the pain and suffering of the patient
      b) Illogical to offer interventions that will, in the long run, only prolong death, not life
  b. Patient preferences:
    1) Issues
      a) The patient has not been consulted as to her wishes vis-á-vis life-support systems.
      b) We have no indication that the wishes of the patient's daughter bear any relationship to the wishes of the patient.
    2) Conclusion to patient preference issue: The patient must, in some manner, be asked about her understanding regarding the disease process and wishes that stem from that knowledge.
  c. Quality of life:
    1) Issues
      a) Objectively, her quality of life appears to be low and decreasing daily.
      b) Again, however, we have no knowledge of how the patient rates her own quality of life.
    2) Conclusion to quality-of-life issue: A discussion with the patient must take place. The information that should be discussed includes the patient's knowledge of the condition and its progress, her own assessment of quality of life, and her wishes concerning treatments that are and are not acceptable.
  d. Contextual features:
    1) Issues
      a) In this case the main contextual feature is the insistence of the daughter to "pull out all the stops" and "spare no effort—no matter what."
      b) No idea as to why the daughter feels this way: is there some unfinished business?
    2) Conclusion regarding contextual features issue:
      a) Talk to the daughter; ask her why she has requested the aggressive interventions.
      b) Discuss with the daughter the concept of "medical futility."
  e. Summary of this case
This is basically an ethical situation in which the concept of indications for medical intervention indicates that aggressive resuscitative attempts are not only not indicated, but also completely futile. This is counterbalanced by the concept of contextual features in which the daughter is insisting that "everything be done."
What is done will be determined by patient preferences in which the patient outlines to all not only her

knowledge of the disease process and its effect on her quality of life but her desires for "heroic measures" to be or not to be undertaken on her behalf.

SUMMARY OF ETHICAL DECISION MAKING ISSUES

1. Ethical decision making can be based on a case analysis method.

2. Case analysis considers four categories:
   a. Indications for medical intervention
   b. Patient preferences
   c. Quality of life
   d. Contextual (or societal) features

3. The most common disagreements involve indications for intervention; patient preferences; and quality-of-life disagreement between individual patient values or autonomy, indications or lack of same for treatment, and one or another of various societal pressures.

4. Golden Rule 1 of Medical Ethics: *Primum non nocere*—first, do no harm (nonmaleficence).

5. Golden Rule 2 of Medical Ethics: Consider first the welfare of the patient (beneficence)

6. Medical futility: A treatment that has no or an extremely remote chance of doing any good whatsoever should not be undertaken. For purposes of security, that really should mean zero chance (as with CPR in a terminal cancer patient with Cheyne-Stokes respiration).

7. There is absolutely no substitute for good doctor-patient communication and good interprofessional health care communication in biomedical ethics.

SUGGESTED READINGS

Goodman MD et al: Effect of advanced directives on the management of elderly critically ill patients, *Crit Care Med* 26(4):701-704, 1998.

Gordon NP, Shade SB: Advanced directives are more likely among seniors asked about end-of-life preferences, *Arch Intern Med* 159(7):701-704, 1999.

Jonsen AR et al: *Clinical ethics*, ed 3, New York, 1992, McGraw-Hill.

Kashiwagi T: Truth telling and palliative medicine, *Intern Med* 38(2):190-192, 1999.

Ott BB: Advanced directives: the emerging body of research, *Am J Crit Care* 8(1):514-519, 1999.

Post SG et al: Physicians and patient spirituality: Professional boundaries, competency, ethics, *Ann Intern Med* 132(7):578-583, 2000.

Sloan RP et al: Religion, spirituality, and medicine, *Lancet* 53(9153):664-667, 1999.

PROBLEM · 116

SENILE DEMENTIA AND DELIRIUM

"Officer, I've Lived in the Same House for the Past 45 Years, but I Can't Seem to Locate It Today. Can You Help Me?"

Case 1 ■ A 78-Year-Old Female with Increasing Confusion, Memory Impairment, and Inability to Look after Herself

A 78-year-old female is brought to the Emergency Department by her daughter. The patient lives alone in an apartment, and her daughter is concerned about her ability to carry on living independently. Her daughter tells you that her mother began having difficulty with her memory 2 years ago, and since that time she has deteriorated in a slow, steady manner.

She is, however, not totally incapacitated. She is able to perform some of the activities of daily living, including dressing and bathing. When she cooks for herself, however, she often leaves burners on, and when she drives the car she often gets lost. She has had four motor vehicle accidents in the past 3 months. Her daughter became alarmed when she learned that her mother had gone to the bank and withdrawn the entire contents of her $80,000 savings account to "give to her new boyfriend." She had asked for the entire amount in $1 bills and argued with the bank teller upon learning that this was impossible.

The daughter states that her mother's memory and confusion have been getting worse. Her personality has changed; she now displays periods of both agitation and aggression.

On examination, the patient's "mini-mental status" examination is 8/30. Her blood pressure is 170/95 mm Hg, and her pulse is 84 and irregular. There is a grade II/VI systolic heart murmur heard along the left sternal edge. Examination of the respiratory system is normal. Examination of the abdomen is normal. Digital rectal examination reveals some hard stool. A detailed neurologic and musculoskeletal examination cannot be carried out.

SELECT THE BEST ANSWER TO THE FOLLOWING QUESTIONS

Q1. Based on this history, what is the most likely diagnosis in this patient?
   a. Alzheimer's disease
   b. multiinfarct dementia
   c. major depressive disorder
   d. hypothyroidism
   e. mixed dementia

Q2. At this time, what would you do?
   a. order an appropriate cost-effective laboratory investigation
   b. arrange for the patient to be admitted to a chronic care facility and placate the daughter
   c. prescribe diazepam for the daughter and haloperidol for the patient
   d. refer the patient for immediate consultation with a geriatrician
   e. begin a trial of a tricyclic antidepressant

Q3. Which of the following diseases is the most common treatable disease confused with Alzheimer's disease in elderly patients?
   a. hypothyroidism
   b. multiinfarct dementia
   c. congestive heart failure
   d. major depressive disorder
   e. normal pressure hydrocephalus

Q4. Which of the following statements regarding Alzheimer's disease is true?
   a. Alzheimer's disease is present to some degree in all persons who are more than 80 years old
   b. Alzheimer's disease is a rapidly progressive dementia
   c. Alzheimer's disease is easy to differentiate from other dementias
   d. Alzheimer's disease is a pathologic diagnosis
   e. Alzheimer's disease usually has a sudden onset

Q5. In contrast to dementia, patients with depression often:
   a. complain about their cognitive deficits
   b. deny that their cognitive deficits exist
   c. try to conceal their cognitive deficits
   d. try to answer questions even if they do not know the answers
   e. perform consistently on tasks of equal difficulty

Q6. In contrast to dementia, the cognitive impairment associated with depression often:
   a. comes on more slowly
   b. comes on more rapidly
   c. is less of an impairment
   d. is not improved with the administration of an antidepressant
   e. none of the above is true

Q7. Reversible causes of confusion in the elderly is (are):
   a. drug intoxication
   b. hypothyroidism
   c. pernicious anemia

   d. hyponatremia
   e. all of the above

Q8. A cost-effective workup of a confused elderly patient does not include:
   a. a complete blood count (CBC)
   b. an electrolyte profile
   c. a plasma glucose level
   d. a computed tomography (CT) scan of the head
   e. all of the above investigations are cost-effective

Q9. After a complete dementia workup, you are unsure whether or not a patient has Alzheimer's disease or a major depressive disorder. At this time, what would you do?
   a. reexamine the patient in 3 months
   b. suggest a trial of electroconvulsive therapy
   c. arrange for the patient to be admitted to a nursing home and begin supportive psychotherapy
   d. prescribe a trial of an antidepressant
   e. none of the above

Q10. Which of the following is (are) important aspects of dementia management?
   a. maintenance of a daily routine
   b. making the environment safe
   c. assessment of family support
   d. minimization of external stimuli
   e. all of the above

Q11. Elderly patients frequently develop "acute confusional states." Acute confusional states are also known as which of the following?
   a. dementia
   b. delusional states
   c. delirium
   d. pseudodementia
   e. pseudodelirium

Q12. Which of the following is (are) associated with acute confusional states in the elderly?
   a. global cognitive impairment
   b. decreased level of consciousness
   c. increased or reduced psychomotor activity
   d. disorganized sleep-wake cycle (rapid eye movement and nonrapid eye movement sleep)
   e. all of the above

Q13. What is the most common cause of dementia in the elderly?
   a. drug-induced dementia
   b. multiinfarct dementia

c. pseudodementia
d. Alzheimer's disease
e. atherosclerotic dementia

Q14. What is the most common symptom and finding in patients with Alzheimer's disease?
a. a progressive decline in intellectual function
b. memory loss
c. impairment in judgment
d. impairment in problem solving
e. impaired orientation

Q15. What is the most important risk factor for a patient acquiring Alzheimer's disease?
a. history of head injury
b. history of thyroid disease
c. a family history of dementia
d. history of psychiatric disease

Q16. Which of the following characteristics regarding the epidemiology of Alzheimer's disease is (are) true?
a. the prevalence of Alzheimer's disease at age 65 varies from a low of 971/100,000 persons in Turku, Finland to 10,300/100,000 persons in East Boston, USA
b. the incidence of acute Alzheimer's disease increases acutely with age
c. in the average American city or town, the prevalence of Alzheimer's disease at age 85 years is 30%
d. there appears to be some cultural and ethnic variation in incidence and prevalence of Alzheimer's disease in the United States
e. all of the above statements are true

Q17. What is (are) the histologic criteria for diagnosing Alzheimer's disease post mortem?
a. senile plaques
b. neuronal loss
c. neurofibrillary tangles (NFTs)
d. a and c
e. all of the above

Q18. What is the treatment of choice for Alzheimer's disease at present?
a. tacrine
b. phosphatidylcholine
c. donepezil
d. physostigmine
e. none of the above

Q19. The main predisposing factors for delirium include which of the following?
a. age over 65 years
b. brain damage

c. chronic cerebral disease
d. b and c only
e. all of the above

Q20. The best-documented hypothesis for delirium suggests which of the following?
a. a serotonin deficiency
b. a norepinephrine deficiency
c. an acetylcholine deficiency
d. a dopamine deficiency
e. a catecholamine imbalance

Q21. What is the most important investigation for patients suspected for having delirium?
a. a CT scan of the head
b. a magnetic resonance imaging scan of the head
c. an electroencephalogram (EEG)
d. a positron emission tomography scan
e. a CBC

SHORT ANSWER MANAGEMENT PROBLEM

Part A: Using the mnemonic DEMENTIA and selecting at least one cause (but in some cases many causes) for each letter, construct a complete differential diagnosis of confusion in the elderly.

Part B: List and briefly describe the distinct disorders that are part of the differential diagnosis of delirium.

ANSWERS

A1. **a.** The most likely diagnosis is Alzheimer's disease. The slow, insidious course of the decline is much more characteristic of Alzheimer's disease than of any other dementive process.

Multiinfarct dementia, in contrast, tends to produce a stepwise decline, with each step (or each decline) being temporally related to a small infarct.

Major depressive disorder tends to come on rather abruptly. This is discussed in detail in Problem 60 and with specific relevance to the geriatric patient in Answers 5 and 6 as well. Hypothyroidism must always be considered as a reversible cause of dementia, but in this case this is an unlikely cause of the symptoms.

Dementia is characterized by evidence of short-term and long-term memory impairment with impaired abstract thinking, impaired judgment, disturbances of higher cortical thinking, and personality changes.

A2. **a.** Alzheimer's disease is a diagnosis of exclusion. Before a patient is labeled as having Alzheimer's disease, a complete history, a complete physical examination, and a cost-effective laboratory evaluation need to be performed. It is inappropriate to arrange care in a chronic care facility and to treat patients (even with an antidepressant) until a dementia workup has been done.

An appropriate cost-effective workup of dementia includes a complete history, a complete physical examination (including a neuropsychiatric evaluation), a CBC, a blood glucose, serum electrolytes, serum calcium, serum creatinine, and serum TSH. Other tests should be done only if there is a specific indication (e.g., vitamin B_{12} and folate if macrocytosis is present). A CT scan should be performed only if there is a specific clinical indication.

A3. **d.** The most common treatable disease confused with Alzheimer's disease in elderly patients is depression. It has been estimated that up to 15% of patients who are labeled with Alzheimer's disease actually have a major depressive disorder. Many more patients with Alzheimer's disease have depression as a clinical feature of the disease itself.

Depression, whether the primary diagnosis or a diagnosis secondary to Alzheimer's disease, will respond to pharmacotherapy and psychotherapy.

A4. **d.** Alzheimer's disease is a pathologic diagnosis.

The prevalence of Alzheimer's disease increases with age to a prevalence level of approximately 30% in patients over the age of 80 years. It is certainly not present in all patients over any age.

The clinical progression of Alzheimer's disease is usually slow and insidious, not rapidly progressive.

It is not easy to differentiate Alzheimer's disease from other conditions or other entities. Because of the slow and insidious onset of the disease, it often goes unnoticed by both friends and family.

A5. **a.** In contrast to patients with dementia, depressed patients often complain about their cognitive deficits.

A6. **b.** Also in contrast to dementia, the cognitive impairment associated with depression usually comes on rapidly. It is apparent that something is wrong. Other features that suggest depression include the following:
   a. A personal or family history of psychiatric illness (especially major depressive disorder), bipolar affective disorder, and alcoholism
   b. Depressive symptoms preceding cognitive changes
   c. Feelings of hopelessness, guilt, and worthlessness
   d. A poor affect on psychologic testing

A7. **e.** Causes of confusion in the elderly, many of which are reversible, may be grouped under the following headings:
   a. Drug intoxication (including alcohol)

   b. Emotional disorders
   c. Metabolic disorders
   d. Sensory disorders
   e. Environmental changes
   f. Neoplasms (benign and malignant)
   g. Trauma
   h. Infectious disorders
   i. Inflammatory disorders
   j. Atherosclerotic disorders
   k. Cardiovascular disorders (not included under atherosclerotic disorders)
   l. Dementia
   m. Anemia
   n. Endocrine disorders

In this scheme (which is expanded in the Short Answer Management Problem), the choices offered in the question fall under the following:
   a. Drug intoxication (item a)
   b. Hypothyroidism (item n)
   c. Pernicious anemia (item m)
   d. Hyponatremia (item c)

A8. **d.** See Answer 2.

A9. **d.**
   a. It can often be difficult to differentiate a dementia from a depression.
   b. A dementia may have, as part of its symptomatology, depressive symptoms.
   c. Depression is reversible; dementia is not.

Thus a cautious trial of an antidepressant can be both a diagnostic test and a therapeutic trial.

Tricyclic antidepressants (especially nortriptyline and desipramine) and the selective serotonin reuptake inhibitors are the most commonly used agents for the geriatric patient. In an elderly patient, you want to do the following:
   a. Maximize the benefit from the antidepressant without producing an adverse drug reaction.
   b. Start low and go slow.
   c. Select an agent that has low anticholinergic, alpha-adrenergic, and antihistaminic side effects.

The tricyclic antidepressant of choice in elderly patients is nortriptyline. The starting dosage in an elderly patient should be 10 mg.

A10. **e.** The management of dementia in the elderly involves both behavioral methods and pharmacologic methods.

Regarding behavioral management, the following four principles apply to all elderly patients with a dementia-like syndrome:
   a. External stimuli (especially external stimuli that may confuse, worry, or upset the elder) should be kept to a minimum.

b. A daily routine that does not vary by any significant degree should be established and maintained.

c. The environmental safety of the particular residence or facility should be maximized. This includes attention to the maximization of lighting in the home or facility; the minimization of significant noise or distractions; the installation of handrails in hallways and rooms and at bathtub edges; and the minimization of stairs in the living accommodations of the patient.

d. Support the elder's family and offer respite care where and when needed.

A11. c. Delirium is also known as an acute confusional state.

A12. e. Delirium represents one of the most common mental disorders seen in the institutionalized elder. Despite its frequency and association with many diseases and disorders, it is frequently misdiagnosed or not diagnosed at all.

Delirium is defined as an organic mental syndrome featuring the following:
a. Global cognitive impairment
b. Disturbances in attention and attention span
c. Reduced level of consciousness
d. Increased or decreased psychomotor activity
e. Disorganized sleep-wake cycles

The onset of delirium is acute (a matter of hours or a few days at the very most) and seldom exceeds 1 month.

The severity of symptoms of delirium fluctuates unpredictably over the course of a day and seems to be most marked during a sleepless night. Delirium can occur at any age but is most common in those individuals over the age of 65 years.

A13. d. The most common cause of dementia in the elderly is Alzheimer's disease.

The wording is important in this question. Drugs do not cause dementia; they cause delirium.

The only other cause of dementia listed in the question is multiinfarct dementia, which is equivalent to atherosclerotic dementia. The latter term is not commonly used.

The other choice in the question, pseudodementia, is really a misnomer. Pseudodementia really represents depression that has been incorrectly diagnosed as an irreversible dementia.

A14. b. Memory loss is the most common presenting feature of Alzheimer's disease, but a personality change or an impairment in the ability to perform intellectual tasks such as calculations may herald the onset.

The five major clinical manifestations of Alzheimer's disease are as follows:
a. Memory loss: Initially the memory loss is a loss for recent events only and is associated with an inability to learn new information. Recall of past events and previously acquired information becomes impaired at a somewhat later stage. Memory loss is the most common presenting feature of Alzheimer's disease.

b. Language impairment: Language impairment is also common among patients with Alzheimer's disease. The term *anomia,* or "word-finding difficulty," often begins with the onset of dementia. This feature usually progresses to a transcortical, sensory-like aphasia.

   Severe language disturbance is a poor prognostic feature of Alzheimer's disease.

c. Visuospatial disturbance: Patients with Alzheimer's disease are often characterized by a difficulty in getting around the neighborhood or house. Practical examples of visuospatial disturbances in patients with Alzheimer's disease include difficulty following directions and getting lost in a familiar place or in familiar surroundings.

d. Loss of interest in activities: The loss of interest in activities such as personal habits or community affairs parallels the intellectual decline already discussed. This may be Alzheimer's disease first and an accompanying depression second or a primary depression manifesting itself as Alzheimer's disease.

e. Delusions and hallucinations: Delusions and hallucinations are prevalent in patients with Alzheimer's disease and tend to indicate a poor prognosis.

A15. d. A family history of Alzheimer's disease is an important risk in acquiring Alzheimer's disease, especially at a younger age. Advanced age is also a risk factor, with more than 30% of those older than 85 developing some degree of Alzheimer's disease.

A16. e. The epidemiology of Alzheimer's disease is fascinating. Because the cumulative incidence of Alzheimer's disease increases rapidly, the prevalence at age 85 in the United States averages 30% of the population (this figure includes both institutionalized and community-based elderly). There is obviously a significant difference depending on the individual's capacity to look after himself or herself, but this really becomes a circular argument.

One excellent review of the literature indicates a significant difference in prevalence depending on geographic location. For example, Turku, Finland has a prevalence of only 971/100,000 population. East Boston has an estimated prevalence of 10,300/100,000 population. This is extremely difficult to explain, and one wonders whether or not there was a significant difference in diagnostic criteria or a significant difference in case assessment criteria.

A17. **d.** As mentioned previously, Alzheimer's disease really is a pathologic diagnosis. The diagnostic criteria of The National Institute on Aging for this disease are as follows:
  a. The quantity of senile plaques (age-specific): Senile plaques are microscopic lesions comprised of a significant percentage of amyloid.
  b. The quantity of NFTs (age-specific): NFTs, initially described in 1907, are neuronal cytoplasmic collections of tangled filaments present in abundance in the neocortex, hippocampus, amygdala, basal forebrain, substantia nigra, locus ceruleus, and other brainstem nuclei.

Although these are the two criteria on which the diagnosis of Alzheimer's disease is based, the following is a complete list of all of the microscopic lesions seen in the brain of a patient with Alzheimer's disease:
  a. Neuritic plaques
  b. NFTs
  c. Amyloid degeneration
  d. Neuronal loss

Most patients with Alzheimer's disease have a slight reduction in total brain weight, with the majority ranging from 900 to 1100 g. Mild to moderate cerebral atrophy is often present.

A18. **c.** The primary treatment for Alzheimer's patients includes the use of the cholinesterase inhibitors tacrine and donepezil. These medications appear to improve cognitive function, and several clinical studies and family assessments suggest they also improve daily living function, which should lead to delay in nursing home placement. Although both are used, donepezil is preferred as a first-line medication because it need only be taken once a day, has shorter introductory period, and lacks the liver toxicity associated with tacrine.

A19. **e.** Delirium (acute confusional state) is caused by one or more organic factors that bring about widespread cerebral dysfunction.

The factors associated with delirium can be divided into the following subcategories:
  a. Predisposing factors
    1) Older than 65 years old
    2) Brain damage
    3) Chronic cerebral disease (such as Alzheimer's disease)
  b. Facilitating factors
    1) Psychologic stress
    2) Sleep loss or sleep deprivation
    3) Sensory deprivation or sensory overload
  c. Precipitating (organic) causal factors
    1) Primary cerebral diseases
    2) Systemic diseases affecting the brain secondarily
      a) Metabolic encephalopathies
      b) Neoplasms
      c) Infections
      d) Cardiovascular diseases
      e) Collagen vascular diseases
    3) Intoxication with exogenous substances
      a) Medical drugs
      b) Recreational drugs
      c) Poisons of plant, animal, or industrial origin
    4) Withdrawal from substances of abuse
      a) Alcohol
      b) Sedative-hypnotic drugs

One of the most common causes of delirium in the elderly is intoxication with anticholinergic drugs, such as tricyclic antidepressants given in doses that would be appropriate for a younger adult but not for a frail elderly patient.

The following are other common causes:
  a. Congestive cardiac failure
  b. Pneumonia
  c. Urinary tract infection
  d. Cancer
  e. Uremia
  f. Hypokalemia
  g. Dehydration
  h. Hyponatremia
  i. Epilepsy
  j. Cerebral infarction (right hemisphere)

Risk factors for delirium in hospitalized elderly patients include the following:
  a. Urinary tract infections
  b. Low serum albumin levels
  c. Elevated white blood cell count
  d. Proteinuria
  e. Prior cognitive impairment
  f. Limb fracture on admission
  g. Symptomatic infective disease
  h. Neuroleptic drugs
  i. Narcotic drugs
  j. Anticholinergic drugs

A20. **c.** The best-documented hypothesis for delirium in the elderly suggests that the syndrome results from a widespread imbalance of neurotransmitters. It is postulated that there is a reduction in brain metabolism that results in diminished cortical function. Impairment of cerebral oxidative metabolism results in reduced synthesis of neurotransmitters, especially acetylcholine, whose relative deficiency in the brain is a common denominator in metabolic-toxic encephalopathies. Hypoxia and hypoglycemia impair acetylcholine metabolism and bring about changes in mental function. The inhibition of acetylcholine metabolism may be caused by calcium-dependent release of the neurotransmitter. Thus the cholinergic deficit is currently the most convincing pathogenic hypothesis of delirium. Numerous experimental studies have shown that the syndrome can be readily induced by anticholinergic agents.

A21. **e.** As discussed in Answer 19, delirium is associated with many different abnormalities. One of the most important factors to rule out in the elderly is an underlying infection. Therefore a CBC would be required. It is a low-cost test that helps rule out infection, a common reversible cause of delirium in the elderly.

SOLUTION TO THE SHORT ANSWER MANAGEMENT PROBLEM

Part A: The following is an all-inclusive mnemonic on confusion in the elderly. This includes both reversible causes and nonreversible causes. The mnemonic is DEMENTIA.

D   **D**rug intoxication (especially anticholinergic agents), but includes alcohol abuse

E   **E**yes and ears (especially cataracts, diabetes mellitus, and sensorineural hearing loss)
Environment (a new environment is a sure trigger for acute confusional state)

M   **M**etabolic, including:
  a. Hyponatremia
  b. Hypokalemia
  c. Hyperkalemia
  d. Hypercalcemia
  e. Elevated blood urea nitrogen
  f. Elevated serum creatinine
  g. Elevated gamma-GT

E   **E**motional, including:
  a. Major depressive disorder
  b. Bipolar affective disorder
  c. Schizoaffective disorder
  d. Chronic schizophrenia
  e. Pseudodementia (depression masking as dementia)
  f. Adverse drug reaction (propranolol causes depression)
Endocrine, including:
  a. Hypothyroidism
  b. Hyperthyroidism
  c. Hyperglycemia
  d. Hypoglycemia

N   **N**eoplasms, including:
  a. Benign neoplasms (rare)
  b. Malignancies
    1) Breast cancer
    2) Lung cancer
    3) Colon cancer
    4) Prostate cancer
    5) Lymphomas
    6) Multiple myeloma
Neurologic
  a. Normal pressure hydrocephalus
  b. Parkinson's disease
  c. Huntington's disease

T   **T**rauma: Chronic subdural hematoma is most common. Burr holes can be life saving in a rural center, if recognized.

I   **I**nfections (in order of frequency as a cause of delirium in three groups of elderly patients)
  a. Infections predominating in hospitalized patients with delirium
    1) Urinary tract infection
    2) Bacterial pneumonia
    3) Surgical wound infections
  b. Infections predominating in nursing home patients who develop delirium
    1) Bacterial pneumonia
    2) Urinary tract infection
    3) Decubitus ulcer
  c. Independent, previously healthy individuals living in the community
    1) Bacterial pneumonia
    2) Urinary tract infection
    3) Intraabdominal infections (appendicitis, diverticulitis)
    4) Infective endocarditis
Inflammatory
  a. New onset/recurrent inflammatory bowel disease (ulcerative colitis or regional enteritis)
  b. Collagen vascular disorders
    1) Rheumatoid arthritis
    2) Systemic lupus erythematosus
    3) Musculoskeletal system
      a) Polymyalgia rheumatica. If not treated properly this can lead to serious consequences, such as blindness. (For a detailed discussion see Problem 117.)
      b) Polymyositis/dermatomyositis
    4) Pericarditis
    5) Pleuritis
    6) Biliary colic
    7) Renal colic
    8) Chronic pancreatitis

A   **A**nemia
  a. Iron-deficiency anemia

b. Anemia of chronic disease

c. Macrocytic anemia (vitamin B_{12} or folate deficiency)

Atherosclerotic vascular disease or cardiovascular disease

a. Myocardial infarction

b. Pulmonary embolism

c. Cerebrovascular accident (stroke)

d. Congestive cardiac failure

e. Alzheimer's and other dementias

    1) Alzheimer's disease

    2) Multiinfarct dementia

    3) Parkinson's disease

    4) Huntington's disease

Part B: The distinct disorders that are part of the complex called *delirium* include the following:

a. Global disorder of cognition: this constitutes one of the essential features of delirium. In this sense, *global* refers to the main cognitive functions including the following:

    1) Memory

    2) Thinking

    3) Perception

    4) Information acquisition

    5) Information processing

    6) Information retention

    7) Information retrieval

    8) Utilization of information

These cognitive deficits and abnormalities constitute an essential diagnostic feature of delirium.

b. Global disorder of attention: disturbances of the major aspects of attention are invariably present. Alertness (vigilance), that is, readiness to respond to sensory stimuli, and the ability to mobilize, shift, sustain, and direct attention at will are always disturbed to some extent.

c. Reduced level of consciousness: This implies a diminished awareness of oneself and one's surroundings to respond to sensory inputs in a selective and sustained manner and to be able to relate the incoming information to previously acquired knowledge.

d. Disordered sleep-wake cycle: Disorganization of the sleep-wake cycle is one of the essential features of delirium. Wakefulness is abnormally increased and the patient sleeps little or not at all or it is reduced during the day but excessive during the night.

e. Disorder of psychomotor behavior: A disturbance of both verbal and nonverbal psychomotor activity is the last essential feature of delirium. A delirious patient can be predominantly either hyperactive or hypoactive. Some patients shift unpredictably from abnormally increased psychomotor activity to lethargy and vice versa.

SUMMARY OF SENILE DEMENTIA AND DELIRIUM

The answer to Part A of the Short Answer Management Problem (the mnemonic for confusion in the elderly) serves as the summary for this problem.

SUGGESTED READINGS

Beardsley T: Putting Alzheimer's to the tests, *Sci Am* 272(2):12-13, 1995.

Fretwell M: Cognitive dysfunction. In Ferri FF, ed: *Practical guide to the care of the geriatric patient,* New York, 1997, McGraw-Hill.

Lipowski ZJ: Delirium (acute confusional states). In Hazzard WR et al, eds: *Principles of geriatric medicine and gerontology,* ed 3, New York, 1994, McGraw-Hill.

Mayeux R, Schofield PW: Alzheimer's disease. In Hazzard WR et al, eds: *Principles of geriatric medicine and gerontology,* ed 3, New York, 1994, McGraw-Hill.

Morris J: Alzheimer's disease: A review of clinical assessment and management issues, *Geriatrics* 52:suppl, 1997.

Tierney LM, Jr, McPhee SJ, Papadakis MA, eds: *Current medical diagnosis and treatment, 2000,* Stamford, Conn, 1999, Appleton & Lange.

PROBLEM · 1 1 7

POLYMYALGIA, RHEUMATICA, AND TEMPORAL ARTERITIS

"Well, Doctor, I Guess Old Age Arthritis Has Finally Caught Up with Me."

Case 1 ■ An 82-Year-Old Female with Aching and Stiffness in the Shoulder and Hip Girdles

An 82-year-old female comes to your office with a 6-month history of "stiffness" and "aching" in the shoulders and hips present for the last 3 months. The onset was quite abrupt. The stiffness and aching are bilateral in both upper and lower limbs. The symptoms are especially severe in the morning. The patient says that it is difficult to get out of a chair and difficult to move her arms above her head.

The patient also mentions significant malaise and fatigue and has experienced a 20-pound weight loss. She mentions a mild fever and also a feeling of "depression."

On examination, the patient's blood pressure and pulse are normal. Although the patient describes "significant weakness," there are no objective findings.

SELECT THE BEST ANSWER TO THE FOLLOWING QUESTIONS

Q1. What is the most likely diagnosis in this patient?

    a. osteoarthritis

    b. rheumatoid arthritis (RA)

c. polymyalgia rheumatica (PMR)
d. polymyositis
e. acute degenerative arthritis

Q2. Which of the following disorders is most closely associated with the geriatric population?
a. PMR
b. osteoarthritis
c. RA
d. degenerative arthritis
e. polymyositis

Q3. Which of the following statements regarding the condition described is (are) true?
a. the cause of the disease is unknown
b. this disease is most likely autoimmune in origin
c. the overall prevalence of this condition is approximately 17/100,000 patients
d. family aggregation of this disorder has been described
e. all of the above statements are true

Q4. Which of the following statements regarding this condition is (are) true?
a. there are no significant complications or related disorders of concern
b. hypothyroidism, hyperthyroidism, and hyperparathyroidism are part of the differential diagnosis
c. systemic lupus erythematosus must be considered a potential diagnostic possibility
d. b and c
e. all of the above statements are true

Q5. What is (are) the major difference(s) between this disorder and polymyositis?
a. marked proximal muscle weakness in polymyositis
b. marked proximal muscle tenderness in polymyositis
c. elevated muscle enzymes such as creatine kinase (CK) in polymyositis
d. a and b
e. all of the above

Q6. Which of the following is the investigation of choice in this condition?
a. muscle CK
b. erythrocyte sedimentation rate (ESR)
c. antinuclear antibody titer
d. rheumatoid factor titer
e. computed tomography scan of the shoulders and hip girdle

Q7. Which of the following is (are) neurologic manifestations of giant cell arteritis (GCA, also known as temporal arteritis)
a. depression
b. deafness
c. amaurosis fugax
d. paralysis
e. all of the above

Q8. Of the symptoms listed in Question 7, which is (are) the most worrisome?
a. depression
b. deafness
c. amaurosis fugax
d. paralysis
e. all of the symptoms are equally worrisome

Q9. The symptom(s) identified in Question 8 as most worrisome can lead to which of the following (greatly feared) complication of GCA?
a. permanent hemiplegia
b. permanent bilateral and complete sensorineural hearing loss
c. permanent monocular or binocular total blindness
d. permanent bilateral and complete sensorineural and conductive hearing losses
e. permanent quadriplegia

Q10. What is the treatment of choice for both PMR and GCA?
a. intravenous pulsed steroids
b. oral prednisone: 20 mg/day for PMR and 60 mg/day for GCA
c. oral methotrexate
d. cyclosporine IV every third day for 4 weeks
e. intravenous dihydroergotamine

Q11. What is the pathophysiologic cause of temporal arteritis?
a. inflammation of the middle meningeal artery
b. inflammation of the temporal artery
c. inflammation of the common carotid artery
d. inflammation of the internal carotid artery
e. inflammation of the external carotid artery

SHORT ANSWER MANAGEMENT PROBLEM
An 82-year-old female comes to your office with a history of shoulder girdle pain and hip pain progressing to involve other joints of the upper and lower extremities. Provide a differential diagnosis for this patient's pain.

ANSWERS

A1. **c.** The diagnosis in this patient is PMR. This is an important diagnosis to make in the elderly.

A2. **a.** Of all of the musculoskeletal conditions, PMR is most closely identified with the geriatric population.

PMR is a diagnosis that is often missed, a diagnosis in which vague symptoms are present, and a diagnosis that is often characterized by the patient's seeing multiple doctors without being correctly diagnosed.

PMR is characterized by aching and stiffness in the shoulder and hip girdles. Profound morning stiffness is especially suggestive of this disorder and should be specifically sought out. The diagnosis of PMR is seldom seen before the age of 50 years; its mean age of onset is 70 years. The onset may be either abrupt or gradual. The stiffness that is present in the hips and the shoulders may become generalized, involving the neck and knees and even extending into the wrists and fingers.

There are also prominent constitutional symptoms. These include symptoms such as malaise, weight loss, low-grade fever, and depression.

A3. **e.** The cause of PMR is unknown, although an autoimmune process appears to be related to the condition. The overall prevalence of PMR is 17/100,000 people. In addition, family aggregation is common.

A4. **d.** The differential diagnosis of PMR in the elderly includes hypothyroidism, hyperthyroidism, hyperparathyroidism, systemic lupus erythematosus, RA, osteoarthritis or degenerative arthritis, and polymyositis.

The single most important complication of concern in PMR is its association with giant cell arteritis (GCA). GCA will be discussed in subsequent questions.

A5. **e.** The differences between PMR and polymyositis on clinical examination are as follows:
   a. There is marked weakness associated with proximal muscle pain in polymyositis
   b. There is marked muscle tenderness associated with the proximal muscle pain in polymyositis
   c. Laboratory examination reveals elevated muscle enzymes only in polymyositis

A6. **b.** Both PMR and GCA are characterized by elevations in the ESR. Elevations to levels greater than 100 mm/hr may be seen in either disease; elevations to levels greater than 50 mm/hr are almost universal.

A7. **e.** Manifestations of temporal arteritis include headache, scalp tenderness, visual symptoms, jaw claudication, constitutional symptoms (fever, weight loss, anorexia, fatigue), polymyalgia symptoms (aching and stiffness of the trunk and proximal muscle groups), cough, and amaurosis fugax.

A8. **c.** Of the neurologic symptoms listed in Answer 7, the most worrisome symptom is amaurosis fugax. Amaurosis fugax, defined as brief visual loss, is related to ischemia of the posterior ciliary branch of the ophthalmic artery.

A9. **c.** The transient visual loss of amaurosis fugax may foretell by days, weeks, or sometimes even months the most dreaded complication, permanent monocular or binocular blindness. If any ocular involvement is present, IV methylprednisolone should be initiated immediately to try to prevent blindness.

A10. **b.** Oral prednisone is the treatment of choice for both PMR and GCA. The dosage is as follows:
   a. PMR: 20 mg/day PO for 4 weeks with gradual reduction thereafter but maintained for at least 1 year
   b. Temporal arteritis: 60 mg/day PO for 4 weeks with gradual reduction beginning at 4 weeks but with maintenance therapy for 1 to 2 years. Dosage should be adjusted by monitoring the ESR.

A11. **b.** From a pathologic point of view, the cause of temporal arteritis is inflammation of the temporal artery. From a local anatomic standpoint, this results in temporal headache (generally unilateral and accompanied by temporal artery swelling and tenderness). Temporal artery biopsy is the definitive diagnostic procedure for GCA and should include a segment at least 2 cm long.

SOLUTION TO THE SHORT ANSWER MANAGEMENT PROBLEM

Differential diagnosis:
a. Nonmusculoskeletal problems:
   1) Hypothyroidism
   2) Hyperthyroidism
   3) Hyperparathyroidism
b. Musculoskeletal problems:
   1) Systemic lupus erythematosus
   2) RA
   3) Osteoarthritis or degenerative arthritis
   4) PMR
   5) Polymyositis
c. Other important systemic conditions:
   1) Metastatic bone cancer
   2) Multiple myeloma

SUMMARY OF THE DIAGNOSIS AND TREATMENT OF POLYMYALGIA RHEUMATICA AND TEMPORAL ARTERITIS

1. PMR:
   a. Epidemiology: Of all the musculoskeletal conditions, none is so closely identified with the geriatric population as PMR.
   b. Prevalence rate: A prevalence rate of 17/100,000 persons over the age of 50 has been established (average age around 70 years old).
   c. Symptoms:
      1) Either sudden onset or gradual onset (gradual implies over a period of months, not years)
      2) Initial manifestation: Pain, aching, and stiffness in the shoulder girdle and hip girdle
      3) Profound morning stiffness
      4) Pain, aching, and stiffness progression to other joints in the upper and lower extremities
      5) Clue: The patient tells you that suddenly he or she can no longer get out of bed in the morning.
   d. Diagnosis: Elevated ESR (almost always greater than 50 mm/hr; frequently greater than 100 mm/hr)
   e. Complication: Temporal arteritis with eventual blindness
   f. Treatment: Prednisone, 20 mg/day for 1 month and taper; maintain for 1 year.
   g. Differential diagnosis: See the Short Answer Management Problem.

2. Temporal arteritis:
   a. Presenting signs and symptoms:
      1) The pain, aching, and stiffness in the shoulder and hip girdles as just described.
      2) Additional systemic signs and symptoms of inflammation include the following:
         a) Fever
         b) Weight loss
         c) Malaise
         d) Jaw claudication
         e) Transient visual complaints leading to blindness if left untreated
         f) Extremity claudication
         g) Aortic aneurysm
      3) Significant local signs and symptoms:
         a) Temporal headache (unilateral)
         b) Temporal artery swelling and tenderness
      4) Significant neurologic symptoms: See Answers 7 to 9.
   b. Diagnosis:
      1) ESR (as mentioned earlier)
      2) Temporal artery biopsy: If you suspect temporal arteritis, do not wait for a surgeon to perform a biopsy. Treat the condition with prednisone immediately.
      c. Complication: Permanent monocular or binocular blindness
      d. Treatment: High-dose prednisone: 60 mg/day for 4 weeks; taper slowly maintain for 1 to 2 years. If symptoms are ocular, use IV methylprednisolone immediately.

SUGGESTED READINGS

Eisenberg G: Polymyalgia rheumatica and giant cell arteritis. In Hazzard WR et al, eds: *Principles of geriatric medicine and gerontology,* ed 3, New York, 1994, McGraw-Hill.

Ferri F, ed: *The care of the geriatric patient,* St Louis, 1997, Mosby.

Tierney LM, Jr, McPhee SJ, Papadakis MA, eds: *Current medical diagnosis and treatment,* 2000, Stamford, Conn, 1999, Appleton & Lange.

PROBLEM · 118

HYPERTENSION MANAGEMENT IN THE ELDERLY

"Doc, Your Pills Don't Do No Good. That Top Number Still Is Always Much More Than 140."

Case 1 ■ An 80-Year-Old Male with Hypertension

An 80-year-old white male, previously healthy, comes to your office for a periodic health examination. He was last seen by a physician 20 years ago. His blood pressure is recorded as 215/95 mm Hg.

A complete history reveals no other cardiovascular risk factors. A complete physical examination reveals no evidence of end organ damage or secondary causes of hypertension.

Basic laboratory investigations, including a complete blood count, urinalysis, electrolytes, serum calcium, fasting blood sugar, plasma cholesterol, uric acid, and an electrocardiogram are all normal.

The patient is on a fixed income and is trying to keep up with payments for his wife's nursing home care.

SELECT THE BEST ANSWER TO THE FOLLOWING QUESTIONS

Q1. Based on the information given, what would you do now?
   a. begin therapy with a thiazide diuretic
   b. begin therapy with a calcium-channel blocker
   c. begin therapy with an angiotensin-converting enzyme (ACE) inhibitor
   d. begin therapy with a beta-blocker
   e. none of the above

Following further investigation and two more visits, appropriate therapy is prescribed for the patient described and he returns in 1 month for follow-up care. His blood pressure remains elevated at 205/92 mm Hg. A visit 1 week later yields the same blood pressure reading.

You also discuss nonpharmacologic treatment with him, and it appears obvious to you that he is not really prepared to alter his "hamburgers and chips (fried in pure lard)" diet. He also states that exercise would kill him.

Q2. What would you do now?
   a. prescribe a thiazide diuretic
   b. prescribe a calcium-channel blocker
   c. prescribe a beta-blocker
   d. prescribe an ACE inhibitor
   e. prescribe a vasodilator

Appropriate therapy is prescribed for the patient, and he returns in 1 month for follow-up care. His blood pressure is now 185/90 mm Hg and his serum potassium level has decreased from 4.0 mEq/L to 3.0 mEq/L.

Q3. At this time, what would you do?
   a. substitute an ACE inhibitor for the present medication
   b. substitute a calcium-channel blocker for the present medication
   c. substitute a beta-blocker for the present medication
   d. substitute a vasodilator for the present medication
   e. review the type and dose of the drug class being prescribed

The patient described has the necessary change to his medication treatment regime made. When he returns next month for follow-up care, his blood pressure is 175/90 mm Hg.

Q4. At this time, what would you do?
   a. add an ACE inhibitor
   b. add a calcium-channel blocker
   c. add a beta-blocker
   d. add a vasodilator
   e. maximize the dose of a beta-blocker

Q5. Which of the following statements regarding the treatment of hypertension in the elderly is (are) true?
   a. elderly patients with hypertension should not be treated
   b. the benefits of treating elderly hypertensive patients have not been established
   c. no change in morbidity or mortality has been demonstrated for elderly patients treated with antihypertensives
   d. elderly patients treated for hypertension are likely to benefit only from a reduction in cere-

brovascular morbidity and mortality, not cardiac morbidity or mortality
   e. none of the above is true

Q6. Regarding the epidemiologic importance of elevations in systolic versus diastolic blood pressure in elderly patients, which of the following statements is true?
   a. elevation of systolic blood pressure is not as important as elevation of diastolic blood pressure
   b. elevation of systolic blood pressure, although important, does not correlate well with cardiovascular morbidity and mortality
   c. elevations of systolic and diastolic blood pressure are equally important
   d. elevated systolic blood pressure is a greater risk for subsequent cardiovascular morbidity and mortality than diastolic blood pressure
   e. the relative importance of elevations in systolic blood pressure in terms of cardiovascular morbidity and mortality remains unclear

Q7. With respect to morbidity and mortality and treatment of systolic hypertension in the elderly, which of the following epidemiologic categories show(s) a significant decrease (compared to placebo) when systolic blood pressure is treated?
   a. total stroke morbidity
   b. total stroke mortality
   c. total coronary artery mortality
   d. a and b only
   e. all of the above
   f. none of the above

Q8. Which of the following drug combinations should be avoided in elderly hypertensive patients?
   a. hydrochlorothiazide (HCT)/amiloride and enalapril
   b. HCT/amiloride and nifedipine
   c. HCT/amiloride and atenolol
   d. HCT/amiloride and hydralazine
   e. HCT/amiloride and reserpine

Case 2 ■ A 75-Year-Old African-American Male with Angina Pectoris

A 75-year-old African-American male with angina pectoris is found, on physical examination, to have a blood pressure of 170/100 mm Hg. His angina is controlled on isosorbide dinitrate, 30 mg qid. His blood pressure reading is repeated on several occasions and remains unchanged.

Q9. At this time, what is the most reasonable treatment for this patient's blood pressure?
a. a calcium-channel blocker
b. a beta-blocker
c. a thiazide diuretic
d. an ACE inhibitor
e. a or c

Case 3 ■ A Hypertensive 72-Year-Old White Female with a Previous Myocardial Infarction and Mild Congestive Heart Failure

A 72-year-old white female with a previous myocardial infarction (MI) and mild congestive heart failure (CHF) (controlled with furosemide 40 mg qid) comes to your office for a routine assessment. She is found to have a blood pressure of 190/100 mm Hg. This reading is repeated on two occasions.

Q10. What would be the most appropriate treatment for her hypertension?
a. an ACE inhibitor
b. a calcium-channel blocker
c. a beta-blocker
d. a thiazide diuretic
e. none of the above

Case 4 ■ A Hypertensive 72-Year-Old White Male with Diabetes

A 72-year-old white male with a 20-year history of non-insulin–dependent diabetes mellitus is found to have a blood pressure of 170/105 mm Hg. He has no history of angina pectoris or other significant vascular disease. He had never been diagnosed as hypertensive.

His blood pressure is repeated on two additional occasions and the readings remain the same. Laboratory evaluation reveals microalbuminuria.

Q11. At this time, what would be the most appropriate treatment for this patient's blood pressure?
a. a thiazide diuretic
b. a beta-blocker
c. a calcium-channel blocker
d. an ACE inhibitor
e. a vasodilator

Q12. What is the recommended dosage of HCT for the treatment of hypertension in the elderly?
a. 12.5 to 25 mg
b. 25 to 50 mg
c. 50 to 75 mg
d. 75 to 100 mg
e. whatever you want

SHORT ANSWER MANAGEMENT PROBLEM

Part A: An 80-year-old African-American male with systolic hypertension (210/85 mm Hg) is a new patient to your practice. He says he has been healthy all of his life. From three consecutive readings you determine that the patient is truly hypertensive.

Discuss your approach to this patient with respect to education and counseling regarding his hypertension. Include lifestyle advice, medication advice, and other pertinent advice that you consider important.

Part B: Discuss the medication efficacy differences that have been demonstrated with respect to race and age in the following types of patients:
a. Young African-American patients
b. Young Caucasian patients
c. Elderly African-American patients
d. Elderly Caucasian patients

ANSWERS

A1. **e.** Even though this patient has a systolic blood pressure of 215 mm Hg, you should consider that this is only one reading and it cannot be assumed to represent his "true blood pressure," and that even if you were able to make the diagnosis of hypertension at this time, you would still want to begin with nonpharmacologic therapy.

This patient should have his blood pressure rechecked on two other occasions before the diagnosis of hypertension is made.

A2. **a.** Recent studies have clearly demonstrated the importance of treating systolic hypertension in the elderly, treating it, in fact, with the same rigor and aggressiveness as diastolic hypertension.

Because of the patient's fixed income and the proven efficacy of thiazide diuretics in reducing morbidity and mortality from cardiovascular disease, a low-dose (25-mg) thiazide diuretic would be the agent of choice.

A3. **e.** At this time, the most reasonable alternative would be to review both the dose and the drug class.

On the positive side, this patient's systolic blood pressure has dropped significantly (from 205 to 185 mm Hg). On the negative side, his potassium has also dropped (from 4.0 to 3.0 mEq/L). This is a significant drop and furthermore puts this patient into the danger zone for hypokalemia, at ¾ the level at which dysrhythmias begin to be a serious concern.

The most reasonable strategy in this case would likely be as follows:
a. Reduce the dose of the thiazide diuretic to an absolute minimum (12.5 mg).
b. Add a beta-blocker (such as atenolol). This combination of drugs (thiazide and beta-blocker) was

selected because of recommendations made in the JNC-VI (also discussed in Problem 5), which documented the reduction in cardiovascular morbidity and mortality induced by thiazides and beta-blockers. A cardioselective beta-blocker should be used in the elderly because of side effects caused by beta-blockers in this population.

c. Potassium supplementation should also be considered.

A4. **e.** The most appropriate strategy at this time would be an increase in the dose of the beta-blocker to its maximum.

At this time, even though the systolic blood pressure has been further reduced to 175 mm Hg, further lowering of his blood pressure should take place.

A5. **e.** There is ample evidence to show that antihypertensive therapy prevents cerebrovascular accidents, congestive cardiac failure, and other blood pressure–related complications. Recently, the Systolic Hypertension in the Elderly Program (SHEP) showed a reduction in MI and other coronary events in older patients with moderate to severe ischemic heart disease. Other studies confirm this.

A6. **c.** The single most important advance in the treatment of hypertension in the elderly is the clear and unequivocal recognition that systolic hypertension is as important as diastolic hypertension as a risk factor for cardiovascular morbidity and mortality and should be aggressively treated. The goal of systolic blood pressure reduction is a reading not exceeding 160 mm Hg.

A7. **e.** See Answer 5.

A8. **a.** Of the choices provided, the drug combination that should clearly be avoided in elderly patients is HCT/amiloride and enalapril. Both amiloride and enalapril are potassium-sparing drugs. In an elderly patient with decreased renal function, this can lead to profound and rapid hyperkalemia with subsequent complications.

A9. **e.** Calcium-channel blockers and thiazide diuretics have been shown to be more effective than beta-blockers in controlling hypertension in elderly African-American patients; thus a calcium-channel blocker (particularly diltiazem) and/or HCT would appear to be the agents of choice in this case. Be aware that verapamil may cause constipation and nifedipine may cause peripheral edema.

A10. **a.** Considering that this elderly female has CHF as well as hypertension, the treatment of choice is an ACE inhibitor. ACE inhibitors reduce both preload and afterload in hypertensive patients and thus are the drug class of choice for the management of CHF. ACE inhibitors have minimal side effects, primarily cough with enalapril and taste disturbances with captopril.

A11. **d.** Patients with diabetes mellitus and resulting renal impairment or microalbuminuria should definitely be treated with ACE inhibitors as the drug class of choice. There is some evidence that ACE inhibitors can be "renal protective agents" in patients with diabetes mellitus and can even be indicated as a prophylactic measure.

A12. **a.** The recommended, or "right," dose of HCT or other thiazide diuretic is the lowest dose that effectively controls the blood pressure and at the same time minimizes all of the metabolic side effects associated with thiazide diuretics.

SOLUTION TO THE SHORT ANSWER MANAGEMENT PROBLEM

Part A: Provide advice for an 80-year-old African-American male with documented systolic hypertension.

a. Review the patient's diet with him. Attempt to have the patient's spouse present (if available) while discussing this.

b. Encourage the patient to adopt the general recommendations of the American Heart Association's type I diet. This includes no more than 300 mg of cholesterol per day, no more than 30% of calories from fat, and no more than 10% of calories from saturated fat.

c. Encourage the patient to begin a "gentle" aerobic exercise program. The most reasonable exercise for a man of this age would be a walking program.

d. Advise the patient to decrease his alcohol intake to no more than two drinks per day.

e. Encourage the patient to stop smoking (cutting down might be more reasonable) if he is a smoker.

f. Start "nonpharmacologic maneuvers" along with treatment.

Part B: Discuss age- and race-related medication efficiency.

The differentiation of efficacy of antihypertensive drugs based on age and race is extremely interesting. Interdrug differences are particularly apparent in black patients. The following results are from a major review article on hypertension in the elderly by Massie (1994). The agents used in this study included atenolol, captopril, clonidine, diltiazem, HCT, and prazosin.

   a. African-American patients less than 60 years old: diltiazem was shown in one major study to be superior to all other agents.

   b. African-American patients more than 60 years old: diltiazem and HCT were the most effective agents. Captopril and atenolol were the least effective.

   c. White patients less than 60 years old: all of first-line agents (thiazides, beta-blockers, calcium-channel blockers, and ACE inhibitors) were equally effective.

   d. White patients more than 60 years old: atenolol is the most effective agent.

SUMMARY OF THE DIAGNOSIS, TREATMENT, AND OUTCOME OF HYPERTENSIVE MANAGEMENT IN ELDERLY PATIENTS

1. Single most important point: Systolic hypertension in the elderly (and in the young as well) is as important as diastolic hypertension.

2. Diagnosis of hypertension in the elderly: New criteria established by JNC-VI (see Problem 5).

3. Treatment of hypertension in the elderly reduces the following:
   a. Cerebrovascular morbidity
   b. Cerebrovascular mortality
   c. Cardiovascular morbidity
   d. Cardiovascular mortality

4. A substantial proportion of patients with mild and moderate hypertension can be controlled with a single agent, and in most this control will be maintained in the long term.

5. Overall, and with specific reference to the study previously quoted (Massie, 1994) the calcium-channel blocker produced the greatest number of positive responses. This should be balanced against the recommendation of JNC-VI (1997) that therapy be started with a thiazide diuretic or a beta-blocker.

6. Captopril was ineffective in African-American patients in this study (Massie, 1994).

SUGGESTED READINGS

Massie B: First-line therapy for hypertension: Different patients, different needs, *Geriatrics* 49(4):22-30, 1994.

The sixth report of the Joint National Committee on prevention, evaluation, and treatment of high blood pressure (JNC-VI), *Arch Intern Med* 157(21):2413-2446, 1997.

PROBLEM · 119

PARKINSON'S DISEASE

"Doctor, My Hand Just Sits There and Quivers on Its Own."

Case 1 ■ A 75-Year-Old Male with a Slow, Shuffling Gait, Tremors, and Depression

A 75-year-old male is brought to your office by his wife. She states that he has just been "staring into space" for the last 2 months. He has been unable to move around the house without falling over. Also, his movements appear to be very slow. According to his wife, he has been very depressed.

On examination, the patient has a slow, shuffling gait and walks in a "stooped-over" position. His blood pressure (lying) is 140/90 mm Hg. His standing blood pressure is 100/70 mm Hg. He has marked rigidity of his upper extremities. He also has a tremor that appears to be present only at rest.

SELECT THE BEST ANSWER TO THE FOLLOWING QUESTIONS

Q1. What is the most likely diagnosis in this patient?
   a. Alzheimer's disease
   b. major depressive disorder with psychomotor retardation
   c. degenerative orthostatic hypotension
   d. Parkinson's disease
   e. multiple sclerosis

2. What is the most common presenting symptom in this disorder?
   a. orthostatic hypotension
   b. depression
   c. gait disturbance
   d. tremor
   e. rigidity

Q3. Where is the lesion associated with the described disorder located?
   a. the caudate nucleus
   b. the substantia nigra
   c. the hypothalamus
   d. the putamen
   e. the globus pallidus

Q4. The disorder described is associated with a central nervous system neurotransmitter deficiency. What is that neurotransmitter?
   a. acetylcholine
   b. serotonin
   c. gamma-aminobutyric acid

d. dopamine

e. norepinephrine

Q5. Many drugs are associated with side effects that mimic some of the symptoms of the described disorder. Which one of the following drugs would not produce these symptoms?

a. diazepam

b. haloperidol

c. chlorpromazine

d. perphenazine

e. reserpine

Q6. Which one of the following statements regarding the condition described is false?

a. there is marked heterogeneity in disease presentation

b. there are at least two major subgroups of this disorder

c. patients who have marked postural instability have a better prognosis than those who have a tremor

d. personality changes commonly appear in the course of this disorder

e. significant depression and dementia appear in one third to one half of patients with this condition.

Q7. What is (are) the drug(s) of choice for mild cases of the condition described (mild meaning that the main or only symptom is tremor)?

a. amantadine

b. trihexyphenidyl

c. levodopa

d. carbidopa

e. selegiline (Deprenyl)

f. a or b

Q8. If the symptoms progress to the point where another agent is needed, dose-limiting side effects develop from the drugs being used, or the drugs being used begin to lose their effectiveness, what is the next step in the treatment of the disorder described?

a. selegiline

b. trihexyphenidyl

c. amantadine

d. all of the above

e. none of the above

Q9. Which of the following drugs may be indicated in the treatment of the disorder described?

a. bromocriptine

b. pergolide

c. amitriptyline

d. all of the above

e. none of the above

Q10. Which of the following symptoms is not characteristic of this disorder?

a. unilateral onset of tremor

b. unilateral onset of bradykinesia

c. impaired balance

d. muscle rigidity

e. psychomotor agitation

Q11. Which of the following statements regarding levodopa is false?

a. levodopa in combination with carbidopa remains the primary drugs for the treatment of most patients with the condition described

b. levodopa is unlikely to lose its effectiveness over time when being used to treat the disorder described

c. levodopa is likely to produce an "on-off" phenomenon during treatment of the disorder described

d. nausea is a frequent side effect of levodopa

e. centrally mediated dyskinesia, hallucinations, dystonia, and motor fluctuations are common in levodopa-treated patients

Q12. Which of the following conditions is most closely associated with the condition described?

a. major depressive disorder

b. cerebrovascular disease

c. epilepsy

d. schizophrenia

e. schizoaffective disorder

Q13. Which of the following statements regarding benign essential tremor is (are) correct?

a. benign essential tremor is often familial

b. a nodding head and tremulousness of speech are often observed with benign essential tremor

c. benign essential tremor is a resting tremor rather than an action tremor

d. a and b only

e. all of the above statements are correct

Q14. Benign essential tremor is frequently treated with which of the following agents?

a. propranolol

b. alcohol

c. atenolol

d. all of the above

e. none of the above

Q15. What illicit drug produces symptoms closely resembling the symptoms of the condition described?
a. a meperidine analog (MPTP)
b. crack cocaine
c. lysergic acid diethylamide
d. apomorphine
e. diamorphine (heroin)

SHORT ANSWER MANAGEMENT PROBLEM

Discuss the therapeutic choices available to treat the condition described in the patient presented in Case 1. Describe a logical approach to instituting these therapeutic choices in any patient with this disorder.

ANSWERS

A1. **d.** This patient has Parkinson's disease. The most common presenting symptoms in Parkinson's disease include tremor, bradykinesia, rigidity, impaired postural reflexes, gait disturbance, autonomic dysfunction (causing orthostatic hypotension), and depression. A "masked facies" expression is typical of the disease.

Other presenting symptoms can be constipation, vague aches and pains, paresthesia, decreased smell sensation, vestibular symptoms, pedal edema, fatigue, and weight loss.

The other choices listed in this question do not explain the constellation of presenting symptoms.

A2. **d.** The most common presenting symptom in Parkinson's disease is a resting tremor. This symptom is seen in 70% of patients with the disease. It may initially be confined to one hand, but it usually extends to involve all limbs.

A3. **b.** The principal pathologic feature in Parkinson's disease is degeneration of the substantia nigra. Degenerative changes are also found in other brainstem nuclei.

A4. **d.** Parkinson's disease is associated with a depletion of dopamine in the substantia nigrostriatal pathway system.

A5. **a.** Parkinsonian-like side effects are common side effects of the neuroleptic drug class. This drug class includes chlorpromazine, haloperidol, and perphenazine. In addition, the prokinetic agent metoclopramide can also produce this side effect.

Reserpine, an older antihypertensive agent, may also produce these extrapyramidal symptoms. This is relevant because many elderly individuals who were started on reserpine are still on it. Diazepam does not produce any such side effects.

A6. **c.** There is marked heterogeneity in Parkinson's disease. There are at least two major subtypes of Parkinson's disease. In one group the symptom of tremor is the most predominant clinical symptom. In the second group, postural instability and gait difficulty (PIGD) are the predominant symptoms. There is some overlap, but most patients fit into only one subgroup. Patients with tremor-predominant Parkinson's disease have slower progression of disease and have fewer problems with bradykinesia. They are also less likely to develop significant mental symptoms.

Personality changes usually occur in the early stages, and patients often become withdrawn, apathetic, and dependent on their spouses. Significant depression occurs in one half of patients, and dementia occurs in one third of patients. As mentioned previously, these personality and mental changes are more common in patients who present with the PIGD subtype of Parkinson's disease.

A7. **e.** Research from three studies has supported the use of selegiline (Deprenyl) early in the course of the disease to delay the onset of the disability and the need for initiation of levodopa therapy. The combination of levodopa and carbidopa are effective and are still considered for primary treatment, but their use should be delayed as long as possible because of their side effect profile and the eventual development of tolerance to these medications.

A8. **e.** The next step in the pharmacologic treatment of Parkinson's disease is the combination of levodopa-carbidopa. Levodopa is a precursor of dopamine synthesis in the substantia nigra. The drug is usually administered in combination with carbidopa, which is a decarboxylase inhibitor. Obviously, treatment must be individualized: a good general rule to follow is to start low and go slow.

A9. **d.** Bromocriptine and pergolide are two dopaminergic agonists. Pergolide and bromocriptine can be useful for sudden episodes of hesitancy or immobility, which Parkinsonian patients describe as "freezing." This can be an intermittent event or a regular event. The freezing often occurs when Parkinsonian patients begin to walk or they pass through a structure such as a doorway. Dyskinesias and other types of involuntary movements are also treated by these drugs. Newer dopaminergic agents include pramipexole and ropinirole.

Amitriptyline is useful in the treatment of Parkinson's disease both as an anticholinergic agent and as an antidepressant.

A10. **e.** The unilateral onset of tremor or bradykinesia is common in patients with Parkinson's disease. Muscle rigidity and impaired balance are other important symptoms. Psychomotor agitation (although one of the characteristic symptoms of major depressive disorder) is rare. Patients with Parkinson's disease have instead psychomotor retardation.

A11. **b.** Levodopa does lose its effectiveness over time in the treatment of Parkinson's disease. That is why, in patients who have mild symptoms, it is best to begin therapy with selegiline (Deprenyl).

Levodopa does exhibit a marked "on-off" phenomenon during treatment of Parkinson's disease. This is characterized by periods of "drug working" and "drug not working."

Side effects of levodopa include nausea and vomiting, dystonias, hallucinations, dyskinesias, and motor fluctuations. Hallucinations become the most common side effect, limiting the titration of carbidopa-levodopa.

A12. **a.** Depression is a common problem in patients with Parkinson's disease. The association between depression and Parkinson's disease generally follows this pathway: when depression occurs, the symptoms of Parkinson's disease become worse; the patient then believes that his or her disease has progressed quickly. This leads to a cycle that is difficult to break.

A13. **d.** Benign essential tremor is the major differential diagnostic possibility when considering tremor. Benign essential tremor is familial. Typical features include generalized tremulousness, including tremulousness of speech, and a "head-nodding" motion. Benign essential tremor is, in contradistinction to the tremor of Parkinson's disease, an action tremor.

A14. **d.** The agents of choice for treating benign essential tremor are as follows:
a. Propranolol
b. Atenolol
c. Alcohol (in moderation)
d. Diazepam

A15. **a.** The illicitly made MPTP produces symptoms that are Parkinson-like in presentation. This agent appears to act as a poison on the substantia nigra. Also, the symptoms appear to be irreversible, and the individual is left with a lifetime disability.

SOLUTION TO THE SHORT ANSWER MANAGEMENT PROBLEM

A reasonable therapeutic approach to the treatment of Parkinson's disease is as follows:
a. Patients with minor symptoms (not significantly impairing function):
1) No pharmacologic treatment
2) Selegiline (Deprenyl)
3) Anticholinergic medications (trihexyphenidyl, benztropine)
4) Amantadine
b. Patients with moderate symptoms: Levodopa-carbidopa (Sinemet) is the drug of choice. Levodopa is a precursor of dopamine; carbidopa is a decarboxylase inhibitor. Although selegiline is not considered the drug of first choice, its use will increase if current research continues to support the idea that it decreases the rate of progression of Parkinson's disease.
c. Patients with moderate to severe symptoms (or patients in whom the effect of levodopa has worn off):
1) Deprenyl (a monoamine oxidase [MAO] B inhibitor); in patients with a significant depressive component because of the MAO activity
2) Bromocriptine and pergolide (dopamine agonists); in patients in whom dyskinesias and other involuntary movements are prominent
d. Patients with Parkinson's disease with significant depression: amitriptyline or another tricyclic antidepressant with or without anticholinergic properties (balance the benefits of the anticholinergic properties of amitriptyline against the risks of increased orthostatic disturbance and imbalance)

SUMMARY OF THE DIAGNOSIS AND TREATMENT OF PARKINSON'S DISEASE

1. Epidemiology: After stroke and Alzheimer's disease, Parkinson's disease is the most commonly encountered neurologic disorder in the elderly population.

2. Pathologic condition: Depigmentation of the substantia nigra, which results in a decrease in brain synthesis of dopamine

3. Major symptoms:
a. Resting tremor
b. Bradykinesia
c. Rigidity

d. Impaired postural reflexes
e. Gait disturbance
f. Autonomic dysfunction
g. Depression

4. Major subtypes:
   a. Parkinson's disease (group A): This group exhibits tremor (resting) as the major symptom and sign.
   b. Parkinson's disease (group B): This group exhibits PIGD as the major symptom. Progression of the disease is usually more rapid in this group; neurobehavioral changes are also more common in this group.

5. Treatment: See the Solution to the Short Answer Management Problem

6. Other related disease entity: Benign essential tremor: benign essential tremor is an action tremor (as opposed to the resting tremor of Parkinson's disease). It is most often seen in the extremities and is sometimes associated with head nodding and tremulousness of speech. It is familial. The drug treatment of this entity includes a beta-blocker, diazepam, or alcohol (in moderation).

SUGGESTED READINGS

McDowell FH: Parkinson's disease and related disorders. In Hazzard WR et al, eds: *Principles of geriatric medicine and gerontology,* ed 3, New York, 1994, McGraw-Hill.

Pruitt A: *Approach to the patient with Parkinson's disease: Primary care medicine,* ed 3, Philadelphia, 1995, JB Lippincott.

Tierney LM, Jr, McPhee SJ, Papadakis MA, eds: *Current medical diagnosis and treatment, 2000,* Stamford, Conn, 1999, Appleton & Lange.

PROBLEM · 120

CONSTIPATION IN THE ELDERLY

"Doctor, I Am Terribly Constipated. I Only Go Two or Three Times a Week."

Case 1 ■ A 78-Year-Old Female with Constipation

A 78-year-old female comes to your office with a 5-year history of "constipation." The patient, who has had significant difficulties with ischemic heart disease, is currently on atenolol and verapamil.

On examination, the patient's blood pressure is 180/95 mm Hg. Her pulse is 72 and regular. Upon examination the head and neck, the lungs, the cardiovascular system, and the abdomen are all normal. Digital rectal examination (DRE) reveals impacted stool.

SELECT THE BEST ANSWER TO THE FOLLOWING QUESTIONS

Q1. Constipation is best defined as which of the following:
a. only one bowel movement in 7 days
b. only two bowel movements in 7 days
c. only three bowel movements in 7 days
d. only four bowel movements in 7 days
e. none of the above

Q2. What is the most accurate elderly patient definition of constipation?
a. anything less than one bowel movement per day
b. any defecation difficulty
c. anything less than two bowel movements per day
d. any straining at stool
e. any of the above: constipation to the elderly means almost anything vaguely associated with bowel movements

Q3. Which of the following is (are) associated with constipation in the elderly?
a. impaired general health status
b. increased medication use
c. decreased level of exercise
d. all of the above
e. none of the above

Q4. Which of the following drug classes is (are) associated with constipation?
a. tricyclic antidepressants
b. anticholinergic agents
c. calcium-channel blockers
d. all of the above
e. none of the above

Q5. Concerning the history and physical examination of elderly patients with constipation, which of the following should be performed?
a. a DRE
b. a complete medication review
c. a functional inquiry of the gastrointestinal (GI) system
d. all of the above
e. a and b only

Q6. Which of the following is (are) complications associated with constipation in the elderly?
a. fecal impaction
b. diarrhea
c. anal fissures
d. sigmoid volvulus
e. a and c
f. all of the above

Q7. Which of the following is not a recommended treatment for constipation in the elderly?
   a. a bowel training regime
   b. an exercise program
   c. chronic laxative use
   d. a high-fiber diet
   e. an above-average consumption of fluids

Q8. Which of the following drugs is most closely associated with constipation in the elderly?
   a. hydrochlorothiazide
   b. verapamil
   c. atenolol
   d. acetaminophen
   e. fluoxetine

Q9. Constipation in the elderly is most closely associated with which of the following?
   a. fecal impaction
   b. diarrhea
   c. crampy back pain
   d. a and c
   e. all of the above

Q10. What is the self-reported percentage incidence of constipation in elderly Americans?
   a. 10%
   b. 20%
   c. 30%
   d. 40%
   e. 50%

Q11. What is the laxative group most closely associated with long-term side effects in the elderly?
   a. the stimulant laxatives
   b. the hyperosmolar laxatives
   c. the saline laxatives
   d. the emollient laxatives
   e. the stool softeners

Case 2 ■ An 86-Year-Old Male with Stage IV Carcinoma of the Prostate

An 86-year-old male with stage IV carcinoma of the prostate comes to your office seeking "pain relief." He has bony metastatic disease and his pain was well controlled on a combination of diclofenac and morphine sulfate. With the morphine his pain decreased from 9/10 to 2/10. However, 5 days after morphine was started he began to experience more severe pain. You decide to increase the morphine dose and see him in a week. He returns after that week with worse pain than before. Now 13/10. You increase the morphine dose even further and ask him to return in another week.

He returns a week later doubled over in pain that he describes as 15/10.

Q12. At this time, what would you do?
   a. switch the patient to hydromorphone
   b. switch the patient to methadone
   c. switch the patient to fentanyl (patch)
   d. switch the patient to oxycodone
   e. none of the above

Q13. At this time your physical examination maneuver of choice for the patient described in Case 2 is which of the following?
   a. none; you do not believe in the sensitivity, specificity, and positive predictive value of physical examination techniques any more
   b. palpation of the abdomen
   c. percussion of the abdomen
   d. auscultation of the abdomen for bowel sounds
   e. none of the above

Q14. At this time which of the following is the investigation of choice for the patient described in Case 2?
   a. a magnetic resonance imaging scan
   b. a repeat bone scan
   c. a computed tomography scan of the pelvis
   d. a serum calcium level to "look for that ever-elusive entity, hypercalcemia"
   e. none of the above

Q15. What is the single most common cause of abdominal pain in the elderly?
   a. angiodysplasia
   b. diverticulitis
   c. spastic colon of the elderly syndrome
   d. the aging gut syndrome
   e. none of the above

SHORT ANSWER MANAGEMENT PROBLEM
Name the drug in each of the drug classes listed below that is most commonly responsible for constipation in the elderly.
   a. antihypertensive agent: _____
   b. antianginal agent: _____
   c. medical diagnostic agent: _____
   d. antacid: _____
   e. nutritional supplement: _____
   f. analgesic: _____
   g. antipsychotic: _____
   h. antidepressant: _____
   i. anticholinergic: _____
   j. inexpensive osteoporotic therapy agent: _____

ANSWERS

A1. e. Constipation is usually medically defined as fewer than three bowel movements per week. It is a major problem for elderly patients in developed countries of the world. This is substantiated by the rise in the use of laxative therapies. Approximately 30% of patients over the age of 65 are regular laxative users.

A2. e. Physicians tend to define constipation on the basis of the frequency of stooling and the consistency of stooling. To the elder, on the other hand, constipation can mean almost anything, including any difficulties in defecation such as straining at stool, anything less than one to two completely-normal-in-every-way (shape, caliber, diameter, length, color) bowel movements, and anything else vaguely related to the bowel movement. The point is, you must ask the elder what he or she means by constipation. It's almost a guarantee that the patient's definition will not match yours.

Again, it is important to realize that there is a significant discrepancy between what physicians define as constipation in the elderly and what the elderly themselves define as constipation. For many elderly patients, the daily bowel movement is somehow a significant mark of health.

A3. d. The factors that appear to be associated with constipation in the elderly include an impaired general health status, an increased number of medications other than laxatives, diminished mobility, and diminished physical activity.

It is unclear what the true effect of diet on bowel habits is. There is epidemiologic evidence from the developed countries that greater amounts of crude dietary fiber are associated with a lesser prevalence of various GI disorders, including diverticular disease, colorectal cancer, and constipation. There may be, however, intervening variables that account for some of this difference.

A4. d. There are a significant number of drug classes that are associated with constipation, and especially constipation in the elderly.
  a. Antacids:
    1) Aluminum hydroxide
    2) Calcium carbonate
  b. Anticholinergic agents: trihexyphenidyl
  c. Antidepressants:
    1) Tricyclic antidepressants
    2) Lithium carbonate
  d. Antihypertensive-antiarrhythmics: calcium-channel blockers, especially verapamil
  e. Metals:
    1) Bismuth
    2) Iron
    3) Heavy metals
  f. Narcotic analgesics: any narcotic analgesic, but especially codeine
  g. Nonsteroidal antiinflammatory drugs: all may produce constipation in the elderly
  h. Sympathomimetics: pseudoephedrine

A5. d. When an elderly patient complains of constipation, a careful history is the most important aspect of the evaluation. Sometimes all that is required is reassurance from the physician that there is a broad range of normal bowel frequency.

Symptoms of disorders that impair the motility of the large bowel should be sought. These general medical conditions include hypothyroidism, hyperparathyroidism, scleroderma, Parkinson's disease, cerebrovascular accidents, and diabetes mellitus.

Localized colorectal diseases, such as tumors or other constricting lesions that may cause constipation, are often accompanied by other symptoms. Thus the history must include questions concerning abdominal pain and bleeding per rectum. In idiopathic, dietary, and drug-related constipation, there are usually no symptoms other than constipation, although a complaint of an abdominal bloating sensation is common with severe constipation.

A DRE is a sensitive screening tool in detecting anal lesions, although fissures and hemorrhoids, unless they are thrombosed or large, are found more reliably on anoscopy. Anoscopy should be performed routinely in constipated elderly patients. DRE of the anal canal and rectum is useful in assessing the tone of the internal anal sphincter and also the strength of the external sphincter and the puborectalis muscle.

The amount and the consistency of stool felt in the rectum may, in fact, indicate what type of constipation is present. Patients with a failure of the defecation mechanism tend to have much stool in the rectal vault, whereas those patients with colonic atony or irritable bowel syndrome have little or no stool in the rectum between defecations.

A6. f. Although for most elderly patients, constipation is just a minor annoyance, for some elders it is much more than that. The elders that are most susceptible to constipation are those who are institutionalized or bedridden.

Complications of constipation in the elderly are as follows:
  a. Fecal impaction is heralded by crampy, lower abdominal and lower back pain
  b. Stercoral ulcers are common in the bedridden patient. They are caused by pressure necrosis of the rectal or sigmoid mucosa due to a fecal mass. In some cases the ulcer may present as rectal bleeding.

c. Anal fissures may result from excessive straining at stool and the subsequent complications that develop, including tears and passive congestion of the tissues near the dentate line. The problem is enhanced by the irritating effect of hard stools and toilet paper. Intraabdominal pressures of up to 300 mm Hg are generated during straining. Excessive straining at stool may cause prolapse of the anal mucosa, venous distention, and internal hemorrhoids.

d. Megacolon in the elderly is almost always idiopathic. Chronic use of cathartics over a period of years may lead to an acquired degeneration of the colonic myenteric plexus and subsequent megacolon. Bacterial overgrowth may occur and further complicate matters.

e. Volvulus, especially of the sigmoid colon, occurs most commonly in institutionalized, bedbound, elderly patients and carries a high mortality rate.

f. Carcinoma of the colon: There is some evidence that chronic constipation is a risk factor for the development of carcinoma of the colon, particularly in women. This might be related to increased exposure time of susceptible mucosa to potentially carcinogenic substances.

A7. **c.** The treatment of constipation is primarily non-pharmacologic. In large part, it involves inducing the patient to adopt a healthier lifestyle. This includes a bowel training regime (a schedule of regular times for attempting defecation), regular exercise (bedfast patients are at great risk of constipation and often respond poorly to treatment), dietary adjustment to increase the amount of fiber in the diet and an increased consumption of liquids, particularly water. Some foods that are exceptionally high in fiber include 100% bran cereal, beans (baked, kidney, lima, and navy), canned peas, raspberries, and broccoli.

It is not recommended that a regular or chronic laxative regime be part of a routine prophylactic and treatment protocol for constipation.

A8. **b.** The drug that is most closely associated with the development of constipation in the elderly is verapamil.

Verapamil is a calcium-channel blocker commonly used to treat angina. Constipation develops in approximately 16% of patients who take verapamil for any length of time, and this percentage may be significantly higher in the elderly, especially in institutionalized and bedridden patients. The development of constipation-related complications already discussed may follow.

Constipation may also occur as a side effect of the use of hydrochlorothiazide, atenolol, or fluoxetine, but it does not appear to be what would be called a major side effect with those drugs.

A9. **e.** Constipation is often associated with fecal impaction, diarrhea, and crampy, lower abdominal and lower back pain.

Fecal impaction is the result of prolonged exposure of accumulated stool to the absorptive forces of the colon and rectum. The stool may become rocklike in consistency in the rectum (70%), in the sigmoid colon (20%), and in the proximal colon (10%).

Symptoms of crampy, lower abdominal and lower back pain are common. Diarrhea may paradoxically follow the constipation, which leads to the impaction (watery material making its way around the impacted mass of stool). The impaction can sometimes be evacuated by the patient after the oral administration of polyethylene glycol (GoLYTELY), but manual disimpaction is usually required.

A10. **c.** A recent survey in the United States of community-dwelling persons over age 65 found that 30% of men and 29% of women considered themselves constipated. In the month preceding the survey, 24% of the men and 20% of the women had used laxatives.

A11. **a.** The laxative group used to treat constipation can be divided into six major categories:

a. The bulk-forming laxatives: The bulk-forming laxatives include the various fiber-containing preparations and are thought to act in two major ways. First, they are hydrophilic and tend to increase the stool mass and soften the stool consistency. They are the safest laxatives and are generally well tolerated by elderly patients when introduced gradually.

b. The emollient laxatives: Emollients, or stool softeners, include mineral oil, as well as the newer docusate salts such as dioctyl sodium sulfosuccinate (Colace). Mineral oil is generally not recommended because safer, more effective agents are available. The newer agents lower surface tension, allowing water to enter the stool more readily. They are generally well tolerated and may be particularly useful in bed-bound elderly patients who are at risk for fecal impaction.

c. The saline laxatives: Saline laxatives and enemas are salts of magnesium and sodium. Those in most common use are oral milk of magnesia, oral magnesium citrate, and sodium phosphate (Fleet's enema). All of these agents function as hyperosmolar agents and cause net secretion of fluid into the colon. Colonic motility is increased by these agents via release of the hormone cholecystokinin. Chronic use of magnesium-containing saline laxatives in elderly patients may contribute to hypermagnesemia (especially when there is associated impaired renal function). The phosphate-containing preparations may also induce hypocalcemia when high doses are used. The phosphate-containing enemas may cause damage to the rectum; this may occur via the nozzle part of the instrument itself, or a direct toxic effect exerted by the hypertonic saline on the rectal mucosa.

d. The hyperosmotic laxatives: Hyperosmolar laxatives such as lactulose draw water into the gut lumen by an osmotic action. Lactulose is an undigestible agent that is metabolized by bacteria to hydrogen and organic acids. This causes acidification of the colon, and this, in addition to its osmotic effect, may alter electrolyte transport and colonic mobility.

e. The stimulant laxatives: The stimulant laxatives include the anthraquinone derivatives cascara, senna, and aloe; phenolphthalein; and bisacodyl (Dulcolax) tablets. Complications of the stimulant laxatives include melanosis coli from the anthraquinone group and complications such as Stevens-Johnson syndrome, dermatitis, and photosensitivity reactions from the phenolphthalein group. Although bisacodyl tablets probably are safer than the rest of the stimulant laxatives, all of the agents can cause electrolyte imbalance and precipitate hypokalemia, fluid and salt overload, and diarrhea. Thus the stimulant laxatives are the laxatives most closely associated with long-term side effects.

f. The lavage laxatives: The lavage laxatives are the newest group of laxatives. They include the agents GoLYTELY and COLyte. They work by stimulating neither secretion nor motility but by passing unimpeded through the GI tract. They are the most commonly used agents for bowel preparation before flexible sigmoidoscopy and colonoscopy.

A12. **e.** In this patient the increasing and different abdominal pain was caused by constipation. This patient had actually not had a bowel movement for 34 days. Thus the increasing severe abdominal pain (caused by increasing doses of morphine) completely overshadowed his previous pain (the pain caused by metastatic bone disease). Therefore switching to another painkiller is not a logical response.

A13. **e.** The physical examination maneuver of choice in this patient is a DRE to confirm impacted stool.

A14. **e.** The investigation of choice is an x-ray of the kidneys, ureter, and bladder (KUB) to confirm stool throughout the colon.

A15. **e.** Remember, constipation is the single most common cause of abdominal pain in the elderly.

This patient's problem was treated by manual disimpaction, tap water enemas, and lactulose. To reduce the possibility of severe constipation, you should treat patients who you start on narcotic analgesics by following these two rules:

a. Start a bowel regimen at the same time as you start the narcotic.
b. Maintain the bowel regimen for as long as you maintain the patient on the narcotic.

SOLUTION TO THE SHORT ANSWER MANAGEMENT PROBLEM

The drug classes and their most common offenders are as follows:

DRUG CLASS	MOST COMMON OFFENDER
Antihypertensives	Verapamil
Antianginal agents	Verapamil
Medical diagnostic agent	Barium sulfate
Antacids	Aluminum hydroxide
Nutritional supplement	Iron
Narcotic analgesics	Codeine
Antipsychotics	Thioridazine
Antidepressants	Amitriptyline
Anticholinergics	Trihexyphenidyl
Cheap osteoporosis therapy	Calcium carbonate

SUMMARY OF THE DIAGNOSIS AND TREATMENT OF CONSTIPATION IN THE ELDERLY

1. Prevalence of constipation: The reported prevalence of constipation in the elderly is 30%.

2. Definition: Constipation is usually defined as fewer than three bowel movements per week.

3. Cause of constipation: The cause of constipation includes declined or impaired general health status in the elderly, increasing number of medications (remember verapamil), and diminished mobility and physical activity.

4. Diagnosis and investigation: The patient's complete medical history is the most important part of the evaluation (remember to include complete functional inquiry of the GI tract). DRE is the most important part of the physical examination; anoscopy should accompany DRE. DRE and anoscopy may detect fissures, fistulas, strictures, carcinoma, or hemorrhoids.

5. Complications: The complications of constipation in the elderly include the following:
   a. Fecal impaction, crampy abdominal and back pain, and overflow diarrhea
   b. Stercoral ulcers
   c. Anal fissures and anal fistulas
   d. Hemorrhoids (internal and external)
   e. Megacolon
   f. Sigmoid volvulus
   g. Risk factor for carcinoma of the colon

6. Treatment:
   a. Nonpharmacologic:
      1) Bowel training
      2) Exercise
      3) High-fiber diet
      4) Increased fluid intake
   b. Pharmacologic: The laxatives:
      1) Bulk laxatives: recommended
      2) Emollient laxatives: mineral oil is not recommended, but Colace is recommended
      3) Saline laxatives and enemas: not recommended on long-term basis
      4) Hyperosmolar laxatives: recommended
      5) Stimulant laxatives: not recommended

7. Golden rules summary section:
   a. Always ask yourself the question, "Why?" Why is the patient constipated? Constipation is not part of the normal aging process.
   b. Cancer is a common diagnosis in elderly patients. Most elderly patients with cancer will eventually require a narcotic analgesic. When that time comes, always start a constipation-correcting bowel regime at the same time.

SUGGESTED READING

Cheskin L, Schuster M: Constipation. In Hazzard WR et al, eds: *Principles of geriatric medicine and gerontology*, ed 3, New York, 1994, McGraw-Hill.

PROBLEM · 1 2 1

PNEUMONIA MANAGEMENT

"I Feel That Nursing Home Is Responsible for My Father's Death from Pneumonia."

Case 1 ■ An 81-Year-Old Male Who Lives by Himself and Has Increasing Confusion and Shortness of Breath

A previously healthy 81-year-old male is brought to the Emergency Department by his daughter. He lives by himself. He was well until 3 days ago. At that time, he became somewhat confused and began wandering aimlessly around the house and muttering incoherently. For the last 3 days he has had both nausea and anorexia. In addition, he became short of breath last night.

On physical examination, his blood pressure is 100/70 mm Hg. His pulse is 96 bpm and regular. His respiratory rate is 28 breaths/min and his respirations appear slightly labored. On auscultation of his lung fields there are a few rales bilaterally but no other abnormalities. His WBC is 11,000/mm^3. His chest x-ray reveals right lower lobe consolidation. His PO$_2$ is 65 mm Hg and his PCO$_2$ is 40 mm Hg.

SELECT THE BEST ANSWER TO THE FOLLOWING QUESTIONS

Q1. What is the most likely diagnosis in this patient?
   a. bacterial pneumonia
   b. viral pneumonia
   c. fungal pneumonia
   d. aspiration pneumonia
   e. obstructive pneumonia

Q2. What is the most likely pathogen in this patient's pneumonia?
   a. *Klebsiella pneumoniae*
   b. *Haemophilus influenzae*
   c. influenza type B
   d. *Escherichia coli*
   e. *Streptococcus pneumoniae*

Case 2 ■ An 84-Year-Old Female Who Is Currently Residing in a Long-Term Care Facility and Has Increasing Confusion and Shortness of Breath

A presentation with almost identical symptoms and signs as the patient in Case 1 occurs in an 84-year-old female who is currently residing in a long-term care facility and who has many chronic medical conditions. Compare her presentation to the presentation of the patient described in Case 1.

Q3. Which of the following statements is (are) true?
   a. the prognosis is likely to be similar in both individuals
   b. the responsible organism is likely to be the same
   c. the treatment is likely to be the same
   d. all of the above statements are true
   e. none of the above statements is true

Q4. What is the treatment of choice for the patient described in Case 1?
a. amoxicillin
b. erythromycin
c. gentamicin
d. cefixime
e. amphotericin B

Q5. Which of the following is (are) risk factors for the development of urinary tract infections in elderly patients?
a. advanced age
b. decreased bladder emptying
c. prostatic hypertrophy
d. decreased host defense mechanisms
e. all of the above

Q6. What is the most common pathogen in urinary tract infections in noncatheterized elderly patients?
a. *Serratia* sp.
b. *Proteus mirabilis*
c. *Klebsiella* sp.
d. *E. coli*
e. *Pseudomonas aeruginosa*

Case 3 ■ An 81-Year-Old Female with Dysuria, Frequency, Urgency, and Incontinence

An 81-year-old female comes to your office with a 5-day history of dysuria, frequency, urgency, and incontinence. She has no other symptoms, including no cardiovascular accident (CVA) tenderness or other symptoms. The patient lives at home by herself and has had no major medical problems.

On examination, her temperature is 37° C. Her blood pressure is 150/80 mm Hg and her pulse is 84 bpm and regular. No other abnormalities are found on physical examination.

Q7. Which of the following statements concerning this patient is (are) true?
a. the most likely diagnosis is acute bacterial cystitis
b. the most likely organism is *P. aeruginosa*
c. amoxicillin is a reasonable first-choice antibiotic
d. this patient should be treated for 14 days
e. all of the above statements are true

Q8. Concerning chronic prostatitis in elderly patients, which of the following statements is (are) true?
a. chronic prostatitis is the most common cause of relapsing urinary tract infections in elderly males

b. prostatic massage is not helpful in establishing a diagnosis
c. *Klebsiella* is the most common pathogen in this condition
d. with prolonged therapy, relapse becomes unlikely
e. all of the above statements are true

Case 4 ■ A 75-Year-Old Female with Fever, Chills, Confusion, Dysuria, and Diarrhea

A 75-year-old female comes to your office with a 2-day history of fever, chills, confusion, dysuria, and diarrhea. There are no other symptoms, including no back pain.

On examination, the patient's temperature is 38.5° C. Her blood pressure is 120/75 mm Hg, and her pulse is 96 bpm and regular. There is no demonstrable CVA tenderness.

Q9. What is the most likely diagnosis in this patient?
a. acute bacterial cystitis
b. viral gastroenteritis
c. acute pyelonephritis
d. bacterial gastroenteritis
e. none of the above

Q10. Regarding the use of antibiotics in elderly patients with indwelling catheters, which of the following statements is (are) true?
a. indwelling urinary catheters are the leading cause of nosocomial infections
b. indwelling urinary catheters are the most common predisposing factor in hospital-acquired, fatal, gram-negative sepsis
c. by the time a urinary catheter has been in place for 2 weeks, 50% of catheterized patients have significant bacteriuria
d. all of the above statements are true
e. none of the above statements is true

Q11. What is the leading cause of death caused by infection in hospitalized elderly patients?
a. bacterial pneumonia
b. urinary tract infection
c. pressure ulcers
d. diverticulitis
e. septic arthritis

Q12. What is the leading cause of death caused by infection in institutionalized elderly patients?
a. bacterial pneumonia
b. urinary tract infection
c. pressure ulcers
d. diverticulitis
e. septic arthritis

Q13. What is the leading cause of death caused by infection in elderly individuals living in the community?
   a. bacterial pneumonia
   b. urinary tract infection
   c. pressure ulcers
   d. diverticulitis
   e. septic arthritis

Q14. In considering acute appendicitis in elderly patients, which of the following statements is (are) true?
   a. the presenting signs and symptoms are similar to younger patients
   b. gangrene of the appendix is uncommon
   c. morbidity and mortality are much higher than in younger patients
   d. all of the above statements are true
   e. none of the above statements is true

Q15. Which of the following statements concerning fever in elderly patients is (are) true?
   a. fever in elderly patients is more likely to be the result of a serious pathologic condition than in younger patients
   b. when compared to younger patients, older adults often fail to show a temperature elevation despite having a serious infectious disease
   c. in elderly patients with fever of undetermined origin (FUO), a localized infection (such as an abscess) is often found
   d. all of the above statements are true
   e. none of the above statements is true

SHORT ANSWER MANAGEMENT PROBLEM

Consider the following functional states or levels of care in elderly patients and the following primary considerations in infectious or inflammatory disease. Fill in the three most common primary infectious diseases in each group, in order of frequency.
   a. Independent healthy elderly individuals living in the community:
      1)
      2)
      3)
   b. Hospitalized elderly patients:
      1)
      2)
      3)
   c. Nursing home or institutionalized elderly residents:
      1)
      2)
      3)

ANSWERS

A1. **a.** The most likely diagnosis in this patient is a bacterial pneumonia. The presentation of bacterial pneumonia in elderly patients is usually much more subtle and nonspecific than in younger patients. As illustrated in this case presentation, confusion is a very common early sign. Other nonspecific early signs include disorientation and a change (decrease) in the elder's interest level. A fall is often part of the presenting symptoms and signs of elder infectious illness.

Findings on physical examination are also nonspecific. Signs of consolidation are often absent. Rales are common but not specific. An increased respiratory rate (as in this patient) may precede other signs and symptoms.

The specificity of laboratory abnormalities found in elders with bacterial pneumonia is low. An increased white blood cell count (WBC less than 10,000 mm^3) is commonly found, but as well as being nonspecific, the WBC also suffers from low sensitivity. Hypoxemia is a common finding. In elderly patients with bacterial pneumonia the correlation between clinical findings and radiologic findings is poor.

A2. **e.** The most likely pathogen associated with community-acquired pneumonia is *S. pneumoniae*. *H. influenzae*, *K. pneumoniae*, and gram-negative bacilli are much less common unless there is associated chronic obstructive pulmonary disease (COPD) or an immune-compromising condition.

In summary, the difference between younger adults and older adults in community-acquired bacterial pneumonia is that *S. pneumoniae* is the responsible organism in 60% to 80% of younger patients but only 40% to 60% of elderly patients.

A3. **b.** The most important differences between the two presentations are as follows:
   a. Patient 1: The patient presented in Case 1 resides in the community.
      Patient 2: The patient presented in Case 2 resides in a long-term care facility.
   b. Patient 1: This patient is otherwise healthy and has no significant medical problems.
      Patient 2: This patient has many other chronic health problems.
   c. The organism found in patient 1 is likely to be the most common cause of bacterial community-acquired pneumonia.

The most likely organism to be found in patient 2 is still *S. pneumoniae*, but other candidates should be thought of, such as *H. influenzae*, *K. pneumoniae*, or another gram-negative organism.
   d. Because it is more likely to find gram-negative organisms in patient 2, the treatments may be different.

e. The virulence of the organism on the host in patient 2 is likely to be significantly greater than the virulence of the organism in patient 1. Thus the prognosis in patient 2 is significantly less favorable than the prognosis in patient 1.

A4. **b.** The treatment of choice for a community-acquired bacterial pneumonia in an elderly patient is an agent that is active against *S. pneumoniae, H. influenzae, Mycoplasma pneumoniae, Chlamydia pneumoniae,* and *Legionella* spp. The current recommendation is a macrolide such as erythromycin, azithromycin or clarithromycin or one of the newer quinolones such as levofloxacin.

A5. **e.** Urinary tract infections in the elderly are second only to respiratory tract infections as causes of febrile illness in patients over the age of 65 years. The risk factors for urinary tract infections in the elderly include the following:
a. Advanced age: the older the patient, the greater the risk (this appears to be immune-system dependent).
b. Decreased functional ability: resulting from cerebral vascular accidents, dementia, neurologic deficits, functional ability, and other chronic underlying illness
c. Decreased bladder emptying: results from neurogenic bladder, bladder-outlet obstruction (such as prostatic hypertrophy), and drugs with anticholinergic side effects
d. Nosocomial spread of organisms: spread from hospitalized patients with asymptomatic bacteriuria, the use of indwelling urinary catheters
e. Physiologic changes: decreased vaginal glycogen and increased vaginal pH in women, decreased prostatic secretions and increased prostatic calculi in men

A6. **d.** The most common organism responsible for urinary tract infections in elderly patients who do not have indwelling urinary catheters is *E. coli.* Other gram-negative organisms responsible include *Klebsiella, Enterococcus, Pseudomonas,* and *Proteus mirabilis.* However, in the absence of a complication (such as an indwelling catheter), *E. coli* still predominates. In summary, the difference between younger adults and older adults with respect to the cause of uncomplicated urinary tract infections is that although *E. coli* is the most common agent in both younger adults and older patients, the percentage of infections caused by *E. coli* is lower in older patients; that is, in older patients with an acute uncomplicated urinary tract infection there is more of a chance of an infection caused by *Klebsiella, Enterococcus, Proteus mirabilis,* or *Pseudomonas.*

A7. **a.** Regarding Case 3, the following facts can be stated:
a. This appears to be an uncomplicated urinary tract infection.
b. The most likely infecting organism is *E. coli.* As well, *Klebsiella, Proteus mirabilis,* and *Pseudomonas aeruginosa* must also be considered.
c. The most likely diagnosis is acute bacterial cystitis, which is confirmed when there are no signs or symptoms of upper urinary tract infection, and the bacterial count is greater than 105 organisms per milliliter of urine. The most common symptoms encountered in acute bacterial cystitis are lower abdominal or pelvic pain, dysuria, increased frequency of urination, and recent episodes of urinary incontinence.
d. The first-line drug in this case would be trimethoprim-sulfamethoxazole (TMP-SMX). A cephalosporin or quinolone (such as ciprofloxacin or levofloxacin) would also be reasonable first-line therapy. Although treatment with a single dose of TMP-SMX is reasonable for younger adults, it cannot be recommended for the elderly. For elders in the same situation, a 7-day course would be the best choice.

A8. **a.** Chronic bacterial prostatitis is the most common cause of relapsing urinary tract infection in elderly males.

The diagnosis of chronic bacterial prostatitis is established by culturing prostatic secretions obtained by prostatic massage. The most common causative organism is *E. coli. K. pneumoniae, Proteus,* and *Enterococcus* spp. are other organisms associated with the condition. The preferred antibiotic treatment is TMP-SMX or a quinolone antibiotic such as ciprofloxacin or levofloxacin. Relapses are common, even with prolonged therapy. This condition may be ameliorated by transurethral resection of the prostate (TURP).

In summary, the difference between younger adult males and older adult males with respect to prostatitis is that acute bacterial prostatitis is much more common in younger males and chronic bacterial prostatitis is much more common in older patients.

A9. **c.** The patient in Case 4 has acute pyelonephritis. Elderly patients who develop a syndrome of fever, chills, and irritating voiding symptoms likely have acute pyelonephritis in spite of the absence of CVA tenderness. In fact, not more than half of elders who develop pyelonephritis have the back pain and CVA tenderness that is so classic in younger patients with the disease. Some elders do not even have fever. Geriatric patients often also have gastrointestinal symptoms such as diarrhea or pulmonary symptoms.

Bacteremia is much more common in elderly patients who develop pyelonephritis, and the urinary tract is the source of bacteremia in over one third of elders admitted to the hospital with generalized sepsis. Thus blood cultures are mandatory before initiating treatment. From sepsis follows septic shock in up to 20% of elders with acute pyelonephritis. As with lower urinary tract infections, the most common organisms involved are *E. coli, Klebsiella, Proteus,* and *Pseudomonas.*

For elderly patients, the best initial antibiotic choice for suspected pyelonephritis is a combination of a beta-lactamase—resistant cephalosporin and an aminoglycoside (the latter to be used with extreme caution and with careful monitoring of serum levels).

In summary, the difference between younger adults and elderly patients with respect to complicated urinary tract infections such as acute pyelonephritis is that older patients frequently do not manifest the same symptoms and signs of complicated urinary tract infections as do younger adults. Specifically, they are less likely to manifest CVA tenderness and even fever and chills. This infection must be suspected in elderly patients who are immunocompromised and incapacitated (hospitalized patients and long-term care facility patients).

In addition, the probability of septicemia/generalized sepsis is greatly increased in elderly patients who develop urinary tract infections.

A10. **d.** By 2 weeks 50% of catheterized patients have significant bacteriuria, and after 1 month virtually all patients do.

Indwelling urinary catheters are the leading cause of nosocomial infection and the most common predisposing factor in hospital-acquired, gram-negative sepsis. Patients who have asymptomatic bacteriuria should not be treated with antibiotics. This applies to catheterized patients as well.

A11. **b.** In the hospitalized elder, the most common cause of morbidity and mortality is septicemia from a urinary tract infection.

A12. **a.** Elderly patients living in long-term care facilities are susceptible to bacterial pneumonia, which is their most common cause of death from an infective source.

A13. **a.** The leading infective causes of morbidity and mortality in elderly patients vary depending on location of the elder's habitation.

The most common cause of death from an infective source is bacterial pneumonia in elderly patients living in the community as well as those living in long-term care facilities. This serves to illustrate the importance of preventive services designated for this age group. The United States Task Force on the Periodic Health Examination recommends the following:
  a. All individuals over the age of 65 years should receive annual influenza vaccinations.
  b. All individuals over the age of 65 years should receive the Pneumovax vaccination.

Although bacterial pneumonia is discussed as the primary cause of morbidity and mortality, it must be understood that viral pneumonia frequently predates bacterial pneumonia (that is, influenza produces a viral pneumonia that leads to a secondary bacterial pneumonia).

A14. **c.** Acute appendicitis is primarily a disease of younger patients in their second or third decade of life. However, it also occurs with increasing frequency in males over the age of 80 years. The mortality in this age group is 10%. As with other abdominal infections such as acute cholecystitis, the increased severity of disease is largely caused by the atypical presentation of the signs and symptoms of acute inflammation (or more appropriately the lack of signs and symptoms of acute inflammation). Instead of the classic time sequence of periumbilical pain; anorexia, nausea, and vomiting; and movement of the pain to the right lower quadrant seen in younger patients, the elderly male with acute appendicitis usually has a prolonged period of vague abdominal discomfort.

There may be mild nausea and anorexia, but vomiting is unusual. As localized peritonitis develops, pain may appear in the right lower quadrant. Rebound tenderness and abdominal guarding, so common in younger adults, are uncommon in the elderly.

Perforation of the appendix is much more common in the elderly because of the narrowing of the lumen and the atherosclerotic changes in the artery supplying the appendix. In elderly patients, approximately 70% of cases of acute appendicitis rupture compared with 20% in younger patients.

In summary, critical differences between younger adults and older adults with appendicitis are that the elderly have atypical symptoms, have a high rate of perforation, and have a high mortality rate (10%).

A15. d. In children and in young and middle-aged adults, fever is often the result of a relatively benign disease. Such is not the case with the elderly. The rapid development of an elevated body temperature in an older adult is almost invariably the result of a serious infection such as pneumonia, urinary tract infection, or an intraabdominal abscess. Although the presence of fever in an older adult usually indicates a serious infection or other serious disease process (such as neoplasia and connective tissue disorders), elderly patients are two to three times as likely to demonstrate a lack of febrile response to the presence of serious disease.

In older adults who have FUO, the probability of a localized infection such as an abscess is high.

In summary, elders with a fever usually have a serious rather than a benign disease process going on. Always take this seriously.

SOLUTION TO THE SHORT ANSWER MANAGEMENT PROBLEM

Primary considerations in infectious diseases in the elderly depending on the habitation status of the elder are as follows:

a. Primary considerations for elders living in a community setting:
   1) Bacterial pneumonia
   2) Urinary tract infections
   3) Intraabdominal infections
      a) Cholecystitis
      b) Diverticulitis
      c) Appendicitis
b. Primary considerations for hospitalized elders:
   1) Urinary tract infections
   2) Bacterial pneumonia
   3) Surgical wound infections
c. Primary considerations for nursing home or other institutionalized elders:
   1) Bacterial pneumonia
   2) Urinary tract infection
   3) Decubitus ulcers

Although tuberculosis and intraabdominal infections are not as common as bacterial pneumonia, urinary tract infection, and decubitus ulcers, they do occur at high rates among institutionalized elders.

Because the summaries are provided throughout the answers, a detailed summary will not be repeated for this chapter.

SUGGESTED READING
Yoshikawa TT: Approach to the diagnosis and treatment of the infected older adult. In Hazzard WR et al, eds: *Principles of geriatric medicine and gerontology*, ed 3, New York, 1994, McGraw-Hill.

PROBLEM · 122

URINARY INCONTINENCE IN THE ELDERLY

"I'm So Embarrassed. I Haven't Done That Since I Was 5 Years Old."

Case 1 ■ An 88-Year-Old Institutionalized Female with Urinary Incontinence

An 88-year-old female patient whom you care for and who resides in a chronic care facility is having increasing difficulties with "bed-wetting." She is embarrassed to talk about this, but the nurses inform you that it is a problem and is getting progressively worse.

On your last weekly visit, the charge nurse requested permission from you to insert an indwelling urinary catheter. At that time, the patient had been incontinent continuously for 6 days. The charge nurse clearly tells you, "I haven't got enough staff to keep changing sheets 10 times a day—please do something."

SELECT THE BEST ANSWER TO THE FOLLOWING QUESTIONS

Q1. At this time, what should your instructions to the charge nurse be?
   a. insert the indwelling catheter; call me if there are any more problems
   b. begin intermittent 4-hour catheterization to avoid the necessity of inserting an indwelling catheter
   c. wait and see what happens over the next couple of weeks
   d. order some routine blood work to attempt to determine the cause of the problem
   e. clearly indicate that you will begin investigation of this problem now; ask the charge nurse, in return, to attempt to manage the current situation for only a short time longer

Q2. Regarding urinary incontinence in the elderly, which of the following statements is false?
   a. 50% of elderly patients in nursing homes have established urinary incontinence
   b. 5% to 15% of elderly patients in a community setting have developed urinary incontinence
   c. women are twice as likely as men to have urinary incontinence
   d. humiliation and embarrassment are significant life problems for the patient with urinary incontinence
   e. none of the above statements is false

Q3. What is the most common type of urinary incontinence in elderly patients?
a. urge incontinence
b. stress incontinence
c. complex incontinence
d. overflow incontinence
e. functional incontinence

Q4. Which of the following statements regarding incontinence in the elderly is (are) true?
a. stress incontinence is usually manifested by loss of small amounts of urine as intraabdominal pressure increases
b. overflow incontinence occurs through bladder distention
c. prostatic obstruction is a common cause of overflow incontinence
d. functional incontinence is characterized by an involuntary loss of urine despite normal bladder and urethral functioning
e. all of the above statements are true

Q5. Which of the following is (are) contributing factors to urinary incontinence in the elderly?
a. a loss of the ability of the elderly to concentrate urine
b. a decreased bladder capacity
c. decreased urethral closing pressure
d. decreased mobility
e. all of the above

Q6. Which of the following classes of drugs has not been implicated in the pathogenesis of urinary incontinence in the elderly?
a. thiazide diuretics
b. neuroleptics
c. sedatives
d. antibiotics
e. hypnotics

Q7. Which of the following nonpharmacologic treatments may be effective in the management of urinary incontinence in the elderly?
a. Kegel exercises
b. biofeedback
c. behavioral toilet training
d. clean intermittent catheterization
e. all of the above

Q8. Which of the following cause(s) acute (reversible) urinary incontinence in the elderly?
a. delirium
b. restricted mobility
c. infection
d. drugs
e. all of the above

Q9. Anticholinergic and narcotic drugs are most commonly associated with which of the following types of urinary incontinence?
a. urge incontinence
b. stress incontinence
c. overflow incontinence
d. complex incontinence
e. functional incontinence

Q10. Which of the following components of the diagnostic evaluation of urinary incontinence is not necessary in every elderly patient with the disorder?
a. complete history
b. focused physical examination
c. renal ultrasound
d. complete urinalysis
e. postvoiding residual (PVR) urine determination

Q11. PVR urine is considered definitely abnormal when it exceeds which of the following?
a. 50 ml
b. 200 ml
c. 75 ml
d. 100 ml
e. 150 ml

Q12. What is (are) the drug(s) of choice for the pharmacologic management of stress incontinence?
a. supplemental estrogen
b. alpha-adrenergic agonists
c. cholinergic agents
d. a and b
e. all of the above

Q13. Which of the following types of urinary incontinence is most amenable to surgical intervention?
a. urge incontinence
b. stress incontinence
c. overflow incontinence
d. complex incontinence
e. functional incontinence

Q14. Which of the following are indications for the use of a chronic indwelling catheter in elderly patients with incontinence?
a. urinary retention causing persistent overflow incontinence
b. chronic skin wounds or pressure ulcers that can be contaminated by incontinent urine

c. terminally ill or severely impaired elderly patients for whom bed and clothing changes are uncomfortable

d. urinary retention that cannot be controlled medically or surgically

e. none of the above statements is true

f. all of the above statements are true

Q15. Alzheimer's disease, Parkinson's disease, and cerebrovascular disease are usually associated with which of the following types of urinary incontinence?

a. urge incontinence

b. stress incontinence

c. overflow incontinence

d. complex incontinence

e. functional incontinence

SHORT ANSWER MANAGEMENT PROBLEM
List the patient-dependent (4) and caregiver-dependent (2) behaviorally oriented training procedures that may be beneficial in the management of urinary incontinence in the elderly.

ANSWERS

A1. **e.** In an elderly patient who has just become incontinent, it is inappropriate to insert a Foley catheter or do anything else until you have established the cause. The pathophysiology of urinary incontinence in the elderly population is complex, even among patients with dementia. Elderly patients deserve the same intensive investigation of the cause of incontinence as you would perform in a younger individual.

A2. **e.** Of elderly patients in nursing homes, 50% have urinary incontinence. Of elderly patients in the community, 5% to 15% have urinary incontinence.

Women are twice as likely as men to develop urinary incontinence.

Humiliation and embarrassment are important consequences of urinary incontinence in elderly patients. This embarrassment leads to social isolation and subsequent anxiety and depression. Incontinence is the second leading cause of admission of elderly patients to long-term care facilities.

In North America it is estimated that the total health care costs associated with urinary incontinence are over $8 billion per year.

Physical consequences, such as predisposition to skin irritations and subsequent skin ulcers and infections, are also a major problem.

A3. **a.** The most common type of urinary incontinence in the elderly population is urge incontinence. Urge incontinence (also known as detrusor hyperreflexia) is characterized by leakage of urine caused by strong and sudden sensations of bladder urgency. Patients with urge incontinence may also experience frequency, urgency, and nocturia. Urge incontinence is also called *unstable bladder, uninhibited bladder,* and *hyperreflexic bladder.* Many conditions may predispose to urge incontinence; these include cerebrovascular accidents, Parkinson's disease, Alzheimer's disease, spinal cord injury or tumor, multiple sclerosis, prostatic hypertrophy, and interstitial cystitis.

Urge incontinence may also be present in patients in whom no neurologic or genitourinary abnormality is present.

A4. **e.** Stress incontinence (urethral incompetence) is characterized by loss of small amounts of urine secondary to increases in intraabdominal pressure. Stress incontinence is most commonly associated with pelvic floor weakening through childbirth, obesity, injury, menopause and aging, and sphincter damage.

Overflow incontinence occurs with bladder overdistention. Overdistention results in a constant leakage of small amounts of urine or "dribbling," a physiologic situation in which the intracystic pressure exceeds the intraurethral resistance. Bladder overdistention is usually caused by an enlarged prostate, urethral stricture, or fecal impaction. A hypotonic bladder secondary to diabetes mellitus, syphilis, spinal cord compression, or anticholinergic medications may also result in overflow incontinence.

Complex incontinence refers to incontinence that has both urge and stress components.

Functional incontinence refers to involuntary loss of urine despite normal bladder and urethral functioning. This is most commonly seen with severe dementia and closed head injuries.

A5. **e.** Many factors are associated with the development and maintenance of urinary incontinence in the elderly. These include a loss of the ability of the kidney to concentrate urine, a decreased bladder capacity, decreased urethral closing pressure following menopause, decreased mobility, decreased vision, depression and secondary inattention to bladder cues, and an inadequate environmental setting.

The importance of drugs in the causation of elderly incontinence is discussed in Answer 6.

A6. **d.** Drug use is a common cause of incontinence in the elderly. The major drugs implicated as a cause of urinary incontinence in the elderly and the pathology involved are summarized below:

DRUG CLASS	PATHOLOGY
Diuretics	Polyuria, frequency, urgency
Anticholinergics	Urinary retention, overflow incontinence, impaction
Antidepressants	Anticholinergic actions, sedation
Antipsychotics	Anticholinergic actions, sedation, rigidity, immobility
Sedative-hypnotics	Sedation, delirium, immobility, muscle relaxation
Narcotic analgesics	Urinary retention, fecal impaction, sedation, delirium
Alpha-adrenergic	Urethral relaxation blockers, urinary retention agonists
Beta-adrenergic	Urinary retention blockers
Calcium-channel blocker	Urinary retention
Alcohol	Polyuria, frequency, urgency, sedation, delirium, immobility

A7. **e.** Nonpharmacologic treatments are both available and useful in the treatment of all forms of urinary incontinence in the elderly. The treatments include the following:

a. Stress incontinence:
   1) Pelvic muscle (Kegel) exercises
   2) Biofeedback
   3) Behavioral therapies (prompted voiding, habit training, scheduled toileting)
   4) Transcutaneous electrical nerve stimulation (TENS)
b. Urge incontinence:
   1) Biofeedback
   2) Behavioral therapies (as previously listed)
   3) TENS
c. Overflow incontinence:
   1) Intermittent catheterization
   2) Indwelling catheterization (if no other options are possible)
d. Functional incontinence:
   1) Behavioral therapies (as previously listed)
   2) Environmental manipulations
   3) Incontinence undergarments and pads
   4) External collection devices
   5) Indwelling catheters (if necessary)
   6) TENS

In the past, TENS has been used successfully to treat chronic pain syndromes. An exciting new development provides another opportunity to avoid both surgery and pharmacologic agents in treatment of incontinence. The use of a pessary TENS unit has recently been shown to be effective for stress incontinence and urge incontinence. More trials need to be carried out before definitive conclusions can be made, but initial results are promising.

A8. **e.** Causes of acute and reversible forms of urinary incontinence are provided by the DRIP mnemonic:
   a. **D**elirium
   b. **R**estricted mobility, retention
   c. **I**nfection (urinary tract), inflammation (urethritis or atrophic vaginitis), impaction (fecal)
   d. **P**olyuria (diabetes mellitus, diabetes insipidus, congestive heart failure, and venous insufficiency), pharmaceuticals

A9. **c.** Urinary retention with overflow incontinence must be considered when any patient, who was previously completely continent, suddenly becomes incontinent. The causes include the following:
   a. Immobility
   b. Anticholinergic drugs
   c. Narcotic analgesic drugs
   d. Calcium-channel blockers
   e. Beta-blockers
   f. Fecal impaction
   g. Spinal cord compression resulting from metastatic cancer

A10. **c.** The evaluation of urinary incontinence in the elderly should be undertaken with the same precision and care as evaluation and investigation of other urinary problems in younger patients.

All elderly patients who present with urinary incontinence should have the following procedures performed:
   a. A complete history
   b. A complete medication review (ideally, every elderly patient on more than one drug should have this done every 3 months)
   c. An age-specific focused physical examination (U.S. Preventive Services Task Force)
   d. A complete urinalysis
   e. A urine culture
   f. A PVR urine determination

A renal ultrasound needs to be done only if problems such as urinary obstruction (a renal tumor), uremia, or the inability of the kidneys to concentrate urine is suspected.

A11. **b.** A PVR urine should be performed on every elderly patient with incontinence to exclude significant degrees of urinary retention. Neither the history nor the physical examination is sensitive or specific enough for this purpose in elderly patients. The PVR urine can be done either by itself as a simple one-test procedure or in conjunction with other simple urodynamic investigations.

To maximize the accuracy of PVR urine, the measurement should be performed within a few minutes of voiding. A postvoiding residual volume of 100 ml or less in the absence of straining reflects adequate bladder emptying in elderly patients; a PVR urine value of 200 ml, on the other hand, is definitely abnormal.

A12. **d.** The ideal combination of pharmacologic agents for certain patients with stress incontinence involves supplemental estrogen and an alpha-adrenergic agonist.

For patients with stress incontinence, pharmacologic management is appropriate if the following is true:
  a. The patient is motivated.
  b. The degree of stress incontinence is "mild to moderate."
  c. There is no major associated anatomical abnormality (such as a large cystocele).
  d. The patient does not have any contraindications to the use of these drugs.

Pharmacologic treatment of stress incontinence is as efficacious as, but not more efficacious than, nonpharmacologic treatment. Approximately 75% of patients improve with each. Combining the two modalities improves the efficacy of treatment.

Supplemental estrogen has not been found, by itself, to be as effective as when used in combination with an alpha-adrenergic agonist. If either oral or vaginal estrogen is used for a prolonged period of time (greater than a few months), then cyclic progesterone should be added to protect the endometrium. A combination of oral Premarin (0.3 mg/day) and oral pseudoephedrine (Sudafed) 30 to 60 mg tid would be a good starting point for pharmacologic treatment of stress incontinence.

A13. **b.** The type of incontinence that is most amenable to surgical intervention is stress incontinence. The indication for surgery in stress incontinence is continued significant bothersome leakage that occurs after attempts at nonsurgical treatment and patients who, along with their stress incontinence, also have a significant degree of pelvic prolapse.

The second most amenable subtype of incontinence that may be significantly improved with surgery is outflow obstruction caused by prostatic hypertrophy or prostatic carcinoma in men. With benign prostatic hypertrophy it would be prudent to reduce the size of the prostate and decrease obstruction by use of a 5-alpha-reductase inhibitor or an alpha-adrenergic blocker (doxazosin, terazosin, prazosin) before contemplating surgery.

A14. **f.** The indications for chronic indwelling catheter use include the following:
  a. Urinary retention, That is:
    1) Causing persistent overflow incontinence
    2) Causing symptomatic infections

    3) Producing renal dysfunction
    4) Unable to be corrected surgically or medically
    5) Not practically managed with intermittent catheterization
  b. Skin wounds, pressure sores, or irritations that are being contaminated by incontinent urine
  c. Care of terminally ill or severely impaired patients for whom bed and clothing changes are uncomfortable or disruptive
  d. Preference of patient or caregiver when a patient has failed to respond to more specific treatments

A15. **a.** Central nervous system disorders such as cerebrovascular accidents (stroke), dementia, Parkinson's disease, and suprasacral spinal cord injury are associated with detrusor motor or sensory instability resulting in urge incontinence.

SOLUTION TO THE SHORT ANSWER MANAGEMENT PROBLEM

Following are examples of behaviorally oriented training procedures for urinary incontinence.
  a. Patient-dependent procedures:
    1) Pelvic muscle (Kegel) exercises
    2) Biofeedback
    3) Behavioral training
    4) Bladder retraining
  b. Caregiver-dependent procedures:
    1) Scheduled toileting or prompted voiding
    2) Habit training

SUMMARY OF THE DIAGNOSIS AND MANAGEMENT OF URINARY INCONTINENCE IN THE ELDERLY

1. Definition: The involuntary loss of urine in sufficient amount or frequency to be a social or health problem
2. Subtypes of urinary incontinence: Acute (reversible) versus persistent urinary incontinence
3. Acute (reversible) urinary incontinence: DRIP mnemonic: **D**elirium; **R**estricted mobility, retention; **I**nfection, inflammation, impaction; **P**olyuria, pharmaceuticals
4. Persistent urinary incontinence:
  a. Stress: Involuntary loss of urine (usually small amounts) with increases in intraabdominal pressure (such as cough, laugh, or exercise). Common causes include weakness and laxity of pelvic floor musculature and bladder outlet or urethral sphincter weakness.
  b. Urge: Leakage of urine (often larger volumes, but variable) because of inability to delay voiding after sensation or bladder fullness is per-

ceived; also known as *detrusor hyperreflexia.* Common causes include detrusor motor or sensory instability, isolated or associated with one or more of the following: cystitis, urethritis, tumors, stones, diverticula, or outflow obstruction; also central nervous system disorders such as stroke, dementia, Parkinson's disease, and suprasacral spinal cord injury.

c. Overflow: Leakage of urine (usually small amounts) resulting from mechanical forces on an overdistended bladder or from other effects of urinary retention on either bladder or sphincter function. Common causes include anatomic obstruction by prostate, stricture, and cystocele; hypotonic bladder associated with diabetes mellitus or a spinal cord injury; neurogenic (detrusor-sphincter dyssynergy) associated with multiple sclerosis, or supraspinal cord lesions.

d. Functional: Urinary leakage associated with the inability to toilet because of impairment of cognitive or physical functioning, psychologic unwillingness, or environmental barriers. Common causes include severe dementia and other neurologic disorders or psychologic factors such as depression, regression, anger, and hostility.

5. Prevalence of urinary incontinence in the elderly:
   a. Institutionalized elderly: 50%
   b. Elderly patients living in the community: 5% to 15%

6. Investigations:
   a. Basic investigations for all elderly patients with urinary incontinence:
      1) Complete history
      2) Complete physical examination
      3) Complete medication review (every 3 months)
      4) Complete urinalysis
      5) Urine for culture and sensitivity
      6) PVR urine determination

7. Primary treatments for different types of geriatric urinary incontinence:
   a. Stress incontinence:
      1) Pelvic muscle (Kegel) exercises
      2) Alpha-adrenergic agonists
      3) Supplemental estrogen (oral or vaginal)
      4) Biofeedback, behavioral training
      5) Surgical bladder neck suspension
      6) Periurethral injections
   b. Urge incontinence:
      1) Bladder relaxants
      2) Estrogen (if vaginal atrophy is present)
      3) Behavioral procedures (biofeedback and behavioral therapy)
      4) Surgical removal of obstructing or other irritating pathologic lesions
   c. Overflow incontinence:
      1) Surgical removal of obstruction
      2) Intermittent catheterization (if practical)
      3) Indwelling catheterization
   d. Functional incontinence:
      1) Behavioral therapies (prompted voiding, habit training, or scheduled toileting)
      2) Environmental manipulations
      3) Incontinence undergarments and pads
      4) External collection devices
      5) Bladder relaxants (selected patients)
      6) Indwelling catheters (selected patients)

SUGGESTED READINGS

AHCPR Urinary Incontinence in Adults Guideline Update Panel: Managing acute and chronic urinary incontinence *Am Fam Physician* 54(5):1661-1672, 1996.

Ouslander JG: Incontinence. In Hazzard WR et al, eds: *Principles of geriatric medicine and gerontology* ed 3, New York, 1994, McGraw-Hill.

Rosenthal AJ, McMurtry CT: Urinary incontinence in the elderly, *Postgrad Med* 92(5):1099-1121, 1995.

Tierney LM, Jr, McPhee SJ, Papadakis MA, eds: *Current medical diagnosis and treatment, 2000,* Stamford, Conn, 1999, Appleton & Lange.

PROBLEM·123

DEPRESSION IN THE ELDERLY

"I'm Dead. They Just Haven't Buried Me Yet!"

Case 1 ■ An 85-Year-Old Female Nursing Home Resident Who Simply "Stares into Space" and Cries Almost All of the Time

You are called to see an 85-year-old patient who moved into a nursing home 9 months ago. Previously, she was living on her own and had managed by herself since the death of her husband 6 years ago. During the past year she has become increasingly disabled with congestive heart failure and osteoarthritis.

During the past 9 months the patient has lost 15 pounds, has not been hungry, has lost interest in all of her social activities, and has been crying almost every day.

You are aware that before moving into the nursing home she was quite active.

Her mental status examination is difficult. She does, however, describe her mood as being worse in the morning. Her short-term memory, according to the staff, is also impaired. She is currently taking furosemide and enalapril for her congestive heart failure and plain acetaminophen for the pain associated with osteoarthritis.

SELECT THE BEST ANSWER
TO THE FOLLOWING QUESTIONS

Q1. What is the most likely diagnosis in this patient?
   a. major depressive illness
   b. Alzheimer's disease
   c. multiinfarct dementia
   d. hypothyroidism
   e. none of the above

Q2. Regarding the diagnosis of the patient described, which of the following statements is false?
   a. this condition occurs less often in older patients than in younger patients
   b. elderly patients are less likely to recover from this illness than young adults
   c. this condition is more common among institutionalized elders than elders living at home
   d. this condition may be related to physical illness
   e. this condition may be related to the move into the nursing home itself

Q3. Which of the following investigations and/or assessments should be performed in the patient described?
   a. a medication review
   b. a complete blood count (CBC)
   c. a serum thyroid-stimulating hormone (TSH) level
   d. all of the above
   e. none of the above

Q4. Which of the following antidepressants is considered an agent of first choice for the treatment of depression in the elderly?
   a. imipramine
   b. nortriptyline
   c. desipramine
   d. amitriptyline
   e. fluoxetine

Q5. Which of the following antidepressants specifically blocks serotonin reuptake?
   a. imipramine
   b. desipramine
   c. nortriptyline
   d. amitriptyline
   e. fluoxetine

Q6. You decide to treat the patient described in Case 1 with nortriptyline. In a patient of this age, at what daily dosage would you start her?
   a. 10 mg
   b. 25 mg

   c. 50 mg
   d. 75 mg
   e. 100 mg

Q7. Regarding the treatment for the condition described, which of the following statements is (are) true?
   a. electroconvulsive therapy (ECT) is unlikely to be of any benefit in the treatment of this condition
   b. socialization, music therapy, and pet therapy have no role to play in the treatment of this condition
   c. cognitive and behavioral therapy may significantly improve this condition
   d. all of the above statements are true
   e. none of the above statements is true

Q8. Which of the following features is most commonly associated with this diagnosis in geriatric patients?
   a. acute mania
   b. hypomania
   c. extreme anxiety
   d. psychomotor agitation or retardation
   e. hypersomnia

Q9. The signs and symptoms of the condition described include all except which of the following?
   a. impaired concentration
   b. guilt
   c. hopelessness
   d. suicidal ideation
   e. violent or aggressive behavior

Q10. The length of time recommended for the pharmacologic treatment of this condition with the drug selected is at least
   a. 1 month
   b. 3 months
   c. 6 months
   d. 12 months
   e. 18 months

Q11. An elderly institutionalized patient is put on nortriptyline. The dose is increased up to 100 mg but no improvement is noted. You decide to substitute fluoxetine. Which of the following side effects might you anticipate?
   a. constipation
   b. blurred vision
   c. urinary retention
   d. dry mouth
   e. agitation

Q12. If the side effect selected in Question 11 occurred, which of the following courses of action would be the most reasonable?
   a. increase the dose of the drug
   b. decrease the dose of the drug
   c. stop the drug
   d. elect ECT as your next option
   e. c and d

SHORT ANSWER MANAGEMENT PROBLEM
Part A: Discuss the differential diagnosis of depressive symptoms in the elderly.
Part B: List the three most common physical illnesses that present or manifest depression in the elderly.
Part C: Name the most common drug associated with depression in the elderly.
Part D: Name the most common drug class associated with depression as a psychoactive substance use disorder.

ANSWERS

A1. **a.** This patient has a major depressive illness. The criteria for major depressive illness are summarized in Problem 60. A mnemonic that is very helpful for diagnosing depression is A SIG: E CAPS:

   A = **A**ffect: At least a 2-week period of a depressed mood or a depressed affect
   S = **S**leep disturbance (hyposomnia, insomnia, hypersomnia)
   I = **I**nterest (lack of interest of life)
   G = **G**uilt or hopelessness
   E = **E**nergy level (decreased) or fatigue
   C = **C**oncentration decreased
   A = **A**ppetite disturbance (decreased or increased with or without weight gain or weight loss)
   P = **P**sychomotor retardation or agitation
   S = **S**uicidal ideation

Major depressive illness is diagnosed when there are 4 of 8 criteria present and at least a 2-week period of a depressed mood or depressed affect.

Despite these criteria, depression in elderly patients is more likely to occur with weight loss and less likely to occur with feelings of worthlessness and guilt. Elderly patients are no more likely than persons in midlife to report cognitive problems, although they do have more difficulties with cognition during an episode of depression.

The other choices listed in this question are discussed in other sections of this book.

A2. **b.** Elderly patients are just as likely to recover from a major depressive illness as are younger adults.

Major depression is less prevalent among those aged 65 and older than in younger groups. Suicide, however, is not; it continues to rise in elderly patients at a rather alarming rate.

The prevalence of major depression in elderly patients in the community is between 1% and 2%. The majority of depressed elderly patients, however, do not fit the DSM-IV criteria but rather have depressive symptoms that are associated with an adjustment reaction (as in this patient who has just had to leave her own home) or that are associated with significant physical illness (as this patient also demonstrates).

In long-term chronic care facilities, the prevalence of major depressive illness may be as high as 10% to 20%.

A3. **d.** The elderly patient with depressive symptoms should have the following evaluations: a complete history, a complete physical examination, and a complete medication review (both prescribed and over-the-counter medications). Some of the most common pharmacologic agents that contribute to depression include antihypertensive agents such as propranolol and methyldopa as well as cimetidine and sedative hypnotic drugs.

In addition to the complete history and physical examination, the elderly patient should also have the following laboratory investigations: CBC, vitamin B_{12}, serum folate level, serum TSH, chest x-ray, electrocardiogram (ECG), complete urinalysis, and serum electrolytes.

A4. **b.** Nortriptyline is the tricyclic of choice in treating geriatric depression because of its relatively low risks of orthostatic hypotension (low alpha blockade) and low anticholinergic side effects (dry mouth, urinary retention, blurred vision, constipation, and sedation). As well, it has a high therapeutic window.

The selective serotonin reuptake inhibitors (SSRIs) such as fluoxetine are not yet considered the drugs of first choice in elderly patients, even though they may well be the agents of first choice in younger patients. As well, some of these agents, especially fluoxetine, actually increase the probability or state of agitation in the elderly.

A5. **e.** The group of antidepressant agents known as SSRIs includes fluoxetine (Prozac), sertraline (Zoloft), and paroxetine (Paxil). These drugs, as indicated, are not the agents of first choice for the treatment of depression in the elderly. They do, however, offer some significant theoretic advantages in that the common tricyclic antidepressant side effects such as dry mouth, blurred vision, tachycardia, constipation (anticholinergic), orthostatic hypotension (alpha-adrenergic blockade), and weight gain may be averted by their use. As well, they do not increase the cardiac risk caused by blockade of impulse conduction through the atrioventricular node.

As experience is gained with the SSRIs in younger patients, they may very well "move up the ladder" and become drugs of first choice for treating depression in the elderly.

A6. **a.** The patient described in this case, an 80-year-old female, should be started on as low a dose of tricyclic antidepressant as possible. A dose of 10 mg would be an ideal starting dose. This dose could be increased slowly as needed.

A7. **c.** Elderly patients with depressive illness may be significantly improved with cognitive or behavioral psychotherapy.

Attempts at increased socialization (especially in chronic care facilities), music therapy, pet therapy, and other therapies that serve to redirect the attention of the elderly patient appear to be effective in the treatment of depression in the elderly.

ECT may be the only effective therapy for severe depression in elderly patients, especially in patients with psychotic depression. ECT is well tolerated in geriatric patients and lacks the side effects associated with the tricyclic antidepressants. Contraindications to ECT include an intracranial mass, recent myocardial infarction, or a recent cardiovascular accident.

A8. **d.** Although acute mania, hypomania, extreme anxiety, and hypersomnia may all be associated with depression in elderly patients, by far the most common symptom of those listed in elderly patients is psychomotor agitation or retardation. Psychomotor agitation is the more common presentation of the two.

A9. **e.** The diagnostic symptoms of depressive illness have been covered in Answer 1. They do not include violent or aggressive behavior. If violent or aggressive behavior is found in a patient who has an underlying depression, there is likely another major diagnosis that would explain the symptom. In an elder the most common diagnosis in this case would be Alzheimer's disease.

A10. **c.** Geriatric patients should be treated with antidepressants for at least 6 months. After 6 months, if the patient is improved, the drug can be tapered and eventually discontinued.

A11. **e.** The side effects of blurred vision, dry mouth, urinary retention, and constipation are all anticholinergic side effects that do not occur with the new SSRIs.

Agitation, however, is a side effect that may be anticipated with these drugs, especially with fluoxetine.

A12. **e.** The most reasonable course of action would be to discontinue the drug and to use ECT. Two failed drug courses (with drugs of different classes) would be a reasonable indication for the use of ECT.

SOLUTION TO THE SHORT ANSWER MANAGEMENT PROBLEM

Part A: The differential diagnosis of depressive symptoms in the elderly is lengthy. It includes four major categories: mood disorders, adjustment disorders, psychoactive substance-use disorders, and somatoform disorders.
  a. Mood disorders:
    1) Major depression (single episode or recurrent)
    2) Dysthymia (or depressive neurosis)
    3) Bipolar affective disorder, depressed
    4) Depressive disorder not otherwise specified (atypical depression with mild biogenic depression)
  b. Adjustment disorders:
    1) Primary degenerative dementia with associated depression
    2) Organic mood disorder, depressed
    3) Secondary to physical illness:
      a) Hypothyroidism
      b) Carcinoma of the pancreas
      c) Stroke
      d) Parkinson's disease
    4) Secondary to pharmacologic agents: methyldopa, propranolol
  c. Psychoactive substance use disorders:
    1) Alcohol use or dependence
    2) Sedative, hypnotic, or anxiolytic abuse or dependence
  d. Somatoform disorders:
    1) Hypochondriasis
    2) Somatization disorder

Part B: The three most common physical illnesses that present or manifest depression in the elderly are hypothyroidism, carcinoma of the pancreas, and cerebrovascular accident (stroke).

Part C: The most common drug associated with depression in the elderly is propranolol.

Part D: The most common drug class associated with depression as a psychoactive substance use class is the drug class that includes all of the sedative-hypnotics. Sedatives and hypnotics are vastly overused in the elderly; this appears to be especially true in institutionalized elderly patients. It is much easier for nursing home staff to prescribe a sedative-hypnotic or both than to recognize and help an elder adjust to altered sleep patterns.

SUMMARY AND DIAGNOSIS OF DEPRESSION IN THE ELDERLY

1. Diagnosis: Follow DSM-IV criteria, except recognize that the elderly are more likely to experience weight loss and cognitive problems and less likely to experience feelings of guilt and hopelessness.

2. Recognize that depression is often an adjustment reaction to life stress, environment change (especially having to leave home), and the realization of the effects of aging itself.

3. Prevalence: Depression prevalence is 1% to 2% in community environment and 10% to 20% in an institutional environment.

4. Differential diagnosis includes mood disorders, adjustment disorders, organic mental disorders, psychoactive substance use, and somatoform disorders.

5. Investigations include mini-mental status examination; complete medication review; and laboratory evaluation including CBC, electrolytes, TSH, vitamin B_{12}, serum folate, ECG, and chest x-ray.

6. Treatment strategies:
   a. Nonpharmacologic strategies:
      1) Relaxation techniques and mind-occupying techniques such as frequent visitors, pet therapy, and music therapy
      2) Cognitive, supportive, and behavioral psychotherapy
   b. Pharmacologic strategies:
      1) Drugs of first choice: Tricyclics antidepressants: the tricyclic of choice is nortriptyline at a starting dosage of 10 mg. Side effects with amitriptyline are often too severe, and this medication should be used judiciously in the elderly.
      2) Drugs of second choice are SSRIs: Use fluoxetine with caution because of potential side effect of agitation.
      3) Drugs of third choice are MAOA inhibitors.
      4) ECT: If two drug classes fail, ECT should be considered. ECT has much more of a role to play in geriatric depression than it does in depression associated with younger patients.
      5) Most importantly, depression in the elderly must not be treated with pharmacologic agents only; treatment should, instead, include an equal contribution from nonpharmacologic treatments and pharmacologic agents.

SUGGESTED READINGS

American Psychiatric Association, Task Force on DSM IV. *Diagnostic and statistical manual of mental disorders*, ed 4, Washington, DC, 1994, American Psychiatric Association Press.

Blazer D: Depression. In Hazzard WR et al, eds: *Principles of geriatric medicine and gerontology*, ed 3, New York, 1994, McGraw-Hill.

Cadieux RJ: Practical management of treatment-resistant depression, *Am Fam Physician* 58(9):2059-2062, 1998.

Fretwell M: Depression. In Ferri FF et al, eds: *Practical guide to the care of the geriatric patient*, ed 2, St Louis, 1997, Mosby.

Mulsant BH, Pollock BG: Treatment-resistant depression in late life, *J Geriatr Psychiatr Neurol* 11(4):186-193, 1998.

Rakel RE: Depression: Primary care, *Clin Office Pract* 26(2):211-224, 1999.

PROBLEM · 124

PRESSURE ULCERS

"Doctor, the Care in This Place Must Be Terrible. Look, My Mother Has a Big Sore on Her Back."

Case 1 ■ An 80-Year-Old Female Nursing Home Resident with a Pressure Ulcer

You are called to a nursing home to see an 80-year-old female with a fever of 40° C. The patient is disoriented and confused. The nursing home staff has had difficulty treating her pressure ulcers, especially one on her sacrum.

On physical examination, the patient's blood pressure is 110/80 mm Hg and her pulse is 72 and regular. There is a 10 cm × 5 cm pressure ulcer on her sacrum. As well, there is a purulent, foul-smelling discharge coming from that ulcer.

SELECT THE BEST ANSWER TO THE FOLLOWING QUESTIONS

Q1. Which of the following diseases or conditions is (are) risk factors for the development of pressure ulcers?
   a. immobility
   b. dementia
   c. Parkinson's disease
   d. congestive heart failure
   e. a, b, and c
   f. all of the above

Q2. Which of the following nutritional or physiologic variables increase(s) the risk of pressure ulcers?
   a. hypoalbuminemia
   b. moist skin
   c. increased pressure
   d. a and b
   e. all of the above

Q3. Regarding the pathophysiology of pressure ulcers, which of the following factors has (have) been implicated in their cause?
   a. the pressure of the body weight itself
   b. shearing forces
   c. friction
   d. moisture
   e. a, b, and d
   f. all of the above

Q4. Which of the following statements concerning the prevention and cause of pressure ulcers is false?
   a. pressure ulcers are impossible to prevent in immobilized elderly patients
   b. good nutrition in the elderly will help prevent pressure ulcers
   c. anemia in the elderly patient predisposes to the formation of pressure ulcers
   d. incontinence in the elderly increases the risk of pressure ulcers by a factor of five
   e. patients who sit for long periods are just as likely to develop pressure ulcers as bed-ridden patients

Q5. Concerning the patient described in Case 1, what amount of time would it take the large ulcer to develop from a small, untreated ulcer?
   a. 28 days
   b. 21 to 28 days
   c. 14 to 20 days
   d. 7 to 10 days
   e. 1 to 2 days

Q6. Which of the following anatomic sites is the least common site for the development of a pressure ulcer?
   a. the ischial tuberosity
   b. the lateral malleolus
   c. the medial malleolus
   d. the sacrum
   e. the greater trochanter

Q7. With respect to pathophysiology, which of the following factors contributes to the formation of pressure ulcers?
   a. blood and lymphatic vessel obstruction
   b. plasma leakage into the interstitial space
   c. hemorrhage
   d. bacterial deposition at the site of the pressure induced injury
   e. muscle cell death
   f. all of the above

Q8. Which of the following statements concerning pressure ulcers and mortality in elderly patients is (are) true?
   a. there appears to be no increase in mortality among elderly individuals who develop pressure ulcers
   b. failure of a pressure ulcer to heal or improve has not been associated with a higher death rate in institutionalized elderly
   c. in-hospital death rates for patients with pressure ulcers range from 23% to 36%
   d. all of the above statements are true
   e. none of the above statements is true

Q9. Patients at high risk for the development of pressure ulcers should be repositioned how frequently?
   a. every 2 hours
   b. every 4 hours
   c. every 6 hours
   d. every 8 hours
   e. every 12 hours

Q10. Which of the following descriptions best illustrate(s) the nature of bacteria usually found in an infected pressure ulcer?
   a. gram-positive aerobic cocci alone
   b. gram-negative aerobic rods alone
   c. anaerobic bacteria alone
   d. a and c
   e. all of the above

Q11. What are the best initial antibiotic treatments for an infected pressure ulcer?
   a. tetracycline and gentamicin
   b. clindamycin and gentamicin
   c. cephalexin and doxycycline
   d. penicillin and gentamicin
   e. trimethoprim-sulfamethoxazole

Q12. What is the most common and serious complication of pressure ulcers in elderly patients?
   a. anemia
   b. hypoproteinemia
   c. infection
   d. contracture
   e. bone resorption

Q13. Bacterial sepsis leading to septic shock in pressure ulcers is most closely associated with which of the following bacteria?
   a. *Bacteroides fragilis*
   b. *Pseudomonas aeruginosa*
   c. *Proteus mirabilis*
   d. *Staphylococcus aureus*
   e. *Providencia* spp.

Case 2 ■ A 78-Year-Old Immobilized Male with a 1-cm Area of Erythema and Bruising on His Heel

A 78-year-old immobilized male is seen with a 1-cm area of erythema and bruising on his left heel.

Q14. Which of the following is the most important aspect of the treatment of this pressure ulcer at this time?
a. application of a full-thickness skin graft
b. extensive débridement of the area and cleansing with an iodine-based solution
c. application of a foam pad to protect the heel from further damage
d. application of microscopic beaded dextran to the lesion
e. elevation of the left leg by 30 degrees

Q15. Which of the following statements concerning the use of pressure-reducing devices in the prevention and treatment of pressure ulcers is true?
a. with the proper use of pressure-reducing devices, all pressure ulcers can be prevented
b. there is consensus regarding the pressure-reducing devices of first choice
c. sheepskin can be considered a pressure-reducing device of first choice
d. there appears to be little difference between the products indicated for the prevention and treatment of pressure ulcers
e. none of the above is true

Q16. Which of the following factors has (have) been associated with a more favorable outcome in the prevention and treatment of pressure ulcers?
a. educational programs for health professionals
b. educational programs for families and caregivers
c. multidisciplinary health care
d. b and c
e. all of the above

Q17. Concerning local wound care in superficial pressure ulcers, which of the following is (are) acceptable for cleaning the ulcer and disinfecting the ulcer?
a. povidone-iodine
b. hydrogen peroxide
c. hypochlorite solutions
d. all of the above
e. none of the above

Q18. Which of the following pressure-reducing devices should not be used for the prevention and treatment of pressure ulcers?

a. an air-fluidized bed
b. a sheepskin mattress
c. a conventional foam pad
d. an air mattress
e. a water mattress

Q19. The débridement of moist, exudative wounds originating from the formation of pressure ulcers may be augmented by the use of which of the following?
a. hydrophilic polymers
b. enzymatic agents
c. acetic acid
d. a and b
e. all of the above

Q20. Which of the following statements concerning the use of occlusive dressings for treating pressure ulcers is (are) true?
a. hydrocolloid dressings and transparent films improve the healing rate of superficial pressure ulcers
b. hydrocolloid has proven to be effective in treating deep pressure ulcers as well as superficial pressure ulcers
c. hydrocolloid dressings and transparent films may remain in place for several days
d. a and c only
e. all of the above statements are true

SHORT ANSWER MANAGEMENT PROBLEM
Pressure ulcers can be classified into four stages dependent on the degree of thickness of penetration of the epidermis and deeper tissues. As the therapy varies depending on the stage of the ulcer, it is important to understand the difference between the four stages. Provide the definition of each of stages I, II, III, and IV pressure ulcers.

ANSWERS

A1. **f.** See Answer 2.

A2. **e.** Risk factors for pressure ulcers include the following:
a. Any disease process leading to immobility and limited activity levels, such as a spinal cord injury, dementia, Parkinson's disease, severe congestive heart failure, and chronic obstructive pulmonary disease.
b. Other factors including urinary incontinence and nutritional factors such as a decreased lymphocyte count, hypoalbuminemia, inadequate dietary intake, decreased body weight,

and a depleted triceps skinfold thickness. Poor nutrition status may be secondary to immobility, poor financial status, isolation, or poor dentition.

c. Potential risk factors identified in prospective studies include moist skin, increased body temperature, decreased blood pressure, increased age, and an altered level of consciousness. Cardiovascular disease fractures, bed or wheelchair confinement, impaired level of consciousness, and hypotension are all independently associated with pressure ulcers.

A3. **f.** The pathophysiology of pressure ulcers include the interaction of all of the following:

a. Pressure: contact pressures of 60 to 70 mm Hg for 1 to 2 hours lead to degeneration of muscle fibers. Repeated exposures to pressure will cause skin necrosis because of decreased oxygen tension, vessel leakage, and lack of nutrients. Pressure is considered the most significant risk factor for developing pressure ulcers.

b. Shearing forces: shearing forces are tangential forces that are exerted when a person is seated or when the head of the bed is elevated and the person slides toward the floor or foot of the bed. Shearing forces disrupt subcutaneous vessels and cause ischemia and subsequent necrosis.

c. Friction: friction has been shown to cause intraepidermal blisters. When unroofed, these lesions result in superficial erosions. This kind of injury can occur when a patient is pulled across a sheet or when the patient has repetitive movements that expose a bony prominence to such frictional forces.

d. Moisture: intermediate degrees of moisture increase the amount of friction produced by the rubbing interface, whereas extremes of moisture or dryness decrease the frictional forces between the two surfaces rubbing against each other. Moisture macerates skin tissue predisposing the skin to breakdown.

A4. **a.** Pressure ulcers are not impossible to prevent in immobilized elderly patients. It is true that it is difficult to prevent all pressure ulcers, but many of those that do develop in immobilized elderly patients are, in fact, preventable.

Good nutrition in elderly patients will help prevent pressure ulcers.

Anemia and incontinence are predisposing factors to the development of pressure ulcers.

Elderly patients who sit for long periods of time are just as likely to develop pressure ulcers as bedridden patients.

A5. **e.** Erythema may progress to ulceration quickly. A small ulcer can progress to a large ulcer within 24 to 48 hours. The progression is caused by local edema or infection, the former being the most important factor. As in the patient described in Case 1, severe infection can lead to septicemia, which must be recognized and treated with appropriate systemic antibiotic therapy.

A6. **c.** The most common sites for pressure ulcers to develop are as follows:

a. The sacrum
b. The trochanters
c. The heels
d. The lateral malleoli
e. The buttocks over the ischium

The least common site of those listed for the formation of pressure ulcers is the medial malleoli.

A7. **f.** The ultimate chain of pathophysiologic events involved in the formation of pressure ulcers is as follows:

a. Ischemia is associated with the occlusion of blood and lymphatic vessels.

b. As plasma leaks into the interstitium, diffusing substances increase between the cellular elements of skin and blood vessels.

c. Ultimately hemorrhage occurs and leads to erythema of the skin that is unable to be blanched.

d. Bacteria are deposited at sites of pressure-induced injury and set up a deep suppurative process.

e. The accumulation of edema fluid, blood, inflammatory cells, toxic wastes, and bacteria ultimately and progressively lead to the death of muscle, subcutaneous tissue, and epidermal tissue.

The damage caused by shearing forces probably is mediated by pressure-induced ischemia in deep tissues as well as by direct mechanical injury to the subcutaneous tissue.

A8. **c.** Increased death rates have been consistently observed in elderly patients who develop pressure ulcers. In addition, failure of an ulcer to heal or improve has been associated with a higher rate of death in nursing home residents. In-hospital death rates for patients with pressure ulcers range from 23% to 36%. Most of these deaths are in debilitated patients; in many cases it is difficult to separate what contribution the actual pressure ulcer makes to the process. The development of a pressure sore quadruples the risk of death for institutionalized patients.

A9. **a.** Data support the recommendation that high-risk patients should be repositioned every 2 hours to prevent pressure ulcers from forming and minimizing the size, thickness, and infectivity rate of pressure ulcers that have already formed.

A10. **e.** Infected pressure ulcers are usually associated with *P. aeruginosa*, *Providencia* spp., *Proteus* spp., *S. aureus*, and anaerobic bacteria (particularly *B. fragilis*). The best combination of antibiotics, therefore, is one that will treat gram-positive aerobic cocci (present in 39% of isolates), gram-negative aerobic rods, and anaerobic bacteria.

A11. **b.** One realizes the risk of using a powerful agent such as gentamicin in a debilitated elder; on the other hand, the debilitated elder has most likely by that time acquired a serious bacteremia/septicemia. Check creatinine clearance and adjust the gentamicin dose accordingly.

A12. **c.** Sepsis is the most common and most serious complication of pressure ulcers in elderly patients. Contraction and bone resorption are also complications of pressure ulcers.

Anemia and hypoproteinemia are risk factors for the formation of pressure ulcers.

A13. **a.** With respect to infection, bacteremia, septicemia, and death:
  a. Most infected pressure ulcers are polymicrobial.
  b. Most infected polymicrobial pressure ulcers have *B. fragilis* as one of the major organisms involved.
  c. Infected pressure ulcers also lead to other infectious complications, such as bacterial cellulitis, osteomyelitis, and septic arthritis.

A14. **c.** The short time interval between the formation of a small area of erythema and a true pressure ulcer has already been described.

The single most important therapy at this time in this patient is to try to protect the patient's heel from progressing to any further stage of damage. This is best done by using a foam pad or other piece of protective apparatus.

A15. **b.** Regarding the formation of pressure ulcers, the prevention of pressure ulcers, and the pressure-reducing devices available, the following facts have emerged:
  a. Despite nurses' best efforts, the use of proper positioning alone is not sufficient to prevent all pressure ulcers. Even with pressure-reducing devices, this is not always possible.
  b. The use of water mattresses or alternating air mattresses decreased the incidence of pressure ulcers by 50% compared with the conventional hospital mattresses.
  c. Although sheepskin products are very popular, it has been demonstrated that sheepskins and 2-inch convoluted foam pad products do not have the capability of decreasing pressure enough to eliminate the risk of cutaneous injury.
  d. The following have been demonstrated to have superior efficacy in preventing pressure ulcers: a foam mattress, a static air mattress, an alternating air mattress, and a gel or water mattress. In addition, the use of air-fluidized and low-air-loss beds are recommended (especially for stage III and stage IV ulcers).

A16. **e.** Several studies have demonstrated a significant decrease in pressure-ulcer incidence after an educational program and a multidisciplinary team approach to the problem of pressure ulcers. Such educational programs should be directed at all levels of health care professionals, patients, family, and caregivers.

A17. **e.** Topical antiseptics such as hypochlorite solutions, povidone-iodine, acetic acid iodophor, and hydrogen peroxide should be avoided in cleaning and débriding a pressure ulcer because of the potential of these compounds for inhibiting wound healing. The preferred alternative is normal saline.

A18. **b.** A sheepskin mattress should not be used for the prevention and treatment of pressure ulcers. See the critique in Answer 15 for further details.

A19. **d.** The débridement of moist, exudative wounds may be augmented by using hydrophilic polymers such as dextranomer. Enzymatic agents such as collagenase, fibrinolysin, deoxyribonuclease, streptokinase, and streptodornase may be helpful in aiding débridement.

A20. **d.** Once an ulcer is clean and granulation or epithelialization begins to occur, then a moist wound environment should be maintained without disturbing the healing tissue. Superficial lesions heal by migration of epithelial cells from the borders of an ulcer; deep lesions heal as granulation tissue fills the base of the wound. Controlled studies have shown that the use of occlusive dressing such as transparent films and hydrocolloid dressings improves healing of stage II pressure ulcers. These dressings remain in place for several days and allow a layer of serous exudate to form underneath the dressing. This facilitates the further migration of epithelial cells. Although these dressings have not been shown to improve the effective healing rate of deep ulcers, they do reduce the nursing time needed for treatment.

Clean stage III and clean stage IV ulcers should be dressed with a gauze dressing kept moistened with normal saline. Moist dressings should be kept off surrounding skin to avoid macerating normal tissues. Unless there are symptoms or signs of infection, these dressings can stay in place for several days.

SOLUTION TO THE SHORT ANSWER MANAGEMENT PROBLEM

The classification of pressure ulcers in elderly patients is as follows:
a. Stage I: Stage I pressure ulcers present as erythema of intact skin that is unable to be blanched.
b. Stage II: Stage II pressure ulcers involve partial-thickness skin loss involving the epidermis or the dermis.
c. Stage III: Stage III pressure ulcers extend from the subcutaneous tissues to the deep fascia and typically show undermining.
d. Stage IV: Stage IV pressure ulcers involve muscle or bone. Full-thickness injury is often manifested by eschar, frequently involving muscle and bone, but cannot be staged until the eschar is removed.

SUMMARY OF THE DIAGNOSIS AND TREATMENT OF PRESSURE ULCERS

a. Terminology:
1) The term *pressure ulcer* is the preferred term at this time.
2) Previous terms included the following:
a) Decubitus ulcers
b) Bedsores
c) Pressure sores
b. Prevalence:
1) The prevalence of pressure ulcers among patients in acute care hospitals ranges from 3% to 14% and from 15% to 25% in long-term care facilities.
2) Among patients expected to be hospitalized and confined to bed or chair for at least 1 week, the prevalence of stage II and greater pressure ulcers is as high as 28%.
3) The prevalence of pressure ulcers in nursing homes is similar to that reported in acute care hospitals. As many as 20% to 33% of patients admitted to nursing homes have stage II or greater pressure ulcers. Less than 20% of pressure ulcers develop in the nursing home and

in the home care setting: more than 60% develop in the acute care setting.
4) Pressure ulcers affect 3 million persons annually, at a cost of 5 billion dollars a year.
c. Complications:
1) Sepsis is the most serious complication of pressure ulcers.
2) Other complications include local infections, cellulitis, and osteomyelitis. As well, infected pressure ulcers may be deeply undermined and lead to podarthritis or penetrate into the abdominal cavity and cause peritonitis. Infected pressure ulcers lead to nosocomial reservoirs for antibiotic-resistant bacteria.
3) Pressure ulcer infections have the following characteristics:
a) They are polymicrobial.
b) Gram-positive anaerobic cocci, gram-negative anaerobic rods, and aerobic bacteria are the most common organisms found.
c) Specific organisms commonly found include: *P. aeruginosa, Providencia* spp., *Proteus* spp., *S. aureus,* and *B. fragilis*
d. Mortality:
1) Failure of a pressure ulcer to heal is associated with a higher rate of death in nursing home residents.
2) In-hospital death rates for patients with pressure ulcers range from 23% to 36%. Most of these deaths are patients with severe underlying disease.
e. Risk factors:
1) Disease processes leading to immobility or reduced activity
2) Spinal cord injury
3) Dementias
4) Parkinson's disease
5) Congestive cardiac failure
6) Incontinence
7) Nutritional factors: Inadequate intake of protein, vitamins, minerals, calcium, or calories leading to cachexia, hypoalbuminemia, decreased body weight, and decreased triceps skinfold thickness
f. Pathophysiology: Four factors have been implicated in the pathogenesis of pressure ulcers:
1) Pressure
2) Shearing forces
3) Friction
4) Moisture
g. Pathophysiologic series of events in pressure-ulcer formation:
1) Pressure on tissues overlying bone prominence

2) Ischemia produced by occlusion of blood vessels and lymphatic vessels

3) Endothelial cell swelling and vessel leak

4) Plasma leakage into the interstitium

5) Increased distance between cellular elements of skin and blood vessels

6) Hemorrhage

7) Erythema of the skin that is unable to be blanched

8) Continued accumulation of edema fluid, blood, inflammatory cells, toxic wastes, and bacteria

9) Death of muscle, subcutaneous tissue, and epidermal skin

h. Prevention of pressure ulcers:

1) Formal risk assessment: A formal "risk assessment" for the development of pressure ulcers should be done on all patients.

2) Frequent repositioning:
   a) Patients at highest risk should be repositioned every 2 hours.
   b) Lower risk patients should be repositioned two to four times a day.

3) Technique of repositioning: repositioning should be performed so that a person at risk is repositioned without pressure on vulnerable bony prominences. Most of these sites are avoided by positioning patients with the back at a 30-degree angle to the support surface, alternatively from the right to the left sides and to the supine position.

4) Pressure-reducing devices:
   a) Although sheepskins and 2-inch convoluted foam pads are popular, they do not have the capability to decrease pressure enough to eliminate risk of cutaneous injury.
   b) Preferred devices include static air mattresses, alternating air mattresses, gel mattresses, and water mattresses.
   c) Lifting devices or bed linen movement (not bed linen drag) will minimize friction and shear-induced injuries during transfers and position changes.

i. Education:

1) There is a significant decrease in pressure ulcer incidence after an educational program and a multidisciplinary team approach to the problem of pressure ulcers is implemented.

2) Educational interventions should be targeted to all levels of health care providers, patients, families, and caregivers.

j. Assessment of patients with pressure ulcers:

1) Appropriate assessment and treatment of underlying diseases and conditions that have put the person at risk for developing pressure ulcers

2) Nutritional assessment particularly important

3) Assessment of associated infections (as discussed)

k. Treatment of pressure ulcers:

1) Systemic treatment:
   a) Vitamin C: The patient should take 500 mg bid (84% reduction in pressure ulcer surface area in patients taking this vitamin).
   b) Drug combination of choice: clindamycin and gentamicin; monitor and watch renal function carefully while the patient is on gentamicin.
   c) Air-fluidized bed therapy is much of an improvement over the conventional bed.

2) Local wound care:
   a) Normal saline is the agent of choice for cleaning and for gentile débridement. Avoid povidone-iodine, hypochlorite, mild acetic acid, and hydrogen peroxide.
   b) Surgical débridement is augmented with wet-to-dry dressings using normal saline.
   c) The débridement of moist, exudative lesions is facilitated by using hydrophilic polymers such as dextranomer. Enzymatic agents should be used only until the ulcer bed becomes clean.
   d) Once clean and granulation or epithelialization begins to occur, a moist wound environment should be maintained. Occlusive dressings and hydrocolloid dressings improve healing rates for stage II ulcers. Stage III and stage IV ulcers should be dressed with a gauze soaked in normal saline.
   e) Surgical therapies should be used to remove necrotic tissue that cannot be removed any other way and that if not removed will cause septicemia and death. Surgical flaps (a more elective procedure) should be carefully considered, especially on debilitated, cachectic patients. Rule out osteomyelitis if clinically suspected.

SUGGESTED READINGS

Allman R: Pressure ulcers. In Hazzard WR et al, eds: *Principles of geriatric medicine and gerontology*, ed 3, New York, 1994, McGraw-Hill.

Ferri FF et al, eds: *Practical guide to the care of the geriatric patient*, ed 2, St Louis, 1997, Mosby.

PROBLEM·125

POLYPHARMACY AND DRUG REACTIONS IN THE ELDERLY

"Gee Mom, Do You Know What All These Different Kinds of Pills Are For?"

Case 1 ■ A 75-Year-Old Female with a Bagful of Pills

A 75-year-old female comes to your office with her daughter. Her daughter describes her mother as having undergone "a marked personality change." Apparently, her elderly mother began seeing "pink rats coming out of the wall" and she began "hearing and seeing people from outer space" floating down into her field of vision.

The patient's daughter brings in her mother's medications in a bag. She describes a visit to her mother's physician 1 week ago. At that time the doctor prescribed a number of medications including pills for her blood pressure, pills for her heart, pills for her arthritis, pills for her stomach, pills for her anxiety, pills for her depression, and pills for her insomnia.

On further questioning, the daughter states that her mother had been fairly well before the physician visit but had (unfortunately) mentioned "a few minor ailments." In response to the patient's complaints the physician prescribed hydrochlorothiazide, propranolol, nifedipine, digoxin, ibuprofen, cimetidine, Maalox, amitriptyline, and triazolam.

You are well aware of the fact that medications in the elderly can often produce significant side effects. You suspect that there is a connection between the pink rats, the space men, and the pills.

On examination, the patient is agitated and confused. She points to the ceiling and yells "pink rats, spacemen, pink rats, spacemen." Her blood pressure is 100/70 mm Hg and her pulse is 54 and regular. She has a bruise on her head from a fall 3 days ago. Examination of the cardiovascular system reveals a normal S1 and S2 with a grade VI systolic murmur heard along the left sternal edge. There are no other abnormalities on physical examination.

SELECT THE BEST ANSWER TO THE FOLLOWING QUESTIONS

Q1. Which of the following statements regarding this patient's acute medical problem is true?
   a. this patient's problem is unlikely to be related to her medications
   b. this patient's presentation is unusual following the initiation of medications in the elderly
   c. this patient's problem is unlikely to lead to hospitalization
   d. this patient's problem is likely to be transient
   e. none of the above statements is true

Q2. Which of the following statements regarding the use of drugs in the elderly is true?
   a. elderly patients should be treated the same way as younger patients with respect to drug initiation
   b. elderly patients generally need the same dose of medications as younger patients
   c. psychotropic drugs are unlikely to produce significant side effects in elderly patients
   d. elderly patients on multiple medications should be reassessed on a yearly basis
   e. none of the above statements is true

Q3. Regarding elderly patients in chronic care facilities, which of the following statements regarding medication use is (are) true?
   a. elderly patients in chronic care facilities are usually on fewer medications than elderly patients living on their own
   b. elderly patients in chronic care facilities are usually on between 8 and 13 different medications at any one time
   c. elderly patients in chronic care facilities are likely to experience iatrogenic side effects from medications at one time or another
   d. b and c
   e. all of the above statements are true

Case 2 ■ An 85-Year-Old Female with a Dangerously High Blood Pressure of 150 mm Hg

An 85-year-old female patient of yours was placed on a combination of hydrochlorothiazide and clonidine because of a "dangerously high" blood pressure of 150/95 mm Hg. When you hear this story you are concerned about possible adverse side effects. Your worst fear comes true when you find yourself attending her in the Emergency Department with a serious adverse event you believe is directly related to the medications on which she was placed.

Q4. Which of the following specialists will you be calling to manage this adverse event?
   a. a rheumatologist
   b. a general surgeon or a general internist
   c. a gerontologist
   d. an orthopedic surgeon
   e. a psychiatrist

Q5. The patient becomes acutely short of breath. The adverse effect that you feared has now lead to a feared complication. What is that complication?
   a. a deep venous thrombosis (DVT) leading to a pulmonary embolus
   b. a splenic infarct
   c. a cerebrovascular accident
   d. aplastic anemia
   e. a drug-induced psychosis

Q6. What is the most likely medication causing the pink rats and the people from outer space in the patient described in Case 1?
   a. propranolol
   b. hydrochlorothiazide
   c. ibuprofen
   d. cimetidine
   e. digoxin

Q7. Consider the possibility that the adverse event and its complication just described did not occur. Considering the rapid introduction of multiple medications that took place on the visit to the other physician, what would be the most appropriate course of action at this time?
   a. discontinue the digoxin
   b. discontinue the hydrochlorothiazide
   c. discontinue the propranolol
   d. discontinue the triazolam
   e. discontinue all medications, observe in a geriatric day hospital environment, and reevaluate the patient continuously for the first few weeks

Q8. Of the drug combinations listed, which is the most likely to result in a drug-drug interaction in the elderly?
   a. cimetidine and propranolol
   b. digoxin and hydrochlorothiazide
   c. ibuprofen and captopril
   d. triazolam and amitriptyline
   e. haloperidol

Q9. What is the most common potentially serious side effect of tricyclic antidepressants in elderly patients?
   a. dry mouth
   b. constipation
   c. bladder spasm
   d. orthostatic hypotension
   e. sedation

Q10. Which of the following combinations of pharmacologic agents is most commonly associated with adverse drug reactions (ADRs) in the elderly?
   a. cardiovascular drugs, psychotropics, and antibiotics
   b. cardiovascular drugs, psychotropics, and analgesics
   c. gastrointestinal drugs, psychotropics, and analgesics
   d. gastrointestinal drugs, psychotropics, and antibiotics

Q11. Which of the following pharmacologic parameters may be associated with ADRs in the elderly?
   a. altered free serum concentration of drug
   b. altered volume of distribution
   c. altered renal drug clearance
   d. altered tissue sensitivity of the drug
   e. all of the above

Q12. Which of the following is (are) examples of ADRs in the elderly?
   a. drug side effects
   b. drug toxicity
   c. drug-disease interaction
   d. drug-drug interaction
   e. all of the above

Q13. What is the recommended starting dose of a tricyclic antidepressant in an elderly patient?
   a. 10 to 25 mg
   b. 50 to 75 mg
   c. 100 to 150 mg
   d. 150 to 225 mg
   e. 250 to 300 mg

Q14. Some pharmacologic agents are excreted virtually unchanged by the kidneys. The dosages of these drugs must be carefully titrated in any elderly patient with renal impairment or potential renal impairment. Drugs in this category include the following:
   a. cimetidine
   b. gentamicin
   c. lithium
   d. all of the above
   e. none of the above

Q15. Regarding antipsychotic drug therapy in the elderly, which of the following statements is (are) true?
   a. antipsychotic drugs are often prescribed for behavior that chronic care staff find objectionable
   b. tardive dyskinesia is a frequent side effect of antipsychotic drug use in the elderly

c. antipsychotic drugs are prescribed much more frequently in institutionalized patients than in noninstitutionalized patients
d. all of the above statements are true
e. none of the above statements is true

SHORT ANSWER MANAGEMENT PROBLEM
List 10 rules that will minimize ADRs in the elderly.

ANSWERS

A1. **e.** This patient's problem can be characterized in the following manner:
a. It is likely to be related to the bagful of medications on which she was started.
b. It is very common following the initiation of medication in the elderly, especially multiple medications.
c. It is very unlikely to be transient unless some or all of the medications are discontinued.
d. It will commonly lead to hospitalization. It is believed that up to 20% of hospitalizations, and perhaps significantly more in the elderly, are a result of iatrogenic disease. Iatrogenic disease is almost always associated with multiple medication use.

A2. **e.** The following are some helpful thoughts on the initiation of drugs in the elderly:
a. Drug initiation in the elderly should be done extremely cautiously. The general rule should be to start very low and go very slow.
b. The elderly patient usually needs a considerably lower dose of drug than does the young adult. This is, of course, especially true of drugs that are renally excreted. The general rule on drug initiation in elderly patients is "no more than 50% of the usual adult dose; no more than one drug at the time. Increases not any more quickly than once a week."
c. Psychotropic drugs should be used with special caution. Psychotropic medications are frequently misused in the elderly and dosing should be monitored closely.
d. All elderly patients should have a formal drug review performed at least every 3 months. At that time, all drugs and the drug doses should be seriously considered for reduction or discontinuation, especially if the elderly patient has symptoms that suggest an ADR to one or more of the drugs that he or she is presently taking.

A3. **d.** Patients in chronic care facilities have the following characteristics with respect to medication use:
a. They are usually on multiple medications. The average number of medications used by the institutionalized elderly is 8 per day. Standard orders may increase this to 13 medications per day.
b. It has been found that the most usual scenario is that medications always are added but never subtracted. Thus the number simply continues to increase.
c. Iatrogenic side effects from medication use in chronic care facilities are extremely common. Considering the number of medications that these senior citizens are taking, they are actually far more likely to experience at least one ADR per year than not.
d. In comparison to senior citizens living on their own in the community, the number of medications used by institutional-based elderly patients is greater.

A4. **d.** The combination of hydrochlorothiazide and clonidine is likely to produce significant orthostatic hypotension in the elderly patient. The most "adverse effect of the adverse effect" is a fall in the elder leading to a fracture of the neck of the femur. Thus the specialist that you most likely will call will be an orthopedic surgeon.

A5. **a.** The most serious complication from a hip fracture is immobility leading to DVT. The development of a DVT is, of course, directly correlated with a subsequent pulmonary embolus.

The mortality of elders in the first year following a hip fracture approaches 25%. Prevention is the best treatment.

Prevention is best accomplished by significantly limiting the number of medications an elder is on, especially medications that tend to produce orthostatic hypotension. It should be noted that sedative hypnotics increase the risk for hip fractures considerably.

A6. **a.** The most common medication-induced cause of hallucinations in elderly patients is propranolol. Many elderly patients who are started on propranolol develop visual or auditory hallucinations. Unfortunately, many of these patients are then started on antipsychotic medications to treat the hallucinations, rather than evaluating their medication list.

A7. **e.** The most reasonable course of action at this time is to stop everything and start again. The rapid introduction of the nine medications listed was a recipe for disaster. In an attempt to counteract the imminent disaster, this logically should take place in the supervised setting of at least a geriatric day hospital. Many geriatric assessment units do exactly that when an elder is admitted for the assessment of any medical problem. With elders who have been on multiple medications for long periods of time, the safest place to accomplish this is in the hospital under close observation. Of elderly hospital admissions, 10% to 17% are a result of inappropriate medication use. Use these hospitalizations to properly assess medications and to develop appropriate treatment plans.

A8. **b.** Patients who develop ADRs are more likely to be taking six or more drugs than those who do not develop an ADR. The most commonly identified combination likely to result in a drug-drug interaction is digoxin with a diuretic. In this case the ADR most likely to be produced is hypokalemia. The hypokalemia produced will often lead to digoxin toxicity in the susceptible elder. These combinations are considered secondary drug reactions, which require at least two drugs to cause an interaction.

A9. **d.** All of the side effects listed are common side effects of tricyclic antidepressant medications. The side effects that are caused by an anticholinergic mechanism include dry mouth, blurred vision, constipation, bladder spasm and urinary retention, and sedation.

The orthostatic hypotension is caused by an alpha-adrenergic blockade and is potentially the most serious due to the association described previously between the following series of events:

a. Orthostatic hypotension
b. Falls in the elder
c. Fractured neck of the femur
d. DVT
e. Pulmonary embolism

Excess morbidity and mortality is associated with events c, d, and e in the chain. In addition, always follow cardiac status when using digoxin, evaluating for bradycardia and dysrhythmias.

A10. **b.** The three most common drug classes associated with ADRs in the elderly are cardiovascular drugs, psychotropic drugs, and analgesics (especially the nonsteroidal antiinflammatory drugs [NSAIDs]). Unfortunately, many of the drugs used in the treatment of geriatric patients are prescribed for symptoms related to the effects and the diseases of aging and not necessarily for a specific acute disease where function can be restored. This results, of course, in the elder's being on the particular agent for a longer period.

A11. **e.** Many physiologic and social variables increase the incidence of ADRs in elderly patients. They include the number of drugs, compliance, absorption of drug, concentration of free drug in the serum, volume of distribution, tissue sensitivity, metabolic clearance, renal drug clearance, general homeostasis, and concentration of serum albumin.

A12. **e.** An ADR is defined as any unintended or undesired effect of a drug in a patient. This may include abnormal laboratory values, patient symptoms, and signs on physical examination.

ADRs can be divided into side effects (dry mouth from tricyclic antidepressants and hypokalemia from diuretics), drug toxicity (daytime sedation from hypnotics, diarrhea from laxatives, and syncope from antihypertensive agents), drug-disease interaction (benzodiazepine and drugs with anticholinergic properties may effect the cognitive function in Alzheimer's patients), drug-drug interaction (digoxin from diuretics), and secondary effects (haloperidol causing drug-induced Parkinsonism).

A13. **a.** The recommended starting dose for a tricyclic antidepressant in elderly patients is 10 to 25 mg. The older and more frail the elder, the lower the dose that should initially be used. We recommend nortriptyline be started on a dose of 10 mg. Amitriptyline may have significant side effects in the elderly. It should be used judiciously and probably not be considered a first-line medication.

A14. **d.** The kidney is the major source of elimination of many commonly prescribed drugs. Drugs that undergo extensive renal clearance and that are therefore likely to accumulate in the elderly include digoxin, gentamicin and other aminoglycosides, lithium, cimetidine, cotrimoxazole, disopyramide, nadolol, procainamide, and sulfonamides. Always remember that NSAIDS may increase renal toxicity, especially in high-risk patients.

A15. **d.** Psychotropic drugs are commonly prescribed for geriatric patients. Indications for the use of these drugs are not well established. In nursing home situations, psychotropic drugs are often prescribed for behaviors that staff members find objectionable (that is, for the benefit of the staff, not the patient); the patient may, in fact, remain on this (these) drug(s) for long periods. The institutionalized elderly are 10 times as likely to receive antipsychotic agents as age-matched noninstitutionalized controls.

Double-blind, randomized, controlled trials have not established the efficacy of antipsychotic drug use in Alzheimer's disease. Tardive dyskinesia, rigidity, and excessive sedation are frequent side effects of antipsychotic drug use. In many states the use of psychotropic medication must be well documented with specific goals for behavior. The use of chemical restraints through the use of psychotropic medications is not justified.

It should be noted that the use of newer antipsychotic agents such as risperidone has been shown to be effective in the treatment of psychotic behavior and neurobehavioral manifestations in severe Alzheimer's patients.

SOLUTION TO THE SHORT ANSWER MANAGEMENT PROBLEM

The following are a good set of rules for prescribing medication in geriatric patients:

a. Recognize that there is no drug to treat senescence.
b. Recognize that mere prolongation of life is not a valid reason for using medications that decrease the quality of life.
c. Make sure that the effects of treatment outweigh the risks.
d. Establish a priority order for treatment.
e. Keep the number of drugs administered concurrently to a minimum.
f. Know your patient well. Consider renal and hepatic impairment. Consider what else (including over-the-counter medications) is being taken and who else is prescribing drugs.
g. Always begin with nonpharmacologic therapy first if possible.
h. If you decide to prescribe a drug, know it well. Consider using a few drugs often rather than a lot of drugs infrequently.
i. Select the dose carefully: Start very low and go very slow.
j. Anticipate and minimize ADRs by considering side-effect profiles.
k. Determine whether or not the patient needs help using the medication.
l. Educate the patient and family.
m. Continually reevaluate whether or not your patient needs a specific drug.
n. Perform a drug review every 3 months on every elder on more than one medication.
o. Use medication diaries: Have patients bring in all medications and over-the-counter and herbal medications used.
p. Check serum levels when indicated.
q. Destroy old medications.
r. Use medication cards.

SUMMARY OF THE DIAGNOSIS AND MANAGEMENT OF DRUG REACTIONS IN THE ELDERLY

a. Prevalence: Drug reactions are common, especially in institutionalized elderly who are on an average of 12 to 20 medications. ADRs are at least twice as common in elderly patients as in younger patients.
b. Types of ADRs:
   1) Side effects
   2) Drug toxicity
   3) Drug-disease interaction
   4) Drug-drug interaction
c. Most common drugs associated with ADRs:
   1) Cardiovascular drugs
   2) Psychotropic drugs
   3) Analgesics
d. Set of reasonable rules: Follow the set of rules listed in the Solution to the Short Answer Management Problem.
e. Types of ADRs:
   1) Primary ADR (one drug with one side reaction)
      a) Cimetidine causes psychosis.
      b) Propranolol induces depression.
   2) Secondary ADR (requires at least two drugs to cause an interaction): Erythromycin and theophylline used together are toxic.
   3) Drug withdrawal syndromes
      a) Beta-blocker withdrawal leads to angina.
      b) Addictive drugs cause withdrawal syndromes (benzodiazepines).
   4) Tertiary ADR: Benzodiazepines resulting in a higher incidence of falls
f. Physician factors implicated in ADRs
   1) The physician gives a high-risk drug to a vulnerable host (NSAID for a patient with peptic ulcer disease).
   2) The physician gives a highly interactive drug to a pharmacologically vulnerable patient (e.g., captopril given to patient on a potassium-sparing agent).
   3) The physician prescribes an inappropriate drug to treat an unrecognized drug side effect (e.g., antidepressant given to treat beta-blocker depression).
g. Automatic or standard drug orders in intensive care unit, chronic care unit, or chronic care facilities.
h. Lack of appropriate follow up.

SUGGESTED READINGS

Chutka D et al: Drug prescribing for elderly patients, *Mayo Clin Proc* 70:634-640, 1995.

Fretwell MD: Optimal pharmacotherapy. In Ferri FF et al, eds: *Practical guide to the care of the geriatric patient*, ed 2, St Louis, 1997, Mosby.

Hazzard WR et al, eds: *Principles of geriatric medicine and gerontology,* ed 3, New York, 1994, McGraw-Hill.

McEvoy GK, ed: *The American hospital formulary service,* Bethesda, Md, 1996, American Society of Health-System Pharmacists.

PROBLEM·126

THE PROPENSITY AND CONSEQUENCES OF FALLS AMONG THE ELDERLY

It's No Longer Just Oopsy Daisy.

Case 1 ■ An 81-Year-Old Female Who Is Repeatedly Falling

An 81-year-old female is brought to your office by her daughter. The elderly mother has been falling repeatedly for at least 3 months. The falling has been getting progressively worse, and the patient's daughter is very concerned about the possibility of her mother "breaking her hip."

On examination, the patient is a frail, elderly female in no acute distress. She appears somewhat depressed, but her mini-mental status examination score is 27. The patient's blood pressure is 180/75 mm Hg. Her pulse is 84 and irregular. No other abnormalities are found.

SELECT THE BEST ANSWER TO THE FOLLOWING QUESTIONS

Q1. What is the prevalence of falls among community-based elderly patients?
   a. 5% per year
   b. 10% per year
   c. 20% per year
   d. 30% per year
   e. 50% per year

Q2. Which of the following statements regarding falls in the elderly is (are) true?
   a. the prevalence of falling in the elderly increases with advancing age
   b. elderly patients who are physically active may be at greater risk of falling than those who are not
   c. approximately 50% of elderly patients who fall once will fall again
   d. falling in the elderly may not necessarily be a marker of functional decline
   e. all of the above statements are true

Q3. Which of the following is the most feared morbid outcome of falling among elderly patients?
   a. fracture of the hip
   b. fracture of the radius

   c. subdural hematoma
   d. epidural hematoma
   e. cervical fracture

Q4. Potential reversible causes of falling in the elderly include which of the following?
   a. medications
   b. postprandial hypotension
   c. alcohol use
   d. urinary urgency
   e. all of the above

Q5. Which of the following are predisposing risk factors for falls in the elderly?
   a. visual impairment
   b. cerebrovascular accidents
   c. Alzheimer's disease
   d. normal pressure hydrocephalus
   e. all of the above

Q6. Regarding the incidence of falling and medication use in the elderly, which of the following statements is (are) true?
   a. multiple drug use is associated with an increased incidence of falling in the elderly
   b. the higher the drug dosage, the greater the probability of falling
   c. drug interactions are a major contributing factor to an increased incidence of falling in the elderly
   d. a and b only
   e. all of the above statements are true

Q7. Falling in the elderly is most commonly associated with which of the following pathophysiologic factors?
   a. orthostatic hypotension
   b. decreased left ventricular output
   c. decreased cerebral circulation
   d. increased left ventricular output
   e. none of the above

Q8. Which of the following medications is most likely to lead to a serious fall in an elderly patient?
   a. amitriptyline
   b. hydrochlorothiazide
   c. enalapril
   d. nifedipine
   e. fluoxetine

Q9. What is the prevalence of falling among institutionalized elderly patients?
   a. 50% per year
   b. 40% per year
   c. 30% per year

d. 20% per year

e. 10% per year

Q10. Which of the following statements regarding the use of restraints in elderly patients as a means to prevent falls is (are) true?

a. restraints have been shown to reduce the incidence of falling in the elderly

b. no study has ever shown a decrease in falls with restraint use in the elderly

c. potential complications of restraint use in the elderly include strangulation, vascular damage, and neurologic damage

d. a and c

e. b and c

SHORT ANSWER MANAGEMENT PROBLEM

Describe the preventive measures that may result in a reduction in falls in the elderly.

ANSWERS

A1. **d.** According to several community-based surveys, about 30% of persons over the age of 65 experience falls each year in situations where there are no overwhelming intrinsic causes (such as syncope).

A2. **e.** Approximately 50% of these elders have multiple falling episodes. The likelihood of falling increases with age. As illustrated by this very high prevalence of 30% among community-based persons, falling is not just confined to the frail elderly; healthy elderly patients fall as well during ordinary daily activities. This suggests that falling is not merely a marker of functional decline in the elderly. While the elder we all picture as falling is the frail elder with multiple medical problems, it may well be the case that falling is more prevalent among the more healthy elders who are more, not less, physically active.

A3. **a.** The most feared outcome of falls in the elderly is a fracture of the hip. This is especially common among elderly women who have significant osteoporosis.

The escalating cost of health care has resulted in increased expectations and demands concerning cost-effective health care. Hip fracture results in the death of at least 12,000 elderly Americans per year. In elderly females with hip fractures, the mortality is approximately 20% in the first year.

A4. **e.** Potential reversible causes of falling include medication, alcohol, postprandial hypotension (30 to 60 minutes after a meal), urinary urgency, insomnia, peripheral edema, and environmental factors.

A5. **e.** Vision, hearing, vestibular function, and proprioception are the major sensory modalities related to stability. Thus declines in vision, hearing, imbalance leading to vertigo and dizziness, peripheral neuropathies, and cervical degenerative disease are the most common causes of falls in elderly patients.

Other associated diseases or conditions associated with falls in the elderly include cerebrovascular accidents, Parkinson's disease, normal-pressure hydrocephalus, dementia (Alzheimer's disease), severe osteoarthritis or rheumatoid arthritis, and medications causing orthostatic hypotension (discussed in Problem 125).

A6. **e.** Iatrogenic disease is a major cause of falls in the elderly. This iatrogenic disease, which is almost completely related to medication use, is a serious problem in elders. As discussed in Problem 125, the average number of medications per elder (especially in the institutionalized setting) is anywhere from 8 to 13.

Multiple drugs, increased drug dosage, and drug-drug interactions are all reasons for orthostatic hypotension (an alpha-blockade phenomenon) and sedation (the two most common predisposing pathophysiologic mechanisms associated with falling in the elderly).

A7. **a.** Decreased left ventricular output, most closely associated with congestive heart failure, may also play a prominent role in some cases of falling, but orthostatic hypotension is the most common.

A8. **a.** Amitriptyline, hydrochlorothiazide, enalapril, and nifedipine may all be associated with falling in the elderly. Enalapril and hydrochlorothiazide are more likely to be associated with falling when given concomitantly. As well, the first-dose hypotensive effect of an angiotensin-converting enzyme (ACE) inhibitor should be remembered; that is, it is much safer to give the first dose of an ACE inhibitor to an elder in your office, where this possible side effect can be monitored.

Of the four medications listed, however, the most prominent predisposing to falls in the elderly is amitriptyline, a tricyclic antidepressant. Amitriptyline predisposes to falls by a combination of two mechanisms: its anticholinergic mechanism and its alpha-blockade mechanism. This drug should be used judiciously in the elderly. Starting very low and going very slowly will minimize falling as a result of drug use in elderly patients.

A9. a. Over half of ambulatory nursing home patients fall each year. The estimated annual incidence is 1600 falls per 1000 beds. The higher frequency of falling among institutionalized elderly patients results both from the greater frailty of these patients compared to community-based elderly patients and the greater reliability of reporting in an institutional setting.

A10. e. No study has confirmed or suggested that the risk of falling in the elderly is lessened because of the use of restraining devices. Restraining devices have, on the other hand, been shown to result in significant morbidity and mortality from strangulation, neurologic damage, and vascular damage.

In some countries in the world (such as the United Kingdom), restraints are almost forbidden. In North America the situation appears to be the opposite. In some institutions they are completely routine.

Restraints have other side effects, including anxiety, anger, agitation, and paranoia.

SOLUTION TO THE SHORT ANSWER MANAGEMENT PROBLEM

A preventive program for minimizing falls in the elderly should include the following:
a. Identification of intrinsic risk factors:
  1) A thorough clinical evaluation aimed at identifying all contributing risk factors for falling is the first, most important step. Directly observing balance and gait has been proven to be effective in identifying residents at risk for falling.
  2) A careful review of all situations may identify problem situations to be avoided in the future.
  3) A complete medication review with elimination of all unnecessary medications and a decrease in the dose of all others will minimize falls.
b. Environmental prevention:
  1) General environmental measures include ensuring adequate lighting without glare; having dry, nonslippery floors that are free of obstacles and contamination; having high, firm chairs; and having raised toilet seats.
  2) Restraints should be used only when there appears to be no other alternative. Restraints should not take the place of close supervision and attention to the risk factors discussed earlier. Alternatives to restraints, including wedges in chairs for maintenance of position

and organized walking and grid barriers for prevention of wandering, may afford the necessary protection.

SUMMARY OF THE DIAGNOSIS AND PREVENTION OF FALLS IN THE ELDERLY

a. Prevalence:
  1) 30%/year in community-based elders
  2) 50%/year in institutionalized elders
b. Major complication: Fracture of the femur: resulting morbidity and mortality from surgery, deep venous thrombosis, and pulmonary embolus
c. Major predisposing conditions precipitating major complication:
  1) Vision, hearing, vestibular function, and proprioception impairments
  2) Other conditions associated with increased risk include Alzheimer's disease, Parkinson's disease, and iatrogenic disease (mainly medication use, including the psychotropic agents and the cardiovascular agents, the agents with the greatest probability of producing sedation and other anticholinergic side effects and alpha-blockade side effects [orthostatic hypotension]).
  3) 1 or 2 (above) associated with significant osteoporosis increases the risk.
d. Elder populations at greatest risk:
  1) Active elderly patients who are at increased risk because of significant activity levels in whom even a minor impairment may be enough to cause significant problems
  2) The "frail elderly" who have concomitant chronic medical conditions
  3) The institutionalized elderly
  4) This list may, in fact, include most elders.
e. Prevention:
  1) Prevent the development of osteoporosis in postmenopausal women whenever possible (estrogens, calcitonin, calcium, alendronate) (see Problem 50).
  2) Look carefully at identifying intrinsic risk factors and environmental protection methods in helping to prevent falls.
  3) Medications:
    a) Provide a medication review to every elder every 3 months.
    b) Keep the number of medications to a minimum.
    c) In starting medications, start very low and go very slow.
    d) To minimize falls, minimize adverse drug reactions. This is covered extensively in Problem 125.

SUGGESTED READINGS

Fuller GF: Falls in the elderly, *Am Fam Physician* 61(7):2159-2168, 2000.

Tierney LM, Jr, McPhee SJ, Papadakis MA, eds: *Current medical diagnosis and treatment, 2000*, Stamford, Conn, 1999, Appleton & Lange.

Riggs J: Mortality from accidental falls among the elderly in the United States, 1962-1988: Demonstrating the impact of improved trauma management, *J Trauma* 35(2):212-219, 1993.

Tinetti M: Falls. In Hazzard W et al, eds: *Principles of geriatric medicine and gerontology*, ed 3, New York, 1994, McGraw-Hill.

CHAPTER 8

Epidemiology and Public Health

PROBLEM·127

RECOMMENDATIONS OF THE U.S. PREVENTIVE SERVICES TASK FORCE ON THE PERIODIC HEALTH EXAMINATION

What to Test for and When

Case 1 ■ A 45-Year-Old Male with No Specific Complaints or Concerns

A 45-year-old male presents for a periodic health maintenance visit. He has no specific complaints or concerns.

SELECT THE BEST ANSWER TO THE FOLLOWING QUESTIONS:

Q1. Which of the following is (are) definitely indicated in the health assessment that you would perform on this individual?
   a. measurement of blood pressure
   b. measurement of body mass index
   c. electrocardiogram (ECG)
   d. a and b
   e. all of the above

Q2. Considering the individual described in Case 1, which of the following is (are) indicated in this individual's health assessment?
   a. serum cholesterol
   b. auscultation for carotid bruits
   c. palpation of peripheral pulses
   d. serum triglycerides
   e. all of the above

Case 2 ■ A 66-Year-Old Male for Whom You Wish to Reduce the Chance of Death from Colorectal Cancer

A 66-year-old male comes to your office for a periodic health maintenance examination.

Q3. In this patient, which of the following procedures has (have) been shown to be effective screens in the reduction of colorectal cancer mortality?
   a. rectal examination
   b. sigmoidoscopy
   c. fecal occult blood testing
   d. all of the above
   e. b or c

Case 3 ■ A 26-Year-Old Asymptomatic Sexually Active Female

A 26-year-old female comes to your office for a health maintenance assessment. She is sexually active and asymptomatic.

Q4. Which of the following is (are) indicated in this young lady's health examination?
   a. palpation of the ovaries
   b. Pap smear
   c. breast examination
   d. all of the above
   e. b and c only

Case 4 ■ A 53-Year-Old Male with a 20-Year History of Smoking Two Packs of Cigarettes Per Day

A 53-year-old male with a 20-year history of smoking two packs of cigarettes per day comes to your office for a health maintenance examination.

Q5. Which of the following is (are) definitely indicated in this patient's examination?
   a. ultrasound of the abdomen to screen for pancreatic cancer
   b. chest x-ray to screen for carcinoma of the lung
   c. glaucoma screening
   d. all of the above
   e. none of the above

Case 5 ■ A 32-Year-Old Male Who Presents for a Health Maintenance Examination

A 32-year-old male comes to your office for a health maintenance examination.

Q6. Which of the following is (are) definitely indicated in this man's assessment?
   a. body mass index
   b. inquiry about smoking

c. inquiry about alcohol intake

d. inquiry into regular aerobic exercise activity

e. all of the above

Case 6 ■ A 45-Year-Old South-Vietnamese Woman with Hot Flashes

A 45-year-old South-Vietnamese woman comes to your office for a routine physical. She claims to be 5 feet tall but only measures 4 feet 10 inches. She weighs 90 pounds. She has a 35-year history of smoking two packs of cigarettes per week, is lactose intolerant, and has a sedentary lifestyle. Her only complaint is frequent hot flashes.

Q7. Which of the following statements regarding estrogen prophylaxis pertain(s) to the patient described in Case 6?

a. routine postmenopausal estrogen replacement is recommended as it would be for all women

b. estrogen therapy can be recommended despite the fact that she is asymptomatic because she is at increased risk for osteoporosis

c. spinal compression fractures are unlikely because she is not yet 60 years old

d. estrogen replacement therapy should be started at 0.3 mg/day

e. all of the above statements are true

Case 7 ■ A 28-Year-Old Pregnant Woman Seeking Prenatal Counseling

A 28-year-old female who recently discovered she was pregnant comes to your office and is concerned about which test she should have performed during the course of her pregnancy.

Q8. Which of the following statements concerning prenatal screening is (are) true?

a. all pregnant women should receive at least one ultrasound in the third trimester

b. all pregnant women should be screened for preeclampsia periodically throughout pregnancy with sophisticated tests

c. all pregnant women should be screened at least once for gestational diabetes mellitus (GDM)

d. all of the above statements are true

e. none of the above statements is true

Q9. The patient described in Case 1 asks about the need for urinary protein analysis. Which of the following is (are) true regarding the performance

of a routine urinalysis to detect the presence of protein in adults?

a. there is good evidence to support the recommendation that the condition be specifically considered in a health maintenance examination

b. there is fair evidence to support the recommendation that the condition be specifically considered in a health maintenance examination

c. there is poor evidence regarding the inclusion of the condition in a health maintenance examination, but recommendations may be made on other grounds

d. there is fair evidence to support the recommendation that the condition be excluded from the health maintenance examination

e. there is good evidence to support the recommendation that the condition be excluded from the health maintenance examination

Case 8 ■ A 20-Year-Old Male with Hay Fever

A 20-year-old male comes to your office complaining about terrible bouts of sneezing and red, tearing, and itching eyes. After examining him, you prescribe an antihistamine. In addition, you counsel him about motor vehicle accidents.

Q10. Regarding counseling to prevent motor vehicle injuries, which of the following statements is (are) true?

a. all patients should be encouraged to use seat restraints for themselves and others

b. all patients should be urged to wear safety helmets when riding bicycles

c. all patients should be urged to refrain from driving while under the influence of alcohol or other drugs

d. all of the above statements are true

e. none of the above statements is true

Case 9 ■ A 65-Year-Old Bisexual Male with Gonorrhea

A 65-year-old male comes to your office complaining of a urethral discharge. You determine that he has gonorrhea. He also tells you that he has had sexual relations with both male and female prostitutes during the past 6 months. You recommend that he be screened for human immunodeficiency virus (HIV) infection.

Q11. Screening for infection with HIV should be offered periodically to which of the following groups?

a. persons seeking treatment for sexually transmitted diseases
b. intravenous drug users
c. homosexual and bisexual men at risk
d. a, b, and c
e. none of the above groups

SHORT ANSWER MANAGEMENT PROBLEM
Summarize the 70 major recommendations of the U.S. Preventive Task Force on the Periodic Health Examination for routine screening.

ANSWERS

A1. **d.** This patient's periodic health examination should include measurement of body mass index and measurement of blood pressure. An ECG is not routinely recommended as part of the periodic health examination of a 45-year-old male.

A2. **a.** The U.S. Preventive Services Task Force recommends the following screening procedures in a 45-year-old male:
a. History: Dietary intake; physical activity; tobacco, alcohol, and drug use; and sexual practices
b. Physical examination: height and weight (body mass index) and blood pressure measurement
c. Laboratory and diagnostic procedures: Nonfasting total blood cholesterol
d. Counseling:
1) Diet and exercise: Fat (especially saturated fat and cholesterol), complex carbohydrates, fiber, sodium, calcium, caloric balance
2) Selection of exercise program
3) Substance use: Tobacco cessation, treatment for abuse of alcohol and other drugs
4) Sexual practices: Sexually transmitted diseases; partner selection, condoms, and intercourse; unintended pregnancy and contraceptive options
5) Injury prevention: Safety belts; safety helmets; smoke detectors; and dental health, including regular tooth brushing, flossing, and dental visits
6) Immunizations: Tetanus-diphtheria booster every 10 years

A3. **e.** There is now sufficient evidence to recommend either annual fecal occult blood testing or periodic (every 2 to 3 years) flexible sigmoidoscopy or both for the screening of the American population for colorectal cancer. Screening with either method is recommended to begin at age 50.

A4. **b.** The only intervention that is recommended by the U.S. Preventive Services Task Force as a screening test in a patient of this age is the Papanicolaou (Pap) smear.

Regular Pap testing is recommended for all women who are or who have been sexually active. Pap smears should begin at the onset of sexual activity and should be repeated every 1 to 3 years at the physician's discretion. They may be discontinued at age 65 if the previous smears have been consistently normal.

In summary, a low-risk patient who has had three normal smears in a row should have Pap smears every 3 to 5 years. A high-risk patient should have a Pap smear every 6 months or every year depending on the specific or degree of risk (see also Problem 52).

A5. **e.** There is insufficient evidence to recommend routine screening for lung or pancreatic cancer in an asymptomatic 53-year-old person or for performance of tonometry by primary care physicians as an effective test for glaucoma. It may be clinically prudent, however, to advise patients aged 65 or older to be tested periodically by an eye practitioner.

A6. **e.** A 32-year-old male, who is otherwise healthy, should have his health assessment concentrate on lifestyle issues. The same issues that were raised in the 45-year-old male should be raised in the 32-year-old male with the lifestyle emphasis being placed on diet (cholesterol, saturated fat); regular aerobic exercise; and inquiry and counseling regarding smoking, regular aerobic exercise, and alcohol and drug use.

The only physical examination maneuvers that have been recommended by the U.S. Preventive Services Task Force in a 32-year-old male include body mass index and blood pressure measurement.

A7. **b.** Although routine postmenopausal estrogen replacement is not recommended for all women, estrogen therapy should be considered for asymptomatic women who are at increased risk for osteoporosis, who lack known contraindications, and who have received adequate counseling regarding the potential benefits and risks. There is also most certainly a role for increased aerobic exercise and dietary calcium supplementation.

Estrogen therapy should be considered in asymptomatic women who are of Caucasian or Asian decent with a low bone mineral content, have a history of early menopause or bilateral oophorectomy before menopause, and do not have any known contraindications, have poor skeletal musculature, have a sedentary lifestyle, smoke cigarettes, and have an excessive alcohol intake (see also Problem 50).

A8. **e.** Although trials of a single prenatal ultrasound (PNU) in the second trimester have not shown a statistically significant effect on the rate of live births or on the Apgar score, the clinical trials that have been conducted have indicated that a single PNU early in pregnancy results in lower rates of induction (presumably through better estimates of gestational age), earlier detection of twin pregnancies, increased birth weight in singletons, and higher rates of therapeutic abortion for fetal abnormalities. Based on these clinical effects the Canadian Task Force on the Periodic Health Examination includes a single PNU examination in routine prenatal care (recommendation B). However, this recommendation has not been adopted by the U.S. Preventive Health Services Task Force because of lack of effect on perinatal morbidity or mortality.

The available evidence does not support a recommendation for or against universal screening for GDM. Women have varying degrees of glucose intolerance during pregnancy and a certain proportion will have adverse outcomes. The value of screening is unclear given potential clinical and financial costs. Women with risk factors for GDM should be carefully followed and prudently screened throughout their pregnancies.

Screening for preeclampsia is not associated with any "sophisticated tests." The accepted screening method is the routine assessment by blood pressure measurement, which in itself should be consistent. Although some studies have documented the efficacy of aspirin prophylaxis as a primary preventive measure, there is not enough evidence to recommend it on a routine basis, even among women at high risk for preeclampsia and intrauterine growth retardation.

A9. **e.** There is good evidence to recommend that routine urinalysis not be performed to detect the presence of proteinuria.

A successful screening program is predicated on the principle that efficacious, nonharmful treatment is available early in the disease course. Thus it is not recommended that dipstick screening for proteinuria in the general adult population for the prevention of end stage renal disease be part of a routine periodic health examination.

A10. **d.** Safety is a major focus of the health maintenance examination. All patients are encouraged to use seat belts in motor vehicles at all times, use safety helmets for bicycles and motorcycles at all times, and refrain from operating any kind of motor vehicle while under the influence of alcohol or other drugs.

These seem reasonable and self-explanatory, but the third point deserves emphasis. When we talk about drugs, we are talking about all drugs, not just illicit drugs. There are many prescription medications that can impair concentration and reaction time, and patients should always be cautioned about driving while using these medications. A good example of the latter would be antihistamines. Antihistamines are commonly prescribed, but seldom do we caution patients about operating motor vehicles while taking them.

A11. **d.** Patients who should be offered screening for HIV infection include all of the high-risk groups for the infection, including individuals with other sexually transmitted diseases, homosexual men, and heterosexuals with multiple partners. Some recommend screening all pregnant women, prisoners, and prostitutes. Sexually active individuals should be counseled.

SOLUTION TO THE SHORT ANSWER MANAGEMENT PROBLEM

Summary of the Health Maintenance Examination: The 70 recommendations of the U.S. Preventive Services Task Force on the Periodic Health Examination

a. The periodic health examination replaces the routine annual complete examination as the most cost-effective regular examination.

b. The task force began by preparing a list of important diseases and injuries in the United States that might be prevented through clinical intervention. The target conditions were selected on the basis of the following important criteria:

1) Burden of suffering from the target condition: Consideration was given to both the prevalence and the incidence of the condition.

2) Potential effectiveness of the preventive intervention: Conditions were excluded from analysis if the task force panel could not identify a potentially effective preventive intervention that could be performed by clinicians.

3) Selection of preventive services: For each target condition, the task force used two criteria to select the preventive services to be evaluated. First, in general, only preventive services carried out on asymptomatic persons were reviewed. Thus only primary and secondary preventive measures were addressed.

4) The maneuver had to be able to be performed in the clinical setting.

5) The criteria for determining effectiveness included the efficacy of the screening test, including the sensitivity and specificity of the maneuver; the reliability (reproducibility) of the test; and the effectiveness of early detection.

c. The task force emphasizes prevention, counseling, and lifestyle changes. It deemphasizes routine history, routine physical examination, and routine laboratory testing. Only procedures that have shown to make a difference are included. The major procedures include measurement of body mass index, measurement of blood pressure, Pap smear, mammography, nonfasting serum cholesterol, lifestyle counseling, and immunizations.

d. A summary of the 70 recommendations of the U.S. Preventive Services Task Force follows.

Recommendation 1: Screening for Asymptomatic Coronary Artery Disease

Clinicians should emphasize the primary prevention of coronary artery disease (CAD) by periodically screening for high blood pressure and high serum cholesterol and by investigating behavioral risk factors for CAD such as tobacco use, dietary fat intake, cholesterol intake, and inadequate physical exercise. There is insufficient evidence to recommend for or against the use of a routine ECG to screen asymptomatic middle-aged or older adults. It may be clinically prudent to perform screening ECGs in certain high-risk groups. Routine resting or exercise ECG screening before entering athletic programs is not recommended for asymptomatic children, adolescents, or young adults.

Recommendation 2: Screening for High Blood Cholesterol

Periodic measurement of total serum cholesterol is most important for middle-aged men, and it may also be clinically prudent in young men, women, and the elderly. All patients should receive periodic counseling regarding dietary intake.

Recommendation 3: Screening for Hypertension

Blood pressure should be measured regularly in persons aged 3 and older.

Recommendation 4: Screening for Carotid Artery Stenosis

There is currently insufficient evidence to recommend for or against auscultation for carotid bruits or noninvasive testing for carotid artery stenosis as effective screening strategies to prevent cerebrovascular disease in asymptomatic persons. It may be clinically prudent to include cervical auscultation in the physical examination of patients with established risk factors for cerebrovascular or cardiovascular disease. All patients should be screened for hypertension and some persons should be tested for high blood cholesterol. Clinicians should also provide counseling about smoking, exercise, and dietary fat consumption.

Recommendation 5: Screening for Peripheral Arterial Disease

Routine screening for peripheral arterial disease in asymptomatic persons is not recommended. Clinicians should be alert to signs of peripheral arterial disease in persons at increased risk and should thoroughly evaluate those patients for clinical evidence of vascular disease.

Recommendation 6: Screening for Abdominal Aortic Aneurysm

There is insufficient evidence to recommend for or against routine screening of asystematic adults for abdominal aortic aneurysm with either abdominal palpation or ultrasound.

Recommendation 7: Screening for Breast Cancer

All women over age 40 should receive an annual clinical breast examination. Mammography every year is recommended for all women beginning at age 50. It may be prudent to begin mammography at an earlier age for women at high risk for breast cancer. Although the teaching of breast self-examination is not specifically recommended at this time, there is insufficient evidence to recommend any change in current breast self-examination practices.

Recommendation 8: Screening for Colorectal Cancer

There is now sufficient evidence to recommend either annual fecal occult blood testing or periodic (every 2 to 3 years) flexible sigmoidoscopy or both for the screening of the American population for colorectal cancer. Screening with either method is recommended to begin at age 50.

Recommendation 9: Screening for Cervical Cancer

Regular Pap testing is recommended for all women who are or have been sexually active. Pap smears should begin with the onset of sexual activity and should be repeated every 1 to 3 years at the physician's discretion. They may be discontinued at age 65 if previous smears have been consistently normal.

Recommendation 10: Screening for Prostate Cancer

There is insufficient evidence to recommend for or against digital rectal examination as an effective screening test for prostate cancer in asymptomatic men. Transrectal ultrasound and serum tumor markers are not recommended for routine screening in asymptomatic men.

Recommendation 11: Screening for Lung Cancer

Screening asymptomatic persons for lung cancer by performing routine chest x-rays or sputum cytology is not recommended.

Recommendation 12: Screening for Skin Cancer

Routine screening for skin cancer is recommended for persons at high risk. Clinicians should advise all patients with increased outdoor exposure to use sunscreen preparations and other measures to protect their skin from ultraviolet rays. Currently there is not evidence for or against counseling patients to perform skin self-examination or for or against routine screening.

Recommendation 13: Screening for Testicular Cancer
Periodic screening for testicular cancer by testicular examination is recommended for men with a history of cryptorchidism, orchiopexy, or testicular atrophy. There is insufficient evidence of clinical benefit or harm to recommend for or against routine screening of other asymptomatic men for testicular cancer. Clinicians should advise adolescent and young males to seek prompt medical attention for testicular symptoms such as pain, swelling, or heaviness.

Recommendation 14: Screening for Ovarian Cancer
Screening of asymptomatic women for ovarian cancer is not recommended. It is prudent to examine the uterine adnexa when performing gynecologic examinations for other reasons.

Recommendation 15: Screening for Pancreatic Cancer
Routine screening for pancreatic cancer in asymptomatic persons is not recommended.

Recommendation 16: Screening for Oral Cancer
Routine screening of asymptomatic persons for oral cancer by primary care clinicians is not recommended. It may be prudent for clinicians to perform careful examinations for cancerous lesions of the oral cavity in patients who use tobacco or excessive amounts of alcohol, as well as in those with suspicious symptoms or lesions detected through self-examination. All patients should be counseled to receive regular dental examinations, and to limit consumption of alcohol. Persons with increased exposure to sunlight should be advised to take protective measures to protect their lips and skin from the harmful effects of ultraviolet rays.

Recommendation 17: Screening for Bladder Cancer
Routine screening for bladder cancer with urine dipstick, microscopic urine analysis, or urine cytology is not recommended in asymptomatic persons. All patients who smoke tobacco should be routinely counseled to stop.

Recommendation 18: Screening for Thyroid Cancer
Routine screening for thyroid cancer using neck palpation or ultrasonography is not recommended for asymptomatic children or adults. Patients with a history of external head or neck radiation in infancy or childhood may be examined periodically by palpation.

Recommendation 19: Screening for Diabetes Mellitus
There is insufficient evidence to recommend for or against routine screening for GDM. If screening is to be performed, it should be performed between 24 and 28 weeks of gestation with a 50-g glucose load. There is insufficient evidence to recommend for or against routine screening for diabetes in asymptomatic adults.

Recommendation 20: Screening for Thyroid Disease
Screening for congenital hypothyroidism is recommended for all neonates during the first week of life.

Routine screening for thyroid disorders is otherwise not warranted in asymptomatic adults or children. Persons with a history of upper-body radiation may benefit from regular physical examination of the thyroid gland.

Recommendation 21: Screening for Obesity
All children and adults should receive periodic height and weight measurements (body mass index).

Recommendation 22: Screening for Iron Deficiency Anemia
Screening using hemoglobin or hematocrit is recommended for pregnant women and for high-risk infants. Breast feeding should be encouraged, as should the inclusion of iron-rich foods in the diet of infants and young children. There is insufficient evidence to recommend for or against routine screening for iron deficiency anemia in other asymptomatic persons or for the routine use of iron supplements for healthy infants or pregnant women.

Recommendation 23: Screening for Elevated Lead Levels in Childhood and Pregnancy
Screening for elevated lead levels by measuring blood lead at least once at age 12 months is recommended for all children at increased risk of lead exposure. There is insufficient evidence to recommend for or against routine screening for lead exposure in asymptomatic pregnant women.

Recommendation 24: Screening for Hepatitis B
All pregnant women should be tested for hepatitis B surface antigen at their first prenatal visit. The test may be repeated in the third trimester in women at increased risk of exposure during pregnancy. Vaccination against hepatitis B is recommended for high-risk groups.

Recommendation 25: Screening for Tuberculosis
Tuberculin skin testing of asymptomatic persons should be performed on those at high risk of acquiring tuberculosis.

Recommendation 26: Screening for Syphilis
Routine screening for syphilis in asymptomatic persons is recommended for those in high-risk groups and for pregnant women.

Recommendation 27: Screening for Gonorrhea
Routine screening for gonorrhea in asymptomatic persons is recommended for persons at high risk and for pregnant women. An ophthalmic antibiotic should be applied topically to the eyes of all newborns after birth to prevent ophthalmia neonatorum.

Recommendation 28: Screening for HIV Infection
Screening for HIV infection should be offered periodically to persons seeking treatment for other sexually transmitted diseases, to intravenous drug users, to homosexual and bisexual men, and to others who may be at increased risk of infection. Testing should also be offered to pregnant women (or women contemplating pregnancy) who are at increased risk of HIV infection.

Recommendation 29: Screening for Chlamydial Infection

Routine testing for Chlamydia trachomatis is recommended for asymptomatic persons at high risk of infection including all sexually active female adolescents. Pregnant women in high-risk categories should be tested at the first prenatal visit. Ophthalmic antibiotics should be applied topically to the eyes of all newborns immediately after birth to help prevent ophthalmic neonatorum.

Recommendation 30: Screening for Genital Herpes Simplex

Screening for genital herpes simplex virus infection is recommended for pregnant women with active lesions.

Recommendation 31: Screening for Asymptomatic Bacteriuria

Urine culture testing of asymptomatic persons is recommended for pregnant women. It is not recommended routinely for asymptomatic adults. Insufficient evidence exists for or against testing diabetic or elderly ambulatory women.

Recommendation 32: Screening for Rubella

Testing for rubella antibodies should be performed at the first clinical encounter with all pregnant and nonpregnant women of childbearing age lacking evidence of immunity. Susceptible nonpregnant women who agree not to become pregnant for 3 months following immunization can be vaccinated. Susceptible pregnant women should not be vaccinated until immediately after delivery.

Recommendation 33: Screening for Visual Impairment

Vision screening is recommended for all children once before entering school, preferably at age 3 or 4. Routine vision testing is not recommended as a component of the periodic health examination of asymptomatic schoolchildren. Clinicians should be alert for signs of ocular misalignment when examining all infants and children. Vision screening of adolescents and adults is not recommended but may be appropriate in the elderly. Screening for glaucoma is discussed in Recommendation 34.

Recommendation 34: Screening for Glaucoma

There is insufficient evidence to recommend for or against routine performance of tonometry by primary care physicians as an effective screening test for glaucoma. It may be clinically prudent, however, to advise patients at high risk, such as those aged 65 and older, to be tested periodically for glaucoma by an eye specialist.

Recommendation 35: Screening for Hearing Impairment

Screening should be performed on all neonates at high risk for hearing impairment. High-risk children not tested at birth should be screened before age 3, but there is insufficient evidence of accuracy to recommend routine audiologic testing of all children in this age group. There is also insufficient evidence of benefit to recommend for or against hearing screening of asymptomatic children beyond the age of 3 years. Screening is not recommended for asymptomatic adolescents or adults not exposed routinely to excessive noise. Elderly patients should be evaluated regarding their hearing, counseled regarding the availability and use of hearing aids, and referred appropriately when abnormalities are detected.

Recommendation 36: Screening for Ultrasonography in Pregnancy

Women at increased risk for delivering a growth-retarded infant should receive ultrasound examinations early in the second trimester to determine gestational age and in the third trimester to measure the size of critical fetal structures. Routine ultrasound screening is otherwise not recommended in normal pregnancies, although physicians may wish to consider ultrasound dating in pregnant women with uncertain menstrual histories. All pregnant women should receive appropriate counseling regarding smoking, alcohol, and other drug use.

Recommendation 37: Screening for Preeclampsia

All pregnant women should receive systolic and diastolic blood pressure measurements at the first prenatal visit and periodically throughout the pregnancy.

Recommendation 38: Screening for Rh Incompatibility

All pregnant women should receive ABO/Rh blood typing and testing for anti-Rh(D) antibody at their first prenatal visit. Unsensitized Rh-negative women should receive Rh(D) immune globulin at 28 to 29 weeks' gestation and within 72 hours of delivery. Other indications for giving Rhogam include spontaneous or therapeutic abortion, ectopic pregnancy, amniocentesis, antepartum placental hemorrhage, or transfusion of Rh-positive blood products.

Recommendation 39: Screening by Electronic Fetal Monitoring

Fetal heart rate should be measured by auscultation in all women in labor to detect signs of fetal distress. Electronic fetal monitoring should not be performed routinely on all women in labor. It should be reserved, instead, for pregnancies at increased risk of fetal distress.

Recommendation 40: Screening for Home Uterine Activity Monitoring

There is insufficient evidence to recommend for or against home uterine activity monitoring in high-risk pregnancies as a screening test for preterm labor.

Recommendation 41: Screening for Down Syndrome

Amniocentesis for karyotyping should be offered to women aged 35 and older who are at high risk for Down syndrome. Ultrasound examination is not recommended as a routine screening test for this congential condition.

Recommendation 42: Screening for Neural Tube Defects

Maternal alpha-fetoprotein should be measured on all pregnant women during weeks' 16 to 18 in centers that have adequate counseling and follow-up services. Daily multivitamins with folic acid to reduce the risk of neural tube defects are recommended for all women who are planning or capable of pregnancy.

Recommendation 43: Screening for Hemoglobinopathies

Hemoglobin analysis is recommended for all newborns at risk for hemoglobin disorders. Hemoglobin analysis should also be discussed and offered to adolescents and young adults at risk for hemoglobinopathies and should be performed routinely at the first prenatal visit on all pregnant black women. All screening efforts should be accompanied by comprehensive counseling and treatment services.

Recommendation 44: Screening for Phenylketonuria

Screening for phenylketonuria is recommended for all newborns before discharge from the nursery. Infants who are tested before 24 hours of age should receive a repeat screening test before the third week of life. Routine prenatal screening for maternal PKU is not recommended.

Recommendation 45: Screening for Congenital Hypothyroidism

Screening for congenital hypothyroidism with thyroid function tests is recommended with all newborns in the first week of life.

Recommendation 46: Screening for Postmenopausal Osteoporosis

There is insufficient evidence to recommend for or against routine radiologic screening to detect low bone mineral content in postmenopausal women. Estrogen replacement therapy is discussed in Recommendation 68.

Recommendation 47: Screening for Adolescent Idiopathic Scoliosis

There is insufficient evidence to recommend for or against routine screening of asymptomatic adolescents for idiopathic scoliosis.

Recommendation 48: Screening for Dementia

There is insufficient evidence to recommend for or against screening for cognitive impairment among asymptomatic elderly persons.

Recommendation 49: Screening for Depression

There is insufficient evidence to recommend for or against the performance of routine screening tests for depression in asymptomatic persons. Clinicians should maintain an especially high index of suspicion for depressive symptoms in those persons who are believed to be at increased risk of suicide.

Recommendation 50: Screening for Suicidal Risk

Routine screening for suicidal intent is not recommended. Clinicians should be alert to signs of suicidal ideation in persons with established risk factors. Persons suspected of suicidal intent should be questioned regarding the extent of preparatory actions and referred for further evaluation if evidence of suicidal behavior is detected. Clinicians should be alert to symptoms of depression and should routinely ask patients about their use of alcohol and other drugs.

Recommendation 51: Screening for Family Violence

There is insufficient evidence to recommend for or against the use of specific screening instruments to detect family violence. However, questions about physical abuse may be prudent as part of a health maintenance examination in adults. Children and adults presenting with unusual injuries should be examined with attention to the possibility of abuse or neglect. Counseling and referral should be offered to those persons at high risk of becoming victims or perpetrators of violence.

Recommendation 52: Screening for Problem Drinking

All adolescents and adults should be asked to describe their use of alcohol and other drugs. Routine measurement of biochemical markers and drug testing are not recommended as the primary method of detecting alcohol and other drug abuse in asymptomatic persons. Persons in whom alcohol or other drug abuse or dependence is confirmed should receive appropriate counseling, treatment, and referrals. All persons who use alcohol, especially pregnant women, should be encouraged to quit drinking alcohol, and all persons who use alcohol or other intoxicating drugs should be counseled about the dangers of operating a motor vehicle or performing other potentially dangerous activities while intoxicated.

Recommendation 53: Screening for Drug Abuse

There is insufficient evidence to recommend for or against screening for drug abuse with standardized questionnaires or biologic assays. As with alcohol, all pregnant women should be advised of the potential adverse effects of drug use on the development of the fetus.

Recommendation 54: Counseling to Prevent Tobacco Use

Tobacco cessation counseling should be offered on a regular basis to all patients who smoke cigarettes, pipes, or cigars and to those who use smokeless tobacco. The prescription of nicotine gum or nicotine patches or bupropion may be appropriate adjuncts for some patients. Adolescents and young adults who do not currently use tobacco products should be advised not to start.

Recommendation 55: Exercise Counseling

Clinicians should counsel all patients to engage in a program of regular physical activity that is tailored to their health status and personal lifestyle.

Recommendation 56: Counseling to Promote a Healthy Diet

Clinicians should provide periodic counseling regarding the dietary intake of calories (especially saturated fat), cholesterol, complex carbohydrates (starches), fiber, and sodium. Women and adolescent girls should receive specific information on nutritional guidelines during pregnancy. Parents should also be counseled about nutritional requirements of infancy and early childhood. Counseling regarding alcohol consumption and breast feeding has already been discussed.

Recommendation 57: Counseling to Prevent Motor Vehicle Accidents

All patients should be urged to use occupant restraints (safety belts and safety seats) for themselves and others, to wear safety helmets when riding motorcycles and bicycles, and to refrain from driving under the influence of alcohol or other drugs.

Recommendation 58: Counseling to Prevent Household and Recreational Injuries

Patients who use alcohol or other drugs should be warned about engaging in potentially dangerous activities while intoxicated. It may also be clinically prudent to provide counseling on other measures to reduce the risk of unintentional household or environmental injuries from falls, drownings, fires or burns, poisoning, and firearms.

Recommendation 59: Counseling to Prevent Youth Violence

There is insufficient evidendence to recommend for or against clinician counseling of asymptomatic adolescents and adults to prevent morbidity and mortality from youth violence. Adolescent and adult patients should be screened for problem drinking.

Recommendation 60: Counseling to Prevent Low Back Pain

There is insufficient evidence to recommend for or against counseling patients to exercise to prevent low back pain, but recommendations for regular physical activities can be made based on other proven benefits.

Recommendation 61: Counseling to Prevent Dental Disease

All patients should be encouraged to visit a dental care provider on a regular basis. Primary care clinicians should counsel patients regarding daily tooth brushing and dental flossing, the appropriate use of fluoride for caries prevention, avoiding sugary foods, and risk factors for developing baby bottle tooth decay. Children living in communities with inadequate water fluoridation should receive appropriate dietary fluoride supplements. While examining the mouth, clinicians should be alert for the obvious signs of oral disease.

Recommendation 62: Counseling to Prevent HIV Infection and Other Sexually Transmitted Diseases

Clinicians should take a complete sexual and drug use history on all adolescent and adult patients. Sexually active patients should be advised about most effective strategies to prevent infection with the HIV virus or with other STDs. Patients should also receive counseling regarding the indications and proper methods for the use of condoms and spermicides in sexual intercourse and about the health risks associated with anal intercourse. Intravenous drug users should be encouraged to enroll in drug treatment programs and should be warned about sharing drug equipment or using nonsterile needles and syringes. All patients should be offered testing in accordance with recommendations on screening for the STDs previously discussed.

Recommendation 63: Counseling to Prevent Unintended Pregnancy

Clinicians should obtain a complete sexual history from all adolescent and adult patients. Sexually active women who do not want to become pregnant and men who do not want to have a child should receive detailed counseling on methods to prevent unintended pregnancy. Sexually active patients should also receive information on measures to prevent STDs.

Recommendation 64: Counseling to Prevent Gynecologic Cancers

There is insufficient evidence to recommend for or against routine counseling of women about measures for the primary prevention of gynecologic cancers. However, clinicians should counsel women about contraceptive practices and risk reduction with respect to specific gynecologic cancers.

Recommendation 65: Childhood Immunizations

All children should receive immunizations that are currently recommended by the American Committee on Immunization Practices of the Center for Disease Control and Prevention in Atlanta. These recommendations have been updated significantly since the U.S. Preventive Services Task Force published its second book, and the latest recommendations are included in Problem 81. In brief, the immunizations that are currently recommended in children are the following:

   a. Hepatitis B
   b. Polio
   c. Diphtheria, pertussis, tetanus
   d. *Haemophilus influenza*
   e. Measles, mumps, and rubella
   f. Varicella

Recommendation 66: Adult Immunizations

Pneumococcal vaccine should be administered at least once and influenza vaccine should be administered to all persons aged 65 and older in addition to persons in other high-risk groups on a yearly basis. Hepatitis B vaccine should be offered to homosexually active men, intravenous drug users, and others at high risk of infection. All adults should receive tetanus-diphtheria toxoid boosters at least once every 10 years. Vaccination against measles and mumps should be provided to all adults who lack evidence of immunity.

Recommendation 67: Postexposure Prophylaxis

Postexposure prophylaxis should be provided to selected persons with exposures to *H. influenzae* type b, meningococcal infection, hepatitis A, hepatitis B, tuberculosis, rabies, or tetanus.

Recommendation 68: Postmenopauseal Hormone Prophylaxis

Routine postmenopausal estrogen replacement counseling is recommended. Estrogen therapy should be considered for asymptomatic women who are at increased risk for osteoporosis, who lack known contraindications, and who have received adequate counseling about potential benefits and risks. The role of exercise and dietary calcium supplementation in preventing osteoporosis has been discussed.

Recommendation 69: Aspirin Prophylaxis

Low-dose aspirin should be considered for men over age 40 who are at significantly increased risk of myocardial infarction and who lack contraindications to the drug. Patients should understand the potential benefits and risks of aspirin therapy before beginning treatment.

Recommendation 70: Aspirin Prophylaxis in Pregnancy

There is insufficient evidence to recommend for or against the use of aspirin to prevent preeclampsia or intrauterine growth retardation in pregnant women including those who are at high risk."

SUGGESTED READINGS

Anonymous: Periodic health examination, 1992 update 2. Routine prenatal ultrasound screening. Canadian Task Force on the Periodic Health Examination, *Can Med Assoc J* 147(8):627-633, 1992.

Centers for Disease Control and Prevention: *ACIP recommended immunization schedule*, Atlanta, 1993, CDC.

http://cancernet.nci.nih.gov/clinp, 1990.

http://www.cdc.gov/nchswww/fastats/deaths.htm.

U.S. Preventive Task Force on the Periodic Health Examination: *Guide to clinical preventive services*, Baltimore, 1996, Williams & Wilkins.

PROBLEM·128

THE ROUTINE COMPLETE PHYSICAL EXAMINATION VS. THE FOCUSED PERIODIC HEALTH MAINTENANCE EXAMINATION

"Doctor, Why Do Your Physical Exams Seem Less Thorough? Is It Because You Became Part of an HMO?"

Case 1 ■ A 51-Year-Old Male Who Presents for a Complete Physical Examination

A 51-year-old male comes to your office for a complete physical examination. He has been in the habit of "coming in for the once-over" every year. The patient has been told that "a complete physical—head to toe" is the best method of ensuring good health.

SELECT THE BEST ANSWER TO THE FOLLOWING QUESTIONS

Q1. With regard to the relative effectiveness of the routine complete physical examination, which of the following statements is most accurate?
   a. the effectiveness of the routine complete physical examination has been confirmed in clinical trials
   b. the effectiveness of the routine complete physical examination has been confirmed with anecdotal evidence
   c. the effectiveness of the routine complete physical examination has been demonstrated in case-control trials
   d. the effectiveness of the routine complete physical examination has been confirmed in some studies but not in others
   e. none of the above statements is true

Q2. Which of the following is (are) criteria for effective periodic health screening?
   a. the condition tested must have a significant effect on quality of life
   b. the disease must have an asymptomatic phase during which detection and treatment significantly reduce morbidity and mortality
   c. acceptable treatment methods must be available
   d. tests must be available at a reasonable cost
   e. all of the above are true

Q3. Good reasons to consider performing a health maintenance examination on an asymptomatic adult independent of routine screening include which of the following?
   a. the establishment of a good doctor-patient relationship
   b. to augment history taking
   c. to maximize your income
   d. a and b
   e. all of the above

Q4. Which of the following statements regarding the performance of a routine health maintenance examination is (are) true?
   a. the examination may in itself be therapeutic
   b. the examination may provide the patient with reassurance
   c. the examination may produce benefit to the patient through therapeutic touch

d. the examination may play an important role in development and maintenance of the clinical skills in the physician

e. all of the above are true

Q5. Which of the following statements regarding the sensitivity and specificity of a routine physical examination is (are) true?

a. routine physical examination is neither highly sensitive nor highly specific

b. routine physical examination is both highly sensitive and highly specific

c. routine physical examination is high in sensitivity but low in specificity

d. routine physical examination is high in specificity but low in sensitivity

e. none of the above statements is true

Q6. Which of the following is (are) valid reasons not to rely significantly on a routine complete physical examination in asymptomatic adults?

a. routine complete physical examination may offer a false sense of security

b. routine complete physical examination is an inefficient use of time

c. routine complete physical examination reinforces misperceptions about physician capabilities

d. routine complete physical examination may detract from time that could be spent on other preventive interventions

e. all of the above are true

Q7. Which of the following statements is (are) true regarding false-positive findings on routine complete physical examination?

a. false-positive findings create needless patient anxiety

b. false-positive findings often initiate an "intervention cascade"

c. false-positive findings place a substantial burden on the entire health care system

d. a and b

e. all of the above statements are true

Q8. Which of the following statements is true regarding patient perceptions of the routine complete physical examination and related laboratory tests?

a. many patients believe that a routine complete physical examination, along with a complete laboratory profile, will diagnose the majority of illnesses

b. most patients understand the meaning of the term *periodic health examination*

c. many patients fail to understand the importance of a focused, regional examination

d. patients are generally sensitive to the costs of routine physical examinations and routine laboratory tests

e. none of the above statements is true

Case 2 ■ A 35-Year-Old Female Who Presents for a Health Maintenance Examination

A 35-year-old female has come to your office for a health maintenance examination. The physician examines the skin in an effort to identify dysplastic nevi, other unusual nevi, or other skin lesions.

Q9. Which of the following statements is true?

a. the examination for skin cancer in a health maintenance examination is highly sensitive and highly specific

b. the examination for skin cancer in a health maintenance examination is highly sensitive but of low specificity

c. the examination for skin cancer in a health maintenance examination is neither sensitive nor specific

d. the examination for skin cancer in a health maintenance examination is highly specific but of lower sensitivity

e. the examination for skin cancer is of variable sensitivity and specificity depending on the skill of the examiner

---

SHORT ANSWER MANAGEMENT PROBLEM

A 51-year-old male comes to your office in an acutely agitated state. Last week he saw your partner for his usual annual examination. Instead of his regular checkup, he states he was given a "very cursory examination." He tells you that his lungs were not checked, his heart was not checked, his reflexes were not tapped, a light was not shone in his eyes, and so on.

You determine your partner had performed a focused periodic health examination, a concept you also believe in. You have just begun to introduce this concept into your own practice. Discuss how you would respond to this patient at this time.

ANSWERS

A1. **e.** Although the routine physical examination has been a primary diagnostic tool throughout the twentieth century, there is little, if any, evidence in the literature to support its efficacy.

The routine physical examination should not be confused with the health maintenance examination, for which there is evidence supporting its efficacy. The health maintenance examination is a comprehensive examination targeted at specific age and gender causes of morbidity and mortality. Recommendations for the periodic health maintenance examination are derived from epidemiologic data that assess population risk and intervention benefit.

A2. **e.** The criteria for effective periodic health screening are as follows:
  a. The condition for which the physician is testing must have a significant effect on the quality of the patient's life.
  b. Acceptable treatment methods must be available for that particular condition.
  c. The disease must have an asymptomatic phase during which detection and treatment significantly reduce morbidity and mortality.
  d. Treatment during the asymptomatic phase must yield a result superior to that obtained by delaying treatment until symptoms appear.
  e. Tests must be available at a reasonable cost.
  f. Tests must be acceptable to the patient.
  g. The prevalence of the condition must be sufficient to justify the cost of screening.

A3. **d.** See Answer 4.

A4. **e.** Reasons to perform a periodic health maintenance examination in asymptomatic adults, independent of routine screening, include the following:
  a. To establish a good doctor-patient relationship
  b. To augment history taking
  c. To fulfill patient expectations
  d. To provide the therapeutic benefit of touch
  e. To maintain the physician's clinical skills
  f. To reinforce patient education, especially self-examination
  g. To realistically reassure the patient (and the physician)
  h. To establish the patient's baseline health status
  i. To determine if the patient is indeed asymptomatic
  j. To avoid giving the patient the impression that he or she must have symptoms to be examined

A5. **a.** See Answer 6.

A6. **e.** The procedures entailed in the routine complete physical examination are neither sensitive nor specific. Because of this, physicians may provide false reassurance on the basis of the findings. Consider statements such as "Your heart sounds great" or "You've got a complete, 100% perfect bill of health." Next week you hear from the Emergency Department doctor that your patient has just had a heart attack. Your next phone call probably will come from his lawyer. Such grandiose statements reinforce misperceptions regarding physicians' capabilities and may certainly result in legal action.

Excessive concentration on physical examination detracts from time that could be spent in more productive pursuits, such as patient education and counseling about health risk behaviors.

A7. **e.** The same excessive compulsiveness that serves as a survival skill in medical training is often dysfunctional in medical practice. False-positive findings are common in the face of low-test sensitivity and specificity and low prevalence of the condition in the population tested. Even if a test has a high sensitivity and specificity, the more tests or maneuvers that are performed on the same individual, the higher the likelihood of a false-positive result. Also, the likelihood that a positive test is true positive (positive predictive value) is directly related to the prevalence of the condition in the target population. Performing examinations in populations in which the condition has a low prevalence will thus generate a high false-positive rate.

False-positive test results create needless anxiety in both patients and physicians. More important, such results often lead to an "intervention cascade," initiating further testing of greater invasiveness, which increases the potential for iatrogenic harm. A good example of this is the finding of a slightly enlarged ovary (you think) on pelvic bimanual examination, a situation in which a benign cause is much more likely than a malignant cause. From that may result routine ultrasound, followed perhaps by laparoscopy to rule out a malignant tumor of very low prevalence.

We must all ask ourselves, "Has this procedure really done the patient any good?"

A8. **a.** Many patients believe that a complete physical examination, along with a complete laboratory profile, will diagnose the majority of illnesses. This is obviously a mistaken impression. Despite efforts aimed at increasing public awareness and understanding, many patients do not understand the concept of the periodic health examination or of focused regional examination.

As well, patients are still not very sensitive about costs of routine examinations and routine tests. Further patient education efforts will be necessary to inform patients regarding these important issues.

A9. **e.** The clinical examination of the skin has significant variability in terms of sensitivity and specificity.

The major reason for the variability is the expertise of the examiner. The greater the training and expertise in skin lesion diagnosis and treatment, the higher the sensitivity and specificity of the examination. Another excellent example of this phenomenon is radiologists reading mammograms. The more training the radiologist has and the more mammograms the radiologist reads, the higher the sensitivity and specificity of mammograms.

SOLUTION TO THE SHORT ANSWER MANAGEMENT PROBLEM

This is a relatively difficult situation and requires both patience and diplomacy. The following may be a reasonable manner in which to approach this problem.

a. Listen to the patient. Have the patient articulate concerns to you regarding the nature and performance of the examination.

b. Explain the rationale for the change in examination technique and procedure. Explain to the patient that the probability of producing a better outcome from this new process (the focused periodic health maintenance examination) is actually significantly higher than with the old process.

c. If the patient appears receptive to the new approach, then it is reasonable to follow up the conversation with some appropriate literature.

d. If the patient does not appear receptive to the new approach, it is important to convey the message that the "old way" may, in fact, be the best for this particular patient and that you will respect his wishes and continue to carry out your assessments for him in the manner of the complete routine checkup. Answer 4 expands on the reasons why this approach may be preferable for other patients as well.

SUMMARY OF THE ROUTINE COMPLETE PHYSICAL EXAMINATION VS. THE FOCUSED PERIODIC HEALTH MAINTENANCE EXAMINATION

1. There is little, if any, evidence that the routine complete physical examination is effective or addresses the issues and conditions that can be prevented or can be addressed or treated while in an asymptomatic phase.

2. In addition to the lack of established efficacy, there are significant risks to performing a routine complete physical examination, not the least of which is labeling someone as healthy when, in fact, he or she is not healthy.

3. There are reasons and situations in which it may be reasonable to perform a routine complete checkup, reasons that, when balanced against the reasons not to perform the same, come out in favor of doing a routine physical examination. These are outlined in Answer 4.

4. Significant misperceptions concerning the routine physical examination often result in excess procedures and excess laboratory tests. If carried to the extreme, this is a sure-fire way to end up on a wild goose chase. This wild goose chase may very well end up in a previously well person now becoming ill from worry regarding a false-positive test result, for example. Thus on many occasions one would not be overstating the case by stating, "Everything was fine until the patient went to the doctor."

SUGGESTED READINGS

Breslow L, Somers AR: The lifetime health-monitoring program, *New Engl J Med* 296(11):601-608, 1997.

Frame PS: A critical review of adult health maintenance. Part 4. Prevention of metabolic, behavioral, and miscellaneous conditions, *J Fam Pract* 23(1):29-39, 1986.

Frame PS: A critical review of adult health maintenance. Part 3. Prevention of cancer, *J Fam Pract* 22(6):511-520, 1986.

Frame PS: A critical review of adult health maintenance. Part 2. Prevention of infectious diseases, *J Fam Pract* 22(5):417-422, 1986.

Frame PS: A critical review of adult health maintenance. Part 1. Prevention of atherosclerotic disease, *J Fam Pract* 22(4):341-346, 1986.

Frank SH et al: The focused physical examination: Should records be tailor-made?, *Postgrad Med* 92(2):171-186, 1992.

PROBLEM · 1 2 9

EPIDEMIOLOGY

"Is It Sensitivity, Specificity, or What?"

Case 1 ■ A 26-Year-Old Medical Student Who Is Having Panic Attacks Regarding His Upcoming Epidemiology Examination

A 26-year-old medical student comes to your office in a state of extreme anxiety manifested by panic attacks throughout the previous week. His physical symptoms include sweating and palpitations.

On physical examination his blood pressure is 120/70 mm Hg, and no thyroid enlargement is noted. You order a thyroid-stimulating hormone test to exclude hyperthyroidism.

Table 129-1 ■ Relationship between Test A and Disease B

	Disease B Present	Disease B Absent
Test A positive	30	50
Test A negative	10	80

In an attempt to deal with his symptoms, you decide to spend some time tutoring the student regarding basic epidemiologic concepts. You begin by explaining the basics of a 2 × 2 table that relates positive and negative test results to the presence or absence of disease in a specific population (Table 129-1).

SELECT THE BEST ANSWER TO THE FOLLOWING QUESTIONS

Use the data from Table 129-1 for Questions 1 to 6.

Q1. What is the sensitivity of test A for disease B?
    a. 25%
    b. 37.5%
    c. 75%
    d. 62.5%
    e. 11%

Q2. What is the specificity of test A for disease B?
    a. 25%
    b. 37.5%
    c. 75%
    d. 61.5%
    e. 11%

Q3. What is the positive predictive value (PPV) of test A in the diagnosis of disease B?
    a. 37.5%
    b. 25%
    c. 75%
    d. 61.5%
    e. 11%

Q4. What is the negative predictive value (NPV) of test A in the diagnosis of disease B?
    a. 37%
    b. 89%
    c. 25%
    d. 75%
    e. 61.5%

Q5. What is the likelihood ratio for test A in disease B?
    a. 0.39
    b. 1.95
    c. 3.80

Table 129-2 ■ Prevalence of Disease X in Certain Populations

Setting	Prevalence (Cases/100,000)
General population	50
Women, age 50 years old and older	500
Women, age 65 years old and older with a suspicious finding on clinical examination	40,000

    d. 0.79
    e. 1.51

Q6. What is the prevalence of disease A in this population?
    a. 15.5%
    b. 23.5%
    c. 40.0%
    d. 10.5%
    e. 18.4%

Consider the data in Table 129-2 illustrating the prevalence of disease X in various populations. Based on this information about disease prevalence and assuming the sensitivity of test A for disease X is 80% and the specificity of test A for disease X is 90%, answer Questions 7 to 10.

Q7. What is the PPV of test A in the diagnosis of disease X in the general population?
    a. 0.4%
    b. 1.3%
    c. 5.4%
    d. 15.7%
    e. 39.6%

Q8. What is the PPV of test A in disease X in women aged 50 and older?
    a. 0.4%
    b. 3.9%
    c. 10.7%
    d. 23.6%
    e. 52.7%

Q9. What is the PPV of test A in disease X in women older than 65 years of age with a suspicious finding on clinical examination?
    a. 0.4%
    b. 5.6%
    c. 34.7%
    d. 84.2%
    e. 93.0%

Table 129-3 ■ Sensitivity and Specificity of Blood Sugar Levels in the Diagnosis of Diabetes Mellitus

Blood Sugar Level 2 Hours after Eating	Sensitivity	Specificity
140 mg/100 (7.8 mmol/L)	57.1%	99.4%

Q10. If the PPV of a test for a given disease in a given population is 4%, how many true positive test results are there in a sample of 100 positive test results?
   a. 4
   b. 10
   c. 40
   d. 96
   e. none of the above

Consider the data in Table 129-3 concerning the sensitivity and specificity in the diagnosis of diabetes mellitus in the population to answer Question 11.

Q11. Given that the data are correct, if the sensitivity of the test for a given blood sugar level was 38.6%, which of the following would be the most likely value for specificity?
   a. 99.2%
   b. 98.7%
   c. 92.4%
   d. 87.3%
   e. 100.0%

Q12. The validity of a test is best defined as which of the following?
   a. the reliability of the test
   b. the reproducibility of the test
   c. the variation in the test results
   d. the degree to which the results of a measurement correspond to the true state of the phenomenon
   e. the degree of biological variation of the test

Q13. Which of the following terms is synonymous with the term reliability?
   a. reproducibility
   b. validity
   c. accuracy
   d. mean
   e. variation

Q14. Which of the following is not a measure of central tendency?
   a. mean
   b. median

Table 129-4 ■ Blood Pressure Readings vs. Visit Number

Visit Number	Mean Diastolic Blood Pressure (MM/HG)
1	99.2
2	91.2
3	90.7

   c. mode
   d. standard deviation
   e. none; all of the above are measures of central tendency Gaussian distribution

Consider the following experimental data: in a trial of the effect of reducing multiple risk factors on the subsequent incidence of coronary artery disease, high-risk patients were selected for study. Elevated blood pressure was one of the risk factors that caused people to be considered. People were screened for inclusion in the study on three consecutive visits. Blood pressure at those visits, before any therapeutic interventions were undertaken, were as listed in Table 129-4.

Use the data in Table 129-4 to answer Question 15.

Q15. Which of the following statements regarding these data is true?
   a. these results are very strange; consider publication in any journal specializing in irreproducible results
   b. this is an example of regression to the mean
   c. this is an example of natural variation
   d. the most likely explanation is either interobserver or intraobserver variation
   e. we are likely dealing with faulty equipment in this case; the most likely reason for this would be failure to calibrate all of the blood pressure cuffs

Consider the following experimental data: a population of heavy smokers (men smoking more than 50 cigarettes per day) is divided into two groups and followed for a period of 10 years.

Use the data from Table 129-5 to answer Question 16.

Q16. Regarding these results, which of the following statements is true?
   a. these results prove that screening chest x-rays improve survival time in lung cancer
   b. these results prove that screening chest x-rays should be considered for all smokers
   c. these results are most likely an example of lead-time bias

Table 129-5 ■ 10-Year Mortality Data

		Diagnosed with Lung Cancer	Average Survival Time from Diagnosis
Group 1 (experimental group)	490 individuals with annual chest x-rays	37	14 months
Group 2 (control group)	510 individuals with no annual chest x-ray	39	8 months

    d. these results are most likely an example of length-time bias

    e. these results do not make any sense; the experiment should be repeated

Q17. Length-time bias with respect to cancer diagnosis is defined as which of the following?

    a. bias resulting from the detection of slow-growing tumors during screening programs more often than fast-growing tumors

    b. bias resulting from the length of time a cancer was growing before any symptoms occurred

    c. bias resulting from the length of time a cancer was growing before somebody got on the ball and started to ask some questions and perform some laboratory investigations

    d. bias resulting from the length of time between the latent and more rapid growth phases of any cancer

    e. none of the above

Q18. Concerning population and disease measurement, prevalence is defined as which of the following?

    a. the fraction (proportion) of a population having a clinical condition at a given point in time

    b. the fraction (proportion) of a population initially free of a disease but that develop the disease over a given period

    c. equivalent to incidence

    d. defined mathematically as $a + b/a + b + c + d$ in a 2×2 table relating sensitivity and specificity to PPV

    e. none of the above

Q19. Concerning population and disease measurement, incidence is defined as which of the following?

    a. the fraction (proportion) of a population having a clinical condition at a given point in time

    b. the fraction (proportion) of a population initially free of a disease but that develop the disease over a given period

    c. equivalent to prevalence

    d. of little use in epidemiology

    e. none of the above

Q20. Regarding clinical epidemiology in relation to the practice of family medicine, which of the following statements is true?

    a. clinical epidemiology is higher mathematics that bears little relation to the world in general, much less the specialty of family medicine

    b. clinical epidemiology was invented to create anxiety and panic attacks that mimic hyperthyroidism in medical students and residents

    c. clinical epidemiology is unlikely to contain any useful information for the average practicing family physician

    d. clinical epidemiology is a passing fad; fortunately for all concerned, its time has passed

    e. none of the above statements about clinical epidemiology is true

SHORT ANSWER MANAGEMENT PROBLEM

A medical resident who is not the least bit interested in clinical epidemiology, admits an 86-year-old woman to the hospital with congestive heart failure. He decodes that "we'd better make sure we're complete here—we sure don't want to miss anything" and orders almost every laboratory test listed on the nursing station computer screen as available. You, a young medical student following behind him, regard him as a truly excellent role model and desire to practice like him when you become a resident. Thus on your next admission (a 37-year-old male with acute gastroenteritis) you throw the book at him—the 100% complete laboratory workup, no ifs, ands, or buts and no test missed."

Unfortunately for yourself, the attending physician in charge of the patient's care is less than impressed by your attentiveness to detail and completeness and asks you to explain yourself. As it turns out, you have ordered a total of 100 different laboratory tests (many of them disguised in chemical panels to give only the appearance of a few brief panels). He asks you if you are aware of the probability of labeling someone who truly is normal as normal if you order 100 tests. Discuss your answer to this question.

ANSWERS

The 2×2 table in Table 129-6 illustrates the answers to Questions 1-6.

Table 129-6 ■ Disease X

	Disease X Present	Disease X Absent
Test A positive	30 (a) TP	50 (b) FP
Test A negative	10 (c) FN	80 (d) TN

TP, True positive; *TN,* true negative; *FP,* false positive; *FN,* false negative.

A1. **c.**

A2. **d.**

A3. **a.**

A4. **b.**

A5. **b.**

A6. **b.**

Sensitivity is defined as the proportion of people with the disease that have a positive test result. A sensitive test will rarely miss patients who have the disease. In Table 129-6, sensitivity is defined as the number of true positives (TPs) divided by the number of true positives plus the number of false negatives (FNs). That is:

$$\text{Sensitivity} = \frac{\text{TP}}{\text{TP} + \text{FN}}$$

$$\text{Sensitivity} = \frac{a}{a + c} = \frac{30}{40} = 75\%$$

A sensitive test (one that is usually positive in the presence of disease) should be selected when there is an important penalty for missing the disease. This would be so, for example, when you had reason to suspect a serious but treatable condition such as using a chest x-ray for a patient with suspected tuberculosis or Hodgkin's disease. In addition, sensitive tests are useful in the early stages of a diagnostic workshop of disease, when several possibilities are being considered, to reduce the number of possibilities. Thus, in situations like this, diagnostic tests are used to rule out diseases.

Specificity is defined as the proportion of people without the disease who have a negative test result. A specific test rarely incorrectly classifies people without the disease as having the disease. In Table 129-6, specificity is defined as the number of true negatives (TNs) divided by the number of true negatives plus the number of false positives (FPs). That is:

$$\text{Specificity} = \frac{\text{TN}}{\text{TN} + \text{FP}}$$

$$\text{Specificity} = \frac{d}{d + b} = \frac{80}{130} = 61.5\%$$

A specific test is useful to confirm, or rule in, a diagnosis that has been suggested by other tests or data. Thus a specific test is rarely positive in the absence of disease, that is, it gives very few false positive test results. Tests with high specificity are needed when false positive results can harm the patient physically, emotionally, or financially. Thus a specific test is most helpful when the test result is positive.

There is always a trade-off between sensitivity and specificity. In general, if a disease has a low prevalence, choose a more specific test; if a disease has a high prevalence, choose a more sensitive test.

PPV is defined as the probability of disease in a patient with a positive (abnormal) test result. In Table 129-6, the PPV is as follows:

$$\text{PPV} = \frac{a}{a + b} = \frac{30}{80} = 37.5\%$$

NPV is defined as the probability of not having the disease when the test result is negative. In Table 129-6, the NPV is as follows:

$$\text{NPV} = \frac{d}{c + d} = \frac{80}{90} = 89\%$$

The likelihood ratio of a positive test result is the probability of that test result in the presence of disease divided by the probability of the test result in the absence of disease. In Table 129-6, the likelihood ratio is as follows:

$$\text{Likelihood ratio (+) test results} \frac{\dfrac{a}{a + c}}{\dfrac{b}{b + d}}$$

The prevalence of a disease in the population at risk is the fraction or proportion of a group with a clinical condition at a given point in time. Prevalence is measured by surveying a defined population containing people with and without the condition of interest (at a given point in time). Prevalence can be equated with pretest probability. In Table 129-6, prevalence is defined as follows:

$$\text{Prevalence} = \frac{a + c}{a + b + c + d}$$

As prevalence falls, PPV must fall along with it and NPV must rise.

A7. **a.**

A8. **b.**

A9. **d.** The respective PPVs for test A in the diagnosis of disease X in the general population, women greater than 50 years, and women older than 65 with a suspicious finding on clinical examination are 0.4%, 3.9%, and 84.2%, respectively.

To perform the calculations necessary to arrive at these answers the following steps are recommended:

Step 1: Identify the sensitivity and specificity of the sign, symptom, or diagnostic test that you plan to use. Many of these are published. If you are not certain, consider asking a consultant with special expertise in the area.

Step 2: Using a 2 × 2 table, set your total equal to an even number (consider, for example, 1000 as a good choice). Therefore,

$$a + b + c + d = 1000$$

Step 3: Using whatever information you have about the patient before you apply this diagnostic test, estimate his or her pretest probability (prevalence) of the disease in question. Next, put appropriate numbers at the bottom of the columns ($a + c$ and $b + d$). The easiest way to do this is to express your pretest probability (or prevalence) as a decimal three places to the right. This result is ($a + c$), and 1000 minus this result is ($b + d$).

Step 4: Start to fill in the cells of the 2 × 2 table. Multiply sensitivity (expressed as a decimal) by ($a + c$) and put the result in cell a. You can then calculate cell c by simple subtraction.

Step 5: Similarly, multiply specificity (expressed as a decimal) by ($b + d$) and put the result in cell d. Calculate cell b by subtraction.

Step 6: You can now calculate PPVs and NPVs for the test with the prevalence (pretest probability) used.

For example, to calculate the PPV for test A in the diagnosis of disease in women older than 65 years old with a suspicious finding on clinical examination, use the following equation:

$$\text{Prevalence} = \frac{40,000 \text{ cases}}{100,000} = \frac{400}{1000}$$

Setting the total number equal to 1000,

$$\frac{a + c}{a + b + c + d} = \frac{400}{1000}$$

Table 129-7 ■ Calculations Involved in a General 2 × 2 Table

	Target Disorder	
	Present	Absent
Test positive	Cell a Sensitivity X ($a + c$)	Cell b Column total − d
Test negative	Cell c Column total − a $a + c - a$	Cell d Specificity X ($b + d$)
Column totals	$a + c$	$b + d$

Therefore $a + c = 400$ and $b + d = 600$. Thus,

$$\text{Cell a} = \text{Sensitivity} \times 400$$
$$= 0.8 \times 400 = 320$$

and

$$\text{Cell c} = 400 - 320 = 80$$

Similarly,

$$\text{Cell d} = \text{Specificity} \times 600$$
$$= 0.9 \times 600 = 540$$

Therefore

$$\text{Cell b} = 600 - 540 = 60$$

$$\text{PPV} = \frac{a}{a + b}$$

$$= \frac{320}{320 + 60} = 84.2\%$$

Similar calculations can be made for the general population (prevalence = 50/100,000) and for women greater than 50 years (prevalence = 500/100,000).

A10. **a.** If the PPV of a test for a given disease is 4%, then only 4 of 100 positive test results will be TPs; the remainder will be FPs. Further testing (often invasive) and anxiety will be inflicted on the 96% of the population with a positive test result but without disease.

Thus careful consideration should be given to the PPV of any test for any disease in a given population before ordering it.

A11. **e.** Remember the inverse relationship between sensitivity and specificity: if the sensitivity goes down, the specificity goes up, and if the sensitivity goes up, the specificity goes down. The only value that is greater than the previous specificity of 99.4% is 100%; therefore it is the most likely correct value of the values listed for the cospecificity of the test. This is actually the case at a cutoff blood sugar level of 180 mg/100 ml 2 hours after eating; if we use this value for the cutoff, there will be even more false negatives than at 140 mg/100 ml (that is, we will incorrectly label more individuals who actually have diabetes as being normal), whereas we will not label anyone who does not have diabetes as having diabetes.

A12. **d.** Validity is the degree to which the results of a measurement of a test actually correspond to the true state of the phenomenon being measured.

A13. **a.** Reliability is the extent to which repeated measurements of a relatively stable phenomenon fall closely to each other. *Reproducibility* and *precision* are other words for this characteristic.

A14. **d.** A normal, or Gaussian, distribution is characterized by the following measures of central tendency:
   a. A mean: the sum of values for observations divided by the number of observations
   b. A median: the point where the number of observations above the mean equals the number of observations below the mean
   c. A mode: the most frequently occurring value

In the same normal, or Gaussian, distribution, expressions of dispersion are the following:
   a. The range: from the lowest value to the highest value in a distribution
   b. The standard deviation: the absolute value of the average difference of individual values from the mean
   c. The percentile: the proportion of all observations falling between specified values

The most valuable measure of dispersion in a normal, or Gaussian, distribution is the standard deviation (SD). It is defined as follows:

$$SD = \frac{\sqrt{\Sigma(x - \bar{x})^2}}{n - 1}$$

In a normal, or Gaussian, distribution 68.26% of the values lie within ±1 SD from the mean; 95.44% of values lie within ±2 SD from the mean; and 99.72% of values lie within ±3 SD from the mean.

A15. **b.** As can be seen in this trial, there was a substantial fall in mean blood pressure between the first and third visits. The explanation for this is called *regression to the mean*. The following is the best explanation of regression to the mean.

Patients who are singled out from others because they have a laboratory test that is unusually high or low can be expected, on the average, to be closer to the center of the distribution (normal, or Gaussian) if the test is repeated. Moreover, subsequent values are likely to be more accurate estimates of the true value (validity), which could be obtained if the measurement were repeated for a particular patient many times.

A16. **c.** This is an example of lead-time bias. Lead time is the period between the detection of a medical condition by screening and when it ordinarily would have been diagnosed as a result of symptoms.

In lung cancer there is absolutely no evidence that chest x-rays have any influence on mortality. However, if, as in this case, the experimental group had chest x-rays done, their lung cancers would have been diagnosed at an earlier time and it would appear that they were longer survivors. The control group would most likely have had their lung cancers diagnosed when they developed symptoms. In fact, however, the

survival time would have been exactly the same; the only difference would have been that men in the experimental group would have known that they had lung cancer for a longer period.

A17. **a.** Length-time bias occurs because the proportion of slow-growing lesions diagnosed during a cancer screening program is greater than the proportion of those diagnosed during usual medical care. The effect of including a greater number of slow-growing cancers makes it seem that the screening and early treatment programs are more effective than they really are.

A18. **a.** Prevalence is defined as the fraction (proportion) of a population with a clinical condition at a given point in time. Prevalence is measured by surveying a defined population in which some patients have and some patients do not have the condition of interest at a single point in time. It is not the same as incidence, and, as previously discussed in relation to sensitivity, specificity, and PPV in a 2 × 2 table, it is defined in mathematic terms as $a + c/a + b + c + d$.

A19. **b.** Incidence in relation to a population is defined as the fraction (proportion) initially free of a disease or condition that go on to develop it over a given period.

A20. **e.** Clinical epidemiology is a specialty that will assume increasingly more importance in the specialty of family medicine. Clinical epidemiology allows us to understand disease, to understand laboratory testing, and to understand why we should do what we should do and why we should not do what we should not do. More importantly, as family physicians in the future are called on by governments, patients, licensing bodies, and boards to justify clinical decisions and treatments, it will allow us to understand the difference between defensive medicine and defensible medicine (the latter being what we are trying to achieve) in the interest of optimizing the health care of patients.

SOLUTION TO THE SHORT ANSWER MANAGEMENT PROBLEM

Although 100 may be a bit of an exaggeration, it may not be. At some hospitals, patients have complete blood counts done routinely every second or third day. With a few chemistry panels thrown in for good measure every week or so, it does not take that long to add up to 100 individual tests. The relationship between the number of tests ordered and the percentage of normal people with at least one abnormal test result is shown in Table 129-8.

Table 129-8 ■ Testing and Positive Predictive Value: An Example of False Positivity

Number of Tests	Percent of People Having at Least One Abnormality
1	5
5	23
20	64
100	99.4

Thus if you did order 100 laboratory tests and the patient was truly well (no evidence of disease), there is less than a 1% chance that you would come to that conclusion. Using the fundamentals of Logic 100 we could justifiably say that a normal patient is defined as someone who has not been sufficiently investigated.

The answer to this short answer management problem is to say as little as possible. Offer to read a short textbook on epidemiology before you see your attending physician again.

SUMMARY

1. Remember the importance of sensitivity, specificity, and especially PPV; understand that the lower the prevalence (or likelihood) of a condition in the patient about to be tested, the lower the PPV of the test.

2. Understand the importance of false negatives and especially false positives in the laboratory tests that you order.

3. Be prepared to draw a 2 × 2 table and calculate the PPV of a test given the sensitivity, specificity, and prevalence of the condition in the population.

4. Misinterpretations that may result in survival statistics in cancer are caused by lead-time bias and length-time bias.

5. Apply the principle of regression to the mean in the diagnosis of certain conditions, hypertension being a prime example.

6. Remember the dictum *primum non nocere:* first do no harm.

7. Sensitivity and specificity are inversely related: as sensitivity of a test goes up, the specificity of the test goes down.

8. Sensitive tests should be used to rule out disease; specific tests should be used to rule in disease.

9. Although a test may be reliable, it may not have any validity.

10. Remember the definition of a normal patient: someone who has not been sufficiently investigated.

SUGGESTED READINGS

Fletcher R et al: *Clinical epidemiology: The essentials,* ed 2, Baltimore, 1988, Williams & Wilkins.
Sackett D et al: *Clinical epidemiology: A basic science for clinical medicine,* Boston, 1985, Little, Brown.

PROBLEM · 130

PHYSICIAN INTERVENTION IN SMOKING CESSATION

"My Father Lived to Be 90 Years Old and He Smoked Like a Chimney. Why Should I Quit?"

Case 1 ■ A 40-Year-Old Executive Who Smokes Three Packs of Cigarettes a Day

A 40-year-old executive who smokes three packs of cigarettes a day comes to your office for his routine health assessment. He states that he would like to quit smoking but is having great difficulty. He has tried three times before, but he says, "Pressures at work mounted up and I just had to go back to smoking."

The patient has a history of mild hypertension. His blood cholesterol level is normal. He drinks only 1 or 2 ounces of alcohol per week. His family history is significant for premature cardiovascular disease and death.

SELECT THE BEST ANSWER TO THE FOLLOWING QUESTIONS

Q1. Current evidence suggests that coronary artery disease (CAD) is strongly related to cigarette smoking. What percentage of deaths from congenital heart disease (CHD) is thought to be directly related to cigarette smoking?
  a. 5%
  b. 10%
  c. 20%
  d. 25%
  e. 30% to 40%

Q2. Which of the following diseases has not been linked to cigarette smoking?
  a. carcinoma of the larynx
  b. hypertension

c. abruptio placenta
d. carcinoma of the colon
e. Alzheimer's disease

Q3. Which of the following statements with respect to passive smoking is false?
a. spouses of patients who smoke are not at increased risk of developing carcinoma of the lung
b. sidestream smoke contains more carbon monoxide than mainstream smoke
c. infants of mothers who smoke absorb measurable amounts of their mothers' cigarette smoke
d. children of parents who smoke have an increased prevalence of bronchitis and pneumonia
e. the most common symptom arising from passive smoking is eye irritation

Q4. Of the following factors listed, which is the most important factor in determining the success of a smoking cessation program in an individual?
a. the desire of the patient to quit smoking
b. a pharmacologic agent as a part of the smoking cessation program
c. the inclusion of a behavior modification component to the program
d. physician advice to quit smoking
e. repeated office visits

Q5. Which of the following agents is now the pharmacologic agent of choice for inclusion in a smoking cessation program?
a. clonidine
b. propranolol
c. nicotine-containing chewing gum
d. transdermal nicotine
e. mecamylamine (a nicotine antagonist)

Q6. Which of the following smoking cessation methods results in the highest percentage of both short-term and long-term success?
a. transdermal nicotine
b. a patient education booklet
c. physician counseling and advice
d. a contract for a "quit date"
e. a combination of all of the above

Q7. What is the approximate percentage of patients who relapse following successful cessation of smoking?
a. 10%
b. 50%

c. 75%
d. 85%
e. 99%

Q8. What is the most modifiable risk factor for increased morbidity and mortality in the United States in 1994?
a. hypertension
b. hyperlipidemia
c. cigarette smoking
d. occupational burnout
e. alcohol consumption

Q9. Nicotine replacement is especially important in which group of cigarette-smoking patients?
a. those patients who smoke when work-related stressors become unmanageable
b. those patients who smoke more than 20 cigarettes a day
c. those patients who smoke within 30 minutes of awakening
d. those patients who experience withdrawal symptoms
e. all of the above
f. b, c, and d

Q10. Which of the following statements regarding the economic burden of smoking is (are) true?
a. the economic burden of smoking is placed not only on the individual but also on society
b. in the United States in 1995 the costs related to cigarette smoking (directly and indirectly) exceeded $65 billion
c. smoking has no significant effect on work-related productivity
d. a and b
e. all of the above statements are true

SHORT ANSWER MANAGEMENT PROBLEM
A 41-year-old male comes to you with an expressed desire to quit smoking. He is smoking three packs of cigarettes per day and has done so for the past 20 years. Discuss your use of nicotine replacement (how, for how long, specific instructions) along with other possible pharmacologic interventions in helping this patient achieve his goal of complete smoking cessation.

Although this question asks you specifically to discuss pharmacologic management, it must be emphasized that this is only one component of a multicomponent program.

ANSWERS

A1. d. Of deaths from CHD, 25% are directly attributable to smoking. The incidence of myocardial infarction and death from CHD is 70% higher in cigarette smokers than in nonsmokers. In the United States 18% of all deaths are caused by cigarette smoking.

A2. d. The health consequences of smoking are enormous. The major processes involved include active smoking, passive smoking, addiction, and accelerated aging.

The following disease categories have been directly linked to smoking: cancer, respiratory diseases, cardiovascular diseases, pregnancy and infant health, and other miscellaneous conditions.

The actual diseases involved include the following:

a. Cancer:
1) Carcinoma of the lung
2) Carcinoma of the larynx
3) Carcinoma of the mouth
4) Carcinoma of the pharynx
5) Carcinoma of the stomach
6) Carcinoma of the liver
7) Carcinoma of the pancreas
8) Carcinoma of the bladder
9) Carcinoma of the uterine cervix
10) Carcinoma of the breast
11) Carcinoma of the brain
b. Respiratory diseases:
1) Emphysema
2) Chronic bronchitis
3) Asthma
4) Bacterial pneumonia
5) Tubercular pneumonia
6) Asbestosis
c. Cardiovascular diseases:
1) CAD
2) Hypertension
3) Aortic aneurysm
4) Arterial thrombosis
5) Stroke
6) Carotid artery atherosclerosis
d. Pregnancy and infant health:
1) Intrauterine growth retardation
2) Abortion
3) Fetal and neonatal death
4) Abruptio placenta
5) Bleeding in pregnancy not yet discovered
6) Placenta previa
7) Premature rupture of the membranes
8) Prolonged rupture of the membranes
9) Preterm labor
10) Preeclampsia
11) Sudden infant death syndrome
12) Congenital malformations
13) Low birth weight
14) Frequent respiratory and ear infections in children
15) Higher incidence of mental retardation
e. Other miscellaneous conditions:
1) Peptic ulcer disease
2) Osteoporosis
3) Alzheimer's disease
4) Wrinkling of the skin ("crow's feet" appearance on the face)
5) Impotence

The mechanisms whereby the linkage between smoking and the aforementioned diseases occur are multifactorial and are beyond the scope of this chapter. What is striking, however, is the number of medical disease categories that smoking affects and the number of diseases within each category that smoking affects. Carcinoma of the colon has not been causally associated with cigarette smoking. It should be noted that research is currently being conducted with smoking and associated leukemia, colon cancer, and prostate cancer, and these too may prove to be associated with an increased risk.

A3. a. Tobacco smoke in the environment is derived from either mainstream smoke (exhaled smoke) or sidestream smoke (smoke arising from the burning end of a cigarette). As well, there is an increased prevalence of bronchiolitis, asthma, bronchitis, ear infections, and pneumonia in infants and children whose parents smoke.

The most common symptom arising from exposure to passive smoking is eye irritation. Other significant symptoms include headaches, nasal symptoms, and cough. Exposure to tobacco smoke also precipitates or aggravates allergies.

Spouses of patients who smoke are at increased risk of developing lung cancer and CAD. For lung cancer, the average relative risk is 1.34 compared to persons not exposed to passive smoke. This risk, in comparison, is more than 100 times higher than the estimated effect of 20 years' exposure to asbestos while living or working in asbestos-containing buildings. It is estimated that of the 480,000 smoking-related deaths each year, 53,000 are associated with passive smoking.

A4. a. The most important factor in determining the success of a smoking cessation program is the desire of the individual to quit. If the individual is not interested in quitting, the probability of success is very low. Physician advice to quit, behavior-modification aids, nicotine replacement, and repeated office visits are all important. However, without the will to quit, they will not be effective.

A5. d. The pharmacologic agent of choice for inclusion in a smoking cessation program is transdermal nicotine. Until a transdermal system was developed for the delivery of nicotine, the agent of choice was nicotine-containing chewing gum (Nicorette). Although the gum is still recommended by some physicians, the transdermal nicotine delivery system has both fewer adverse physiologic effects and fewer side effects. The unpleasant side effects that are avoided by prescribing nicotine in a transdermal system rather than in a gum include bad taste, nausea, dyspepsia, and singultus. In addition, there is no unsightly chewing or the inconvenience of the need for frequent administrations.

Clonidine has proven efficacy in the relief of symptoms of opiate and alcohol withdrawal. It has, in some studies, been shown to be superior to placebo in helping patients remain abstinent from smoking for periods up to 1 year. Thus it may still be considered to be a useful adjunct. It has significant side effects, however, and is certainly not routinely recommended.

Mecamylamine is a nicotine receptor antagonist that is analogous to naloxone for the treatment of opiate abuse. Mecamylamine may be useful as a method of smoking cessation in the recalcitrant smoker. It has not been extensively studied in such a population.

Propranolol has been shown to relieve some of the physiological changes associated with alcohol withdrawal–induced anxiety, but it has been shown to be ineffective in smoking cessation and has no effect on reducing subjective satisfaction and extinction of smoking behavior.

The recent use of the antidepressant bupropion (Zyban) has been proven to be effective in the treatment of cigarette smokers. The aim is to stop smoking within 1 to 2 weeks after starting the medication with the duration of treatment between 7 and 12 weeks. This treatment modality helps address both the psychologic and physiologic aspects of smoking addiction. It acts by boosting brain levels of dopamine and norepinephrine, thus mimicking the effects of nicotine.

A6. **e.** A metaanalysis of controlled trials of smoking cessation compared the effectiveness of smoking cessation counseling, self-help booklets, nicotine replacement, and establishing a contract and setting a quitting date. The study found that each modality was effective, but no single modality worked significantly better than the others. When treatment modalities were combined, however, the following results were obtained:

   a. Two treatment modalities were more effective than one.
   b. Three treatment modalities were more effective than two.
   c. Four treatment modalities were more effective than three.

A mnemonic for the smoking cessation protocol that you should employ with patients is BAD NICOTINE:

   B = Education **b**ooklet
   A = **A**dvice, counseling, specific suggestions for patient behavior modification
   D = **D**ate of quitting (establish a contract and a date that is convenient for the patient)
   NICOTINE = Nicotine replacement (transdermal nicotine)

A7. **d.** Arranging follow-up appointments for the patient is extremely important. This, in effect, prepares the patient for the support and surveillance of the physician. At the follow-up visits there is an opportunity to review concerns, review continuing plans, and discuss relapses. This last issue is extremely important because lapses occur in 85% of those who quit. The reaction and counseling of the physician following a lapse is crucial and should be framed in the context of a positive learning experience. One of the key points that needs to be reinforced by the physician is that learning to live without cigarettes is like learning any new skill—you learn from mistakes until your action becomes a new habitual behavior. Most patients take a few trials before they quit completely.

A8. **c.** Cigarette smoking continues to be the most prevalent modifiable risk factor for increased morbidity and mortality in the United States. Not only does the smoker incur medical risks attributable to cigarette smoking, but passive smokers and society also bear the ill effects and the increased economic costs attributable to the smoker's habit.

Hypertension and hyperlipidemia have already been modified to some degree (hypertension more than hyperlipidemia).

Alcohol consumption and abuse is also an important problem and is addressed in Problem 63.

Although this problem is focused on smoking, its risks, and the importance and means to quit, one of the choices in Question 8 offers a short detour to stress and burnout. Occupational stress and burnout might, to some, seem like a lightweight compared to the other choices listed. While that may be true, relatively speaking, the effect that the move to a global economy is having on the workers in our countries should not be underestimated. Although the terms downsizing and rightsizing make good business talk and are reasonable business jargon (as far as anything in business is reasonable in this age), health care professionals may contend that wrongsizing is the more appropriate word, in the sense of what the new economy is doing to employment (or, more correctly, stable employment), relative standard of living, and the family. In health (as defined by the World Health Organization as "not just the absence of disease but the presence of physical, emotional, and social well-being"), one could argue that the effect of this entity on morbidity in North America is underestimated and should always be addressed by primary care physicians when the opportunity arises.

A9. **f.** Nicotine replacement is especially important for the following smokers:
  a. Smokers who smoke more than 20 cigarettes a day
  b. Smokers who smoke within 30 minutes of waking up
  c. Smokers who experience withdrawal symptoms
Smokers who smoke when exposed to extremely stressful work situations should be managed mainly by behavior modification techniques, although bupropion may be a consideration for therapy.

A10. **d.** The individual smoker and society in general incur enormous economic costs as a result of smoking. Health care costs, lost work, and productivity are important and often forgotten hazards of smoking. With the inclusion of the last two factors, the costs associated with cigarette smoking are estimated to exceed $65 billion per year in the United States.

SOLUTION TO THE SHORT ANSWER MANAGEMENT PROBLEM

This patient is one who certainly will potentially benefit (potentially because we are not sure whether he will be successful in quitting altogether and maintain that status) from a pharmacologic component to his smoking cessation program.

The agent of choice, as described earlier, is transdermal nicotine. I will select a specific agent and describe the method in which it could best be used.

Agent: Habitrol

Dosage: 21 mg nicotine per day, 14 mg nicotine per day, 7 mg nicotine per day
  a. Before starting the nicotine replacement, the patient must quit smoking completely (not just cut down). If the patient has been unable to maintain or otherwise reestablish abstinence with the aid of Habitrol after 1 month, then treatment should be discontinued.
  b. Begin with one patch per day of the 21 mg nicotine Habitrol. Instruct the patient to apply one system (patch) daily and have him leave it on the skin for 24 hours.
  c. Continue with the 21 mg nicotine system for at least 4 weeks (the greater the previous amount

per day smoked, the longer you should treat with the transdermal nicotine). The preferred range seems to be from about 8 weeks to about 16 weeks.
  d. Switch after 4 weeks to the 14-mg/day nicotine system. Continue for 4 weeks.
  e. Switch after a total of 8 weeks to the 7-mg/day nicotine system. Continue for at least another 4 weeks.
  f. Discontinue the Habitrol at that time or shortly thereafter. As of the time of writing of this book, clonidine has not been approved by the Food and Drug Administration for use in smoking cessation. You may wish to consider this agent if that status changes or consider discussing the issue with a physician who has expertise in smoking cessation. If clonidine were to be used, the dosage would be between 0.2 mg/day and 0.4 mg/day. Also consider bupropion as an alternate for smoking cessation.
  g. See the patient at least once every 2 weeks while he or she is maintained on Habitrol.
  h. Following cessation of Habitrol, see the patient every 4 weeks to follow up his continued cessation.
  i. For patients using the nicotine patches, start at 14 mg/day for those who have CAD, smoke more than 14 cigarettes a day, or weigh more than 100 pounds.
  j. Patients must stop smoking to prevent nicotine toxicity and the increase risk of a myocardial infarction.

SUMMARY OF PHYSICIAN INTERVENTION IN SMOKING CESSATION

1. Identify all patients in your practice who smoke.

2. Present all the health consequences of smoking.

3. Present the health benefits of smoking cessation.

4. Assess and develop the desire to modify smoking behavior.

5. Develop and formalize a patient-centered plan for change.

6. Establish a quitting date and have the patient sign a contract.

7. Use transdermal nicotine as an adjunct, especially in patients who smoke more than 20 cigarettes a day, who smoke within 30 minutes of awakening, and who experience withdrawal symptoms.

8. Use behavior modification techniques as part of counseling and advice. Have the patient keep a journal of at-risk times for smoking.

9. Consider using all of the following to improve the chance of quitting permanently: obtain smoking-cessation patient education booklets from the American Lung Association or the American Cancer Society and give one to every patient; establish a quit date and a contract; advise and counsel the patient at regular intervals and incorporate behavior modification techniques; and use a transdermal nicotine replacement for 8 to 12 weeks. Consider bupropion.

10. Have the patient consider times at which he or she may relapse (which will happen in 85% of patients); for example, triggers such as having a drink with friends at the end of a stressful week should be avoided for the first few months.

11. Continue surveillance for relapse prevention and plan modifications as needed. Identify alternative behaviors such as chewing gum, projects to use their hands, a walking program.

12. Establish a reward system (i.e., take a trip with all the money you saved from no longer smoking).

SUGGESTED READINGS

Brosky G: Smoking cessation counseling: A practical protocol, *Can J CME* 43-60, 1994.
Jayanthi V et al: Smoking and prevention, *Respir Med* 85:179-183, 1991.
Kottke T et al: Attributes of successful smoking cessation interventions in medical practice, *JAMA* 259:2882, 1988.
Lee E, D'Alonza G: Cigarette smoking, nicotine addiction, and its pharmacologic treatment, *Arch Intern Med* 153:34-48, 1993.
The Smoking Cessation Clinical Practice Guideline: The Agency for Health Care Policy and Resource, *JAMA* 1275:80, 1996.
Tierney LM, Jr, McPhee SJ, Papadakis MA, eds: *Current medical diagnosis and treatment, 2000,* Stamford, Conn, 1999, Appleton & Lange.

PROBLEM · 131

TRENDS IN CANCER EPIDEMIOLOGY

"Hell, Doctor, It Seems Like Everything Causes Cancer! So Why Worry?"

Case 1 ■ A 74-Year-Old Farmer with Abdominal Pain

A 74-year-old grain farmer comes to your office for assessment of abdominal pain of 6 months' duration.

The pain is located in the central abdomen with radiation through to the back. It is a dull, constant pain with no significant aggravating or relieving factors. It is not affected in any way by food. It is rated by the patient as a 5/10 baseline with occasional increases to 7/10. It has been getting worse for the last 2 months.

On examination, the abdomen is scaphoid. There is the suggestion of hepatomegaly, with the liver palpated 2 cm below the right costal margin. No other masses are felt.

Abdominal ultrasound reveals a solid mass lesion in the area of the head of the pancreas measuring 4 cm. There are also two or three small densities (<1 cm) in the liver.

SELECT THE BEST ANSWER TO THE FOLLOWING QUESTIONS

Q1. What is the most likely diagnosis in this patient?
a. benign pseudocyst of the pancreas
b. adenocarcinoma of the pancreas
c. squamous cell carcinoma of the pancreas
d. pancreatitis
e. malignant pseudocyst of the pancreas

Q2. With regard to the diagnosis in this patient, which of the following statements is true?
a. the death rate from this disease has remained constant over the last 20 years in the United States
b. the death rate from this disease has decreased significantly over the last 20 years in the United States
c. the survival rate from this disease has greatly increased over the last 20 years in the United States
d. there are no accurate data on death rates from this disease in the United States over the last 20 years
e. none of the above is true

Q3. With regard to cancer mortality in the United States over the last 20 years, which of the following statements is true?
a. during the last 20 years, the death rate from all cancers has decreased significantly in children
b. during the last 20 years, the death rate from prostate cancer has decreased by 20%
c. during the last 20 years there has been no significant change in the death rate from lung cancers
d. during the last 20 years, the death rate from all cancers has increased by 20%
e. during the last 20 years, the death rate from breast cancers has increased by 15%

Q4. With respect to the reason(s) for the death rates discussed in Question 3, which of the following statements is true?
  a. the major cause of the changing mortality rates is an increase in the American life span
  b. the major cause of the change in mortality rates is likely a result of improved diagnostic techniques
  c. the major cause of the change in mortality rates is better treatments for the majority of cancers
  d. the major cause of the change in mortality rates is increased prevention
  e. there is no one clear answer as to the cause of the change in cancer death rates

Q5. With respect to pesticide application and the patient described in Case 1, which of the following statements is true?
  a. there is no definite link between this disease and environmental carcinogens
  b. there is some suggestion of a link between pesticide application and the disease described in Case 1
  c. there is clear evidence that there is a link between pesticide application and the disease described in Case 1
  d. environmental carcinogens are not thought to play a role in the disease described in the patient in Case 1
  e. there is no evidence either way to suggest a link between environmental carcinogens and the disease described in the patient in Case 1

Q6. With respect to the disease described in the patient in Case 1, which of the following statements is the most accurate?
  a. cigarette smoking has been implicated as a cause of the disease
  b. alcohol abuse has been implicated as a cause of the disease
  c. both cigarette smoking and alcohol abuse have been implicated as causes of the disease
  d. neither cigarette smoking nor alcohol abuse has been implicated as a cause of the disease
  e. nobody really knows for sure

Q7. The death rate from which of the following cancers has increased to the greatest extent over the last 20 years?
  a. breast cancer
  b. lung cancer
  c. pancreatic cancer
  d. stomach cancer
  e. malignant melanoma

Q8. What is the most common cause of cancer death in women in the United States today?
  a. breast cancer
  b. colon cancer
  c. lung cancer
  d. brain cancer
  e. liver cancer

Q9. Which of the following cancers has (have) demonstrated an increased 5-year survival rate in the last 20 years?
  a. cancer of the stomach
  b. cancer of the ovary
  c. cancer of the lung
  d. cancer of the liver
  e. a, b, and d

SHORT ANSWER MANAGEMENT PROBLEM

Discuss the preventive measures your patients may undertake to lower their risk of cancer from all causes.

ANSWERS

A1. **b.** The most likely diagnosis in this patient is adenocarcinoma of the pancreas. With the clinical history of progressive pain, the finding of hepatomegaly (which suggests liver metastases), and the finding of a mass lesion on ultrasound, the diagnosis is almost certainly confirmed.

None of the other choices are reasonable. Pseudocysts do not show solid mass lesions. Squamous cell carcinoma does not occur in the pancreas. The history, physical findings, and ultrasound findings are not compatible with a diagnosis of pancreatitis.

A2. **e.** Over the last 20 years, the survival rate from carcinoma of the pancreas has increased slightly by 2%. Pancreatic cancer remains one of the most lethal forms of cancer with a dismal 5-year survival rate of approximately 3%.

A3. **a.** During the last 20 years, the overall death rate from all cancers has decreased by 40% in children in the United States. The 15- to 44-year-old age group has also experienced a drop, but not as large. Older individuals have experienced an increased mortality from cancer during the last 20 years. Lung and prostate mortality have risen; stomach, cervix, and colorectal cancer mortality have fallen. Lung cancer mortality now surpasses breast cancer mortality in woman. With the advent of mammography, the death rate from breast cancer has decreased.

A4. **e.** There is no clear answer as to reason(s) for the increase in cancer death rates in the last 20 years despite a combination of increased diagnostic ability, better prevention, and treatment. It is not because the population is living longer; rates are age-adjusted. The change may be a result of a variety of environmental factors (increased or new exposures) or host factors (increased susceptibility). For example, there is a definite cancer link to smoking, a possible link to dietary fat, and a definite link to multiple environmental carcinogens, all of which may play a role in this increased death rate.

A5. **a.** There is no suggestion of a link between pesticide application and pancreatic cancer in farmers. The types of cancer that are more common in farmers include Hodgkin's disease, multiple myeloma, leukemia, malignant melanoma, cancer of the lip, and cancer of the prostate.

A6. **a.** Cigarette smoking has been implicated as a cause of pancreatic cancer.

A7. **b.** Death rates from lung cancer, especially among women, have increased significantly over the past 20 years. This is mainly because of a significant increase in smoking among women, which started some four decades ago.

A8. **c.** Lung cancer is now the most common cause of cancer death in American women. This is primarily associated with the significantly increased risk as a result of smoking, as previously discussed.

A9. **e.** Cancers that have shown an increased 5-year survival rate over the past 20 years include cancer of the stomach, ovary, liver, brain, testicles, breast, bladder, thyroid, and prostate. Racial disparities exist however, with African-Americans trailing Caucasian-Americans in almost all areas. The number one cause of cancer deaths for both sexes in the United States is lung cancer.

SOLUTION TO THE SHORT ANSWER MANAGEMENT PROBLEM

The most important preventive measures that your patients may undertake to lower their risk of cancer from all causes are as follows:

  a. Discontinue cigarette, pipe, and cigar smoking.
  b. Decrease the amount of alcohol consumed.
  c. Decrease the amount of dietary fat, especially saturated fat.

  d. Maintain a normal weight (to be accomplished by a decrease in dietary fat, a decrease in overall caloric intake, and an exercise program).
  e. Decrease exposure to environmental carcinogens whenever possible (protect yourself when applying pesticides, herbicides, and related chemicals).
  f. Avoiding sun exposure without a sunscreen with a sun protective factor of at least 15 or greater.
  g. Follow the recommendations of the U.S. Preventive Services Task Force on the Periodic Health Examination.

SUMMARY OF TRENDS IN CANCER EPIDEMIOLOGY

1. The overall mortality rate from all cancers has leveled off in the United States during the past 5 years.

2. Lung cancer is now the number one cause of cancer deaths in both sexes (overtaking breast cancer in women).

3. Although the overall mortality rate from all cancers has leveled off, the overall incidence has increased. This increase in overall incidence has not been completely explained but may result from a combination of better diagnostic techniques, or an increase in smoking (during a life time), alcohol use, and exposure to new pesticides or herbicides and other environmental carcinogens, or a longer life span.

4. Prevention remains the best strategy. The most important preventive measures include discontinuing tobacco smoking, discontinuing or significantly decreasing alcohol consumption, decreasing the amount of dietary fat in the diet, increasing the fiber in the diet, avoiding exposure to the sun without a sunscreen, and avoiding exposure to other environmental carcinogens.

SUGGESTED READING

http://www.nci.nih.gov

PROBLEM·132

CARDIOVASCULAR EPIDEMIOLOGY

"Doctor, I'm African-American, Male, I Smoke, I'm Too Fat, and I Have High Cholesterol and Uncontrollable Hypertension. I Guess I Better Write My Will Now."

Case 1 ■ A 52-Year-Old Male with Coronary Artery Disease Who Has Had Both Coronary Artery Bypass Grafting and Percutaneous Transluminal Angioplasty Procedures Done

A 52-year-old male with a history of coronary artery disease (CAD) treated by a coronary artery bypass grafting procedure following three percutaneous transluminal angioplasty procedures and who currently is on "triple angina therapy" comes to your office for a discussion of his condition and of the implications of his condition for his children. He has recently read that family history is a strong risk factor for CAD.

SELECT THE BEST ANSWER TO THE FOLLOWING QUESTIONS

Q1. During the past 15 years, the death rate from cardiovascular disease in the United States has
   a. increased by 15%
   b. decreased by 15%
   c. decreased by 35%
   d. increased by 10%
   e. remained unchanged

Q2. During the past 15 years, the death rate from CAD in the United States has
   a. increased by 15%
   b. decreased by 40%
   c. decreased by 25%
   d. increased by 20%
   e. remained unchanged

Q3. During the past 15 years, the death rate from stroke in the United States has
   a. decreased by 50%
   b. decreased by 25%
   c. increased by 15%
   d. increased by 25%
   e. remained unchanged

Q4. What has been the major reason for the change in death rate from cardiovascular disease in the United States?
   a. new technology
   b. improved pharmacology
   c. better surgical techniques
   d. risk factor reduction
   e. nobody really knows for sure

Q5. The risk of developing cardiovascular disease in hypertensive patients compared to nonhypertensive patients is
   a. three to four times as high for CAD and seven times as high for stroke
   b. twice as high for CAD and five times as high for stroke
   c. six times as high for CAD and eight times as high for stroke
   d. the same for CAD and twice as high for stroke
   e. the same for CAD and the same for stroke

Q6. Regarding cigarette smoking and the risk of developing CAD, which of the following statements is true?
   a. cigarette smokers have a 70% greater risk of developing CAD than nonsmokers
   b. cigarette smokers have a 50% greater risk of developing CAD than nonsmokers
   c. cigarette smokers have a 25% greater risk of developing CAD than nonsmokers
   d. cigarette smokers have a 10% greater risk of developing CAD than nonsmokers
   e. there is no difference in the risk of developing CAD between smokers and nonsmokers

Q7. Regarding serum cholesterol and the incidence of CAD, which of the following statements is true?
   a. for each 1% reduction in serum cholesterol there is a 6% reduction in the risk of heart disease death
   b. for each 1% reduction in serum cholesterol there is a 4% reduction in the risk of heart disease death
   c. for each 1% reduction in serum cholesterol there is a 2% reduction in the risk of heart disease death
   d. for each 1% reduction in serum cholesterol there is a 1% reduction in the risk of heart disease death
   e. there is no established relationship between serum cholesterol and the risk of heart disease death

Q8. Which of the following statements regarding the influence of race on mortality from CAD, stroke, and diabetes is true?
   a. the death rate in blacks from CAD and stroke is higher than whites; conversely, the death rate from end-stage renal failure secondary to hypertension is higher in whites than in blacks

b. the death rate from CAD and end-stage renal failure caused by hypertension is higher in blacks than in whites

c. the death rate in blacks from diabetes is higher than in whites; conversely, the death rate from stroke is higher in whites than in blacks

d. the death rates in blacks from CAD, stroke, and diabetes is higher than in whites

e. the death rate in whites from CAD, stroke, and diabetes is higher than in blacks

Q9. Regarding the risk of obesity in relation to cardiovascular disease, which of the following statements is (are) true?

a. obesity is a risk factor for hypertension

b. obesity is a risk factor for hypercholesterolemia

c. obesity is a risk factor for diabetes

d. obesity is an independent risk factor for CAD

e. all of the above statements are true

Q10. What is the definition of obesity?

a. a weight 40% above normal weight for height

b. a weight 30% above normal weight for height

c. a weight 20% above normal weight for height

d. a weight 15% above normal weight for height

e. a weight 10% above normal weight for height

Q11. Body mass index (BMI) is defined as which of the following?

a. the weight in pounds divided by the square of the height in meters

b. the weight in kilograms divided by the square of the height in meters

c. the square of the height in meters divided by the weight in pounds

d. the square of the height in meters divided by the weight in kilograms

e. none of the above

Q12. With respect to physical inactivity (sedentary lifestyle) and the risk of cardiovascular disease, which of the following statements is (are) true?

a. sedentary lifestyle is an independent risk factor for cardiovascular disease

b. sedentary lifestyle is associated with an increased death rate from cardiovascular disease

c. sedentary lifestyle may be as strong a risk factor for cardiovascular disease as several other risk factors combined

d. sedentary lifestyle is strongly correlated with obesity

e. all of the above statements are true

Q13. With regard to the level of serum cholesterol in the American population, which of the following statements is true?

a. serum cholesterol levels are increasing in the United States

b. serum cholesterol levels are decreasing in the United States

c. serum cholesterol levels are higher in blacks than in whites

d. serum cholesterol levels are higher in whites than in blacks

e. the "target" serum cholesterol for the U.S. population for the year 2000 is 240 mg%

Q14. What is the estimated percentage of hypertensive Americans whose blood pressure is under good control?

a. 50%

b. 75%

c. 25%

d. 10%

e. 5%

Q15. What is the percentage of total calories consumed as fat by the average American?

a. 10%

b. 20%

c. 25%

d. 30%

e. 36%

SHORT ANSWER MANAGEMENT PROBLEM

A 63-year-old male comes to your office for his periodic health examination. You check his serum cholesterol and find it to be 225 mg%. Describe what you would do at this time considering what you know about standardization of serum cholesterol levels in clinical laboratories in the United States.

ANSWERS

A1. **c.** During the past 15 years, the death rate for cardiovascular disease in the United States has decreased significantly. Overall, for all cardiovascular disease, there has been a 35% decrease in the death rate.

A2. **b.** The death rate from CAD has decreased by 40%.

A3. **a.** The death rate from stroke has decreased by 50%.

A4. **d.** The major reasons for the significant decrease in cardiovascular mortality in the United States are changes in lifestyle and risk factor reduction. Other contributing reasons include new technology, improved pharmacology, better surgical techniques, and more effective medical managements.

A5. **a.** Americans with hypertension have three to four times the risk of developing CAD and as much as seven times the risk of stroke as do those with normal blood pressure.

A6. **a.** Cigarette smoking is a major risk factor for cardiovascular disease. Cigarette smokers are at increased risk for fatal and nonfatal myocardial infarctions and for sudden cardiac death. Smokers have a 70% greater CAD rate, a twofold to fourfold greater incidence of acquiring CAD, and a twofold to fourfold greater risk for sudden death than nonsmokers.

A7. **c.** Elevated serum cholesterol levels are associated with an increased risk of CAD. Epidemiologic work in this area has suggested that for each 1% reduction in serum cholesterol there is an associated 2% reduction in the risk of heart disease death.

A8. **c.** Death rates for heart disease and stroke are higher in whites than in blacks. In 1997 the age-adjusted rate per 100,000 for heart disease was 288 for whites vs. 227 for blacks. The age-adjusted death rates for strokes were 62 for whites and 53 for blacks.

Diabetic death rates, however, were higher for blacks than for whites, being 32 and 22, respectively. Blacks also experience higher homicide and human immunodeficiency virus death rates, but lower suicide rates than do whites.

A9. **e.** Being obese is a risk factor for hypertension, hypercholesterolemia, and diabetes mellitus. It is also an independent risk factor for CAD. Being obese and being physically inactive increase all risks.

A10. **c.** The definition of obesity is a weight 20% that expected for (or defined as normal) for height.

A11. **b.** BMI is defined as the weight of a person in kilograms over the height of the person in meters squared. Tables are available that allow the calculation of BMI to be made easily in the office.

A12. **e.** Physical inactivity, or a sedentary lifestyle, is becoming quickly recognized as a powerful risk factor for cardiovascular disease. It is recognized as an independent risk factor for cardiovascular disease and cardiovascular death. There is some evidence that a vigorous exercise program may, in fact, counteract some or all other risk factors when it comes to both the car-

diovascular death rate and the cardiovascular disease prevalence rate.

Physical inactivity is also associated with being obese, and these two risk factors are additive.

Weight reduction programs are rarely successful in the absence of a reasonable exercise program. Most authorities suggest that to make a significant difference to the cardiovascular system, aerobic exercise must occur three times per week and last at least 30 minutes per session.

A13. **b.** Mean serum cholesterol levels in the United States are declining. Values for men and women from 1960 to 1962 averaged 217 mg% and 233 mg%, respectively. By 1980 the same mean serum cholesterol levels were 211 mg% and 215 mg%, respectively. By the year 2000 the U.S. Department of Health and Human Services has targeted a value of no more than 200 mg% for both men and women in the United States. Blacks and whites have similar serum cholesterol values.

A14. **c.** The percentage of hypertensive Americans whose blood pressure is under good control is estimated to be no more than 25%. One of the major targets for the years to come is to increase that figure to at least 50%. The U.S. Department of Health and Human Services has set that 50% target for the year 2000.

A15. **e.** At the present time, the average percentage of calories derived from fat in the typical American's diet is 36%. Of this 36%, 13% is saturated fat. The American Heart Association has set the upper limit of fat intake calories at 30% and the upper limit of saturated fat intake calories at 10%.

A significant reduction in the intake of total fat and saturated fat will be necessary if the 200 mg% of total serum cholesterol is to be met by the year 2000.

SOLUTION TO THE SHORT ANSWER MANAGEMENT PROBLEM

The College of American Pathologists has determined that no more than 53% of American clinical laboratories have established an accuracy standard of ±5% for total serum cholesterol. Thus one reading of a serum cholesterol that is high is certainly not enough to act on. First, the serum cholesterol should be repeated. If at all possible, inquiries should be made that will allow you to determine whether or not the laboratory to which you are sending your serum cholesterol has established the ±5% accuracy standard.

If, in this patient, the total serum cholesterol level on repeat is found to be high, a fractionation is indicated. To rely on and base your judgment and advice to a patient on a single reading of the total serum cholesterol level is unwise. You may, in fact, be giving the patient misinformation that could contribute to cardiac neurosis or other serious problems. Make sure you know what the true value of serum cholesterol is before you share this information with the patient.

SUMMARY OF IMPORTANT CONCEPTS IN CARDIOVASCULAR EPIDEMIOLOGY

1. Unlike the mortality from cancer, there has been a significant decrease in cardiovascular mortality in the United States during the last 15 years.

2. Death rates from CAD and stroke, the two major causes of cardiovascular mortality, are down by 40% and 50%, respectively, in the last 15 years.

3. The major reasons for the decrease in cardiovascular mortality rates in the United States are lifestyle modification and risk factor reduction.

4. Lifestyle modification, particularly weight loss and physical activity, are particularly important in efforts to further reduce cardiovascular mortality.

5. Hypertension, hypercholesterolemia, cigarette smoking, obesity, and physical inactivity are all independent risk factors for cardiovascular disease.

6. A vigorous exercise program may be enough to counteract several other cardiovascular risk factors and prevent cardiovascular morbidity and mortality.

7. Death rates from diabetes (a cardiovascular disease risk factor) is significantly higher in blacks than in whites.

8. Cigarette smoking is estimated to account for 40% of deaths from CAD in Americans under the age of 65.

9. The U.S. Department of Health and Human Services has set a number of objectives, or targets, for the year 2010. Many of these targets include a further decrease in modifiable risk factors for cardiovascular disease.

10. The continuing education of the American population with respect to what they can do themselves to decrease risk from cardiovascular disease remains our number-one priority. Aggressive intervention with risk factors through lifestyle modification, education, and counseling will remain one of the greatest and most rewarding challenges for family physicians in the next century.

SUGGESTED READINGS

Hoxert DL et al: Deaths: Final data for 1997, *Natl Vit Stat Rep* 47:19, 1999.

Smith SC: The challenge of risk reduction therapy for cardiovascular disease, *Am Fam Physician* 55:491-498, 1997.

U.S. Department of Health and Human Services: *Heart disease and stroke: The healthy people 2000.* National Health Promotion and Disease Prevention Objectives, Boston, 1992, Jones & Bartlett. *http://www.cdc.gov.*

PROBLEM·133

USE AND ABUSE OF LABORATORY MEDICINE FOR ROUTINE SCREENING

Having Too Much Laboratory Data May Be Perilous.

Case 1 ■ A 45-Year-Old Male Who Requests a Complete Laboratory Workup

A 45-year-old "high-powered executive" (self-described) comes to your office for "the old once-over." He further tells you that he would like you to perform "every test known to man." From the history and physical examination of this gentleman, you construct the following problem list:

1. Obesity (body mass index 36)
2. Nicotine addiction (two packs of cigarettes per day)
3. Workaholic: married to his work
4. Essential hypertension (last blood pressure was 175/95 mm Hg)
5. Sedentary lifestyle
6. History of gouty arthritis

You get the feeling that one day soon you will be testing his "cardiac enzymes" in a coronary care unit. You recall some of the basic principles regarding routine laboratory screening procedures—their usefulness, cost-benefit ratio, and positive predictive value.

SELECT THE BEST ANSWER TO THE FOLLOWING QUESTIONS

Q1. On the basis of the information provided, what would you do next?
   a. order a complete battery of investigations to get rid of the patient
   b. order selected investigations
   c. tell the patient that you do not specialize in his type of problems and give him the name of one of your physician friends down the street

d. discuss the advantages and disadvantages of screening for various conditions with the patient
e. none of the above

Case 2 ■ A 53-Year-Old Male with a Slightly Elevated Serum Bilirubin Value

A 53-year-old male comes to your office for his annual checkup. The following tests were performed: complete blood count (CBC), electrolytes, blood urea nitrogen (BUN)/creatinine, liver enzymes, proteins and fractionation of same, cholesterol (fractionated) and triglycerides, prostate-specific antigen (PSA), blood sugar, serum calcium, serum phosphate, and serum uric acid.

The patient finds out that one of his liver function tests (serum bilirubin) is slightly elevated and starts to worry about it. His physician then orders an abdominal ultrasound, a computed tomography scan of the abdomen, a repeat liver enzymes test, and a consultation with a gastroenterologist. As the patient is waiting for these tests to be performed and waiting to see the gastroenterologist, he becomes more and more anxious. When he finally sees the specialist, the consultant states, "Well, I can't really find anything wrong. It's probably of no consequence, but we probably should check it every 6 months."

Q2. Which of the following statements is (are) true?
a. because of the number of laboratory tests ordered, there was approximately a 40% chance that a positive test result (if found) would be a false-positive result rather than a true-positive result
b. the patient who was previously healthy has now lost that status because of anxiety-creating psychologic distress
c. even after the testing and consultations are complete, the patient may still be worried (that is, his health is negatively affected) because of the rather inconclusive remarks by the consultant
d. the testing and consultation process was very costly in terms of patient health
e. all of the above statements are true

Q3. The percentage of routine laboratory tests performed in asymptomatic persons that result in a change in management strategy is estimated to be which of the following?
a. 0.3%
b. 3.0%
c. 13.0%

d. 33.3%
e. 63.3%

Q4. The measure of the ability of a test to discriminate between normal and diseased states is known as which of the following?
a. the sensitivity of the test
b. the specificity of the test
c. the likelihood ratio (LR) of the test
d. the positive predictive value of the test
e. the negative predictive value of the test

Q5. Which of the following is (are) justifiable reasons for ordering a laboratory or radiologic investigation?
a. screening
b. confirmation of clinical findings
c. disease treatment and follow-up
d. patient and doctor reassurance
e. all of the above

Q6. Which of the following questions is (are) important to ask before implementing a screening program for a particular disorder?
a. does the current burden of suffering justify a screening program?
b. has the program's effectiveness been demonstrated in a clinical trial?
c. can the health care system cope with the screening program?
d. will people who screen positive accept advice and intervention for the condition?
e. all of the above are important

Q7. Which of the following is (are) possible disadvantages of some screening laboratory tests?
a. the direct costs of the tests
b. the direct costs of physician visits at the time of screening or to discuss results
c. the danger of the costs of being labeled as having a disease as a result of a test
d. the direct costs of any consultant's fees when a patient is referred to him or her for evaluation following a false positive test
e. all of the above

Q8. In one large Canadian city, there are 45 walk-in clinics. The walk-in clinic phenomenon has spread through many areas of North America. Walk-in clinics do not maintain, in many situations, the fundamental principles of family medicine. Which of the following best explains the popularity of treatment at a walk-in clinic?
a. convenient care
b. comprehensive care

c. compassionate care
d. continuous care
e. coordinated care

Q9. Which of the following appears to reflect the major focus of care at a walk-in clinic?
   a. primary prevention
   b. secondary prevention
   c. tertiary prevention
   d. acute, episodic care
   e. comprehensive preventive care

Cost-effectiveness in the delivery of medical care services is becoming a crucial issue for health care providers, health care consumers, and health care funders (government and private insurance plans, in particular).

Q10. Which of the following statements regarding routine laboratory testing in asymptomatic individuals and the standard measure of quality of care, (namely quality of adjusted life years [QALY]) best describe(s) the contribution of diagnostic laboratory services in this situation?
   a. routine laboratory testing in asymptomatic patients improves QALY
   b. routine laboratory testing in asymptomatic patients decreases QALY
   c. in a randomized asymptomatic population where 50% receive routine testing and 50% did not, there was no difference in QALY
   d. in the same randomized asymptomatic population, a larger proportion of the laboratory screened group ended up in a hospital
   e. c and d

One of the reasons for significant confusion among physicians regarding routine laboratory test ordering is that there are so many different and contradictory recommendations from many different societies and organizations.

A case in point is screening of the male population over the age of 40 with PSA for the detection of cancer of the prostate. The recommendations of various groups on this issue are as follows:
   1. The U. S. Preventive Services Task Force: PSA is not recommended for routine screening.
   2. The Canadian Task Force on the periodic health examination: PSA is not recommended for routine screening.
   3. The United States National Cancer Institute: there is insufficient evidence to recommend PSA for routine screening.
   4. A certain expert American association: annual PSA determination should be performed on all men over the age of 50 years.

You have just started out in practice and are trying to establish your guidelines and protocols for practicing medicine.

Q11. Keeping the above in mind, which of the following would you recommend for an asymptomatic 55-year-old male at the time of his periodic health examination?
   a. follow the recommendation of the certain expert American association; they are the experts, and they should know
   b. follow the recommendation of the United States National Cancer Institute; it gives you a little more leeway in what you order in this patient
   c. follow the recommendations of the U.S. Preventive Services Task Force and The Canadian Task Force on the Periodic Health Examination
   d. flip a coin: heads—determine the level of PSA; tails—do not determine the level of PSA
   e. forget the whole thing; this is far too complicated

Q12. *Screening* is defined as which of the following?
   a. any health service attempt to measure a variable that may be linked to primary prevention of a disorder
   b. any health service attempt to measure a variable that may be linked to secondary prevention of a disorder
   c. any health service attempt to measure a variable that may be linked to tertiary prevention of a disorder
   d. all of the above
   e. none of the above

Q13. *Case finding* is defined as which of the following?
   a. the presumptive identification of an unrecognized disease or defect by the application of tests, examinations, or other procedures in patients who happen to be in your clinical setting
   b. the presumptive identification of an unrecognized disease or defect by the application of tests, examinations, or other procedures in a non–health care setting
   c. the presumptive identification of an unrecognized disease or defect by use of a screening test among patients who are consulting the physician for unrelated symptoms
   d. a or b
   e. a and b

Q14. Which of the following routine laboratory tests is (are) indicated in an asymptomatic 54-year-old male who comes to your office for a periodic health examination?
a. routine urinalysis
b. routine CBC
c. serum PSA
d. nonfasting cholesterol
e. a, b, and d

Q15. Which of the following routine laboratory tests is indicated in the periodic health examination of an asymptomatic 23-year-old female?
a. serum BUN
b. serum creatinine
c. serum glucose
d. serum uric acid
e. none of the above

Q16. For purposes of laboratory medicine and in recognition of the "zealous overtesting syndrome" that many physicians seem to have acquired, a *normal patient* is defined as which of the following?
a. a patient who has had "the works"
b. a patient who has had all of the laboratory tests performed that he or she has specifically requested
c. a patient who has not been sufficiently investigated
d. a patient who has only had the absolute minimum number of tests performed
e. it all depends

SHORT ANSWER MANAGEMENT PROBLEM
As a primary care physician, you make extensive use of laboratory services. Discuss the difference between *defensive medicine* and *defensible medicine*.

ANSWERS

A1. **d.** Routine laboratory testing and the costs associated with same are increasing at an alarming rate. Although one individual test is not expensive, when taken together laboratory tests are responsible for an ever-increasing percentage of the total health care budget.

There is no evidence that physicians' increased use of laboratory testing has improved the care of their patients. There is also no evidence to suggest an increase in QALY, a measurement that at present is the "gold standard" for macro cost-effectiveness. The concepts of appropriate use of the laboratory at all levels of care must be introduced and emphasized to patients.

A2. **e.** Routine laboratory testing in asymptomatic patients rarely has anything to do with either quality of care or clinical practice guidelines. The most commonly cited reason for routine laboratory testing being performed on patients by their physicians is simply "because we have always done it."

Physicians are extremely concerned about "missing something" in their patients and thus tend to overinvestigate when there is no real reason for doing so. Many patients request or demand testing and will not be satisfied unless it is performed. What these patients seek is an absolute or objective form of reassurance that they wrongly believe testing provides. The physician's responsibility is to educate themselves and their patients about the reliability, validity, predictive value, and proper place of testing in clinical decision making. Concepts relating to sensitivity, specificity, positive predictive value, and negative predictive value are detailed in Problem 129.

A3. **a.** The percentage of routine laboratory tests performed in asymptomatic patients that result in a change in management strategy is estimated to be between 0.3% and 0.5%. Thus 99.5% to 99.7% of routine laboratory tests are a complete waste of both time and money and may (as just illustrated) actually produce disease.

A4. **c.** The LR is a measure of the ability of a test to discriminate between a normal and a diseased state. The LR ratio is the likelihood of finding a positive test result in a person with, rather than in a person without, the disease. The higher the LR, the more likely is the case that the disease is present if the test result is positive.

A5. **e.** Screening for disease, case-finding for disease, confirmation of clinical findings, and patient and doctor reassurance are all valid reasons for ordering a laboratory or radiologic investigation, to some extent. However, the last reason (patient and physician reassurance) must only be taken so far. For example, if you believe that, by not ordering the test, the patient will suffer from significant anxiety and worry and the request is reasonable, you may choose to order the test. A good example of this would be a serologic test for hepatitis B in an unimmunized asymptomatic man who had unprotected intercourse with at least eight different partners in a 2-year period. On the other hand, limitations of the test must be explained regarding recent exposures, and patient education and immunization are more important than any reassurance a test may bring.

A6. **e.** When trying to decide whether a screening program does more harm than good, you should consider asking the following questions:

a. Has the program's effectiveness been demonstrated in a clinical trial? Was this trial double-blind?

b. Are there effective treatments or effective preventive measures for the disorder?

c. Does the current burden of suffering warrant screening?

d. Is there a good screening test available?

e. Can the health care system cope with (afford in terms of financial and nonfinancial resources) the screening program?

f. Will individuals who screen positive accept advice and intervention for the condition?

If you decide to perform a screening test, the following criteria must also be met:

a. The condition must have a significant effect on the quality or quantity of life in the population.

b. Treatment for the condition must be available.

c. The condition should have an asymptomatic period during which detection and treatment significantly reduce morbidity and mortality.

d. Treatment in the asymptomatic period should result in an outcome that is superior to delaying treatment until symptoms occur.

e. Tests to detect the condition in the asymptomatic period must be readily available and affordable.

f. Tests to detect the condition in the asymptomatic period must be acceptable to patients.

g. There must be a high enough prevalence of the condition to justify screening.

A7. **e.** There are many possible direct and indirect costs to the performance of laboratory tests for screening purposes:

a. Direct costs of laboratory tests:

1) The direct cost of the laboratory test as determined by the laboratory charges

2) The direct cost of the physician's visit at which time the test is ordered or discussed

3) The direct cost of any repeat laboratory test if an abnormal result is obtained

4) The direct cost of additional laboratory and radiologic tests that are ordered because of the presence of one false-positive test result

5) The direct cost of a referral to a consultant in the area of concern

6) The direct cost of repeat and additional laboratory and radiologic tests that are ordered by the consultant

7) The direct cost of the repeat office visit to either the consultant or the family physician following the completion of consultant-ordered tests

b. Indirect costs of laboratory tests:

1) The patient stress and anxiety caused by an abnormality found on routine laboratory testing

2) The patient stress and anxiety of waiting to complete the diagnostic testing and consultations

3) The patient's family stress and anxiety caused by the thought of what the diagnosis could be

4) The lost time from productive employment caused by physician appointments and waiting in physicians' offices

5) The possible inability to obtain life insurance or disability insurance following one abnormal and possibly erroneous result

A8. **a.**

A9. **d.** The walk-in clinic phenomenon has spread across North America like an epidemic. Although it is established much more so in Canada, it is growing in the United States as well.

The reason that patients seem to seek treatment for health-related conditions in a walk-in clinic is, in most cases, convenience. The walk-in clinic phenomenon is geared, from a physician's perspective, to acute, episodic care rather than preventive medical care. Generally speaking, a walk-in clinic does not offer all the five "C" principles of family medicine:

a. Continuous care

b. Comprehensive care

c. Coordinated care

d. Compassionate care

e. Competent care

A10. **e.** Routine laboratory screening is, for all intents and purposes, completely devoid of any benefits to QALY. It does, however, result in a significantly higher percentage of people who end up in community and secondary care hospitals.

A11. **c.** The most solid, most scientific sources of evidence regarding PSA screening are provided by the U.S. Preventive Services Task Force and the Canadian Task Force on the Periodic Health Examination. It is rare, as well, that these two important task forces disagree on any recommendation. Of course, always discuss conflicting recommendations with patients, and seek your patients input into decision making.

A12. **e.**

A13. **c.** The distinction between screening, on the one hand, and case finding, on the other, is:
   a. *Screening* is defined as the presumptive identification of tests, examinations, or other procedures that can be applied to a population. Screening tests sort out apparently well persons who have a disease from those who probably do not. A screening test is not intended to be diagnostic. Persons with positive or suspicious findings must be referred to their physician for diagnosis and treatment.
   b. *Case finding* is defined as the identification by testing following the clinician's search for disease with screening tests among patients who are consulting them for unrelated reasons.
   The distinction between screening and case finding is subtle.

A14. **d.** The only test that is indicated from those listed is the nonfasting cholesterol in a middle-aged male. This recommendation is made by the U.S. Preventive Services Task Force and the Canadian Task Force on the Periodic Health Examination.

A15. **e.** Serum creatinine, BUN, serum glucose, or serum uric acid analyses are not indicated in the periodic health examination of an asymptomatic 23-year-old female.

A16. **c.** Although somewhat tongue-in-cheek, it was suggested by the scientific editor of a prominent North American family medicine journal that "a normal patient is defined as someone who has not been sufficiently investigated."

The point is that the zealous overtesting syndrome is a serious and costly problem. The major problem appears to be that physicians are not aware of the epidemiologic implications of overtesting. Epidemiologic principles will confirm that if 20 laboratory tests are done, there is a high probability that at least one of those will be abnormal and that will most likely be a false positive (99%). What happens from there, of course, really amounts to a wild goose chase. The goose is never caught, the patient (who was previously well) is now unhealthy because of worry caused by the condition, and the physician is frustrated (in not being able to diagnose something that is not there).

This could all be avoided if every time you ordered a laboratory test you asked yourself two simple questions:
   a. "Why am I doing this test?"
   b. "Is there a reasonable chance that the result of this test may change my patient management?"

If the answer to the first question is valid and able to be substantiated by scientific evidence and the answer to the second question is yes, perform the test. If not, do not perform the test.

SOLUTION TO THE SHORT ANSWER MANAGEMENT PROBLEM

The major difference between defensive medicine and defensible medicine is as follows:
   a. *Defensive medicine:* a physician who practices defensive medicine practices in a manner in which he or she is afraid of possible litigation and thus orders every possible test (to avoid missing something, however esoteric). The problems with defensive medicine are as follows:
      1) It does not offer you the protection you think it does.
      2) It results in a pathway of decision making that has really nothing to do with hypothetic deductive or inductive reasoning. Rather, it is really a blind shot in the dark with a tremendously big gun.
      3) Because of all of the false-positive test results that are generated, you end up spending most of your life chasing geese that you will never catch.
      4) It is a tremendously expensive and wasteful process.
   b. *Defensible medicine:* a physician who practices defensible medicine practices medicine that is based on a sound approach to clinical reasoning and an inherent knowledge of the following concepts:
      1) Sensitivity
      2) Specificity
      3) Negative predictive value
      4) Positive predictive value
      5) Prevalence
   Each decision that the physician makes should be a well-thought out, reasoned decision that could, with the help of a local epidemiologist, be defended from the point of optimal patient outcome.
   The advantages of defensible medicine are as follows:
   a. Improved quality of care
   b. Improved physician and ultimately patient satisfaction (although the latter may be somewhat more difficult to attain)
   c. A sense of being in the "innovative group" of physicians who feel confident enough to believe in themselves and in their clinical diagnosis and clinical management

SUMMARY OF USE AND ABUSE OF LABORATORY MEDICINE FOR ROUTINE SCREENING OF ASYMPTOMATIC PATIENTS

1. Estimate of abuse of laboratory medicine:
   a. Conservative estimate of abuse: at least 50% of all laboratory tests performed in a primary care setting are unnecessary and cost-ineffective.
   b. Estimates suggest that only 0.3% to 0.5% of all laboratory tests make any difference to the patient or have any chance of changing the patient's management.

2. Appropriate use of the laboratory:
   a. Must follow the criteria described in Answer 6
   b. Key questions: the following two questions must be answered in the affirmative or with a specific answer:
      1) "Why am I doing this test?"
      2) "Is there reasonable chance that the result of this test will change my patient's management?"

3. Laboratory medicine and epidemiology:
   a. Screening versus case finding:
      1) Screening: Testing a non-self−identified population
      2) Case finding: Testing a self-identified population in a health care setting
   b. Major epidemiologic concepts:
      1) Prevalence: The lower the prevalence in the population in question, the lower the positive predictive value and the higher the number of false positives
      2) Positive predictive value: The percentage of all positive test results that are actually true positives

4. Guidelines to follow (task force recommendations): The best guidelines to follow with respect to screening and case finding for all disorders are contained in the following two task force recommendations:
   a. The U.S. Preventive Services Task Force
   b. The Canadian Task Force on the Periodic Health Examination

5. The dangers of inadequate knowledge of the epidemiologic principles of effective laboratory testing:
   a. The wild goose chase
   b. The definition of a normal patient as a patient who has not been sufficiently investigated
   c. The complete wasting of resources in an already difficult-to-manage (costwise) health care system
   d. The creation of disease in patients who were previously well before their physician visit. In one controlled study of routine screening versus non-

routine screening, the only difference in the two populations was the excessive hospitalizations in the screened group. There was no effect on QALY (quality of adjusted life years).

SUGGESTED READINGS

Feldman W: On ordering tests, *Ann R Coll Phys Surg Can* 26(5):269-270, 1993.

Guide to Clinical Preventive Services: *Report of the U.S. Preventive Services Task Force*, ed 2, Baltimore, 1996, Williams & Wilkins.

PROBLEM · 134

HUMAN IMMUNODEFICIENCY VIRUS AND ACQUIRED IMMUNODEFICIENCY SYNDROME

"Now with the Discovery of These New Drugs I Can Have Sex with No Worries, Right?"

Case 1 ▪ A 24-Year-Old Male with a Nonproductive Cough

A 24-year-old male comes to your office with a 2-month history of a dry, nonproductive cough accompanied by shortness of breath. He has felt tired and has had intermittent fevers for the past 6 weeks.

On physical examination, the patient appears pale. He has significant cervical, axillary, and inguinal lymphadenopathy. Examination of the respiratory system reveals rales bilaterally. His respiratory rate is 32 per minute.

You suspect human immunodeficiency virus (HIV) infection and question him carefully. He states that he is bisexual. He has a wife and one child but also has two other regular male partners.

His chest x-ray reveals a significant bilateral infiltrate. His HIV serology comes back positive.

SELECT THE BEST ANSWER TO THE FOLLOWING QUESTIONS

Q1. What is the most likely diagnosis in this patient?
   a. infectious mononucleosis
   b. acquired immunodeficiency syndrome (AIDS)
   c. community-acquired pneumonia
   d. hepatitis B prodromal syndrome
   e. none of the above

Q2. What is the most likely pulmonary diagnostic possibility based on the limited information provided?
   a. viral pneumonia
   b. streptococcal pneumonia
   c. *Klebsiella* pneumonia

d. *Mycoplasma* pneumonia

e. PCP

Q3. Based on a correct diagnosis in Question 2, what is the treatment of choice for prevention of this patient's respiratory tract infection?

a. dapsone

b. ampicillin

c. trimethoprim-sulfamethoxazole

d. atovaquone

e. none of the above

Q4. Which of the following is not a common life-threatening opportunistic infection in patients with AIDS?

a. PCP

b. *Toxoplasma gondii* central nervous system (CNS) infection

c. *Cryptosporidium* gastroenteritis

d. *Mycobacterium avium* complex

e. none of the above

Q5. What is the most common malignancy associated with the condition described in Case 1?

a. Kaposi's sarcoma

b. non-Hodgkin's lymphoma

c. primary lymphoma of the brain

d. acute lymphoblastic leukemia

e. Hodgkin's disease

Case 2 ■ A 32-Year-Old African-American Female with Fever, Lymphadenopathy, a Rash, and Pharyngitis

A 32-year-old African-American female comes to your office with a fever, lymphadenopathy, a rash, and pharyngitis. You have reasons to suspect that this patient has acute retroviral syndrome.

Q6. Which of the following signs and symptoms occur(s) with a frequency of greater than 50% in this syndrome?

a. diarrhea

b. myalgia or arthralgia

c. oral thrush

d. facial palsy

e. a and b

Q7. The rash associated with the condition described in Case 2 is best described as which of the following?

a. linear streaks

b. bullae

c. confluent plaques

d. erythematous macular papular lesions

e. none of the above

Case 3 ■ A 31-Year-Old Patient with Full-Blown AIDS

A 31-year-old patient comes to your office with A 10-day history of severe dysphagia. The dysphagia has been getting progressively worse, and the patient's oral intake is limited to liquids.

Q8. Based on the history, what is the most likely cause of this patient's dysphagia?

a. herpes simplex esophagitis

b. Kaposi's sarcoma of the esophagus

c. esophageal candidiasis

d. *P. carinii* esophagitis

e. none of the above

Q9. What is the most common cause of sight-threatening infectious disease in patients with AIDS?

a. cytomegalovirus

b. herpes simplex

c. cryptococcosis

d. toxoplasmosis

e. histoplasmosis

Q10. Reasons to perform plasma HIV-RNA testing include all of the following except:

a. to establish diagnosis

b. to help decide when to begin antiviral therapy

c. to assess drug efficacy

d. to help decide whether to change therapy

e. to assess a baseline viral load

Case 4 ■ A 28-Year-Old Male Who Recently Tested HIV Positive

A 28-year-old male comes to your office. He has recently tested HIV positive but is asymptomatic. He wishes to discuss the pros and cons of early initiation of antiretroviral therapy with you. His CD4 T cell count is less than 500/mm^3, and his plasma HIV RNA is less than 10,000.

Q11. You tell him possible potential benefits of early initiation of therapy include all but which of the following:

a. delayed progression to AIDS

b. control of viral replication and mutation

c. decreased selection of resistant virus
d. potential maintenance of a normal immune system
e. extended duration of current antiviral therapies

Q12. You also counsel the patient in Case 4 that the potential risks of early initiation of antiviral therapy include all but which of the following:
a. quality of life reductions from adverse drug effects
b. earlier development of drug resistance
c. unknown long-term drug toxicities
d. unknown duration of effectiveness of current therapies
e. suppression of natural immune system response to infection

Q13. The antiviral regimen that is recommended for treatment of established HIV infection under most circumstances is:
a. monotherapy in non-pregnant females
b. two nucleoside reverse transcriptase inhibitors (NRTIs) and a protease inhibitor (PI)
c. two NRTIs
d. two nonnucleoside reverse transcriptase inhibitors (NNRTIs)
e. two NRTIs and Saquinavir-HCG

Q14. Which of the following is (are) common side effects of zidovudine (ZDV)?
a. nausea
b. headache
c. dyspepsia
d. myalgias and myositis
e. all of the above

Q15. Which of the following classes of drugs is (are) generally contraindicated in patients on antiviral medication?
a. HMG coenzyme reductase inhibitors
b. sulfa antimicrobials
c. oral antihistamines
d. ergot alkaloids
e. a, c, and d

Q16. Neurologic manifestations of AIDS include which of the following?
a. peripheral neuropathy
b. meningitis
c. encephalitis
d. cognitive impairment
e. all of the above

Q17. In the transmission of AIDS from mother to newborn, which of the following statements is (are) true?
a. the baby may test negative and continue to test negative throughout its life
b. only 20% to 30% of babies born to HIV-positive mothers seroconvert to an HIV-positive state
c. HIV infection in infants and children has a better prognosis than HIV infection in adults
d. all of the above statements are true
e. none of the above statements is true

Q18. What is the test most frequently used to screen for HIV infection?
a. CD4 T-cell count
b. plasma HIV-RNA
c. enzyme-linked immunosorbent assay (ELISA) test
d. Western blot test
e. none of the above

Q19. A 39-year-old male tests positive for HIV infection during a routine insurance medical examination. What should be your next step in testing?
a. do nothing
b. perform ELISA testing for HIV
c. perform a Western blot test for HIV
d. perform a p-24 antigen level for HIV
e. perform a CD4 T-cell count

Q20. Which of the following patient groups are considered at potentially higher risk for exposure to the HIV virus?
a. male homosexuals engaging in unprotected intercourse
b. intravenous drug users sharing needles
c. heterosexual females with multiple male sexual partners using nonbarrier protection
d. a and b only
e. all of the above

SHORT ANSWER MANAGEMENT PROBLEM
Discuss the general principles of HIV counseling and testing services in terms of the general goals and objectives and the important aspects of counseling patients before HIV testing.

ANSWERS

A1. **b.** This patient has AIDS. Although it remains speculation at this point, the most likely cause of the "bilateral infiltrates" is *Pneumocystis carinii* pneumonia

(PCP), an AIDS-defining illness. None of the other entities fully explain the presenting picture.

A2. **e.** As just mentioned, *Pneumocystis carinii* is the most likely cause of this patient's symptoms based on the limited diagnostic information provided.

The most characteristic symptoms of PCP are a dry cough, dyspnea, fever, and night sweats. The most characteristic signs are increased respiratory rate, acute shortness of breath at rest, rales or rhonchi heard in both lung fields, and a general look of ill health.

Diagnostically, apart from a chest x-ray, which reveals bilateral diffuse interstitial infiltrates or airspace infiltrates, a PO_2 and PCO_2 saturation level should also be done. Optional investigations, depending on the patient, include a transbronchial biopsy and a computed tomography scan of the chest.

A3. **c.** The drug of choice for prevention of PCP is trimethoprim-sulfamethoxazole. Alternatives include (1) dapsone, pyrimethamine, and leucovorin; (2) pentamidine; or (3) atovaquone. The latter is extremely expensive. Delivery issues abound. Check the Centers for Disease Control and Prevention (CDC) web site referenced at the end of this problem for the latest recommendations.

A4. **e.** All the conditions listed are common life-threatening opportunistic infections in patients with AIDS.

A5. **a.** The most common malignancy associated with patients with AIDS is Kaposi's sarcoma. The characteristics of Kaposi's sarcoma are reddish/purplish skin lesions anywhere, and complications including gastrointestinal obstruction causing nausea and vomiting, dyspnea from intrapulmonary lesions, or lymphatic system lesions causing lymphedema and swelling of the extremities.

The second most common malignancy is lymphoma (usually non-Hodgkin's). The non-Hodgkin's lymphoma may occur as a primary tumor in the CNS or as a primary non-CNS tumor (frequently beginning in the gut).

A6. **b.** The most common signs and symptoms that occur with a frequency of more than 50% in acute retroviral syndrome are fever (96%), lymphadenopathy (74%), pharyngitis (70%), rash (70%), and myalgia and arthralgia (54%). Almost any other symptoms and signs are possible, but they occur at a much lower rate.

A7. **d.** The rash is typically distributed on the face and trunk and sometimes is on the extremities including the palms and the soles. Mucocutaneous ulceration can also occur involving the mouth, esophagus, and genitals.

A8. **c.** This patient, on the basis of the history alone, has esophageal candidiasis. This is a common opportunistic infection that often progresses from the pharynx to the esophagus. Although thrush that is limited to the pharyngeal area is well treated with a relatively simple remedy such as nystatin or clotrimazole, esophageal candidiasis should be treated aggressively. See Suggested Readings at the end of this problem for current guidelines. Patients with esophageal candidiasis should be considered for maintenance therapy because of the significant risk of recurrence.

A9. **a.** The major infectious disease that produces loss of sight in patients with AIDS is cytomegalovirus. Symptoms include blurring of vision or altered vision. Sight can, however, be lost quickly with this disease.

A10. **a.** Indications for plasma HIV-RNA testing include all of those listed except to establish a diagnosis. For this, an HIV antibody test is preferred. However, in the face of a syndrome consistent with acute HIV infection, the HIV-RNA viral load may be used to confirm the diagnosis if the HIV antibody test is negative or indeterminant.

A11. **e.** Extended duration of antiviral therapies is a doubtful benefit. While all the others listed are potential benefits, many of these benefits need to be proven by further research.

A12. **e.** Similarly, many of the potential risks need further study. However, a careful risk benefit discussion should take place with all patients in whom early antiviral therapy is contemplated. Such discussion builds trust and keeps the patient informed of the realities of treatment.

A13. **b.** Current evidence suggests that combination therapy with different classes of agents is best in most circumstances. Because recommendations change quickly, please consult the Selected Readings listed at the end of this problem, especially the CDC web site which is updated frequently. Monotherapy is contraindicated in virtually all instances.

A14. **e.** ZDV has both early and late side effects. The early side effects of ZDV are frequent but are usually limited to the first 12 weeks of therapy. They include headache, nausea, and dyspepsia. The late side effects (which occur in 5% of patients on ZDV, 600 mg/day) include hepatic dysfunction, bone marrow suppression, neutropenia, and myositis and myopathy.

A15. **e.** Multiple drug interactions are common in patients on antiviral therapy. In general, HMG-coenzyme reductase inhibitors, nonsedating oral antihistamines, and ergot alkaloids are contraindicated. Although sulfas may interact with ZDV and other agents, they may be used with caution in most instances.

A16. **e.** Neurologic complications of AIDS include cognitive impairment, AIDS dementia, encephalitis, meningitis, primary lymphoma formation, and peripheral neuropathy. Peripheral neuropathy is more often associated with the treatment of AIDS (particularly NRTIs) than the primary disease process itself.

A17. **d.** The transmission of HIV infection from pregnant mother to infant is certainly not universal. Moreover, extremely effective prophylaxis exists and should be used. Nevertheless, it is extremely important that all health care personnel involved in delivery of the infant take meticulous precautions to avoid the transfer of blood and blood products to themselves. From the point of view of the newborn, several scenarios may occur.

a. The transmission rate from infected mother to infant is thought to be in the range of approximately 20% to 30%. Thus 70% to 80% of infants born to mothers infected with the HIV virus will not, even in the absence of prophylaxis, become infected themselves. They will continue to test negative for the rest of their lives.

b. The prognosis for HIV infection progression and the development of AIDS and AIDS-related complications is somewhat more favorable in infants than in adults, even in those whose mothers were not given prophylaxis. However, it may take up to a year for them to test positive.

A18. **c.** HIV diagnostic testing is based on an ELISA test. This is the initial screening test. If a patient has a positive ELISA test, a confirmation test known as the Western blot needs to be carried out to confirm positivity.

A19. **c.** See Answer 18.

A20. **e.** High-risk behaviors include unprotected intercourse and the sharing of needles used for intravenous (IV) drug use. Groups historically at higher risk include homosexual males, IV drug users, and bisexual males. Available data strongly suggest that the

heterosexual female with many male sexual partners who uses nonbarrier methods of birth control is also at substantial risk.

Such behaviorally associated risk factors are modifiable, which is why patient education is so important for the physician to undertake.

SOLUTION TO THE SHORT ANSWER MANAGEMENT PROBLEM

Much has changed in the past decade regarding the treatment and prognosis in individuals with HIV infection. The advent of protease inhibitors and other antiviral agents has meant what was once a death sentence has been transformed into a problem of living with a chronic illness. Although drug resistance remains a problem, the focus has shifted to how to maintain health; in essence, secondary and tertiary prevention for those infected. Nevertheless, primary prevention should be the emphasis, as in the long term for society, it is far easier to prevent this illness than to deal with its consequences. Physicians have an obligation to support prevention of this illness in all its forms and to speak out for the compassionate care of those afflicted.

HIV counseling and testing are extremely important. HIV counseling and testing services are meant to achieve the following:

a. Provide an opportunity for individuals to determine their current HIV serostatus

b. Provide behavioral counseling to prevent infection in those who are not infected in a continued effort to avoid infection and in those who are infected but can transmit the infection to others

c. Help those who are infected to obtain appropriate services

d. Help partners of infected individuals to receive proper preventive services

Individuals have various degrees of understanding and knowledge about HIV transmission, testing, and risky behaviors. The physician should view all requests for HIV testing as an educational opportunity, an opportunity that cannot be missed. Among the important issues that all health care professionals associated with the counseling, testing, diagnosis, and treatment of HIV-positive patients face are sensitivity to sexual identity, sensitivity to culture, sensitivity to socioeconomic conditions, and an awareness of the individual's previous mental and physical conditions. The language used by the health care professional should be appropriate to the patient. An example of this last issue is the term *HIV-positive*. Frankly, patients who have the HIV virus see nothing "positive" about this at all.

Once risk factors have been identified, the decision to test for HIV seropositivity should be made by the patient. The physician has an ethical responsibility to explain the following tests:
   a. Nominal test: This test directly uses the patient's name.
   b. Nonnominal test: The patient identifier is known only to the physician and to the patient.
   c. Anonymous: This has an identifier known only by the patient.

Given the biologic, psychologic, and economic consequences of HIV disease, it is essential that the patient be made aware of the reasons for the test and the consequences of the test.

The following should be done before the test:
   a. Ask the patient directly why he or she wants to be tested.
   b. Explain the test. Explain the "window period." The body takes time to produce antibodies, usually 6 to 12 weeks. During this time the individual will continue to test negative.
   c. Explain that a positive ELISA test suggests but does not prove that the patient has been infected. Also explain that a positive confirmatory Western blot test means that the patient has been infected and that sexual contacts need to be notified by the patient, the doctor, or the public health authorities. Requirements vary from state to state.
   d. Clarify the difference between HIV infection and AIDS.
   e. Discuss the benefits of testing.
   f. Discuss the risks and disadvantages of testing, including insurance issues, false positives, false negatives, and indeterminate test results.
   g. Obtain informed consent before testing.
   h. Discuss confidentiality and the circumstances under which the result must be disclosed by law or ethical obligation.

SUGGESTED READINGS

Goldschmidt RH, Dong BJ: Treatment of AIDS- and HIV-related conditions, 1999, *J Am Board Fam Pract* 12(1):71-94, 1999.
Minkoff HL: Human immunodeficiency virus infection in pregnancy, *Semin Perinatol* 22(4):293-308, 1998.
Shearer WT: HIV infection and AIDS, *Prim Care* 25(4):759-774, 1998.
Smith C et al: AIDS-related malignancies, *Ann Med* 30(4):323-344, 1998.
Tulpule A, Matheny SC: AIDS-related malignancies, *Prim Care* 25(2):473-482, 1998.
Weber J: HIV and sexually transmitted diseases, *Br Med Bull* 54(3):717-729, 1998.
http://www.cdc.gov. Search under AIDS. (Frequently updated; the best source of current information.)

PROBLEM · 135

ADVICE FOR TRAVELERS

"Oh! I Didn't Drink the Water, but I Never Thought About the Ice."

Case 1 ■ A 51-Year-Old Male Who Is Planning on Traveling to Africa

A 51-year-old male comes to your office for a periodic health examination. He is planning on traveling to equatorial Africa in the near future and wishes to discuss immunizations and prophylaxis against malaria.

He is feeling well. He has had no major medical problems in the past, nor has he had any surgeries. He has no known allergies.

SELECT THE BEST ANSWER TO THE FOLLOWING QUESTIONS

Q1. What is the prophylactic agent of choice for the prevention of malaria in most areas of the world?
   a. chloroquine
   b. mefloquine
   c. pyrimethamine
   d. dapsone
   e. proguanil

Q2. The drug of choice you selected in Question 1 should be given for the following length of time:
   a. 1 week before travel and for at 6 weeks after return from travel
   b. 1 month before travel and for at least 1 month after return
   c. 2 weeks before travel and for at least 2 weeks after return
   d. 1 week before travel and for 1 week after return
   e. 6 weeks before travel and for at least 4 weeks after return

Q3. The drug of choice you selected in Question 1 was chosen primarily for its activity against which of the following?
   a. *Plasmodium falciparum*
   b. *P. vivax*
   c. *P. ovale*
   d. *P. malariae*
   e. none of the above

Q4. Which of the following symptoms is (are) common in clinical malaria?
   a. fever or chills
   b. diarrhea
   c. headache

d. myalgias

e. all of the above

Q5. What is the most common cause of traveler's diarrhea?

a. *Campylobacter jejuni*

b. *Shigella*

c. enterotoxigenic *Escherichia coli*

d. *Clostridium difficile*

e. rotavirus

Q6. What is (are) the prophylactic drug(s) of choice for the prevention of traveler's diarrhea?

a. bismuth subsalicylate

b. trimethoprim-sulfamethoxazole

c. ciprofloxacin

d. any of the above

e. none of the above

Q7. Which of the following should only be used for the treatment of moderate or severe traveler's diarrhea?

a. bismuth subsalicylate

b. loperamide hydrochloride

c. ciprofloxacin

d. oral rehydration

e. none of the above

Case 2 ■ **A 73-Year-Old Farmer Who Punctured His Foot on a Rusty Nail**

A 73-year-old farmer comes to the Emergency Department after having punctured his foot on a rusty nail while cleaning out a pig barn. You consider tetanus immunization. The patient is not sure that he has ever received a tetanus shot in the past.

Q8. Which of the following regimens should be administered to this patient for the prevention of tetanus?

a. tetanus toxoid is not indicated at this time

b. a single dose of tetanus toxoid

c. three doses of tetanus toxoid, with the first dose now and subsequent ones 2 months apart

d. three doses of tetanus toxoid, with the first dose now and subsequent ones 2 months apart, and a single dose of tetanus immunoglobulin

e. three doses of tetanus toxoid, with the first dose now and subsequent ones 2 months apart and three doses of tetanus immunoglobulin

Q9. Diphtheria and tetanus boosters should be a routine part of preventive health care in adults. How often should routine diphtheria and tetanus boosters be administered?

a. every year

b. every 2 years

c. every 3 years

d. every 5 years

e. every 10 years

Q10. Pneumococcal vaccine is an effective agent for prophylaxis against pneumococcal pneumonia. Which of the following is (are) indication(s) for the administration of pneumococcal vaccine?

a. chronic cardiopulmonary disease

b. chronic renal disease

c. age greater than 65 years

d. Hodgkin's disease

e. all of the above

SHORT ANSWER MANAGEMENT PROBLEM
List the immunizations and other prophylactic measures and treatments that a patient traveling from the United States to Central Africa should receive before departure.

ANSWERS

A1. **b.** Mefloquine 250 mg once/week is the drug of choice for travel to areas with chloroquine-resistant malaria. Because chloroquine-resistant malaria is now found throughout the world, mefloquine has become the preferred drug.

A2. **a.** The usual recommendation is that treatment begins 1 week before traveling to the malaria-infected area and continues for 6 weeks after the return home.

A3. **a.** There are several strains of malaria: that caused by *P. falciparum, P. ovale, P. vivax,* and *P. malariae.* Most of the concern arises over *P. falciparum;* it is crucial that treatment be directed to the most virulent and morbidity-producing strain. In addition, drug resistance has been seen primarily in *P. falciparum,* with only a few exceptions the others remain sensitive to chloroquine.

A4. **e.** Typical symptoms of malaria include fever, chills, myalgia, arthralgias, and headache. Abdominal pain, cough, and diarrhea may also occur.

Frequent clinical and laboratory findings include hepatosplenomegaly, anemia, and thrombocytopenia. Pulmonary or renal dysfunction (in the absence of dehydration) and changes in mental status may complicate *P. falciparum* malaria.

A5. **c.** The most common cause of traveler's diarrhea, usually a self-limited illness lasting several days, is enterotoxigenic *E. coli. Campylobacter, Shigella, Salmonella,* viruses, and parasites are less common causes of this condition. In areas where hygiene is poor, travelers should be advised to avoid foods that are not steaming hot, raw vegetables, and fruit they have not peeled themselves, as well as tap water and ice.

A6. **e.** It is generally not recommended to prescribe drugs to provide prophylaxis against traveler's diarrhea. On the rare occasions when prophylaxis is indicated, the prophylactic agent of choice is a quinolone, such as norfloxacin or ciprofloxacin.

A7. **c.** Treatment of traveler's diarrhea should consist of oral rehydration solutions, loperamide hydrochloride (a synthetic opioid), and, when diarrhea is moderate or severe, ciprofloxacin or trimethoprim-sulfamethoxazole.

A8. **d.** Because this wound is classified as a dirty wound and it is unknown if the patient has completed a primary tetanus series, the patient should receive both tetanus toxoid and a single dose of tetanus immunoglobulin at the time of presentation. Because his primary immunization status is unsure, a total of three doses of tetanus toxoid should be administered to complete a primary series. Tetanus immunoglobulin should be administered intramuscularly (250 units).

A9. **e.** Adults should be given a booster dose of tetanus-diphtheria (Td) every 10 years unless contraindicated.

A10. **e.** Pneumococcal vaccine is recommended in the following patients: all patients over age 65, patients with asplenia or splenic dysfunction, sickle-cell disease, hepatic cirrhosis, chronic cardiorespiratory disease, chronic alcoholism, chronic renal disease, Hodgkin's disease, and other conditions associated with immunosuppression.

SOLUTION TO THE SHORT ANSWER MANAGEMENT PROBLEM

The immunizations and other prophylactic measures and treatments include the following:
- a. Immunizations:
    1) Immunization with hepatitis A vaccine
    2) Polio vaccine (if immunization status not up to date; adults should receive one dose in adulthood)
    3) Tetanus-diphtheria (if immunization status not up to date)
    4) The live oral typhoid vaccine
    5) Yellow fever vaccine (if traveling to an endemic area such as Central and South America or Africa)
    6) Measles vaccine (if not up to date)
- b. Prophylactic measures and treatments:
    1) Traveler's diarrhea:
        a) Enterotoxigenic *E. coli* is the most common cause.
        b) Prophylaxis is not indicated in most cases: treatment with oral rehydration, loperamide (2 mg orally after each loose stool up to maximum of 16 mg), and ciprofloxacin or another quinolone is indicated if the diarrheal illness is severe.
    2) Malaria: Mefloquine is now the drug of choice for the prevention of malaria in most areas of the world. Treatment begins 1 week before travel and continues for 6 weeks after returning.

SUMMARY OF ADVICE FOR TRAVELERS

See the Solution to the Short Answer Management Problem

SUGGESTED READINGS

Advice for travelers, *Med Lett Drugs Therapeutics,* 41(1051):39-42, 1999.
McCarthy A: Malaria. In Rakel R, ed: *Conn's current therapy,* Philadelphia, 1994, WB Saunders.
www.cdc.gov/Traveler's Health

PROBLEM·136

DIAGNOSIS AND TREATMENT OF INFLUENZA

"Doctor, I Heard That the Flu Shot Caused Guillain-Barré Syndrome, a Very Bad Disease. Why Risk That to Prevent Ordinary, Everyday, Old-Fashioned Flu?"

Case 1 ■ A 73-Year-Old Male with Fever, Headache, and Myalgias

You are called to see a 73-year-old nursing home resident who has a temperature of 103° F, headache, myalgias, cough, rhinorrhea, sore throat, and malaise. In this case, seven other nursing home residents have come down with similar symptoms. It is December, and there has been a significant outbreak of respiratory illness in the community. On examination, the patient appears acutely ill. Apart from the aforementioned fever, the patient also has prominent pharyngeal erythema. There are a few expiratory rhonchi heard and the occasional bilateral rales.

SELECT THE BEST ANSWER
TO THE FOLLOWING QUESTIONS

Q1. What is the most likely diagnosis in this patient?
a. influenza A
b. bronchiolitis
c. bacterial pneumonia
d. septicemia secondary to an unknown focus of infection
e. peritonsillar abscess

Q2. Which of the following investigations may be indicated in this patient?
a. complete blood count (CBC)
b. blood cultures
c. chest x-ray
d. all of the above
e. none of the above

Q3. Which of the following statements regarding the influenza virus(es) is (are) true?
a. influenza epidemics occur annually and are of major public health importance worldwide
b. influenza viruses are subclassified as influenza A, influenza B, and influenza C
c. excess morbidity and mortality are consistently reported during influenza epidemics
d. all of the above
e. none of the above

Q4. Concerning the use of antibiotics for influenza infection in the elderly, which of the following statements most accurately describes a high practice standard?
a. no elderly patients with influenza should receive prophylactic antibiotics
b. all elderly patients with influenza should receive prophylactic antibiotics
c. the benefit of prescribing prophylactic antibiotics must be weighed against the risk: in most cases of uncomplicated influenza the risk/benefit ratio favors withholding antibiotics
d. basically, give the patient antibiotics if they ask for them; if they don't ask, don't give them
e. nobody really knows for sure

Q5. What is the most common complication of the illness described in this patient?
a. meningitis
b. pneumonia
c. serum sickness

d. agranulocytosis
e. brain abscess

Q6. Which of the following types of influenza is responsible for most of the world pandemics?
a. influenza A
b. influenza B
c. influenza C
d. influenza D
e. influenza E

Q7. What is the drug of choice for treating the symptoms of the patient described in Case 1?
a. acetylsalicylic acid
b. acetaminophen
c. amantadine
d. meperidine
e. ibuprofen

Q8. What is the primary mode of transmission of the illness described?
a. transfer via blood and blood products
b. oral-fecal contamination
c. sneezing and coughing
d. fomites
e. kissing

Q9. What is the most reliable method for preventing influenza?
a. gamma globulin
b. beta-interferon
c. activated influenza vaccine
d. inactivated influenza vaccine
e. amantadine hydrochloride

Q10. Regarding influenza vaccine, which of the following statements is true?
a. influenza vaccine is effective only against influenza A
b. the efficacy of influenza vaccine is approximately 95%
c. influenza vaccine should be administered every 2 years
d. the ideal time for administration of influenza vaccine is in the late spring
e. none of the above is true

Q11. Regarding influenza vaccination, which of the following statements is (are) true?
a. influenza vaccination typically produces no adverse drug reactions
b. the recommended dosage of influenza vaccine is 0.5 ml for adults
c. influenza vaccination reduces the severity of illness in vaccinated persons who become infected

d. b and c

e. all of the above statements are true

Q12. Which of the following statements regarding amantadine prophylaxis of influenza is (are) false?
   a. amantadine prophylaxis is effective against both influenza A and influenza B
   b. amantadine prophylaxis has been shown to reduce the duration of fever and other symptoms
   c. amantadine prophylaxis has been shown to reduce the duration of viral shedding
   d. amantadine prophylaxis should be used in high-risk individuals in whom vaccine is contraindicated
   e. all of the above statements are false

Q13. Amantadine should be administered for how long in unvaccinated individuals?
   a. 1 week
   b. 2 weeks
   c. 3 weeks
   d. 4 weeks
   e. for the duration of the particular outbreak

Q14. Which of the following groups should be considered for vaccination against influenza on a yearly basis?
   a. healthy adults over the age of 65 years
   b. children and adolescents receiving chronic aspirin therapy
   c. health care workers
   d. adults and children in chronic care facilities
   e. all of the above

Q15. Which of the following diseases shares a therapeutic agent with influenza?
   a. bronchial asthma
   b. congestive cardiac failure
   c. ulcerative colitis
   d. Parkinson's disease
   e. pulmonary thromboembolism

SHORT ANSWER MANAGEMENT PROBLEM

You have just assumed the role of medical director of a long-term care facility. It is now the end of November and it appears that the residents were not vaccinated when they should have been.

Two residents have just developed symptoms suggestive of influenza. Discuss your management of the long-term care facility residents and staff.

ANSWERS

A1. **a.** This patient most likely has influenza A. Influenza A strains usually predominate in adults; influenza B strains tend to infect children.

Bacterial pneumonia and a secondary septicemia may follow influenza, but at this time, with the history and physical examination reported, the most likely diagnosis is influenza.

A common symptom of influenza is a severe generalized or frontal headache, often accompanied by retroorbital pain. Other early symptoms of influenza include diffuse myalgias, fever, and chills. Respiratory symptoms especially tend to follow the occurrence of the early symptoms.

The term *flu* is used loosely by both physicians and patients. True influenza has a specific set of symptoms that can usually be used to differentiate it clinically from other viral infections.

In children the signs and symptoms of influenza are more subtle; they may simply appear as another upper respiratory tract infection or a cold.

A2. **d.** At this time, it would be reasonable to perform a CBC, blood cultures, and a chest x-ray. The chest x-ray is indicated because rales are heard in the lung fields. A CBC, blood culture, and a chest x-ray will rule out a secondary bacterial pneumonia, most often caused by *Streptococcus pneumoniae* and the bacteremia that may accompany it.

A3. **d.** Influenza epidemics occur annually and are of major public health importance worldwide. The epidemics are usually associated with a less serious antigenic drift or a more serious antigenic shift. The antigenic drifts (a shift in the hemagglutinin and neuraminidase antigens) provide, in most cases, the next year's challenge for public health practitioners. The antigenic shifts are responsible for the major "pandemics" that have occurred with influenza. They are also responsible for the major epidemics seen each year. Influenza epidemics and influenza pandemics are almost always associated with influenza A.

Both morbidity and mortality are definitely associated with influenza epidemics. This is true especially of the very old and the very young. Those with chronic disease are at even greater risk.

There are three major influenza viruses, designated influenza A, influenza B, and influenza C. By far the most virulent and most significant is the influenza A virus.

A4. **c.** In uncomplicated influenza viral infections, as in uncomplicated viral infections in general, there is no indication for the prescription of antibiotics. One could argue that those patients at high risk for the development of complications, such as those patients with chronic bronchitis, should be treated. This, and any other chronic cardiopulmonary condition, may very well be a reasonable exception to the no-antibiotics rule.

A5. **b.** The most common complication of influenza is pneumonia. This pneumonia is initially a viral pneumonia but often develops, especially in susceptible elderly patients, into a double pneumonia, with *S. pneumoniae* as the most common pathogen. Others include *Staphylococcus aureus* and *Haemophilus*. This is the reason for the recommendations of the U.S. Preventive Services Task Force on the Periodic Health Examination with respect to influenza:
   a. Immunize all patients who are over the age of 65 each year with the influenza vaccine.
   b. Immunize all patients who are over the age of 65 and high risk with the pneumococcal vaccine.

A6. **a.** All of the world's pandemics (caused by major antigenic shifts) are associated with influenza A. Influenza B and influenza C are associated neither with epidemics nor pandemics.

A7. **c.** Amantadine and rimantadine are approved in the United States for the specific prophylaxis and treatment of influenza A.

Amantadine can be used during the influenza season as an adjunct to late vaccination, as a supplement to preseason vaccination in immunodeficient persons, and as chemoprophylaxis in the absence of vaccination.

Amantadine can also be used to reduce the spread of the virus and to minimize disruption of patient care both in the community and in the institutional setting. It can be prescribed as a prophylaxis for healthy unvaccinated persons who simply want to avoid illness during an outbreak.

Amantadine is 70% to 90% effective in preventing influenza A infections. It is also the treatment of choice once influenza A is contracted. When given 24 to 48 hours after the onset of infection, amantadine reduces both the severity and duration of symptoms. The standard dose of amantadine is 200 mg/day. Elderly patients should receive 100 mg/day.

A8. **c.** The influenza virus is transmitted through respiratory secretions and thus is easily spread to susceptible persons. Sneezing, coughing, and close contact while talking are thought to be the major modes of transmission.

A9. **d.** The most effective method for preventing influenza A is by immunizing patients before the influenza season begins with inactivated (or killed) influenza vaccine. Influenza vaccine confers approximately 70% protection against the development of influenza and an even greater rate of protection against death from influenza.

A10. **e.** Influenza vaccine is effective against both influenza A and influenza B, has an efficacy rate of approximately 85%, and should be administered yearly and ideally 1 to 2 months before the influenza season begins in the late fall.

A11. **d.** Influenza vaccine typically produces some minor side effects such as a sore arm, redness at the injection site, and a low-grade fever. A history of anaphylactic hypersensitivity to eggs or egg products is a contraindication to receiving influenza vaccine.

Details of vaccine dose are discussed in a later question, but the usual dose of whole virus vaccine for adults is 0.5 ml.

In those patients in whom immunization fails and in whom influenza does develop, influenza vaccine still reduces both the severity and the duration of symptoms.

A12. **a.** Amantadine is effective only against influenza A. Amantadine reduces viral shedding, reduces the duration and severity of influenza A symptoms (such as headache, fever, chills, myalgias, and cough) once the virus is established, and should be used as treatment in high-risk patients in whom the vaccine is contraindicated.

A13. **e.** Patients who cannot take the vaccine and are at high risk can be protected by using a prophylactic during the local outbreak. Rimantadine (Flumadine) can also be used. The drug should be started as soon as possible after the outbreak is recognized and continued until it ends, usually in about 6 weeks. The usual dosage of amantadine is 200 mg/day, but this depends on renal function. In many elderly patients a dosage of 100 mg/day is safer.

A14. **e.** Individuals who should receive influenza vaccine include the following:
   a. Persons of any age with cardiovascular or pulmonary conditions that necessitate regular medical follow-up
   b. Residents of nursing homes and other chronic care facilities regardless of age
   c. Medical personnel who have contact with and can therefore transmit the influenza virus to high-risk patients
   d. Healthy adults over age 65

e. Children with chronic diseases (diabetes mellitus, renal dysfunction, anemia, immunosuppression, or asthma) or those on aspirin therapy. Split-dose vaccine should be used in children in a dose of 0.5 ml for children ages 3 to 8 years and 0.25 ml for those 6 to 35 months old. A second dose 4 weeks or more after the first dose is needed if the child has never received influenza vaccine. Children 9 to 12 years of age should receive one 0.5-ml dose of split-virus vaccine. Adults can be given either whole- or split-virus vaccine as a 0.5-ml dose.

f. HIV patients can be safely vaccinated but the vaccination is less effective when CD4 counts are less than 100/ml.

A15. **d.** Parkinson's disease shares a therapeutic agent with influenza. The therapeutic agent is, of course, amantadine. Treatment of Parkinson's disease is discussed in Problem 119.

SOLUTION TO THE SHORT ANSWER MANAGEMENT PROBLEM

As the new medical director of the chronic care facility, it is your job to minimize both the morbidity and mortality from influenza by immunization. Obviously the first job is to blunt the effect of the influenza outbreak that appears to be hitting your facility.

First, in those patients who have come down with influenza, treatment with amantadine or rimantadine should begin immediately. Although resistant strains are already developing, both amantadine and rimantadine are about 70% to 90% effective against strains of type A influenza virus. Rimantadine is preferred in patients with renal failure and has fewer central nervous system effects, which, in either case, are usually mild. Although those patients are unlikely to benefit from vaccine with respect to the current illness, vaccination should be undertaken in any case to prevent against further infections with a different influenza strain that year.

All noninfected residents and health care workers associated with the nursing home should be vaccinated immediately. Because the development of antibodies takes some 2 weeks after vaccination in adults (up to 6 weeks in children), chemoprophylaxis is started for all.

SUMMARY OF THE DIAGNOSIS AND TREATMENT OF INFLUENZA

1. Epidemiology: Influenza A is responsible for all epidemics and pandemics of influenza. It is also the most virulent of the influenza types, which include A, B, and C. Yearly outbreaks result mostly from antigenic drift in the H and N antigens. Influenza outbreaks begin in the late fall and can last until early into the new year.

2. Signs and symptoms: Headache is a common symptom, particularly in the forehead. Other symptoms include fever, chills, and myalgias, followed by the symptoms of cough and congestion.

3. Prevention: Influenza vaccine should be given to all high-risk groups discussed. Ideally, immunization should take place in September or October. Vaccine efficacy averages around 85% and is effective for both influenza A and influenza B.

4. Prophylaxis: Amantadine and rimantadine are prophylactic agents that can be used as an adjunct to vaccination in high-risk situations (especially in chronic care facilities). Amantadine is 70% to 90% effective in preventing influenza A. It is not effective against influenza B. Amantadine not only prevents influenza A, but also reduces the severity and duration of symptoms in persons who have already contracted the virus.

In late 1999 two new antiinfluenza drugs zanamivir (Relenza) and oseltamivir (Tamiflu) were approved by the Food and Drug Administration. Both of these drugs are neuraminidase inhibitors and are active against the influenza B virus as well as the influenza A virus. Zanamivir is administered orally and oseltamivir by oral inhalation. For these new drugs to be effective, they must be administered as soon as possible following the onset of influenza symptoms.

SUGGESTED READINGS

Recommendations of the Advisory Committee on Immunization practices: *Prevention and control of influenza,* MMWR 48:RR-4, 1999.

Ruben F: Influenza. In Rakel R, ed: *Conn's current therapy,* Philadelphia, 1994, WB Saunders.

Tierney LM, Jr, McPhee SJ, Papadakis MA, eds: *Current medical diagnosis and treatment, 2000,* Stamford, Conn, 1999, Appleton & Lange.

CHAPTER 9

Emergency and Sports Medicine

CARDIOPULMONARY RESUSCITATION AND EMERGENCY CARDIAC CARE

"You Are Looking at a Man Who Died Twice."

Case 1 ■ A 55-Year-Old Male Found Collapsed in the Street

A 55-year-old male is found collapsed in the street by a passerby. The passerby begins cardiopulmonary resuscitation (CPR) and is joined shortly by another citizen. Emergency 911 is called, and CPR is continued until the paramedics arrive and initiate advanced cardiac life support (ACLS).

Despite complete ACLS maneuvers, the patient remains pulseless and breathless as the paramedics hand over care to the Emergency Department doctor on duty at the closest hospital.

SELECT THE BEST ANSWER TO THE FOLLOWING QUESTIONS

Q1. What is the most common rhythm initially responsible for cardiac arrest?
   a. ventricular tachycardia
   b. ventricular fibrillation
   c. ventricular standstill
   d. asystole
   e. complete heart block

Q2. What is the most common rhythm leading directly to death in cardiac arrest?
   a. ventricular tachycardia
   b. ventricular fibrillation
   c. second-degree heart block (Mobitz type II)
   d. ventricular asystole
   e. complete heart block

Q3. A "quick-look paddles" is performed on the patient in Case 1. You diagnose ventricular fibrillation. What should be your first step?
   a. defibrillate with 200 joules
   b. administer sodium bicarbonate 50 mEq IV bolus and epinephrine 10 cc (1:1000 solution) and follow by countershock

   c. administer sodium bicarbonate 500 mEq IV bolus and calcium chloride 500 ml of a 10% solution IV bolus and countershock after drug infusion
   d. defibrillate with 400 joules
   e. administer atropine 1.0 mg IV bolus and epinephrine 10 cc (1:10,000 solution) and wait for the response

Q4. What is the antiarrhythmic of choice in the management of ventricular arrhythmias?
   a. bretylium
   b. lidocaine
   c. procainamide
   d. verapamil
   e. amrinone

The patient above is successfully converted to sinus rhythm. Unfortunately, on the way to the coronary care unit he arrests again. The rhythm strip reveals asystole. CPR is restarted.

Q5. Which of the following is the next logical step in treatment?
   a. administer epinephrine 1.0 mg IV push (1:10,000 solution)
   b. administer calcium chloride 10 cc of a 10% solution IV push
   c. administer sodium bicarbonate 1 mEq/kg IV push
   d. administer isoproterenol 2 to 20 µg/kg/min
   e. administer lidocaine 75 mg IV push

With appropriate treatment the patient again converts to sinus rhythm. He is stabilized in the coronary care unit. Unfortunately, 2 hours later he develops ventricular tachycardia. His blood pressure is 100/60 mm Hg and he has a palpable pulse.

Q6. Your next step should be to administer which of the following?
   a. lidocaine 1 to 1.5 mg/kg IV push
   b. procainamide 20 mg/min up to a maximum of 1000 mg/min
   c. bretylium 5 mg IV bolus
   d. verapamil 5 mg IV bolus
   e. none of the above

Sinus rhythm is restored again and the patient's condition returns to satisfactory. Unfortunately, he develops a second-degree atrioventricular (AV) block (Mobitz type II). His pulse is 40 bpm and his blood pressure drops to 70/40 mm Hg.

Q7. Given this change, what would you do now?
   a. only observe the patient
   b. administer isoproterenol 2 to 10 µg/min
   c. administer atropine 0.5 to 1.0 mg
   d. administer epinephrine 0.5 to 1.0 mg
   e. none of the above

Q8. What is the definitive therapy for the dysrhythmia described in Question 7?
   a. a constant infusion of isoproterenol 2 to 20 µg/min
   b. a constant infusion of lidocaine 2 to 4 mg/min
   c. a constant infusion of procainamide 2 to 4 mg/min
   d. a transvenous pacemaker
   e. none of the above

Case 2 ■ A 70-Kg Man Who Collapsed in the Street

CPR is in progress on a 70-kg man who collapsed in the street (witnessed arrest). Basic life support (BLS) was begun, as was ACLS, when the paramedics arrived. He was brought immediately to the Emergency Department and a blood gas sample was drawn. The following were the results:

pH	7.10
PCO_2	60 mm Hg
PO_2	75 mm Hg
HCO_3^-	15 mEq/L

Q9. Which of the following do these results represent?
   a. metabolic acidosis with respiratory alkalosis
   b. respiratory acidosis with metabolic alkalosis
   c. pure metabolic acidosis
   d. pure respiratory acidosis
   e. mixed respiratory and metabolic acidosis

Q10. What is the most appropriate treatment of the patient described in Case 2?
   a. sodium bicarbonate 1 mEq/kg
   b. sodium bicarbonate 0.5 mEq/kg
   c. increased ventilation

   d. both a and c
   e. both b and c

Q11. Which of the following should be treated first in this patient?
   a. the respiratory acidosis
   b. the metabolic acidosis
   c. the respiratory alkalosis
   d. the metabolic alkalosis
   e. all of the above

Case 3 ■ A 53-Year-Old Male with a Rapid Heartbeat, Nausea, and Dizziness

A 53-year-old male comes to the Emergency Department with a 2-hour history of a rapid heartbeat, nausea, and dizziness.

A 12-lead electrocardiogram (ECG) shows atrial flutter with variable AV conduction. As you are taking his history he becomes disoriented. You are only able to obtain his systolic blood pressure (40 mm Hg).

Q12. At this time, what should you do?
   a. administer epinephrine 1.0 mg IV
   b. administer isoproterenol 2 to 20 µg/min IV
   c. defibrillate with 300 joules
   d. cardiovert with 300 joules
   e. cardiovert with 100 joules

Q13. What is the first step in initiation of resuscitation following a witnessed or unwitnessed cardiac arrest?
   a. begin rescue breathing
   b. begin rescue compression
   c. initiate a call to 911
   d. check pulse
   e. go for help

Q14. Which of the following statements concerning BLS is false?
   a. prompt administration of BLS is the key to success
   b. mouth-to-mouth resuscitation is the recommended method of respiratory exchange in performing BLS
   c. BLS is most commonly used in family situations (one family member resuscitating another)
   d. BLS succeeds no more frequently than in 15% of out-of-hospital attempts
   e. infectious diseases such as acquired immunodeficiency syndrome (AIDS) and serum hepatitis pose little, if any, risk to rescuers

Q15. What is the recommended BLS compression/ventilation rescue sequence in one-person CPR?
   a. 15:2
   b. 15:1
   c. 20:4
   d. 10:1
   e. 10:3

Q16. The National Heart, Lung, and Blood Institute in the United States recommends that to minimize permanent cardiac muscle damage in patients with ST-segment elevation acute myocardial infarction, the ideal upper limit of time from onset of symptoms to start of treatment is:
   a. 60 minutes
   b. 90 minutes
   c. 120 minutes
   d. 240 minutes
   e. none of the above

Q17. The National Heart, Lung and Blood Institute in the United States recommends that to minimize permanent cardiac muscle damage, the "Emergency Department door-to-needle" time for clot-dissolving drugs should not exceed:
   a. 30 minutes
   b. 60 minutes
   c. 90 minutes
   d. 120 minutes
   e. 240 minutes

SHORT ANSWER MANAGEMENT PROBLEM
Part A: Describe the importance and sequence for performing a "critical incident debriefing" among emergency room personnel or emergency rescue staff involved in an unsuccessful resuscitation. This "critical incident debriefing" is especially important if there is an unusual feature to the case such as a patient of young age, a victim known to some or all of the rescuers, or rescue personnel who are not accustomed to failure.
Part B: Explain the importance of the "chain of survival" in out-of-hospital cardiac arrest.

ANSWERS

A1. **b.** The most common initial rhythm diagnosed in patients who suffer a cardiac arrest is ventricular fibrillation.

A2. **d.** The usual course of events is as follows: coarse ventricular fibrillation to fine ventricular fibrillation to ventricular asystole. If BLS and ACLS are available within the recommended 4- and 8-minute time intervals, the probability of successfully converting ventricular fibrillation before ventricular asystole occurs is significantly increased. The best survival rate is when CPR is started within 3 minutes of cardiac arrest and defibrillation is delivered soon after. Even in the best of community coronary care units, the survival rate of out-of-hospital cardiac arrest rarely exceeds 15%. Higher rates have been reported but are extremely rare. Once ventricular asystole develops, the probability of successful resuscitation is virtually zero. Thus although ventricular fibrillation is the most common initial rhythm, ventricular asystole is the most common arrhythmia leading directly to death.

A3. **a.** The first step in the treatment of ventricular fibrillation is defibrillation with an energy level of 200 joules. If the first attempt is unsuccessful, two further defibrillations (200 to 300 joules and 360 joules) should follow immediately (before pharmacologic therapy is initiated). If defibrillation is unsuccessful, IV access should be established, epinephrine given, intubation performed, and antiarrhythmic drugs administered. Sodium bicarbonate is given if the patient has known preexisting hyperkalemia. Atropine is indicated in the management of symptomatic bradycardia or asystole, not ventricular fibrillation. Calcium chloride is no longer recommended for the management of any arrhythmia or dysrhythmia. It is used in certain situations, namely hypocalcemia, hyperkalemia, and calcium channel blocker toxicity.

A4. **b.** The antiarrhythmic agent of choice is lidocaine. Lidocaine should be administered in a dosage of 1.5 mg/kg IV push up to a maximum of 3 mg/kg. When spontaneous circulation returns, a lidocaine drip of 2 to 4 mg/kg should be started.

Bretylium and procainamide are second-line agents. Bretylium is administered in a dose of 5 mg/kg IV and repeated in 5 minutes at 10 mg/kg to a maximum dose of 30 mg/kg.

Bretylium is the drug of choice in the presence of hypothermia. Procainamide is administered in a dose of 20 mg/min until one of the following is observed:
   a. The arrhythmia is suppressed.
   b. Hypotension ensues.
   c. The QRS complex is widened by 50% of its original width.
   d. A total of 17 mg/kg of drug has been administered.

Procainamide is especially useful when having difficulty distinguishing the origin of a wide complex tachycardia. Verapamil may be used for rate control in atrial fibrillation or flutter and refractory paroxysmal supraventricular tachycardia (PSVT).

Amrinone is a rapid-acting inotropic agent that is useful in the treatment of patients with severe congestive heart failure refractory to diuretics, vasodilators, and conventional inotropic agents.

A5. **a.** The next step in the management of the original patient is the administration of epinephrine 1.0 mg IV push (1:10,000). This should be repeated every 5 minutes. If intubation has not been performed, it should be. Atropine in a dose of 1.0 mg IV push should be given as well and repeated every 3 to 5 minutes to a total of 0.04 mg/kg.

If used, transcutaneous cardiac pacing should be performed early. Sodium bicarbonate is used in certain situations.

A6. **a.** The treatment of choice for patients with ventricular tachycardia who are hemodynamically stable is lidocaine 1 to 1.5 mg/kg. This can be repeated in a dose of 0.5 to 0.75 mg/kg every 5 to 10 minutes until the ventricular tachycardia resolves or until a total of 3 mg/kg has been given.

The second-line drug in this case is procainamide in a dose of 20 to 30 mg/min until the ventricular tachycardia resolves or a total of 17 mg/kg has been given.

Bretylium can be used but is recommended for use after procainamide in stable ventricular tachycardia.

When hemodynamically unstable ventricular tachycardia is diagnosed (pulseless or hypotensive), the treatment of choice is synchronized cardioversion. The initial energy recommended is 100 joules. This should be followed by repetitive shocks of 200 joules, 300 joules, and finally 360 joules. If ventricular tachycardia is recurrent, lidocaine should be given as an IV bolus and cardioversion again attempted (at the energy level that was previously successful).

A7. **c.** Second-degree heart block (Mobitz type II) occurs below the level of the AV node either at the bundle of His (uncommon) or at the bundle branch level (more common). It is usually associated with an organic lesion in the conduction pathway. Its usual progression is to a third degree (complete) heart block.

Initial treatment is aimed at increasing the heart rate in an attempt to increase cardiac output. Thus atropine in a dose of 0.5 to 1.0 mg is the drug of choice. The maximum dose of atropine is 0.04 mg/kg

A8. **d.** If signs or symptoms persist, an external pacemaker can be placed and dopamine and epinephrine can be given. Epinephrine and observation are in appropriate treatment options for this patient. The definitive treatment in this patient is a transvenous pacemaker.

A9. **e.** Most patients who have arrested and who are undergoing CPR have a mixed respiratory and metabolic acidosis. Normal P_{CO_2} is 40 mm Hg.

The patient in this case has a markedly elevated P_{CO_2} of 60 mm Hg and thus is being hypoventilated. The patient's bicarbonate level of 15 mEq/L is below the normal range of 21 to 28 mEq/L and thus he has a metabolic acidosis as well.

A10. **c.** Recent recommendations suggest that bicarbonate should be used with caution. Although cardiac function is depressed by acidosis, the determining factor is intracellular pH, not extracellular pH, as is measured by arterial pH. Hypoxia, not acidosis, accounts for most of the cardiac depression. Moreover, respiratory acidosis produces immediate and profound depression, thus increasing ventilation should be used as the primary means of correcting acidosis and hypoxia.

A11. **a.** The respiratory acidosis should be treated first. By contrast, the use of bicarbonate has long been known to present risks that are not limited to alkalosis but include hypernatremia and hyperosmolarity. The accumulation of metabolic by-products, not bicarbonate deficits, produces the acidosis. Giving bicarbonate to buffer the arterial pH will not benefit the patient.

A12. **e.** The treatment of choice for acute unstable atrial flutter is synchronized cardioversion. The initial energy chosen should be 100 joules. If unsuccessful, this should be followed by cardioversion at 200, 300, and 360 joules. If the patient is stable, vagal maneuvers can be attempted first, followed by medications (diltiazem, beta-blockers, and verapamil).

A13. **c.** When witnessing a collapse or seeing an unresponsive victim, the first step in the adult BLS protocol is to access the Emergency Medical Service (EMS) system by dialing 911 or the emergency number in your area. This now precedes opening the airway by the head-tilt-chin-lift or the jaw-thrust maneuver.

In children, however, 1 minute of CPR should follow initial assessment before calling EMS.

A14. **b.** Until recently, the recommended method of BLS ventilation was mouth-to-mouth. However, because increased fear of contact of infectious diseases (especially AIDS), the recommendation has been changed to a primary recommendation of mouth-to-mask ventilation. However, if masks are unavailable, mouth-to-mouth resuscitation must be immediately begun. The risk of contacting an infectious disease through mouth-to-mouth resuscitation is extremely remote.

A15. **a.** For one-rescuer CPR, the compression/ventilation ratio recommended is 15:2 (compressions to ventilations). When a second rescuer arrives, a 5:1 compression/ventilation ratio should begin. The compression rate for one-rescuer and two-rescuer CPR remains at 80 to 100/min.

A16. **a.**

A17. **a.** The National Heart, Lung, and Blood Institute in the United States has made recommendations for the maximum time intervals to initiate thrombolytic therapy to salvage heart muscle and improve a patient's chance of survival from an acute myocardial infarction. The maximum times are as follows:

    a. The onset of cardiac symptoms (including prodromal symptoms of nausea, vomiting, and dizziness) to start of thrombolytic treatment in Emergency Department is 60 minutes.

    b. The time of admission to the Emergency Department to injection of thrombolytic agents is 30 minutes.

If these guidelines are followed, the greatest probability for preserving cardiac muscle will be attained.

SOLUTION TO THE SHORT ANSWER MANAGEMENT PROBLEM

Part A: Following an unsuccessful resuscitation attempt, a therapeutic intervention should be undertaken. This is known as a critical incident debriefing. Critical incident debriefing helps the rescuer deal with possible feelings of grief or guilt associated with the patient's death. Suggested guidelines include the following:

    a. The debriefing should occur as quickly as possible after the cardiac arrest with all team members present.

    b. Call the group together, preferably in the resuscitation room. State that you want to have a code debriefing.

    c. Review the scenario and conduct of the code. Include the contributory pathophysiology leading to the code, the decision tree followed, and any variations present.

    d. Analyze the things that were done wrong and especially the things that were done right. Allow free discussion.

    e. Ask for recommendations/suggestions for future resuscitations.

    f. Encourage all team members to share their feelings of anxiety, anger, and possible guilt.

    g. Any team member unable to be present should be informed of the process followed, the discussion generated, and the recommendations made.

    h. The team leader should encourage any team member to contact him or her if unanswered questions arise later.

Part B: The effectiveness of community with emergency cardiac care depends very much on what is called the *chain of survival.*

In simplest terms the chain of survival requires four basic steps being performed in a specific order. If these four steps are instituted quickly, the probability of a successful outcome is increased:

    a. Early access to EMS personnel

    b. Early CPR (maximum 4 minutes from victim down)

    c. Early defibrillation

    d. Early advanced care (maximum 8 minutes)

SUMMARY OF THE TREATMENT OF THE CARDIAC ARREST PATIENT

1. Ventricular fibrillation:
    a. Defibrillation: 200, 300, and 360 joules
    b. Epinephrine 1.0 mg IV push every 3 to 5 minutes
    c. Defibrillate again
    d. Lidocaine 1.5 mg/kg IV push
    e. Second-line antiarrhythmic (procainamide or bretylium)

2. Asystole:
    a. Consider immediate transcutaneous pacing
    b. Epinephrine 1.0 mg IV push every 3 to 5 minutes
    c. Atropine 1.0 mg IV push every 3 to 5 minutes up to total 0.04 mg/kg
    d. Consider bicarbonate

3. Ventricular tachycardia: Stable ventricular tachycardia:
    a. Lidocaine 1.0 to 1.5 mg/kg IV push, then lidocaine 0.5 to 0.75 mg/kg IV push every 5 to 10 minutes (maximum 3 mg/kg)
    b. Procainamide 20 to 30 mg/min until ventricular tachycardia resolves or a maximum 17 mg/kg
    c. Bretylium 5 to 10 mg/kg over 8 to 10 minutes (maximum of 30 mg/kg over 24 hours)
    d. Cardiovert as in unstable ventricular tachycardia:
       1) Consider sedation
       2) Cardiovert 100, 200, 300, and 360 joules

4. Second-degree heart block (Mobitz type II) and third-degree heart block:
    a. Atropine 0.5 to 1.0 mg IV every 3 to 5 minutes up to 0.04 mg/kg

   b. Dopamine 5 to 20 μg/kg/min
   c. Epinephrine 2 to 10 μg/min

5. Supraventricular tachycardia
   a. Vagal maneuvers
   b. Adenosine 6 to 12 mg rapid IV push
   c. Verapamil, diltiazem, cardioversion, digoxin, beta-blockers

SUMMARY OF AMERICAN HEART ASSOCIATION CHANGES ON THE BASIS OF THE 1992 NATIONAL CONFERENCE ON CARDIOPULMONARY RESUSCITATION AND EMERGENCY CARDIAC CARE

1. BLS: Dial 911 first

2. Chain of survival in CPR:
   a. Early access to EMS
   b. Early CPR
   c. Early defibrillation
   d. Early ACLS

3. Esophageal obturator airway: no longer recommended

4. Increased restrictions on use of sodium bicarbonate

5. Use of calcium chloride: Essentially eliminated

6. Adenosine: 6 to 12 mg (drug of choice for PSVT in adults)

7. Interosseous administration of drugs in infants and children recommended up to the age of 6 years

8. Glucose-containing fluids discouraged in resuscitation attempts because of deleterious effects on cerebral perfusion

9. Thrombolytic agents: t-PA and streptokinase administered within 6 hours of onset of chest pain in patients under age of 70 who have an ECG pattern indicative of acute myocardial infarction

10. Ethical issues and critical incident debriefing now considered part of ACLS courses

SUGGESTED READINGS

American Heart Association: Guidelines for cardiopulmonary resuscitation and emergency cardiac care. Recommendations of the 1992 National Consensus Conference, *JAMA* 16:2125-2302, 1992.

Pousada L et al: *Emergency medicine*, Baltimore, 1996, Williams & Wilkins.

P R O B L E M · 1 3 8

DIAGNOSIS AND MANAGEMENT OF TRAUMA

"I Wish I Had Fastened the Safety Belt!"

Case 1 ■ A 27-Year-Old Female Injured in a Motor Vehicle Accident

A 27-year-old female is injured in a two-car, head-on collision. She is transported to your Emergency Department in critical condition. You are the duty doctor in a small, rural hospital. The nearest trauma center is 180 miles away.

On examination, the patient is in acute respiratory distress. Her respiratory rate is 32 bpm. Breath sounds are absent in the right lung field. She is pale and her blood pressure is 90/60 mm Hg. Her pulse is 106 bpm. Her heart sounds are distant and muffled. Her jugular venous pressure (JVP) appears elevated.

When you touch her abdomen she pulls back in pain. This appears to be maximal over the left upper quadrant. Her right hip is in a posture of external rotation. As she is wheeled through the Emergency Department doors, her cervical spine appears to be adequately immobilized.

Her neurologic examination reveals a dilated right pupil. She is responsive to deep pain and pressure, as well as deep palpation of the abdomen. There is blood and pink-tinged fluid leaking from her nose. There is blood present at the urethral meatus, and her pelvis appears to be in an "odd position." A large scalp laceration is present.

SELECT THE BEST ANSWER TO THE FOLLOWING QUESTIONS

Q1. At this time, what should be your first priority?
   a. carry on with the rest of the complete assessment
   b. establish an intravenous (IV) infusion
   c. send the patient to x-ray for an immediate chest x-ray
   d. send the patient to x-ray for a lateral x-ray of the cervical spine
   e. none of the above

Q2. What is the most likely cause of this patient's respiratory distress?
   a. flail chest
   b. tension pneumothorax
   c. acute pulmonary embolus
   d. pericardial tamponade
   e. none of the above

Q3. After establishing an airway and dealing with the patient's respiratory status, what should you do?
   a. complete the neurologic examination
   b. perform a Glasgow coma scale
   c. establish a central venous pressure (CVP) line or two large peripheral IV lines
   d. perform a diagnostic paracentesis
   e. perform an immediate electrocardiogram (ECG)

Q4. What is the most likely cause of this patient's dilated right pupil?
   a. a middle meningeal artery tear
   b. a chronic subdural hematoma
   c. an acute subdural hematoma
   d. a or c
   e. none of the above

The patient's neurologic status is as follows:
Eyes: closed; no response to verbal commands but a response to pain
Best verbal response: none
Best motor response: flexion withdrawal to pressure on the brachial plexus

Q5. What is the patient's Glasgow coma scale?
   a. 12
   b. 8
   c. 7
   d. 4
   e. 2

A paracentesis is performed and draws bloody fluid. On examination, pain is maximal in the left upper quadrant.

Q6. What is the most likely cause of this patient's abdominal pain?
   a. liver laceration
   b. duodenal rupture
   c. renal hematoma
   d. splenic rupture
   e. pancreatic tear

Case 2 ■ A 31-Year-Old Male Who Was Involved in a Car-Motorcycle Accident

A 31-year-old male is brought to the Emergency Department after having been involved in a car-motorcycle accident.

On examination, he is drowsy but conscious. His respiratory rate is 32 breaths/min. His blood pressure is 70/50 mm Hg. His heart sounds are muffled. He has significant elevation of the JVP. He has a large contu-sion over the sternal area. There is a laceration seen over the precordial region. No other significant abnor-malities are noted on primary survey.

Q7. What is the most likely diagnosis in this patient?
   a. myocardial contusion
   b. pericardial tamponade
   c. aortic rupture
   d. pulmonary contusion
   e. pneumothorax

Q8. What is the treatment of choice for the patient described in Case 2?
   a. regular observation
   b. increased rate of crystalloid infusion
   c. crystalloid infusion and blood
   d. pericardiocentesis
   e. chest tube insertion

Q9. What is the minimal gauge of a peripheral IV catheter that should be inserted in a patient in shock?
   a. #25 gauge
   b. #22 gauge
   c. #18 gauge
   d. #16 gauge
   e. #12 gauge

Q10. What is the most common error in Emergency Department trauma stabilization?
   a. inadequate airway management
   b. inadequate cervical spine immobilization
   c. failure to recognize or decompress pneumo-thorax
   d. inadequate shock therapy
   e. distracting visually impressive but not life-threatening maxillofacial trauma

SHORT ANSWER MANAGEMENT PROBLEM
Part A: List the major mandatory interventions that should be immediately undertaken in someone who presents with traumatic shock.
Part B: Describe, in order of frequency, the major mistakes in treating patients with trauma.

ANSWERS

A1. **e.** Your first priority is to attend to the ABCs of resuscitation (airway, breathing, circulation). Thus the establishment of an airway is first. Following that, breathing should be assessed (this includes assess-ment of breath sounds in both lung fields as well as re-spiratory rate). Finally, the patient's circulatory status must be attended to with the establishment of either a CVP line or two large-bore IV lines.

A2. **b.** The most likely cause of this patient's respiratory distress is a tension pneumothorax. Tension pneumothorax is a common life-threatening injury that needs to be assessed and treated immediately. In this patient, the clue to the high probability of this being a tension pneumothorax is the complete absence of breath sounds in the right lung field.

The most common error in this situation would be to transport the patient to x-ray without a physician. In fact, with the history and physical findings it would be entirely appropriate to treat the patient on the basis of your presumed diagnosis without an x-ray. A needle can be inserted into the chest wall cavity to decompress the potentially life-threatening tension pneumothorax. A "rush of air" will confirm the diagnosis. Subsequent management requires a chest tube thoracostomy.

A3. **c.** As mentioned previously, the priority following A and B is C (circulation). A CVP line or two large-bore (#16 gauge) IV catheters should be inserted to maximize the ability to replace intravascular volume.

A4. **d.** The dilated right pupil is most likely caused by an initial skull fracture producing tearing of either veins (subdural hematoma) or the middle meningeal artery (epidural hematoma). If computed tomography (CT) scanning is unavailable and the patient is comatose with decerebrate or decorticate posturing that is unresponsive to mannitol or hyperventilation, a burr hole should be placed. The burr hole is placed in the temporal region on the ipsilateral side of the dilated pupil.

A5. **c.** This patient's Glasgow coma scale is 7.
The Glasgow coma scale rating is as follows:
a. Eyes
   1) Open: Spontaneously 4
   2) To verbal command 3
   3) To pain 2
   4) No response: 1
b. Best verbal response:
   1) Orientated and converses 5
   2) Disoriented and converses 4
   3) Inappropriate words 3
   4) Incomprehensible sounds 2
   5) No response 1
c. Best motor response:
   1) To verbal command: Obeys 6
   2) To painful stimulus: Localizes pain 5
   3) Flexion withdrawal 4
   4) Abnormal flexion (decorticate rigidity) 3
   5) Extension (decerebrate rigidity) 2
   6) No response 1
   TOTAL POSSIBLE 15

A6. **d.** A paracentesis that draws bloody fluid suggests an intraabdominal bleed most likely caused by organ laceration or organ rupture. Pain maximal in the left upper quadrant suggests that this is most likely caused by splenic rupture, one of the most common abdominal injuries seen in multiple-trauma victims.

A7. **b.** This patient has a pericardial tamponade. Pericardial tamponade is an injury that is often missed. It also is a frequent injury in motor vehicle accident victims in which multiple injuries are sustained. It is particularly common in car-motorcycle accident victims in which the motorcyclist is thrown a significant distance.

A8. **d.** Pericardiocentesis (the removal of fluid from around the heart) is the treatment of choice. Pericardiocentesis will remove the constriction that is impeding the ability of the heart to pump blood.

A9. **d.** The minimum gauge of an IV catheter that should be inserted in a patient in shock is #16 gauge. It is recommended two #16 gauge catheters be inserted—one in each arm.

A10. **a.** The most common error in Emergency Department trauma stabilization is inadequate airway management. The common errors that arise from diagnosis and treatment of trauma victims are completely discussed in the Short Answer Management Problem.

SOLUTION TO THE SHORT ANSWER MANAGEMENT PROBLEM

Part A: The major interventions that should be undertaken when a patient presents with traumatic shock are as follows:
a. The ABCs (airway, breathing, circulation); assess and treat these priorities first.
   1) **Airway:** airway management with protection of the cervical spine. Techniques to maintain an airway include chin lift, jaw thrust, artificial airway placement, and suctioning. Supplemental oxygen should be provided to multiple-trauma patients. Intubation is often necessary.
   2) **Breathing:** ensure breath sounds are heard on both sides of the chest.
   3) **Circulation:** establish a CVP line or two large-bore IV lines. Intraarterial catheter is preferable for monitoring vital signs, but, if not, continuous monitoring by other means is necessary. Begin fluid resuscitation with

Ringer's lactate or normal saline. Cross-match for immediate blood.

4) **D**eficits of neurologic function. Perform a brief neurologic examination. Assess the level of consciousness, pupil size and reactivity, and motor and sensory function.

5) **E**xposure: Completely undress all trauma patients.

b. Input and output: urinary catheter, nasogastric tube

c. Perform primary survey of all systems: pay particular attention to the following:

1) Neurologic status (the Glasgow coma scale): Is there any sign of increased intracranial pressure? Consider IV Mannitol, hyperventilation, maintain $O_2 > 80$ mm Hg, and control blood pressure. Burr holes should be used in dire circumstances when indicated.

2) Cardiovascular system: Low blood pressure, elevated JVP, and muffled heart sounds suggest pericardial tamponade; consider other myocardial injuries such as contusion.

3) Respiratory system: is there any evidence of pneumothorax? Is a flail chest present? Are there any other injuries?

4) Abdomen: is there any abdominal tenderness or bruising? Is there any tenderness in the RUQ (possible liver laceration) or LUQ (splenic laceration or rupture)? Are there any other injuries? Is CT scan or ultrasound available in the Emergency department?

5) Reassess ABCs at regular intervals.

6) Musculoskeletal: Are there any obvious fractures, especially open? Is there any evidence of pelvic fracture? Is there blood at the urethral meatus?

7) Maxillary-facial trauma: Do not let injuries that look worse than they are detract your attention from more serious injuries.

8) Perform secondary survey.

9) Contact tertiary care facility and arrange transfer if this has not already been done.

10) Order investigations: Complete blood count (CBC); electrolytes; chest x-ray; cervical spine x-ray; skull x-ray; ECG; amylase; urinalysis; x-ray of the kidneys, ureter, and bladder; three views of the abdomen; abdominal ultrasound; and any other appropriate investigations deemed necessary for the individual patient (x-rays of long bones and so on). If CT or magnetic resonance imaging scanning facilities are available, other investigations may be ordered.

11) Treat non-life-threatening injuries when the patient has been stabilized.

Part B: The major mistakes (in order of frequency) in treating patients with trauma are as follows:

a. Inadequate airway management

b. Inadequate shock therapy

c. Inadequate cervical spine immobilization

d. Failure to recognize and decompress pneumothorax

e. Distracting visually impressive but not life-threatening injuries (maxillofacial trauma, compound fractures)

f. Delay in transfer to tertiary care facility

g. Failure to transfer patients to tertiary care center at all

SUMMARY OF THE DIAGNOSIS AND MANAGEMENT OF TRAUMA

An excellent summary of the diagnosis and management of trauma is found in the Solution to the Short Answer Management Problem, particularly Part A.

Presented in place of the summary is a probable problem list for this patient.

1. Motor vehicle accident: patient in critical condition
2. Cervical spine injury until proven otherwise
3. Hypovolemic shock
4. Tension pneumothorax
5. Pericardial tamponade
6. Skull fracture: acute epidural or subdural hematoma
7. Cerebrospinal fluid leak secondary to item 6
8. Probable splenic rupture or tear
9. Probable pelvic fracture
10. Probable femoral fracture
11. Probable urethral tear secondary to item 9
12. Scalp laceration

SUGGESTED READING

Pousada L et al: *Emergency medicine,* Baltimore, 1996, Williams & Wilkins.

PROBLEM · 139

DIABETIC KETOACIDOSIS

"You Mean My Belly Aches because I Haven't Been Taking My Insulin Shots?"

Case 1 ■ A 17-Year-Old Male with Abdominal Pain

A 17-year-old male comes to the Emergency Department with acute abdominal pain. He describes the pain as follows: (1) *quality:* dull, aching; (2) *quantity:* baseline 8/10, incremental increases to 10/10, decreases to 6/10; (3) *location:* central abdominal; (4) *chronology:* began approximately 4 days ago and has been getting progressively worse, especially over last 18 hours; (5) *constancy/intermittency:* constant; (6) *aggravating factor:* movement; (7) *relieving factor:* relieved by rest; (8) *associated manifestations:* nausea, vomiting, and significantly increased thirst; (9) *radiation:* some radiation through to the back; (10) *previous pain history:* no similar episodes of same; and (11) *provocative maneuver:* superficial palpation to the abdomen reproduces the pain.

On examination, he appears dehydrated. His skin and his tongue are dry. His blood pressure is 140/70 mm Hg, and his pulse 84 bpm and regular. He is hyperventilating and his respiratory rate is 32 breaths/min. His abdomen is tender to touch. The tenderness is generalized. There is no rebound tenderness.

SELECT THE BEST ANSWER TO THE FOLLOWING QUESTIONS

Q1. Which of the following laboratory tests should you order at this time?
a. complete blood count (CBC)/differential (diff)
b. electrolytes
c. urinalysis
d. serum lipase
e. spot blood sugar
f. all of the above

Q2. Of the laboratory tests listed in Question 1, which one is likely to be abnormal to the greatest degree?
a. CBC/diff
b. serum potassium
c. serum sodium
d. serum lipase
e. spot blood sugar

The results of the laboratory investigations are as follows:
CBC = 17,500 with 20% bands
Potassium = 5.7 mEq/L
Chloride = 76 mEq/L
Sodium = 156 mEq/L
Bicarbonate = 12 mEq/L
Urinalysis pH = 4.5; leukocytes +, sugar +, ketones +
Lipase = pending
Blood sugar = 450 mg/dl
Blood pH = 7.1

Q3. What is the most likely diagnosis at this time in this patient?
a. diabetic hyperosmolar state
b. diabetic ketoacidosis
c. acute pancreatitis
d. acute peritonitis
e. none of the above

Q4. At this time, what would you do?
a. rehydrate the patient in the Emergency Room (ER) with oral fluids and discharge him
b. rehydrate the patient in the ER with intravenous (IV) fluids and discharge him
c. observe the patient for 2 hours before discharge
d. admit the patient for active treatment
e. it depends on the patient's condition

Q5. In the condition described, which one of the following situations regarding the serum/body potassium is usually true?
a. the serum potassium is low; total body potassium is low
b. the serum potassium is elevated; total body potassium is low
c. the serum potassium is low; total body potassium is high
d. the serum potassium is low; total body potassium is high
e. neither the serum potassium nor the total body potassium is usually altered

Q6. Electrolyte and fluid replacement in the condition described should initially be which of the following?
a. dextrose 5% normal saline
b. hypertonic saline
c. Ringer's lactate
d. one-half normal saline
e. normal saline

Q7. In this condition, which of the following pathophysiologic abnormalities usually does not occur?
a. elevated serum potassium
b. depressed pH
c. depressed serum glucagon level
d. elevated blood sugar
e. depressed serum bicarbonate level

Q8. Insulin is usually administered in this condition in a recommended dosage of approximately:
a. 0.1 units/kg/hr IV
b. 1.0 units/kg/hr IV
c. 1.5 units/kg/hr IV
d. 2.5 units/kg/hr IV
e. 0.5 units/kg/hr IV

Q9. In this condition, glucose is usually added to the IV solution when the serum glucose is lowered to which of the following?
   a. 600 mg/dl
   b. 500 mg/dl
   c. 400 mg/dl
   d. 250 mg/dl
   e. 125 mg/dl

Q10. Which of the following is not characteristic of the condition described?
   a. Kussmaul's respirations
   b. significant dehydration
   c. decreased respiratory rate
   d. acetone breath
   e. increased sweating

SHORT ANSWER MANAGEMENT PROBLEM
Describe the basic therapeutic principles of treating the condition described in Case 1.

ANSWERS

A1. **f.** This patient presented to the Emergency Department with acute abdominal pain. In addition to either an x-ray of the kidneys, ureter, and bladder or three views of the abdomen, this patient should have a complete blood chemistry workup, including at least CBC/diff, electrolytes, spot blood sugar, serum amylase or serum lipase, blood urea nitrogen (BUN) and creatinine, serum calcium, serum uric acid, and arterial blood gases.

A2. **e.** This patient has the signs and symptoms compatible with diabetic ketoacidosis (DKA). Although the CBC and diff, the serum electrolytes (sodium, potassium, bicarbonate, and BUN), and the pH and the P_{CO_2} may be abnormal, the plasma glucose is likely to be the test that is abnormal to the greatest degree.

A3. **b.** This patient most likely has DKA. A patient with DKA often initially comes to the Emergency Department with abdominal pain as the major symptom. Diabetes may often be overlooked in this situation and the patient not assessed sufficiently. This may result in the patient being discharged without the correct diagnosis being made. Ultimately, this could be catastrophic.

A4. **d.** This patient needs to be hospitalized now. He needs acute, active treatment in a highly monitored area, if not an intensive care unit. At the present time he has severe disturbances of his intravascular volume (he is significantly dehydrated), his electrolyte balance, his arterial blood gases, his blood sugar, and his serum insulin level.

A5. **b.** The serum potassium in a patient with DKA is often significantly elevated. This, however, is deceptive. Although the serum potassium is usually elevated, the total body potassium is usually low and the patient needs potassium added to the IV fluids.

This is true for two basic reasons. First, intra-cellular acidosis displaces potassium from the cells. This results in spillage of potassium into the plasma. Second, in an attempt to secrete hydrogen ions, the kidney tends to retain potassium ion. This prevents serum potassium ion levels from returning to normal. Thus because the cellular compartment normally contains the vast majority of the body's potassium ion, there is a total body deficit, but serum levels are raised.

A6. **e.** The requirements of fluid resuscitation can usually be met if therapy begins with normal saline at a rate of 10 to 20 ml/kg/hr for the first 2 hours. Amounts at the higher end of this range are used in cases with hypotension or severe acidosis. The subsequent rate is calculated from the estimated deficit; a rate of 3 to 6 ml/kg/hr will usually suffice. After the first 2 to 4 hours, normal saline can be replaced by ½ normal saline.

When the serum glucose approaches 250 mg/dl, 5% glucose solutions should be used to maintain glucose between 200 and 300 mg/dl.

A7. **c.** The serum insulin level in DKA is depressed, and, conversely, the glucagon levels are elevated because of the absence of insulin's inhibitory effect on glucagon secretion. Many of the symptoms of type 1 diabetes are caused by this unrestrained effect of glucagon on the target cells.

The basic principles of therapy are to replace deficits of fluid, replace deficits of electrolytes, replace carbohydrate deficits, and to reverse the catabolic state with insulin.

A8. **a.** There are many alternative methods for delivering insulin during the treatment of DKA; probably any method that delivers a dose of at least 0.1 units/kg/hr is acceptable. A constant IV insulin infusion offers many advantages, including simplicity of dosing, predictable insulin effect, and ease of dose adjustment. A convenient way to achieve a dose of 0.1 units/kg/hr in a constant infusion is to add 100 units of regular insulin to 100 ml of saline (1 unit/ml). This solution should be piggybacked onto replacement fluids so that each can be adjusted independently. Before the insulin infusion begins, 10 to 20 ml of insulin-saline mixture should be run through the tubing to saturate insulin binding on the plastic; the infusion is then begun at 0.1 ml/kg/hr. Remember to give potassium via IV infusion when administering insulin.

A9. **d.** As mentioned previously, when the serum glucose level approaches 250 mg/dl, the fluid replacement can be changed from isotonic saline to 5% glucose solutions.

A10. **c.** The respiratory rate in DKA is increased, not decreased.

Kussmaul breathing is a rapid, deep breathing pattern that is usually associated with metabolic acidosis. Increased sweating and dehydration are also common, as is acetone breath, a result of the production of acetone as a byproduct of the pathophysiologic process that produces DKA.

SOLUTION TO THE SHORT ANSWER MANAGEMENT PROBLEM

The basic therapeutic principles of treating DKA are as follows:
  a. Replacement of intravascular fluid volume (often several liters because of dehydration)
  b. Replacement of electrolytes (potassium, magnesium, phosphate, calcium), even though electrolyte panel suggests elevated potassium and sodium levels
  c. Replacement of IV insulin (beginning at 0.1 unit/kg/hr)
  d. Correction of metabolic acidotic state (by actions above the metabolic acidotic state will be corrected in most cases by itself). Bicarbonate administration should probably only be given to patients with a blood pH less than 6.9. Studies have not shown any decrease in morbidity/mortality when bicarbonate is given to patients with a blood pH between 6.9 and 7.1.
  e. Begin IV solution with normal saline; after the first 2 to 4 hours, this can be changed to ½ normal saline. Remember to add 10 to 20 mEq of potassium to the IV solution when administering insulin, even in the face of initial serum hyperkalemia. When the blood sugar reaches 250 mg/dl, ½ normal saline can be switched to dextrose 5% water or dextrose 5%, ½ normal saline.

SUMMARY OF THE DIAGNOSIS AND MANAGEMENT OF DKA

1. Diagnosis: Most often a young person comes to the Emergency Department with the most common complaints being polyuria, polydipsia, abdominal tenderness and rigidity, increased sweating, and, in severe cases, altered levels of consciousness. The most common error in not properly diagnosing DKA is not thinking of the diagnosis because of "concentrating on the abdominal pain" and a failure to associate abdominal pain with diabetes.

2. Pathophysiology: DKA is caused by insulin deficiency. Its development is promoted by an excess of counterregulatory hormones, including glucagon, catecholamines, cortisol, and growth hormone; these hormones act synergistically with insulin deficiency to reduce glucose utilization, increase hepatic glucose production, and increase lipolysis and hepatic ketogenesis.

3. Laboratory evaluation: investigations should include CBC/diff, electrolytes (potassium, magnesium, phosphate, calcium), BUN, creatinine or bicarbonate, serum amylase or lipase, plasma glucose, urinalysis, and arterial blood gases.

4. Management: See the Solution to Short Answer Management Problem.

5. Complications:
  a. Cerebral edema: Cerebral edema is a rare complication that may be caused by too aggressive fluid replacement therapy. This is best prevented by maintaining blood glucose levels between 200 and 300 mg/dl for the initial 24 hours of therapy.
  b. Pancreatitis
  c. Hypoxemia
  d. Hypoglycemia
  e. Hypokalemia
  f. Noncardiogenic pulmonary edema

SUGGESTED READINGS

Kitabchi AE et al: Diabetic ketoacidosis and hyperosmolar nonketotic state. In Rakel R, ed: *Conn's current therapy*, Philadelphia, 1999, WB Saunders.
Tierney LM, McPhee SJ, Papadakis MA, eds: *Current medical diagnosis and treatment, 2000*, ed 39, Stamford, Conn, 1999, Appleton & Lange.

PROBLEM · 1 4 0

EMERGENCY TREATMENT OF ABDOMINAL PAIN IN THE ELDERLY

"In All My Born Days I've Never Had Such a Stomach Ache."

Case 1 ■ An 84-Year-Old Male with Abdominal Pain

An 84-year-old male comes to your office with a 6-hour history of severe abdominal pain. The pain is described as follows: (1) *quality:* dull, aching; (2) *quantity:* severe, baseline 9/10, increases to 10/10 and decreases to 8/10; (3) *location:* epigastric; (4) *chronology:* began suddenly after supper 6 hours ago; (5) *radiation:* radiates through to the back; (6) *aggravating factor:* movement; (7) *relieving factor:* rest; (8) *provocative maneuver:* deep palpation to abdomen; (9) *pain history:* no previous episodes like this, no history of similar pain; (10) *previous significant history:* angina pectoris; (11) *continuous/intermittent:* continuous; (12) *associated manifestations:* faintness and dizziness with nausea.

On examination, the patient's blood pressure is 90/70 mm Hg and his pulse is 96 bpm and regular. His respiratory rate is 16 breaths/min. He is breathing normally. Examination of the abdomen reveals no distention and normal bowel sounds. There is, however, marked central abdominal tenderness on palpation.

SELECT THE BEST ANSWER TO THE FOLLOWING QUESTIONS

Q1. What is the major differential diagnosis in this patient's case?
a. ruptured aortic aneurysm
b. intestinal ischemia or infarction
c. perforated peptic ulcer
d. splenic infarction
e. all of the above

Q2. Given the history and physical examination findings, which of the following diagnostic possibilities is most likely?
a. ruptured aortic aneurysm
b. intestinal ischemia or infarction
c. perforated peptic ulcer
d. splenic infarction
e. myocardial infarction

Q3. The diagnosis of the condition described can best be confirmed by which of the following?
a. real-time ultrasound
b. computed tomography (CT) scan of the abdomen
c. magnetic resonance imaging scan of the abdomen
d. 12-lead electrocardiogram (ECG)
e. laparotomy

Q4. What is the most important diagnostic clue that leads you to arrive at the diagnosis?
a. the patient's hypotension
b. the location of the abdominal pain
c. the symptom of faintness and dizziness associated with hypotension
d. the periumbilical tenderness
e. none of the above

Q5. What is the most critical early intervention that must take place in this patient?
a. the placement of an endotracheal tube
b. the establishment of intravenous access for fluid and blood replacement
c. an abdominal paracentesis
d. the administration of a thrombolytic agent
e. the establishment of an arterial line

Q6. In which of the following conditions do pharmacotherapy and the adverse effects of iatrogenic disease play the greatest role?
a. ruptured aortic aneurysm
b. intestinal ischemia or infarction
c. perforated peptic ulcer
d. splenic infarction
e. diverticulitis

Q7. What is the therapeutic agent most closely associated with a perforated peptic ulcer?
a. ibuprofen
b. piroxicam
c. Naprosyn
d. aspirin
e. sulindac

Q8. What is the treatment of choice for the patient described in the problem?
a. intensive care unit (ICU) monitoring, thrombolytic therapy, aspirin, beta-blockers, and antiarrhythmic therapy
b. laparotomy—oversew perforation
c. laparotomy—removal of ischemic bowel
d. laparotomy—surgical repair of aortic aneurysm
e. laparotomy and splenectomy

Q9. Which of the following statements is (are) true regarding ruptured aortic aneurysm?
a. over 80% of abdominal aortic aneurysms are asymptomatic when first diagnosed
b. the diagnosis is often missed because physicians do not consider it
c. most abdominal aortic aneurysms are atherosclerotic in nature
d. all of the above statements are true
e. none of the above statements is true

Q10. What is the key to reducing morbidity and mortality in the condition described?
a. enhanced tertiary prevention
b. enhanced secondary prevention
c. regular yearly check-ups
d. early diagnosis and intervention
e. early administration of thrombolytic agents

SHORT ANSWER MANAGEMENT PROBLEM
Describe the major differential diagnosis of the elderly patient coming to the Emergency Department with a diagnosis of abdominal pain.

ANSWERS

A1. **e.** The differential diagnosis of abdominal pain in the elderly is extensive. In this case the sudden onset of the pain and the severity of the pain strongly suggests an acute abdomen. At the top of the list would be ruptured aortic aneurysm, perforated peptic ulcer, intestinal ischemia or infarction, a perforated diverticulum, and pancreatitis.

A2. **a.** Given the history and physical findings, the most likely diagnosis is ruptured aortic aneurysm. The tip-off to ruptured aortic aneurysm in this case is the dizziness associated with pain and hypotension that the patient experienced early in the symptomatology. The dizziness, hypotension, and pain suggest at least a leaking aneurysm.

A3. **b.** The working diagnosis can best be confirmed by the performance of a CT scan of the abdomen. The common presentation of abdominal pain in the elderly is a good argument for having a CT scanner in close proximity to the Emergency Room. An ultrasound screen has largely been supplanted by a CT scan in the emergency setting. Although ultrasound is still used in some places as a screen, it is no longer recommended for an emergency situation.

A4. **c.** See Answer 2.

A5. **b.** Remember the ABCs of resuscitation. Since this patient is breathing normally, the next most important step is circulation. You should immediately place either a central venous pressure line or two large-bore intravenous lines of at least #16 gauge.

A6. **c.**

A7. **d.** Iatrogenic disease (in the form of nonsteroidal antiinflammatory drug [NSAID] prescription) is closely associated with perforated peptic ulcer. Many thousands of Americans die each year from perforated and bleeding peptic ulcers caused by the prescription of NSAIDs.

The NSAID (and it really is a nonsteroidal antiinflammatory) that causes more peptic ulcers and is associated with more perforated peptic ulcers than any other agent (on a prevalence/administration rate basis) is acetylsalicylic acid (aspirin).

A8. **d.** The treatment of choice in this patient is surgical repair of the aortic aneurysm.

A9. **d.** Over 80% of aortic aneurysms are asymptomatic when first diagnosed. As previously stated, the diagnosis is often missed because the possibility is not considered.

The vast majority of aortic aneurysms are atherosclerotic in nature and result from a generalized atherosclerotic process.

A10. **d.** The key to reducing morbidity and mortality from aortic aneurysm is early diagnosis and intervention. Although routine screening for aortic aneurysms in the elderly is not recommended by the U.S. Preventive Task Force on the Periodic Health Examination, it is wise to consider this on a risk-factor basis in the patients you see. High-risk patients and patients with symptoms that even vaguely suggest aortic aneurysm should probably be evaluated by both physical examination and CT scan.

SOLUTION TO THE SHORT ANSWER MANAGEMENT PROBLEM

The following is a differential diagnosis of abdominal pain in the elderly as an Emergency Department presentation.
    a. Nonabdominal-related causes:
        1) Myocardial infarction
        2) Pneumonia
        3) Pericarditis
    b. Abdominal-related causes
        1) Constipation (major cause)
        2) Diverticulitis
        3) Cholecystitis/cholelithiasis
        4) Peptic ulcer disease/gastritis
        5) Pancreatitis
        6) Appendicitis
        7) Bowel obstruction—large bowel, small bowel
        8) Inflammatory bowel disease
        9) Carcinoma—stomach, pancreas, colon
        10) Ruptured aortic aneurysm
        11) Intestinal ischemia or infarction
        12) Urinary tract sepsis

SUMMARY OF THE DIAGNOSIS AND EMERGENCY TREATMENT OF ABDOMINAL PAIN IN THE ELDERLY

1. Diagnosis:
    a. Differential diagnosis as previously discussed
    b. Remember that constipation is the single most common cause of abdominal pain in the elderly.

c. When elderly patients come to the Emergency Department with sudden onset of abdominal pain, think of the following:
   1) Nonabdominal causes: Myocardial infarction
   2) Abdominal causes: Ruptured aortic aneurysm, perforated peptic ulcer, and intestinal ischemia

2. Investigations: Basic investigations in an elderly patient with abdominal pain: complete blood count; electrolytes; ECG; x-ray of the kidneys, ureter, and bladder; urinalysis; and either a CT scan or a real-time ultrasound.

3. Treatment:
   a. Treat the cause.
   b. Remember the ABCs of resuscitation in acutely ill elderly patients.
   c. Remember that elderly patients present differently from younger patients—they often lack the classic signs and symptoms of any acute abdominal condition.
   d. A major error in acutely ill elderly patients seen in community or rural hospitals is the failure to transfer to a tertiary care center soon enough.

SUGGESTED READING

Hazzard WR et al, eds: *Principles of geriatric medicine and gerontology,* New York, 1994, McGraw-Hill.

PROBLEM·141

POISON MANAGEMENT

"It Really Was an Accident. I Just Forgot How Many I Took."

Case 1 ■ A 24-Year-Old Female Brought into the Emergency Department with a Suspected Drug Overdose

A 24-year-old female is brought into the Emergency Department of the local hospital with a suspected drug overdose. She was found unconscious beside her bed with a number of unmarked pill containers beside her. Her friend, who found her, does not know any other details. Her friend is hysterical and has to be restrained.

You are called by the first-year resident who is on his first day of service. He asks you, "What should I do now?" You come down immediately and examine the patient. The patient has a Reed Coma scale of stage 1. This includes the following:
1. Conscious level: coma
2. Pain response: decreased

3. Reflexes: normal
4. Respirations: normal
5. Circulation: normal

The patient's blood pressure is 90/70 mm Hg, her pulse is 84 bpm and regular, and her respirations are 16 breaths/min and regular. No other abnormalities are evident. Her pupils are equal and reactive to light and accommodation.

SELECT THE BEST ANSWER TO THE FOLLOWING QUESTIONS

Q1. What is the first step in the management of the potential drug overdose victim?
   a. administration of syrup of ipecac
   b. administration of naloxone
   c. administration of dextrose 5% water
   d. administration of activated charcoal
   e. none of the above

Q2. Accidental poisonings make up what percentage of total poisoning episodes in children and adults?
   a. 20%
   b. 40%
   c. 60%
   d. 70%
   e. 85%

Q3. The majority of drug-related suicide attempts involve which of the following?
   a. central nervous system anxiolytics
   b. central nervous system antidepressant medications
   c. central nervous system antipsychotic medications
   d. over-the-counter analgesics
   e. prescription narcotic analgesics

Q4. What is the most common cause of death in drug overdose patients outside the hospital?
   a. lower airway obstruction
   b. upper airway obstruction
   c. cardiac arrest
   d. ventricular fibrillation
   e. complete heart block

Q5. Which of the following conditions resulting in coma or altered level of consciousness can be treated quickly if recognized immediately?
   a. hypoxia
   b. hypoglycemia
   c. opioid overdose
   d. b and c
   e. all of the above

Q6. Which of the following is not routinely indicated in the initial assessment of the possible overdose patient?
   a. a history from anyone who has knowledge of the patient
   b. physical examination with particular attention to vital signs and neurologic status
   c. complete blood count (CBC) and serum electrolytes
   d. complete toxicology screen
   e. blood glucose

Q7. The anion gap is defined as which of the following?
   a. anion gap = $[K^+ + Cl^-] - [Na^+ + HCO_3^-]$
   b. anion gap = $[Na^+ + K^+] - [Cl^- + HCO_3^-]$
   c. anion gap = $[Cl^-] + [Na^+] + [K^+] - [HCO_3^-]$
   d. anion gap = $[pH] + [Na^+ + Cl^-]$
   e. anion gap = $[HCO_3^-] - [Cl^- + Na^+]$

Q8. Which of the following is not a cause of an increased anion gap?
   a. an accumulation of organic acids
   b. diabetic ketoacidosis
   c. reduced inorganic acid excretion (that is, chronic renal failure)
   d. hypernatremia
   e. lactic acidosis

Q9. Which of the following is (are) associated with an increased anion gap?
   a. salicylates
   b. methanol
   c. ethylene glycol
   d. organic solvents
   e. all of the above

Q10. Following the assessment and maintenance of vital functions, which of the following is (are) the next step(s)?
   a. antidote administration (if poison known)
   b. prevention of absorption
   c. reduction of local damage
   d. b and c
   e. all of the above

Q11. Generally speaking, in poison management, which of the following is the most effective method of gastrointestinal decontamination?
   a. syrup of ipecac
   b. gastric lavage
   c. administration of activated charcoal
   d. dilution of poison with intravenous (IV) fluids
   e. none of the above

Q12. Which of the following should be administered with the first dose of activated charcoal (if not contraindicated)?
   a. magnesium hydroxide
   b. aluminum hydroxide
   c. 70% sorbitol
   d. calcium carbonate
   e. none of the above

Q13. What is the specific antidote for the treatment of acetaminophen poisoning?
   a. N-acetyl coenzyme A
   b. N-acetyl ATPase
   c. N-acetylcysteine
   d. calcium disodium etidronate
   e. atropine

Q14. What is the specific antidote for the treatment of benzodiazepine poisoning?
   a. Antabuse
   b. naloxone
   c. carbamazepine
   d. flumazenil
   e. naltrexone

Q15. What is the specific antidote for the treatment of methanol or ethylene glycol poisoning?
   a. Antabuse
   b. naloxone
   c. ethanol
   d. flumazenil
   e. naltrexone

Q16. What is the specific antidote for the treatment of opioid intoxication (poisoning)?
   a. Antabuse
   b. naloxone
   c. carbamazepine
   d. flumazenil
   e. naltrexone

Q17. What is the specific antidote for the treatment of organophosphate poisoning?
   a. ethanol
   b. naloxone
   c. naltrexone
   d. atropine
   e. arginine

SHORT ANSWER MANAGEMENT PROBLEM
Describe the absolute and relative contraindications to the administration of syrup of ipecac in the induction of emesis in a poisoning victim.

ANSWERS

A1. **e.** The first step in the management of the potential overdose victim is the assessment and support of the ABCs (airway, breathing, circulation) of life support. Before any medications are administered, a secure airway must be established, respiratory and circulatory system function should be assessed and supported, and IV or central venous lines should be inserted.

A2. **e.** The severity of the manifestations of acute poisoning exposures varies greatly with the age and intent of the victims. Accidental poisoning exposures make up 80% to 85% of all poisoning episodes and are most frequent in children under the age of 5. Intentional poisonings constitute 10% to 15% of all poisonings, and often these patients require more intensive therapy. Suicide attempts represent a significant number of these poisonings, and the use of toxic substances is often involved.

A3. **d.** The top drugs used in suicide attempts (all ages and in order of frequency) are as follows:
   a. Over-the-counter analgesics
   b. Prescribed sedative-hypnotics
   c. Prescribed benzodiazepines
   d. Cleaning agents and petroleum products
   e. Alcohol and controlled substances
   f. Pesticides
   g. Tricyclic antidepressants
   h. Plants
   i. Carbon monoxide
   j. Opioids

A4. **b.** The most common cause of death in drug overdose patients outside the hospital is upper airway obstruction. Any patient who is comatose and has absent protective airway reflexes is able to tolerate an endotracheal (ET) tube (cuffed for those over the ages 7) and should have one inserted immediately.

A5. **e.** The second step in the management of the potential overdose victim is the treatment of specific conditions with specific antidotes. Because it is almost impossible to differentiate one from another at this time, give the following:
   a. 2 mg of naloxone (antidote for opioid intoxication)
   b. 100 mg thiamine IV (antidote for Wernicke's encephalopathy)
   c. 50 cc of 50% dextrose (antidote for hypoglycemia—secondary to insulin overdose)
   d. supplemental oxygen

A6. **d.** After you have stabilized the patient, you should attempt to establish the identity of the particular poison.

A physical examination with emphasis on vital signs (and particular attention to pupil size and reaction to light and accommodation), temperature, and a complete neurologic examination should be done.

Although the patient will be unable to supply accurate (if any) information, as much information as possible should be obtained from the family, friends, the patient's physician, or anyone else who knows the patient.

Laboratory testing should include serum electrolytes (and measurement of anion gap), arterial blood gases, blood glucose, CBC, a 12-lead electrocardiogram (ECG), three views of the abdomen, and specific drug levels. Generally, however, a routine toxicology screen is not indicated, nor is it appropriate.

A7. **b.** The term *anion gap* was developed to indicate the difference between the measured sodium plus potassium ion level and the measured chloride and bicarbonate ion level (really the CO_2 content). This is important, especially in diabetic ketoacidosis and toxic acidic chemicals.

A8. **d.** An increased anion gap will be induced by the following:
   a. An accumulation of organic acids, such as that seen in lactic acidosis
   b. An accumulation of organic acids, such as that seen in diabetic ketoacidosis
   c. An accumulation of organic acids, such as that seen in acute renal failure and toxic ingestions
   d. Exogenous anions
   e. Reduced inorganic acid excretion, such as seen in chronic renal failure
   f. An increase in the anionic contribution of unmeasured weak acids
   g. A decrease in unmeasured cations
Hypernatremia causes a decreased anion gap rather than an increased anion gap.

A9. **e.** The determination of the presence or absence of a normal anion gap will help define the cause of a metabolic acidotic episode. The normal anion gap is 8 to 12. An increased anion gap can usually be traced to one of the following:
   a. Toxic amounts of salicylates
   b. Any amount of methanol
   c. Any amount of ethylene glycol
   d. An overdose of iron (as in ferrous sulfate)
   e. Any amount of paraldehyde

f. An overdose of phenformin

g. An overdose of isoniazid

h. Certain organic solvents such as toluene

A10. **e.** The second step after the assessment and maintenance of vital functions includes the prevention of absorption, administration of an antidote (if known), and the reduction of local damage.

Reduction of local damage applies primarily to the eye (with a caustic acid or a caustic base) and the skin (with a significant burn).

A11. **c.** The prevention of absorption is best accomplished by gastrointestinal decontamination. First, to decrease gastrointestinal absorption, emesis should be induced or gastric aspiration and lavage performed. Neither of these methods is completely effective; each removes only 30% to 50% of the ingested substance. These methods are recommended in the time period up to 4 hours after ingestion. In the emergency room, however, there are few indications for the administration of syrup of ipecac or gastric lavage because they delay the more effective treatment of activated charcoal (an exception to this would be a documented very recent ingestion).

A12. **c.** The dose of activated charcoal to give is 1 g/kg/dose orally with a minimum of 15 g. The usual adolescent and adult dose is 60 to 100 g. It is administered as a slurry mixed with water or by orogastric tube.

Dilution of the initial poison is useful but not as useful as the administration of cathartics along with the activated charcoal. The agent of choice is probably 70% sorbitol. It is recommended that 70% sorbitol be given with the first dose of activated charcoal.

A13. **c.** N-acetylcysteine is the specific antidote that should be administered in cases of acetaminophen poisoning. It can be given orally or intravenously. The IV route is the route of first choice.

A14. **d.** Flumazenil (Mazicon) is the first benzodiazepine antagonist to be approved by the Food and Drug Administration. Flumazenil binds competitively and reversibly to the GABA-benzodiazepine receptor complex and inhibits the effects of benzodiazepine. The drug is approved for the treatment of benzodiazepine overdose or for the reversal of benzodiazepine oversedation.

A15. **c.** Ethanol is the antidote for methanol or ethylene glycol poisoning. The first step in the metabolism of both of these poisons is oxidation, using alcohol de-

hydrogenase as the catalyst. Ethanol is a preferred substrate, thereby inhibiting their conversion to toxic metabolites.

A16. **b.** The antidote for opioid overdose is naloxone. Once an opioid user is detoxified, he or she may benefit from opioid antagonist therapy with naltrexone. Naltrexone is a long-acting, orally active opioid antagonist that, when taken regularly, entirely blocks mμ-opioid receptors, thus blocking the opioid's euphoric, analgesic, and sedative properties.

A17. **d.** The specific antidote for organophosphate poisoning is atropine. Organophosphate poisoning is most commonly observed in the ingestion of herbicides and pesticides.

SOLUTION TO THE SHORT ANSWER MANAGEMENT PROBLEM

Specific contraindications to the administration of syrup of ipecac can be divided into absolute contraindications and relative contraindications.

    a. Absolute contraindications:
1) Caustic (alkali) or corrosive (acid) ingestion
2) Convulsions (danger of aspiration and possible induction of laryngospasm)
3) Coma (possibility of aspiration with the loss of protective airway reflexes)
4) Absence of a cough reflex
5) Hematemesis
6) A child less than 6 months of age

    b. Relative contraindications:
1) Petroleum distillate ingestion of high-viscosity agents
2) Agents that are likely to rapidly produce coma (short-acting barbiturates) or convulsions (propoxyphene, camphor, isoniazid, strychnine, tricyclic antidepressants)
3) Significant prior vomiting

SUMMARY OF THE GENERAL MANAGEMENT PRINCIPLES OF POISON MANAGEMENT

1. Assessment and maintenance of vital functions:
    a. The ABCs of resuscitation:
1) **A**irway management (ET tube in unconscious patient)
2) **B**reathing (assisted ventilation if the respiratory rate and depth are inadequate)
3) **C**irculation (assessed by blood pressure, heart rate, and heart rhythm); volume expan-

sion may be indicated if there is hypotension or other measurements of decreased cardiac function: Ringer's lactate or normal saline is preferred for hypovolemia; plasma expanders and vasopressors are indicated if IV fluids are not sufficient.

b. History, physical examination, and laboratory investigations:
  1) History: Attempt to elicit history from any family member or friend who happens to be there. Attempt to search for empty pill containers.
  2) Physical examination: Pay particular attention to vital signs and neurologic examination with emphasis on either the Glasgow coma scale or the Reed coma scale.
  3) Laboratory investigations:
    a) 12-lead ECG
    b) CBC, electrolytes, BUN, creatinine, glucose Calculate the anion gap = $(Na^+ + K^+) - (Cl^- + HCO_3^-)$. Remember that the normal anion gap is 8 to 12.
    c) Arterial blood gases
    d) Chest x-ray
    e) Three views of the abdomen
    f) Aspirin and acetaminophen levels should be checked in all intentional overdoses.

2. Treatment:
  a. Immediate treatment to all victims:
    1) ABCs (may include ET tube, IV fluids)
    2) 2 mg naloxone
    3) 100 mg thiamine IV
    4) 50 cc of 50% glucose
    5) Supplemental oxygen
  b. Decontamination:
    1) Induction of emesis with syrup of ipecac (not usually recommended in hospital setting)
    2) Gastric lavage (if ingestion occurred less than 60 minutes earlier and airway is protected)
    3) Administration of activated charcoal plus sorbitol as a cathartic
  c. Elimination:
    1) Enhance elimination with pH-dependent diuresis
    2) Multidose activated charcoal
    3) Dialysis: Hemodialysis
  d. Specific antidotes:
    1) Substance: Acetaminophen; antidote: N-acetylcysteine
    2) Substance: Opioid analgesics; antidote: naloxone
    3) Substance: Methanol or ethylene glycol; antidote: ethanol
    4) Substance: Benzodiazepines; antidote: flumazenil
    5) Substance: Organophosphates; antidote: atropine

3. Most common drug overdoses:
  a. Over-the-counter analgesics (acetaminophen is number one)
  b. Prescribed hypnotics-sedatives
  c. Prescribed benzodiazepines

4. Prevention of complications: Anticipate and treat complications such as seizures, coma, hypotension, and hyperthermia.

SUGGESTED READINGS

Linden CH., Lovejoy FH Jr: Poisoning and drug overdose. In Fauci AS et al, eds: *Harrison's principles of internal medicine,* ed 14, New York, 1998, McGraw-Hill.

Mofenson HC et al: Acute poisonings. In Rakel R, ed: *Conn's current therapy,* Philadelphia, 1994, WB Saunders.

Pousada L et al: *Emergency medicine,* Baltimore, 1996, Williams & Wilkins.

PROBLEM·142

URTICARIA AND ANGIONEUROTIC EDEMA

"If There Are Shrimp in That Soup, It Will Kill Me. Keep It Away!"

Case 1 ■ A 24-Year-Old Male Who Developed a Skin Rash while Playing Football

A 24-year-old male was playing football with his friends on a hot summer afternoon. Approximately 10 minutes into the game, he began to "feel funny," and he began to itch all over. He sat down, but the itch did not go away; it only got worse. Within 10 minutes he was covered with a raised rash all over his body, with individual lesions varying from 2 cm to 5 cm in diameter. His lips also became very swollen, and he began to have trouble breathing.

His friends called 911, and he was brought to the local hospital, which is located only 3 minutes from the football field. A friend who works with the patient tells you that he is certain that the problem has arisen because of stress; the patient apparently had a bad day at work today.

On examination, his respiratory rate is 42 breaths/min and he is gasping. His lips are swollen, and he has a prominent, raised skin rash with lesions of various sizes covering his entire body. His blood pressure is 75/50 mm Hg.

SELECT THE BEST ANSWER
TO THE FOLLOWING QUESTIONS

Q1. At this time, what is your first priority?
  a. give the patient scopolamine
  b. give the patient oral (PO) steroids
  c. give the patient intravenous (IV) Benadryl
  d. give the patient PO chlorpheniramine
  e. none of the above

Q2. What is the most likely diagnosis in this patient?
  a. ordinary urticaria with angioneurotic edema
  b. exercise-induced bronchospasm
  c. exercise-induced anaphylaxis and urticaria
  d. urticarial vasculitis with angioneurotic edema
  e. stress-induced urticaria with esterase inhibitor deficiency

Q3. What is the first priority in this patient?
  a. establish a large-gauge IV line
  b. establish a central venous pressure (CVP) line if possible; if not possible, establish two large-bore IV lines
  c. intubate the patient
  d. administer 100% oxygen to the patient by nasal specs
  e. draw blood gases

Q4. What is the second priority in the management of this patient?
  a. auscultate both lung fields
  b. forget this "tube and airway" business; get with the IV lines and get with them now!
  c. draw blood gases
  d. perform a chest x-ray to check the position of the endotracheal (ET) tube
  e. administer 100% oxygen by Venturi Mask

Q5. What is the third priority in the management of this patient?
  a. draw blood gases
  b. draw serum electrolytes
  c. put two large-bore peripheral IV lines in
  d. put military antishock trousers (MASTs) on the patient
  e. administer "pretty much every pressor agent you can think of"

Q6. Which of the following is (are) also indicated in the management of this patient?
  a. administer isotonic fluids
  b. administer epinephrine intravenously, subcutaneously (SQ), or intramuscularly (IM)
  c. administer Solu-medrol IV
  d. administer vasopressor agents if blood pressure does not rise with the measures outlined in a, b, and c
  e. all of the above

Q7. With respect to exercise in the future, what should your advice be to this patient?
  a. take an antihistamine before exercise
  b. carry an epinephrine kit during exercise at all times
  c. begin with only short periods of exercise and work up
  d. do not exercise alone
  e. all of the above

Q8. Angioneurotic edema is most likely to occur in which of the following situations?
  a. allergy to peanuts
  b. allergy to chocolate
  c. allergy to milk
  d. allergy to red wine
  e. allergy to monosodium glutamate

Case 2 ■ A 51-Year-Old Farmer with a Nonhealing Ulcer on the Tip of His Nose

A 51-year-old farmer develops a nonhealing ulcer on the tip of his nose. It has been present for the past 6 months and has not gotten any better. His wife brings him to the Emergency Department to have it checked.

On examination, there is a 0.5-cm ulcer "shaped like a crater." There is a depression in the center surrounded by a scaly exterior.

Q9. What is the most likely diagnosis?
  a. squamous cell carcinoma of the nose
  b. basal cell carcinoma of the nose
  c. actinic keratosis
  d. malignant melanoma—atypical
  e. atypical nevus

Q10. What is the treatment of choice for this lesion in this patient?
  a. cryosurgery
  b. electrodesiccation and curettage
  c. excisional surgery
  d. Moh's micrographic surgery
  e. chemotherapy: 5-fluorouracil

Case 3 ■ A 65-Year-Old Male with a Nonhealing Skin Lesion on His Lower Lip

A 65-year-old male comes to the Emergency Department for assessment of a nonhealing skin lesion on his lower lip. He comes into the Emergency Department tonight because his wife has been bugging him about it, and he "finally got tired of all the nagging."

This is 1 cm in diameter and has been growing steadily over the past 4 years. It has been bleeding on and off for the last year. The patient has smoked a pipe for the last 40 years.

Q11 What is the most likely diagnosis in this case?
  a. actinic keratosis
  b. squamous cell carcinoma
  c. basal cell carcinoma
  d. herpes simplex virus
  e. keratoacanthoma

Q12. Which of the following treatments is not contraindicated in the management of this lesion in this patient?
  a. cryosurgery
  b. electrodesiccation
  c. curettage and electrodesiccation
  d. excisional biopsy
  e. all of the above are contraindicated

Case 4 ■ A 45-Year-Old Female with Scaly Patches

A 45-year-old female patient has a 5-year history of erythematous, round, scaly patches on both elbows. She is now beginning to develop one on her left hand.

She comes into the Emergency Department this evening when she noticed the onset of significant pain, tenderness, and swelling in some of the small joints of her hands and feet. She wonders if the two symptoms are related.

Q13. At this time, what would you tell this patient?
  a. there is no relationship
  b. she has "nervous dermatitis" and now has developed "nervous joints"; the two are completely unrelated
  c. yes; the skin lesions sometimes precede a certain type of arthritis
  d. she has Lyme disease
  e. you would not tell her anything; instead you would refer her to the nearest dermatologist

Q14. What would be the treatment of first choice for this patient's skin lesions?
  a. "zap and burn" electrocautery
  b. cryosurgery
  c. medium- to high-potency topical corticosteroids
  d. "freeze and remove": liquid nitrogen
  e. a complex tar solution

Case 5 ■ A 25-Year-Old Female with Pruritic, Polygonal, Flat-Topped Violaceous Papules

A 2-cm skin lesion located on the wrist of a 25-year-old female is best described as "pruritic, polygonal, flat-topped violaceous papules."

Q15. What is the most likely diagnosis of this skin lesion?
  a. pityriasis rosea
  b. pityriasis alba
  c. lichen planus
  d. hairy oral leukoplakia
  e. tinea versicolor

Case 6 ■ A 67-Year-Old Farmer with Skin Lesions on His Ears

A number of skin lesions are present on the ears of a 67-year-old farmer. They are erythematous, scaly, and growing slightly larger in size over time. The largest is 1.0 cm in diameter. The more time the farmer spends in the sun, the more these skin lesions seem to grow. His wife has dragged him into the Emergency Department tonight.

Q16. What is the most likely diagnosis of these skin lesions?
  a. seborrheic dermatitis
  b. keratoacanthomas
  c. actinic keratoses
  d. lichen planus
  e. parapsoriasis

Case 7 ■ A 57-Year-Old Farmer with Greasy, Warty, Heaped-Up Skin Lesions

A 57-year-old farmer has a number of "greasy, warty, heaped-up" skin lesions present on both cheeks. These seem to be growing and are concerning the patient. The largest is 1.0 cm in diameter.

Q17. What is the most likely diagnosis of these skin lesions in this patient?
a. seborrheic dermatitis
b. seborrheic keratosis
c. actinic keratoses
d. lichen planus
e. parapsoriasis

Case 8 ■ A 29-Year-Old Farmer with a Brown Skin Lesion

A 29-year-old farmer has developed a brown skin lesion on the back of his neck. It has expanded significantly over the past 6 months and is beginning to darken in color. The present size of the skin lesion is 4 cm × 3 cm. He finished harvesting this afternoon, so he came into the Emergency Department tonight.

Q18. You are most concerned about which of the following in this patient?
a. superficial spreading squamous cell carcinoma
b. superficial spreading basal cell carcinoma
c. superficial spreading malignant melanoma
d. superficial spreading intraepithelial carcinoma
e. none of the above

Q19. The "herald patch" (solitary lesion, mildly pruritic, oval in shape, young adult) is associated with which of the following diagnoses in young adults?
a. pityriasis alba
b. pityriasis rosea
c. pityriasis rosacea
d. pityriasis versicolor
e. pityriasis multiforme

Q20. The natural evolution of which of these skin lesions to its worst potential is known as the Stevens-Johnson syndrome?
a. erythema marginatum
b. erythema nodosum
c. erythema chronicum migrans
d. erythema multiforme
e. pemphigus vulgaris

Q21. What is the most common drug to cause urticaria and angioedema?
a. acetaminophen
b. sulfonamide antibiotic
c. ampicillin antibiotic
d. aspirin
e. Naprosyn

Q22. Which of the following form(s) part of an allergic triad?
a. nasal polyps
b. asthma
c. aspirin sensitivity
d. all of the above
e. none of the above

SHORT ANSWER MANAGEMENT PROBLEM
Describe the pathophysiology of urticaria and angioneurotic edema.

ANSWERS

A1. **e.** Your first priority is to go through the ABCs of cardiopulmonary resuscitation.

A2. **c.** The diagnosis in this case is exercise-induced anaphylaxis and urticaria. Certain foods and medication can coprecipitate an episode of exercise-induced anaphylaxis.

A3. **c.** Establish an airway. This patient, from the history given, is close to having his airway completely obstructed. Thus the placement of a properly sized ET tube is the first priority.

A4. **a.** Establish proper ventilation. Make sure that the ET tube is in the trachea and not in the esophagus, and establish that there is bilateral airflow through auscultation of both lung fields.

A5. **c.** Circulation: establish access with a CVP line or two large-bore IV lines. Start isotonic fluids (Ringer's lactate or normal saline).

A6. **e.** Treatment should also include SQ epinephrine 0.3 to 0.5 ml (for patients with severe respiratory symptoms or blood pressure <70 mm Hg). IV epinephrine and corticosteroids should be given, and pressor agents (dopamine, dobutamine) should be given only if necessary.

A7. **e.** This patient should be careful in participating in any sports that will bring on physical urticaria; whether he decides to abstain is a personal risk/benefit decision.
If he is going to begin exercise again, however, he should do the following:
a. Begin with only a short period of exercise. The more intense the exercise, the more likely symptoms will occur.
b. Take an antihistamine before exercise.

c. Carry an epinephrine kit during exercise at all times.

d. Do not exercise alone.

e. Do not eat food for at least 4 hours before exercise.

A8. **a.** Angioneurotic edema is life threatening. It occurs most commonly in association with food allergy. The two most common foods implicated in angioneurotic edema are nuts (of all kinds) and fish and shellfish. In the case of the latter, even the odor of the cooking of the fish or shellfish may be enough to set off a life-threatening reaction.

Angioneurotic edema associated with food kills hundreds of Americans each year.

A9. **b.** This patient has the typical description of a basal cell carcinoma.

A10. **c.** The treatment alternatives are as follows:
a. Excisional surgery
b. Electrodesiccation and curettage
c. Cryosurgery
d. Mohs' microscopic surgery
e. Radiation therapy
f. Chemotherapy: 5-fluorouracil

Although all of these procedures can be used to eliminate the cancer, because of the importance of making a pathologic diagnosis without destroying the specimen, all but excisional surgery are contraindicated.

A11. **b.** This patient has what appears by description to be a squamous cell carcinoma of the lip.

A12. **d.** As in Answer 10, the procedure of choice is excisional biopsy. Again, the tissue must not be destroyed. All other treatments provided as options are, therefore, contraindicated.

A13. **c.** This patient has psoriasis with progression to psoriatic arthritis, the latter of which needs to be investigated.

A14. **c.**

A15. **c.**

A16. **c.**

A17. **b.**

A18. **c.** Any change in a pigmented skin lesion, including color, bleeding, scaling, size, or texture, can be a malignant melanoma.

A19. **b.**

A20. **d.**

A21. **d.**

A22. **d.** The most common drug causing angioneurotic edema is aspirin. Many of the patients who develop aspirin anaphylaxis have the following allergic triad:
a. Aspirin sensitivity
b. Asthma
c. Nasal polyps

Any individual who has developed a significant allergic reaction or angioneurotic edema to aspirin should never take another nonsteroidal antiinflammatory agent. There is a very high cross-reactivity.

SOLUTION TO THE SHORT ANSWER MANAGEMENT PROBLEM

Sequence of events producing urticaria and angioneurotic edema:
a. Difference between urticaria and angioneurotic edema:
1) Urticaria: caused by plasma leakage into the skin
2) Angioneurotic edema: caused by plasma leakage into the subcutaneous or submucosal tissue
b. Causes of plasma leakage: plasma leakage is mediated by the release of the following:
1) Histamine from the mast cells
2) Bradykinin from the mast cells
3) Other vasoactive substances from the mast cells
c. Activation of various systems along with the substance release; there is activation of the following:
1) Complement system
2) Fibrinolytic system
3) Kinin system
d. Skin lesions produced by plasma leakage produce:
1) Wheals (dermal edema)
2) Subcutaneous edema (angioedema)
3) Submucosal edema (angioedema)
e. Skin lesion characteristics:
1) Usually total body
2) Begin as "small wheals" and eventually coalesce
3) Pruritic and erythematous
f. Physiologic consequences: serious complications include:
1) Airway edema and airway closure

2) Hypoxemia

3) Hypotension and shock

g. Treatment of angioneurotic edema:

   1) Airway management; intubate if necessary

   2) 100% oxygen

   3) Epinephrine 0.3 to 0.5 ml SQ

   4) Antihistamine

   5) Corticosteroid

   6) Administer isotonic fluids (Ringer's lactate, normal saline)

   7) Vasopressor agents if hypotension is not corrected

SUMMARY OF THE DIAGNOSIS AND TREATMENT OF URTICARIA AND ANGIONEUROTIC EDEMA

1. Seriousness of problem: A life-threatening problem that must be treated both quickly and appropriately

2. Development of condition: Urticaria can develop for many reasons:

   a. Temperature

   b. Exercise

   c. Response to food and exercise together

   d. Stress

   e. Certain foods (sometimes just odors)

   f. Drug allergy (such as aspirin)

3. Most important treatment: prevention

4. Treatment in detail:

   a. Always follow the ABCs of resuscitation.

   b. Patients should do the following:

      1) Carry epinephrine and antihistamines

      2) Never eat a food that they are even remotely concerned may contain what they are allergic to

      3) Follow treatment protocol just discussed

5. Most common foods causing urticaria and angioneurotic edema are as follows:

   a. Peanuts and other nuts

   b. Shellfish and fish

6. Most common drug causing angioneurotic edema: Aspirin

7. Severity of future reactions: Generally speaking, the reactions experienced increases in severity each time.

SUGGESTED READING

Gratten CE: Urticaria and angioedema. In Rakel R, ed: *Conn's current therapy,* Philadelphia, 1994, WB Saunders.

P R O B L E M · 1 4 3

FRACTURE MANAGEMENT

"You Don't Really Expect Me to Wear That Thing for 6 Weeks, Do You?"

Case 1 ■ A 75-Year-Old Female Who Slipped and Fell on Her Outstretched Hand

A 75-year-old female is brought to the Emergency Department after having fallen on her outstretched hand. She complains of pain in the area of the right wrist.

On examination, there is a deformity in the area of the right wrist. The wrist has the appearance of a dinner fork. There is significant tenderness over the distal radius. Both pulses and sensation distally to the injury are completely normal.

SELECT THE BEST ANSWER TO THE FOLLOWING QUESTIONS

Q1. What is the most likely diagnosis in this patient?

   a. fracture of the distal ulna with dislocation of the radial head

   b. fracture of the carpal scaphoid

   c. fracture of the radial styloid

   d. Colles' fracture

   e. fracture of the shaft of the radius with dislocation of the ulnar head

Q2. What is the treatment of choice for the patient described?

   a. internal reduction and immobilization

   b. internal reduction and fixation

   c. external reduction and immobilization

   d. external reduction and fixation

   e. none of the above

Case 2 ■ An 18-Year-Old Basketball Player Who Fell on His Outstretched Hand

An 18-year-old basketball player is brought to the Emergency Department after having fallen on his outstretched hand. He is the league's leading scorer and his coach directs you to "fix it and fix it fast."

On examination, there is slight tenderness and swelling just below the distal radius. No other abnormalities are found. X-ray examination of the wrist and hand are normal.

Q3. What is the most likely diagnosis in this patient?

   a. second-degree wrist sprain

   b. avulsion fracture of the distal radius

   c. fractured scaphoid

d. fractured triquetrum

e. none of the above

Q4. What is the treatment of choice for the patient described in Case 2?
a. active physiotherapy
b. passive physiotherapy
c. ice, compression, and elevation of the extremity
d. surgical exploration of the wrist
e. none of the above

Q5. What is the major complication of the injury described in Case 2?
a. peripheral nerve injury
b. local muscle damage
c. peripheral arterial injury
d. avascular necrosis of the bone
e. septic arthritis of the joint

Case 3 ■ A 25-Year-Old Male with Severe Ankle Pain

A 25-year-old male is brought to the Emergency Department after having been thrown from his motorcycle. He complains of severe pain in the area of the right ankle.

On examination, there is swelling of the entire right ankle, with a more prominent swelling on the lateral side. There is point tenderness over the area of the lateral malleolus. There does not appear to be any other deformity or abnormality.

Q6. What is the most likely diagnosis in this patient?
a. second-degree ankle sprain
b. third-degree ankle sprain
c. fractured distal tibia
d. fractured lateral malleolus
e. fractured talus

Q7. What is the treatment of choice for the patient described in Case 3?
a. internal reduction and fixation
b. external reduction and fixation
c. active physiotherapy
d. ice, compression, and elevation
e. a walking cast or cast boot

Q8. Which of the following statements regarding acute compartment syndrome is (are) true?
a. acute compartment syndrome is caused by increasing pressure within a closed fascial space caused by the effects of the injury
b. acute compartment syndrome is found primarily in the lower leg and the forearm

c. acute compartment syndrome may lead to muscle and nerve ischemia
d. acute compartment syndrome may lead to muscle and nerve death
e. all of the above statements are true

Q9. The emergency treatment of orthopedic injuries includes which of the following?
a. assessment of all injuries, many of which are multiple
b. assessment of arterial injury in the involved region
c. correction of deformities
d. splinting or immobilization of all injured areas
e. all of the above

Q10. Which of the following is (are) part of the Ottawa Ankle Rules for determining the need for x-rays when evaluating ankle injuries?
a. bone tenderness at the posterior edge or tip of the lateral malleolus
b. bone tenderness at the posterior edge or tip of the medial malleolus
c. inability to bear weight both immediately at time of injury and at time of assessment
d. patient is 18 years or older
e. all of the above

SHORT ANSWER MANAGEMENT PROBLEM
Summarize the basics of the treatment of fractures and other orthopedic injuries.

ANSWERS

A1. **d.** This patient has a Colles' fracture, a fracture of the distal radius. It occurs most commonly in elderly patients, especially women. It is most often associated with osteoporosis.

Colles' fracture is almost always caused by a fall on a outstretched hand. The typical displacement is reflected in a characteristic appearance that has been termed the *dinner-fork deformity*.

The clinical history and deformity are not compatible with any of the choices listed in the question.

A2. **c.** The treatment of choice for the patient described in Question 2 is external reduction under a regional block or a local hematoma block, followed by immobilization in a splint or bivalve cast. Because of the age of the patient, the plaster cast will probably have to remain for 6 weeks to ensure complete healing.

A3. **c.** This young man most likely has a fractured scaphoid bone. This is an injury that is significantly more common in younger adults. The most common cause of a scaphoid fracture is a fall on a outstretched hand.

A4. **e.** Fracture of the scaphoid bone should be suspected if there is tenderness in the "anatomic snuff box" and scaphoid tubercle. Radiographs may be negative initially. If a fracture is suspected, in spite of negative x-rays, the region should be immobilized in a thumb Spica cast. After 2 weeks reevaluate the injured area and repeat x-rays. If there is a fracture of the scaphoid, x-rays will be positive at 2 weeks (a bone scan will be positive within 72 hours of a scaphoid fracture). A nondisplaced fracture of the scaphoid requires 8 to 12 weeks of cast immobilization.

A5. **d.** Failure to properly treat a scaphoid fracture will likely lead to complications. The major complication is avascular necrosis.

A6. **d.** The history of trauma, the symptoms elicited, and the signs present suggest a fracture of the lateral malleolus. Although the physical findings of a major (second- or third-degree) ankle sprain may be somewhat similar, the injury (being thrown from a motorcycle) is definitely more suggestive of a fracture injury than a sprain injury.

A7. **e.** The treatment of choice for the patient described in Case 3 is a walking cast for 6 weeks. In the absence of significant deformity and confirmation on x-ray of a nondisplaced fracture to the lateral malleolus, no other treatment is indicated. An x-ray should be repeated in 1 to 2 weeks after the injury to check for any displacement of the fracture.

A8. **e.** Acute compartment syndromes are caused by increasing tissue pressure in a closed fascial space. The fascial compartments of the leg or forearm are most frequently involved. Acute compartment syndromes are usually caused by a fracture with a subsequent hemorrhage, limb compression, or a crushing injury.

In an acute compartment syndrome, fluid pressure is increased. This leads to muscle and tissue ischemia. Severe ischemia for a period of 6 to 8 hours results in subsequent muscle and nerve death, with resulting contractures.

Physical examination reveals swelling and definitive palpable tenseness over the muscle compartment. The signs on physical examination include paresis in the involved area and a sensory deficit over the involved area.

Acute compartment syndrome should be treated with immediate fasciotomy.

A9. **e.** In treating orthopedic injuries in a patient who has been involved in a traumatic event, it is important to remember that these injuries must be seen and treated within the overall context of the patient's condition.

Thus the ABCs of resuscitation, which are discussed in Problems 137 and 138, must take first priority. Associated cardiac dysrhythmias must be treated according to basic life support and advanced cardiac life support protocols. Traumatic injuries must be treated according to basic trauma life support and advanced trauma life support protocols.

First, the trauma patient must be suspected of having multiple injuries rather than a single injury. Cervical spine injuries should be assumed to be present until they have been excluded. Primary and secondary surveys must be performed as per advanced trauma life support protocol.

Second, with any injured extremity, arterial injury must be suspected and pulses assessed quickly. Acute compartment syndromes must be ruled out.

Third, deformities should be corrected as soon as possible under local (hematoma block), regional, or general anesthesia. Ideally, the injured limb(s) should be splinted before the patient arrives in the Emergency Room. Open fractures and surrounding tissue must be thoroughly débrided and cleaned as quickly as possible.

Fourth, after stabilization is complete, tetanus prophylaxis should be given and antibiotics active against coagulase positive staphylococcus must be started.

A10. **e.** The Ottawa Ankle Rules are guidelines to determine the need for ankle radiographs in patients who have sustained an ankle injury. If there is bone tenderness at the posterior edge or tip of the lateral or medial malleolus or an inability to bear weight both immediately at time of injury and at time of assessment, x-rays should be obtained. The Ottawa Ankle Rules do not apply to patients under the age of 18. It is important to also use clinical judgment when deciding when to obtain x-rays.

SOLUTION TO THE SHORT ANSWER MANAGEMENT PROBLEM

The basics of fracture management and other orthopedic and trauma injuries are as follows:
a. Remember the ABCs of resuscitation.
b. Suspect and search for multiple injuries.
c. Suspect and prevent potential spine injuries.

d. Rule out arterial injury in the affected limb.
e. Rule out a compartment syndrome.
f. Recognize and treat open fractures with copious irrigation, débridement, and initiation of intravenous antibiotics.
g. Correct deformities whenever possible.
h. Splint each injured area.
i. If there is significant swelling in a limb, consider either a bivalve cast or splint until swelling has significantly decreased. A full cast can lead to complications such as compartment syndrome if applied when there is significant swelling.
j. If one fracture is found, always check the joint above and the joint below for additional fractures, dislocations, or other injuries.

SUMMARY OF FRACTURE MANAGEMENT

The Solution to the Short Answer Management Problem serves as the summary for this problem.

SUGGESTED READINGS

Liu SH, Nguyen TM: Ankle sprains and other soft tissue injuries, *Curr Opin Rheumatol* 11(2):132-137, 1999.
Strayer SM et al: Fractures of the proximal fifth metatarsal, *Am Fam Physician* 59(9):2516-2522, 1999.
Touliopolous S, Hershman EB: Lower leg pain: Diagnosis and treatment of compartment syndromes and other pain syndromes of the leg, *Sports Med* 27(3):193-204, 1999.
Trumble TE et al: Intraarticular fractures of the distal aspect of the radius, *Instr Course Lect* 48:465-480, 1999.
Ullom-Minnich P: Prevention of osteoporosis and fractures, *Am Fam Physician* 60(1):194-202, 1999.
Wexler RK: The injured ankle, *Am Fam Physician* 57(3):474-480, 1998.

PROBLEM·144

SPRAINS AND STRAINS

"Are You Sure It's Not Broken, Doc?"

Case 1 ■ A 28-Year-Old Female with a Swollen Ankle

A 28-year-old female is brought to the Emergency Department after having fallen down three steps in her new home. She is complaining of a significant amount of pain in her right ankle.

On examination, there is mild ecchymosis and swelling on the lateral side of her right ankle. There is pain with inversion of the right ankle. Ankle tenderness is maximal just anterior to the tip of the lateral malleolus. There is no actual bone tenderness. There is no ligamentous laxity.

SELECT THE BEST ANSWER TO THE FOLLOWING QUESTIONS

Q1. The injury in this patient is most likely which of the following?
    a. a grade I sprain of the ligament complex on the medial side of the right ankle
    b. a grade II or grade III sprain of the ligament complex on the medial side of the right ankle
    c. a grade I sprain of the ligament complex on the lateral side of the right ankle
    d. a strain of the peroneus brevis tendon
    e. a fracture of the distal fibula

Q2. What is the most likely ligament involved in this injury?
    a. anterior inferior tibiofibular ligament
    b. calcaneofibular ligament
    c. anterior talofibular ligament
    d. dorsal calcaneocuboid ligament
    e. interosseous talocalcaneal ligament

Q3. What is the treatment of choice in this patient?
    a. a fiberglass cast
    b. weightbearing as tolerated with active range of motion (ROM) exercises
    c. nonweightbearing with a posterior splint
    d. a corticosteroid injection
    e. surgical repair of the ligament

Case 2 ■ A 26-Year-Old Professional Football Player Whose Knee Buckled

A 26-year-old professional football player is brought to the Emergency Department after being hit on the lateral side of the left knee. His knee buckled and he is now in severe pain.

On examination, there is swelling over the medial aspect of the left knee. There is laxity when a valgus stress test is performed on the knee. There is a negative Lachman's test and McMurray's test.

Q4. What is the most likely injury in this patient?
    a. a tear of the left lateral meniscus
    b. a tear of the left medial meniscus
    c. a tear of the left lateral collateral ligament
    d. a tear of the left medial collateral ligament
    e. a fracture of the intercondylar eminence of the left knee

Q5. You diagnose a grade II sprain of the medial collateral ligament. What is the initial treatment of choice?
    a. corticosteroid injection
    b. knee brace

c. fiberglass cast
d. complete bed rest
e. surgical repair

Case 3 ■ A 22-Year-Old Football Player Who Felt a Sharp Pain at the Anteromedial Aspect of His Knee after Being Hit

A 22-year-old football player is brought to the Emergency Department after having his right leg twisted while carrying the ball. As he was being tackled, he felt a sharp pain at the anteromedial aspect of the right knee joint. He was unable to straighten his knee fully and was carried off the field by his teammates.

On examination, there is significant swelling on the medial side of the right knee joint. As well, there is tenderness at the joint line on the medial side, limitation of the last few degrees of extension by a springy resistance, and sharp anteromedial pain when passive extension is forced.

Q6. What is the most likely diagnosis in this patient?
 a. torn right medial meniscus
 b. torn right lateral meniscus
 c. torn right medial collateral ligament
 d. torn right anterior cruciate ligament
 e. fractured patella

Q7. What is the radiologic procedure of choice in the patient described in Case 3?
 a. a plain anteroposterior and lateral x-ray of the right knee
 b. a cone-view x-ray of the right knee
 c. an arthrogram
 d. a computed tomography scan
 e. a magnetic resonance imaging (MRI) scan

Q8. What is the treatment of choice for the injury to the patient described in Case 3?
 a. nonweightbearing and a half cast
 b. a full cast
 c. ice, elevation, and an elastic bandage
 d. arthroscopic surgery
 e. active physiotherapy

Case 4 ■ A 23-Year-Old Runner with Anterior Thigh Pain

A 23-year-old female comes to your office with right anterior thigh pain. She was running in a 100-m race when the pain started.

On examination, there is tenderness over the midportion of the right quadriceps muscle. There is mild swelling and discoloration. No other injuries are noted.

Q9. What is the most likely diagnosis in this patient?
 a. right quadriceps strain
 b. right quadriceps sprain
 c. right quadriceps hemorrhage
 d. right quadriceps avulsion
 e. none of the above

Q10. What is the initial treatment of choice for the patient described in Case 4?
 a. surgical repair
 b. splint
 c. a full cast
 d. ice, rest, elevation, and compression
 e. none of the above

Case 5 ■ A 14-Year-Old Female Who Sustained a Knee Injury while Pivoting

A 14-year-old female who is a star on her high school basketball team sustains an injury that results from a sudden pivot on her right knee. She collapses to the floor in pain. She is immediately brought to the Emergency Department. By the time she arrives, approximately 45 minutes after the injury, her right knee is swollen. There is significant ligamentous laxity when a Lachman's test is performed.

Q11. What is the most likely diagnosis in this patient?
 a. anterior cruciate ligament tear
 b. posterior cruciate ligament tear
 c. quadriceps tendon tear
 d. lateral collateral ligament tear
 e. medial collateral ligament tear

Q12. The diagnosis of this injury is best confirmed in the Emergency Department by which of the following?
 a. history of the injury
 b. anterior drawer test
 c. the Lachman's test
 d. aspiration of the knee joint
 e. MRI of the knee

Q13. What is the definitive treatment of choice in this patient for her injury?
 a. ice, elevation, and compression
 b. a half cast
 c. corticosteroid injection
 d. reconstruction surgery
 e. none of the above

Q14. Which of the following is the most common cause of chronic low back pain?
 a. vertebral body pain
 b. lumbar muscular pain

c. intervertebral disc pain

d. intervertebral facet joint pain

e. exact cause is unknown

Q15. What is the most common musculoskeletal presenting complaint in primary care?

a. a lower-limb fracture

b. patellofemoral pain syndrome

c. a grade I ankle sprain

d. a grade II ankle sprain

e. low back pain

SHORT ANSWER MANAGEMENT PROBLEM
Discuss the differentiation of a collateral ligament strain from a meniscal tear on physical examination.

ANSWERS

A1. **c.** This patient most likely has a grade I sprain of the ligament complex on the lateral side of the ankle.

A sprain is defined as a complete or partial tear of the ligaments (interligamental or at origin/insertion). Swelling and tenderness over a ligament and pain when it is stretched suggest a sprain. Excessive motion of the joint when the ligament is stretched confirms the diagnosis. Sprains are graded according to the following criteria:

a. Grade I: a tear of a few ligament fibers. The joint is tender and painful, but there is no laxity. Swelling and ecchymosis are usually minimal.

b. Grade II: a tear of a moderate number of ligament fibers. On physical examination, there is a moderate amount of swelling and pain. There is little to no instability of joint.

c. Grade III: total disruption or tear of the ligament involved. No end point is felt when the joint is stressed. Swelling and ecchymosis are prominent.

The most common ankle injury is an inversion injury in which there is partial or complete disruption of the lateral collateral ligament complex.

A2. **c.** Most ankle sprains are secondary to inversion type injuries. The lateral ligaments are most commonly involved. Specifically, the anterior talofibular ligament is the most commonly injured ligament in angle inversion type injuries. Tenderness is maximal anterior to the tip of the lateral malleolus.

A3. **b.** The treatment of choice in this patient is ice, elevation, weightbearing as tolerated, active ROM exercise, and an ankle support brace. A cast is both inappropriate and can lead to complications if the swelling worsens. Surgical intervention is not indicated in most ankle sprains. Corticosteroid injections are not indicated in the acute management of ankle sprains.

A4. **d.** The most likely injury in this patient is a tear of the left medial collateral ligament. The mechanism of injury (a blow to the lateral side of the left knee), the swelling demonstrated on the medial side of the knee, and the laxity with valgus stress testing suggest a sprain of the left medial collateral ligament complex. The Lachman's test is used to diagnose injuries to the anterior cruciate ligament. The McMurray's test is used to diagnose tears of the menisci.

A5. **b.** Initial treatment consists of a knee brace, ice, elevation, and straight leg raise exercises in the brace. The patient may ambulate as tolerated in the brace. It is unnecessary to apply a cast. Surgery is not indicated, and the patient does not need bed rest.

A6. **a.** This patient has a torn right medial meniscus. The history of the injury is characteristic. Usually, a torn meniscus is the result of a significant twisting or squatting type of injury. The patient then falls (or in this case is tackled) and has pain along the joint line. The knee usually swells over the first 12 hours and there is sometimes a sensation of "locking." This locking can be from a displaced fragment or from hamstring spasm ("pseudolocking").

On physical examination, there is joint line tenderness and an effusion may be present. There is a positive McMurray's test and Apley's test.

In cases of a long-standing injury there may be significant wasting of the quadriceps muscle. In addition to meniscal tears, twisting injuries may also (often) give rise to anterior cruciate ligament tears.

A7. **e.** The diagnostic test of choice for suspected medial meniscal tear and locking is an MRI scan.

A8. **d.** The treatment of choice for the patient described in Case 3 is arthroscopic surgery. With the use of the arthroscope, the torn fragment can either be removed or repaired.

A9. **a.** This patient most likely has a right quadriceps muscle strain. A strain is defined as an over-stretching of some portion of muscle or tendon. In a manner analogous to sprains, every degree of strain, ranging from the over-stretching of just a few muscle fibers to the complete rupture of a muscle or tendon, may occur.

A10. **d.** The initial treatment of choice for the patient discussed in Case 4 is ice, rest, elevation, and compression with a tensor bandage. This should be followed by physiotherapy.

A11. **a.** This is a classic description of an injury to the anterior cruciate ligament. The mechanism of injury is usually noncontact: a deceleration, hyperextension, or marked internal rotation. It may also be associated with a medial meniscal tear.

A12. **c.** The diagnosis of injury to the anterior cruciate ligament is made by utilizing the Lachman's test, the anterior drawer test, and the pivot shift. Although the anterior drawer test is a time-honored test, it turns out not to be very sensitive. The Lachman's test is much more sensitive.

In this test, the examiner places the knee in 20 degrees of flexion by resting it on a pillow and stabilizing the femur above the knee with his or her nondominant hand. The dominant hand of the examiner is placed behind the leg at the level of the tibial tubercle, and the examiner introduces an anterior force, attempting to displace the tibia forward. If there is excessive anterior translation of the tibia and lack of a firm end point, a tear in the anterior cruciate ligament has occurred.

Anterior cruciate ligament tears are frequently associated with blood fluid aspirates. Although not diagnostic, this is another clue that, if positive, increases the probability of the diagnosis. Aspiration is rarely necessary for the acutely injured knee.

A13. **d.** The initial treatment includes a knee brace, ice packs, and elevation, followed by isometric and ROM exercises. The definitive treatment in young active patients is most often reconstruction. Surgery is usually delayed 3 weeks postinjury to allow for increased ROM and strength and decreased swelling.

A14. **e.** Chronic low back pain is a difficult diagnostic entity to make a definite diagnosis. Whether the cause is vertebral body bone pain, paravertebral muscle pain, intervertebral disc pain, intervertebral facet joint pain, some other source of pain, or some combination of these pains, nobody really knows for sure.

A15. **e.** The most common musculoskeletal presenting complaint in primary care is low back pain.

SOLUTION TO THE SHORT ANSWER MANAGEMENT PROBLEM

The differentiation of a collateral ligament tear from a meniscal tear includes positive varus or valgus stress testing present on clinical examination when a ligamentous injury is present and the presence of joint line tenderness when a meniscal tear is present.

SUMMARY OF THE DIAGNOSIS AND TREATMENT OF SPRAINS AND STRAINS

1. Definitions:
   a. Sprain: A ligament injury. Sprains are classified as follows:
      1) First-degree: Tear of only a few ligament fibers with no joint instability
      2) Second-degree: Tear of a moderate number of ligament fibers with little or no joint instability
      3) Third-degree: Complete rupture of ligament with joint instability
   b. Strain: A muscle-tendon injury. Strain injuries are classified as follows, ranging from tearing only a few fibers to a complete rupture of the muscle tendon unit:
      1) First-degree
      2) Second-degree
      3) Third-degree

2. Most common sites:
   a. Ankle sprain: Lateral ligamentous complex injured more frequently than medial ligamentous complex (tenderness maximal anterior to tip of lateral malleolus-anterior talofibular ligament)
   b. Knee: Tests:
      1) Medial and lateral collateral ligaments: Varus and valgus stress testing
      2) Anterior cruciate ligament: Lachman's test
      3) Strain: Location, not specific

3. Other significant injury: Medial and lateral meniscal injuries of the knee:
   a. Clinical clue: Joint line tenderness
   b. Diagnosis: If further diagnostic procedure is needed, MRI is the radiologic test of choice.

4. Treatments: Sprain (ankle)—conservative
   Rest: Stop physical activity; protected weight bearing as tolerated
   Ice: Apply ice to the injury for 15 to 20 minutes each hour while awake for the first 24 hours. Wrap the ice in a wet towel or other buffer to prevent skin damage. Ice reduces swelling and pain.
   Compression: Use an elastic bandage or air-filled splint to apply pressure to the injury. Wear it all day long, except when the injury is being iced. Compression keeps swelling down.
   Elevation: Keep the injured area elevated. This allows fluid to drain from the injury site, reducing swelling.

SUGGESTED READING
Mellion MB et al: *The team physician's handbook,* ed 2, Philadelphia, 1997, Hanley & Belfus.

PROBLEM·1 4 5

HEAT- AND COLD-RELATED INJURIES

"He Could Have Won the Race If He Didn't Give Up on the Last Lap."

Case 1 ■ A 51-Year-Old Alcoholic Male Brought into the Emergency Department

A 51-year-old alcoholic male is brought into the Emergency Department after having been found in a snow bank. He is unconscious and no history can be obtained. No family is known.

On physical examination, his blood pressure is 90/60 mm Hg. His pulse is 36 bpm and regular. His core body temperature is 28° C. His electrocardiogram (ECG) reveals sinus bradycardia and an Osborne (J) wave after the QRS complex.

SELECT THE BEST ANSWER
TO THE FOLLOWING QUESTIONS

Q1. Which of the following statements regarding the hypothermia in this patient is false?
   a. most hypothermic patients are intoxicated with ethanol or other drugs
   b. body temperatures from 32° C to 35° C constitute mild hypothermia
   c. the Osborne (J) wave on the ECG is characteristic of hypothermia
   d. arrhythmias and dysrhythmias are common when the core body temperature drops below 30° C
   e. intravascular volume is usually maintained in patients in hypothermia

Q2. What is the treatment of choice for the patient described in Case 1?
   a. passive rewarming
   b. active external rewarming
   c. active core rewarming
   d. a and b
   e. none of the above

Case 2 ■ A 45-Year-Old Male with Blanched Feet

A 45-year-old male is brought into the Emergency Department from his work-site with numbness of both feet after working in 40° F weather for 6 hours.

On examination, both feet are blanched. Sensation is decreased in both feet to the level of the ankles. Both feet are cold to touch and are bloodless. You suspect frostbite.

Q3. What is the most appropriate treatment of this patient at this time?
   a. passive rewarming
   b. vigorous rubbing
   c. immersion in water at 42° C
   d. placement close to a radiant heater
   e. immersion in water at 30° C

Case 3 ■ A 4-Year-Old Male Who Fell through the Ice

A 4-year-old male is brought into the Emergency Department after having fallen through the ice into a lake. He was rescued approximately 15 minutes later. Cardiopulmonary resuscitation (CPR) was begun at the scene and is in progress as the patient is wheeled through the Emergency Department doors.

On examination, there is no spontaneous breathing or cardiac activity. The child's core temperature is 28° C.

Q4. At this time, what would be the most important action?
   a. discontinue CPR
   b. continue CPR while rewarming the patient with active external rewarming
   c. continue CPR while rewarming the patient with inhalation warming therapy
   d. continue CPR while rewarming the patient with peritoneal dialysis
   e. activate the advanced cardiac life support (ACLS) protocol

Q5. Following the initial treatment just selected, what would be your next step?
   a. discontinue CPR
   b. continue CPR while rewarming the patient with active external rewarming
   c. continue CPR while rewarming the patient with inhalation warming therapy
   d. continue CPR while rewarming the patient with active core rewarming
   e. none of the above

Case 4 ■ A 34-Year-Old Male Who Worked in Temperatures Exceeding 100° F

A 34-year-old male is brought into the Emergency Department after having worked outdoors all day in temperatures exceeding 45° C. He complains of painful spasms of the skeletal muscles, most prominent in the lower extremities and the abdomen. No other symptoms are associated with these spasms.

On physical examination, the patient is alert and cooperative. His blood pressure is 120/80 mm Hg and his pulse is 108 bpm. His temperature is 38° C. The remainder of the physical examination is normal.

Q6. Which of the following conditions does this patient have?
   a. heat cramps
   b. heat stroke
   c. heat exhaustion
   d. b or c
   e. none of the above

Q7. What is the treatment of choice for this patient at this time?
   a. oral rehydration therapy
   b. core body cooling
   c. warm intravenous (IV) fluids
   d. intensive care unit monitoring and Swan-Ganz catheterization
   e. none of the above

Case 5 ■ An Exhausted 23-Year-Old Female Marathon Runner

A 23-year-old female marathon runner comes to the Emergency Department after completing a marathon. During the last mile, she began to develop lightheadedness, nausea, vomiting, severe headache, rapid heart rate, and rapid respiratory rate.

On examination, the patient's blood pressure is 90/70 mm Hg. Her pulse is 120 bpm and regular. She is orthostatic. Her temperature is 37.5° C. The rest of the physical examination is normal.

Q8. Which of the following statements regarding this patient's condition is (are) true?
   a. rapid IV volume and electrolyte replacement are indicated in this patient
   b. this patient can be safely discharged without any active treatment; oral fluids will suffice
   c. this patient's temperature will likely go up significantly in the next few hours
   d. serum potassium and serum sodium levels are likely to be normal in this patient
   e. none of the above statements is true

Q9. Which of the following conditions does the patient described in Case 5 have?
   a. heat cramps
   b. heat stroke
   c. heat exhaustion
   d. b or c
   e. none of the above

Q10. What is (are) the treatment(s) of choice for the patient described in Case 5 at this time?
   a. rapid IV volume and electrolyte repletion
   b. rapid external body cooling
   c. rapid internal body cooling
   d. all of the above
   e. none of the above

Case 6 ■ A 34-Year-Old Male Who Collapsed while Running the Marathon

A 34-year-old male is brought to the Emergency Department by paramedics after having collapsed in a marathon. Apparently, at approximately the eighteenth mile he fell to the ground in an unconscious state.

On physical examination, his blood pressure is 90/60 mm Hg. His pulse is 128 bpm. The patient's temperature is 41° C.

Q11. Which of the following statements about this patient is (are) true?
   a. this patient has heatstroke
   b. hepatic and renal abnormalities are common in this condition
   c. treatment should be directed at lowering the core temperature as quickly as possible
   d. all of the above statements are true
   e. none of the above statements is true

SHORT ANSWER MANAGEMENT PROBLEM
Discuss the main risk factors for heat-related illnesses.

ANSWERS

A1. **e.** The majority of hypothermic patients are intoxicated with ethanol or other drugs. Ethanol is a vasodilator, and because of its anesthetic and central nervous system (CNS)-depressant effects, intoxicated subjects do not feel the cold. Hypothermia may be associated with other drugs (including barbiturates, phenothiazines, and insulin), hypothyroidism, sepsis, and other acute illnesses.

Hypothermia is defined as mild if the body temperature is between 32° C and 35° C, moderate if the body temperature is between 27° C and 32° C, and severe if below 27° C. Shivering stops at 31° C.

Hypothermia causes characteristic ECG changes and may induce certain life-threatening dysrhythmias, including ventricular fibrillation and asystole. The Osborne (J) wave, a slow, positive deflection at the end of the QRS complex, is characteristic, although not pathognomonic, of hypothermia. The probability of dysrhythmias increases with decreasing body temperature. Oxygen delivery to the tissues is impaired, and intravascular volume is lost because of a plasma shift to the extravascular space.

Hypothermia produces a depression of CNS function resulting in confusion and lethargy and, in severe cases, coma.

A2. **c.** Because of the severity of the hypothermia (core temperature of 28° C), active core rewarming is the method of choice for the correction of this patient's hypothermia.

Core rewarming will warm all of this patient's internal organs preferentially and at the expense of other areas of the body. Core rewarming will also decrease myocardial irritability and the risk of dysrhythmias, as well as improve cardiac function.

The methods of active core rewarming include inhalation rewarming; heated IV fluids; heated irrigation of the peritoneum, thorax, and gastrointestinal tract; and extracorporeal warming.

Passive rewarming includes removing wet clothing and insulating patients with blankets. Core temperature rises slowly with this method and therefore passive rewarming cannot be recommended in a patient, as presented, with cardiovascular compromise.

Active external rewarming (warm-water immersion, heating blankets, radiant heat, and so on) may be successful in rapidly raising body temperature. The application of external heat, however, may cause peripheral vasodilation and return cold blood to the core. It is thus not appropriate for this patient.

The method of choice for rewarming a patient depends on the duration, degree, and cause of the hypothermia. Cold-water immersion, for example, produces little disturbance of intravascular volume, electrolyte balance, and acid-base status. In these patients, rapid external rewarming, therefore, is usually both safe and successful.

In patients who are in the early phase of hypothermia, improvement usually occurs irrespective of the method chosen. At temperatures above 30° C there is a very low incidence of arrhythmia, and rapid rewarming is unnecessary.

The most important consideration in the choice of rewarming method is the patient's cardiovascular status. Patients who have stable cardiac function do not need rapid rewarming. Passive rewarming and noninvasive internal modalities (moist warm oxygen and warm IV fluids) will suffice.

Patients with cardiovascular compromise, including persistent hypotension and life-threatening dysrhythmias, need to be rewarmed rapidly. The initial management of hypothermic patients always begins with the ABCs of resuscitation.

A3. **c.** The initial clinical response to cold is known as frostnip. Frostnip, a superficial and reversible injury, begins as a blanching and numbness of the involved area followed by a sudden cessation of cold and discomfort. The sudden loss of cold sensation at the injury site is a reliable sign of impending frostbite. If treatment is initiated at this point, frostnip will not progress to frostbite.

The best initial treatment for frostnip and frostbite is rapid rewarming of the involved extremity in a circulating warm (42° C) water bath. Slow rewarming is less effective and may actually increase tissue damage.

A4. **e.** The first step in the resuscitation of this patient should be the activation of the ACLS protocol. Again, remember the ABCs (in that order). The cardiac status of a drowning victim is the first priority. With the activation of the ACLS protocol, CPR should not be stopped until the core temperature is above 32° C.

A5. **d.** Death in hypothermia is confirmed only when the patient has failed to respond to basic cardiac life support and ACLS and the core temperature is above 32° C. In this case, the rewarming recommended is active core rewarming.

A6. **a.** This patient has heat cramps. Heat cramps are usually associated with strenuous physical activity. The painful spasm of skeletal muscles, including muscles of the extremities and abdomen, occurs. Other symptoms include weakness, fatigue, nausea, vomiting, and tachycardia.

On physical examination, the body temperature is normal. The pathophysiology is a total body salt deficiency.

A7. **a.** Heat cramps are benign and respond well to oral electrolyte replacement and mild cooling.

A8. **a.**

A9. **c.** This patient has heat exhaustion. Heat exhaustion is characterized by volume depletion, fluid and electrolyte losses from sweating, and tissue hypoperfusion secondary to the hypovolemia. Heat exhaustion usually presents with fatigue, lightheadedness, nausea, or vomiting, or headache. Significant hypovolemia with associated tachycardia, hyperventilation, and hypotension also occur. The patient's body temperature is usually normal or only slightly elevated. Sweating may be profuse.

A10. **a.** The treatment of choice in this patient is IV fluid replacement (normal saline or Ringer's lactate). Treatment also includes removal to a cool environment, removal of excess clothing, and spraying with lukewarm water and cooling with fans.

A11. **d.** This patient has heatstroke. Heatstroke is defined as the combination of hyperpyrexia (>40° C) with associated neurologic symptoms. Classic heat stroke, seen primarily in the elderly, is characterized by altered mental status and absence of sweating. In exertional heat stroke, seen in younger patients undergoing rigorous exercise, there is profuse sweating. Heatstroke is a medical emergency.

Risk factors for heatstroke include the following:
a. The extremes of age
b. Preexisting cardiovascular disease
c. High environmental temperature and humidity
d. Occupations such as professional athletes, laborers, and military recruits
e. Patients taking certain pharmacologic agents that include anticholinergic drugs, phenothiazines, tricyclic antidepressants, monoamine oxidase inhibitors (MAOIs), and antihistamines

Heatstroke usually presents abruptly, with the rapid onset of neurologic dysfunction.

Hepatic, renal, and hematologic abnormalities are common in heatstroke. Hepatic failure, renal failure, and disseminated intravascular coagulation may occur.

Fluid and electrolyte abnormalities vary with the onset and duration of heatstroke, underlying disease, and the prior use of medications (especially diuretics). Unlike in heat exhaustion, dehydration and volume depletion may not occur in heatstroke. Vigorous fluid replacement may result in pulmonary edema.

Heatstroke is treated by removing all clothing, applying cool water to the entire skin before reaching the Emergency Department, followed by treatment in the Emergency Department that consists of spraying with a mist of lukewarm water while using a high-volume fan, ice packs applied to the groin and axillae, ice water gastric lavage, and iced peritoneal lavage. Ice water immersion makes it difficult to monitor the patient and initiate CPR or defibrillation if necessary. As with all emergencies, the initial treatment begins with the ABCs.

SOLUTION TO THE SHORT ANSWER MANAGEMENT PROBLEM

The risk factors for heat-related illnesses are as follows:
a. The extremes of age: The elderly are especially prone to serious heat syndromes when heat waves and high humidity hit.
b. Underlying chronic disease: Chronic cardiovascular disease and chronic pulmonary disease predispose to exaggerated response to heat. This is especially true for patients in congestive cardiac failure.
c. Occupations and activities: Athletes, laborers, and military recruits are prone to heat syndromes especially when they are exercising vigorously or working in a hot, outside environment.
d. Drugs: Patients on such drugs as diuretics, anticholinergic drugs, phenothiazines, tricyclic antidepressants, MAOIs, and antihistamines are predisposed to heat syndromes.

SUMMARY OF THE DIAGNOSIS AND TREATMENT OF ENVIRONMENTAL HEAT- AND COLD-RELATED SYNDROMES

1. Cold injuries and syndromes:
   a. Frostnip and frostbite:
      1) Frostnip: Superficial, really an "early frostbite" and completely reversible
      2) Frostbite: Superficial or deep but usually associated with some tissue damage
      3) Treatment of both syndromes: Immersion of the extremity in a circulating warm (42° C) water bath
   b. Hypothermia:
      1) Mild hypothermia: Core temperature above between 32° and 35° C
      2) Severe hypothermia: Core temperature below 27° C
      3) Treatment of mild hypothermia: Passive rewarming and active external rewarming
      4) Treatment of severe hypothermia: Active core rewarming
      5) Remember, no one is dead until he or she is warm and dead.

2. Heat syndromes:
   a. Heat cramps: No disturbance of core body temperature; salt deficiency.
      Treatment: Oral electrolyte replacement

b. Heat exhaustion: Volume and electrolyte depletion; core temperature normal or slightly elevated
   Treatment: IV fluids (normal saline/Ringer's lactate), remove excess clothing, cool environment, spray lukewarm water and cool with fans

c. Heatstroke: Hyperpyrexia and neurologic symptoms; characteristic absence of sweating.
   Treatment: Rapid, aggressive, lowering of body temperature, including iced gastric lavage, iced peritoneal lavage, and in some cases ice water immersion

SUGGESTED READING

Pousada L et al: *Emergency medicine,* Baltimore, 1996, Williams & Wilkins.

Index

A

ABCs of resuscitation, 629, 636
  in cold-related injuries, 655
  in fracture management, 648
  for shock, 630-631
Abdomen, acute
  in appendicitis, 459
  in pancreatitis, 471
Abdominal aortic aneurysm, screening for, 579
Abdominal pain
  age-related diagnoses for, 423
  assessment of, 635
  in diabetic ketoacidosis, 631-633
  differential diagnosis of, 636
  in elderly, 634-637
  emergency treatment of, 634-637
    summary of, 636-637
  in pancreatic cancer, 599-601
  pediatric, 421-423
    characteristics of, 421, 422
    giardiasis-related, 422
    summary of, 423
    treatment of, 422-423
  trauma-related, 628
ABO incompatibility, neonatal jaundice and, 372
Abortion
  completed, 227
  euploidic
    alcohol use and, 228
    smoking and, 228
  incomplete, 227
  inevitable, 227
  spontaneous, 226-228
    chromosomal abnormalities in, 227-228
    classification of, 228
    defined, 227
    diabetes and, 228
    precipitating factors in, 227
    recurrent, 227
    summary of, 228
  therapeutic, rubella exposure and, 406, 408
  threatened, 227
    management of, 228
Abruptio placenta, aspirin-associated, 215
Abscess
  as complication of appendectomy, 460
  outpatient surgery for, 469
Absence seizures, 124
  findings in, 125
Absorptiometry, dual-energy x-ray, 236
Abuse; see Child abuse; Drug abuse; Elder abuse; Sexual abuse; Substance abuse
Accutane; see 13-cis-retinoic acid
ACE inhibitors; see Angiotensin-converting enzyme inhibitors
Acebutolol, lipid effects of, 16
Acetaminophen
  for childhood fever/pain, 451
  for fever in children, 378
  for headache, 119
Acetaminophen poisoning, 640

Acetone breath, 634
N-Acetylcysteine for acetaminophen poisoning, 640
Achalasia
  characteristics and treatment of, 56
  dysphagia due to, 56
Acid reflux disease; see also Esophageal motility disorder
  diagnosis of, 55
Acidosis in cardiac arrest, 626
ACLS; see Advanced cardiac life support
Acne, 172-176
  adolescent, 432, 434
  causes of, 174
  myths about, 175-176
  summary of, 175-176
  treatment of, 174-175
Acquired immunodeficiency syndrome; see AIDS
Acromegaly, 99
  causes of, 102
  signs and symptoms of, 101-102
  summary of, 104
  treatment of, 102
Actinic keratoses, skin lesions of, 643
Activated partial thromboplastin time in acute MI, 4
Activity after MI, 5, 7
Actonel; see Risedronate
Acute cor pulmonale, pulmonary embolism and, 35
Acute lymphoblastic leukemia *versus* mononucleosis, 67
Acute lymphocytic leukemia, symptoms of, 143
Acute myeloblastic leukemia, symptoms of, 143
Acute myocardial infarction
  activity after, 5, 7
  of anterior wall, 3
  case study, 1-7
  diagnosis of, 3-4, 6, 7
  followup treatment, 7
  non-Q-wave, 4
  pathophysiology of, 4-5
  signs and symptoms of, 7
  treatment of, 4-5, 7
    adjunctive agents for, 6-7
Acyclovir for herpes simplex infection, 275
Addison's disease, 99
  causes of, 102
  signs and symptoms of, 102
  summary of, 104
  treatment of, 102
Adenocarcinoma
  of cecum, 475
  development of, 476
  esophageal, 56
    dysphagia due to, 57
Adenoidectomy, summary of, 404
Adenoma
  in Conn's syndrome, 102
  development of, 476
  hepatocellular, OCPs and, 267
  hyperthyroidism in, 107
  malignant potential of, 476

Adenomyosis in dysmenorrhea, 255
Adenosine for PSVT, 29
Adenovirus
  in bronchiolitis, 391-392
  conjunctivitis due to, 409
  pneumonia due to, 52, 53
    symptoms and treatment of, 412
Adenovirus infection, ocular, 490
ADHD; see Attention-deficit hyperactivity disorder
Adjustment disorder
  with depressed mood, 282
  in differential diagnosis of depression of elderly, 558
  psychotherapy for, 335-338
  symptoms of, 337
  treatment of, 282-283
Adjustment sleep disorder, 185
Adolescents, 432-436; see also Children/adolescents
  accidental death of, 434
  acne in, 432, 434
  behavioral changes in, 434
  development phases of, 435-436
  drug/alcohol use by, 435
  emotional problems of, 434
  mnemonic for assessing, 435
  pregnancy of, 435
  sexual intercourse and, 434-435
  suicide of, 434
Adrenocortical insufficiency; see Addison's disease
Advance directives, components of, 520
Advanced cardiac life support, 623
  for atrial fibrillation, 28-29
  in cold-related injuries, 655
Adverse drug reactions, in elderly, 566-571
Afterload in congestive heart failure, 20
Agoraphobia
  defined, 324, 326
  symptoms of, 322
AIDS
  antiviral therapies in, 614
  cytomegalovirus infection in, 614
  Kaposi's sarcoma in, 614
  neurologic complications of, 615
  opportunistic infections in, 612, 614
  Pneumocystis carinii pneumonia in, 613-614
  symptoms of, 612
  treatment and prognosis, 615-616
Air travel, fear of, 325
Airway obstruction
  in bronchial asthma, 392
  wheezing in, 393
Albuterol for preventing asthma, 48
Alcohol
  atrial fibrillation and, 28
  coronary artery disease and, 17
  euploidic abortion and, 228
  pancreatic carcinoma and, 486
  during pregnancy, 207
  triglyceride levels and, 17
  urinary incontinence due to, 553
Alcohol abuse; see Alcohol dependence/abuse

Alcohol dependence/abuse, 294-299
  definitions of, 296-299
  diseases related to, 299
  economic costs of, 298
  factors associated with, 297
  hepatomegaly in, 297
  hypertension and, 23
  hypothermia associated with, 653, 654
  laboratory testing for, 299
  memory deficits and, 296, 297, 298
  neurologic effects of, 299
  screening for, 298, 299
  social costs of, 297
  spousal abuse and, 345
  susceptibility to, 297
  symptoms of, 294, 296-297
  treatment of, 298, 299
Alcohol withdrawal, treatment of, 302
Alcohol withdrawal syndrome, defined,
      297
Alcoholic encephalopathy, 297
Alcoholic hepatitis
  summary of, 74
  symptoms of, 71
Alcohol-induced amnestic disorder, 298
Alcoholism; see also Alcohol
      dependence/abuse
  defined, 298
  pancreatitis associated with, 470-473
  pneumonia and, 51, 53, 54
  screening for, 582
Alcohol-related amnestic disorder, 297
Alendronate for treating osteoporosis, 236
Alexithymia, defined, 319
Allergic conjunctivitis, 442, 490
Allergic rhinitis, 439-443
  causes of, 441
  summary of, 442-443
  symptoms of, 439, 441
  treatment of, 441-442
Allergic shiners, 441
Allergy, food, angioneurotic edema due to,
      645
Alpha-adrenergic agents, urinary
      incontinence due to, 553
Alprazolam
  contraindications to, 327
  for panic disorder, 323
Alprostadil for erectile disorder, 334
Alternative complementary care, 340-343
  for cancer, 340-343
  cost of, 342
  guidelines for, 341
  patient control of, 342
  primary physician's role in, 341, 342-343
  side effects of, 342
  summary of, 343
Alzheimer's disease
  versus depression, 525
  diagnosis of, 524-525
  epidemiology of, 526-527
  symptoms of, 524, 526
  treatment of, 527
Amantadine for influenza A, 621
Amaurosis fugax, 130

Amenorrhea
  in hyperprolactinemia, 100
  induced, 255
American Heart Association
  CPR recommendations of, 628
  hyperlipidemia diet guidelines of, 17
American Medical Association,
      recommendations for elderly abuse,
      514-515
Amiodarone, digoxin interaction with, 20
Amitriptyline
  and falls by elderly, 572
  for Parkinson's disease, 539
Amnestic syndrome, alcohol-related, 297,
      298
Amniotomy
  for hypotonic labor, 210
  indications of, 208
Amoxicillin
  for COPD, 43
  for peptic ulcer disease, 64
Amphetamine
  abuse of, 302
  effects of, 301
Ampicillin for COPD, 43
Amrinone, administration of, 626
Amyloid in diabetes, 97-98
Amylophagia, 201
Anabolic steroids, effects of, 302-303
Anal fissure, 543
  outpatient treatment of, 466, 468-469, 469
Analgesia, epidural, 195, 197
  pros and cons of, 196
Analgesics, narcotic; see Narcotic analgesics
Anaphylaxis, exercise-induced, 644-645
Anaprox; see Naproxen sodium
Anemia, 132-138
  of chronic disease, 135, 137
  in chronic renal failure, 166
  classification of, 136
  defined, 135
  fatigue and, 132, 133
  folic acid deficiency, 136
  hemolytic, 137-138
    in sickle-cell disease, 455
  hypochromic-microcytic, 135
  iron deficiency; see Iron deficiency
      anemia
  megaloblastic, 135, 137
  menorrhagia and, 134
  paresthesia and, 133-134
  pernicious, 135-136
    treatment of, 136
  during pregnancy, 133, 135
  in rheumatoid arthritis, 146
  sickle-cell, 454
  summary of, 136-138
  types of, 135
  uterine bleeding and, 132
Aneurysm
  intracranial, causes of, 130
  ruptured aortic, 634-637
Angina pectoris, 7-13
  defined, 12
  diagnosis of, 10, 11
  history of, 8

Angina pectoris—cont'd
  with hypertension, 9, 11
  laboratory evaluation of, 12
  versus MI, 7
  pathophysiology of, 11-12
  Prinzmetal's, 11, 12
  with sharp retrosternal chest pain, 8-9
  signs and symptoms of, 12
  summary of, 12-13
  versus transmural infarction, 6
  treatment of, 10-11
  unstable, 10, 12-13
  variants of, 12-13
Angiodysplasia, pathophysiology and
      symptoms, 478
Angiography, coronary, for angina, 10
Angioneurotic edema
  sequence of events in, 645-646
  summary of, 646
  symptoms of, 644, 645
Angiotensin-converting enzyme inhibitors
  for congestive heart failure, 21
  for hypertension, 25
  indications for, 11
  during pregnancy, 215
  side effects of, 25
  for systolic dysfunction, 20
Anion gap, assessment of, 639-640
Ankle
  fracture of, 648
  sprained, 649, 651
Anorexia nervosa
  coexisting conditions, 305
  complications of, 305, 306-307
  in glomerulonephritis, 162
  infant, 390
  management of, in advanced cancer, 88
  in ovarian cancer, 86
  in palliative care patient, 91
  symptoms of, 305, 306
  treatment of, 307
  types of, 305
  weight loss in, 303
Anorgasmia, primary, 334
Anovulation, dysfunctional uterine
      bleeding and, 258
Anterior cruciate ligament, injury to, 652
Anterior drawer test, 652
Antiarrhythmic agents
  administration of, 625-626
  for MI, 5
Antibiotics
  bacteria resistant to, 42
  for chronic bronchitis, 42
  for common cold, 399-400
  contraindications to, 460-461, 620-621
  for COPD, 43
  diarrhea associated with, 420
  OCP interaction with, 269
  prophylactic, for bacteremia, 416
  for sinusitis, 511
Anticholinergics, urinary incontinence due
      to, 553
Anticoagulation therapy
  endocarditis and, 130
  for MI, 5

Anticonvulsants
  for bipolar disorder, 287
  IUGR and, 220
  OCP interaction with, 269
Antidepressants; *see also* Tricyclic
      antidepressants
  OCP interaction with, 269
  selection of, 282
  urinary incontinence due to, 553
Antihistamines for viral URIs, 451
Antihypertensive agents
  age and race factors, 535-536
  contraindications to, 215
  for elderly, 534-536
  preventive effects of, 535
  sexual dysfunction and, 332
Antinauseants
  neurotransmitter sites for, 90
  in palliative care, 88-89
  during pregnancy, 200
Antipsychotics
  OCP interaction with, 269
  urinary incontinence due to, 553
Antipyretics, indications for, 416
Antisocial personality disorder in
      differential diagnosis of factitious
      disorder, 313
Antiviral therapy
  drug interactions in, 615
  risk-benefit analysis of, 614
Anxiety; *see also* Generalized anxiety
      disorder
  disorders associated with, 308-309
  performance, 323
  in PTSD, 325
  rebound, after sedative-hypnotic
      discontinuation, 188
  in social phobia, 324
Aorta, enlarged, 6
Aortic aneurysm
  abdominal, screening for, 579
  ruptured, 634-637
Apgar score with outlet forceps/vacuum
      extractor, 211
Apnea; *see* Sleep apnea
Appendectomy, complications of, 460
Appendicitis, 458-461
  atypical presentations of, 460
  differential diagnosis of, 460
  in elderly, 549
  pathophysiology of, 460
  retrocecal, 459
  summary of, 461
  symptoms of, 458-459
  treatment of, 459-460
APSAC for acute MI, 4
APTT; *see* Activated partial thromboplastin
      time
Arrhythmia; *see* Dysrhythmia; specific
      dysrhythmias
Arteritis, temporal, characteristics and
      treatment of, 119
Arthritis; *see also* Osteoarthritis;
      Rheumatoid arthritis
  characteristics of, 145
  gouty, 160; *see also* Gout

Ascites
  in cirrhosis, treatment of, 73
  in hepatitis, 69
  malignant
    drug management of, 90
    in palliative care patient, 91
    treatment of, 71-72
Asphyxia
  fetal, prediction of, 224
  in IUGR, 219
Aspirin
  angioneurotic edema due to, 645
  for MI, 5, 6
  MI prophylaxis with, 584
  peptic ulcer disease and, 64
  preeclampsia prophylaxis with, 584
  for preventing preeclampsia, 215
  Reye's syndrome and, 396
Assertiveness training for social phobia, 327
Asterixes, symptoms of, 297
Asthenia; *see also* Fatigue
  in advanced cancer, 89
Asthma, 44-50
  acute, 49
    treatment of, 392
  assessment of, 48
  versus bronchiolitis, 47, 392
  chronic cough in, 44
  clinical findings in, 48-49
  cough variant, 47, 49, 393
  defined, 47
  exacerbation of, 48
  exercise-induced, 391, 392-393
  infant, 390-391
  inherited factors in, 49
  mild chronic, 392
  morbidity/mortality from, 47
  pathophysiology of, 47-48
  pharmacotherapy for, 48
  phases of, 48
  prophylaxis of, 48
  respiratory syncytial virus and, 49
  shortness of breath in, 45
  summary of, 49, 393
  triad, 442
  wheezing in, 45, 393
Asystole, summary of, 627
Ataxia
  in multiple sclerosis, 109-110
  in vestibular neuronitis, 507, 509
Atenolol
  for angina, 11
  constipation associated with, 543
Atheroma in angina, 12
Atherosclerosis, progression of, 4-5
Atopic dermatitis, diaper rash due to,
      444-445
Atorvastatin for hypercholesterolemia, 15
Atrial fibrillation
  chronic, treatment of, 29
  with hemodynamic stability, 28
  with rapid ventricular response, 28
  treatment of, 29
Atrial flutter
  symptoms of, 624
  treatment of, 626

Atrial premature beats
  signs of, 28
  treatment of, 28, 29
Atropine for organophosphate poisoning,
      640
Attention-deficit hyperactivity disorder,
      359-364
  differential diagnosis of, 361
  drug therapy for, 362
  features associated with, 361
  parental behaviors associated with, 363
  psychiatric disorders associated with,
      362
  summary of, 363
  symptoms of, 359, 361
  teacher diagnosis of, 363
Aura, migraine-associated, 117-118
Autonomy, issues in, 520
Azathioprine
  for Crohn's disease, 61
  for MS, 112
Azithromycin for *Legionella* pneumonia,
      53

B

Baby stress, 376
Back pain, 186
  low; *see* Low back pain
  in osteoporosis, 233, 235
  during pregnancy, 198, 201, 202
  treatment of, 188-189
Bacteremia
  in elderly, 549
  in fever without focus, 415-416
  occult, 416
  prophylactic antibiotics and, 416
Bacteria, antibiotic-resistant, 42
Bacterial endocarditis
  causative organism in, 402-403
  summary of, 404
Bacterial vaginosis
  causative organisms, 240
  differential diagnosis of, 240
  symptoms of, 240
  treatment of, 240
Bacteriuria
  asymptomatic, screening for, 581
  in catheterized patients, 549
Bad news
  communicating, 353-358, 486
  patient support system and, 355
  summary for dealing with, 357-358
Barium enema in Crohn's disease, 60-61
Barrett's esophagus, 56
Basal cell carcinoma
  treatment of, 645
  ulcer in, 642
Basic life support, 624
  procedure for, 626
Baycol; *see* Cerivistatin
Behavioral therapy for panic disorder, 322,
      324
Beneficence, defined, 520
Benign positional vertigo
  symptoms of, 507, 509
  treatment of, 509

Benign prostatic hypertrophy
  summary of, 505
  symptoms of, 501-502
  treatment of, 503-504, 505
Benzodiazepine overdose, treatment of,
    302, 640
Benzodiazepines
  contraindications to, 327
  for GAD, 309
  for panic disorder, 323, 324
β-Adrenergic agonists for angina, 10
β-Adrenergic blocking agents
  for acute MI, 6
  for angina, 10, 11
  for atrial fibrillation, 28-29
  for cirrhosis, 73
  for hypertension, 24, 534-535
  lipid effects of, 16
  for MI, 5
  for panic disorder, 323, 324
  for performance anxiety, 323
  for social phobia, 327
  urinary incontinence due to, 553
Bias, types of, 593
Bicarbonate, recommendations for, in
    cardiac arrest, 626
Biguanides, mechanism of action of, 97
Bile acid sequestrants for
    hypercholesterolemia, 18
Biliary colic
  summary of, 464
  symptoms of, 463
Biliary tract disease, 461-465
  symptoms of, 461, 463
Bilirubin
  light absorption by, 373
  permissible range of, 373
  serum, laboratory evaluation of, 606, 608
  toxic levels of, 373
Binge-eating, 304; see also Bulimia
Biofeedback for panic disorder, 324
Biophysical profile testing, components of,
    220
Biopsy in diagnosis of breast disease, 482
Bipolar disorder, 285-289
  classification of, 288-289
  diagnosis of, 287, 289
  in differential diagnosis of
      schizophrenia, 291
  DSM-IV classification of, 287
  genetic factors in, 288, 289
  hypomania in, 288
  mania in, 285, 287, 288
  prevention of relapse, 289
  summary of, 288-289
  treatment of, 287-288, 289
Birth control pills, VLDLs and, 17
Birth plans, 194, 195-196, 197
Birth weight, smoking and, 219
Bladder cancer, screening for, 580
Bleeding
  anovulatory, 257
  dysfunctional uterine; see Dysfunctional
      uterine bleeding
  rectal, 467
    from hemorrhoids, 475

Bleeding—cont'd
  uterine, anemia-related, 132
  vaginal
    hospitalization for, 227
    spontaneous abortion and, 226-228
Blindness; see also Visual loss
  from temporal arteritis, 119
Blood pressure; see also Hypertension;
    Hypotension
  assessing, 23
  classification of, 25t
  home evaluation of, 23
Blood transfusions for sickle-cell disease,
    454
BLS; see Basic life support
Blues, postpartum; see Postpartum blues
BMI; see Body mass index
Body dysmorphic disorder; see
    Dysmorphic disorder
Body mass index, defined, 604
Bone disease, metastatic, in prostate
    cancer, 81-82
Bone pain
  in multiple myeloma, 139, 142
  in prostatic carcinoma, 502-503
Borderline personality disorder in
    differential diagnosis of factitious
    disorder, 313
Borrelia burgdorferi, 409
Bouchard's nodes in osteoarthritis, 149
Bowel disease, irritable; see Irritable bowel
    syndrome
Bowel movements, frequency of, 542; see
    also Constipation
Bowel obstruction in palliative care
    patient, 89, 91
Bowlegs, 428-429
BPH; see Benign prostatic hypertrophy
BPP; see Biophysical profile testing
Bradykinesia in Parkinson's disease, 539
Brain scan, MRI, 123-124
Brain tumor
  gliomas, 125
  seizures and, 123
Breast cancer
  death rate from, 600
  disseminated, 87
  mammography in diagnosis of, 482
  prevalence of, 482
  prevention of, 482
  risk factors for, 482
  summary of, 484
  symptoms of, 479-483
  treatment of, 482-483
  types of, 482
Breast disease, 479-484
  benign, 481
  fibrocystic, diagnosis and treatment, 483
  mammography in diagnosis of, 480
  summary of, 483-484
Breast feeding, 196, 378, 379, 381; see also
    Infant feeding
  advantages of, 385
  characteristics of, 385
  colostrum and, 384
  decreased milk production and, 383-384

Breast feeding—cont'd
  difficulties with, 383
  inadequate milk for, 385
  mastitis and, 381-382, 384
  neonatal jaundice and, 373
  vitamin supplements and, 384
Breast milk jaundice, 372
Breast milk *versus* cow's milk, 384, 385, 386
Breath, shortness of; see Dyspnea;
    Shortness of breath
Breathing, Kussmaul, 634
Bretylium, administration of, 625
Brief psychotic disorder in differential
    diagnosis of schizophrenia, 291
Bromocriptine
  for hyperprolactinemia, 103
  for Parkinson's disease, 538
Bronchial asthma; see Asthma
Bronchiolitis
  versus bronchial asthma, 47, 392
  causes of, 391-392
  diagnosis of, 391
  signs and symptoms of, 389, 391
  summary of, 393
  treatment of, 391
  wheezing in, 393
Bronchitis
  acute, 40
    treatment of, 42
  chronic; see Chronic bronchitis
  pneumonia as complication of, 50, 53
Bronchodilators
  for chronic bronchitis, 41-42
  for COPD, 43
Bronchogenic carcinoma, 87
  and new-onset seizures, 123
Bronze baby syndrome, 373
Bulimia nervosa, 305-306
  complications of, 307
  symptoms of, 304, 305-306, 306
  treatment of, 306, 307
  types of, 305
Bullae, defined, 409
Bupropion for smoking cessation, 597
Burkitt's lymphoma, Epstein-Barr virus
    and, 68
Burns
  classification of, 469
  outpatient surgery for, 466
  outpatient treatment of, 469
BV; see Bacterial vaginosis

C
CABG; see Coronary artery bypass graft
Caffeine, effects of, 302
CAGE questionnaire, 298
Calcaneovalgus foot, 428, 430
Calcimar; see Calcitonin
Calcitonin for treating osteoporosis, 236
Calcium, absorption of, estrogen and, 250
Calcium carbonate
  for preventing osteoporosis, 236
  for treating osteoporosis, 236
Calcium-channel blocking agents
  for achalasia, 56
  for angina, 10, 11

Calcium-channel blocking agents—cont'd
    for atrial fibrillation, 28-29
    for hypertension in elderly, 535
    for MI, 5
    urinary incontinence due to, 553
Caldwell-Moloy classification, 207
Campylobacter in IBS, 76
Campylobacter jejuni, gastroenteritis due to, 419
Cancer; *see also* specific types
    alternative complementary care for, 340-343
    death rate from, 600-601
    epidemiology of, 599-601
    esophageal, dysphagia due to, 57
    lowering risk from, 601
    obesity and, 31
    OCP use and, 267
    palliative care for; *see* Palliative care
    prevention of, 601
    smoking and, 596
    survival rates for, 601
    terminal, ethical decision making and, 516-517
Cancer pain, 78-86; *see also* Pain
    adjuvant analgesics for, 85
    classification of, 85
    management of, 82-83
    neuropathic, 82
    palliative treatment of, 83, 85-86
    pathophysiology of, 85
    prevalence of, 486
    in prostate cancer, 81
    summary of, 84-86
    10 commandments of, 84
    WHO Analgesic Ladder and, 82, 84-85
Candidal dermatitis, diaper rash due to, 445
Candidiasis, 238
    differential diagnosis of, 241
    esophageal, in AIDS, 614
    risk factors for, 239-240
    signs of, 239
    treatment of, 239
Cannabis, effects of, 302
Caps, cervical, characteristics of, 268
Carbamazepine
    for bipolar disorder, 287
    for conduct disorder, 363
Carcinoma; *see* specific types
Cardiac arrest
    critical debriefing after, 627
    summary of, 627-628
    symptoms of, 623-625
    treatment of, 625-627
Cardiac hypertrophy, signs of, 24
Cardiac murmurs, 446-449
    characteristics of, 446-448
    diagnosis of, 448
    explaining to parents, 448
    innocent, 447-448
    pansystolic, 447
    prevalence of, 448
    summary of, 449
    types of, 448
    ventricular septal defect, 447, 448
Cardiogenic shock, 6

Cardiomegaly, PMI in, 296
Cardiopulmonary arrest, ethical decision making and, 517
Cardiopulmonary resuscitation, 623-628; *see also* Cardiac arrest
    one-rescuer, 627
Cardiovascular disease
    death rate for, 603, 604
    in diabetes, 95
    epidemiology of, 602-605
    estrogen replacement therapy and, 250-251
    prevention of, estrogen in, 237
    smoking and, 596
Cardioversion
    for atrial flutter, 626
    for ventricular tachycardia, 626
Carotid artery stenosis, 131
    screening for, 579
Carotid endarterectomy, indications for, 130-131
Carvedilol for systolic dysfunction, 20
Case finding *versus* screening, 610
CAST study, 29
Cataplexy, defined, 184
Catecholaminergic agents, 32
Catheterization for urinary incontinence, 552, 554
CEA; *see* Carotid endarterectomy
CEA antigen, diagnostic significance of, 476-477
Cecum, adenocarcinoma of, 475
Cefoxitin for PID, 274
Celexa; *see* Citalopram
Celiac sprue
    GI complaints in, 61
    summary of, 62
    treatment of, 61
Cephalosporin cefuroxime for pneumonia, 53
Cerebral artery, occlusion of, in stroke, 128-129, 129
Cerebral edema
    as complication of diabetic ketoacidosis, 634
    headache of, 120
    in palliative care patient, 91
Cerebrovascular accident; *see also* Stroke
    in sickle-cell disease, 455, 456
Cerivistatin for hypercholesterolemia, 15
Cervical caps, characteristics of, 268
Cervical carcinoma
    alternative complementary care for, 340-342
    causes of, 245
    condyloma acuminatum and, 275
    death rate from, 600
    human papilloma virus and, 243
    risk factors for, 243-244
    screening for, 243, 579
Cervix
    abnormalities of, 241-246
        summary of, 245-246
    dilatation of, 207
    SIL of, 245
Chain of survival, 627

Charcoal, activated, in poisoning management, 640
Chest pain
    in acute myocardial infarction, 1
    in angina pectoris, 7-8, 10
    in dysrhythmia, 27
    in lymphoma, 138
    in panic disorder, 320, 322
    sharp retrosternal, 8-9
Chicken pox, symptoms of, 409
Child abuse, 364-368
    defined, 366
    failure to thrive and, 364, 366
    family rehabilitation in, 366
    interventions for, 368
    parental prototypes in, 366
    prevalence of, 367
    spousal abuse and, 346-347, 366-367
    summary of, 367-368
    symptoms of, 364-366
Childbirth; *see also* Delivery; Obstetrics
    with forceps/vacuum extractor, 211
    natural, summary of, 197
Children/adolescents, 359-457; *see also* Adolescents; Infant
    abuse of, 364-368
    with adolescent developmental problems, 432-436
    with allergic rhinitis, 439-443
    with attention-deficit hyperactivity disorder, 359-364
    with cardiac murmurs, 446-449
    with common cold, 397-400
    with conduct disorder, 359-364
    with diaper dermatitis, 443-446
    with enuresis, 436-439
    with failure to thrive/short stature, 386-389
    fever in, 378
    with fever without focus, 413-417
    with foot and leg deformities, 428-432
    with gastroenteritis, 417-421
    immunizations for, 377-379, 380
    infant feeding, 379, 381-386
    with infantile colic, 374-377
    with limp, 423-428
    with neonatal jaundice, 368-374
    with oppositional defiant disorder, 359-364
    and OTC drug abuse, 449-453
    with otitis media, 394-397
    with pneumonia, 410-413
    with recurrent abdominal pain, 421-423
    with respiratory syndromes, 389-394
    with sickle-cell disease, 453-457
    with streptococcal infections, 400-405
    with viral exanthems, 405-410
Chiropractic, insurance for, 342
Chlamydia, screening for, 581
Chlamydia trachomatis
    with gonococcal infection, 275
    in PID, 273
Cholangitis, cause and symptoms, 464
Cholecystectomy
    complications of, 464
    laparoscopic, 464
        summary of, 464

Cholecystitis
summary of, 464
symptoms of, 463
treatment of, 463
Choledocholithiasis, prevalence and
treatment, 464
Cholelithiasis, prevalence of, 463
Cholera, gastroenteritis-related death and,
420
Cholesterol
high, 13-17, 18
defined, 15
screening for, 579
home monitoring of, 17
normal values for, 15, 18
serum, cardiovascular disease and, 604
Cholestyramine for hyperlipoproteinemia,
16
Chronic bronchitis, 39, 40
acute exacerbation of, 42
causes of, 40
defined, 43
diagnosis of, 41
pathophysiology of, 43
pulmonary function abnormalities in,
40
smoking and, 41
treatment of, 41-42
Chronic fatigue syndrome, 154-158
CDC definition of, 156
epidemiology of, 157
fatigue in, 153
interventions for, 157-158
versus mononucleosis, 67
risk factors for, 158
signs and symptoms of, 154, 156, 157,
158
summary of, 158
treatment of, 158
Chronic lymphocytic leukemia, symptoms
of, 143
Chronic myelogenous leukemia, symptoms
of, 143
Chronic obstructive pulmonary disease,
37-43; *see also* Chronic bronchitis;
Emphysema
classification of, 40
pneumonia with, 51, 53
pulmonary function abnormalities in, 43
signs and symptoms of, 43
smoking and, 40, 41
summary of, 43
treatment of, 43
Chronic pain of psychogenic origin, 318
Chronic renal failure
anemia in, 166
causes of, 165
death due to, 166
diabetes-induced, 166
summary of, 167-168
treatment of, 166
Cigarette smoking; *see* Smoking
Cimetidine
for peptic ulcer disease, 64-65
side effects of, 65
Ciprofloxacin for *Legionella* pneumonia, 53

Circulation, hyperdynamic, management
of, 25
Cirrhosis, 69-74
alcoholism and, 71
ascites management in, 73
causes of, 71
complications of, 73
findings in, 72-73
hypoalbuminemia in, 72
Laënnec's, 297
prognosis for, 71
stages of, 71
summary of, 73-74, 74
symptoms of, 71
treatment of, 73
13-Cis-retinoic acid, contraindication to,
174
Citalopram for MDD, 281
CK-MB fraction; *see* Creatine kinase
isoenzyme MB fraction
Clarithromycin for *Legionella* pneumonia,
53
Claustrophobia, defined, 326
Clay, craving for, 201
Client; *see* Patient
Clindamycin for PID, 274
Clinical judgment, defined, 520
Clinics, walk-in, limitations of, 609
Clofibrate, OCP interaction with, 269
Clomipramine for panic disorder, 324
Clonidine
with hydrochlorothiazide, and
orthostatic hypotension in elderly,
568
for menopausal symptoms, 252
for opioid withdrawal, 302
for smoking cessation, 597
Clozapine
for GAD, 309
for schizophrenia, 292
side effects of, 292
Cluster headache, symptoms of, 117
Cocaine
aneurysm and, 130
effects of, 302
Cocaine intoxication
complications of, 301
symptoms of, 301
treatment of, 301
Cognition, global disorder of, 529
Cognitive psychotherapy for MDD, 281
Cognitive therapy
advantages of, 338
for GAD, 309
for panic disorder, 322, 324
in primary care, 339
Colchicine
for cirrhosis, 73
for gout, 161
Cold, common; *see* Common cold
Cold-related injuries, 653-657; *see also*
Hypothermia
summary of, 656-657
symptoms of, 653, 654-655
Colestid; *see* Colestipol
Colestipol for hyperlipoproteinemia, 16

Colic, 374-377
biliary
summary of, 464
symptoms of, 463
defined, 375
interventions for, 376
renal, 499-500
summary of, 376-377
versus urinary tract infection, 376
Colitis; *see* Ulcerative colitis
Colles' fracture, management of, 646-647
Colon, polyps of
malignant potential of, 476
summary of, 479
Colon carcinoma; *see also* Colorectal cancer
constipation and, 543
diagnosis of, 476
inflammatory bowel disease and, 61
prevention of, 478
symptoms of, 473-475
terminal, 87-88
treatment of, 476
from ulcerative colitis, 60
Colonic disorders, summary of, 478-479
Colonoscopy, indications for, 59
Colorectal cancer; *see also* Colon carcinoma
Crohn's disease and, 61
death rate from, 600
health maintenance exam and, 575, 577
screening for, 476, 579
summary of, 478-479
Colostrum, components of, 384, 386
Common cold, 398-400
antibiotics and, 399-400
causes of, 399
prevention of, 399
summary of, 400
symptoms of, 398-399
treatment of, 399
Communication
about bad news, 353-358
between family physician and specialist,
352-353
with terminally ill patient, 357
Compartment syndromes, causes and
treatment of, 648
Complex incontinence, 552
Compulsions; *see also*
Obsessive-compulsive disorder
defined, 328
types of, 328
Concentration, lack of, in seizure disorder,
122
Condoms, characteristics of, 268
Conduct disorder
causes of, 362
diagnosis of, 361
summary of, 363
Condyloma acuminatum
causes and symptoms of, 275
summary of, 277
symptoms of, 272
treatment of, 275
Confabulation, 298
Confusion
in Alzheimer's disease, 522
causes of, 525

Confusion—cont'd
  differential diagnosis of, 524
  in pneumonia of elderly, 547
Congestive heart failure, 18-21
  biventricular, 20
  drug therapy for, 20-21
  left-sided, 20
  nonpharmacologic therapy for, 20
  pathophysiology of, 21
  in sickle-cell disease, 455
  summary of, 21
  treatment of, 21
Conjunctivitis
  in adenoviral pneumonia, 412
  allergic, 442, 490
  bacterial, 490
  cause of, 409
  in rubeola, 406, 408
  summary of, 492
  viral, 490
Conn's syndrome, 100
  causes of, 102
  signs and symptoms of, 102
  summary of, 104
  treatment of, 103
Consciousness, loss of
  in delirium, 529
  in grand mal seizures, 124
  sudden, 122
Consent, informed, defined, 520
Constipation
  defined, 542
  in elderly, 540-545
    complications of, 542-543
    factors associated with, 542
    summary of, 544-545
    treatment of, 543-544
  infant, 384
  in irritable bowel disease, 75
  narcotic-induced, 90
  in palliative care patient, 91
  during pregnancy, 200, 202
  preventing, 82
  with prostate carcinoma, 541
Consultants, responsibilities of, 352
Consultations, summary of, 353
Contraception
  barrier methods of, 180, 268, 273-274
  management of, 263-270
    with hypertensive patient, 266
    with multiple sex partners, 264
    with OCPs, 263-264
    postintercourse, 264
    side effects and, 266-267
    with thrombophlebitis history, 264-265
  summary of, 270
Contraceptives, oral; see Oral contraceptive
    pills
Contraction stress test, 218
  assumptions of, 220
Contractions during pregnancy, 209-211
Conversion disorder
  in differential diagnosis of factitious
    disorder, 313
  DSM-IV criteria for, 318
  spousal abuse and, 318-319

Conversion disorder—cont'd
  summary of, 320
  symptoms of, 318
  treatment of, 319
Convulsions
  control of, 215
  febrile, 416
Cor pulmonale, acute, pulmonary
    embolism and, 35
Core rewarming, methods of, 655
Coreg; see Carvedilol
Corneal ulcer, summary of, 492
Coronary angiography in angina pectoris,
    10
Coronary artery bypass graft
  for angina, 12
  indications for, 11
  versus PTCA, 11
Coronary artery disease; see also
    Cardiovascular disease
  alcohol and, 17
  asymptomatic, screening for, 579
  hypertriglyceridemia in, 18
  risk factors for, 16-17
Coronary heart disease, smoking and, 596
Corticosteroids
  for allergic rhinitis, 441-442
  for chronic bronchitis, 42
  for COPD, 43
  for gout, 161
  for MS, 112
  for ulcerative colitis, 59-60
Corynebacterium vaginitis, 240
Coryza in rubeola, 406, 408
Cough
  from ACE inhibitors, 25
  after smoking cessation, 41
  in AIDS, 611
  in childhood pneumonia, 410-411
  chronic, in asthma, 44
  in common cold, 398
  in COPD, 37-38
  infant, 389
  in infants/children, OTC drugs for, 450,
    452
  in pneumonia, 50
  in rubeola, 406, 408
  10-day, 39-40
Cough preparations, side effects of, 452
Coxsackievirus A16, symptoms of, 409
CPR; see Cardiopulmonary resuscitation
Crack cocaine, 301, 302
Cramps, heat, treatment of, 655
Creatine kinase isoenzyme MB fraction
  in acute MI, 7
  in diagnosis of MI, 6
Crepitus in osteoarthritis, 148
Critical incident debriefing, 625, 627
Crohn's disease
  colorectal cancer and, 61
  complications of, 60
  in differential diagnosis of IBS, 76
  extracolonic manifestations of, 61
  pathophysiology of, 60
  radiographic manifestations of, 61
  versus RAP syndrome, 422

Crohn's disease—cont'd
  signs and symptoms of, 60
  summary of, 62
  treatment of, 61
Croup
  cause of, 409
  summary of, 393
  symptoms of, 389, 391
Cryosurgery for plantar warts, 467-468
Cullen's sign in pancreatitis, 471
Cushing's disease
  causes of, 103
  defined, 103
  signs and symptoms of, 103
  treatment of, 103
Cushing's syndrome, summary of, 104-105
CVA; see Cerebrovascular accident
Cyanosis in pulmonary embolism, 33-34
Cyclosporine for ulcerative colitis, 60
Cyclothymic disorder
  defined, 288
  summary of, 289
Cyst
  breast, 483
  defined, 409
  sebaceous, outpatient surgery for, 469
Cystitis, hematuria in, 169, 170
Cytology, sputum, in pneumonia
    diagnosis, 53
Cytomegalovirus infection in AIDS, 614

D

D and C; see Dilatation and curettage
DASH diet, 24
Dawn phenomenon, 96
Death, sudden; see Sudden death
Death/dying, ethical decision making and,
    519, 521-522
Debriefing, critical incident, 627
Decongestants for URI symptoms, 452
Deep venous thrombosis
  assessment of, 36
  diagnosis of, 35, 37
  risk factors for, 36
  summary of, 37
  treatment of, 36-37, 37
Dehydration
  diarrhea-related, 420
  in palliative care patient, 91
  symptoms of, 418
Delirium
  causes of, 527-528
  components of, 529
  differential diagnosis of, 528
  symptoms of, 526
Delivery; see also Childbirth; Obstetrics
  gestational age and, 225
Delta hepatitis; see hepatitis D
Delusional disorder in differential
    diagnosis of schizophrenia, 291
Delusions
  in Alzheimer's disease, 526
  defined, 291
Dementia
  multiinfarct, 524
  screening for, 582

DEMENTIA mnemonic, 524, 528-529
Dental disease, counseling
        recommendations, 583
Depession, adjustment disorder with, 282
Depot-medroxyprogesterone acetate,
        268-269
Deprenyl; *see* Selegiline
Depression, 278-285; *see also* Major
        depressive disorder
    versus Alzheimer's disease, 525
    atypical, 284
    in bipolar disorder, 286
    case studies, 278-280
    in elderly, 555-559
        differential diagnosis of, 558
        drug overuse and, 558-559
        evaluation of, 557
        prevalence and prognosis, 557
        summary of, 559
        symptoms of, 555, 557, 558
        treatment of, 557-558, 559
    in fibromyalgia, 153
    illness and, 283
    masked, 284
    in palliative care patient, 90, 92
    in Parkinson's disease, 539
    in PMS, 247
    postpartum; *see also* Postpartum blues
        risk factors for, 230
        summary of, 232
        symptoms of, 230
        treatment of, 230-231
    prevalence of, 284
    in schizophrenia, 290
    screening for, 582
    suicide risk and, 282-283
    treatment of, 281, 285
Dermatitis, diaper; *see* Diaper rash
Desipramine for ADHD, 362
Detrusor hyperreflexia, 555
DEXA; *see* Dual-energy x-ray
        absorptiometry
Dexamethasone
    in palliative care for lung carcinoma, 90
    in peptic ulcer disease, 65
    for progressive headache, 120
Dextroamphetamine for ADHD, 362
Dextromethorphan, side effects of, 452
Diabetes insipidus, 100
    nephrogenic
        treatment of, 102
        types of, 102
    summary of, 104
Diabetes mellitus, 92-98
    cardiovascular disease in, 95
    chronic renal failure due to, 166
    complications of, 98
    death rate for, 604
    diet for, 95-96
    gestational, 97
        health maintenance exam and, 578
    hyperglycemia in, 94-95
    lipid levels and, 17
    obesity and, 31
    screening for, 580
    spontaneous abortion and, 228

Diabetes mellitus—cont'd
    summary of, 98
    treatment of, 98
    type 1
        diagnosis of, 95
        types of, 96
    type 2, 96, 97
    vascular complications of, 95
Diabetic ketoacidosis, 631-634
    complications of, 634
    pathophysiology of, 634
    summary of, 634
    symptoms of, 631-633
    treatment of, 633-634
*Diagnostic and Statistical Manual of Mental
        Disorders,* 4th ed.
    bipolar disorder in, 287
    conversion disorder in, 318
    enuresis in, 437
    factitious disorder in, 312, 314
    PTSD in, 327
    spousal abuse in, 345
Diagonal conjugate, pelvic, 207
Diaper rash
    after cessation of breast feeding, 443
    from atopic dermatitis, 444-445
    from candidal dermatitis, 445
    from contact dermatitis, 445
    from dirty diapers, 444
    feeding-related, 445
    long-term, 444
    from seborrheic dermatitis, 445
    summary of, 446
Diaphragms, characteristics of, 268
Diarrhea
    antibiotic-associated, 420
    camping-related, 418, 420
    with dehydration, 418
    in infants/children, OTC drugs for, 451,
        452
    in inflammatory bowel disease, 57-58
    in palliative care patient, 91
    pediatric, 417-421
        causes of, 419
        death due to, 420
        investigations of, 420
        summary of, 420-421
        treatment of, 419, 421
    from radiotherapy, 89
    traveler's, 618
Diastole, dysfunction in, 20
Dicyclomine for colic, 376
Diet/diet therapy
    bowel habits and, 542
    for celiac sprue, 61
    DASH, 24
    for diabetic patient, 95-96
    for hypercholesterolemia, 15, 18
    for hyperlipidemia, 17
    for hypertension, 24
    peptic ulcer disease and, 64
    during pregnancy, 206-207
    for weight loss, 32
Digital rectal examination, 540, 542
    for prostatic carcinoma, 504
    for prostatitis, 505

Digoxin
    for congestive heart failure, 21
    drug interactions with, 20
    indications for, 20
    for systolic dysfunction, 20
Dilatation and curettage after completed
        abortion, 227
Dilators, esophageal, 56
Diltiazem for angina, 10
Dimenhydrinate
    abuse of, 452
    side effects of, 452
Dinner-fork deformity, 647
Diphtheria, immunizations against, 617
Discharge
    in otitis media, 394
    urethral
        in *C. trachomatis* infections, 274
        in *C. trachomatis* urethritis, 272
        in nongonococcal urethritis, 271,
            273
    vaginal; *see also* Vulvovaginitis
        differential diagnosis of, 240
        during pregnancy, 200, 202, 203
Disruptive behavior disorders; *see also*
        Attention-deficit hyperactivity
        disorder; Conduct disorder;
        Oppositional defiant disorder
    differential diagnosis of, 363
Disseminated intravascular coagulation,
        symptoms of, 143
Diuretics
    for COPD, 43
    gout and, 161-162
    for hypertension, 24, 534-535
    loop, 21
    potassium-sparing, hyperkalemia due to,
        165
    for systolic dysfunction, 20
    thiazide; *see* Thiazide diuretics
    urinary incontinence due to, 553
Divalproex acid for bipolar disorder, 287
Diverticulitis
    causative organisms, 477
    causes and symptoms of, 477
    summary of, 479
    treatment of, 477
Diverticulosis, summary of, 479
Dizziness; *see also* Vertigo
    in benign positional vertigo, 507
    in Meniere's disease, 506
    in orthostatic hypotension, 506
    in panic disorder, 320
    in vestibular neuronitis, 507, 509
DMPA; *see* Depot-medroxyprogesterone
        acetate
Domestic violence, conversion disorder
        and, 318-319
Down syndrome, screening for, 581
Doxycycline cefaclor for COPD, 43
Doxycycline for *Legionella* pneumonia, 53
DRE; *see* Digital rectal examination
Drinking, problem; *see also* Alcohol
        dependence/abuse; Alcoholism
    screening for, 582
DRIP mnemonic, 553

Drug(s)
  constipation-associated, 542, 544
  over-the-counter; *see* Over-the-counter
    drugs
  and renal toxicity in elderly, 569
  sexual dysfunction and, 332, 335
  urinary incontinence due to, 552-553
Drug abuse, 299-303; *see also* Alcohol
    dependence/abuse; Alcoholism;
    Polypharmacy
  cocaine, 301
  defined, 188
  gateway drugs and, 302
  HIV infection and, 301
  mood swings in, 299-300
  narcotic, 186, 187-188
  of psychoactive agents, 188
  screening for, 302, 582
  spousal abuse and, 345
  summary of, 302-303
  treatment of, 303
Drug overdose
  cause of death in, 639
  management of, 637, 639
Drug reactions in elderly, 566-571
Drug therapy
  in chronic care facilities, 568
  for colic, 376
  in elderly, 568, 570
  and falls by elderly, 572
  for gout, 161-162
  for hypercholesterolemia, 15, 18
  for obesity, 32
  for osteoarthritis, 150-151
  for rheumatoid arthritis, 147
  for somatization disorders, 317
Dual diagnosis, defined, 301
Dual-energy x-ray absorptiometry, 236
DUB; *see* Dysfunctional uterine bleeding
Duodenal ulcer
  H. pylori in, 63-64
  recurrence rate of, 65
  summary of, 65
  symptoms and treatment of, 64
DVT; *see* Deep venous thrombosis
Dysfunctional uterine bleeding, 256-259
  anovulatory, 258
  causes of, 257-258
  conditions associated with, 258
  defined, 258
  ovulatory, 258
  pregnancy and, 257
  secondary causes of, 257
  summary of, 259
  treatment of, 258-259
Dyskinesias, treatment of, 538
Dyslipidemia, 13-17
  risk factors for, 15
Dysmenorrhea, 252-256
  diagnosis of, 255
  pain in, 252-254
  prevalence of, 254
  primary, 254
  secondary, 254-255
  summary of, 255-256
  treatment of, 254-255, 255-256

Dysmorphic disorder
  differential diagnosis of, 317
  summary of, 320
  symptoms of, 317
Dyspareunia
  after episiotomy, 196
  causes of, 334
  defined, 334
Dysphagia
  in AIDS, 612
  cause of, 56
  differential diagnosis of, 56
  malignant, 56
  in stroke, 126
Dyspnea; *see also* Shortness of breath
  infant, 389
  in left ventricular failure, 20
  in palliative care patient, 91
  paroxysmal nocturnal, 21
Dysrhythmia, 27-29
  summary of, 29
  treatment of, 29
  ventricular, treatment of, 5
Dysthymia
  versus MDD, 284
  prevalence of, 284
Dysthymic disorder
  definition of, 282
  symptoms of, 280
Dysuria
  in benign prostatic hypertrophy, 501-502
  in cystitis, 169
  in herpes simplex infection, 272
  in prostatic carcinoma, 502-503
  in prostatitis, 503-504

E

Ear disorders, 506-512
  summary of, 511-512
Earache
  in otitis media, 394
  treatment of, 396
Eating disorders, 303-307; *see also* Anorexia
    nervosa; Bulimia nervosa
  prevalence of, 306
  psychiatric disorders related to, 306
  summary of, 306-307
Echocardiography for obese patient, 32
Eclampsia, seizures with, 215
Ectopic pregnancy, 259-263
  complications of, 262
  death due to, 261
  differential diagnosis of, 261
  dysmenorrhea and, 254
  epidemiology of, 261
  management of, 262
  pain in, 259, 261
  risk factors for, 262
  signs and symptoms of, 261-262
  STDs and, 262-263
  summary of, 263
Edema
  angioneurotic
    sequence of events in, 645-646
    summary of, 646
    symptoms of, 644, 645

Edema—cont'd
  cerebral
    as complication of diabetic
      ketoacidosis, 634
    headache of, 120
    in palliative care patient, 91
  lower extremity, during pregnancy,
    201-202
EES
  for *Legionella* pneumonia, 53
  for pneumonia, 52, 53
EFM; *see* Electronic fetal monitoring
Ejaculation, premature, treatment of, 333
Ejection fraction, low, 20
Elbows, swelling in, in lymphoma, 139
Elder abuse, 513-516
  AMA recommendations for, 514-515
  defined, 515
  management of, 516
  prevalence of, 514-515
  research priorities for, 515-516
  risk factors for, 515
  symptoms of, 513-514
Elderly
  abdominal pain in, 634-637
  adverse drug reactions in, 566-571
Electrocardiogram
  in acute MI, 6, 7
  in angina, 8-9, 10
  in anterior wall MI, 3
  in musculoskeletal chest wall pain, 4
Electronic fetal monitoring, screening with,
    194, 196, 197, 581
ELISA, characteristics of, 403
Embolism
  fat, 35
  pulmonary; *see* Pulmonary embolism
Embolus, cerebral, 130
Emergency medicine, 623-649
  abdominal pain, 634-637
  CPR, 623-628
  diabetic ketoacidosis, 631-634
  fracture management, 646-649
  heat- and cold-related injuries, 653-657
  poison management, 637-641
  trauma, 628-631
  urticaria/angioneurotic edema, 641-646
Eminase; *see* APSAC
Emphysema
  defined, 40, 43
  pathophysiology of, 43
Enalapril
  for angina, 11
  and falls by elderly, 572
  for hypertension, 25
Encainide, contraindication to, 5
Encephalopathy, alcoholic, 297
Endocarditis
  anticoagulation therapy and, 130
  bacterial
    causative organism in, 402-403
    summary of, 404
Endocervical canal, sampling, 243
Endocrine disease, 99-105; *see also* specific
    conditions
  acromegaly, 99
  Addison's, 99

Endocrine disease—cont'd
Conn's syndrome, 100
diabetes insipidus, 100
hyperprolactinemia, 100
summary of, 104-105
thyroid carcinoma, 101
Endolymphatic hydrops, 508-509
Endometriosis
in dysmenorrhea, 255
symptoms and diagnosis, 255
treatment of, 255
Endometrium, estrogen/progesterone
proliferation of, 257-258
Endothelium in atherosclerosis, 5
Enema, barium, in Crohn's disease, 60-61
Enuresis, 436-439
diagnosis and treatment of, 437-438
DSM classification of, 437
mental disorders and, 437, 438
primary *versus* secondary, 437
summary of, 438-439
Enzyme-linked immunosorbent assay,
characteristics of, 403
Epidemiology/public health, 575-622
basic concepts in, 587-594
cancer, 599-601
cardiovascular, 602-605
complete *versus* focused periodic exams
in, 584-587
HIV and AIDS, 611-616
influenza, 618-622
laboratory medicine in, 605-611
smoking cessation, 594-599
summary of, 594
travelers' advice, 616-618
U.S. Preventive Services Task Force
recommendations, 575-584
Epididymis with NGU, 276
Epididymitis
causative organisms, 276
summary of, 277
Epidural analgesia, 195, 197
Epiglottis, acute, 390, 392
summary of, 393
Epilepsy; *see also* Status epilepticus
febrile seizures and, 125
Epinephrine
in social phobia, 327
for ventricular fibrillation, 626
Episcleritis, symptoms of, 490
Episiotomy, 195
indications and contraindications, 197
pain from, 196
summary of, 197
Epstein-Barr virus
in mononucleosis, 67
tests for, 67-68
Erectile disorder, treatment of, 334
Erectile dysfunction, 332, 333
Ergotamine preparations for cluster
headache, 117
Erysipelas
cause and symptoms of, 403
summary of, 404
Erythema, pressure ulcers formation and,
562, 563

Erythema infectiosum, symptoms of, 405,
407
Escherichia coli
gastroenteritis due to, 419-420
pneumonia due to, 53
Esophageal candidiasis in AIDS, 614
Esophageal motility disorder, 54-57
cause of, 55
classification of, 55
differential diagnosis of, 55
treatment of, 56
Esophageal motor disorder, chest pain in,
10
Esophageal rings, dysphagia due to, 56-57
Esophagus
Barrett's, 56
cancer of, 56
spasm of, 56
dysphagia due to, 56
Estrogen
high-dose, for postcoital prevention of
pregnancy, 267
lipid profile and, 251, 266-267
migraine and, 118
for stress incontinence, 554
Estrogen replacement therapy
cardiovascular disease and, 250-251
contraindications to, 251
for preventing osteoporosis, 236, 237, 251
recommendations for, 577
ESWL; *see* Extracorporeal shock wave
lithotripsy
Ethanol
for methanol/ethylene glycol poisoning,
640
neurotransmitter effects of, 297
Ethics
with brain dead newborn, 518-521
contextual factors in, 521
in end of life decisions, 519, 521-522
in geriatric medicine, 516-517, 519
guidelines for, 192
of pharmaceutical companies, 190-193
with referrals and consolations, 348-353
summary of, 193, 522
with terminal illness, 516-517, 519
with unmarried pregnant woman,
517-519
Ethylene glycol poisoning, treatment of,
640
Evista; *see* Raloxifene
Exanthem subitum, symptoms of, 405, 407
Exanthems, viral, 405-410
Exercise
anaphylaxis induced by, 644-645
asthma induced by, 391, 392-393
for hypertension, 24
for osteoarthritis, 150
for osteoporosis, 236
Exercise counseling, recommendations for,
582
Exocervix, sampling, 243
Extracorporeal shock wave lithotripsy for
nephrolithiasis, 500
Eye disorders; *see* Ophthalmologic
problems; specific disorders

F
Factitious disorder, 310-314
differential diagnosis of, 312-313, 314
DSM-IV criteria for, 312, 314
etiology of, 313-314
versus hypochondriasis, 319
prevalence of, 312
risk factors for, 312
summary of, 313
symptoms of, 310, 311-312
treatment of, 313
Failure to thrive, 386-389
disorders manifesting as, 388
followup assessment of, 387-388
maternal neglect and, 388
nonorganic *versus* organic, 387
summary of, 388-389
symptoms of, 364, 366, 386
treatment of, 387
Falls by elderly, 571-574
causes of, 572
in nursing homes, 573
outcomes of, 572
prevalence of, 572
prevention of, 573
risk factors for, 573
summary of, 573
Family physician
advocate role of, 353
versus specialist practices, 352
specialty areas of, 352
Family violence; *see also* Child abuse; Elder
abuse; Sexual abuse; Spousal abuse
screening for, 582
Famotidine for peptic ulcer disease, 64-65
Farmers, cancer in, 601
Fat, dietary, 604
Fat embolism, 35
Fatigue
in advanced cancer, 89
anemia-related, 132, 133
in chronic fatigue syndrome, 154, 156
differential diagnosis of, 153
in glomerulonephritis, 162
in hepatitis, 69
in non-Hodgkin's lymphoma, 139
during pregnancy, 202
Febrile convulsions, 416
Febrile seizures, 125
Fecal impaction
causes of, 543
symptoms of, 542
Fecal occult blood testing,
recommendations for, 577
Feet
blanched, 653, 655
crooked, 428, 429; *see also* Foot/leg
deformities
flat, 429-430
Felty's syndrome in rheumatoid arthritis,
146
Femoral anteversion, excessive, 429, 431
Fentanyl for cancer pain, 82
Fetal alcohol syndrome, 207
intrauterine growth restriction and, 219
prevalence of, 219

Fetal heart rate
  decelerations of, definition and
      significance of, 220-221
  labor termination and, 211
  monitoring of, 196
  nonstress test for assessing, 220
  and termination of labor, 211
Fetal monitoring, electronic, 194, 196, 197
  screening with, 581
Fetal outcome, predictors of, 220
Fetus
  asphyxia of, prediction of, 224
  gestational age of
      versus fundal height, 218
      missing data for, 224
  head engagement of, 207
  intrauterine growth restriction of,
      216-222
  maternal preeclampsia and, 214
  maternal smoking and, 219
  mortality rate versus gestational age, 225
  small for gestational age, 219
      nomenclature for, 221
  testing of, 220
Fever
  after immunizations, 377-378
  antipyretics for, 416
  in childhood pneumonia, 410-411
  in children, 378
      classification of, 415
      OTC drugs for, 449, 451-452
      patterns of, 416
  in exanthem subitum, 405, 407
  in gout, 160
  in infants, OTC drugs for, 449, 451-452
  in influenza, 618-619
  in mononucleosis, 66
  in scarlet fever, 407, 408
  treatment of, 396
      versus nontreatment, 451
  without focus, 413-417
      diagnosis and management of,
          416-417
      summary of, 417
      symptoms of, 413, 415
  in young versus elderly, 550
Fibroadenoma
  of breast, 481
  summary of, 484
Fibrocystic breast disease
  diagnosis and treatment, 483
  summary of, 483-484
Fibromyalgia
  diagnosis of, 154
  differential diagnosis of, 153
  versus mononucleosis, 67
  signs and symptoms of, 151, 152-153
  summary of, 154
  treatment of, 153-154
  trigger points in, 513
Fibrosis in rheumatoid arthritis, 146
Finasteride for BPH, 503, 505
Fish oil, lipid levels and, 17
Flatfeet, 429-430
  flexible, 429-431
      summary of, 432

Flatulence in inflammatory bowel disease,
      58-59
Flecainide, contraindication to, 5
Floxin; see Ofloxacin
Fluconazole for candidiasis, 239
Flumazenil for benzodiazepine overdose,
      302, 640
Fluoride supplements, infant, 384
Fluoxetine
  constipation and, 543
  for eating disorders, 306
  for MDD, 281
Fluvoxamine for MDD, 281
Flying, fear of, 325
Foley catheter for urinary incontinence, 552
Folic acid
  deficiency of, 136
  supplemental, during pregnancy, 207
Food allergy, angioneurotic edema due to,
      645
Food cravings during pregnancy, 201
Foot drop in stroke, 127
Foot/leg deformities, 428-432
  calcaneovalgus foot, 428, 430
  excessive femoral anteversion, 429, 431
  flexible flatfeet, 429-431
  internal tibial torsion, 428-431
  metatarsus adductus, 428, 430
  summary of, 432
  talipes equinovarus, 429, 431
  toeing in, 429, 431
Forceps delivery
  Apgar score and, 211
  classification of, 211
  indications for, 211-212
Formula
  infant constipation and, 384
  infant feeding with, 382-383
Fosinopril, lipid effects of, 16
Fracture management
  ankle, 647
  basics of, 648-649
  scaphoid, 646-647
  wrist, 646
Fractures
  management of, 646-649
  vertebral, in osteoporosis, 235
Fragile X syndrome, 388
Frank-Starling curve in congestive heart
      failure, 21
Friedman labor curve, 207
Frostnip, symptoms of, 655
FTT; see Failure to thrive
Functional incontinence, 552
  summary of, 555
  treatment of, 553
Fungating growths
  in palliative care patient, 91
  treatment of, 90
Furosemide
  for congestive heart failure, 21
  side effects of, 21

G

GAD; see Generalized anxiety disorder
Gallbladder disease, from OCPs, 266

Gallstones; see also Biliary tract disease
  asymptomatic, 463-464, 465
  composition of, 463
  diagnosis of, 463
  pancreatitis and, 472
  treatment of, 463-464
Ganser syndrome in differential diagnosis
      of factitious disorder, 313
Gardnerella vaginitis, 240
Gastric ulcer
  H. pylori in, 64
  summary of, 65
Gastroenteritis
  pediatric; see also Diarrhea, pediatric
      causes of, 419
      death due to, 420
      summary of, 420-421
  Salmonella, 419
Gastroesophageal reflux disease
  in differential diagnosis of IBS, 76-77
  dysphagia due to, 57
  during pregnancy, 199, 201, 203
Gastrointestinal cancer, anemia in, 135
Gastroparesis, diabetic, 96
Gastroplasty, 32
Gaussian distribution, 593
GBBS; see Streptococcus, group ß
GCA; see Giant cell arteritis
Gemfibrozil for hypertriglyceridemia, 17
General surgery; see Surgery
Generalized anxiety disorder, 307-310; see
      also Anxiety
  behavioral treatment of, 309
  defined, 308
  misdiagnosis of, 308-309
  pharmacologic treatment of, 309
  substances associated with, 309
  summary of, 309-310
  symptoms of, 280, 307, 309
  treatment of, 310
Genital herpes simplex virus, screening
      for, 581
Gentamicin in elders, 563
Gentian violet for candidiasis, 239
Geophagia, 201
Geriatric medicine, 513-574
  constipation, 540-545
  depression, 555-559
  elderly abuse, 513-516
  ethics in, 516-522
  falls, 571-574
  hypertension, 532-536
  Parkinson's disease, 536-540
  pneumonia, 545-550
  polymyalgia, rheumatica, temporal
      arteritis, 529-532
  polypharmacy/drug reactions, 566-571
  pressure ulcers, 559-565
  senile dementia and delirium, 522-529
  urinary incontinence, 550-555
German measles; see Rubella
Gestational age
  delivery timing and, 225
  estimating, 196
  versus fundal height, 218
  missing data for, 224
  mortality rate and, 225

Gestational diabetes mellitus, health maintenance exam and, 578
Giant cell arteritis, symptoms of, 531-532
Giardiasis
abdominal pain in, 422
symptoms of, 418, 420
Glasgow coma scale, 630, 631
Glatiramer acetate for MS, 112
Glaucoma
screening for, 581
summary of, 492
symptoms of, 491
Gliomas, 125
Global disorder of cognition, 529
Glomerulonephritis, 162-168
poststreptococcal, 164-165
versus non-poststreptococcal, 166
summary of, 167
Glucagon, serum, in diabetic ketoacidosis, 633
Glucose intolerance from OCPs, 266
Gluten enteropathy; *see* Celiac sprue
Goiter, hyperthyroidism in, 107
Gonococcal urethritis, summary of, 277
Gonorrhea
health maintenance exam and, 576-577
screening for, 580
treatment of, 171
Gout, 158-162
diagnosis of, 160
prevention of, 161
signs and symptoms of, 160-161
summary of, 162
treatment of, 161-162
Grand mal seizures, 124
Graves' disease
causes of, 107
signs and symptoms of, 107
treatment of, 108
Grey-Turner's sign in pancreatitis, 471
Group psychotherapy, 339
Growing pains, 423, 425-426
GUSTO trial for acute MI, 4
Gynecologic cancer, counseling recommendations, 583

H

Habitrol for smoking cessation, 598
Haemophilus influenzae
in community-acquired pneumonia, 547
pneumonia due to, 53
vaccine against, 379
Haemophilus vaginitis, 240
Hairy cell leukemia, symptoms of, 143
Hallucinations
in Alzheimer's disease, 526
hypnagogic, defined, 184
and polypharmacy in elderly, 566, 568
Hallucinogens, effects of, 303
Haloperidol for bipolar disorder, 287
Hand-foot syndrome, 454-455
Hand-foot-mouth disease, 409
Hashimoto's thyroiditis, 107
symptoms of, 108
Hay fever, health maintenance exam and, 576

hCG; *see* Human chorionic gonadotropin
Headache, 113-121
in acromegaly, 99
chronic, 119
second opinion on, 350
classification of, 120-121
cluster, symptoms of, 117
in influenza, 618-619
left-sided, temporal, 116
migraine, 116, 117-119
mixed syndrome, 118
with nausea, vomiting, neck stiffness, 117
with nausea and vomiting, 114
during pregnancy, 202
with progressive course, 120
progressive course of, 116, 119-120
rebound analgesic, 120
recurrent, 114, 115
in scarlet fever, 407, 408
secondary, 120, 121
summary of, 121
tension-type, 119
Health maintenance exam, 584-587; *see also* Physical exam
colorectal cancer in, 575, 577
gestational diabetes in, 578
gonorrhea in, 576-577
hay fever in, 576
hot flashes in, 576, 577
indications for, 586
lung cancer in, 577
menopausal symptoms in, 576, 577
pancreatic cancer in, 577
versus physical exam, 585-586
preeclampsia in, 578
pregnancy in, 576, 578
proteinuria in, 578
safe behavior in, 576, 578
skin cancer in, 585
smoking in, 575
summary of, 587
Health screening, periodic, criteria for, 586
Hearing, tests of, 510
Hearing loss
conductive, 510
intermittent, 507, 509
in labyrinthitis, 510
in mastoiditis, 508, 510
screening for, 581
summary of, 511-512
in vestibular neuronitis, 507, 509
Heart block, second-degree, 626
summary of, 627-628
Heart failure; *see also* Congestive heart failure
in sickle-cell disease, 455
Heart murmurs; *see* Cardiac murmurs
Heart rate, fetal; *see* Fetal heart rate
Heartburn during pregnancy, 201, 203
Heat cramps, treatment of, 655
Heat exhaustion, symptoms and treatment, 655-656
Heat-related injuries, 653-657
risk factors for, 656
summary of, 656-657
symptoms of, 653-656

Heatstroke
risk factors for, 656
symptoms and treatment, 656
Helicobacter pylori
in duodenal ulcer, 63-64
eradication of, 64
Helplessness, learned, 345-346, 347
Hematologic disorders
disease descriptions for, 140
summary of, 143
Hematologic malignancy; *see* Lymphoma; Multiple myeloma
Hematoma, subungual, outpatient treatment of, 469
Hematuria
in cystitis, 169, 170
in sickle-cell trait, 455
Hemianopia, homonymous, in stroke, 127
Hemiplegia in stroke, 126-127
Hemoglobin, normal levels of, 136
Hemoglobin A1c in diabetes, 95
Hemoglobinopathies, screening for, 582
Hemolytic anemia, 137-138
in sickle-cell disease, 455
Hemorrhage, subarachnoid
headache due to, 120
lumbar puncture and, 131
Hemorrhoids
bleeding due to, 475
internal, outpatient treatment of, 470
iron deficiency anemia and, 135
during pregnancy, 199, 201, 202-203
thrombosed, outpatient treatment of, 466, 468, 469
treatment of, 477
Heparin
for acute MI, 4, 6
for angina, 10
for DVT, 35-36, 37
for pulmonary embolism, 35-36, 37
Hepatitis, 69-74
alcoholic, 71
summary of, 74
chronic active, 72
infectious forms of, 73-74
versus mononucleosis, 67
summary of, 73-74
Hepatitis A, 71
antigens/antibodies in, 72
causes of, 72
diagnosis of, 72
signs and symptoms of, 72
summary of, 73
viral, 72
Hepatitis B
progression of, 71
screening for, 580
summary of, 73-74
vaccination against, 72, 378
Hepatitis C, 72
progression of, 71
summary of, 74
Hepatitis D, 72
summary of, 74
Hepatitis E, 722
summary of, 74

Hepatitis G, summary of, 74

Hepatocellular adenoma, OCPs and, 267

Hepatomegaly
in alcohol abuse, 297
in alcoholic hepatitis, 71
in mononucleosis, 67

Herpes genitalis, summary of, 277

Herpes simplex infection
in dendritic ulcer, 490
screening for, 581
symptoms and treatment of, 275
symptoms of, 272, 409

Herpes simplex virus type 2, cervical
carcinoma and, 243

Herpes varicella, symptoms of, 409

Herpesvirus 6 in exanthem subitum, 407

Heterophil antibody test for Epstein-Barr
virus, 67-68

Hip fracture in elderly, 572

Hip replacement, total, pulmonary
embolism and, 34-35

Histrionic personality disorder in
differential diagnosis of factitious
disorder, 313

HIV
in drug users, 301
screening for, 580
spermicides and, 268
testing for, 615-616

HIV infection
asymptomatic, 612-613
counseling and testing, 615
counseling recommendations, 583
high-risk behaviors for, 615
maternal-infant transmission of, 615

HIV RNA testing, indications for, 614

HIV/AIDS infection, 611-616
symptoms of, 611-614

HMG CoA reductase inhibitors for
hypercholesterolemia, 15-16, 18

Hodgkin's disease
chest pain in, 138
histologic typing of, 141
versus non-Hodgkin's lymphoma, 142-143
Reed-Sternberg cells in, 141
staging of, 141
treatment of, 141

Homonymous hemianopia in stroke, 127

Hormone replacement therapy, regimen
for, 250

Hot flashes
health maintenance exam and, 576, 577
menopausal, 249, 250

Household injuries, counseling
recommendations, 583

HPV; *see* Human papilloma virus

H2 receptor antagonists for peptic ulcer
disease, 64-65

Human chorionic gonadotropin in ectopic
pregnancy, 261

Human herpesvirus 6 in exanthem
subitum, 407

Human papilloma virus, cervical
carcinoma and, 243

Human parvovirus B19 in erythema
infectiosum, 407

Hydrochlorothiazide
with clonidine, and orthostatic
hypotension in elderly, 568
constipation associated with, 543
and falls by elderly, 572
lipoprotein effects of, 16

Hyperbilirubinemia
indirect, 373
neonatal, 374

Hypercalcemia
cancer-related, 90
from metastatic malignancy, 103
in palliative care patient, 92

Hypercholesterolemia
screening for, 15
treatment of, 15-16

Hyperdynamic circulation, management
of, 25

Hyperglycemia in diabetic patient, 94, 96

Hyperkalemia, causes of, 165

Hyperlipoproteinemia
drug therapy for, 16
screening for, 17-18
summary of, 17-18

Hyperparathyroidism
characteristics and treatment of, 103-104
primary, summary of, 105

Hyperpigmentation in Addison's disease, 99

Hyperprolactinemia, 100
signs and symptoms of, 103
treatment of, 103

Hypersomnolence, idiopathic, 185
summary of, 186

Hypertension, 21-27
alcohol abuse and, 23
with angina, 9, 11
anorexic drugs and, 32
cardiovascular disease and, 604
chronic, 214
defined, 216
classification of, 25t
in Conn's syndrome, 100
with diabetes, 535
diagnosis of, 23, 25
in elderly, 532-536
with angina, 533-534
with diabetes, 534
with heart disease, 534
summary of, 536
symptoms of, 532-533
treatment of, 534-536
family history of, 13
with heart disease, 535
IUGR and, 219
lacunar infarcts and, 129
malignant, 24-25
mild, 24
obesity and, 32
from OCPs, 266
polypharmacy due to, 566
during pregnancy, 212-216
summary of, 216
treatment of, 214-215, 216
pregnancy-induced, defined, 214, 216
screening for, 579
stroke and, 129, 130

Hypertension—cont'd
summary of, 26
systolic *versus* diastolic, 535
thiazide diuretics and, 213
treatment of, 23-24, 25; *see also*
Antihypertensive agents
nonpharmacologic, 23-24
work-up for, 24

Hypertensive disorders, definition of, 216

Hypertensive emergency
examples of, 24-25
treatment of, 25

Hypertensive urgency, examples of, 25

Hyperthyroidism
causes of, 107
in Graves' disease, 107
summary of, 109

Hypertriglyceridemia
in coronary artery disease, 18
in diabetic patient, 95
drug therapy for, 17

Hyperuricemia, asymptomatic, 162

Hypnagogic hallucinations, defined, 184

Hypnotic agents
OCP interaction with, 269
for sleep disorders, 185

Hypoactive sexual desire disorder, 334

Hypoalbuminemia in cirrhosis, 72

Hypochondriasis
differential diagnosis of, 319
in differential diagnosis of factitious
disorder, 313
DSM-IV criteria for, 319
summary of, 320
treatment of, 319

Hypochromic-microcytic anemia, 135

Hypoglycemic agents, oral, 97

Hypomania
characteristics of, 288
versus mania, 287
theories of, 288

Hypotension
orthostatic, in elderly, 568
shock due to, 6

Hypothalamic set point, mediation of, 416

Hypothermia
death due to, 655
defined, 654
ethanol-associated, 653, 654
symptoms of, 655
treatment of, 655

Hypothyroidism
causes of, 108
congenital, screening for, 582
diagnosis of, 108
in differential diagnosis of spousal
abuse, 345
fatigue in, 153
summary of, 109

Hypovolemia, shock due to, 6

I

Idiopathic hypersomnolence, summary of,
186

Idiopathic thrombocytopenic purpura,
symptoms of, 143

Illness, terminal
  breaking news about, 353-358
  ethical issues in, 516-517, 519
Imidazole for candidiasis, 239
Imipramine
  for panic disorder, 324
  for PTSD, 327
Imitrex; see Sumatriptan
Immunizations
  adverse effects of, 377-378
  contraindications to, 378-379
  guidelines for, 377-379
  influenza, 621
  recommendations for, 380, 583
  against rubella, 408
  tetanus, 617, 618
  for travelers, 616-618, 618
Immunocompromised patient
  COPD in, 53-54
  pneumonia in, 53-54
Impedance plethysmography, 36
Impetigo
  cause and symptoms of, 403
  summary of, 404
Impotence with hypertension, 330, 332
Incest; see also Sexual abuse
  defined, 367
  forms of, 367
Incidence, defined, 593
Incontinence; see Urinary incontinence
Infant
  acceptable weight gain for, 383
  failure to thrive in, 386-389
  health of, smoking and, 596
  regurgitation by, 382, 384-385
Infant feeding, 379, 381-386; see also Breast
    feeding
  on demand, 383
  diaper rash associated with, 443, 445
  fluoride supplementation and, 384
  with formula, 382-383
  mistakes in, 383
  with solid foods, 384
  summary of, 385-386
  technique for, 385
  typical patterns of, 384
Infections, opportunistic, in AIDS, 612,
    614
Infectious disease in elderly, 550
Infectious mononucleosis; see
    Mononucleosis
Infertility, 176-182
  defined, 178
  factors affecting, 178
  female factors in, 178, 180, 181
  male factors in, 178, 180, 181
  pelvic inflammatory disease and, 176
  prevalence, 178-179
  secondary, 178
  summary of, 180-181
  testing for, 179-180
  treatment of, 181
Inflammatory bowel disease, 57-62
  colon cancer and, 61
  summary of, 62
Infliximab for Crohn's disease, 61

Influenza
  complications of, 621
  diagnosis and treatment of, 618-622
  epidemics of, 620
  immunizations against, 621-622
  summary of, 622
Influenza A
  pandemics of, 621
  symptoms of, 618, 620
Informed consent, defined, 520
Ingrown toenail, outpatient procedure for,
    466, 468
Inhalants, effects of, 303
Insomnia, psychophysiologic, 185
Insufficient sleep syndrome, 185, 337
Insulin
  for diabetic ketoacidosis, 633-634
  for diabetic patient, 96
  serum, in diabetic ketoacidosis, 633
Interferon for common cold, 399
Interferon-β for MS, 112
Intestines; see Colon; Small intestine
Intoeing, 428, 429, 431
  summary of, 432
Intrauterine device
  contraindications to, 269
  summary of, 270
Intrauterine growth restriction, 216-222
  antepartum management of, 222
  asymmetric *versus* symmetric, 219,
    221-222
  drugs and, 220
  fetal alcohol syndrome and, 219
  fetal outcome and, 220
  intrapartum management of, 222
  maternal hypertension and, 219
  perinatal death due to, 219
  postpartum management of, 222
  prevalence of, 221
  smoking and, 219
  summary of, 221-222
Intrinsic factor, deficiency of, 136
Ipecac, syrup of
  contraindications to, 640
  indications for, 640
Ipratropium bromide for COPD, 41
Iridocyclitis
  summary of, 492
  symptoms of, 490-491
Iritis, symptoms and treatment of, 491
Iron, supplemental, during pregnancy,
    206
Iron deficiency anemia, 134
  causes of, 135
  diagnosis of, 135
  screening for, 580
  secondary causes of, 134
  summary of, 136-137
Iron supplements, infant, 385
Irritable bowel syndrome, 75-78
  cause of, 76
  differential diagnosis of, 76-77
  second opinion on, 348-350
  sexual abuse and, 77
  summary of, 78
  treatment of, 77

Ischemia
  asymptomatic, management of, 12
  testing of, 12
ISIS-II study of acetylsalicylic acid, 5
Isosorbide dinitrate for angina, 10

J

Jarisch-Herxheimer reaction, 275-276
Jaundice, neonatal; see Neonatal jaundice
Joints, in osteoarthritis, 148-150

K

Kaposi's sarcoma in AIDS, 614
Kawasaki disease, symptoms of, 409
Kernicterus, causes of, 373
Ketoacidosis, diabetic; see Diabetic
    ketoacidosis
Ketoconazole for candidiasis, 239
Kidney stones; see Renal stones
Klebsiella pneumonia, 52
Klebsiella pneumoniae
  in community-acquired pneumonia, 547
  signs and symptoms of, 53
Knee
  injuries to, 649-652
  limping due to, 425, 426
Korsakoff's psychosis, 298
Kussmaul breathing, characteristics of,
    634
Kyphosis, 233

L

La Leche League, 385
Labor
  1st stage of, 209-212
    summary of, 212
  2nd stage of, 209-212
    summary of, 212
  3rd stage of, 207-208
  Friedman curve of, 207
  hypotonic, 210-211
  induced
    with membrane stripping, 212
    protocol for, 212
  intravenous infusions during, 196
  intravenous therapy during, 197
  pain during, 196
  stages and phases of, 207
  support person during, 197
  termination of, fetal heart rate and, 211
Laboratory testing
  in asymptomatic patients, 608
  costs of, 609
  indications for, 608-609
  overuse of, 610
  prostatic carcinoma, 607
  quality of adjusted life years and, 607
  serum bilirubin, 606, 608
  summary of, 611
  use and abuse of, 605-611
Labyrinthitis, symptoms and treatment of,
    510
Lachman's test, procedure for, 652
Lactase deficiency
  summary of, 62
  treatment of, 61

Lactation
  dietary allowances during, 206
  OCPs during, 268
Lactose intolerance
  in differential diagnosis of IBS, 76
  versus RAP syndrome, 422
Lactulose for narcotic-induced
    constipation, 90
Lacunar infarcts, 129
Laënnec's cirrhosis, 297
Lamaze classes, 195
Lamaze technique, 196
Language, impaired, in Alzheimer's
    disease, 526
Laxatives
  recommendations for, 543-544
  types of, 543-544
Lead, elevated blood levels of, screening
    for, 580
Lead-time bias, 593
Learned helplessness, 345-346, 347
LEDO therapy, 334-335
LEEP; *see* Loop electrode excision
    procedure
Left ventricular ejection fraction in acute
    MI, 4
Left ventricular failure, symptoms of, 20,
    21
Legg-Calvé-Perthes disease, symptoms of,
    424, 426
Legionella pneumonia, 52-53
  signs and symptoms of, 53-54
Legs, swollen, during pregnancy, 201-202,
    203
Leiomyomata in dysmenorrhea, 255
Length-time bias, 593
Lethargy in thyroid disease, 107
Leukemia
  acute lymphocytic, symptoms of, 143
  acute myeloblastic, symptoms of, 143
  chronic lymphocytic, symptoms of, 143
  chronic myelogenous, symptoms of, 143
  in differential diagnosis of spousal
      abuse, 345
  hairy cell, symptoms of, 143
Levodopa
  for Parkinson's disease, 538-539
  side effects of, 539
Levofloxacin for *Legionella* pneumonia, 53
Levorphanol for cancer pain, 82
Libido, decreased, in hyperprolactinemia,
    100
Lichen planus, symptoms of, 643
Lidocaine
  administration of, 625
  contraindication to, 5, 7
  for PVCs, 5
  for ventricular tachycardia, 626
Life support, ethical decision making
    about, 519-522
Lifestyle
  cardiovascular disease and, 604
  health maintenance exam and, 577
Ligaments
  ankle, sprain of, 651
  anterior cruciate, tear of, 650, 652

Ligaments—cont'd
  collateral tear *versus* meniscal tear, 652
  knee, tear of, 649-651
Ligation, rubber band, 477-478
Likelihood ratio, defined, 591, 608
Limping child, 423-428
  differential diagnosis in, 427
  with knee pain, 425, 426
  with Legg-Calvé-Perthes disease, 424, 426
  with Osgood-Schlatter disease, 424, 426
  with osteochondritis, 424, 426-427
  with patellofemoral syndrome, 425, 427
  with slipped capital femoral epiphysis,
      424, 426
  summary of, 427-428
  symptoms of, 423, 425-426
  with toxic synovitis, 425, 427
Lipids
  estrogen and, 251
  OCP use and, 266-267
  progestin and, 251
Lipitor; *see* Atorvastatin
Lipoproteins, low-density, elevated, 15
Lithium carbonate
  for bipolar disorder, 287
  for conduct disorder, 363
  in nephrogenic diabetes insipidus, 102
Lithotripsy, extracorporeal shock wave, for
    nephrolithiasis, 500
Liver, cirrhosis of; *see* Cirrhosis
Liver flap, characteristics of, 297
Loop diuretics for congestive heart failure,
    21
Loop electrode excision procedure, 245
Lorazepam for alcohol withdrawal, 302
Lovastatin for hypercholesterolemia, 15
Low back pain, 492-498
  chronic, 492-495
  compensation schemes for, 497-498
  counseling recommendations, 583
  diagnosis of, 496
  disability due to, 495
  incidence of, 494-495
  inflammatory, 495
  mechanical, 495
  pathophysiology of, 495
  patient education about, 496
  radiographic exams of, 496
  summary of, 498
  treatment of, 496-497
Low-density lipoprotein
  elevated, 15
  high values for, 18
LR; *see* Likelihood ratio
Lumpectomy, 482
Lung cancer
  with brain metastasis, palliative care for,
      90
  death rate from, 600, 601
  health maintenance exam and, 577
  screening for, 579
  in women, 601
Luvox; *see* Fluvoxamine
Lyme disease, symptoms and cause of, 409
Lymph nodes
  in Hodgkin's disease, 141
  in non-Hodgkin's lymphoma, 141-142

Lymphadenitis, mesenteric, *versus* RAP
    syndrome, 422
Lymphoblastic leukemia, acute, *versus*
    mononucleosis, 67
Lymphocytic leukemia
  acute, symptoms of, 143
  chronic, symptoms of, 143
Lymphoma, 138-143
  bone pain in, 139
  chest pain in, 138
  neck and elbow swelling in, 139
  non-Hodgkin's; *see* Non-Hodgkin's
      lymphoma
  summary of, 142-143
  in supraclavicular area, 138

M

Macrocytosis, differential diagnosis of, 136
Macrocytosis, *versus* megaloblastosis, 136
Macule, defined, 409
Magnesium pemoline for ADHD, 362
Magnesium sulfate
  for acute MI, 6
  for seizures, 215
Major depressive disorder, 278, 279; *see also*
      Depression
  versus Alzheimer's disease, 524
  diagnosis of, 280
  DSM-IV criteria for, 280
  versus dysthymia, 284
  mnemonic for, 281
  pain disorder and, 318
  pharmacologic management of, 281-282,
      284
  prevalence of, 284
  psychotherapy for, 338
  sexual dysfunction and, 334
  subclassifications of, 284-285
  summary of, 284-285
  treatment of, 338
Malaria
  chloroquine-resistant, 617
  strains of, 617
  symptoms of, 617
Malignant hypertension, 24-25
Malignant melanoma
  metastasis of, 353-358
  symptoms of, 645
  terminal, ethical decision making and,
      517
Malingering
  in differential diagnosis of factitious
      disorder, 313
  summary of, 320
Malleolus, fracture of, 648
Mammography
  in diagnosis of breast cancer, 480, 482
  recommendations for, 483
Mania
  in bipolar disorder, 285, 287
  characteristics of, 288
  versus hypomania, 287
  theories of, 288
  treatment of, 289
MAOIs; *see* Monoamine oxidase inhibitors
Marburg type multiple sclerosis, 111

Marijuana, effects of, 302
Mastectomy, types of, 482
Mastitis, breast feeding and, 381-382, 384
Mastoiditis
    causes, symptoms, and treatment, 510
    symptoms of, 508, 510
Maternity care, family-centered, 194-198
Mazicon; see Flumazenil
MDD; see Major depressive disorder
Medical futility, defined, 520
Medicine, defensive versus defensible, 610
Medispeak, 356
Medroxyprogesterone for menopausal
        symptoms, 250, 252
Mefenamic acid for dysmenorrhea, 248
Mefloquine for malaria prevention, 617, 618
Megacolon, causes of, 543
Megaloblastic anemia, 135, 137
Megaloblastosis versus macrocytosis, 136
Megestrol acetate
    for anorexia in advanced cancer, 88
    for menopausal symptoms, 252
Meglitinides, mechanism of action of, 97
Melanoma, malignant; see Malignant
        melanoma
Memory loss
    alcohol abuse and, 296, 297, 298
    in Alzheimer's disease, 522, 526
    thiamine deficiency and, 298
Meniere's disease, symptoms of, 506, 508
Meningitis
    H. influenzae, 379
    neonatal, streptococcal infection in, 403
Meniscus
    tear of, versus collateral ligament tear, 652
    torn, 650, 651
Menometrorrhagia, defined, 257
Menopause
    diagnosis of, 250
    health maintenance exam and, 576, 577
    hormone replacement therapy for, 250
    summary of, 251-252
    symptom management, 250, 252
    symptoms of, 249-252
Menorrhagia
    with hemodynamic compromise, 134
    secondary causes of, 257
Menstrual cycle; see also Dysfunctional
        uterine bleeding; Dysmenorrhea;
        Premenstrual syndrome
    breakthrough bleeding in, 266
    heavy flow during, OCPs and, 134
    migraine during, 118
    normal duration of, 258
    and side effects of OCPs, 266
Menstrual history, gestational age and, 224
Mental capacity, defined, 520
Meperidine, contraindications to, 81-82
6-Mercaptopurine for Crohn's disease, 61
Mesalamine for ulcerative colitis, 59-60
Mesenteric lymphadenitis versus RAP
        syndrome, 422
Metabolic acidosis
    anion gap and, 639-640
    in cardiac arrest, 626
    in diabetic ketoacidosis, 634

Metamucil, contraindications to, 90
Metatarsus adductus deformity, 428, 430
Metatarsus varus deformity, 428, 430
Methadone
    for cancer pain, 82
    therapeutic use of, 302
Methanol poisoning, treatment of, 640
Methotrexate for ulcerative colitis, 60
Methylphenidate for ADHD, 362
Metoprolol
    for acute MI, 6
    for angina, 11
    lipid effects of, 16
Metronidazole for Crohn's disease, 61
Metrorrhagia, defined, 257
Mevacor; see Lovastatin
Miacalcin; see Calcitonin
Michigan Alcohol Screening Test, 298
Microalbuminuria in diabetes, 95
Microvasive Rigiflex achalasia dilator, 56
Migraine, 116
    with aura, 118
    classification of, 120
    during menstrual cycle, 118
    narcotic analgesics for, 189
    pathophysiology of, 118
    prodromal phase of, 117-118
    prophylaxis of, 119
    with rebound analgesic headache, 120
    treatment of, 119, 120
    triggers of, 118-119
    without aura, 117-118
Milk, breast versus cow's, 384, 385, 386
Mini-mental status exam, 522
MMR vaccine, 378
Mnemonics
    for assessing adolescents, 435
    for assessing major depressive disorder,
        281
    for assessing senile dementia/delirium,
        528-529
    DEMENTIA, 524, 528-529
    SAFE TIMES, 435
    SIG: E CAPS, 557
Mobitz type II heart block, 626
    summary of, 627-628
Molluscum contagiosum, symptoms of,
        409
Monilia during pregnancy, 202
Monoamine oxidase inhibitors
    for MDD, 282
    for panic disorder, 323, 324
    for PTSD, 328
    for social phobia, 327
Mononucleosis, 66-69
    complications of, 68
    Epstein-Barr virus in, 67
    summary of, 68-69
    symptoms of, 67, 68
    treatment of, 68
Mood disorders
    in differential diagnosis of depression of
        elderly, 558
    medical condition-induced, 283
    substance-induced, 282-283
    treatment of, 281

Mood swings, drug abuse and, 299-300
Morphine
    for acute MI, 6
    for cancer pain, 82
    increased tolerance to, 83
Motor vehicle accidents
    counseling recommendations, 583
    health maintenance exam and, 576, 578
    trauma from, 628
Mouth-to-mouth ventilation, 626
MPA; see Medroxyprogesterone
Mucus
    in irritable bowel disease, 75
    secretion of, 40-41
Multiinfarct dementia, 524
Multiple myeloma, 138-143
    bone pain in, 139, 142
    summary of, 142-143
    treatment of, 142
Multiple sclerosis, 109-113
    categories of, 111
    diagnosis of, 111
    etiologic agents in, 112-113
    laboratory findings in, 112
    Marburg type, 111
    MRI in, 111, 112
    pathophysiology of, 112
    risk factors for, 111, 113
    summary of, 113
    symptoms of, 112
    treatment of, 112
Munchausen syndrome
    symptoms of, 310, 311-312
    terms for, 312
Murmurs, cardiac; see Cardiac murmurs
Muscle weakness, narcolepsy and, 182
Mycoplasma
    in bronchiolitis, 391
    in COPD, 53
Mycoplasma pneumonia, 52, 53
    childhood, 412
    diagnosis of, 53
Myeloblastic leukemia, acute, symptoms
        of, 143
Myelofibrosis, symptoms of, 143
Myelogenous leukemia, chronic, symptoms
        of, 143
Myocardial infarction
    acute; see Acute myocardial infarction
    psychological effects of, 6
    risk factors for subsequent infarction, 5
    thrombolytic therapy after, 627
Myoclonus, nocturnal, 185
    summary of, 186
Myofascial pain syndrome in differential
        diagnosis of fibromyalgia, 153
Myringitis, 396

N
Nägele's rule, 206
Naloxone for opioid overdose, 640
Naproxen sodium for dysmenorrhea, 248
Narcolepsy
    summary of, 186
    symptoms of, 182, 184
    treatment of, 184

Narcotic analgesics
  abuse of, 186, 187-188
  conversion of, 85
  dependence on, 188
  guidelines for, 188-189
  headache due to, 120
  for migraine, 189
  in palliative care, 90
  preventing constipation from, 82
  psychotherapy and, 339
  urinary incontinence due to, 553
Nasogastric tubes in cancer patients, 89
National Cholesterol Education Program,
  15
National Heart Lung and Blood Institute,
  DASH diet of, 24
National Institute on Aging, Alzheimer's
  criteria of, 527
National Institutes of Health, alternative
  complementary care guidelines of,
  341
Natural childbirth, summary of, 197
Nausea
  in acute appendicitis, 458-459
  cancer pain management and, 83
  chemotherapy-induced, 83
  with headache, 114, 117
  in infants/children, OTC drugs for,
    450-452
  nonpharmacologic treatment of, 88-89
  from OCPs, 266
  in ovarian cancer, 86
  in palliative care patient, 89, 91
  during pregnancy, 198, 200, 202
Neck, swelling in, in lymphoma, 139
Negative predictive value
  calculation of, 592
  defined, 591
Neisseria gonorrhea
  antibiotic-resistant, 274
  with *C. trachomatis*, 275
  in PID, 273
  symptoms of, 275
Neonatal jaundice, 368-374
  with ABO incompatibility, 372
  breast milk, 372
  cause of, 372
  differential diagnosis of, 371
  exaggerated physiologic, 371-372
  kernicterus and, 373
  pathophysiology of, 374
  phototherapy for, 371
  physiologic, 371
  prevalence of, 372
  summary of, 373-374
  symptoms of, 368-371
  treatment of, 372, 374
Neonatal sepsis, 373
Neonate
  acceptable weight gain for, 383
  brain dead, ethical issues and, 518-521
Nephrolithiasis, treatment of, 500
Nephropathy, diabetic, 95
Nephrotic syndrome
  causes of, 166
  presentation of, 165

Nephrotic syndrome—cont'd
  signs of, 166
  summary of, 167
  treatment of, 166
Neural tube defects, screening for, 582
Neuroleptic agents, Parkinsonian-like side
  effects of, 538
Neurologic status, assessing, 631
Neuronitis, vestibular
  symptoms of, 509
  treatment of, 509-510
Neurotransmitters
  ethanol and, 297
  in social phobia, 327
NGU; *see* Nongonococcal urethritis
Niacin
  for hypercholesterolemia, 18
  for hyperlipoproteinemia, 16
  side effects of, 16
Nicotine; *see also* Smoking
  addiction to, 301, 303
  replacement of, 598
  transdermal, for smoking cessation,
    596-597, 598
Nifedipine
  for achalasia, 56
  for angina, 11
  digoxin interaction with, 20
  and falls by elderly, 572
  lipid effects of, 16
Nitrates
  for angina, 10
  for systolic dysfunction, 20
  for unstable angina, 10
Nitroglycerin for acute MI, 7
Nitroglycerin-enalapril-nifedipine for
  angina, 11
Nizatidine for peptic ulcer disease, 64-65
Nocturia in benign prostatic hypertrophy,
  501-502
Nocturnal dyspnea, paroxysmal, 21
Nocturnal myoclonus, 185
  summary of, 186
Nocturnal penile tumescence, 333
Nodule
  defined, 409
  hot *versus* cold, 106
Nongonococcal urethritis
  with epididymis, 276
  summary of, 277
Non-Hodgkin's lymphoma
  clinical findings in, 141-142
  versus Hodgkin's disease, 142-143
  staging of, 142
  symptoms of, 139
  treatment of, 142
Nonmaleficence, defined, 520
Nonrestorative sleep in fibromyalgia, 153
Nonsteroidal antiinflammatory drugs
  for dysmenorrhea, 248, 254-255
  endometrial bleeding and, 258
  for gout, 161
  for metastatic bone pain, 81
  for osteoarthritis, 150
  peptic ulcer disease and, 64, 65, 636
  toxicity of, 150

Nonstress test, 218
  assumptions of, 220
Noonan's syndrome, 388
Norepinephrine in social phobia, 327
Nortriptyline
  for depression in elderly, 525
  for geriatric depression, 557
NPV; *see* Negative predictive value
Numbness in stroke, 127
Nursing homes, falls by elderly in, 573
Nutrition; *see also* Diet/diet therapy
  during pregnancy, 206-207
Nutrition counseling, recommendations
  for, 583
Nystagmus in stroke, 127

O
Obesity, 30-33
  complications of, 33
  defined, 31, 33, 604
  diabetes mellitus and, 31
  diseases linked with, 31, 604
  drug therapy for, 32
  essential, 31-32
  prevalence of, 31-32, 33
  screening for, 580
  secondary, 33
  summary of, 33
  surgical intervention for, 32
  treatment of, 33
Obsessions, types of, 328
Obsessive-compulsive disorder
  summary of, 329
  symptoms of, 328
Obstetrics, 194-232; *see also* Women's health
  complaints during pregnancy, 198-203
  family-centered maternity care, 194-198
  hypertension during pregnancy, 212-216
  intrauterine growth restriction, 216-222
  labor management, 209-212
  postpartum blues, 228-232
  postterm pregnancy, 222-226
  prenatal care, 203-209
  spontaneous abortion, 226-228
Obstructive sleep apnea; *see* Sleep apnea
OCP; *see* Oral contraceptives
ODD; *see* Oppositional defiant disorder
Ofloxacin for COPD, 43
Olanzapine for schizophrenia, 292
Olsalazine for ulcerative colitis, 59
Omeprazole for peptic ulcer disease, 64
Ondansetron
  for chemotherapy-induced nausea, 83
  in palliative care, 89
Ophthalmologic problems, 488-492
  blurred vision, 489
  conjunctivitis, 490
  dendritic ulcer, 490
  episcleritis/scleritis, 490
  glaucoma, 491
  iridocyclitis, 490-491
  iritis, 491
  painful eyes, 489
  red eyes, 488-490
  summary of, 492
  uveitis, 490-491

Opioid overdose, antidote for, 640
Opioid withdrawal, management of, 302
Opioids
  addiction to, 303
  guidelines for, 189-190
Oppositional defiant disorder
  with ADHD, 361
  characteristics of, 362
  summary of, 363
Oral cancer, screening for, 580
Oral contraceptive pills, 180
  benefits of, 268
  cancer and, 267
  elevated T₄ and, 108
  gonococcal PID and, 273
  heavy menstrual flow and, 134
  for lactating women, 268
  low-estrogen, 267-268
  medications interacting with, 269
  progestin-only, 269
  side effects of, 266
  smoking and, 266
  STDs and, 267
  stroke associated with, 129
  summary of, 270
  thrombosis risk and, 269
Oral rehydration therapy for pediatric
      diarrhea, 419
Organophosphate poisoning, antidote for,
      640
Orgasm, inhibited, 334
Orgasmic disorder, 334
Orthopnea, 21
Orthostatic hypotension
  dizziness in, 509
  in elderly, 568
  management of, 509
  summary of, 511
  symptoms of, 506
Osgood-Schlatter disease, symptoms of,
      424, 426
Osteoarthritis
  exercise therapy in, 150
  pathophysiology of, 148-149
  radiographic changes in, 150
  signs and symptoms in, 148, 149
  summary of, 151
  treatment of, 150
Osteochondritis, symptoms of, 424, 426-427
Osteomalacia
  defined, 235
  diagnosis of, 237
Osteopenia, WHO definition of, 237
Osteoporosis, 233-238
  back pain in, 233, 235
  diagnosis of, 237, 251
  estrogen replacement prophylaxis of,
      251, 584
  postmenopausal, screening for, 582
  prevention of, 236, 237
  risk factors for, 235, 251
  subtypes of, 235-236
  summary of, 237
  treatment of, 236-237, 237
  vertebral fractures in, 235
  WHO definition of, 235

OTC drugs; *see* Over-the-counter drugs
Otitis media, 394-397
  acute, 396
  bacteriology of, 396
  chronic, 394, 396
  complications of, 397, 511
  mastoiditis as complication of, 510
  occult bacteremia and, 416
  prevalence of, 396-397
  recurrent, 397
  summary of, 397
  symptoms of, 394, 396
  treatment of, 396
  without effusion, 396
Otorrhea, 396
Otosclerosis
  hearing loss in, 510
  symptoms of, 507, 509
Ottawa Ankle Rules, 648
Outpatient procedures/surgery
  for ingrown toenail, 466, 468
  for rectal bleeding, 467
  for rectal pain, 466
  for second-degree burns, 466, 468
  for skin lesions, 465-467
  for subungual hematoma, 466, 468
  summary of, 469-470
Ovarian cancer, 86-87
  screening for, 580
Overflow incontinence, 552
  summary of, 555
  treatment of, 553
Over-the-counter drugs for
      infants/children, 449-453
  with cough, 450, 452
  with fever, diarrhea, red cheeks, 451, 452
  with nausea and vomiting, 450-452
  with respiratory tract infection/fever,
      449, 451-452
  summary of, 452-453
Ovulation
  assessing, 179
  disorders of, 181
  inducing, 180
Oxprenolol, lipid effects of, 16
Oxygen
  for acute MI, 7
  humidified, for bronchiolitis, 391
Oxytocin
  for hypotonic labor, 211
  protocol for, 212
  risk-benefit analysis of, 212

P

Pacemaker, external, 626
PACs; *see* Premature atrial contractions
Pain
  abdominal; *see* Abdominal pain
  in acute appendicitis, 458-459
  in angina pectoris *versus* acute MI, 7
  back; *see* Back pain
  in biliary tract disease, 461, 463
  in breast cancer, 481
  cancer; *see* Cancer pain
  chest; *see* Chest pain
  in cholecystitis, 463

Pain—cont'd
  chronic, 318
  in colon carcinoma, 473-474
  costovertebral angle, 168
  in dysmenorrhea, 252-254
  in ectopic pregnancy, 259, 261, 262
  from episiotomy, 196
  in esophageal motility disorder, 54
  in fibrocystic breast disease, 483
  in fibromyalgia, 151
  in gout, 158-159, 160
  in hepatitis, 69-70
  in herpes simplex infection, 272
  in IBS, 76
  in inflammatory bowel disease, 57-59
  in irritable bowel disease, 75
  during labor, 196
  low back; *see* Low back pain
  ocular, 491
  in osteoarthritis, 148
  in pancreatic carcinoma, 484
  in pancreatitis, 471
  in peptic ulcer disease, 62-63
  in polymyalgia, 529-531
  rectal, 466-467
    during pregnancy, 199
  in renal colic, 499, 500
  in rheumatoid arthritis, 144
  in salpingitis, 270
  in sickle-cell disease, 454, 455
  in somatoform disorders, 319
Pain disorder
  differential diagnosis of, 318
  summary of, 320
  symptoms of, 317-318
  treatment of, 318
Pain management, 186-190
  for chronic back pain, 186
  for chronic pain, 189
  with opioids, 189-190
Pain threshold, lowering, 83
Palliative care, 86-92
  antinauseants in, 88-89
  summary of, 91-92
Palpitations
  causes of, 28
  in dysrhythmia, 27-28
  in generalized anxiety disorder, 307
  in thyroid disease, 105
Pancreatic adenocarcinoma, symptoms of,
      599-601
Pancreatic carcinoma, 484-487
  genetic mutations and, 487
  health maintenance exam and, 577
  management of, 487
  prevention of, 487
  risk factors for, 486-487
  screening for, 580, 609
  smoking and, 601
  survival rate, 600
  symptoms of, 484, 486
Pancreatitis
  alcohol-associated, 470-473
  chronic, 472
  Ranson's criteria for, 472
  summary of, 472

Pancreatitis—cont'd
  symptoms of, 470-471
  treatment of, 471
Panic disorder, 320-324
  conditions associated with, 323
  defined, 322
  genetic factors in, 322
  summary of, 323-324
  symptoms of, 322, 324
  treatment of, 322-323, 324
Pap smear
  abnormal, 241-243, 245-246
  classification system for, 243
  cost-effectiveness of, 244, 245
  false-negative rate for, 244
  indications for, 244
  intervals for, 244, 245
  performing, 243
  in postmenopausal women, 243
  reporting system for, 245
  unsatisfactory for evaluation, 244
Pap testing, recommendations for, 577
Papilloma, intraductal, 481-482
  summary of, 484
Papule
  defined, 409
  violaceous, in lichen planus, 643
Parainfluenza 3 virus in bronchiolitis, 391
Parainfluenza virus, croup due to, 409
Paralysis
  sleep, defined, 184
  stroke-related, 126
Paresthesia, anemia-related, 133-134
Parkinson's disease
  differential diagnosis of, 539
  in elderly, 536-540
    symptoms of, 536, 538
  subtypes of, 538
  summary of, 539-540
  treatment of, 538-539, 539
Paronychia, outpatient treatment of, 469
Paroxysmal nocturnal dyspnea, 21
Paroxysmal supraventricular tachycardia
  treatment of, 29
  vagal maneuvers for, 29
Parvovirus B19 in erythema infectiosum,
    407
Patellofemoral syndrome, symptoms of,
    425, 427
Paternalism, defined, 520
Patient
  autonomy of, 520
  communicating bad news to, 353-358,
    486
  support system for, 355
  terminally ill, colleagues' reactions to,
    356-357
Patient rights, 351, 357
Patient Self-Determination Act, 520
Peak expiratory flow rate in asthma, 48
Pelvic inflammatory disease
  barrier contraception and, 273-274
  differential diagnosis of, 273
  in dysmenorrhea, 255
  ectopic pregnancy and, 262
  gonococcal, OCPs and, 273

Pelvic inflammatory disease—cont'd
  infertility and, 176
  organisms associated with, 273
  risk factors for, 276
  summary of, 276-277
  treatment of, 274
Pelvis
  Caldwell-Moloy classification of, 207
  diagonal conjugate of, 207
Penicillin G for streptococcal pneumonia,
    52
Peptic ulcer, 62-66
  differential diagnosis of, 65
  NSAID-related *versus*
    non-NSAID-related, 65
  perforated, 636
  summary of, 65
  treatment of, 65
Percutaneous transluminal coronary
    angioplasty
  versus CABG, 11
  contraindications to, 11
  indications for, 11
  pros and cons of, 11
Performance anxiety, 323
Pergolide for Parkinson's disease, 538
Pericarditis
  acute, 3
  in rheumatoid arthritis, 146
  uremic, 21
Periodic limb movement disorder, 185
  summary of, 186
Peripheral artery disease, screening for, 579
Peritonitis
  with acute appendicitis, 459
  with appendicitis, 460
  contraindication to antibiotics in, 460-461
Pernicious anemia, 135-136
  treatment of, 136
Personality disorders in differential
    diagnosis of factitious disorder, 313
Pertussis vaccine, fever due to, 378
Pesticides, pancreatic cancer and, 601
Petit mal seizures, 124
  findings in, 125
Pharmaceutical companies, ethics of,
    190-193
Pharyngitis
  beta-hemolytic streptococcal, 400-402
  streptococcal, summary of, 404
Phenelzine for PTSD, 327
Phenylketonuria, screening for, 582
Phenytoin, IUGR and, 220
Phobias
  school, in RAP syndrome, 422
  social; see Social phobia
  specific, 327
Phototherapy
  complications of, 373
  for hyperbilirubinemia, 373
  for neonatal jaundice, 372
Physical exam; see also Health maintenance
    exam
  versus health maintenance exam, 585-586
  procedures in, 586
  summary of, 587

Pica, 201
PID; *see* Pelvic inflammatory disease
Pigeon-toe, 428
Pindolol, lipid effects of, 16
Pityriasis rosea, symptoms of, 409
Plantar warts
  outpatient surgery for, 465-466, 469
  removal of, 467-468
Plethysmography, impedance, 36
Pleural effusions
  in palliative care patient, 89, 91
  in rheumatoid arthritis, 146
PMR; *see* Polymyalgia rheumatica
PMS; *see* Premenstrual syndrome
Pneumococcal pneumonia, immunizations
    against, 617-618
Pneumocystis carinii pneumonia
  in AIDS, 613-614
  prevention of, 614
Pneumonia, 50-54
  adenoviral, 52, 53
  age-related diagnosis of, 413
  in alcoholic patient, 51, 53, 54
  bacterial *versus* viral, 54
  as bronchitis complication, 53
  causative organisms in, 53
  childhood, 410-413
    adenoviral, 412
    bacterial, 412
    from group B streptococcus, 411-412
    mycoplasmal, 412
    respiratory syncytial virus, 412
    staphylococcal, 412-413
    streptococcal, 412
    symptoms of, 410-412
    viral agents of, 412
  community-acquired, 53
  with COPD, 51, 53
  in elderly, 545-550
    with appendicitis, 549
    bacterial, 547, 549
    in community *versus* institution,
      547-548, 550
    fever in, 550
    in long-term-care facilities, 549
    with pyelonephritis, 548-549
    symptoms of, 545-548
    treatment of, 548
    with urinary tract infections, 548
  in immunocompromised host, 53
  as influenza complication, 621
  Klebsiella, 52
  Legionella, 52-53
    signs and symptoms of, 53-54
  Mycoplasma, 52, 53
    diagnosis of, 53
  nosocomial, 53
  pneumococcal, 52
    immunizations against, 617-618
  Pneumocystis carinii, 613-614
  prevention of, 54
  in renal transplant patient, 51
  Streptococcus, 52-53
  summary of, 53-54
  treatment of, 54

Pneumothorax, tension, trauma-related, 630
Point of maximum impulse, alcohol abuse and, 294, 296
Poison management, 637-641
  anion gap in, 639-640
  in drug overdose, 637, 639
  and preventing absorption, 640
  summary of, 640-641
Poisoning, epidemiology of, 639
Polio vaccines, 378
Polycythemia vera, symptoms of, 143
Polydipsia in diabetes mellitus, 92
Polymyalgia rheumatica, 529-531
  differential diagnosis of, 531
  summary of, 532
  symptoms of, 529
  treatment of, 531
Polymyositis versus polymyalgia rheumatica, 531
Polypharmacy in elderly, 566-571
  symptoms of, 566, 568
Polyps, colonic
  malignant potential of, 476
  summary of, 479
Polyuria in diabetes mellitus, 92
Ponstel; see Mefenamic acid
Positive predictive value
  calculation of, 592
  defined, 591
Postmature, defined, 225
Postmenopausal Estrogen/Progestin Interventions, 250
Postpartum blues
  hormonal factors in, 230
  prevalence of, 230
  summary of, 232
  treatment of, 230
Posttraumatic stress disorder
  DSM-IV criteria for, 327
  summary of, 329
  symptoms of, 327
  treatment of, 327-328
Potassium, serum, in diabetic ketoacidosis, 633
PPV; see Positive predictive value
Pravachol; see Pravastatin
Pravastatin for hypercholesterolemia, 15
Prazosin for angina, 10
Prednisone
  for anorexia in advanced cancer, 88
  for Crohn's disease, 61
  for temporal arteritis, 119
Preeclampsia
  complications of, 214
  defined, 214, 216
  health maintenance exam and, 578
  pathophysiology of, 215
  prevention of, 215
  risk factors for, 215
  screening for, 581
Pregnancy
  alcohol use during, 207
  anemia during, 133, 135
  antepartum events in, 208-209
  aspirin prophylaxis in, 584

Pregnancy—cont'd
  back pain during, 198, 201, 202
  complaints during, 198-203
  constipation during, 200, 202
  dietary allowances during, 206-207
  drugs contraindicated in, 215
  dysfunctional uterine bleeding and, 257
  ectopic; see Ectopic pregnancy
  factors affecting success of, 178
  fatigue during, 202
  food cravings during, 201
  gastroesophageal reflux disease during, 199, 201, 203
  headache during, 202
  health maintenance exam and, 576, 578
  heartburn during, 201
  hemorrhoids during, 199, 201, 202-203
  hypertension during
    summary of, 216
    treatment of, 214-215, 216
  hypertension in, 212-216
  landmarks in, 224
  maternal-infant HIV transmission in, 615
  mean duration of, 206
  nausea and vomiting during, 198, 200, 202
  perinatal morbidity rates and, 211
  peripartum events in, 208-209
  postcoital prevention of, 267
  postpartum blues after, 228-232
  postterm, 222-226
    defined, 224
    guidelines for, 225
    summary of, 225
  preconception care and, 206
  ptyalism during, 202
  rectal pain during, 199
  rubella exposure during, 406
  smoking and, 207, 596
  swollen legs during, 199-202, 203
  thrombophlebitis during, 201
  ultrasound during, 194, 196, 197, 581
  unintended, counseling recommendations, 583
  of unmarried woman, ethical issues for, 517-519
  vaginal discharge during, 200, 202, 203
  varicose veins during, 199, 201, 203
  weight gain during, 206
Preload in congestive heart failure, 20
Premarin for preventing cardiovascular disease, 237
Premature atrial contractions, 28
  treatment of, 29
Premature ejaculation, treatment of, 333
Premature ventricular contractions
  symptoms of, 28
  treatment of, 5, 29
Premenstrual syndrome, 246-249
  defined, 248
  depression and, 248
  diagnosis of, 247
  factors associated with, 247-248
  prevalence of, 248
  summary of, 248
  symptoms of, 247
  treatment of, 248

Prenatal care, 203-209
  drugs and, 205
  first visit, 206
  number of visits during, 205-206
  preconception care and, 206
Prenatal counseling, health maintenance exam and, 576, 578
Pressure ulcers, 559-565
  classification of, 564
  death associated with, 562
  formation of, 563
  in immobilized elder, 561
  infected, 563
  in nursing home residents, 559
  pathophysiology of, 562
  prevention of, 562-563
  risk factors for, 561-562
  sites of, 562
  summary of, 564-565
  treatment of, 563-564
Prevalence, defined, 591, 593
Priapism in sickle-cell disease, 455
Primary care, psychotherapy in, 335-340
Prinzmetal's angina, 11, 12
Problem drinking; see also Alcohol dependence/abuse; Alcoholism
  screening for, 582
Procainamide
  administration of, 625
  digoxin interaction with, 20
  for ventricular tachycardia, 626
Proctitis, ulcerative, 61
Proctocolectomy for ulcerative colitis, 60
Progesterone
  deficiency of, in dysfunctional uterine bleeding, 258
  for menopausal symptoms, 252
  vaginal suppositories of, for PMS, 248
Progestin
  intramuscular, 268-269
  lipid levels and, 251
  lipid profile and, 266-267
  for menopausal symptoms, 250
Prolactinoma, summary of, 104
Propranolol
  for angina, 10, 11
  in differential diagnosis of depression of elderly, 558
  lipoprotein effects of, 16
  for smoking cessation, 597
Proscar; see Finasteride
Prostaglandin inhibitors for dysmenorrhea, 248
Prostaglandin synthetase in dysmenorrhea, 254
Prostate carcinoma
  constipation in, 541
  laboratory testing for, 607
  metastatic bone disease in, 81-82
  pain in, 78, 81
  prevalence and risk factors, 504
  screening for, 579
  summary of, 505
  symptoms of, 502-503
  treatment of, 504
Prostate disorders, 501-506
  summary of, 505-506

Prostatitis
bacterial, in elderly, 548
causes and treatment, 505
summary of, 505-506
symptoms of, 503-504
Proteinuria
in diabetic patient, 93
health maintenance exam and, 578
Provocative maneuvers, example of, 487
Prozac; *see* Fluoxetine
Pruritus in candidiasis, 239
Pseudocyst, pancreatic, 471
Psoriasis, symptoms of, 643
PSVT; *see* Paroxysmal supraventricular tachycardia
Psychoactive drugs, abuse of, 188
Psychomotor agitation in depression of elderly, 558
Psychomotor behavior disorder, delirium and, 529
Psychosis
differential diagnosis of, 292
Korsakoff's, 298
postpartum; *see also* Postpartum blues
and risk of suicide/infanticide, 231
summary of, 232
symptoms of, 231
treatment of, 231
symptoms of, 291-292
Psychotherapy
for adjustment disorder, 335-338
for bulimia, 306
cognitive; *see also* Cognitive therapy
for MDD, 281
for depression, 337
forms of, 339
group, 339
for MDD, 338
narcotic analgesics and, 339
for obsessive-compulsive disorder, 328
in primary care, 335-340
cognitive, 338
for PTSD, 328
summary of, 339
supportive, 337-338, 339
Psychotic disorder
brief, in differential diagnosis of schizophrenia, 291
substance-induced, in differential diagnosis of schizophrenia, 291
Psychotropic drugs in elderly, 569-570
PTCA; *see* Percutaneous transluminal coronary angioplasty
Ptyalism during pregnancy, 202
Public health; *see* Epidemiology/public health
Pulmonary embolism, 33-37
assessment of, 36
diagnosis of, 37
drug therapy for, 35-36
hip surgery and, 35
mortality due to, 35
prevention of, 36
risk factors for, 36
summary of, 37
treatment of, 36-37

Pulmonary function
in asthma, 48-49
in chronic bronchitis, 40
in COPD, 43
Pustules, defined, 409
PVCs; *see* Premature ventricular contractions
Pyelonephritis
in elderly, 548-549
signs and symptoms of, 168, 169
treatment of, 170

Q

QALY; *see* Quality of adjusted life years
Quadriceps muscle, strain of, 650, 651
Quality of adjusted life years, laboratory testing and, 607
Quality of life
defined, 520-521
ethical decision making and, 519, 521-522
Questran; *see* Cholestyramine
Quetiapine for schizophrenia, 292
Quinidine, digoxin interaction with, 20
Quinolone antibiotics
for *Legionella* pneumonia, 53
for urinary tract infection, 170-171

R

Radiation therapy for Hodgkin's disease, 141
Radioiodine therapy, advantages and disadvantages of, 108
Raloxifene for treating osteoporosis, 236
Ranitidine for peptic ulcer disease, 64-65
Ranson's criteria for pancreatitis, 472
RAP syndrome, symptoms of, 421-422
Rape, female sexual dysfunction and, 331, 333
Rash
diaper; *see* Diaper rash
in erythema infectiosum, 405, 407
in exanthem subitum, 405, 407
in rubella, 406, 408
in urticaria, 641
Rectal bleeding from hemorrhoids, 475
Recurrent abdominal pain syndrome
summary of, 423
symptoms of, 421-422
treatment of, 422-423
Red eye, 488-490
differential diagnosis and management of, 491-492
summary of, 492
Reed Coma Scale, 637
Reed-Sternberg cells in Hodgkin's disease, 141
Referrals
benefits of, 351
lateral, 352
patient requests for, 348-350
patient's right to, 351
purpose of, 351
summary of, 353
Regurgitation, infant, 382, 384-385
Reliability, defined, 592

Remicade; *see* Infliximab
Renal cell carcinoma, pain in, 79
Renal colic, 499-500
Renal disease, summary of, 167-168
Renal failure
anorexic drugs and, 32
chronic; *see* Chronic renal failure
Renal stones, 499-501
calcium oxalate, 500, 501
infective, 501
magnesium-ammonium-phosphate, 500-501
metabolic, 500
summary of, 501
symptoms of, 499, 500
uric acid, 500, 501
Renal transplantation, pneumonia following, 51
Reserpine, Parkinsonian-like side effects of, 538
Resins for hyperlipoproteinemia, 16
Respiratory acidosis in cardiac arrest, 626
Respiratory disease, smoking and, 596
Respiratory distress, trauma-related, 628, 630
Respiratory syncytial virus
asthma and, 49
in bronchiolitis, 391
pneumonia due to, 412
Respiratory syndromes
infant/child, 389-393
summary of, 393
Respiratory tract infection
in infants/children, OTC drugs for, 449, 451-452
in otitis media, 394
Resting tremor in Parkinson's disease, 536, 538
Restless legs syndrome
summary of, 186
symptoms of, 185
Restraining devices
and falls by elderly, 573
side effects of, 573
Resuscitation
ABCs of, 629, 630-631, 636
in cold-related injuries, 655
in fracture management, 648
fluid, in diabetic ketoacidosis, 633
Retinopathy, diabetic, 95
Retroviral syndrome, symptoms of, 612, 614
Rewarming, methods of, 655
Reye's syndrome, aspirin and, 396
Rh incompatibility, screening for, 581
Rheumatic fever
diagnosis of, 165
prevention of, 165
Rheumatoid arthritis
anemia in, 146
complications of, 146
pathophysiology of, 145-146, 147
radiologic findings in, 146
signs and symptoms of, 145, 147
spinal instability in, 146
summary of, 147

Rheumatoid arthritis—cont'd
  symptoms of, 144
  treatment of, 146, 147
Rhinitis
  allergic, 439-443
  vasomotor, 442
Rhinitis medicamentosa, 442
Rhinophyma, 175
Rhinorrhea
  in adenoviral pneumonia, 412
  infant, 389
Rhinosinusitis, causes and symptoms,
    510-511
Rhinovirus in common cold, 399
Rhonchi in asthma, 48
Ribavirin for bronchiolitis, 391
Right ventricular failure
  chronic bronchitis and, 40
  signs of, 20, 21
Rimantadine for prophylaxis and
    treatment of influenza A, 621
Ringworm, symptoms and causes of, 409
Rinne test, procedure for, 510
Risedronate for osteoporosis, 236
Risperidone
  for bipolar disorder, 287
  for schizophrenia, 292
Romazicon; see Flumazenil
Rosacea
  signs of, 174-175
  summary of, 176
  treatment of, 175
Rotavirus, diarrhea due to, 419, 420
Rubber band ligation, 477-478
Rubella
  causative agent, 409
  immunizations against, 408
  pregnant woman exposed to, 406
  screening for, 581
  symptoms of, 406, 408
Rubeola
  causative agent, 409
  complications of, 408
  symptoms of, 406, 408

S
Sabin vaccine, 378
SAFE TIMES mnemonic, 435
Safety
  counseling recommendations, 583
  health maintenance exam and, 576, 578
Saint's triad, 442
Salk vaccine, 378
Salmonella
  gastroenteritis due to, 419
  in IBS, 76
Salpingitis
  diagnostic criteria for, 273
  ectopic pregnancy and, 262
  pain in, 270
  signs and symptoms of, 276
Sarcoma, Kaposi's, in AIDS, 614
Scaly patches in psoriasis, 643
Scaphoid bone, fracture of, 648
Scarlet fever, symptoms of, 400, 402, 407,
    408

Schatzki ring, 56
Schizoaffective disorder
  diagnosis of, 292
  in differential diagnosis of
    schizophrenia, 291
Schizophrenia, 289-294
  causes of, 293
  differential diagnosis of, 291, 293
  neurochemical basis of, 292
  psychotic symptoms in, 292
  subtypes of, 293
  summary of, 292-293
  symptoms of, 289-290, 291, 292-293
  treatment of, 292, 293
Schizophreniform disorder, classification
    of, 292
School phobia in RAP syndrome, 422
Scleritis, 490
Sclerosis
  in angina, 12
  systemic, dysphagia due to, 56
Scoliosis, idiopathic, screening for, 582
Screening *versus* case finding, 610
Seborrheic dermatitis, diaper rash due to,
    445
Seborrheic keratosis, skin lesions in, 643
Sedative-hypnotics
  anxiety after discontinuation of, 188
  in differential diagnosis of depression of
    elderly, 558-559
  urinary incontinence due to, 553
Sedatives, OCP interaction with, 269
Seizure disorders, 121-126
  absence (petit mal), 124, 125
  epileptic, 126
  febrile, 125
  grand mal, 124
  laboratory studies of, 124
  lack of concentration in, 122
  neurologic disorders and, 125
  new-onset, 121, 123
    causes of, 123
  nonepileptic, 125-126
    causes of, 124-125
  partial, 123, 125
  simple, 123
  smoking and, 123
  and sudden loss of consciousness, 122
  summary of, 125-126
  treatment of, 124
Seizures
  clozapine-induced, 292
  eclampsia-associated, 215
Selective serotonin reuptake inhibitors
  for eating disorders, 306
  for geriatric depression, 557-558
  for MDD, 281
  mechanism of action of, 281
  for obsessive-compulsive disorder, 328
  for panic disorder, 323, 324
  for postpartum depression, 230-231
  for PTSD, 327, 328
Selegiline for Parkinson's disease,
    538-539
Semen, analysis of, 179

Senile dementia/delirium, 522-529; *see also*
    Alzheimer's disease; Dementia
  causes of, 526
  DEMENTIA mnemonic for, 528-529
  management of, 525-526
  symptoms of, 522, 524-525
Sensitivity, defined, 591
Sepsis
  as complication of pressure ulcer, 563
  neonatal, 373
Septicemia
  neonatal
    streptococcal infection in, 403
  from UTI in elderly, 549
Serotonergic agents, 32
Serotonin, migraine and, 120
Sertaline for eating disorders, 306
Set point, hypothalamic, mediation of, 416
Sexual abuse
  female sexual dysfunction and, 331, 333
  IBS and, 77
  prevalence of, 367
Sexual activity, decisions about, 268
Sexual desire, hypoactive, 334
Sexual dysfunction
  diabetes and, 332
  erectile dysfunction, 332
  female, 333, 334
  male, 332-333
  medication-related, 332
  prevalence of, 332
  psychologic factors in, 332-333, 334
  summary of, 335
Sexual function disorders, 330-335
  with history of rape, 330
  impotence, 330, 332
Sexual intercourse after MI, 5, 7
Sexually transmitted disease, 270-277
  counseling recommendations, 583
  ectopic pregnancy and, 262-263
  OCPs and, 267
  patient education about, 180
  summary of, 276-277
  treatment of, 171-172
  urinary tract infections and, 171
Shearing forces, pressure ulcers and, 562
Shigella, in IBS, 76
Shiners, allergic, 441
Shock
  in acute MI, 6
  cardiogenic, 6
  traumatic, interventions for, 629, 630-631
Short stature
  causes of, 388
  diagnosis of, 387, 388
  summary of, 389
Shortness of breath, 18; *see also* Dyspnea
  in asthma, 45
  in generalized anxiety disorder, 307
  in panic disorder, 320
Sickle-cell disease, 453-457
  complications of, 455-456
  genetic factors in, 454
  hand-foot syndrome, 454-455
  sickle cell anemia, 454
  summary of, 456-457

Sickle-cell disease—cont'd
    symptoms of, 453-454
    treatment of, 456-457
Sickle-cell trait, 454
SIG: E CAPS mnemonic, 557
Sigmoidoscopy for Crohn's disease, 61
SIL; see Squamous intraepithelial lesion
Sildenafil for erectile disorder, 334
Simvastatin for hypercholesterolemia, 15
Sinusitis
    causes and symptoms, 510-511
    summary of, 512
    treatment of, 511
Skin cancer, screening for, 579, 586-587
Skin lesions
    of actinic keratoses, 643
    in angioneurotic edema, 644, 645
    changes in, 645
    outpatient surgery for, 465-467, 469
    in seborrheic keratosis, 643
    in squamous cell carcinoma, 643
Skull fracture, assessment of, 630
Sleep
    behaviors harming, 184
    investigations of, 185
    nonrestorative, in fibromyalgia, 153
    phases of, 185
    types of, 186
Sleep apnea
    COPD and, 40
    management of, 184
    pathophysiology of, 183
    predisposing factors, 184
    summary of, 186
    symptoms of, 181, 183-184
Sleep disorders, 181-186
    adjustment, 185
    hypnotic agents for, 185
    insufficient sleep syndrome, 337
    summary of, 185-186
Sleep disturbance, delirium and, 529
Sleep paralysis, defined, 184
Sleepiness, daytime, 184
Slipped capital femoral epiphysis
    pathophysiology of, 426
    symptoms of, 424
    treatment of, 426
Small for gestational age, 219, 221
Small intestine, lactase deficiency in, 61
Smoke, second-hand, 39
Smoking
    cardiovascular disease and, 604
    cervical carcinoma and, 244
    chronic bronchitis and, 40, 41
    chronic obstructive pulmonary disease
        and, 41
    as contraindication to OCPs, 266
    coronary heart disease and, 596
    counseling to prevent, 582
    economic costs of, 598
    ectopic pregnancy and, 262
    euploidic abortion and, 228
    health consequences of, 596
    health maintenance exam and, 575
    IUGR due to, 219
    pancreatic carcinoma and, 486, 601

Smoking—cont'd
    passive, 596, 597
    peptic ulcer disease and, 64-65
    pregnancy outcomes and, 207
    seizures due to, 122, 123
    stroke associated with, 129
Smoking cessation, 594-599
    for COPD, 43
    coughing and, 41
    factors affecting, 596
    for hypertension, 24
    methods for, 597
    pharmacologic aids to, 596-597
    summary of, 598-599
Snoring, sleep apnea and, 181
Social drinking, 297
Social phobia
    chemical basis of, 327
    performance anxiety as, 323
    summary of, 328-329
    symptoms of, 324, 326, 327
Sodium cromoglycate for allergic rhinitis,
        441-442
Sodium restriction for ascites, 73
Somatization disorders
    assessment and treatment of, 317
    conversion disorder, 318-319
    in differential diagnosis of factitious
        disorder, 313
    dysmorphic disorder, 317
    hypochondriasis, 319
    versus medical disorders, 318
    pain disorder, 317-318
    somatothymia, 319
    summary of, 319
    symptoms of, 317
Somatoform disorders, 314-320
    in differential diagnosis of factitious
        disorder, 313
    pain in, 319
    summary of, 319-320
Somatothymia, defined, 319
Somogyi effect, 96
Sore throat
    in adenoviral pneumonia, 412
    in common cold, 398
    in mononucleosis, 66
    in streptococcal infection, 400
Spasm, esophageal, 56
Specialists
    communication with, 352-353
    responsibilities of, 352
Specificity, defined, 591
Speech, impaired, in Alzheimer's disease,
        526
Sperm, normal analysis of, 180
Spermicides, vaginal, characteristics of, 268
Spironolactone for cirrhotic ascites, 73
Spitting up, infant, 382, 384-385
Sponges, characteristics of, 268
Sports medicine, 649-657
    fracture management, 646-649
    sprains/strains, 649-652
Spousal abuse, 343-348
    child abuse and, 346-347, 366-367
    conversion disorder and, 318-319

Spousal abuse—cont'd
    differential diagnosis of, 345
    epidemiology of, 345
    interventions for, 347
    learned helplessness and, 345-346
    perpetrator characteristics, 345, 347
    physician-patient communication and,
        346
    prevalence of, 345
    summary of, 347-348
    symptoms of, 345, 346
Sprain/strain, 649-652
    ankle, 649, 651
    defined, 651, 652
    quadriceps, 650, 651
    summary of, 652
    treatment of, 652
Sprue; see Celiac sprue
Sputum cytology in pneumonia diagnosis,
        53
Squamous cell carcinoma
    esophageal, 56
        dysphagia due to, 57
    skin lesions in, 643
    treatment of, 645
Squamous intraepithelial lesion, treating,
        245
Squamous metaplasia, 245
SSRIs; see Selective serotonin reuptake
        inhibitors
Staphylococcal infections, pneumonia,
        412-413
Staphylococcus aureus
    in nosocomial pneumonia, 53
    pneumonia due to, 53
Starch, craving for, 201
Status epilepticus, causes and treatment of,
        124
Status migrainous, defined, 120
STDs; see Sexually transmitted diseases
Steam for nasal congestion, 452
Stercoral ulcers, 542
Sterilization
    advantages/disadvantages of
        female, 269
        male, 269-270
    summary of, 270
Steroids
    anabolic, effects of, 302-303
    for asthma, 48, 49
Still's murmur, 447-448
Stimulants
    for ADHD, 362
    for oppositional defiant disorder, 363
Stomach cancer, death rate from, 600
Stomatitis, 409
Stool, altered, in IBS, 76
Strain; see Sprain/strain
Streptococcal infection, 400-405
    beta-hemolytic, 400-402
    in endocarditis, 402-403
    in erysipelas, 403
    group A beta-hemolytic, treatment of,
        409
    in impetigo, 403
    in neonatal septicemia/meningitis, 403

Streptococcal infection—cont'd
  pneumonia, 412
  in scarlet fever, 400, 402
  summary of, 404-405
  symptoms of, 400-402
  in tonsillitis, 403
  treatment of, 404-405
Streptococcus
  group A β-hemolytic, complications due
      to, 165
  group β, preventing infant mortality
      from, 208
Streptococcus pneumonia, 52-53
Streptococcus pneumoniae, 53
  in community-acquired pneumonia, 547
  pneumonia due to, 53
Streptokinase
  for acute MI, 4
  for pulmonary embolism, 37
  versus t-PA, for acute MI, 4
Stress, baby, 376
Stress incontinence, 552
  summary of, 554
  surgical treatment of, 554
  treatment of, 553, 554
Stroke, 126-132; *see also* Cerebrovascular
      accident
  carotid endarterectomy and, 130-131
  cerebral artery occlusion in, 128-129
  classification of, 131
  completed, defined, 131
  CT scan of, 130
  death rate for, 603, 604
  diagnosis of, 130
  embolic, conditions associated with, 129
  incidence of, 130
  in-evolution, 128
  lacunar, 129
  pathophysiology of, 129
  in region of anterior cerebral artery, 129
  risk factors for, 129, 130, 131
  summary of, 131
  thrombotic, *versus* embolic, 129
  vertebral-basilar, 130
  visual loss in, 128
Stroke-in-evolution, defined, 131
Subarachnoid hemorrhage
  headache due to, 120
  lumbar puncture and, 131
Substance abuse; *see also* Alcohol
      dependence/abuse; Drug abuse
  in differential diagnosis of factitious
      disorder, 313
  dual diagnosis with, 301
  sexual dysfunction and, 332
  susceptibility to, 297
  treatment of, 301
Sudden death
  from acute MI, 6
  calorie-restricted diets and, 32
Suicide attempts, drugs used in, 639
Suicide risk, assessing, 282-283, 582
Sulfasalazine
  for Crohn's disease, 61
  for ulcerative colitis, 59
Sulfonylureas, mechanism of action of, 97

Sumatriptan for cluster headache, 117
Support system, 355, 357
Supraventricular tachycardia, paroxysmal;
      see Paroxysmal supraventricular
      tachycardia
Surgery, 458-512
  for acute appendicitis, 458-461
  for biliary tract disease, 461-465
  for breast disease, 479-484
  for colonic disorders, 473-479
  for ear, nose, and throat problems, 506-512
  family physician's role in, 352-353
  in-office, 465-470
  for low back pain/whiplash injuries,
      492-498
  outpatient; *see* Outpatient
      procedures/surgery
  for pancreatic carcinoma, 484-487
  for pancreatitis, 470-473
  for prostate disorders, 501-506
  for renal stones, 498-501
Sweating in thyroid disease, 105
Synovial fluid in osteoarthritis, 148
Synovitis, toxic, symptoms of, 425, 427
Syphilis
  diagnosis of, 275-276
  screening for, 580
  summary of, 277
  treatment of, 276
Syrup of ipecac
  contraindications to, 640
  indications for, 640
Systole, dysfunction in, 20

T
T₄; *see* Thyroxine
Tachycardia
  paroxysmal supraventricular; *see*
      Paroxysmal supraventricular
      tachycardia
  ventricular
    summary of, 627
    treatment of, 626
Talipes equinovarus deformity, 429, 431
TCAs; *see* Tricyclic antidepressants
Teething, treatment of, 452
Temporal arteritis
  characteristics and treatment of, 119
  summary of, 532
  symptoms of, 531-532
Tension pneumothorax, trauma-related, 630
Terminal illness
  breaking news about, 353-358
  ethical issues in, 516-517, 519
Test results, false-positive, 586, 591
Testicles, varicocele of, 180
Testicular cancer, screening for, 580
Tetanus-diphtheria immunization, boosters
      for, 618
Therapeutic abortion, rubella exposure
      and, 406, 408
Thiamine, memory loss and, 298
Thiazide diuretics
  for hypercalciuria, 500
  for hypertension, 24, 534-535
  hypertension due to, 213

Thiazide diuretics—cont'd
  during pregnancy, 215
  side effects of, 24
Thiazolindinediones, mechanism of action
      of, 97
Thirst in diabetes insipidus, 100
Thrombocytopenia, neonatal, thiazide
      diuretics and, 215
Thrombocytopenic purpura, idiopathic,
      symptoms of, 143
Thrombolytic therapy
  for acute MI, 5, 6
  after myocardial infarction, 627
  contraindications to, 4
  criteria for, 4
  underutilization of, 5
Thrombophlebitis
  from OCPs, 266
  during pregnancy, 201
Thrombosis
  deep vein; *see* Deep venous thrombosis
  OCPs and, 269
Thrush, oral, in palliative care patient, 89,
      91
Thyroid, measurement of, 107
Thyroid carcinoma, 101, 109
  characteristics of, 108
  screening for, 580
Thyroid disease, 105-109
  asymptomatic, 106
  screening for, 580
  summary of, 109
Thyroiditis, 106
  Hashimoto's, 107, 108
  types of, 108
Thyroid-stimulating hormone,
      measurement of, 107
Thyroxine
  elevated, 106
    causes of, 108
    oral contraceptives and, 108
  measurement of, 107
TIA; *see* Transient ischemic attack
Tibial torsion, internal, 428-430
Tinea corporis, symptoms and cause of, 409
Tinea versicolor, symptoms and cause of,
      409
Tissue protein activator; *see* t-PA
TMP-SMX
  for COPD, 43
  for *Legionella* pneumonia, 53
Tobacco; *see also* Smoking
  addiction to, 301
Tobacco use, counseling to prevent, 582
Toeing in; *see* Intoeing
Toenail, ingrown, outpatient procedure for,
      466, 468
Tonic-clonic seizures, 124
Tonsillectomy
  complications of, 403
  indications for, 404
Tonsillitis
  cause and symptoms of, 403
  summary of, 404
Total hip replacement, pulmonary
      embolism and, 34, 35

Toxic synovitis, symptoms of, 425, 427
t-PA
  for acute MI, 4
  for pulmonary embolism, 37
  regimens for, 4
Transcutaneous electrical nerve stimulation
    for incontinence, 553
Transdermal nicotine for smoking
    cessation, 598
Transfusions, blood, for sickle cell anemia,
    454
Transient ischemic attack
  defined, 131
  symptoms of, 130
Transurethral resection of the prostate, for
    BPH, 504
Trauma, 628-631
Traumatic shock, interventions for, 629,
    630-631
Travelers
  advice for, 616-618
  immunizations for, 618
Traveler's diarrhea, 618
Tremor
  benign essential
    versus Parkinson's disease, 539
    treatment of, 539
  in Parkinson's disease, 536, 538, 539
  in thyroid disease, 105
Treponema pallidum
  diagnosis of, 275-276
  infection rate, 275
Triad asthma, 442
Trichomonas, 241-242
  Pap smear detection of, 243
  treatment of, 243
Trichomoniasis
  differential diagnosis of, 241
  symptoms of, 240
  treatment of, 240
Tricyclic antidepressants
  for depression in elderly, 525
  in elderly, 569
  for geriatric depression, 558
  for MDD, 281-282
  orthostatic hypotension and, 509
  for panic disorder, 323
  for PTSD, 328
  side effects of, 281-282
Trigger points in fibromyalgia, 151-152
Triglycerides
  in diabetes mellitus, 17
  elevated
    defined, 15
    in diabetic patient, 95
Trimethadione, IUGR and, 220
Trimethoprim-sulfamethoxazole for
    preventing PCP, 614
Trisomy 21, 388
Tubal ligation, ectopic pregnancy and, 262
Tuberculosis, screening for, 580
Tumors; *see* specific types
Turner's syndrome, 388
  symptoms of, 387
TURP; *see* Transurethral resection of the
    prostate

U
Ulcer; *see also* Peptic ulcer; Pressure ulcers
  in basal cell carcinoma, 642
  corneal, summary of, 492
  dendritic, 490
  duodenal; *see* Duodenal ulcer
  gastric, *H. pylori in*, 64
  stercoral, 542
Ulcerative colitis
  complications of, 60
  in differential diagnosis of IBS, 76
  prognosis for, 60
  refractory, 60
  signs and symptoms of, 59
  summary of, 62
  treatment of, 59-60
Ulcerative proctitis, 61
Ultrasound
  for monitoring fetal growth, 218-219
  during pregnancy, 194, 196, 197
  for pregnancy dating, 206
U. S. Preventive Services Task Force on the
    Periodic Health Examination,
    recommendations of, 575-584
Uremic pericarditis, 21
Urethritis
  C. trachomatis, 275
  gonococcal, summary of, 277
  nongonococcal, 276, 277
Urge incontinence, 552
  causes of, 554
  summary of, 554-555
  treatment of, 553
Uric acid in gout, 160-161
Urinary incontinence
  defined, 554
  in elderly, 550-555
    catheterization for, 552
    causes of, 552-553
    epidemiology of, 552
    evaluation of, 553-554
    summary of, 554-555
    surgical management of, 554
    treatment of, 553, 554
    types of, 552
Urinary tract infection, 168-172
  causative organisms in, 548
  versus colic, 376
  diagnosis of, 170
  in elderly, 548
  in females, 171
  in males, 171
  signs of, 170
  summary of, 171-172
  treatment of, 170-171
  uncomplicated, 170
Urine
  bloody, 162
  protein in, in diabetic patient, 93
Urticaria, 641-646
  exercise-induced, 644-645
  sequence of events in, 645-646
  summary of, 646
  symptoms of, 641
Uterine activity, home monitoring of,
    screening for, 581

Uterine bleeding, anemia-related, 132
Uveitis
  anterior, 490-491
  summary of, 492

V
Vaccines; *see also* Immunizations; specific
    vaccines
  against *H. influenzae*, 379
  hepatitis B, 72, 378
  polio, 378
Vagal maneuvers
  for PSVT, 29
  types of, 29
Vagina, pH of, 245
Vaginal discharge; *see also* Vulvovaginitis
  differential diagnosis of, 240
  during pregnancy, 200, 202, 203
Vaginismus, 331
  defined, 333
Vaginitis; *see also* Bacterial vaginosis
  terminology for, 240
Vaginosis, bacterial; *see* Bacterial
    vaginosis
Validity, defined, 592
Varicella vaccine, 379
Varicocele, testicular, 180
Varicose veins during pregnancy, 199, 201,
    203
Vasculitis in rheumatoid arthritis, 146
Vasomotor rhinitis, 442
Venereal warts, treatment of, 468
Ventilation, mouth-to-mouth, 626
Ventricular failure
  left; *see* Left ventricular failure
  right; *see* Right ventricular failure
Ventricular fibrillation
  course of, 625
  sudden death due to, 6
  summary of, 627
  treatment of, 625-626
Ventricular premature beats, treatment of,
    29
Ventricular septal defect, murmur due to,
    447, 448
Ventricular tachycardia
  summary of, 627
  treatment of, 626
Verapamil
  for angina, 11
  constipation associated with, 543
  digoxin interaction with, 20
Vertebrae, fracture of, in osteoporosis, 235
Vertebral-basilar stroke, 130
Vertigo; *see also* Dizziness
  benign positional, symptoms of, 507,
    509
  summary of, 511
Very-low-density lipoprotein
  in diabetes mellitus, 17
  high values for, 18
Vesicle, defined, 409
Vestibular neuronitis
  symptoms of, 507, 509
  treatment of, 509-510
Viagra for erectile disorder, 334

Violence; *see also* Rape; Sexual abuse; Spousal abuse
  cycle of, 346, 347
  family, screening for, 582
  youth, counseling recommendations, 583
Viral exanthems, 405-410
  summary of, 410
Viral infections, diarrhea, 419
Visual impairment, screening for, 581
Visual loss
  cytomegalovirus infection and, 614
  in multiple sclerosis, 109-110
  in stroke, 128
Vitamin C, common cold and, 399
Vitamin D
  supplemental, for breast-fed baby, 384
  for treating osteoporosis, 236
Vitamin supplements
  breast feeding and, 384
  infant, 385
Vomiting
  in acute appendicitis, 458-459
  with headache, 114, 117
  in infants/children, OTC drugs for, 450-452
  nonpharmacologic treatment of, in advanced cancer, 88-89
  from OCPs, 266
  in palliative care patient, 89, 91
  during pregnancy, 198, 200, 202
  in scarlet fever, 407, 408
von Willebrand's disease, symptoms of, 143
Vulvovaginitis, 238-240
  with curdy-white discharge, 238, 239-240
  differential diagnosis of, 240-241
  with gray malodorous discharge, 238

Vulvovaginitis—cont'd
  risk factors for, 239-240
  signs of, 239
  summary of, 241
  treatment of, 239

W
Walk-in clinics, limitations of, 609
Warfarin
  for acute MI, 7
  for atrial fibrillation prophylaxis, 29
  for pulmonary embolism, 37
Warts
  plantar
    outpatient surgery for, 465-466, 469
    removal of, 467-468
  venereal, treatment of, 468
Weakness
  in Addison's disease, 99
  in multiple sclerosis, 109-110
Weber test, procedure for, 510
Weight gain
  in acromegaly, 99
  maternal, IUGR and, 219
  during pregnancy, 206
Weight loss
  in anorexia nervosa, 303
  calorie intake for, 31
  in diabetes mellitus, 92
  programs for, 32
  short-term, rebound effect of, 32
Weight reduction for hypertension, 24
Wheals, defined, 409
Wheezing
  in asthma, 45, 48
  differential diagnosis of, 393
  infant, 389

Whiplash injuries, 497-498; *see also* Low back pain
  summary of, 498
Women's health, 233-277; *see also* Obstetrics
  cervical abnormalities, 241-246
  contraception, 263-270
  dysfunctional uterine bleeding, 256-259
  dysmenorrhea, 252-256
  ectopic pregnancy, 259-263
  osteoporosis, 233-238
  postmenopausal symptoms, 249-252
  premenstrual syndrome, 246-249
  sexually transmitted disease, 270-277
  vulvovaginitis, 238-241
World Health Organization
  Analgesic Ladder of, 82, 84-85
  osteopenia defined by, 237
  osteoporosis defined by, 235
Wounds, dirty, tetanus prophylaxis and, 618

Y
Yersinia, in IBS, 76
Youth violence, counseling recommendations, 583

Z
ZDV; *see* Zidovudine
Zidovudine, side effects of, 614-615
Zocor; *see* Simvastatin
Zoloft; *see* Sertraline
Zyban; *see* Bupropion

CONTINUING MEDICAL EDUCATION CREDIT

An added asset of the fourth edition of *Swanson's Family Practice Review* is the potential for the reader to earn Continuing Medical Education (CME) credits. This has become possible insomuch as this edition was planned and produced by the National Medical School Review (NMSR), a CME division of Kaplan Medical, in accordance with the Essentials of the Accreditation Council for Continuing Medical Education (ACCME).

NMSR is accredited by the ACCME to sponsor continuing medical education for physicians and designates this educational activity for up to 75 hours in Category 1 credit toward the American Medical Association Physician's Recognition Award. Each physician should claim only those hours of credit that he or she actually spent completing the educational activity.

TARGET AUDIENCE

As described in the introduction, this text presents the core knowledge required by the contemporary primary care physician. Moreover, the previous editions have gained wide acceptance as books of premiere value to the family practice physician preparing for certification or recertification, as well as for physicians, physician assistants, and other primary care health delivery professionals desiring an up-to-date review of the essentials of primary care.

OBJECTIVES

1. A primary goal is to help family practice physicians prepare for the certification and recertification examinations. Previous readers have informed us, time and again, that this goal was realistic; studying the third edition helped them prepare for their examination. To this end, the book contains over 2000 multiple-choice questions. The third edition has also been of proven value for physicians preparing for the SPEX examination and for the United States Medical Licensing Examination, Step 3.

2. The second basic goal is to provide a platform that will assist the primary care practitioner in updating their understanding of diagnostic and therapeutic methodologies. Achievement of this goal is enhanced by the structure of the text wherein each problem describes a set of symptoms, illuminated by different cases that cover the various relevant aspects of the differential. The dominant role of family practitioners in preparing this edition assures that the cases provide realistic, practical examples, whereas participation of specialists ensures that the information includes the most recent concepts.

3. Still additional goals are to assist the physician to recognize the most cost-efficient, yet appropriate means of arriving at a definitive diagnosis and to increase the physician's awareness of effective communication techniques that enable the practitioner to solicit essential information in the minimum amount of time. These have become particularly sensitive issues in this time of increasing health costs and changing practice models. Once again, these are achieved through the use of realistic case scenarios.

Whereas the above represent overall goals, each chapter has a specific focus. This arrangement permits the reader to concentrate on areas of specific interest. This may be of particular importance to the family practice physician preparing for recertification, as well as the primary care practioner who limits his or her practice to certain areas.

Chapter 1 **Adult Medicine**
The goal of this chapter is to provide relevant updates in the major areas of general internal medicine, emphasizing problems typically seen by the practioner and tested for by the American Academy of Family Physicians in the subdisciplines of cardiology, pulmonary disease, infectious disease, gastroenterology, endocrinology, rheumatology neurology, nephrology, dermatology, and hematology.

Chapter 2 **Obstetrics**
The goal of this chapter is to provide contemporary thought concerning health problems associated with pregnancy and childbirth.

Chapter 3 **Women's Health**
This chapter provides the contemporary medical thought of particular concern regarding the adult female patient.

Chapter 4 **Psychiatry, Behavioral Science, and Communication**
The aim of this chapter is to lead the practioner through behavioral and psychologic problems commonly encountered by a primary care physician, emphasizing communication skills and drug therapy.

Chapter 5 **Children and Adolescents**
The goal of this chapter is to provide the primary care practioner with further insight into the health care needs of children and adolescents with their unique problems and metabolism.

Chapter 6 **General Surgery and Surgical Specialties**
This chapter is designed to help the physician recognize when surgery is needed and to provide a review of the special

needs of the perioperative patient. It is not intended to provide an evaluation or review of surgical techniques.

Chapter 7 **Geriatric Medicine**
This chapter is designed to highlight the special needs of elderly patients, with particular emphasis on distinguishing between truly chronic conditions requiring institutional care and acute problems that can be modulated effectively by conservative care, permitting the patient to maintain an independent lifestyle.

Chapter 8 **Epidemiology and Public Health**
This chapter is designed to refresh the physician's training with respect to some basic epidemiologic concepts and to review community-based health problems.

Chapter 9 **Emergency and Sports Medicine**
The goal of this chapter is to review conundrums faced, in particular, by practitioners caring for patients with emergencies and sports-related injuries and illnesses, including how to decide when to admit and ethical issues sometimes arising from the need for immediate treatment.

CREDIT AND FEE SCHEDULE

Physicians requesting CME credit may do so upon completion of each individual chapter, or alternatively, elect to request the credit after completing the full text. The maximum number of credit hours* and the associate administrative fee of seven dollars per CME credit hour is listed below.

Chapter	Maximal credit hours	Fee
1. Adult Medicine	18.5	$130
2. Obstetrics	4.0	$ 28
3. Women's Health	4.5	$ 32
4. Psychiatry, Behavioral Science, and Communication	15.0	$105
5. Children and Adolescents	11.5	$ 80
6. General Surgery and Surgical Specialties	6.0	$ 42
7. Geriatric Medicine	5.5	$ 38
8. Epidemiology and Public Health	5.5	$ 38
9. Emergency and Sports Medicine	4.5	$ 32
The whole book (10% discount)	75.0	$472

*These are the average number of hours reported by five different readers.

OBTAINING CONTINUING MEDICAL EDUCATION CREDIT

Physicians wishing to earn CME credit for this educational tool should complete the following steps:

1. Read the chapter(s) relevant to your educational needs.
2. Fill out the attached registration form with a nonrefundable $25 registration fee, which, however, will be applied to the total administrative fee.
3. You will then receive the CME package, which consists of a brief evaluation instrument for each chapter in which you expressed an interest.
4. Return the completed evaluation instrument indicating the number of CME hours you have earned and wish to be credited for, along with the appropriate payment, based on hours spent in completing the relevant educational activity. However, the minimal net fee will be $25.
5. Your CME certificate will be mailed to you upon our receipt of your completed evaluation questionnaire(s).

For additional information contact Kenneth H. Ibsen, Ph.D., Director, CME Kaplan Medical, and Academic Editor:

Phone 800-533-8850, ext. 4420
E-Mail Ken__Ibsen@Kaplan. com
Or post: 4500 Campus Dr, Suite 201
Newport Beach, CA 92660

Registration Form for CME Credits

Swanson's Family Practice Review, ed 4

Name _____   Degree _____

Address _____
                Street   City   State   Zip

Day Phone _____   Fax _____

E-Mail _____   Social Security Number _____

Specialty _____

A nonrefundable fee of $25 must be included with this registration form:

Method of Payment:

Visa _____   MasterCard _____   Check _____

Credit Card Number _____   Expiration Date _____

I agree to pay the above amount according to credit card agreement.

Signature _____

Either mail or fax the completed form or e-mail the pertinent information to:
Dr. Kenneth H. Ibsen, Ph.D.
Director of Continuing Medical Education
Kaplan/NMSR
4500 Campus Drive
Suite 201
Newport Beach, CA 92660

Fax: 949-476-6286; e-mail: Ken__Ibsen@Kaplan.com; phone: 800-533-8850, ext 4420